CURRENT
Diagnosis and Treatment: Pediatric Emergency Medicine

Edited by

C. Keith Stone, MD, FACEP
Professor and Chairman
Department of Emergency Medicine
Texas A&M University Health Science Center
College of Medicine
Scott & White Healthcare
Temple, Texas

Dorian Drigalla, MD, FACEP
Associate Professor and Residency Director
Department of Emergency Medicine
Texas A&M University Health Science Center
College of Medicine
Scott & White Healthcare
Temple, Texas

Roger L. Humphries, MD
Professor and Chair
Department of Emergency Medicine
University of Kentucky College of Medicine
Lexington, Kentucky

Maria Stephan, MD, FAAP
Associate Professor of Emergency Medicine
University of Kentucky College of Medicine
Lexington, Kentucky
Richmond Emergency Physicians, Inc.
Bon Secours Health System
St. Mary's Hospital
Richmond, Virginia

Mc
Graw
Hill
Education

New York   Chicago   San Francisco   Athens   London   Madrid   Mexico City
Milan   New Delhi   Singapore   Sydney   Toronto

Current Diagnosis and Treatment: Pediatric Emergency Medicine

1 2 3 4 5 6 7 8 9 0   DOC/DOC   19 18 17 16 15 14

ISBN 978-0-07-179945-4
MHID 0-07-179945-1

Notice

Medicine is an ever-changing science. As new research and clinical experience broaden our knowledge, changes in treatment and drug therapy are required. The authors and the publisher of this work have checked with sources believed to be reliable in their efforts to provide information that is complete and generally in accord with the standards accepted at the time of publication. However, in view of the possibility of human error or changes in medical sciences, neither the authors nor the publisher nor any other party who has been involved in the preparation or publication of this work warrants that the information contained herein is in every respect accurate or complete, and they disclaim all responsibility for any errors or omissions or for the results obtained from use of the information contained in this work. Readers are encouraged to confirm the information contained herein with other sources. For example and in particular, readers are advised to check the product information sheet included in the package of each drug they plan to administer to be certain that the information contained in this work is accurate and that changes have not been made in the recommended dose or in the contraindications for administration. This recommendation is of particular importance in connection with new or infrequently used drugs.

This book was set in Minion Pro by Cenveo® Publisher Services.
The editors were Anne M. Sydor and Christie Naglieri.
The production supervisor was Catherine Saggese.
Project Management was provided by Anupriya Tyagi, Cenveo Publisher Services.
The cover designer was Thomas De Pierro.
Cover Image: Swallowed Nail; Credit: Edward Kinsman.
Cover Image: Doctor Looking at X-Ray on Digital Tablet; Credit: Cavan Images.
RR Donnelley was printer and binder.

This book is printed on acid-free paper.

Library of Congress Cataloging-in-Publication Data

Current diagnosis and treatment. Pediatric emergency medicine / edited,
    C. Keith Stone, Roger Humphries, Dorian Drigalla, Maria Stephan.
        p. ; cm.
    Pediatric emergency medicine
    Includes bibliographical references.
    ISBN 978-0-07-179945-4 (pbk. : alk. paper)—ISBN 0-07-179945-1 (pbk. : alk. paper)
    I. Stone, C. Keith, editor of compilation.   II. Humphries, Roger L., editor of compilation.
III. Drigalla, Dorian, editor of compilation.   IV. Stephan, Maria, editor of compilation.
V. Title: Pediatric emergency medicine.
    [DNLM: 1. Emergency Treatment—methods. 2. Pediatrics—methods. 3. Child.
4. Emergency Medical Services—methods. 5. Infant. 6. Wounds and Injuries—therapy. WS 205]
RJ370
618.92'0025—dc23

               2014003879

International Edition ISBN 978-1-25-925520-5; MHID 1-25-925520-4. Copyright © 2015. Exclusive rights by McGraw-Hill Education, for manufacture and export. This book cannot be re-exported from the country to which it is consigned by McGraw-Hill Education. The International Edition is not available in North America.

I dedicate this first edition to my late mother. I remain eager to learn and believe anything is possible from your courage and dedication to my youth. Your premature passing reminds me to live for every day. Your love is the foundation of my life as a husband, father, and physician.

Dorian Drigalla

To my husband, James, for his persistent support in all my endeavors. And in honor and memory of my parents, Tim and Thomai, who provided the opportunity for my becoming a physician.

Maria Stephan

Contents

Authors

Brian Adkins, MD
Associate Professor
Department of Emergency Medicine
University of Kentucky College of Medicine
Lexington, Kentucky
Chapter 30

Brit Anderson, MD
Pediatric Emergency Medicine Fellow
Department of Emergency Medicine
Cincinnati Children's Hospital Medical Center
Cincinnati, Ohio
Chapter 18

Timothy E. Brenkert, MD
Assistant Professor of Clinical Pediatrics
Division of Emergency Medicine
Cincinnati Children's Hospital Medical Center
Cincinnati, Ohio
Chapter 29

Corinne L. Bria, MD
Assistant Professor of Clinical Pediatrics
Division of Emergency Medicine
Cincinnati Children's Hospital Medical Center
Cincinnati, Ohio
Chapter 16

C. J. Buckley, MD
Assistant Professor
Department of Emergency Medicine
Texas A&M University Health Science Center
College of Medicine
Scott & White Healthcare
Temple, Texas
Chapter 5

Craig T. Carter, DO
Associate Professor
Department of Emergency Medicine and Pediatrics
University of Kentucky College of Medicine
Chandler Medical Center
Lexington, Kentucky
Chapter 47

Jason N. Collins, MD, FACEP
Assistant Professor
Department of Emergency Medicine
Texas A&M University Health Science Center
College of Medicine
Scott & White Healthcare
Temple, Texas
Chapter 33

Christopher Colvin, MD
Emergency Service Partners
Austin, Texas
Chapter 4

Thomas Cunningham, MS IV
University of Kentucky College of Medicine
Lexington, Kentucky
Chapter 13

Matt Dawson, MD, RDMS, RDCS
Associate Professor
Department of Emergency Medicine
University of Kentucky
Lexington, Kentucky
Chapter 2

Sameer Desai, MD
Associate Professor
Department of Emergency Medicine
University of Kentucky
Lexington, Kentucky
Chapter 13

Dorian Drigalla, MD, FACEP
Associate Professor and Residency Director
Department of Emergency Medicine
Texas A&M University Health Science Center
College of Medicine
Scott & White Healthcare
Temple, Texas
Chapters 5, 24, 45

Michelle Eckerle, MD
Clinical Fellow
Division of Emergency Medicine
Cincinnati Children's Hospital Medical Center
Cincinnati, Ohio
Chapter 40

Cristina M. Estrada, MD
Fellowship Director, Pediatric Emergency Medicine
Assistant Residency Director, Emergency Medicine
Department of Pediatrics
Vanderbilt Children's Hospital
Division of Pediatric Emergency Medicine
Nashville, Tennessee
Chapters 41 & 49

LeeAnne Feher, MS III
Texas A&M School of Medicine
College Station, Texas
Chapter 11

Michael Feldmeier, MD
Resident Physician
Department of Emergency Medicine
University of Kentucky College of Medicine
Lexington, Kentucky
Chapter 43

Sing-Yi Feng, MD
Assistant Professor of Pediatrics
Medical Toxicologist
Division of Emergency Medicine
Department of Pediatrics
Children's Medical Center of Dallas
University of Texas Southwestern
    Medical Center
Dallas, Texas
Chapter 46

Ruqayya Gill, MBS, DO
Attending Emergency Physician
Kaweah Delta Medical Center
Visalia, California
Chapter 42

Jenny Glover, MS
Texas A&M School of Medicine
College Station, Texas
Chapter 9

Collin S. Goto, MD
Associate Professor of Pediatrics
Medical Toxicologist
Division of Emergency Medicine
Department of Pediatrics
Children's Medical Center of Dallas
University of Texas Southwestern Medical Center
Dallas, Texas
Chapter 46

Matthew N. Graber, MD, PhD, FAAEM
Institutional Research Director and Attending Emergency
    Physician
Kaweah Delta Medical Center
Visalia, California
Chapter 42

Robert D. Greenberg, MD, FACEP
Associate Professor and Vice-Chair
Director, Division of Prehospital Medicine
Department of Emergency Medicine
Texas A&M Health Science Center
College of Medicine
Scott & White Healthcare
Temple, Texas
Chapter 32

Mary Greiner, MD
Assistant Professor of Pediatrics
Department of Pediatrics
University of Cincinnati College of Medicine
Mayerson Center for Safe and Healthy Children
Cincinnati Children's Hospital Medical Center
Cincinnati, Ohio
Chapter 6

Selena Hariharan, MD, MHSA
Assistant Professor of Pediatrics
Division of Emergency Medicine
Cincinnati Children's Hospital Medical Center
Cincinnati, Ohio
Chapter 48

Blake D. Hatfield, MSIV
Department of Emergency Medicine
Texas A&M Health Science Center College of Medicine
Scott & White Memorial Hospital
Temple, Texas
Chapter 19

Jendi Haug, MD
Assistant Professor of Pediatrics
Department of Pediatrics
Division of Pediatric Emergency Medicine
University of Texas Southwestern, Children's Medical Center of
    Dallas
Dallas, Texas
Chapter 39

Brian Hawkins, MD
Assistant Professor
Department of Emergency Medicine
University of Kentucky College of Medicine
Lexington, Kentucky
Chapter 8

Joseph W. Heidenreich, MD, FACEP
Emergency Service Partners
Austin, Texas
Chapter 7

Halim Hennes, MD, MS
Professor of Pediatrics and Surgery
Department of Pediatrics
Division of Pediatric Emergency Medicine
University of Texas Southwestern Medical Center
Dallas, Texas
Chapter 26

Shawn Horrall, MD, DTM&H
Assistant Professor
Department of Emergency Medicine
Texas A&M University Health Science Center
College of Medicine
Scott & White Healthcare
Temple, Texas
Chapter 31

Timothy R. Howes, MD
Resident Physician
Department of Emergency Medicine
University of Kentucky College of Medicine
Lexington, Kentucky
Chapter 47

Craig J. Huang, MD
Associate Professor
Division of Pediatric Emergency Medicine
University of Texas Southwestern Medical Center
Children's Medical Center
Emergency Services
Dallas, Texas
Chapter 25

Roger L. Humphries, MD
Professor and Chair
Department of Emergency Medicine
University of Kentucky College of Medicine
Lexington, Kentucky
Chapter 37

Nicholas Irwin, MD
Resident Physician
Department of Emergency Medicine
University of Kentucky College of Medicine
Lexington, Kentucky
Chapter 37

Jon Jaffe, MD
Assistant Professor
Department of Emergency Medicine
Texas A&M University Health Science Center
College of Medicine
Scott & White Healthcare
Temple, Texas
Chapter 17

Anthony James, MD
Resident Physician
Department of Emergency Medicine
Texas A&M University Health Science Center
College of Medicine
Scott and White Healthcare
Temple, Texas
Chapter 12

Thomas R. Jones, MD, Mdiv, FAAEM
Associate Professor
Department of Emergency Medicine
Texas A&M University Health Science Center
College of Medicine
Scott & White Healthcare
Temple, Texas
Chapter 1

Andrew L. Juergens II, MD
Assistant Professor and Assistant Residency Director
Department of Emergency Medicine
Texas A&M University Health Science Center
College of Medicine
Scott & White Healthcare
Temple, Texas
Chapter 9

Ian D. Kane, MD
Division of Pediatric Emergency Medicine
Department of Pediatrics
Vanderbilt Children's Hospital
Nashville, Tennessee
Chapter 41

Jessica Kanis, MD
Fellow, Pediatric Emergency Medicine
Division of Emergency Medicine
Cincinnati Children's Hospital Medical Center
Cincinnati, Ohio
Chapter 29

Brooks Keeshin, MD
Fellow, Child Abuse Pediatrics
Mayerson Center for Safe and Healthy Children
Cincinnati Children's Hospital Medical Center
Cincinnati, Ohio
Chapter 6

Jakob Kissel, MD
Resident Physician
Department of Emergency Medicine
University of Kentucky College of Medicine
Lexington, Kentucky
Chapter 23

Heather Kleczewski, MD
Assistant Professor of Pediatrics
Division of Emergency Medicine
Department of Pediatrics
University of Texas Southwestern Medical Center
Division of Emergency Medicine
Dallas, Texas
Chapter 22

Sophia A. Koen, MD
Dallas Regional Medical Center
Mesquite, Texas
Chapter 21

Sandy Y. Lee, BS
Medical Student-IV
Texas A&M University Health Science Center
College of Medicine
Temple, Texas
Chapter 33

Scott A. Letbetter, MD
Resident Physician
Department of Emergency Medicine
Texas A&M Health Science Center
College of Medicine
Scott & White Memorial Hospital and McLane Children's
    Hospital
Temple, Texas
Chapter 38

Dominic Lucia, MD
Assistant Professor
Department of Emergency Medicine
Texas A&M University Health Science Center
College of Medicine
Medical Director
McLane Children's Hospital of Scott & White
Scott & White Healthcare
Temple, Texas
Chapter 12

Kathi Makoroff, MD
Associate Professor of Pediatrics
Department of Pediatrics
University of Cincinnati College of Medicine
Mayerson Center for Safe and Healthy Children
Cincinnati, Ohio
Chapter 6

Julia Martin, MD, FACEP
Associate Professor
Department of Emergency Medicine
University of Kentucky College of Medicine
Lexington, Kentucky
Chapter 23

Constance M. McAneney, MD, MS
Professor of Clinical Pediatrics
Division of Emergency Medicine
Cincinnati Children's Hospital Medical Center
Cincinnati, Ohio
Chapter 16

Scott A. McAninch, MD, FACEP
Assistant Professor
Department of Emergency Medicine
Texas A&M Health Science Center
College of Medicine
Scott & White Memorial Hospital and McLane Children's
    Hospital
Temple, Texas
Chapter 38

Stephen McConnell, MD
Emergency Service Partners
Austin, Texas
Chapters 3 & 24

Khylie McGee, MD
Resident, Department of Emergency Medicine
Texas A&M University Health Science Center, College of
    Medicine
Scott & White Healthcare
Temple, Texas
Chapter 44

Ian Taylor McGraw, MS, MS1
Texas A&M College of Medicine
Temple, Texas
Chapter 44

Tyler McSpadden, MD
Resident, Department of Emergency Medicine
Texas A&M University Health Science Center, College of
    Medicine
Scott & White Healthcare
Temple, Texas
Chapter 45

Robert K. Minkes, MD, PhD
Professor, Division of Pediatric Surgery
University of Texas, Southwestern Medical School
Children's Medical Center of Dallas
Dallas, Texas
Chapter 36

Evan Moore, MS IV
Medical Student
University of Kentucky College of Medicine
Lexington, Kentucky
Chapter 47

Andrew Morris, DO
Resident Physician
Department of Emergency Medicine
Texas A&M Health Science Center
College of Medicine
Scott & White Healthcare
Temple, Texas
Chapter 7

James E. Morris, MD, MPH
Associate Professor
Department of Emergency Medicine
Texas A&M Health Science Center
College of Medicine
Scott & White Healthcare
Temple, Texas
Chapter 19

Ryan P. Morrissey, MD
Assistant Professor
Department of Emergency Medicine
Medical Director, Central Texas Poison Center
Texas A&M University Health Science Center
College of Medicine
Scott & White Healthcare
Temple, Texas
Chapter 15

Dhriti Mukhopadhyay, MD
Resident, Department of Surgery
Texas A&M University Health Science Center
College of Medicine
Scott & White Healthcare
Temple, Texas
Chapter 27

Jo-Ann O. Nesiama, MD, MS
Assistant Professor
Division of Pediatric Emergency Medicine
University of Texas Southwestern Medical Center
Children's Medical Center
Dallas, Texas
Chapter 25

Pamela J. Okada, MD, FAAP, FACEP
Associate Professor of Pediatrics
Division of Pediatric Emergency Medicine
University of Texas
Southwestern Medical School
Children's Medical Center of Dallas
Dallas, Texas
Chapter 36

Brandon Pace, MD
Resident Physician
Department of Emergency Medicine
University of Kentucky College of Medicine
Lexington, Kentucky
Chapter 8

Douglas Patton, MD
Resident Physician
Department of Emergency Medicine
Texas A&M University Health Science Center
College of Medicine
Scott & White Healthcare
Temple, Texas
Chapter 35

Jullie Phillips, MD
Clinical Instructor, Pediatric Emergency Medicine
Department of Pediatrics
Vanderbilt Children's Hospital
Division of Pediatric Emergency Medicine
Nashville, Tennessee
Chapter 49

Emily A. Porter, MD
Metropolitan Methodist Hospital
San Antonio, Texas
Chapter 15

Taylor Ratcliff, MD, EMT-P
Assistant Professor
Department of Emergency Medicine
Texas A&M University Health Science Center
College of Medicine
Scott & White Healthcare
Temple, Texas
Chapter 11

Manoj P. Reddy, BS
Texas A&M School of Medicine
College Station, Texas
Chapter 9

Richard M. Ruddy, MD
Director, Division of Emergency Medicine
Cincinnati Children's Hospital Medical Center
Professor of Pediatrics
University of Cincinnati College of Medicine
Cincinnati, Ohio
Chapter 40

Patrick Russell, MD
Department of Emergency Medicine
University of Kentucky College of Medicine
Lexington, Kentucky
Chapter 2

Susan M. Scott, MD
Associate Professor of Pediatrics
Division of Emergency Medicine
Department of Pediatrics
University of Texas Southwestern Medical Center
Dallas, Texas
Chapter 22

Adam Scrogham, MD
Resident Physician
Department of Emergency Medicine
University of Kentucky College of Medicine
Lexington, Kentucky
Chapter 30

Alicia Shirakbari, MD
Assistant Professor
Department of Emergency Medicine
University of Kentucky College of Medicine
Lexington, Kentucky
Chapter 43

David A. Smith, MD
Assistant Professor
Department of Emergency Medicine
Texas A&M University Health Science Center
College of Medicine
Scott & White Healthcare
Temple, Texas
Chapter 34

Eric William Stern, MD
Assistant Professor
Department of Emergency Medicine
Texas A&M University Health Science Center
    College of Medicine
Scott & White Healthcare
Temple, Texas
Chapters 27 & 35

Charles Tad Stiles, MD, FACEP
Assistant Professor
Department of Emergency Medicine
Texas A&M University Health Science Center
College of Medicine
Scott & White Healthcare
Temple, Texas
Chapter 14

C. Keith Stone, MD, FACEP
Professor and Chairman
Department of Emergency Medicine
Texas A&M University Health Science Center
College of Medicine
Scott & White Healthcare
Temple, Texas
Chapters 20 & 21

Margaret Strecker-McGraw, MD, FACEP
Assistant Professor
Texas A&M University Health Science Center, College of
    Medicine
Scott & White Healthcare
Temple, Texas
Chapter 44

Ryun Summers, DO
Resident, Department of Emergency Medicine
Texas A&M University Health Science Center
College of Medicine
Scott & White Healthcare
Temple, Texas
Chapter 27

Terren Trott, MD
Resident Physician
Department of Emergency Medicine
University of Kentucky College of Medicine
Lexington, Kentucky
Chapter 30

Brett Trullender, MS, PT, MSIV
Texas A&M School of Medicine
College Station, Texas
Chapter 11

Irma Ugalde, MD
Assistant Professor
Baylor College of Medicine
Texas Children's Hospital
Houston, Texas
Chapter 10

Mercedes Uribe, MD
Assistant Professor of Pediatrics
Department of Pediatrics
Division of Pediatric Emergency Medicine
University of Texas Southwestern
Dallas, Texas
Chapter 26

Brian Wagers, MD
Fellow in Pediatric Emergency Medicine
Division of Emergency Medicine
Cincinnati Children's Hospital Medical Center
Cincinnati, Ohio
Chapter 48

Mary Wardrop, MD
Resident Physician
Department of Emergency Medicine
University of Kentucky College of Medicine
Lexington, Kentucky
Chapter 13

Jonathan Wheatley, MD
Resident, Department of Emergency Medicine
Texas A&M University Health Science Center
College of Medicine
Scott & White Healthcare
Temple, Texas
Chapter 31

Richard Whitworth, MD
Chief Resident
Department of Emergency Medicine
Texas A&M University Health Science Center
College of Medicine
Scott & White Healthcare
Temple, Texas
Chapter 17

J. Scott Wieters, MD
Assistant Professor
Department of Emergency Medicine
Texas A&M Health Science Center
College of Medicine
Scott & White Healthcare
Temple, Texas
Chapter 7

Kenneth Yen, MD, MS
Associate Professor of Pediatrics
Department of Pediatrics
Division of Pediatric Emergency Medicine
University of Texas Southwestern Medical Center
Dallas, Texas
Chapter 39

Cassandra Zhuang, BS
Medical Student
Round Rock, Texas
Chapter 32

Preface

Current Diagnosis and Treatment Pediatric Emergency Medicine, first edition is designed to present concise, easy-to-read, practical information for the diagnosis and treatment of a spectrum of pediatric conditions that present to the emergency department. The chapters emphasize immediate management of life-threatening problems and then present the evaluation and treatment of specific disorders. We trust that this text will aid all students, residents, and practitioners of emergency medicine in providing care to pediatric patients.

OUTSTANDING FEATURES

In keeping with the tradition of the Current series, *Current Diagnosis and Treatment Pediatric Emergency Medicine* strives to provide the reader with a broad-based text written in a clear and succinct manner. Our goal is to provide practicing emergency physicians quick access to accurate and useful information that will aid in their everyday practice of emergency medicine.

Because this text focuses on the practical aspects of emergency care, there is little discussion of the basic science or pathophysiology of disease processes. In addition, discussion of management restricts the material presented to treatments routinely provided in the emergency department.

INTENDED AUDIENCE

The book will be useful to all practitioners of emergency medicine, including physicians, residents, medical students, as well as physician extenders. It will also provide valuable information for emergency nurses and prehospital care providers.

ORGANIZATION

The book is organized in priority-based and problem-oriented fashion. Chapters in Section I, Special Aspects of Pediatric Emergency Medicine, are written in a nonstructured text format. Chapters in Section II, Management of Common Emergency Problems, are presented in a problem-based format. Life-threatening disorders are discussed first, followed by a presentation of specific disorders. This format is carried out in the remainder of the book in Section III, Trauma Emergencies, and in Section IV, Nontrauma Emergencies.

ACKNOWLEDGMENTS

We would like to thank the staff at McGraw-Hill, Anne Sydor, Christie Naglieri, and Christine Barcellona for their patience and support throughout the preparation of the manuscript. We would also like to thank our families, Gail and Chase; Jessica, Luke, and Cash, for their love and support that allowed us to commit the time needed to work on this first edition.

C. Keith Stone, MD
Dorian Drigalla, MD
November 2014

Approach to the Pediatric Emergency Department Patient

Thomas R. Jones, MD, Mdiv

It is important for the emergency physician to be capable of managing pediatric emergencies when they present. Children are a unique and significant subset of patients presenting to the emergency department. In 2010 the Center for Disease Control (CDC) database reported a total of 129.8 million emergency department visits in the United States: 25.5 million visits were patients younger than 15 years, and an additional 20.7 million visits were patients between 15 and 24 years. The emergency physician should be prepared to care for pediatric emergencies, whether they present to a children's hospital, tertiary referral center, or community hospital. Additionally, the presenting child at an adult hospital may develop an airway problem, acute allergic reaction, or other life-threatening event.

▼ INITIAL ASSESSMENT

What is the best way for the physician to assess a pediatric emergency department patient? The challenges are to simultaneously obtain a history, perform a physical examination, and determine if the child requires an intervention immediately or whether treatment can wait.

Evaluation of a child in the emergency department begins with an assessment of mental status. Children naturally investigate their environment. A child that does not track the examiner could have a visual deficit or other neurologic issue. A child that is sleeping normally at the time of the encounter would be expected to be less attentive when awoken, whereas a somnolent or lethargic child is a potential emergency.

Respiratory function should be assessed in the initial moments when the physician enters the room. Evaluation of respiratory effort, rate, and oxygen saturation should be made. Stridor is an indication of a potentially obstructed airway and should elicit concern. Acquired upper airway obstruction can be systematically evaluated and should be treated accordingly.

Temperature should be measured at the onset of the visit. Infants younger than 2 months are particularly vulnerable because their immunity has not developed fully and transplacental immunity provided by the mother is declining. Preterm infants are at even greater risk. Fever may prompt a sepsis workup.

HISTORY

The emergency physician needs to obtain a history as well, and should be particularly interested in what prompted the current visit, including what caregivers know and suspect. Past medical history will primarily focus on the conditions, workups, or admissions the child has experienced, which may lend important insight to the visit. Immunization status will also be important to determine if the child is at risk for preventable illnesses.

Review of family history is important. Open-ended questions are most helpful and often raise differential diagnostic possibilities. Close family members may have had atypical presentations of common disease processes. For example, the wise physician will pay attention when family states the child's father had the same symptoms and was later discovered to have appendicitis.

Other sources of information such as emergency medical services (EMS) personnel, grandparents, or siblings may be important to question, as the parents that present the child for care may have been at work or at another location when the event or symptoms occurred. The physician may need to gain this important information by phone or EMS radio in the event these individuals are not in the emergency department.

Review of past medical history in the child's chart, if available, is also important. Electronic records have revolutionized the speed at which this information may be reviewed. The parent or caregiver may have misunderstood past diagnoses, especially when acronyms or eponyms were used by providers or in the documentation. The emergency physician should compare the current history with the medical diagnoses in the medical record, and clarify any confusion.

The physician should inquire about the use of electronic media. Yahoo, Google, and other online search engines have been used increasingly by many parents in attempt to "self-diagnose" their child's current condition. Parents may suspect their child has a condition they found on the Internet, and the physician who does not address this issue may have dissatisfied parents at the end of the visit.

PHYSICAL EXAMINATION

Assessment of the pediatric patient is different from that of the adult patient, in that it is often prudent to evaluate the presenting part. The physical examination is not typically conducted from head to toe. The majority of the examination is possible in a parent's arms or lap, provided it is done in a nonthreatening, nonrestraining way. Save uncomfortable parts of the examination for last. Sleeping children should have lungs auscultated as they may cry when disturbed and obscure useful physical examination findings. The examination of the abdomen of a sleeping child is preferred to the examination of a squirming apprehensive patient.

Infants tend to be less difficult to examine as they have yet to develop stranger anxiety and often enjoy the human interaction. Additionally, infants have limited vision. The examiner who smiles, opens eyes widely, and gets closer to the infant will often be met with positive results, especially when associated with cooing or soft verbal tones.

Inspection of an active toddler's ears and oropharynx may require some restraint assistance to adequately evaluate these sensitive areas. Aligning the ear canal with traction on the pinna may require minimal or no contact of the otoscope speculum with the ear canal and decrease discomfort. Likewise, a child may be coaxed into opening the mouth more easily if a tongue depressor is not involved.

The genitourinary examination is important to complete the examination. If an external vaginal examination is required, generally the child will feel less threatened by a knee-to-chest position, even when evaluating injuries. The physician must not cause pain or else this will not be effective.

ADDITIONAL CONSIDERATIONS

The emergency physician at this time will usually discuss pertinent findings on the examination with the parents and then describe what further testing, if indicated, will be forthcoming. It would be wise to provide details about any procedures needed, including any expected associated discomfort, and what may be done to minimize that discomfort. The discriminating physician may determine that it is best for certain family members to leave the area, which may or may not be congruent with parent or caregiver preference. A caregiver who is the physician's ally will lessen the burden of the examination, treatment plan formulation, and ultimate plan for disposition.

It is imperative that the physician considers child abuse as a reason for the encounter. The constantly crying child may be associated with a parent at wits end. History that does not fit the examination should arouse suspicion and prompt further questions and consideration. Two or more bruises in a precruising (nonwalking) child should also prompt concern.

Learning how to assess the pediatric patient involves knowledge and skills that a physician will continue to perfect and modify with experience. Each presenting patient's condition will dictate a specific pediatric assessment approach, and determine whether stabilization, history, or examination takes priority.

Centers for Disease Control: National Hospital Ambulatory Medical Care Survey: 2010 Emergency Department Summary Tables. Bethesda, MD; 2010. Also available at http://www.cdc.gov/nchs/data/ahcd/nhamcs_emergency/2010_ed_web_tables.pdf. Accessed May 17, 2013.

Claudius I, Baraff LJ: Pediatric emergencies associated with fever. *Emerg Med Clin North Am* 2010;28(1):67 [PMID: 19945599].

Kellogg ND: Evaluation of suspected child physical abuse. *Pediatrics* 2007;119(6): 1232 [PMID: 17545397].

Pfleger A, Eber E: Management of acute severe upper airway obstruction in children. *Paediatr Respir Rev.* 2013;14(2):70-7 [PMID: 23598067].

van den Berg JP, Westerbeek EA, van der Klis FR, et al: Transplacental transport of IgG antibodies to preterm infants: A review of the literature. *Early Hum Dev* 2011;87(2):67.

Emergency Bedside Ultrasound

Matt Dawson, MD, RDMS, RDCS

Patrick Russell, MD

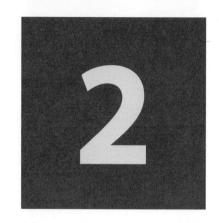

Bedside ultrasound has revolutionized the practice of emergency medicine. It has allowed physicians to diagnose and treat patients more efficiently and safely. One of the main benefits of ultrasound is that it does not expose the patient to ionizing radiation. This is especially important for pediatric patients, who are the most vulnerable individuals to radiation risk. The number of computed tomography (CT) scans in the United States has increased from 2 million in 1980 to 72 million in 2007. This is despite the fact that radiation from two to three abdominal scans gives the same amount of radiation exposure that survivors of the Hiroshima nuclear bombing received, and 1–2% of all cancers in the United States may be attributable to the radiation from CT examinations.

One of the limitations of ultrasound is that as the ultrasound beam penetrates further into the body, resolution is diminished, making diagnosis more difficult. However, children are on average smaller than adults, making this less of a problem.

These two factors, that children are small with less soft tissue to penetrate, and that they are the individuals with the most to gain from decreased radiation make them an ideal population for this modality.

Bedside ultrasound applications useful in a pediatric population include the following: EFAST for trauma, nerve blocks, lung, cardiac, soft tissue, appendicitis, testicular, rapid ultrasound in shock and hypotension (RUSH), heart, gallbladder, pyloric stenosis, intussusception, vascular access, MSK, and ocular.

There are a number of additional applications for bedside ultrasound, but these are the ones that we will focus on.

EXTENDED FOCUSED ASSESSMENT WITH SONOGRAPHY FOR TRAUMA (EFAST)

One of the most well-known uses of bedside ultrasound is in the evaluation of trauma with multiple studies over the last 30 years showing the great utility of this examination.

The majority of the studies are in adults, and the pediatric literature had historically been less promising. Recent studies had sensitivities of 81% and 92.5%, specificities of 100% and 97.2%, and accuracies of 97% and 95.5%. The acronym FAST stands for Focused Assessment with Sonography for Trauma and comprises four windows. However, the term may be outdated as now the pleural window is routinely added looking for pneumothorax. This is now referred to as EFAST with the E standing for Extended Ultrasound. The pleural window has been shown to be much more sensitive than chest radiography for pneumothorax in the supine patient. In one study the sensitivity was 76% for radiography compared with 98% for sonography. Ultrasound for pneumothorax in children has been reported.

The EFAST windows are the RUQ, LUQ, cardiac, pelvic, and pleural windows. The goals of the EFAST are to identify hemodynamically significant intraperitoneal bleeding, pericardial tamponade, hemothorax, and pneumothorax.

The probes used are quite variable. Some practitioners prefer the phased array probe, while others prefer the curvilinear probe. There are smaller curved probes designed specifically for pediatric patients. It is sometimes possible to use the linear, high-frequency probe for the entire scan on a very small patient.

The RUQ, or Morrison pouch, is the area between the liver and kidney. It is the most sensitive view for intraperitoneal fluid and fluid appears as a dark stripe between these two structures. The window used, the liver, is a very large structure that allows the practitioner some variability in the successful placement of the probe. (Figures 2–1, 2–2, 2–3).

The LUQ view, or splenorenal recess, is the area between the spleen and kidney. This is a more difficult view for many to obtain because of the small window, the spleen. It is atypical to have an isolated positive LUQ than RUQ as fluid tends to drain to the RUQ more readily. Frequently there will be fluid above the spleen instead of between the spleen and kidney (Figures 2–4, 2–5, 2–6).

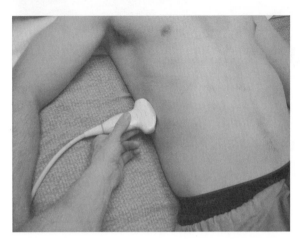

▲ **Figure 2–1.** RUQ hand placement. (Reproduced with permission from Dawson M, Mallin M. Introduction to Bedside Ultrasound. Lexington, KY: Emergency Ultrasound Solutions, 2012.)

The cardiac view is traditionally obtained via the subxiphoid approach using the liver as the window (Figures 2–7, 2–8). The goal is to identify pericardial tamponade. Pericardial tamponade is defined by the effect of the pressure on the chambers of the heart, and not simply the presence of pericardial fluid, as there are causes of chronic pericardial effusions. However, in a pediatric trauma patient it would be very rare for a pericardial effusion (Figure 2–9) not to be acute and pathologic. If the subxiphoid approach is not possible, then a quick parasternal view is an option.

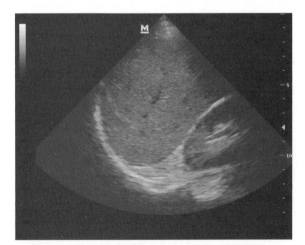

▲ **Figure 2–2.** Normal RUQ. (Reproduced with permission from Dawson M, Mallin M. Introduction to Bedside Ultrasound. Lexington, KY: Emergency Ultrasound Solutions, 2012.)

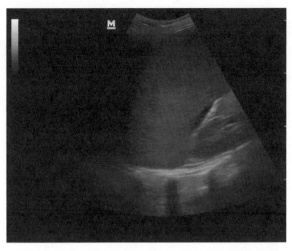

▲ **Figure 2–3.** Positive RUQ. (Reproduced with permission from Dawson M, Mallin M. Introduction to Bedside Ultrasound. Lexington, KY: Emergency Ultrasound Solutions, 2012.)

The pelvic view is obtained by using the bladder as the window to view the area posterior to the bladder that is intraperitoneal. In order to view the intraperitoneal area posterior to the bladder, it is very important to hold the probe completely perpendicular to the patient, not at an angle, as the angled view will give you an extraperitoneal view (Figures 2–10, 2–11). A positive view in this window will look like the following (Figure 2–12).

Hemothorax is evaluated at the same time as evaluation of the RUQ and LUQ views. The view of the hemithorax is obtained by simply tilting or sliding the probe slightly more

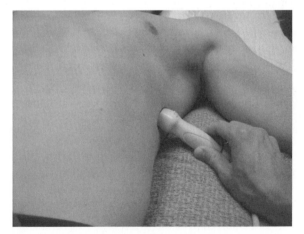

▲ **Figure 2–4.** LUQ. (Reproduced with permission from Dawson M, Mallin M. Introduction to Bedside Ultrasound. Lexington, KY: Emergency Ultrasound Solutions, 2012.)

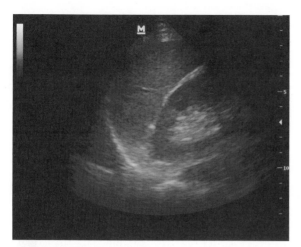

▲ **Figure 2–5.** Normal LUQ. (Reproduced with permission from Dawson M, Mallin M. Introduction to Bedside Ultrasound. Lexington, KY: Emergency Ultrasound Solutions, 2012.)

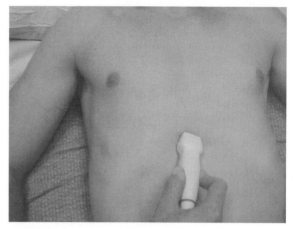

▲ **Figure 2–7.** Subxiphoid view. (Reproduced with permission from Dawson M, Mallin M. Introduction to Bedside Ultrasound. Lexington, KY: Emergency Ultrasound Solutions, 2012.)

cephalad. Ultrasound is more sensitive than chest radiography for hemothorax (Figure 2–13).

The pleural windows are assessed by moving the probe up onto the chest and identifying the pleural line between the ribs. The presence of lung sliding is normal, and the absence of lung sliding signifies a pneumothorax. M mode allows documentation of lung sliding with a single image. A pneumothorax will have a "bar code" appearance and normal lung will have a "sandy beach" appearance. With pneumothoraces, because lung sliding is absent, flat lines are above and below the pleura (bar code), in contrast to normal lung which appears as grainy on M mode (sandy beach) (Figures 2–14, 2–15). Several rib interspaces should be

assessed when looking for pneumothorax, although almost any rib interspace should have the sign of pneumothorax on the anterior chest in a supine patient if the pneumothorax is large enough to cause hemodynamic instability.

The goal in the initial evaluation of pediatric trauma patients is to rapidly identify life-threatening issues, which EFAST achieves. Although it will not identify every intraperitoneal bleed or small hemothorax, it certainly has a very important role in the evaluation of the pediatric trauma patient.

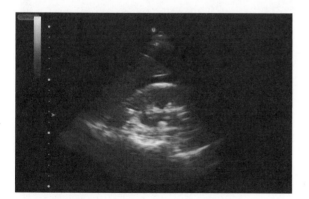

▲ **Figure 2–6.** Positive LUQ. (Reproduced with permission from Dawson M, Mallin M. Introduction to Bedside Ultrasound. Lexington, KY: Emergency Ultrasound Solutions, 2012.)

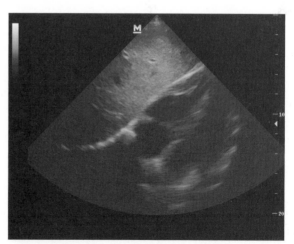

▲ **Figure 2–8.** Normal subxiphoid. (Reproduced with permission from Dawson M, Mallin M. Introduction to Bedside Ultrasound. Lexington, KY: Emergency Ultrasound Solutions, 2012.)

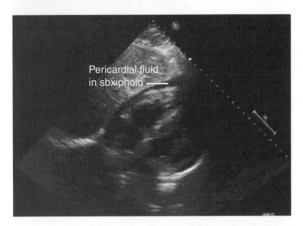

▲ **Figure 2–9. Pericardial effusion.** (Reproduced with permission from Dawson M, Mallin M. Introduction to Bedside Ultrasound. Lexington, KY: Emergency Ultrasound Solutions, 2012.)

Au AK, Rotte MJ, Grzybowski RJ, Ku BS, Fields JM: Decrease in central venous cathether placement due to use of ultrasound guidance for peripheral intravenous catheters. Am J Emerg Med. 2012;30:1950-4 [PMID: 22795988].

2007 CT Market Summary Report. International Marketing Ventures. Rockville, MD: International Marketing Ventures; 2008. Available at http://www.imvinfo.com.

Brenner DJ, Hall EJ: Computed tomography–An increasing source of radiation exposure. N Engl J Med. 2007;357:2277. [PMID: 18046031].

Hall EJ, Brenner DJ: Cancer risks from diagnostic radiology. Br J Radiol. 2008;81:362. [PMID: 18440940].

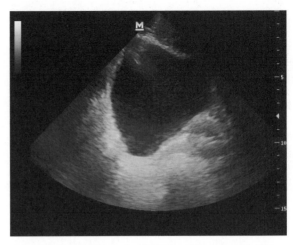

▲ **Figure 2–11. Normal pelvic view.** (Reproduced with permission from Dawson M, Mallin M. Introduction to Bedside Ultrasound. Lexington, KY: Emergency Ultrasound Solutions, 2012.)

Berrington de González A, Mahesh M, Kim KP, et al: Projected cancer risks from computed tomographic scans performed in the United States in 2007. Arch Intern Med. 2009;169:2071. [PMID: 20008689].

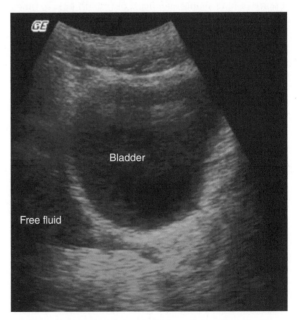

▲ **Figure 2–12. Positve pelvic view.** (Reproduced with permission from Dawson M, Mallin M. Introduction to Bedside Ultrasound. Lexington, KY: Emergency Ultrasound Solutions, 2012.)

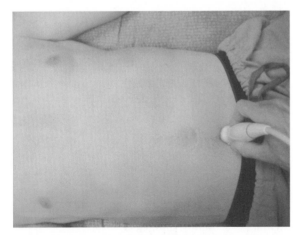

▲ **Figure 2–10. Pelvic view.** (Reproduced with permission from Dawson M, Mallin M. Introduction to Bedside Ultrasound. Lexington, KY: Emergency Ultrasound Solutions, 2012.)

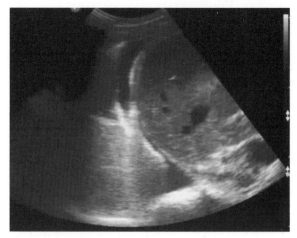

▲ **Figure 2–13.** Hemothorax. (Reproduced with permission from Dawson M, Mallin M. Introduction to Bedside Ultrasound. Lexington, KY: Emergency Ultrasound Solutions, 2012.)

Grimberg A, Shigueoka DC, Atallah AN, Ajzen S, Lared W: Diagnostic accuracy of sonography for pleural effusion: A systematic review. Sao Paulo Med J. 2010;128:90. [PMID: 20676576].

NERVE BLOCKS

Multiple studies have shown ultrasound guided nerve blocks to be safe and effective when performed by emergency physicians. Furthermore, ultrasound guidance has been shown

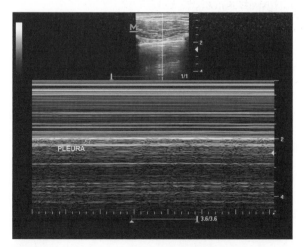

▲ **Figure 2–14.** Sandy beach sign. (Reproduced with permission from Dawson M, Mallin M. Introduction to Bedside Ultrasound. Lexington, KY: Emergency Ultrasound Solutions, 2012.)

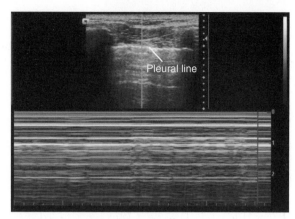

▲ **Figure 2–15.** Bar code sign. (Reproduced with permission from Dawson M, Mallin M. Introduction to Bedside Ultrasound. Lexington, KY: Emergency Ultrasound Solutions, 2012.)

to be safer and more efficacious than traditional landmark or nerve stimulator techniques in children. These blocks can aid emergency physicians in controlling acute pain from injuries and facilitate successful completion of painful procedures. The ability of ultrasound guided nerve blocks to allow success with less anesthetic make them particularly useful in children.

Commonly performed pediatric nerve blocks in the emergency department are the femoral block, sciatic block, brachial plexus blocks, and peripheral arm blocks, including the radial, median, and ulnar nerves. The linear, high-frequency 5–10 MHz probe can be used for most blocks. Or if a "hockey-stick" probe is available, it is very useful for some of these blocks.

A "femoral nerve 3-in-1" block is a procedure that can be used to control pain related to a femoral fracture. The three nerves involved are the femoral, obturator, and lateral cutaneous femoral nerve. For this block, use the linear high-frequency probe and place it parallel and just inferior to the inguinal ligament. In this orientation you will identify the neurovascular bundle with the nerve, artery, and vein from lateral to medial. The needle can be placed in long or short axis to the probe with a lateral approach to the nerve in order to avoid the artery and vein. It is important to remember that you must keep the needle tip in view at all times and you must inject the anesthetic deep to the fascia iliaca. By injecting beneath this fascial plane you will anesthetize the femoral nerve and have a successful block. In general 5–20 mL of anesthetic will be sufficient depending on the size of the child. To perform this procedure, sterile technique should be maintained at all times. Prepare the skin in usual fashion once landmarks have been identified. Cover the ultrasound probe with a sterile sheath. A 10-cc syringe and 21-gauge,

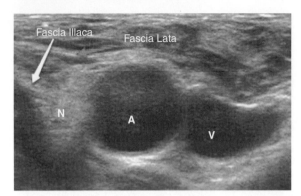

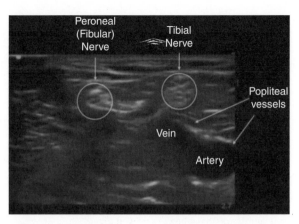

▲ Figure 2–16. Femoral nerve. (Reproduced with permission from Dawson M, Mallin M. Introduction to Bedside Ultrasound. Lexington, KY: Emergency Ultrasound Solutions, 2012.)

▲ Figure 2–17. Tibial and common peroneal nerves.

1.5-in needle can be used in smaller patients, 3.5-in spinal needle in larger patients. For the purpose of peripheral nerve blocks in the emergency department, it is preferable to use plain 1.0% lidocaine (Figure 2–16).

The femoral nerve block is useful for the upper leg, but inferiorly it anesthetizes only the patella and the medial part of the lower leg. Therefore, painful procedures such as lower leg fracture reductions require a separate block. The sciatic nerve block can be accomplished with ultrasound guidance in pediatric patients with a posterior approach, which has been shown to be more reliable than an anterior approach. This block has been described extensively in pediatric patients and is safe and effective. The posterior approach can be accomplished with a patient either prone or supine. Either way, the high-frequency probe is placed in the popliteal fossa and the popliteal artery is visualized. From this landmark one can identify the tibial nerve just superficial and lateral to the popliteal artery. As this nerve is traced proximally, the common peroneal nerve will be seen joining the tibial nerve to form the sciatic nerve (Figure 2–17). This is the point where 5–20 mL of anesthetic, depending on patient size, will be injected to anesthetize the lower leg. The needle should be inserted laterally on the leg, in plane with the ultrasound probe, at a depth determined by the depth of the nerve (Figures 2–18, 2–19).

Brachial plexus blocks can be very useful to facilitate pain management for injuries or procedures of the upper extremity. There are multiple approaches to the brachial plexus including interscalene, supraclavicular, infraclavicular, and axillary. In children it is sometimes helpful to use a small amount of sedation for this procedure because of the anxiety associated with an injection in the neck or upper extremity region. The initial minimal sedation can frequently avoid a deeper sedation that would have been required for the procedure. The most common of the brachial plexus approaches

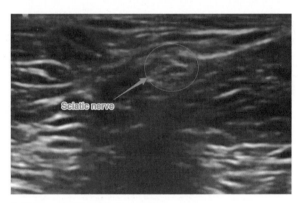

▲ Figure 2–18. Sciatic nerve.

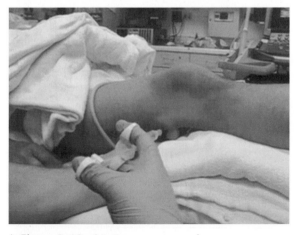

▲ Figure 2–19. Sciatic nerve approach.

is the axillary approach, which we will describe. It allows blockade of the radial, median, ulnar, and musculocutaneous nerves. However, the axillary nerve itself is frequently not blocked with this approach. This means that anesthesia from this block is best distal to the elbow. If anesthesia of the upper arm is necessary, then blockade from one of the more proximal blocks would be more appropriate.

The patient should be positioned with the affected arm abducted and flexed to 90 degrees in a "high-five" position. In this position the high-frequency probe should be placed in the axillary crease to visualize the axillary artery. Surrounding the axillary artery one can see the median, radial, and ulnar nerves. To perform this procedure, sterile technique should be maintained at all times. Prepare the skin in usual fashion once landmarks have been identified. Cover the ultrasound probe with a sterile sheath. A 10-cc syringe and 21-gauge, 1.5-in needle can be used in smaller patients, 3.5-in spinal needle in larger patients. For the purpose of peripheral nerve blocks in the emergency department, it is preferable to use plain 1.0% lidocaine. The musculocutanous nerve can be visualized more inferior within the coracobrachialis muscle. Each nerve should be surrounded with 2–4 cc of anesthetic for an adequate block. By injecting near the median nerve as illustrated, anesthetic will follow fascial planes and engulf radial and ulnar nerves. When performing this block it is advisable to collapse the axillary vein to reduce the chance of intravascular injection. This can be accomplished with minimal pressure (Figures 2–20, 2–21).

In conclusion, nerve blocks can be a very useful adjunct for pain control in pediatric patients. Nerve blocks can reduce the risks associated with sedation for procedures, and allow for more adequate pain control in general.

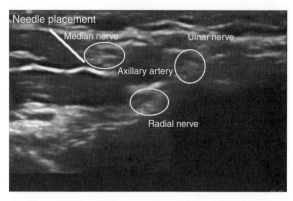

▲ **Figure 2–21. Axillary nerve block.** (Reproduced with permission from Dawson M, Mallin M. Introduction to Bedside Ultrasound. Lexington, KY: Emergency Ultrasound Solutions, 2012.)

Antonis MS, Chandwani D, McQuillen K: Ultrasound-guided placement of femoral 3-in-1 anesthetic nerve block for hip fractures. Acad Emerg Med. 2006;13:S122.
Oberndorfer U, Marhofer P, Bosenberg A, et al: Ultrasonographic guidance for sciatic and femoral nerve blocks in children. Br J Anaesth. 2007;98(6):797. [PMID: 17449890].

LUNG ULTRASOUND

As described in the EFAST section, ultrasound has been used in pediatric patients and shown to be more sensitive than chest radiography for both pneumothorax and hemothorax. The technique for diagnosing pneumothorax and hemothorax was discussed in that section. However, there are a number of other applications of ultrasound when evaluating a patient for lung pathology. While lung sonography is performed with multiple different probes in adults, the high frequency, linear probe is generally sufficient for all but the largest pediatric patients. In a very large pediatric patient a curvilinear or phased array probe may be more appropriate when evaluating for consolidation, effusion, pleural edema, or pathologies other than pneumothorax.

Pleural effusion can be evaluated in a similar manner to hemothorax (see Figure 2–13). The effusion will be seen as a dark stripe just superior to the diaphragm. Fluid, whether it is blood or effusion, will appear anechoic (black). In addition to identifying pleural effusions, ultrasound can also be very helpful in guiding a thoracentesis to make it safer. The pleural effusion can be identified and the size of the effusion can be measured by measuring the width of the fluid stripe. This information can be used, as well as the measurement from the skin to the lung to help guide the thoracentesis. Real-time guidance and visualization of the needle tip can make the procedure even safer.

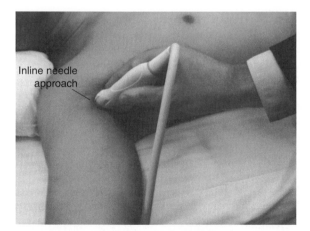

▲ **Figure 2–20. Axillary nerve position.** (Reproduced with permission from Dawson M, Mallin M. Introduction to Bedside Ultrasound. Lexington, KY: Emergency Ultrasound Solutions, 2012.)

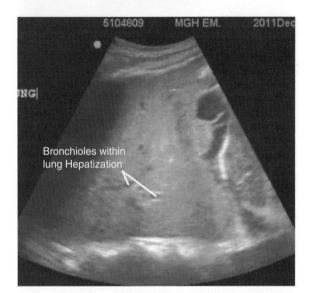

▲ **Figure 2–22. Lung hepatization.** (Reproduced with permission from Dawson M, Mallin M. Introduction to Bedside Ultrasound. Lexington, KY: Emergency Ultrasound Solutions, 2012.)

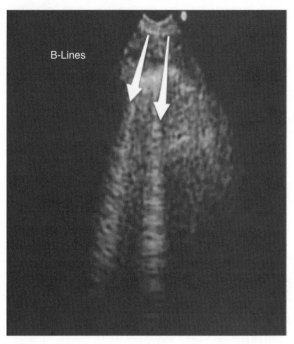

▲ **Figure 2–23.** B lines. (Reproduced with permission from Dawson M, Mallin M. Introduction to Bedside Ultrasound. Lexington, KY: Emergency Ultrasound Solutions, 2012.)

Pneumonia and lung consolidation are evaluated readily with lung sonography. Multiple studies have shown it to be much better than chest radiography and comparable to chest CT. As the interstitial space consolidates, the density changes and becomes more like that of the liver. This is referred to as hepatization of the lung and gives the lung a very similar appearance to the liver (Figure 2–22). With lung ultrasound, it is also possible to distinguish consolidation and atelectasis. Consolidation will have mobile, dynamic air bronchograms as the bronchi are usually not obstructed. However, bronchial obstruction is present in atelectasis and results in what appears as static, nonshimmering bronchograms.

Bronchiolitis is a clinical disorder that is usually treated without imaging. However, frequently in more severe cases a chest radiograph is ordered. Ultrasound has not historically been a part of this workup, but a recent study showed that ultrasound is more accurate and correlates better with clinical severity than radiography. In this study ultrasound showed subpleural consolidations, numerous "B lines," and pleural line abnormalities that correlated with disease severity. B lines are a kind of comet tail artifact indicative of pleural interstitial edema. "A lines" are a horizontal artifact indicating normal lung surface.

Interstitial disease in general can be appreciated on ultrasound. It is seen as B lines and can represent pulmonary edema, pulmonary fibrosis, and infection or tumor (Figure 2–23). In pulmonary edema the number of B lines can be followed to evaluate the success of therapeutic maneuvers such as CPAP. Although clinical correlation is necessary when B lines are present to determine the exact etiology, the severity of each of the previously mentioned pathologic processes correlates with the number of B lines present.

Ultrasound has been shown to be effective for diagnosis and as a tool to follow the disease process for pneumothorax, hemothorax, pleural edema, pneumonia, bronchiolitis, and other diseases of the lung. Some authors have gone as far as to suggest that ultrasound can basically replace the standard chest x-ray. When this is adopted as a widespread practice, significant amounts of time and radiation in the evaluation of pediatric lung pathology will be saved.

Parlamento S, Copetti R, Di Bartolomeo S: Evaluation of lung ultrasound for the diagnosis of pneumonia in the ED. Am J Emerg Med. 2009;27(4):379. [PMID: 19555605].

Reissig A, Kroegel C: Sonographic diagnosis and follow-up of pneumonia: A prospective study. Respiration. 2007;74(5):537. [PMID: 17337882].

Cortellaro F, Colombo S, Coen D, Duca P: Lung ultrasound is an accurate diagnostic tool for the diagnosis of pneumonia in the emergency department. Emerg Med J. 2012;29(1):19. [PMID: 21030550].

Caiulo VA, Gargani L, Caiulo S, et al: Lung ultrasound in bronchiolitis: Comparison with chest x-ray. Eur J Pediatr. 2011;170(11):1427. [PMID: 21468639].

Liteplo AS, Marill KA, Villen T, et al: Emergency thoracic ultrasound in the differentiation of the etiology of shortness of breath: Sonographic B-lines and N-terminal probrain type natriuretic peptide in diagnosing congestive heart failure. Acad Emerg Med. 2009;139:1140. [PMID: 19183402].

Gargani L, Doveri M, D'Errico L, et al: Ultrasound lung comets in systemic sclerosis: A chest sonography hallmark of pulmonary interstitial fibrosis. Rheumatol. 2009;48:1382. [PMID: 19717549].

Dawson M, Mallin M: Introduction to Bedside Ultrasound. Lung Ultrasound chapter. (this is an ebook published on-line; Editors Malin and Dawson)

CARDIAC ULTRASOUND

Ultrasound of the heart can be a very useful and sometimes life-saving tool. Its use in penetrating trauma has been shown to increase survival in patients. This was due to faster time to diagnosis and operative treatment in patients with pericardial effusions (see discussion in the EFAST section). Basic echocardiography is also a key element of the Rapid Ultrasound for Shock and Hypotension (RUSH) examination for patients with undifferentiated hypotension (see discussion in the RUSH examination section). In addition to trauma and undifferentiated hypotension, cardiac ultrasound is useful in the evaluation of dyspnea, chest pain, syncope, and cardiac arrest.

In patients presenting in cardiac arrest, a quick look at the heart during ACLS can be beneficial. It can identify a reversible cause of arrest such as pericardial tamponade. It can also give very good prognostic information by assessing the global function of the heart. If the patient is in cardiac standstill, this is a very poor prognostic sign. In a study of 136 patients arresting who had cardiac standstill on the initial bedside ultrasound, no patients survived. Although most physicians use cardiac standstill to definitively end a code in adult patients, it may be less clear in pediatric patients. It is certainly a strong prognostic indicator and gives the team more resolve and objective evidence that it is time to call the code when they already feel that is the right decision.

If pericardial tamponade is diagnosed, ultrasound can make the pericardiocentesis easier, safer, and with a higher success rate. One study found a complication rate of 1% for major and 3% for minor, which compares to 7–50% with the blind approach (Figure 2–24).

The basic windows for performing cardiac ultrasound are the subxiphoid, parasternal long axis, parasternal short axis, and apical view (Figure 2–25). The subxiphoid is frequently the most sensitive for picking up pericardial tamponade. However, other views can be used as well. The apical view can be improved by rolling the patient into the left lateral decubitus position.

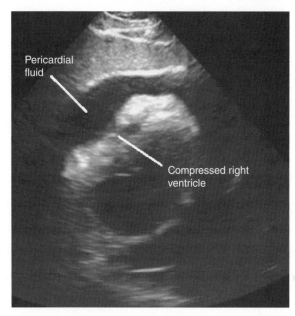

▲ **Figure 2–24. Pericardial tamponade.** (Reproduced with permission from Dawson M, Mallin M. Introduction to Bedside Ultrasound. Lexington, KY: Emergency Ultrasound Solutions, 2012.)

Although the level of evidence for pediatric cardiac ultrasound has not been as developed as for adult bedside cardiac ultrasound, it is certainly a useful examination. It can give very valuable information in patients with trauma, undifferentiated hypotension, dyspnea, cardiac arrest, and other diseases.

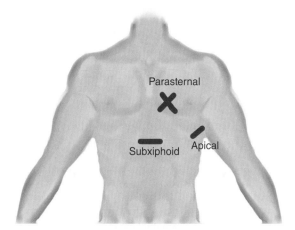

▲ **Figure 2–25. Cardiac views.** (Reproduced with permission from Dawson M, Mallin M. Introduction to Bedside Ultrasound. Lexington, KY: Emergency Ultrasound Solutions, 2012.)

Dawson M, Mallin M: Introduction to Bedside Ultrasound. Lung Ultrasound chapter. (this is an ebook published on-line; Editors Malin and Dawson)

Labovitz AJ, Noble VE, Bierig M, et al: Focused cardiac ultrasound in the emergent setting: A consensus statement of the American Society of Echocardiography and American College of Emergency Physicians. J Am Soc Echocardiogr. 2010;23(12):1225. [PMD: 21111923].

Tibballs J, Russell P: Reliability of pulse palpation by healthcare personnel to diagnose paediatric cardiac arrest. Resuscitation. 2009;80(1):61. [PMID: 18992985].

SOFT TISSUE ULTRASOUND

Soft tissue ultrasound is one of the most common applications in pediatric patients. Cellulitis and abscess are very common complaints and can frequently be hard to differentiate from one another. The treatment regimens are different and if an abscess is treated as cellulitis with antibiotics alone, it will most likely fail treatment. Furthermore, the treatment of an abscess, which is incision and drainage, can be very painful and should not be performed on a patient who has cellulites only. This makes ultrasound very useful for patients with skin infections.

In one study, bedside ultrasound changed the physicians' treatment plan for a soft tissue skin infection 57% of the time. Even when the clinician knows that an abscess is present, it can be helpful to visualize the size and exact location to guide drainage.

An abscess will appear as a hypoechoic or anechoic area whereas cellulitis will have a cobblestone appearance due to edema. (Figures 2–26, 2–27). An abscess will also be fluctuant under pressure, which can help discriminate it from a lymph node. It is also helpful to place color flow on the anechoic structure to determine there is no flow, which would suggest that it is a blood vessel rather than an abscess.

Tayal VS, Hasan N, Norton HJ, Tomaszewski CA: The effect of soft-tissue ultrasound on the management of cellulitis in the emergency department. Acad Emerg Med. 2006;13(4):384. [PMID: 16531602].

APPENDICITIS

Approximately 80,000 patients are diagnosed with appendicitis each year in the United States. Although many patients may be diagnosed clinically, a number of patients have no classic presentation, specifically women and children too young to express themselves. Therefore, testing is the norm for pediatric patients suspected of having appendicitis. White blood counts (WBC) and radiography are not sensitive or specific, and CT scanning has the downside of radiation exposure.

Ultrasound has been used for evaluation of appendicitis for 30 years and is reported to have sensitivities ranging from 76 to 100% and specificities from 88 to 100%. Sensitivity and

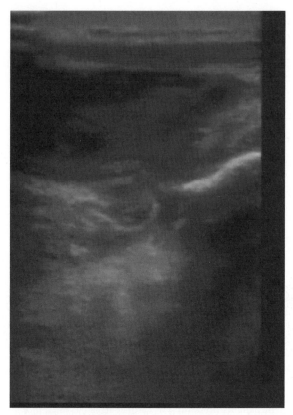

▲ **Figure 2–26.** Abscess.

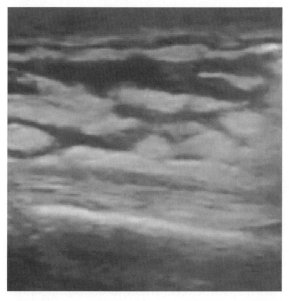

▲ **Figure 2–27.** Cellulitis. (Photo used with permission of Sonocloud.org).

specificity of CT scanning has been shown to be in a similar range, but it is generally thought to be slightly higher. In 2011 study at Stanford University, sensitivity and specificity of the protocol at 98.6% and 90.6%, respectively. The negative appendectomy rate was 8.1% with a missed appendicitis rate of 0.5%. This was accomplished while avoiding CT in 53% of patients.

Evaluation of the appendix by ultrasound is accomplished by graded compression looking for the appendix in the right lower quadrant. In the pediatric patient, the high-frequency linear probe is usually the most appropriate probe to use, but in an obese patient the curvilinear probe is sometimes more appropriate. This graded compression in the area of maximal tenderness is very important as it moves bowel, and the gas that accompanies it, out of the way. Slow, gentle movements, as well as adequate pain control, are necessary as the patient will have exquisite pain and not tolerate the procedure otherwise. The iliac artery is a good landmark as the appendix frequently lies just medial to it or sometimes superficial to it.

The normal appendix will be less than 7 mm and compressible. In contrast, an inflamed appendix will be greater than 7 mm, noncompressible, and have a "target" appearance caused by edema of the mucosal walls. A perforated appendix, however, will not appear as a target, but there will sometimes be an anechoic or hypoechoic structure representing an abscess (Figures 2–28, 2–29).

It is important to remember that a high percentage of patients do not need any imaging or further testing after a thorough history and physical. It is also important to keep in mind that ultrasound for appendicitis is a very operator-dependent modality. With use and experience, skill with the examination will improve. Furthermore, it has potential to

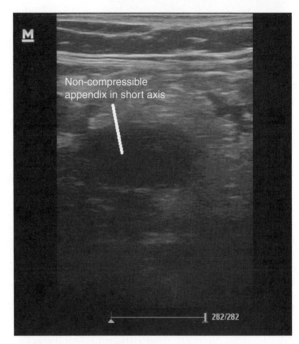

▲ **Figure 2–29. Appy-free fluid.** (Photo used with permission of Sonocloud.org.)

decrease costs and radiation from CT scans if used in the appropriate context.

Krishnamoorthi R, Ramarajan N, Wang N, et al: Effectiveness of a staged US and CT protocol for the diagnosis of pediatric appendicitis: Reducing radiation exposure in the age of ALARA. Radiology. 2011;259(1):231. [PMID: 21324843].

TESTICULAR TORSION

Testicular complaints, such as torsion, epididymitis, orchitis, trauma, hydrocele, and hemorrhage, are common emergency department complaints. However, physical examination findings are not always very sensitive or specific for the emergent causes of testicular pain. Ultrasound is an ideal modality to assess the testicle as it is a very superficial organ. Furthermore, most of the pathologic processes affecting the testicle, such as torsion, epididymitis, and orchitis, can be readily assessed based on increased or decreased flow on ultrasound.

Torsion is a time-dependent process that can lead to loss of testicle or testicular function. Ultrasound will show decreased flow to the affected testicle and heterogeneity compared to the unaffected testicle. The affected testicle is more hypoechoic because of the edema and venous lymphatic obstruction. The sensitivity and specificity of

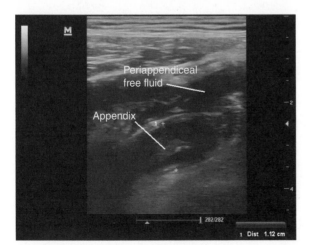

▲ **Figure 2–28. Appy-long axis measured linear.** (Photo used with permission of Sonocloud.org.)

emergency physician performed ultrasound for testicular torsion has been shown to be 95% and 94% in one study. The major limitation of ultrasound for testicular torsion is that it is user dependent. Until a provider is sure of their competence, it is probably safest to use bedside ultrasound to rule in torsion but not rule it out. If the clinical suspicion for testicular torsion is high, the urologist should be called immediately so definitive surgical management is not delayed by the ultrasound procedure. There exists the possibility of "intermittent torsion" where there would be flow on ultrasound between episodes of torsion. This is another reason to call the urologist in cases of high clinical suspicion regardless of the ultrasound results.

To perform the procedure, the patient should be situated in a comfortable frog-legged position with a towel sling underneath the scrotum to maximize comfort. The unaffected testicle can be scanned first and color flow can be adjusted while scanning this testicle to pick up blood flow. Once this is achieved, the other testicle can be scanned and evaluated for flow with the same settings. Power Doppler can be used to assess for flow if it is difficult to assess with normal color Doppler. If possible, imaging both testicles at the same time can be helpful to compare flow. No flow or decreased flow are both suggestive of torsion and are indications for emergent surgery (Figure 2–30).

Additional pathologic processes that can be seen on ultrasound of the scrotum are orchitis and epididymitis, which appear as increased flow to the testicle and epididymis, respectively. A testicular rupture will appear as a grossly misshapen, heterogenous testicle. A hydrocele will appear as an anechoic mass in the scrotum. It is easy to confuse a hematocele or pyocele for a hydrocele, so clinical correlation is important. Varicoceles will appear as an extratesticular

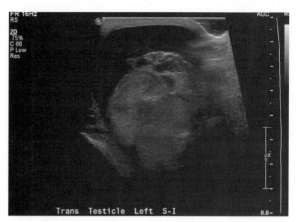

▲ **Figure 2–31.** Testicular rupture. (Reproduced with permission from Dawson M, Mallin M. Introduction to Bedside Ultrasound. Lexington, KY: Emergency Ultrasound Solutions, 2012.)

bundle of tubular structures. It is easy to confuse this with an inflamed epididymis or bowel from a hernia, but color flow can help differentiate a varicocele from these other processes. Color flow Doppler performed will diagnose varicocele by demonstrating backflow in the spermatic veins (Figures 2–31, 2–32, 2–33).

While the position of the testicles make it very easy to ultrasound them, it is important to remember that this is a user-dependent procedure. Practice is important to establish sufficient skill, and physicians must be cognizant of their own limitations with the procedure.

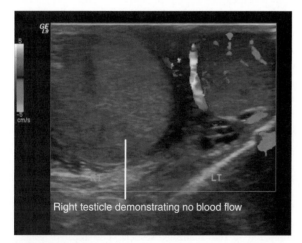

▲ **Figure 2–30.** Torsion. (Photo used with permission of Sonocloud.org.)

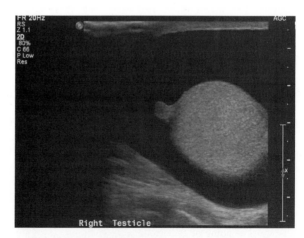

▲ **Figure 2–32.** Hydrocele. (Reproduced with permission from Dawson M, Mallin M. Introduction to Bedside Ultrasound. Lexington, KY: Emergency Ultrasound Solutions, 2012.)

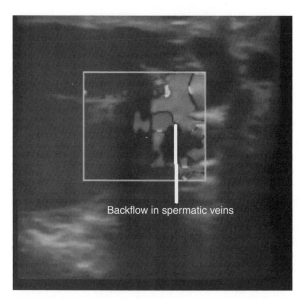

▲ **Figure 2–33.** Varicocele. (Reproduced with permission from Dawson M, Mallin M. Introduction to Bedside Ultrasound. Lexington, KY: Emergency Ultrasound Solutions, 2012.)

RAPID ULTRASOUND FOR SHOCK AND HYPOTENSION (RUSH)

The use of bedside ultrasound in the evaluation of trauma patients is standard of care. Though equally important and effective, the use of bedside ultrasonography in the evaluation of critically ill medical patients has historically been less common. This lack of utilization was addressed by Weingart et al. with their development of the RUSH examination in 2006. This revolutionary paper combined the most recent research on various ultrasound modalities in the evaluation of hypotensive patients.

The RUSH examination was designed to be a rapid, easily performed examination, using portable machines found in most emergency departments. The examination consists of scans of the heart, inferior vena cava (IVC), Morison pouch (right upper quadrant), aorta, and bilateral lung fields (pneumothorax). The components and sequence of the examination can be recalled using the mnemonic HI-MAP.

▶ Heart

The starting point of the RUSH examination is directed toward identifying pathology that could contribute to hypotension (eg, pericardial effusion, tamponade, right ventricular failure, and left ventricular function). For full details of the cardiac examination, see cardiac section of this chapter.

▶ Inferior Vena Cava

Evaluating the inferior vena cava (IVC) with bedside ultrasound can estimate the intravascular volume in a noninvasive manner. The findings of the examination should be interpreted based on whether the patient is spontaneously breathing or mechanically ventilated. This is an important consideration as mechanical ventilation will cause a dilation of the IVC during inspiration instead of collapse. In general the IVC should be evaluated for compressibility as well as response to respiration. A completely compressible IVC with large inspiratory collapse (spontaneously breathing patients only) suggests volume depletion, whereas a noncompressible IVC with no inspiratory collapse suggests no response to fluid challenge (Figure 2–34).

▶ Morison Pouch

As in trauma, free fluid anywhere in the abdomen can give clinical clues as to possible sources of hypotension. Ultrasonography of the right upper quadrant, left upper quadrant, and suprapubic area can provide information suggesting diagnoses such as ruptured viscus, spontaneous intraabdominal bleeding, and ectopic pregnancy. In completing a rapid evaluation, Morison pouch with the patient in the Trendelenburg position is the most sensitive for intraperitoneal free fluid.

While evaluating upper quadrant views, the probe can be angled toward the thorax to allow visualization of the lung bases. These views can assess for pleural effusion or hemothorax. This modality is further described in the lung section of this chapter.

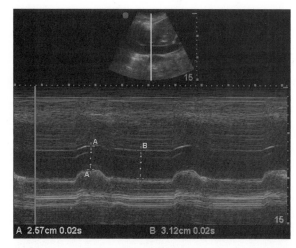

▲ **Figure 2–34.** IVC collapsibility. (Reproduced with permission from Dawson M, Mallin M. Introduction to Bedside Ultrasound. Lexington, KY: Emergency Ultrasound Solutions, 2012.)

Aorta

The evaluation of the abdominal aorta is a fundamental indication for the use of bedside ultrasonography. As a component of the RUSH examination, the abdominal aorta should be evaluated at four levels. Scanning in a transverse fashion, the aorta should be evaluated just below the heart, suprarenal, infrarenal, and just proximal to the iliac bifurcation. Moving the probe down the abdomen in a continuous stroke, one can follow the aorta through these areas. In an adult, an aorta greater than 5 cm, in the presence of shock, suggests a ruptured aneurysm. Though far less likely in the pediatric patient, the assessment could provide further clues to the etiology of hypotension.

Pneumothorax

Though more probable in trauma patients, tension pneumothorax is a possible source of hypotension in medical patients. Central line placement or other instrumentation of the thorax makes this more likely. Full details of this evaluation are covered in the lung section of this chapter.

With the probe in the hands of a competent emergency physician, the RUSH examination is easily completed in less than 2 minutes and can provide valuable details in the assessment of the hypotensive patient. This rapid evaluation, using the HI-MAP sequence, can provide invaluable information and quickly direct clinical action (Figure 2–35).

Weingart, Scott, Daniel Duque, Bret Nelson: The RUSH exam–Rapid ultrasound for shock/hypotension. Available at http://www.webcitation.org/5vyzOaPYU. Accessed July 30, 2012.

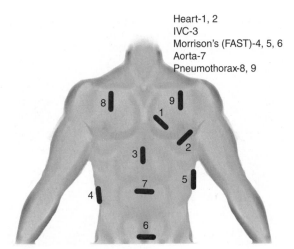

Heart-1, 2
IVC-3
Morrison's (FAST)-4, 5, 6
Aorta-7
Pneumothorax-8, 9

▲ **Figure 2–35.** RUSH sequence. (Reproduced with permission from Dawson M, Mallin M. Introduction to Bedside Ultrasound. Lexington, KY: Emergency Ultrasound Solutions, 2012.)

Hernandez C, Shuler K, Hannan H, Sonyika C, Likourezos A, Marshall J: CAUSE: Cardiac arrest ultrasound exam–A better approach to managing patients in primary non-arrhythmogenic cardiac arrest. Resuscitation. 2008;76(2):198. [PMID: 17822831].

Weekes AW: Symptomatic hypotension: ED stabilization and the emerging role of sonography. EM Practice. 2007;9(11).

Jardin F, Veillard-Baron A: Ultrasonographic examination of the vena cava.

GALLBLADDER ULTRASOUND

Though less common than in adults, symptomatic cholelithiasis and complicated obstructive biliary disease are the most common indications for pediatric cholecystectomy. Bedside ultrasound can be diagnostic in acute cholecystitis. As in adults, sonographic criteria include gallbladder wall thickening (> 3 mm), pericholecystic fluid, gallstones, dilatation of the common bile duct (CBD), and sonographic Murphy sign. In comparison with imaging specialists, emergency physicians demonstrated similar sensitivities and specificities for detecting gallstones (86–96% and 88–97% compared with 84 and 99% respectively). On average, an experienced clinician can perform a focused examination of the gallbladder in about 2–3 minutes. This quick and effective assessment has been shown to expedite treatment and decrease emergency department length of stay.

Acute cholecystitis is a disease process that can present with a myriad of physical and laboratory findings. Rarely will a patient present with fever, leukocytosis, and right upper quadrant pain. The variety of clinical presentations makes the diagnosis heavily reliant on imaging modalities, specifically right upper quadrant ultrasound. Ultrasonography of the right upper quadrant generally has a sensitivity and specificity of 94% and 84%, respectively. To make the diagnosis of acute cholecystitis, it is generally accepted that the emergency physician can rely on the presence of gallstones, gallbladder wall thickening, sonographic Murphy sign, and physical examination. The presence of gallstones in combination with a sonographic Murphy sign alone had a positive predictive value of 92.2%. Gallbladder wall thickening in the presence of gallstones had a positive predictive value of 95.2% (Figure 2–36).

To perform a focused ultrasound evaluation of the right upper quadrant, the patient should be placed in the left lateral decubitus position (Figure 2–37). Imaging in the recumbent position is possible, however technically more difficult. Positioning in the left lateral decubitus position causes the liver to shift downward pulling the gallbladder away from interfering rib shadows. If visualization is still insufficient, a large inspiration can further depress the liver and gallbladder. For most patients the curvilinear probe will be the best option for gallbladder evaluation. Begin with the probe placed sagittally under the costal margin just right of midline. From this point

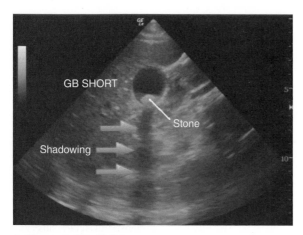

▲ **Figure 2–36.** Gallstone.

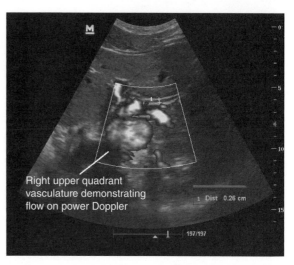

▲ **Figure 2–38.** Color flow. (Reproduced with permission from Dawson M, Mallin M. Introduction to Bedside Ultrasound. Lexington, KY: Emergency Ultrasound Solutions, 2012.)

the probe should be fanned through the right upper quadrant until an image of the gallbladder is obtained. Using color flow can help distinguish the cystic structure from large abdominal vasculature (Figure 2–38). Once identified, the gallbladder should be evaluated for presence of stones, wall thickening, and pericholecystic fluid, as well as a sonographic Murphy sign. Wall thickening should be measured on the anterior wall, with a normal finding of less than 3 mm (Figure 2–39). From

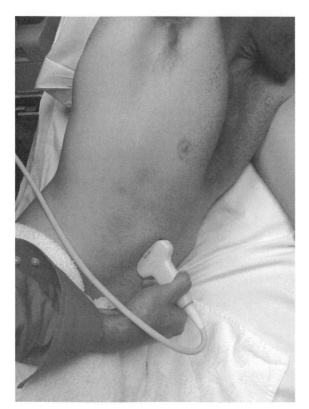

▲ **Figure 2–37.** Gallbladder position. (Reproduced with permission from Dawson M, Mallin M. Introduction to Bedside Ultrasound. Lexington, KY: Emergency Ultrasound Solutions, 2012.)

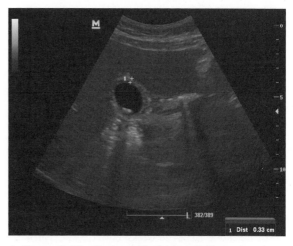

▲ **Figure 2–39.** Cholecystitis thick wall. (Reproduced with permission from Dawson M, Mallin M. Introduction to Bedside Ultrasound. Lexington, KY: Emergency Ultrasound Solutions, 2012.)

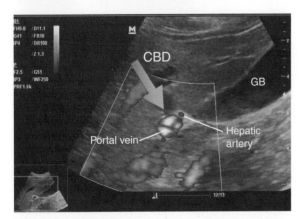

▲ **Figure 2–40.** Common bile duct. (Reproduced with permission from Dawson M, Mallin M. Introduction to Bedside Ultrasound. Lexington, KY: Emergency Ultrasound Solutions, 2012.)

this point the CBD should also be evaluated. In the sagital plane, one can track the gallbladder in a cephalad direction, bringing the hepatic triad and classic "Mickey Mouse" sign into view. The Mickey Mouse sign consists of the portal vein as Mickey's face and ears made up of hepatic artery and CBD. Color flow will differentiate the CBD from the hepatic artery and portal vein. The CBD will also represent Mickey's left ear (Figure 2–40). A normal CBD measures less than 7 mm from inner wall to inner wall dilation suggest biliary disease.

Mehta S, Lopez ME, Chumpitazi BP, et al: Clinical characteristics and risk factors for symptomatic pediatric gallbladder disease. Pediatrics. 2012;129:e82. [PMID: 22157135].
Tsung JW, Raio CC, Ramirez-Schrempp D, Blaivas M: Point-of-care ultrasound diagnosis of pediatric cholecystitis in the ED. Am J Emerg Med. 2010;28:338. [PMID: 20223393].

PYLORIC STENOSIS

Pyloric stenosis is a serious condition encountered in pediatric patients. The condition results from hypertrophy of the musculature of the gastric pylorus. Though often idiopathic, the condition has been associated with elevated levels of gastrin and dysfunction of the pyloric ganglion. The hypertrophied pylorus obstructs gastric outflow, causing persistent, classically projectile, vomiting. The disease has been shown to occur at a rate of 1:200–300 births. Pyloric stenosis has been diagnosed as early as 10 days postnatal and as late as 20 weeks; however, the typical age of presentation is 4–6 weeks. The prevalence in males is 3–6 times that of females, and is the most common surgical condition in infants. In most patients pylorotomy is curative with relatively few sequelae. If left untreated, the disease

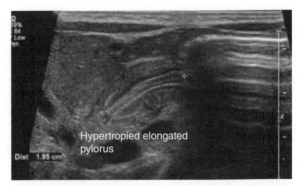

▲ **Figure 2–41.** Pyloric stenosis.

process can be fatal as a result of profound dehydration and metabolic abnormalities.

Pyloric stenosis is classically diagnosed by means of either fluoroscopic upper gastrointestinal series or ultrasound. Neither study is superior; however, ultrasound offers similar sensitivities and specificities, 85% and 100%, without the use of ionizing radiation.

The examination should be performed by experienced ultrasonographers only, as it is one of the more challenging bedside examinations to perform. The key aspects of the examination include identifying hypertrophied musculature of the pylorus as well as evaluating the dynamic function of the musculature over a 5–10 minute period. The examination should be completed with the linear probe, patient in the supine position. From an anterior approach, the pylorus will be located between the gastric antrum and duodenum. If pyloric stenosis is present, the stomach may be filled by the obstructed gastric contents. Measurement should be made at a perpendicular cross section in the midline of the longitudinal axis. A normal pylorus will have a muscle wall thickness (MWT) of less than 3 mm and a normal pyloric channel length less than 15 mm. At this location the pylorus should be observed for a period of 5–10 minutes to confirm the measurements. A changing MWT or passage of fluid through the pylorus can indicate pylorospasm rather than pyloric stenosis (Figures 2–41, 2–42). Although there are many variants, as well as further measurements that can confirm or refute the diagnosis of pyloric stenosis, the longitudinal MWT is the most accurate and widely accepted. As pyloric stenosis is an acute surgical emergency, diagnosis should prompt immediate surgical consultation.

INTUSSUSCEPTION

The telescoping and invagination of one piece of bowel into a more distal segment is known as intussusception. This diagnosis can be life threatening if left untreated and occurs

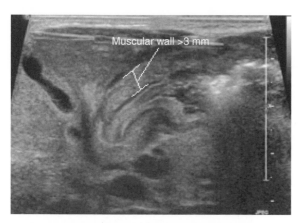

▲ **Figure 2–42.** Pyloric stenosis.

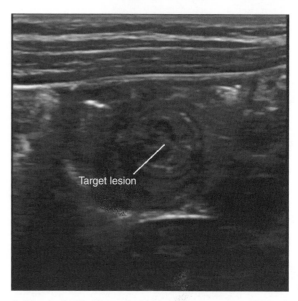

▲ **Figure 2–43.** Target lesion in intussusception. (Photo used with permission of Sonocloud.org.)

at a rate of 50 per 100,000 children per year. The ailment may result from an anatomical anomaly. A "lead point" such as a lymphoma or Meckel diverticulum can be pushed from the proximal bowel into the distal segment by peristalsis. Though identified in approximately 20% of patients, a lead point, such as a Peyer patch, is thought to be present even when not radiographically appreciated. Although there are reported patients as old as 7 years, the ailment is usually found in patients aged 6 months to 1 year. In a recent study of novice sonographers in an emergency department, a sensitivity of 87% and specificity of 97% was achieved with bedside ultrasound with minimal training.

The usual presentation is that of a child in the aforementioned age group with intermittent severe abdominal pain with pain-free intervals. Up to 75% of patients may have some blood present in the stool. However, the classic triad of "currant jelly stool," abdominal pain, and emesis is found in approximately 20% of confirmed diagnoses. Of confirmed cases, up to 50% of patients will have a palpable abdominal mass on initial presentation. Once diagnosed, intussusception can usually be reduced with either hydrostatic or pneumatic enema under ultrasound or fluoroscopic guidance. If the patient presents with bowel ischemia, evidence of perforation, or clinical instability, surgical intervention should be made.

The evaluation of intussusception is multifaceted. If there is clinical concern for perforation or obstruction, plain films should be obtained. Plain films will reveal free air and obstructive gas patterns. Plain films can also reveal patterns consistent with intussusceptions such as "target lesions" or "crescent lucencies" in 45–73% of patients (Figure 2–43). The gold standard for evaluation of intussusception has classically been contrasted enema, as it is both diagnostic and therapeutic. Ultrasound has been gaining popularity in recent years as it is noninvasive, and does not carry the risk of perforation associated with contrasted enemas. The exami-

nation also uses no ionizing radiation, and can be performed at the bedside if needed. The use of bedside ultrasound has demonstrated sensitivities 98–100%. Ultrasonography also has the advantage of diagnosing lead points that are not evident on contrasted enema studies.

Similar to pyloric stenosis, the bedside ultrasound examination can be a challenging examination. As such, it can be reliably performed by a skilled ultrasonographer only. As in the evaluation of pyloric stenosis the linear, high-frequency probe should be utilized. The examination should be performed in the supine position. The entire path of the colon should be evaluated, beginning at the cecum. Once located, the bowel should be followed from the cecum/distal ileum in a clockwise fashion, from the left lower quadrant through the right lower quadrant. If the patient is found to have a palpable abdominal mass, the area should be examined in multiple planes. The normal bowel will have a hyperechoic ring surrounding the hypoechoic bowel contents. If a segment of intussuscepted bowel is present, it may appear as multiple hypoechoic layers in contrast to the normal segments. This appearance has often been compared to the appearance of a normal kidney, the "pseudo kidney sign" (Figure 2–44). The appearance of an intussusception has also been described as the target sign. This is visualized as a hyperdense center surrounded by concentric hyperdense rings.

Demonstration of such findings should prompt emergent contrasted enema as well as pediatric surgical consultation. Surgical consultation should be present at time of contrasted enema in preparation for possible complications, including perforation.

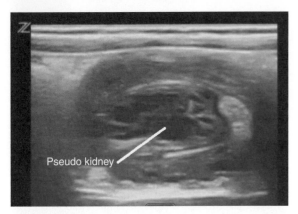

▲ **Figure 2–44.** Pseudo kidney. (Photo used with permission of Sonocloud.org.)

Riera A, Hsiao A, Langhan M, Goodman R, Chen L: Diagnosis of intussusception by physician novice sonographers in the emergency department. Ann Emerg Med. 2012;60(3):264. [PMID: 22424652].

VASCULAR ACCESS

As in the adult patient, vascular access can be of critical importance in the treatment of patients in the emergency department. Obtaining reliable vascular access is often most challenging in patients who are in the most desperate need. The use of bedside ultrasound has revolutionized the practice of obtaining both central as well as peripheral vascular access.

Classically obtained through the use of anatomic landmarks, the advances in bedside ultrasound have allowed the visualization of central vasculature in real time. By means of real-time visualization, the complication rates of central venous access have been minimized. Problems caused by distorted anatomy, lack of identifiable landmarks, and anatomical variations can be reduced with the use of bedside ultrasonography.

There are many risks such as pneumothorax, hemorrhage and injury to vessels and nerves associated with central venous line placement. With the use of ultrasound, peripheral vessels that would otherwise be difficult to see or palpate can be visualized and cannulated.

In both central and peripheral access, the use of bedside ultrasound has reduced complications and increased rates of successful cannulation. The Agency for Healthcare Research and Quality (AHRQ) and the National Institute for Clinical Excellence have advocated for the use of bedside ultrasonography to obtain central vascular access. Research and subsequent publications support vascular access guidance as a crucial indication for bedside ultrasonography performed by emergency physicians. A brief discussion of approaches to central access and a general overview of peripheral intravenous line placement follows.

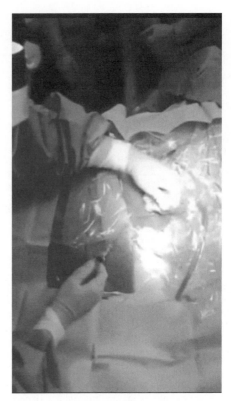

▲ **Figure 2–45.** Internal jugular. (Reproduced with permission from Dawson M, Mallin M. Introduction to Bedside Ultrasound. Lexington, KY: Emergency Ultrasound Solutions, 2012.)

The most common locations for central venous cannulation are the internal jugular, subclavian, and femoral veins. The internal jugular artery is generally found deep to the sternocleidomastoid muscle, lateral and superficial to the carotid artery (Figures 2–45, 2–46). The subclavian and axillary veins are easily located from an infraclavicular approach at the lateral aspect of the clavicle, and the femoral vein is found just inferior to the inguinal canal midway between the iliac crest and the pubic symphysis. Properties of the vasculature should be evaluated at each site. The vein will generally be more easily compressed, have thinner walls, and lack arterial pulsations. Color flow can be utilized to differentiate further between the venous and arterial vasculature.

To perform the task of dynamic vascular access guidance, the linear transducer should be utilized. Before draping the patient, the area should be scanned to determine the viability of the site. This survey can reveal anatomic anomalies that may present a challenge as well as clots within the targeted vessel (Figure 2–47). Once visualized and determined to be an appropriate site, the patient should be prepped and draped in a sterile fashion, including the use of sterile ultrasound probe

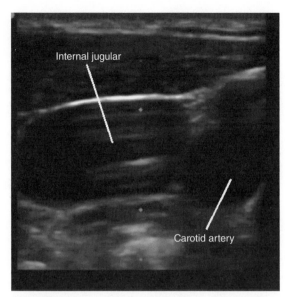

▲ **Figure 2–46. Internal jugular.** (Reproduced with permission from Dawson M, Mallin M. Introduction to Bedside Ultrasound. Lexington, KY: Emergency Ultrasound Solutions, 2012.)

cover. The skin should then be punctured with the transducer over the desired vasculature in the transverse plane. In this orientation, the operator should be able to visualize the needle tip as well as look for secondary signs of proper alignment (eg, ring down artifact), which is a solid streak or series of

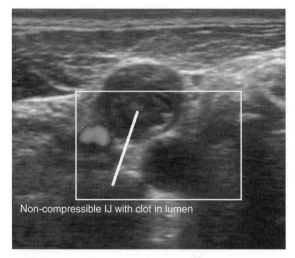

▲ **Figure 2–47. Internal jugular thrombus.** (Reproduced with permission from Dawson M, Mallin M. Introduction to Bedside Ultrasound. Lexington, KY: Emergency Ultrasound Solutions, 2012.)

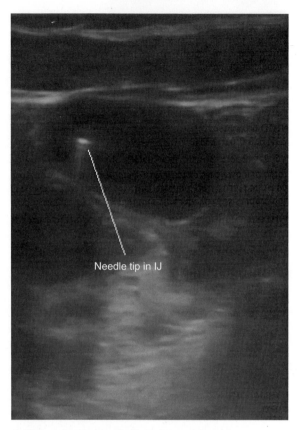

▲ **Figure 2–48. Needle tip in internal jugular.** (Reproduced with permission from Dawson M, Mallin M. Introduction to Bedside Ultrasound. Lexington, KY: Emergency Ultrasound Solutions, 2012.)

parallel bands radiating away from the object, or indentation of vasculature and surrounding structures. Once alignment has been established, the operator can choose from two methods in which to proceed. The tip of the needle can either be followed to venipuncture in the transverse plane, or the operator can switch to the longitudinal plane, tracking the needle progression to venipuncture (Figure 2–48). Once successful cannulation is confirmed by flash in the syringe, cannulation proceeds using the Seldinger technique.

Similar to the benefits provided with the use of bedside ultrasound in the placement of central venous access, its use in peripheral line placement offers profound advantages. Real-time ultrasonography allows visualization of peripheral vasculature not readily visible, palpable, or found in a routinely used anatomic location. Peripheral access is achieved using the same basic concepts as in central catheterization; however, peripheral veins are more superficial and more easily compressible. To obtain the best visualization very light pressure should be placed on the transducer, and in extremities, tourniquets should be utilized to minimize compression.

Bedside ultrasonography utilization in the guidance of arterial puncture or cannulation follows the same basic guidelines, conversely targeting the thick-walled, pulsatile, noncompressible vessel. Once the target is visualized, standard technique for arterial puncture/cannulation is followed.

Whether placing a central, peripheral, or arterial line, the use of bedside ultrasound can be utilized to increase success and decrease complications.

> Rothschild JM: Ultrasound guidance of central vein catheterization: Making healthcare safer: A critical analysis of patient safety practices. Available at http://www.ahrq.gov/clinic/ptsafety/ch21.htm.

MUSCULOSKELETAL (MSK) ULTRASOUND

Bedside ultrasound has demonstrated sensitivity and specificity in the diagnosis of long bone fractures and other disorders of the musculoskeletal system. In the evaluation of long bone fractures studies have shown sensitivity and specificity of 91% and 100%, respectively. Further, bedside ultrasound has shown to be beneficial in the reduction and treatment of long bone fractures. Its use in the evaluation of pediatric musculoskeletal disorders is not limited to fractures. Significant evidence proves the use of bedside ultrasound in the diagnosis of hip effusions to be sensitive (85%), specific (93%), and to decrease emergency department length of stay. Multiple case reports have demonstrated the ability of emergency medicine physicians to diagnose hip effusions using bedside ultrasound. Further, ultrasound has been proven to be effective in guiding aspiration in the evaluation of transient synovitis versus septic arthritis.

Performance of musculoskeletal ultrasonography is one of the simpler bedside ultrasound procedures performed by the emergency physician. As in most superficial indications, the linear probe should be utilized, but the curvilinear probe can be used for deeper structures. To evaluate for an acute fracture of long bones, two basic principles are used: scan at the location of pain and scan in two planes. Visualization of the bone will illustrate a hyperechoic bone cortex beneath the hypoechoic soft tissue and periosteum. Any defect in this cortex will be readily visualized (Figure 2–49).

Ultrasonography of long bone fractures has challenges in the pediatric population that may limit success. The examination can be painful with pressure applied directly to fracture sites, thus limiting compliance. Also, in the pediatric patient, immature growth plates will be visualized as a hypoechoic area within the hyperechoic cortex. The demonstration of growth plates has been shown to account

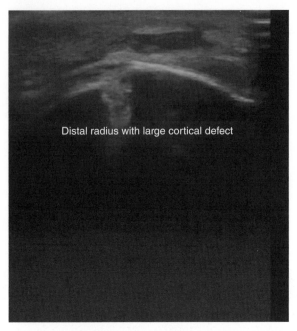

Distal radius with large cortical defect

▲ **Figure 2–49.** Distal radius fracture. (Photo used with permission of Sonocloud.org.)

for the majority of errors in bedside ultrasonography in the evaluation for fractures in the pediatric patient.

Evaluation of the pediatric hip follows a similar pattern as found in the evaluation for fracture. The patient should be supine, legs extended in neutral position. Because the pediatric hip is a superficial structure in most patients, the liner transducer will produce the best imaging. Begin with the probe sagittally, parallel to the long axis of the femoral neck. This view will demonstrate the femoral head, femoral neck, capsule, and iliopsoas muscle (Figure 2–50). With these structures in view, the capsular-synovial thickness can be measured from the anterior concavity of the femoral neck to the posterior surface of the iliopsoas. When this measurement is obtained, it should be compared to the unaffected side to determine the presence of an effusion (Figure 2–51). Parameters that define an effusion are generally a capsular-synovial measurement of greater than 5 mm, or greater than 2 mm difference from the unaffected side. Once diagnosed, ultrasonography can also be utilized in the aspiration of the effusion for the evaluation of synovial fluid.

Bedside ultrasound can be utilized additionally in the diagnosis of acute ailments of tendons and ligaments. The most relevant example is the evaluation of acute Achilles tendon rupture. In conjugation with the physical examination, evaluation of the Achilles tendon is both sensitive and specific. The examination, as most musculoskeletal examinations are, is

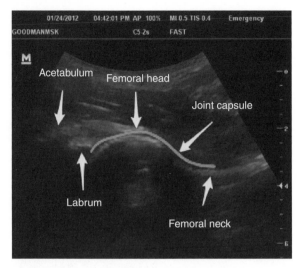

▲ **Figure 2–50.** Hip joint.

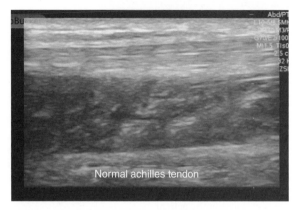

▲ **Figure 2–52.** Normal Achilles tendon. (Photo used with permission of Sonocloud.org.)

performed with the high-frequency linear probe. The Achilles tendon should be scanned with the probe in both the short and long axis. Normal tendon will demonstrate a homogenous structure with intermediate echogenicity. A pathological tendon will demonstrate heterogeneity of the tissue with associated edema and free fluid. The tendon can also be examined in a dynamic fashion with the patient attempting to plantarflex the foot (Figures 2-52 and 2-53).

Chinnock B, Khaletskiy A, Kuo K, Hendey GW: Ultrasoundguided reduction of distal radius fractures. J Emerg Med. 2011;40(3):308. [PMID: 19959315].

Shavit I, Eidelman M, Galbraith R: Sonography of the hip joint by the emergency physician: Its role in the evaluation of children presenting with acute limp. Pediatr Emerg Care. 2006;22(8):579. [PMID: 16912625].

Minardi JJ, Lander OM: Septic hip arthritis: Diagnosis and arthrocentesis using bedside ultrasound. J Emerg Med. 2012;43:316-8 [PMID: 22284975].

Tsung JW, Blaivas M: Emergency department diagnosis of pediatric hip effusion and guided arthrocentesis using point-of-care ultrasound. J Emerg Med. 2008;35(4):393. [PMID: 18403170].

Vieira RL, Levy JA: Bedside ultrasonography to identify hip effusions in pediatric patients. Ann Emerg Med. 2010;55(3):284. [PMID: 19695738].

Weinberg ER, Tunik MG, Tsung JW: Accuracy of clinician-performed point-of-care ultrasound for the diagnosis of fractures in children and young adults. Injury. 2010;41(8):862. [PMID: 20466368].

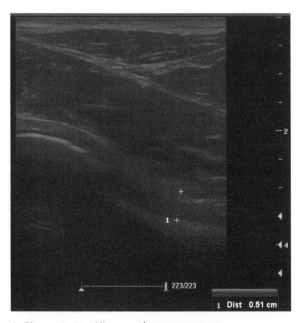

▲ **Figure 2–51.** Hip capsule measurement.

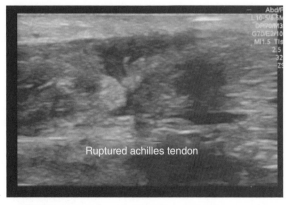

▲ **Figure 2–53.** Achilles tendon rupture. (Photo used with permission of Sonocloud.org.)

OCULAR ULTRASOUND

A number of properties of the eye make it an ideal subject for ultrasonic evaluation. Its superficial location and high fluid composition make for easily obtainable quality images. The ease of examination using bedside ultrasound offers a noninvasive evaluation of the anterior chamber, globe, and posterior eye (including the optic nerve).

Specific to the pediatric patient, this noninvasive examination can aid in the diagnosis of globe rupture, foreign body, retinal detachment, or elevated intracranial pressure (ICP). The indications for ocular ultrasound are vast. This section will by no means cover all the indications for ocular ultrasound, but will briefly cover the most important indications in the pediatric patient.

To perform the bedside ultrasound evaluation of the pediatric patient's eye, the high-frequency linear probe should be selected. Ultrasound should be placed on the ocular setting, or power setting set to 20–30% on linear high-frequency probe to avoid theoretical damage to sensitive structures. The patient should be either in the recumbent or supine position. A large volume, or "pillow" of gel should be placed over the closed eyelid. If there is concern that the child will open the eye, a Tegaderm dressing can be placed over the eye prior to gel placement. The scanning hand should be placed on the nasal bridge or forehead to avoid unintended pressure on the eye. If a globe rupture is obvious or highly suspected, this examination is contraindicated. The eye should be kept in a neutral position throughout the entire examination. From this point the eye should be scanned through both the transverse and longitudinal planes, creating a mental three-dimensional image of the eye. From this simple technique a number of common pathologies can be evaluated (Figure 2–54).

Perhaps the greatest concern in the evaluation of eye trauma is globe rupture. Of note, if this diagnosis is evident or highly suspected, ultrasound should be deferred and ophthalmology consultation should be obtained. In this evaluation, the emergency physician should take extreme caution to put no direct pressure on the eye. Maintenance of an echolucent stripe from the gel pillow will avoid unintentional pressure on the globe. Findings consistent with globe rupture include decreased size of the globe, anterior chamber collapse, and buckling of the sclera (Figure 2–55).

Intraocular foreign body is classically difficult to diagnose and a missed diagnosis can carry profound morbidity. Negative Siedel test or small entry sites can lead to false diagnoses such as corneal abrasion. Furthermore, objects such as glass and organic material may not be visualized on x-ray or CT. If present, intraocular foreign bodies generally appear as an echogenic structure with shadowing or tail artifact.

In suspected cases of retinal detachment, direct funduscopy presents multiple challenges and often inconclusive findings. Utilization of bedside ultrasound by the emergency physician has shown to have a sensitivity of 97% and specificity

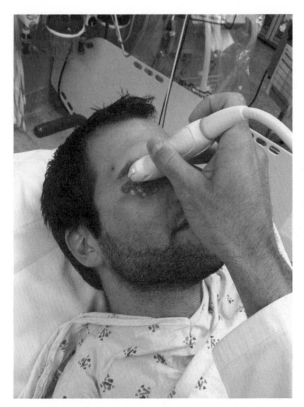

▲ **Figure 2–54.** Ocular scan.

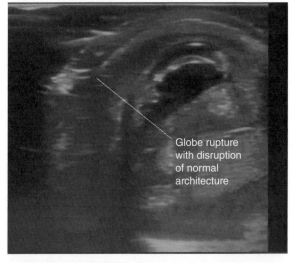

▲ **Figure 2–55.** Globe rupture.

Globe rupture with disruption of normal architecture

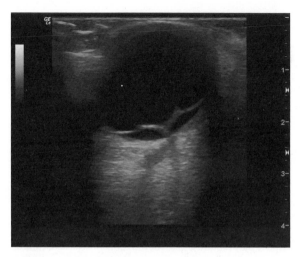

▲ **Figure 2–56.** Retinal detatchment.

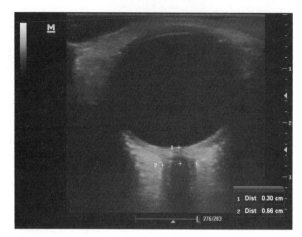

▲ **Figure 2–57.** Optic nerve measurement.

of 92% in the evaluation of possible retinal detachment. If present, the detached retina will appear as a highly reflective, thin structure that seems to float through the vitreous (Figure 2–56). The retina will maintain fixed points to the choroid, which may distinguish it from other vitreous pathologies. A complete tear may maintain attachment only at the optic nerve and ora serrata. These fixed points will cause the retina to produce a v-shape within the globe. All retinal detachments should prompt emergent ophthalmology consultation.

A key indication for the use of bedside ultrasonography of the eye is the measurement of ICP. To assess ICP, the optic nerve sheath should be measured in both eyes and averaged. The sheath should be measured perpendicularly, 3 mm behind the globe. An averaged value greater than 5 mm represents an ICP greater than 20 with sensitivity of 90% and specificity of 85% (Figure 2–57).

Ma J: Ocular ultrasound. In: Emergency Ultrasound. 2nd ed. New York, NY: McGraw-Hill; 2008.

Sawyer, NA: Ultrasound imaging of penetrating ocular trauma. J Emerg Med. 2009;36(2)181. [PMID: 17976814].

Shinar Z, Chan L, Orlinski M; Use of ocular ultrasound for the evaluation of retinal detachment. J Emerg Med. 2011;40(1):53. [PMID: 19625159].

Moretti R: Ultrasonography of the optic nerve in neurocritically ill patients. Acta Anaesthesiol Scand. 2011;55(6):644. [PMID: 21463263].

Dubourg J, Javouhey E, Geeraerts T, Messerer M, Kassai B: Ultrasonography of optic nerve sheath diameter for detection of raised intracranial pressure: A systematic review and meta-analysis. Intensive Care Med. 2011;37(7):1059. [PMID: 21505900].

Rajajee V: Optic nerve ultrasound for the detection of raised intracranial pressure. Neurocrit Care. 2011;15(3):506. [PMID: 21769456].

The use of bedside ultrasonography continues to revolutionize the practice of emergency medicine. Diagnoses traditionally made by common x-ray, CT, and radiology-analyzed ultrasonography are now being made by emergency physicians using bedside ultrasonography. Pediatric patients in the emergency department stand to benefit the most as emergency physicians become more comfortable and confident with ultrasound.

Jardin F, Veillard-Baron A: Ultrasonographic examination of the vena cava. *Intensive Care Med.* 2006;32:203. [PMID: 16450103].

Ramirez-Schrempp D, Dorfman DH, Tien I, Liteplo AS: Bedside ultrasound in pediatric emergency medicine fellowship programs in the United States: Little formal training. *Pediatr Emerg Care.* 2008;24:664. [PMID: 19242134].

Marin JR, Zuckerbraun NS, Kahn JM: Use of emergency ultrasound in Unites States pediatric emergency medicine fellowship programs in 2011. *J Ultrasound Med.* 2012;31(9):1357. [PMID: 22922615].

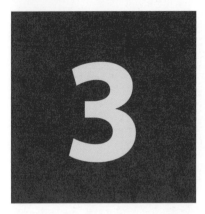

Emergency Procedures

Stephen McConnell, MD

Successful performance of a variety of procedures may prove critical in management of patients throughout the pediatric age spectrum. Although the frequency of procedures performed in clinical practice will vary, the physician should feel confident in performance of the procedures, and have knowledge of the indications, contraindications, and alternative procedures. When possible and circumstances allow, obtain appropriate informed consent prior to beginning a procedure. The following procedures are described in detail: tube thoracostomy, cardioversion and defibrillation, cardiac pacing, pericardiocentesis, peripheral intravenous catheter placement, umbilical vessel catheterization, central venous access, venous cutdown, intraosseous access, arterial catheter placement, gastrostomy tube replacement, abscess incision and drainage, external auditory canal foreign body removal, nasal canal foreign body removal, epistaxis management, common dislocation reductions, arthrocentesis, lumbar puncture, and subprapubic bladder catheterization.

AIRWAY MANAGEMENT

Management of a patient's airway is paramount in the emergency clinical setting. Identification of the patient who may benefit from simple or advanced airway management is not always straightforward. A number of methods and techniques described below may be employed in order to appropriately care for the patient in need of airway interventions. See Chapter 9, Compromised Airway, for further discussion.

CHEST PROCEDURES

TUBE THORACOSTOMY

Indications

Insertion of a tube thoracostomy may be indicated to relieve the accumulation of fluid or air from the pleural space. The patient may require a tube thoracostomy because of trauma, spontaneous pneumothorax, iatrogenic causes, or other systemic disease processes. Parapneumonic effusions may also require placement of a tube thoracostomy to assist in patient management.

Contraindications

Chest tube thoracostomy is often a lifesaving procedure and has few contraindications, which are typically relative, such as coagulopathy or overlying skin infection. The need for lung re-expansion typically takes priority over relative contraindications. There are no alternative procedures for most indications for tube thoracostomy. The clinician should always ensure that the correct side is affected prior to procedure initiation.

Equipment and Supplies

Gather all needed supplies and materials before performing the procedure. Many facilities provide a standardized tube thoracostomy tray with all essential supplies for the procedure; it is prudent to check the supply list on the tray to assure all needed elements are provided. In the absence of a prepackaged tray, determine that the following supplies and equipment are present and ready for use:

- Skin sterilization supplies
- Sterile technique operator equipment and personal protective equipment: mask, cap, gown, and sterile gloves
- Local anesthetic, syringe, and appropriate needles
- Sterile towels and drape
- Appropriate chest tube
- Scalpel, #11 or #15 blade is preferred
- Kelly and Mayo clamps
- Size 0 silk suture
- Needle holder
- Petrolatum-impregnated gauze
- Sterile gauze 4-inch squares

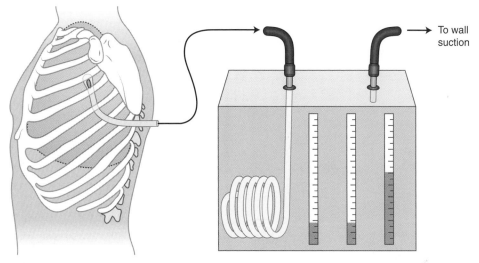

▲ **Figure 3–1. Commercial thoracostomy tube drainage system** with three chambers (from left to right): collection, water seal, and water column. Each chamber is filled with sterile water based on manufacturer's specifications. The collection chamber is directly connected to the tubing from patient and chest tube to the device, and allows for any drainage to accumulate. The middle chamber (water seal) allows air to exit the pleural space during exhalation, and prevents backflow of air into the pleural space during inhalation. Bubbling of air in the water seal chamber indicates an air leak. The water column chamber is used to regulate suction strength. The height of the water column indicates amount of suction relative to the water seal chamber. Adjusting the wall suction device should affect the water column, which in term is used to clinically manage the amount of desired suction. (Reproduced, with permission, from Dunphy JE, Way LW (eds): *Current Surgical Diagnosis & Treatment*, 5th ed. Lange, 1981. Copyright © McGraw-Hill Education LLC.)

- 2- or 3-inch wide silk or plastic adhesive tape
- Suction device, typically a commercially available prepackaged device that includes connection tubing (Figure 3–1)

Identify the appropriate approach path, and select the appropriate size chest tube. Chest tube size recommendations may be found on a Broselow tape. In the emergency setting, the diagnosis of pneumothorax versus fluid in the pleural space may not be clear. In general, insertion of the largest possible tube will minimize risk of clotting or clogging with accumulated fluid or blood. A summary of usual chest tube sizes is listed in Table 3–1. Ensure that the proximal air port of the selected chest tube will be in the pleural cavity after placement is complete by placing the tube over the patient for an approximated comparison. Keep a sterile field and abide by sterile technique throughout the procedure. Anesthetize a sufficient area to ensure adequate analgesia, paying close attention to the skin incision site and intended tube path. Depending on clinical status, the patient may benefit from systemic medication administration, or procedural sedation in order to allow the procedure to be performed comfortably.

The majority of chest tubes should be inserted in the, third, fourth, or fifth intercostal space in the midaxillary line. Rarely, an anterior approach may be taken to place a small-bore chest tube in the second intercostal space, midclavicular line. The technique is primarily utilized for a pneumothorax; however, the location is utilized less in clinical practice because of potential complications and decreased patient satisfaction with an anterior chest tube.

Table 3–1. Chest tube size.

Patient Age	Neonate	0-1 y	1-2 y	2-5 y	5-10 y	> 10 y	Adult
Patient weight	< 5 kg	5-10 kg	10-15 kg	15-20 kg	20-30 kg	30-50 kg	~50 kg
Approximate chest tube size (French)	8-12	10-14	14-20	20-24	20-28	28-40	32-40

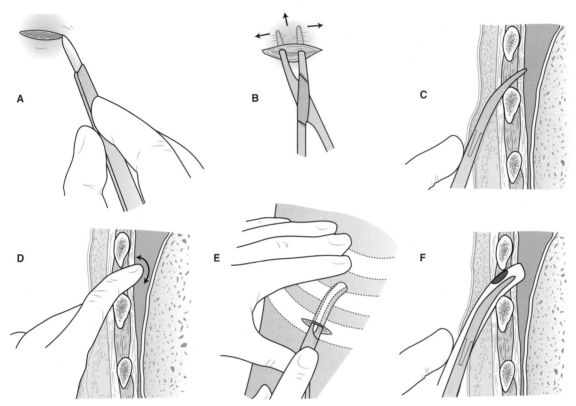

▲ **Figure 3–2. Tube thoracostomy.** A. Incise the skin at the chosen site. B. Use blunt dissection from the incision to the intercostal muscles. C. Enter the pleural space with a closed Kelly clamp. D. Palpate the tract with a single finger to assure entry into the pleural space. E. Guide the tube with a Kelly clamp through the opening in the subcutaneous tissue. F. Guide the chest tube into the pleural cavity. (Reproduced, with permission, from Reichman EF, Simon RR: *Emergency Medicine Procedures*. New York, McGraw-Hill, 2004. Copyright © McGraw-Hill Education LLC.)

Procedure

Figure 3–2 illustrates the tube thoracostomy procedure.

Prepare all equipment including the suction device, and connect it to wall suction.

1. Position the patient with the ipsilateral arm overhead or raised away from the field.

2. Prepare the sterile instruments and gown in sterile fashion.

3. Sterilize the skin at the appropriate predetermined site and several centimeters around the intended incision site.

4. Determine the interspace and palpate the rib above and below the intended site of insertion. Anesthetize the area over the interspace and the area inferior (Figure 3–3).

5. Drape the surrounding chest wall with sterile towels, leaving an exposed window approximately 10 cm wide over the insertion site.

6. Make an incision with the scalpel through the skin one or two rib spaces below where the chest tube will insert into the pleural space. Ensure that the incision is large enough to allow both the tube and the operator's finger or other device (eg, Kelly clamp) to be inserted through the skin. Making the incision one or two rib spaces below where the chest tube will insert into the pleural space will allow tunneling to occur in the subcutaneous tissue and help to guide the chest tube to its appropriate final destination. The incision should be parallel to the adjacent rib.

7. Use blunt dissection with the Mayo clamp in a cephalad direction to identify the pleural space where the chest tube will insert. Blunt dissection should also be directed anterior or posterior, depending on the intention of the chest tube. In the supine patient, air preferentially will be located anterior, while fluid will be located posterior. Insertion of the chest tube above the lower rib

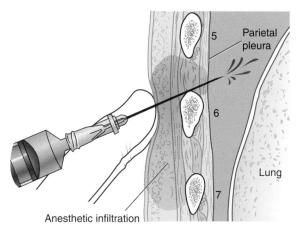

▲ Figure 3–3. Local anesthetic infiltration into the chest wall for tube thoracostomy. (Reproduced, with permission, from Reichman EF, Simon RR: *Emergency Medicine Procedures*. New York, McGraw-Hill, 2004. Copyright © McGraw-Hill Education LLC.)

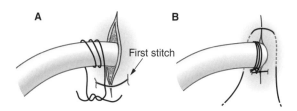

▲ Figure 3–4. Silk suture is used to secure the chest tube to the skin of the chest wall. (Reproduced, with permission, from Reichman EF, Simon RR: *Emergency Medicine Procedures*. New York, McGraw-Hill, 2004. Copyright © McGraw-Hill Education LLC.)

will help to minimize the possibility of damaging the neurovascular bundle running along the inferior edge of the upper rib.

8. Enter the pleural space just over the inferior rib of the interspace with the closed blunt tips of the Kelly clamp by maintaining steady pressure, and then spread the tips wide once past the parietal pleura and inside the pleural space. This will open the space wide enough to pass the tube. Many operators underestimate the amount of force needed to pass through the intercostal muscles and chest wall; use steady pressure and be prepared to release pressure when the clamp suddenly enters the pleural space. A sudden rush of air or fluid is to be expected.

9. If the intercostal space is of the appropriate size, the operator should insert one finger into the pleural space and sweep 360 degrees to confirm location.

10. Clamp the distal end of the chest tube prior to insertion; this will ensure that a rapid escape of blood or fluid does not cause unneeded exposure to bodily fluids. Guide the tube as it is inserted into the pleural space in a superior and anterior or posterior fashion, depending on the clinical situation.

11. Connect the distal chest tube to the suction device and evaluate for variance of the water columns with respiration. Improper placement will result in no water movement with inhalation and exhalation.

12. Secure the tube in place with silk suture. This is commonly performed by sewing a horizontal mattress suture around both sides of the tube, which aids in closing the incision on either side of the tube. Use the tails of the silk suture to wind around the tube from opposing directions (4–5 passes each) and tie the ends securely (Figure 3–4).

13. Wrap petrolatum gauze around the tube over the incision site to prevent leakage. Cut the 4-inch gauze squares and secure them around the tube, over the petrolatum gauze. Tape the gauze to the patient's chest wall, and secure the tube by taping it directly inferior to the insertion site to the chest wall. Secure the chest tube to suction device tubing connection with additional tape (Figure 3–5).

14. Evaluate tube placement by an upright chest radiograph, paying specific attention to lung re-expansion and improvement of fluid collection (if an initial radiograph was obtained).

Alternative techniques for evacuating air include the following: needle decompression (usually performed in the second intercostal space, midclavicular line), small-bore Seldinger-technique placed chest tube, and needle aspiration.

Disposition

Most patients who have a chest tube placed emergently should be admitted to the hospital for further care, usually to a surgical or intensive care department. Consider transfer to a facility with appropriate consultants as indicated.

Complications

Damage to the neurovascular bundle including the thoracic nerve or intercostal arteries may occur while dissecting the tissue, prior to insertion of the chest tube. Inappropriately placed chest tubes may damage intra-abdominal or mediastinal structures. Damage to the lung tissue may also occur during tube thoracostomy placement. Hemodynamic

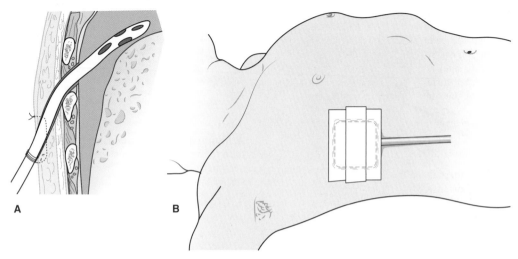

A   B

▲ **Figure 3–5. Chest tube dressing** is placed after securing the chest tube with suture. (Reproduced, with permission, from Reichman EF, Simon RR: *Emergency Medicine Procedures*. New York, McGraw-Hill, 2004. Copyright © McGraw-Hill Education LLC.)

instability may also be encountered due in part to rapid evacuation of an effusion or by direct compression of the heart. Infection may also occur when sterile technique is not followed during insertion of the chest tube or in maintenance of a placed chest tube.

Lin CH, Lin WC, Chang JS: Comparison of pigtail catheter with chest tube for drainage of parapneumonic effusion in children. *Pediatr Neonatol.* 2011;52(6):337 [PMID: 22192262].

Yadav K, Jalili M, Zehtabchi S: Management of traumatic occult pneumothorax. *Resuscitation.* 2010;81(9):1063 [PMID: 20619952].

CARDIAC PROCEDURES

Cardiac interventions are performed infrequently in the pediatric patient. However, proper knowledge and timely implementation may be the difference in outcome for the patient. The majority of indications for cardiac intervention depend on the hemodynamic stability of the patient. See Cardiac Emergencies, Chapter 35, for further discussion.

CARDIOVERSION & DEFIBRILLATION

Cardioversion and defibrillation use an external source of energy with the goal of restoring a perfusing rhythm. With synchronized cardioversion, the current of energy is passed during the QRS complex and avoids the relative refractory period when a shock could cause refractory ventricular fibrillation. In defibrillation, usually a larger amount of energy is passed through the heart at a time that is not synchronized with the intrinsic electrical cardiac cycle.

Synchronized cardioversion may take place in the hemodynamically unstable patient, or in the patient where medical management has been unsuccessful in managing the patient's condition. Synchronized cardioversion should be started at 0.5 joules/kg and then doubled every 1–2 minutes up to 2 joules/kg. It is imperative that the monitor be synchronized to the patient prior to delivering a shock.

When performing defibrillation on a pediatric patient, synchronization is not necessary. Begin the first defibrillation attempt at 2 joules/kg; each subsequent debrillation should be 4 joules/kg.

CARDIAC PACING

Cardiac pacing is rarely performed in the pediatric patient; however, its appropriate use may change the patient's outcome. Two forms of pacing are available in the emergency setting: transthoracic and transvenous. Each form provides unique challenges until definitive management is provided. Administer analgesia or anxiolysis when appropriate.

Indications

Asystole and symptomatic bradycardia are the most common indications in children.

▶ Transthoracic Pacing

Transthoracic, or external cardiac pacing, utilizes similar electrodes to performing cardioversion or defibrillation. Place the pacing pads on the patient with one over the left anterior chest and one over the posterior chest wall, typically adjacent to the left scapula. Some clinicians prefer to place the second pad directly posterior or on the left lateral chest wall. Ensure that the pads do not touch. Prior to turning the pacing function on, set the desired rate (usually based upon the patient's age) and turn the output to its lowest possible level. After turning the pacemaker function on, gradually increase the output until mechanical capture is obtained. Consult with cardiologic physician for definitive management.

▶ Transvenous Pacing

Transvenous, or internal cardiac pacing, utilizes central venous access to allow insertion of a pacing wire. Most pediatric patients will require a 6 French sheath, which can allow a 4 French pacer wire to be inserted. Although nearly any central vein can be accessed to allow for pacer wire insertion, ideally the right internal jugular vein (adolescents and children over 8 years) or the femoral vein (children 8 years and younger) is accessed. Avoiding the left subclavian vein, if possible, will allow for an easier approach if a permanent pacemaker is required.

One of the challenges in placing transvenous pacer wires is appropriate placement. This may be especially challenging if one of the femoral veins is accessed. Some catheters come with a balloon, which may be inflated to help "float" the wire into the appropriate place. However, in low-flow states, this is often ineffective. One means to ensure appropriate placement is the use of fluoroscopy or electrocardiogram (ECG) guidance. Although fluoroscopy is routinely available in the operating room or cardiac catheterization laboratory, the technology is not usually available in the emergency department. Utilizing one of the V leads from the ECG machine (with the limb leads attached) and attaching it directly to the pacer wire, the clinician can "see," based on the electrical activity through the V lead, where the tip of the pacemaker is located.

More commonly, insertion of the pacer wire in the emergency department is performed in a "blind" method. This involves insertion of the catheter through the sheath and having the pacer in full-demand mode. This allows the pacer to sense the intrinsic cardiac activity, but does not allow the pacer to generate an electric current. When the clinician notices the pacemaker is sensing appropriately, the output should be increased and the pacer wire slowly advanced until mechanical capture is obtained.

Complications

Complications from pacing may occur with the transvenous approach, although burns to the skin have been noted with continued transthoracic approach. The use of rigid pacer wires has been associated with ventricular rupture. The balloon on the end of the pacer wire may rupture and cause an air embolism. Ventricular dysrhythmias may also occur with the transvenous approach.

Disposition

Regardless of the method used to pace a patient, clinical scenarios that require cardiac pacing warrant hospital admission and cardiology consultation.

PERICARDIOCENTESIS

The ability to perform a pericardiocentesis may be lifesaving in the appropriate clinical scenario. Not all effusions require emergent pericardiocentesis in the emergency department.

Indications

The patient who has a pericardial effusion with hemodynamic instability, such as cardiac tamponade, benefits from timely pericardiocentesis. The patient with a more chronic pericardial effusion may have a diagnostic pericardiocentesis performed in order to evaluate the condition as an inpatient.

Contraindications

There are no absolute contraindications to performing emergent pericardiocentesis in the setting of cardiac tamponade. Relative contraindications (relevant for non–life-threatening tamponade) are overlying skin infection and known or suspected bleeding disorders.

Equipment and Supplies

Gather all supplies including:

- Skin sterilization supplies
- Sterile technique operator equipment and personal protective equipment: mask, cap, gown, and sterile gloves
- Local anesthetic, syringe, and appropriate needles
- Assorted syringes (two each) including 50 mL size
- Pericardiocentesis needle 14–18 gauge; spinal needles are often used. A needle up to 5–6 inches long may be needed for larger adolescents
- Sterile towels/drape
- Electrocardiographic monitor or ECG machine capable of continuous monitoring strip
- Ultrasound machine, if available, with sterile sheath for the probe

If a catheter is to be left in place for continued drainage, ensure that all appropriate support supplies are present. Commercially available kits are often used to leave a pericardial drain in place.

Bedside ECG machines may be used to inform the practitioner if the tip of the needle comes into contact with the ventricular wall. This may reduce the complication of ventricular puncture. Real-time bedside ultrasound makes it possible to watch the needle penetrate the pericardium. Ultrasound may also help the practitioner assess for cardiac

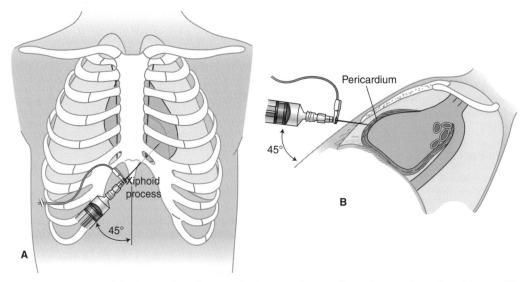

▲ **Figure 3–6. Angles used during pericardiocentesis. A.** Insert the needle 45 degrees from the midsagittal line, and **B.** 45 degrees over the abdominal surface. (Reproduced, with permission, from Reichman EF, Simon RR: *Emergency Medicine Procedures*. New York, McGraw-Hill, 2004. Copyright © McGraw-Hill Education LLC.)

compromise and the presence of tamponade prior to performance of the procedure.

Procedure

Appropriate analgesia or procedural sedation should be administered when possible. Pericardiocentesis is a sterile procedure. The patient may require airway management prior to performance of pericardiocentesis. The use of real-time bedside ultrasound may improve success and reduce potential complications.

1. After ensuring appropriate analgesia and observing sterile technique (when possible), position the patient in slight reverse Trendelenburg.

2. Select the appropriate size syringe and needle for the patient, or have the pericardial drain set at bedside.

3. Sterilize the proposed field for the procedure in a wide area over the subxiphoid space; drape the surround chest and abdominal walls.

4. Attach the needle to one of the V leads on the ECG machine with the limb leads attached. Utilize real-time bedside ultrasound, if available, to help assist in the procedure.

5. Identify landmarks: 1 cm to the left of the inferior margin of the xiphoid process. Alternatively, consider a parasternal approach in the fifth intercostal space.

6. Advance the needle, with negative pressure through the syringe, through the skin. Xiphoid approach: 45-degree angle to the anterior plane of the skin, and 45 degrees to

the midline aiming toward medial to the left shoulder (Figure 3–6). Parasternal approach: perpendicular to the skin through the fifth intercostal space.

7. Withdraw as much pericardial fluid as possible, or insert the pericardial drain.

8. When a drain is not utilized, remove the needle and cover the wound with a sterile dressing.

9. Obtain chest x-ray to evaluate for potential complications.

Disposition

Patients who undergo pericardiocentesis in the emergency department should be admitted for further evaluation and management. Cardiothoracic surgery or cardiology should be consulted depending on the clinical scenario.

Complications

Infection is a known complication. In addition, complications may include hemothorax or pneumothorax, damage to vasculature including the coronary vessels, as well as the potential for damage to peritoneal structures such as the liver.

Arya SO, Hiremath GM, Okonkwo KC, et al: Central venous catheter-associated pericardial tamponade in 6-day old: a case report. *Int J Pediatr.* Epub 2010 [PMID: 20169087].

Berul CL, Cecchin F, American Heart Association, et al: Indications and techniques of pediatric cardiac pacing. *Expert Rev Cardiovasc Ther.* 2003;1(2):165 [PMID: 15030277].

Manole MD, Saladino RA: Emergency department management of the pediatric patient with supraventricular tachycardia. *Pediatr Emerg Care.* 2007;23(3):176 [PMID: 17413437].

Weil BR, Ladd AP, Yoder K: Pericardial effusion and cardiac tamponade associated with central venous catheters in children: an uncommon but serious and treatable condition. *J Pediatr Surg.* 2010;45(8):1687 [PMID:20713221].

VASCULAR PROCEDURES

Most emergency clinicians will encounter an appropriate clinical scenario when IV access is required for patient care. It is important for the clinician to understand and be proficient at obtaining peripheral venous access, and when a vein is not identifiable of obtaining access via a different route.

PERIPHERAL INTRAVENOUS CATHETER PLACEMENT

Peripheral intravenous (IV) access is most commonly obtained in the emergency department. Although the task and difficulty may be increased because of patient size, volume status, and cooperation, the relative technique remains the same. There are four main sites where peripheral IV access commonly occurs: upper extremity, lower extremity, scalp, and external jugular vein in the neck.

Indications

There are a number of indications for obtaining peripheral IV access. For patients requiring diagnostic laboratory studies, blood may be obtained during or immediately after catheter placement. For patients requiring IV systemic medications or fluid resuscitation, a peripheral IV catheter is suitable for these clinical situations.

Contraindications

A small number of contraindications exist for peripheral access placement. Avoid areas of infection and inflammation, such as overlying cellulitis or apparent phlebitis. Also avoid thrombosis and previous skin breakdown, including burns. Choose an alternative site if there is lymphedema or trauma proximal to the insertion site. Evaluate for perfusion prior to application of a tourniquet and if there is evidence of poor perfusion, the practitioner should attempt to find an alternative location.

Equipment & Supplies

The peripheral IV access procedure is similar in all age groups, although the equipment size will vary. One of the keys to success in peripheral IV catheter placement is rapport with the patient and family members. Building trust can decrease anxiety for the patient and family members, as well as for the clinician who will perform the procedure. The use of tourniquets may be helpful, although should not be used when attempting to place an IV catheter in the external jugular vein.

The use of an assistant may prove beneficial to help stabilize and immobilize the extremity where the IV access will occur.

- Skin cleansing supplies/alcohol swabs
- Tourniquet
- IV catheter and needle of appropriate size
- Preprepared and flushed IV fluid bag or saline flush

Procedure

1. Discuss with the patient (if appropriate) and family members about what will happen.
2. After evaluation and vein selection, immobilize the extremity and apply a tourniquet proximal to the vein site, if appropriate.
3. Clean the area of IV access thoroughly.
4. Insert the needle through the skin approximately 0.5–1 cm distal to the site of venous entry, at an angle of approximately 15 degrees to the skin surface. Keeping the skin taught may improve success to help immobilize the vein.
5. After receiving a flash of blood in the catheter, advance additional 1–2 mm to ensure that both the needle tip and catheter are in the vein.
6. Advance the catheter into the vein smoothly while keeping the needle in place.
7. Once the catheter is in the vein, withdraw the needle and place in an appropriate sharps container immediately.
8. If blood is needed for laboratory analysis, draw blood sample(s).
9. Remove tourniquet and flush the IV with saline, ensuring that the catheter remains in the vein and there is no extravasation.
10. Secure the IV catheter in place. It may be helpful in younger children to apply a brace or splint to secure the patient's extremity to reduce movement.

Special Considerations

Not all patients require an indwelling IV catheter. If a blood sample is all that is needed, consider using a butterfly needle, which is smaller in diameter. If there is difficulty identifying a suitable vein, consider darkening the room and use a flashlight to illuminate the vein from the opposite side of the extremity. Commercially devices are also available to illuminate a vein.

Consider use of topical anesthetics or injection of local anesthetics to relieve pain for the patient. However, some topical medications may take up to 1 hour to be effective and may not be practical in an emergency department setting. There is evidence that distraction of the child (playing videogames or watching television) and oral sucrose in infants may decrease pain during IV catheter placement.

Scalp veins may be used for peripheral IV access in patients aged 6–9 months, or when hair precludes visualization. An advantage to scalp veins for access is that they are generally more superficial. A tourniquet may be used when accessing the veins and, at times, a rubber band may serve this purpose well. Ensure that there is a piece of tape or other tag to assist in removal of the tourniquet after it is used. The tourniquet should never be placed around the patient's neck. Catheterization occurs in the technique as outlined previously, and once the catheter is placed, gauze or other material should be fashioned to support the catheter so it does not move.

Complications

Damage to the vessel may result in hematoma formation. Other structures near the vein, including arteries or nerves, may be inadvertently damaged. Local areas of inflammation or infection occur. When placing an external jugular catheter, extreme care should be taken to avoid damage to any of the deeper structures, including the carotid artery.

UMBILICAL VESSEL CATHETERIZATION

Umbilical artery catheterization is primarily performed in the first 24 hours of life of a patient. This usually occurs in a neonatal intensive care unit, but may be required in the emergency department. Accessing the umbilical artery allows for frequent blood draws including arterial blood gas, and provides a route for fluid and medication administration. Exchange transfusion may also be performed via this route. Most, but not all, infants have two umbilical arteries, which appear similar to each other, and have thicker walls than the single vein. The arteries are typically located inferiorly or toward the 6-o'clock position.

Umbilical vein catheterization is most successful in the neonate, but may be attempted in infants up to 2 weeks of age. Fluids and medications may be given via this route, but other access sites should be exhausted prior to cannulating the umbilical vein. The umbilical vein often appears flat rather than round, and is usually superior at the 12-o'clock position.

Equipment & Supplies

Umbilical catheters are commercially supplied in a kit with most of the required materials. The clinician should be familiar with the kit at their institution as well as other required materials. This is a sterile procedure, and strict adherence to sterile technique is paramount. The patient undergoing umbilical vessel catheterization is generally critically ill and may require other interventions such as airway management prior to the procedure.

Procedure

1. Measure the appropriate distance that the catheter will be inserted. Use appropriate guide or nomogram for arterial or venous catheter insertion and the shoulder to umbilicus length. Most procedures performed in the emergency department will be emergent, and the clinician may not have time to determine ideal insertion length.

2. Loosely secure the base of the umbilical cord with either a purse-string suture or umbilical tape.

3. Using a scalpel, transversely cut the umbilical cord stump 0.5–2 cm from the base and identify the vessels.

4. Using hemostats, evert the umbilical stump edges.

5. Dilate the appropriate vessel using smooth-edged forceps.

6. Insert the appropriate catheter either to the depth suggested by the nomogram, or until blood flow is noted.

7. Secure the catheter in place and review a postprocedure x-ray to confirm placement.

Figures 3–7 and 3–8 show umbilical artery and vein cannulation.

Complications

Because there are a number of complications for umbilical vessel catheterizations, routine use of the procedure is not recommended. Ischemia of the lower extremity or bowel, or

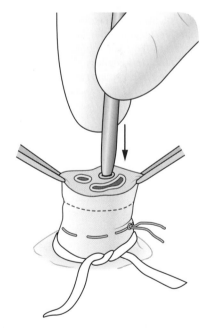

▲ **Figure 3–7. Umbilical artery catheter insertion.** The catheter is placed into one of the two umbilical arteries. (Reproduced, with permission, from Reichman EF, Simon RR: *Emergency Medicine Procedures*. New York, McGraw-Hill, 2004. Copyright © McGraw-Hill Education LLC.)

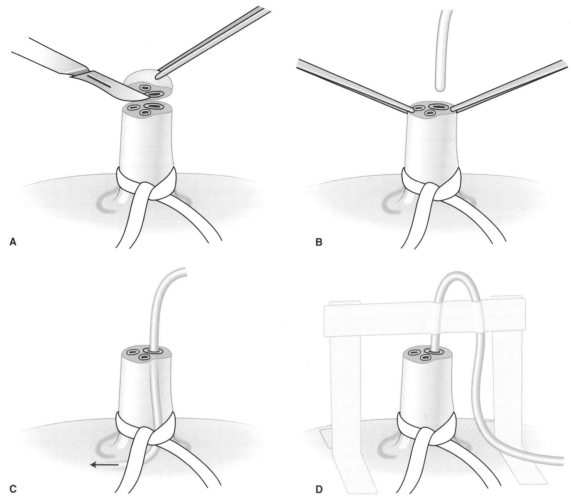

▲ **Figure 3–8.** Umbilical vein catheter insertion. (Reproduced, with permission, from Tintinalli JE, Stapczynski JS, Ma OJ, Cline DM, Cydulka RK, Meckler GD: *Tintinalli's Emergency Medicine: A Comprehensive Study Guide*, 7th ed: New York, McGraw-Hill, 2011. Copyright © McGraw-Hill Education LLC.)

thrombus formation may be seen. Infection is also a complication of any invasive procedure, and specifically necrotizing enterocolitis may be seen with umbilical vessel catheterization.

Disposition

Patients who have an umbilical vessel catheter placed will need to be admitted to a neonatal or pediatric intensive care unit.

CENTRAL VENOUS ACCESS

Although commonly less performed than peripheral venous access, understanding the unique challenges and complexities of central venous access is crucial. Central venous access

is accomplished through the internal jugular vein, subclavian vein, or femoral vein.

Site Selection

The clinician must have a complete understanding of the anatomy related to the site of central venous catheterization prior to beginning the procedure. Many clinicians are able to use real-time ultrasonography to help guide them during the procedure, as discussed in Chapter 2.

The femoral vein lies medially to the femoral artery in the proximal thigh. This site is often considered a top choice for emergent central venous access. It is readily identified by anatomic landmarks, is able to have pressure applied in the event of bleeding, and does not interfere with other procedures such as airway management that may be ongoing. Also, complications present at the other sites (eg, pneumothorax) are not be encountered in this approach.

The internal jugular vein runs within the carotid sheath with the carotid artery and vagus nerve. Preferentially, the right internal jugular vein should be catheterized because it is a more direct route to the superior vena cava. This site allows for central venous pressure monitoring, which is not possible from a femoral route.

The subclavian vein is the least common site to place a central venous catheter in the pediatric patient. Anatomic landmarks are not as well defined in children as they are in adults or adolescents. Similar to the internal jugular vein, the right subclavian vein should preferentially be chosen because of a lower cupola on the right as well as a more direct route to the superior vena cava.

Indications

Indications for central venous access include administration of IV fluids or medications, measuring central venous pressures, or for access of a Swan-Ganz catheter or transvenous pacemaker placement.

Contraindications

There is no absolute contraindication for central venous access, although care should be taken to select the most appropriate site for the patient. Avoid the femoral route if there is a femoral hernia, abdominal trauma, or if the catheter is being placed for transvenous pacer placement. Avoid the subclavian route in patients receiving positive-pressure ventilation or those with known or suspected bleeding disorders because of the noncompressible nature of this site.

Equipment & Supplies

Most of the materials needed are included in a commercially available pediatric central line kit. A single lumen catheter

Table 3–2. Central venous access French catheter diameter.

Age	0-6 mo	6 mo-2 y	3-6 y	7-12 y
Internal jugular	3	3	4	4-5
Subclavian	3	3	4	4-5
Femoral	3	3-4	4	4-5

allows rapid infusion of fluid or blood products, while a multiple lumen catheter allows for simultaneous administration of medications/fluids. Choose the appropriate size catheter for the specific patient. Tables 3–2 and 3–3 summarize expected catheter sizes for different access sites and pediatric age groups. Some adolescents may require an adult central line kit because of their body size. The most common technique for central line placement is the Seldinger technique (Figure 3–9). This is a sterile procedure, and strict adherence to sterile technique is crucial. Attempt to obtain informed consent prior to beginning procedure, if the clinical situation allows.

Procedure

1. Position the patient appropriately for the site into which the catheter will be inserted. Subclavian and internal jugular vein catheter placement benefit from the patient in Trendelenburg position, whereas femoral vein catheter placement benefits from the patient in reverse Trendelenburg.

2. Use appropriate analgesia or sedation, as appropriate, to minimize patient discomfort.

3. Sterilize the surrounding skin and site of insertion, and surround the area with sterile drape or towels. Observe sterile technique including personal sterile attire.

4. If available, use real-time ultrasound guidance (see Chapter 2).

Table 3–3. Average catheter length in centimeter.

Age	1 mo	3 mo	6 mo	9 mo	1 y	1.5 y	2 y	4 y	6 y	8 y	10 y	12 y	14 y	16 y
Average weight (kg)	4.2	5.8	7.8	9.2	10.2	11.5	12.8	16.5	20.5	26	31	39	50	62.5
Average height (cm)	55	61	68	72	76	83	88	103	116	127	137	149	165	174
IJ	6.0	6.6	7.3	7.6	8.0	8.7	9.2	10.6	11.8	12.9	13.8	15.0	16.5	17.3
SC	5.5	6.0	6.6	6.9	7.3	7.9	8.3	9.6	10.7	11.7	12.5	13.5	14.9	15.7
Fem	15.7	17.3	19.1	20.1	21.1	22.9	24.2	28.1	31.4	34.2	36.8	39.9	44.0	46.3

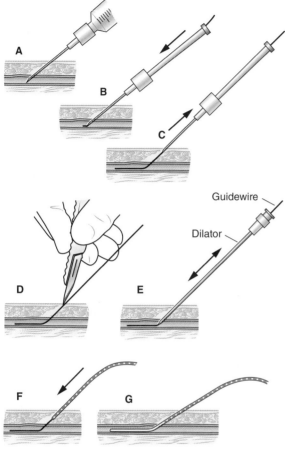

▲ **Figure 3–9. Seldinger technique.** A. An introducer needle is used to puncture the vein and aspirate blood. B. With the syringe removed, the guidewire is passed through the needle and into the vein. C. Remove the needle over the guidewire. D. Use a scalpel to widen the skin puncture site adjacent to the guidewire. E. Advance the dilator over the wire, through the skin opening, and to the depth of its hub; remove the dilator. F. Insert the catheter over the wire and into the vein. G. Remove the guidewire while holding the catheter in place. (Reproduced, with permission, from Reichman EF, Simon RR: *Emergency Medicine Procedures.* New York, McGraw-Hill, 2004. Copyright © McGraw-Hill Education LLC.)

5. Anesthetize the site of insertion with local injection of anesthetic.

6. Insert the entry needle through the skin, applying negative pressure from an attached syringe.

7. Advance needle 1–2 mm after the initial flash of blood to ensure the needle tip is in the vein.

8. Remove the syringe from the needle, taking care not to move the needle during this process. Ensure that the blood return is dark and nonpulsatile.

9. Insert the guide wire through the needle into the vessel. Do not force the guide wire; reposition the needle if the wire does not advance freely.

10. Remove the needle over the guide wire while leaving the guide wire in place. Always have the guide wire secured with a grasp when it is in the vessel.

11. Use an 11-blade scalpel to create a nick in the skin at the site of entry, adjacent to the wire.

12. Advance a dilator over the guide wire and into the vessel. Once the dilator is inserted, remove the dilator, holding pressure over the skin where the dilator was located and maintaining the position and grasp of the wire.

13. Insert the catheter over the guide wire and into the vessel. Make note of the length of the catheter inserted.

14. Secure the catheter in place with suture.

15. Obtain and review a postprocedure chest x-ray for confirmation of placement (internal jugular and subclavian sites).

▶ Femoral Vein

Position the patient's hip in abduction and external rotation. Palpate the femoral artery approximately 1–2 cm below the inguinal ligament. Approximately 1–2 cm medial to this site is where the femoral vein is located. Ultrasound guidance has improved success rates in femoral vein catheterization and should be utilized when possible. Insert the needle at a 45-degree angle to the skin and advance toward the ischial tuberosity. Once the needle has entered the vessel, consider flattening the angle toward the skin (20–30 degrees) if the guide wire does not freely advance. Do not allow the needle to pass beyond the inguinal ligament and into the peritoneal cavity (Figure 3–10).

▶ Internal Jugular Vein

The median approach is the most popular in pediatric patients. Position the patient so that the head is rotated 30 degrees from midline, facing the contralateral side. Identify the junction of the two heads of the sternocleidomastoid muscle, which will form an apex where the internal jugular vein is located. Palpate the carotid artery and note that the internal jugular vein is lateral to the artery. Whenever possible, real-time ultrasound guidance should be used. Insert the needle at a 30-degree angle to the skin, and advance in the direction of the ipsilateral nipple (Figure 3–11).

▶ Subclavian Vein

There are two approaches to cannulating the subclavian vein: supraclavicular and infraclavicular. For the supraclavicular

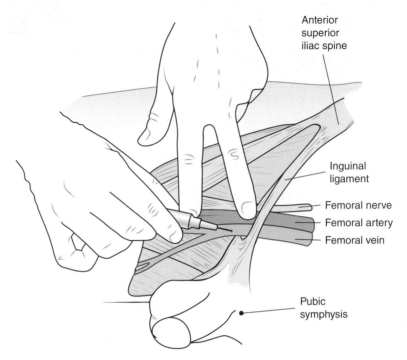

Anterior superior iliac spine

Inguinal ligament

Femoral nerve
Femoral artery
Femoral vein

Pubic symphysis

▲ **Figure 3–10. Central line placement: femoral vein.** The puncture should occur approximately 1-2 cm inferior to the inguinal ligament and 1 cm medial to the pulse of the femoral artery. Enter the skin at 45 degrees. (Reproduced, with permission, from Reichman EF, Simon RR: *Emergency Medicine Procedures.* New York, McGraw-Hill, 2004. Copyright © McGraw-Hill Education LLC.)

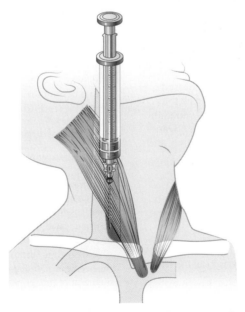

▲ **Figure 3–11. Central line placement: internal jugular vein, median approach.** Enter the skin at 30 degrees between the heads of the sternocleidomastoid muscle, aiming at the ipsilateral nipple. (Reproduced, with permission, from Dunphy JE, Way LW (eds): *Current Surgical Diagnosis & Treatment,* 5th ed. Lange, 1981. Copyright © McGraw-Hill Education LLC.)

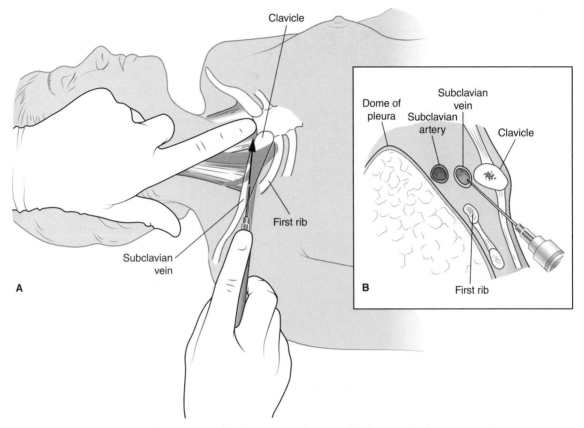

▲ **Figure 3–12. Central line placement: subclavian vein, infraclavicular approach.** A. Illustrates the operator's view of the patient as the needle is inserted. B. Illustrates a cross-sectional view as the needle passes deep to the clavicle and enters the subclavian vein. (Reproduced, with permission, from Reichman EF, Simon RR: *Emergency Medicine Procedures.* New York, McGraw-Hill, 2004. Copyright © McGraw-Hill Education LLC.)

approach, locate the lateral border of the clavicular head of the sternocleidomastoid muscle and the superior aspect of the clavicle at this junction. Insert the needle about one fingerbreadth laterally to this site at the superior margin of the clavicle, and advance the needle toward the suprasternal notch. For the infraclavicular approach, identify the mid-clavicular line and the inferior border of the clavicle. Insert and advance the needle under the clavicle aimed toward the suprasternal notch (Figure 3–12).

Complications

There are a number of identified complications to central venous catheter placement. The catheterized vessel can become thrombosed, lacerated, or perforated. Cardiac dysrhythmias may occur when advancing the guide wire. Infection may occur as well. With internal jugular and subclavian catheter placement, pneumothorax and hemothorax are known complications. Femoral catheters have been associated with damage to the peritoneal contents as well as retroperitoneal hematomas.

Disposition

Patients with central venous catheters placed in the emergency department are typically admitted for further evaluation and management of the clinical condition requiring catheter placement.

VENOUS CUTDOWN CATHETERIZATION

Venous catheterization using a cutdown technique allows direct visualization of the vessel being catheterized. Several techniques and locations have been described, however, the basilic and distal saphenous veins are most commonly performed.

Indications

Venous cutdown catheterization is primarily done when other peripheral techniques have not produced suitable vascular access. This may be true in patients with significant burns.

Contraindications

There are no absolute contraindications to the procedure. Alternative methods or sites should be considered if there is trauma to the region or to a region proximal to where the intended access site will be. The operator should consider an alternative location if there is evidence of infection, underlying pathology such as a fracture, or compartment syndrome.

Equipment and Supplies

This is a sterile procedure and all efforts to maintain sterile technique should be employed. The practitioner should prepare an 11-blade scalpel, hemostats, forceps, silk suture, and syringes. The appropriate size vascular catheter should be selected based on the patient's size and location. The vascular anatomy should be well reviewed by the phsician.

Procedure

▶ Distal Saphenous Vein

The procedure is illustrated in Figure 3–13.

1. Make a 1–2 cm superficial incision perpendicular to the distal saphenous vein, approximately 1 cm superior to the medial malleolus. The incision should be deep enough to go through the dermis, but should not damage the underlying tissue.
2. Bluntly dissect the subcutaneous tissue and identify the distal saphenous vein.
3. Insert the silk suture material to form two ligatures on the vein.
4. Tie the distal ligature of the vessel.
5. Lift the proximal suture ligature and make a small venotomy.
6. Insert the catheter into the venotomy site and secure the proximal ligature. This should secure the catheter inside the vein.
7. Close the skin with suture and secure the extremity.

▶ Basilic Vein

1. Position the patient's arm with the elbow extended and the forearm supine.
2. Approximately 2 cm proximal to the flexor crease, create a 2–3 cm incision perpendicular to the basilic vein. Determine that this incision is anterior to the medial epicondyle.

3. Bluntly dissect the subcutaneous tissue and identify the basilic vein.
4. Insert the silk suture material to form two ligatures on the vein.
5. Tie the distal ligature of the vessel.
6. Lift the proximal suture ligature and make a small venotomy.
7. Insert the catheter into the venotomy site and secure the proximal ligature. This should secure the catheter inside the vein.
8. Close the skin with suture and secure the extremity.

Complications

The majority of complications arise with the initial incision or with the venotomy, including transection of the vessel or surrounding structures. Infection may occur locally or spread systemically.

Disposition

Consider admission of all patients who require a venous cutdown in the emergency department. The venous cutdown should be considered temporary vascular access. Once the intravascular volume status is restored, continue to evaluate for other suitable peripheral venous access.

INTRAOSSEOUS ACCESS

An alternative option for initial vascular access is the intraosseous route. This technique is utilized in both hospital and prehospital settings for providing quick and reliable vascular access in the care of critically ill pediatric patients.

Indications

Intraosseous devices should be placed only when immediate vascular access is required and other routes deemed difficult or impossible. The routine use of intraosseous devices for patient care is not recommended. Intraosseous devices are not considered definitive vascular access.

Contraindications

Contraindications include recent fractures (at the chosen site), referred to as osteogenesis imperfecta, or evidence of overlying infection or burn.

Equipment & Supplies

Intraosseous needles are commercially available; the needle is a heavy-gauge trocar with an internal obturator associated cannula. Manual needles as well as power drill needles exist in the commercial market. Additionally, a local anesthetic or systemic analgesic should be administered whenever the clinical situation warrants and time allows.

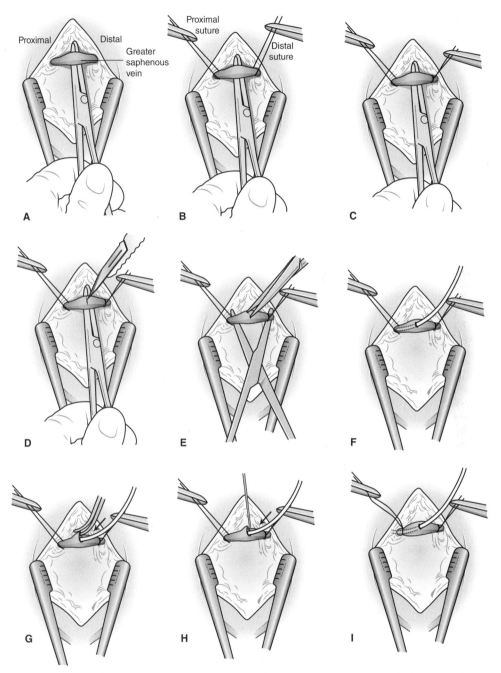

▲ **Figure 3–13. Venous cutdown.** A. Isolate the vein. B. Place silk suture ties on either side of the cannulation site. C. Tie the distal suture. D. Using a scalpel, incise the vein with enough room to place the IV catheter. E. An alternate method uses a hemostat and scissors to create the opening. F. Advance the catheter in the proximal direction. G. A small hemostat may aid in maintaining patency of the vein during cannulation. H. Maintain control and visibility of the vein until the catheter is fully inserted. I. Tie the proximal suture to secure the catheter in place. (Reproduced, with permission, from Reichman EF, Simon RR: *Emergency Medicine Procedures*. New York, McGraw-Hill, 2004. Copyright © McGraw-Hill Education LLC.)

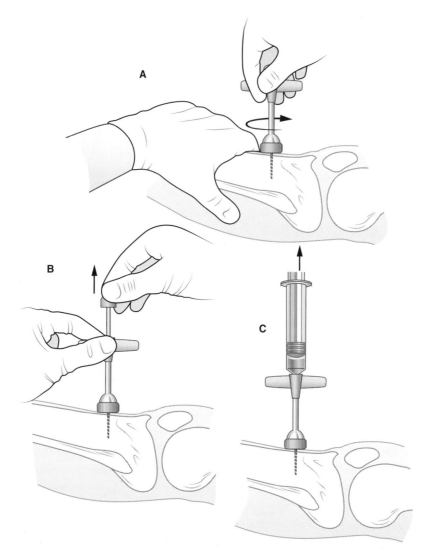

▲ **Figure 3–14. Placing an intraosseous line.** A. Support the extremity with one hand, and use a twisting effort to place the line at the appropriate site. B. Remove the handle and obturator. C. Use a syringe to connect to the intraosseous needle and aspirate bone marrow to ensure correct placement. (Reproduced, with permission, from Reichman EF, Simon RR: *Emergency Medicine Procedures.* New York, McGraw-Hill, 2004. Copyright © McGraw-Hill Education LLC.)

Procedure

The most common location for insertion of the intraosseous needle is the proximal or distal tibia. Attempt to maintain sterile technique throughout the procedure (Figure 3–14).

▶ Proximal Tibia

1. Identify the tibial tuberosity and palpate the area just distal and medial to the tibial tuberosity. Locate the flattest area in the region. Sterilize the skin in a wide margin around the area.

2. Place the tip of the intraosseous needle perpendicular to the cortex of the tibia.

3. With constant and firm pressure, advance the intraosseous needle. Twisting of the needle improves the rate of penetration. Do not rock the needle.

4. There will be a sudden release of pressure, signifying that the tip of the needle is in the marrow space.

5. Withdraw the obturator, leaving the cannula portion of the intraosseous needle in place.

6. Attach a syringe to the catheter and aspirate bone marrow to confirm correct placement. If no marrow can be aspirated, attempt to flush the catheter gently and look for evidence of extravasation. Flushing the catheter with saline should be simple if the catheter is successfully placed.

7. Secure the catheter in place, by enclosing with gauze sponges and an overlying dressing.

▶ Distal Tibia

1. Identify the medial malleolus. Approximately one fingerbreadth proximal to the superior margin of the medial malleolus, locate the flattest portion of the distal tibia in this region. Sterilize the skin in a wide margin around this area.

2. Place the tip of the intraosseous needle perpendicular to the cortex of the tibia.

3. With constant and firm pressure, advance the intraosseous needle. The operator may find twisting the needle improves the rate of penetration. Do not rock the needle.

4. There will be a sudden release of pressure, signifying that the tip of the needle is in the marrow space.

5. Withdraw the trocar, leaving the catheter in place.

6. Attach a syringe to the catheter and aspirate bone marrow to confirm correct placement. If no marrow can be aspirated, attempt to flush the catheter gently and look for evidence of extravasation. Flushing the catheter with saline should be simple if the catheter is successfully placed.

7. Secure the catheter in place, by enclosing with gauze sponges and an overlying dressing.

Complications

Several complications are associated with intraosseous catheters. Infection such as osteomyelitis or cellulitis may develop. If the catheter is not placed correctly, a fracture may occur, and cause damage to growth plates. Placement of the intraosseous needle completely through a bone has been reported, with resultant extravasation of administered fluids.

Compartment syndrome may occur in patients who have an unrecognized misplaced intraosseous catheter.

Disposition

Patients with an intraosseous catheter placed should be admitted to the hospital. Depending on the response of the patient, a pediatric intensive care unit may be needed. Additional vascular access should be sought when the clinical situation allows.

ARTERIAL CATHETER PLACEMENT

Although placement of a venous catheter is routine in the management of many pediatric patients, arterial catheterization is reserved for those patients who are critically ill. The radial and femoral arteries are most frequently chosen as the site for arterial catheter placement.

Indications

Arterial catheter placement will allow for real-time monitoring of blood pressure and allow for blood gas sample draws. Both options may prove beneficial in the care of critically ill pediatric patients.

Contraindications

There are a number of contraindications to arterial catheter placement. The clinician should avoid sites with underlying fractures, absent pulse or vascular compromise in the chosen extremity (or a positive Allen test), or evidence of overlying infection.

Equipment & Supplies

Commercially available kits contain most of the equipment needed for arterial catheterization. Arterial cannulation is either performed with a catheter-over-needle approach or a modified Seldinger method. Ensure that the size of the needle or catheter is appropriate for the patient (Table 3–4). Have an assistant prepare the appropriate arterial monitoring device. Obtain consent prior to the procedure being performed, and

Table 3–4. Arterial catheter equipment sizes.

Artery	Radial, posterior tibial, dorsalis pedis, or brachial	Femoral or axillary umbilical	Umbilical
<10 kg patient	Needle size: 25 or 23 Catheter size: 24 or 22	Needle size: 23 Catheter size: 20 or 18 French size: 3.0-4.0	French size: 3.5-5.0
10-40 kg patient	Needle size: 23 Catheter size: 22	Needle size: 23 or 21 Catheter size: 18 or 16 French size: 4.0-5.0	
>40 kg patient	Needle size: 23 or 21 Catheter size: 22 or 20	Needle size: 21 Catheter size: 18, 16, or 14 French size: 5.0-6.0	

consider analgesia or sedation for patient comfort. This procedure is performed while observing sterile technique.

Procedure

▶ Radial Artery

Prior to performing a radial artery catheterization, perform an Allen test to ensure adequate collateral flow through the ulnar artery. The Allen test is performed by applying pressure to both the radial and ulnar arteries just proximal to the wrist, allowing blood to exit the hand. After pallor is achieved, release pressure over the ulnar artery and observe for a prompt return of color to the hand. Absence of return to the radial side of the hand indicates a lack of collateral flow and is a contraindication to catheter placement in the radial artery.

1. Position the patient's hand, slightly extended with ulnar deviation to expose the radial artery.
2. Palpate the arterial pulse throughout the procedure.
3. Insert the needle through the skin at a 30–45-degree angle aiming cephalad and toward the pulse.
4. Slowly advance the needle until arterial blood is returned in the syringe.
5. Advance the wire through the needle and then the catheter over the wire if performing a Seldinger technique. Advance the catheter into the vessel if performing a catheter-over-needle approach.
6. Ensure pulsatile flow and attach to arterial monitor tubing.
7. Secure the arterial catheter and consider a splint to keep the patient from moving or dislodging the catheter.

▶ Femoral Artery

The femoral artery is commonly used in the pediatric patient because of its larger size.

1. Position the patient with external rotation and abduction of the ipsilateral hip.
2. Palpate the arterial pulse throughout the procedure.
3. Insert the needle through the skin at a 30–45-degree angle aiming cephalad and toward the pulse.
4. Slowly advance the needle until arterial blood is returned in the syringe.
5. Advance the wire through the needle and then the catheter over the wire if performing a Seldinger technique. Advance the catheter into the vessel if performing a catheter-over-needle approach. Because of the deeper location of the femoral artery, compared with the radial artery, most clinicians use a Seldinger technique.
6. Ensure pulsatile flow and attach to arterial monitor tubing.
7. Secure the arterial catheter and consider a splint to keep the patient from moving or dislodging the catheter.

Complications

The most serious complication associated with arterial catheterization includes damage to the artery and subsequent insufficient blood flow to the distal extremity. Recheck after 10–15 minutes to ensure adequate distal blood flow to the affected extremity. Injury may also occur to other surrounding structures. Hematoma and thrombus formation are known complications. On failed attempts, apply direct pressure over the puncture site for 10 minutes.

Alten JA, Borasino S, Gurley WQ, et al: Ultrasound-guided femoral vein catheterization in neonates with cardiac disease. *Pediatr Crit Care Med.* 2012;13(6):654 [PMID: 22791091].

Biran V, Gourier E, Cimerman P, et al: Analgesic effects of EMLA cream and oral sucrose during venipuncture in preterm infants. *Pediatrics.* 2011;128(1):e63 [PMID: 21669894].

Bothur-Nowacka J, Czech-Kowalska J, Grusfeld D, et al: Complications of umbilical vein catherisation. Case Report. *Pol J Radiol.* 2011;76(3):70 [PMID: 22802847].

Brzezinski M, Luisetti T, London MJ: Radial artery cannulation: A comprehensive review of recent anatomic and physiologic investigations. *Anesth Analg.* 2009;109(6):1763 [PMID: 19923502].

Chappell S, Cilke GM, Chan TC, et al: Peripheral venous cutdown. *J Emerg Med.* 2006;31(4):411 [PMID: 17046484].

DiCarlo JV, Auerbach SR, Alexander SR: Clinical review: Alternative vascular access techniques for continuous hemofiltration. *Crit Care.* 2006;10(5):230 [PMID: 16989669].

Haumont D, de Beauregard VG, Can Herreweghe I, et al: A new technique for transumbilical insertion of central venous silicone catheters in newborn infants. *Acta Paediatr.* 2008;97(7):988 [PMID: 18422804].

Jimenez N, Bradford H, Seidel KD, et al: A comparison of needle-free injection system for local anesthesia versus EMLA for intravenous catheter insertion in the pediatric patient. *Anesth Analg.* 2006;102(2):411 [PMID:16428534].

Khouloud AS, Julia G, Abdulaziz B, et al: Ultrasound guidance for central vascular access in the neonatal and pediatric intensive care unit. *Saudi J Anaesth.* 2012;6(2):120 [PMID: 22754436].

Kim do K, Choi SW, Kwak YH: The effect of SonoPrep on EMLA cream application for pain relief prior to intravenous cannulation. *Eur J Pediatr.* 2012;171(6):985 [PMID: 22350285].

Lewis GC, Crapo SA, Williams JG: Critical skills and procedures in emergency medicine: vascular access skills and procedures. *Emerg Med Clin North Am.* 2013;31(1):59 [PMID: 23200329].

Minute M, Badina L, Cont G, et al: Videogame playing as distraction technique in course of venipuncture. *Pediatr Med Chir.* 2012;34(2):77 [PMID: 22730632].

Schindler E, Kowald B, Suess H, et al: Catheterization of the radial or brachial artery in neonates and infants. *Paediatr Anaesth.* 2005;15(8):677 [PMID: 16029403].

Voigt J, Waltzman M, Lottenberg L: Intraosseous vascular access for in-hospital emergency use: a systematic clinical review of the literature and analysis. *Pediatr Emerg Care.* 2012;28(2):185 [PMID: 22307192].

Watchko JF: Route of exchange transfusion in neonates with hyperbilirubinemia. *Pediatr Crit Care Med.* 2011;12(1):110 [PMID: 21209575].

Weiser G, Hoffmann Y, Glabraith R, et al: Current advances in intraosseous infusion-a systematic review. *Resuscitation.* 2012;83(1):20 [PMID: 21871243].

Yigiter M, Arda IS, Hicsonmez A: Hepatic laceration because of malpositioning of the umbilical vein catheter: case report and literature review. *J Pediatr Surg.* 2008;43(5):e39 [PMID: 18485935].

GASTROINTESTINAL PROCEDURES

GASTROSTOMY TUBE REPLACEMENT

Patients who have had a percutaneous endoscopic gastrostomy (PEG) procedure performed will present to the emergency department for a variety of reasons, including dislodgment of the PEG tube. The clinician should understand the risks and benefits of replacing the tubes, or inserting another device.

Indications

Patients without means of adequate nutritional intake require replacement of the feeding tube or appropriate consultation to have the tube replaced.

Contraindications

There are few contraindications to replacing a dislodged gastrostomy tube. Primarily, as long as the tract is matured, and the patient presents soon after tube dislodgement, reinsertion of a gastrostomy tube is not difficult. However, if the gastrostomy tube was placed less than 2 or 3 weeks prior to the patient presentation, the tract has not had time to mature and attempting to replace the gastrostomy tube in the emergency department is contraindicated.

Materials & Supplies

If possible, replace a dislodged gastrostomy tube with the same size and manufacturer. This may not be feasible in all emergency departments, depending on availability of equipment. If an identical device is not available, attempt to locate a Foley catheter of the same size as the dislodged gastrostomy tube.

Procedure

Gastrostomy tube replacement procedure is illustrated in Figure 3–15. It is not a sterile procedure. Consider placing a topical anesthetic, such as viscous lidocaine, over the gastrostomy site to help alleviate discomfort.

1. Locate the appropriate size gastrostomy tube or Foley catheter. Test the device prior to insertion to ensure adequate function.

2. Place a water-based lubricant over the skin where the gastrostomy site is located.

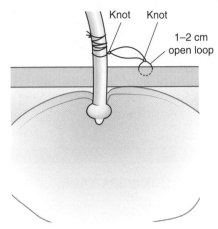

▲ **Figure 3–15. Gastrostomy tube replacement.** Diagram illustrates the correctly replaced gastrostomy tube, secured in place with silk suture. (Reproduced, with permission, from Reichman EF, Simon RR: *Emergency Medicine Procedures.* New York, McGraw-Hill, 2004. Copyright © McGraw-Hill Education LLC.)

3. Apply gentle pressure while inserting the gastrostomy tube through the mature tract.

4. Inflate the balloon of the gastrostomy tube or Foley catheter, and secure the catheter in place. Silk suture may be used to secure the tube if a commercially available bolster is not available.

5. Confirm placement in the stomach with clinical examination, and by injecting water-soluble contrast followed by a confirmatory x-ray.

Complications

There are few complications if the gastrostomy site is mature. However, sites that are less than 2–3 weeks old require endoscopic or surgical intervention. Bleeding may occur in some patients, but is usually self-limited. Local cauterization around the site may be needed in cases of persistent leakage of blood. Cases of peritonitis have occurred when attempting to provide nutrition through a misplaced gastrostomy tube.

Disposition

The patient may return home after the tube has been replaced. If a Foley catheter is utilized, it is possible to provide nutrition until a permanent PEG tube can be placed at follow-up.

Minchff TV: Early dislodgement of percutaneous and endoscopic gastrostomy tube. *J S C Med Assoc.* 2007;103(1):13 [PMID: 17763821].

Saavedra H, Losek JD, Shanley L, et al: Gastrostomy tube-related complaints in the pediatric emergency department: identifying opportunities for improvement. *Pediatr Emerg Care.* 2009;25(11):728 [PMID: 19864965].

Showalter CD, Kerrey B, Spellman-Kennebeck S, et al: Gastrostomy tube replacement in a pediatric ED: Frequency of complications and impact of confirmatory imaging. *Am J Emerg Med.* 2012;30(8):1501 [PMID: 22306396].

Wu TS, Leech SJ, Rosenberg M: Ultrasound can accurately guide gastrostomy tube replacement and confirm proper tube placement at the bedside. *J Emerg Med.* 2009;36(3):280 [PMID: 18614327].

SOFT TISSUE PROCEDURES

ABSCESS INCISION & DRAINAGE

Cutaneous abscesses are a common presenting concern to emergency departments. Understanding their pathology as well as management is crucial in clinical practice.

Indications

The patient who presents to the emergency department with a cutaneous abscess should undergo incision and drainage. Depending on the location and the patient's age and medical history, it may or may not be a simple procedure.

Contraindications

Contraindications to incision and drainage in the emergency department may include the following: concern for deep space tissue infection, perineal or perianal location, facial or orbital cellulitis, abscesses involving the anterior neck, and abscesses that involve the genitalia or breast tissue. The appropriate surgeon should be consulted in such cases. Avoid draining an abscess believed to be communicating with a joint space, or one where the resultant scar will be unacceptable.

Equipment and Supplies

Supplies required for incision and drainage are an 11-blade scalpel and hemostats. Irrigation saline is useful as well as packing material, depending on the abscess size and preference of the operator. Local anesthetics or systemic analgesics may be required. Depending on the patient and clinical circumstance, consider procedural sedation for abscess drainage. The clinician may consider bedside ultrasound to help delineate an abscess.

Procedure

1. Anesthetize the area around the abscess. Using a buffered lidocaine infusion will ease the pain.
2. Incise the abscess cavity with an 11-blade scalpel.
3. Remove loculations by using hemostats for blunt dissection. Spread the tips of the hemostats throughout the cavity to ensure all loculations have been disrupted.
4. Irrigate the abscess cavity with copious amounts of saline.
5. Consider packing the abscess cavity to ensure continued drainage of additional or newly formed purulent material.

Complications

Complications are encountered rarely while draining an abscess. Early closure of the wound may prompt recurrence of fluctuance. The incision must be large enough, or packing used to wick away recurrent purulence. When loculations are not completely disrupted, individual remaining pockets are isolated and may grow into recurrent abscesses. Similarly, if the abscess is located near vital structures, there is risk of vascular or nerve damage. Cosmetic defects may occur at the site of drainage.

Disposition

The patient who undergoes abscess management in the emergency department is rarely admitted to the hospital. Patients who may benefit from consultation or admission include those with significant systemic effects, complicated abscesses, and those who may have underlying immunosuppression.

Baumann BM, Russo CJ, Pavlik D: Management of pediatric skin abscesses in pediatric, general academic, and community emergency departments. *West J Emerg Med.* 2011;12(2):159 [PMID: 21691519)].

OTORHINOLARYNGOLOGY PROCEDURES

EXTERNAL AUDITORY CANAL FOREIGN BODY

External auditory canal (EAC) foreign bodies are a common presenting concern to the emergency department by patients. Common objects that get lodged in the EAC include beads, toys, paper, and insects. Removal of foreign bodies from the EAC is a skill that emergency clinicians should have. The patient may present to the emergency department with ear pain, decreased hearing from one side, or knowledge that a foreign body is in the ear. A thorough examination is crucial.

Indications

Removal of EAC foreign bodies may be performed in the emergency department.

Contraindications

Contraindications are rare. The uncooperative patient may require procedural sedation to ensure the operator can safely remove the foreign body without causing trauma to the tympanic membrane or EAC. Foreign bodies surrounded by significant swelling, erythema, or drainage should prompt ENT consultation. If the foreign body cannot be appropriately visualized, consultation is appropriate.

Equipment and Supplies

There are a host of commercially available products to help remove foreign bodies from the EAC. Alligator forceps, hooks, curettes, suction catheters, and other devices may be employed in order to make foreign body removal as quick and painless as possible.

Procedure

Identify the site of the foreign body. It is important to have a cooperative patient, and on occasion anxiolysis or analgesia is required. Consider having a specialist remove the foreign body if procedural sedation is required. Visualize the foreign body on physical examination and determine the best method to remove the object.

▶ Irrigation

Irrigation is a technique that can be used without full visualization of the foreign body and with minimal risk to damaging the ear canal or tympanic membrane. Use an 18- or 20-gauge catheter attached to a syringe to instill room-temperature water directed at the posterior, superior wall of the ear canal. Do not use water on an object that may swell, as this could make its removal difficult.

▶ Suction

Foreign bodies that have a regular and a flat surface may be removed from the EAC with suction catheter. Place the suction catheter flush with the foreign body, taking care not to push the object deeper into the EAC. Apply suction and gently remove the foreign body.

▶ Instruments

Foreign bodies with irregular surfaces may be removed from the EAC with the use of alligator forceps, or a right angle hook. Do not attempt foreign body removal in a blind fashion as it can lodge the object deeper into the EAC, causing trauma to the canal or tympanic membrane.

Complications

Regardless of the method used to attempt foreign body removal, it is important to examine the ear after removal or attempted removal of the object to evaluate for a complication. If the practitioner is not successful at removing the foreign body, otolaryngology consultation is indicated.

Most complications occur when attempting to remove the foreign body with rigid instruments. These may cause abrasions or lacerations to the auditory canal, or may penetrate through the tympanic membrane. Extreme caution

should be practiced when placing something into the EAC to remove a foreign body. Evaluate the EAC after removal of the foreign body to ensure complete resolution.

Disposition

Patients may be safely discharged from the emergency department after successful removal of the foreign body. Some patients may be discharged with referral to follow-up with a specialist. Most foreign bodies can be removed during normal business hours in the office of the otolaryngologist. Emergent consultation should be obtained in the setting of bleeding or signs of severe systemic infection.

NASAL FOREIGN BODY REMOVAL

As in the EAC, foreign bodies may also become lodged in the nare. Identification of a nasal foreign body may be challenging as the parent or caregiver may have not witnessed insertion of the object, and the patient may not admit or describe the event.

Indications

Removal of a foreign body in the nose should be attempted while protecting the patient's airway. Foul, purulent discharge from a unilateral nare in the toddler or young child is a possible clue to foreign body.

Contraindications

Bleeding disorders are a relative contraindication; therefore, consider specialist consultation in these patients. Do not attempt to remove foreign bodies superior to the middle turbinate as the cribriform plate may be inadvertently damaged.

Equipment & Supplies

As with commercial products available for EAC foreign body removal, a number of commercial products exist for nasal foreign body removal. The blood supply to the nares is substantially higher than the EAC, and the risk of epistaxis is notable. Clinicians should have vasoconstrictors available, such as oxymetazoline or phenylephrine. An appropriate size nasal speculum is also required.

Procedure

A number of procedures have been described on the successful removal of nasal foreign bodies. A cooperative patient will yield the best results. Provide anxiolysis as well as analgesics when appropriate. Consider specialist consultation if procedural sedation is required.

▶ Positive-pressure Techniques

Several techniques have been described using positive pressure. Occlude the patient's unaffected nostril, and request the patient to blow the nose. Sometimes, foreign bodies that are lodged in the vestibule may be removed. A technique that may work for younger children is to have a parent provide positive pressure through the patient's mouth while occluding the unaffected nostril. This has a similar effect in the patient who cannot blow the nose on command. Remember, nasal foreign bodies can become tracheal or esophageal foreign bodies, so caution is recommended.

▶ Instrumentation

A number of instruments are available to aid in the removal of nasal foreign bodies. Utilizing a nasal speculum, identify the foreign body's presenting surface. Consider alligator forceps if the surface can be grasped or a suction catheter if the surface is smooth and regular. A catheter with balloon tip can be inserted beyond the foreign body, followed by inflation of the balloon and then withdrawn, causing the foreign body to be removed. The foreign body may dislodge down the nasopharynx that could result in a tracheal or esophageal foreign body.

Complications

There are several complications with nasal foreign body removal. Dislodged objects may be aspirated, swallowed, or lodged in the trachea. Instrumentation may cause damage to the vasculature of the nasal mucosa resulting in epistaxis. Evaluate the nose after removal of the foreign body to identify any potential complication.

MANAGEMENT OF EPISTAXIS

Epistaxis is a common presenting symptom to the emergency department with a variety of etiologies and levels of severity. Most episodes resolve prior to the patient's arrival, although some may persist despite the clinician's efforts.

The source of epistaxis in a majority of patients is in the anterior aspect of the nose, in Kiesselbach plexus. This is an area rich in capillary beds that may begin bleeding with minimal irritation or manipulation. Illnesses, such as upper respiratory infections with associated localized inflammation, may predispose the patient to epistaxis. Dry climate can also contribute. Rarely, epistaxis is caused from a posterior source, which may be from a venous source (Woodruff plexus), or from the sphenopalatine or ethmoidal arteries. Posterior bleeds are usually caused by trauma, and are rarely spontaneous.

Indications

Epistaxis management should be employed to varying degrees in pediatric patients. Simple maneuvers such as external pressure may fully resolve the patient's symptoms.

Contraindications

There are no absolute contraindications.

Materials & Supplies

There are various ways to manage epistaxis. The clinician should have the selected equipment available, including topical vasoconstrictors (oxymetazoline or phenylephrine). Cautery should be available as well as suction. Nasal speculums help to visualize the area that is bleeding. Packing, both anterior and posterior, should be available. Commercially available packing may be used in the adolescent patient, whereas the younger patient may require different tools.

Procedure

The clinician should wear a gown and face mask during examination in addition to other personal protective equipment. The patient will often gag and expectorate blood during assessment.

▶ Anterior Bleeding

1. Identify the area of bleeding. Consider having the patient blow the nose to evacuate loose blood and clot.

2. Consider application of a topical vasoconstrictor.

3. If there is a local area of bleeding, consider cautery. Avoid prolonged cauterization of the septal surface to avoid permanent damage and poor healing.

4. If all methods have failed and bleeding is still occurring, consider anterior nasal packing. Commercial devices available include nasal tampons of various sizes that may be used. The clinician should be familiar with devices available prior to initiating epistaxis management.

▶ Posterior Bleeding

Posterior packing can be performed in the emergency department, and is a relatively uncomfortable procedure. Consider specialist consultation for these patients, and ensure airway protection when appropriate.

1. Identify area of bleeding if possible. Most posterior bleeds are difficult to visualize in detail.

2. Consider application of a topical vasoconstrictor.

3. If these methods have failed, consider a posterior nasal packing. This may be with a commercially available product or by using another technique, such as:

Gauze Pad Posterior Packing

1. Roll 2 × 2-inch or 4 × 4-inch gauze to create a cylindrical shape. Suture the gauze roll allowing for long tails at each end. There should be four tails: right and left nare tails, and a tail to be secured to each cheek.

2. Insert a flexible catheter in the right nostril, and grasp the catheter tip from the posterior oropharynx. Topical anesthetics work well to prevent the patient's gag reflex.

3. Affix one of the tails of the gauze roll to the catheter and withdraw through the right nare.

4. Repeat steps 2 and 3 for the left nare.

5. Pull the gauze pack through the oropharynx to occlude the passage from the nasopharynx to the oropharynx. There should be a suture tail through the right nare, the left nare, and two suture tails left coming through the mouth.

6. Secure the right and left nare suture tails to another gauze roll. This gauze roll will serve to keep pressure off of the nasal septum.

7. Affix the two suture tails from the mouth to the cheek.

8. Pack the nose as securely as possible.

Foley Posterior Packing

1. Obtain a Foley catheter of the same diameter as the nare. Inflate the balloon to ensure integrity and cut the distal tubing from the Foley.

2. Coat the Foley catheter in an antibiotic ointment, and insert into the affected nare.

3. Once the catheter is visible in the posterior pharynx, inflate the balloon and withdraw the proximal end of the Foley catheter until the balloon becomes seated.

4. Pack the anterior nares and secure the Foley catheter.

Treatment for a posterior nosebleed may compromise the patient's airway. It is recommended that airway management take priority. Furthermore, insertion of catheters or commercial devices into the nasal cavity is not recommended in the setting of trauma. There could be bony disruption at the cribriform plate and insertion of catheters could cause intracranial damage.

Complications

Complications from anterior epistaxis management are rare. If packing is placed, it is imperative that the patient have the packing removed within 24 hours. Posterior nosebleeds are higher risk in management, and may be accompanied by other traumatic findings. Ischemia, infection, and trauma are leading complications of epistaxis management. Also, airway compromise has been recorded for both anterior and posterior nasal packings.

Disposition

Most patients who present to the emergency department have anterior nosebleeds, which can be managed in the emergency department. If anterior packing is placed, urgent specialty follow-up is indicated, usually within 24 hours. If a posterior bleed is encountered, or the clinician is unable to get bleeding controlled, consider specialty consultation in the emergency department or transfer patient to a facility with specialist availability.

Damrose JF, Maddalozzo J: Pediatric epistaxis. *Laryngoscope.* 2006;116(3):387 [PMID: 16540895].

Heim SW, Maughan KL: Foreign bodies in the ear, nose and throat. *Am Fam Physician.* 2007;76(8):1185 [PMID: 17990843].

Kumar S, Kumar M, Lesser T, et al: Foreign bodies in the ear: a simple technique for removal analysed in vitro. *Emerg Med J.* 22(4):2005;266 [PMID: 15788826].

Marin JR, Trainor JL: Foreign body removal from the external auditory canal in a pediatric emergency department. *Pediatr Emerg Care.* 2006;22(9):630 [PMID: 16983246].

MUSCULOSKELETAL PROCEDURES

The pediatric musculoskeletal system is different from that of the adult, as it is still maturing. Having a clear understanding of the anatomy of the pediatric skeletal structure is useful in the management of musculoskeletal procedures.

DISLOCATIONS & SUBLUXATIONS

The pediatric patient may present to the emergency department after a traumatic injury results in a limb or digit deformity. Imaging is important to identify fractures as well as dislocations or subluxations. The clinician should be able to reduce common dislocations in the emergency department. Successful reduction will likely depend on adequate analgesia and possibly sedation. A complete neurovascular examination is required before and after any attempt at reduction.

▶ Radial Head Subluxation (Nursemaid Elbow)

Generally, the history and physical examination are sufficient to diagnose a radial head subluxation. The injury commonly occurs in patients aged 1 to 4 years. The mechanism is usually an abrupt pull on the patient's arm with the elbow in extension and the forearm in pronation. Anatomically, the annular ligament becomes lodged within the radiocapitellar joint causing the subluxation. The patient will usually present refusing to move the affected arm. If imaging is obtained, the radiographs may appear normal. There should be no posterior fat pad, and the radiocapitellar line should be maintained. If either of these is present, consider an alternative diagnosis such as occult suprachondylar humerus fracture.

Reduction of a radial head subluxation requires no special equipment. Gently apply pressure on the radial head with the nondominant hand. Simultaneously, apply traction on the forearm while supinating the forearm and flexing the elbow in one motion. A gentle "click" is frequently felt during reduction. After reduction, no special treatment or immobilization is necessary. The patient will typically begin moving the affected arm soon after reduction, if not immediately.

Shoulder Dislocation

Anterior shoulder dislocation is common in adolescents, whereas younger children rarely dislocate the shoulder joint. The primary mechanism is direct trauma from a sporting-related incident. Reduction of the dislocated joint should be performed in the emergency department. Often, adequate analgesia may be obtained with intra-articular medications or systemic medication. Some patients may require sedation for the dislocation reduction to be performed. The key to success is adequate pain management and relaxation of the affected musculature.

There are a number of described techniques to reduce a dislocated shoulder. Traction/countertraction is one of the more common methods and may be improved with scapular manipulation. In this procedure, the patient is placed supine, and two sheets are used to assist in the reduction. The first sheet is passed under the patient's affected axilla with one side passing anterior to the chest, and the other under the back. The second sheet is wrapped around the proximal forearm. Constant and steady pressure is applied until the muscles of the shoulder begin to relax. Pushing the scapular tip medially while the superior aspect of the scapula is pushed laterally may help the reduction. In addition, internal and external rotation of the shoulder may facilitate the reduction. After reduction, imaging should be obtained and the patient placed in a shoulder immobilizer. Follow-up with an orthopedic physician is recommended.

Digit Dislocation

Both the proximal and distal interphalangeal joints may become dislocated, usually with the distal segment being dorsally displaced. Axial load trauma to the digit is responsible for most dislocations. Because of the intricacies of the finger, a thorough examination is required.

For reduction, the patient will usually benefit from systemic analgesia or by performing a digital block. Once adequate pain management has been achieved, reduction should be attempted. Hyperextend the affected joint to re-create the injury. Apply steady and constant axial traction to the affected joint, and press the dislocated phalanx back into anatomic alignment. Once reduction has been achieved, the clinician should document ligamentous stability. Immobilize the digit and obtain postreduction imaging. Refer patient for follow-up, either to the primary care physician or to an orthopedic hand specialist.

Patellar Dislocation

Patellar dislocations are common injuries that occur to adolescents participating in athletic events. The typical mechanism

is a twisting injury or direct injury to the knee. Neurovascular injuries do not occur in the setting of patellar dislocation.

Reduction is usually simple and easily performed. Extend the affected knee while providing slight pressure on the patella back to a neutral alignment. Pain medication may be given systemically. Postprocedure imaging should be obtained, and the patient should have the affected knee placed in a knee immobilizer for 6 weeks. The patient should be referred to an orthopedic physician for follow-up.

ARTHROCENTESIS

Arthrocentesis is performed in a sterile fashion and involves the removal of synovial fluid for analysis. This is performed by inserting a needle into the joint space and aspirating an amount of fluid. The more common sites to perform the procedure on are the knee, ankle, and elbow. Informed consent should be obtained, when feasible.

Indications

Pain, redness, swelling, and warmth in a joint are clinical symptoms that may warrant evaluation for a septic or inflammatory arthropathy.

Contraindications

Caution should be taken in performing this procedure on a patient with a coagulopathy. The clinician should not perform this procedure in a site where overlying cellulitis is present.

KNEE

There are two common approaches to performing an arthrocentesis of the knee: superior lateral and medial. Local anesthesia should be administered prior to the procedure. Sterilize the skin surface prior to insertion of the needle.

In the superior-lateral approach, the knee is extended and the needle is inserted lateral to the superior-lateral border of the patella. The tract of the needle should be guided to aim for the intercondylar fossa.

In the medial approach, the knee should be fully extended or flexed at 45 degrees. Providing support with blankets will help the patient maintain the desired angle of the knee joint. The needle is inserted medial to the middle of the patella and guided to aim for the intercondylar fossa.

Regardless of the method, gentle traction on the syringe to provide negative pressure will allow for identification when the needle has entered the joint space. The synovial fluid will range from clear, to straw-colored, to purulent or bloody, and typically be viscous in nature.

ANKLE

There are two common approaches to performing an arthrocentesis of the ankle: tibiotalar joint and subtalar joint. Local anesthesia should be administered prior to the procedure. The clinician should be aware of all landmarks, and be able to identify them on the patient.

The tibiotalar approach is most successful with the foot in slight plantar flexion. Insert the needle anterior to the medial malleolus and medial to the tibialis anterior tendon. Guide the needle posterolateral applying negative pressure on the syringe as the practitioner advances the needle.

The subtalar joint is best accessed with the ankle at 90 degrees. Insert the needle just distal to the lateral malleolus, in the same horizontal plane as the subtalar joint, and direct the needle medially.

▶ ELBOW

The elbow has one approach caused by the path of the neurovascular bundle on the medial side. Position the patient's elbow at 90 degrees, and identify the radial head, lateral epicondyle, and the olecranon tip. In the middle of this triangle, insert the needle directed toward the coronoid process of the ulna.

Complications

Arthrocentesis procedures have possible complications. Damage may occur to the internal structure of the joint, to neurovascular structures that run near the joint, and to connective tissue such as ligaments or tendons. Infection is a complication that may also occur.

Disposition

Depending on the results of the fluid analysis, the patient may be discharged or admitted. If fluid analysis results in concern for septic arthropathy, immediate orthopedic consultation should be obtained.

Bettencourt RB, Linder MM: Arthrocentesis and therapeutic joint injection: an overview for the primary care physician. *Prim Care.* 2010;37(4):691 [PMID: 21050951].

Bishop JY, Flatow EL: Pediatric shoulder trauma. *Clin Orthop Relat Res.* 2005;432:41 [PMID: 15738802].

Carson S, Woolridge DP, Colletti J: Pediatric upper extremity injuries. *Pediatr Clin North Am.* 2006;53(1):41 [PMID: 16487784].

Tsung JW, Blaivas M: Emergency department diagnosis of pediatric hip effusion and guided arthrocentesis using point-of-care ultrasound. *J Emerg Med.* 2008;35(4):393 [PMID: 18403170].

NEUROLOGIC PROCEDURES

LUMBAR PUNCTURE

A lumbar puncture allows the clinician to evaluate the cerebrospinal fluid for evidence of inflammation, infection, or the presence of blood, as in a subarachnoid hemorrhage.

Indications

Most lumbar punctures are performed in pediatric patients to rule out infection. Evaluation for pseudotumor cerebri and other neurologic disorders may include the need for lumbar puncture.

Contraindications

Contraindications include suspicion for increased intracranial pressure, evidence of infection over the site where the lumbar puncture would be performed, as well as a coagulopathy. Patients may have a spinal column formation that precludes the clinician from performing the procedure. Bedside ultrasound has demonstrated to be beneficial in some patients.

Equipment & Supplies

Performing a lumbar puncture is a sterile procedure. Informed consent should be obtained, whenever possible. Commercially available kits contain most items needed for performance of the procedure. Depending on patient size, a spinal needle of different gauge or length may be more appropriate than the standard size spinal needle contained in the kit. Consider applying a transdermal analgesic if time permits.

Procedure

There are two positions in which the patient can be placed for the lumbar puncture: sitting upright or lying in the lateral decubitus position. With the patient lying on the side, measuring the opening pressure may be easily and more accurately performed. The most critical step is patient alignment. Ensuring that the hips and shoulders are parallel is crucial to help the operator determine the true midline of the patient's spinal canal.

1. Palpate the posterior superior iliac crest, which should be at the approximate level of the L3-L4 interspace.

2. Cleanse the area with a betadine solution and allow it to dry completely.

3. Inject a local anesthetic at the planned site of puncture.

4. Identify the L3-L4 interspace again, and insert the needle in the midline, perpendicular to the skin at the level of the interspace.

5. Guide the needle through the skin and the interspace toward the umbilicus.

6. Advance the needle with the stylet in place.

7. Once a sudden release of pressure is felt, withdraw the stylet.

8. Repeat steps 6 and 7 until cerebrospinal fluid (CSF) is returning. Consider slight repositioning of the needle if it will not pass and stops at bone. Withdraw the needle to its tip on each reposition attempt.

9. Attach the manometer to measure the opening pressure, if the lying position is used.

10. Collect approximately 1 mL of CSF in each CSF collection tube.

11. Replace stylet and withdraw the needle. Place an appropriate dressing at the needle insertion site.

Complications

Rarely, permanent neurologic complications occur with a lumbar puncture. Risk of damage to the spinal cord is minimal caused by the insertion site in the L3-L4 region. Pain and occasionally parasthesias may be noticed by the patient. A persistent CSF leak and headache may also be complications associated with a lumbar puncture. Infection or epidural hematoma may also result.

Disposition

Disposition depends on the indication for performing the lumbar puncture as well as the results of the fluid analysis. If there is clinical concern for infection, the clinician should initiate antibiotic therapy while awaiting results of the lumbar puncture.

Bruccoleri RE, Chen L: Needle-entry angle for lumbar puncture in children as determined by using ultrasonography. *Pediatrics.* 2011;127(4):e921 [PMID: 21444601].

Gorchynski J, McLaughlin T: The routine utilization of procedural pain management for pediatric lumbar punctures: are we there yet? *J Clin Med Res.* 2011;3(4):164 [PMID: 22121399].

Greenberg RG, Smith PB, Cotton CM, et al: Traumatic lumbar punctures in neonates: test performance of the cerebrospinal fluid white blood cell count. *Pediatr Infect Dis J.* 2008; 27(12):1047 [PMID: 18989240].

UROLOGIC PROCEDURES

SUPRAPUBIC BLADDER CATHETERIZATION

A suprapubic bladder catheterization allows the clinician an alternative means to obtain a urine sample, or to relieve urinary obstruction caused by urethral injury or other urologic concern. This is a sterile procedure, which is aided with the use of real-time bedside ultrasound.

Indications

Patients with urethral injury or trauma who are unable to void may require urgent bladder decompression. Performing a suprapubic bladder catheterization or aspiration allows the clinician an alternative means of obtaining an uncontaminated urine specimen. Most patients and families prefer a urethral catheterization over the suprapubic approach.

Contraindications

Contraindications include acceptable alternative means to obtain a urine sample or concern for bowel interference with the procedure.

Equipment & Supplies

Commercially available suprapubic bladder catheterization kits exist. If the clinician requires only a sample of urine, it may be obtained with a small-gauge needle and 20-cc syringe. Sterile technique should be maintained throughout the procedure.

Procedure

1. Place the patient in the frog-leg position. Use of an assistant may be required if the patient will not cooperate.

2. Identify landmarks: midline, 1–2 cm superior to the pubic symphysis.

3. Use a betadine solution to cleanse the area, allowing the solution to dry completely, and drape the area in a sterile fashion.

4. Approximately 1–2 cm superior to the pubic symphysis, insert and advance the needle. Angle the needle about 10–20 degrees off of vertical in a cephalad direction. If available, use an ultrasound machine to help guide the needle trajectory.

5. Once urine is obtained, either withdraw the needle or continue to insert the bladder catheter by Seldinger technique or catheter-over-needle technique.

6. Apply a bandage or secure the catheter in place.

Complications

Hematuria may be noted after suprapubic catheterization. In addition, penetration of the intestinal tract may occur if a loop of bowel overlies the bladder. Ultrasound may be beneficial in reducing this complication. Infection may also occur, as with other invasive procedures.

Disposition

Consider admitting the patient who has a suprapubic bladder aspiration or catheterization performed. Most patients who require this procedure are critically ill or have sustained significant trauma, and will require specialty care.

Mohammed A, Khan A, Shergill IS, et al: A new model for suprapubic catheterization: The MediPlus Seldinger suprapubic catheter. *Expert Rev Med Devices.* 2008;5(6):705 [PMID: 19025347].

Procedural Sedation

Christopher Colvin, MD

▼ GENERAL CONSIDERATIONS

Procedural sedation and analgesia has proven safe and effective in the emergency department, and should be utilized when patients undergo painful procedures. In addition to facilitating painful procedures, a number of agents are utilized in pediatrics to facilitate diagnostic studies (CT, MRI, lumbar punctures). The most important step in addition to monitoring the patient involves extensive preparation and, at conclusion of sedation, the patient should return to mental and physiologic baseline. In scenarios where the patient's severity of illness questions the applicability of emergency department sedation, the physician must review the risks, and consider consultation with the anesthesiologist. Although degrees of sedation can at times be ambiguous, observation of the patient's progression, and remaining vigilant for respiratory depression can diminish untoward effects and facilitate successful recovery and disposition.

The nomenclature "procedural sedation and analgesia" (PSA) has replaced the previous term "conscious sedation" following recent guideline recommendations, and is defined by The American College of Emergency Physicians (ACEP) as the "administration of sedatives or dissociative agents with or without analgesics to induce a state that allows the patient to tolerate unpleasant procedures while maintaining cardiorespiratory function." The ACEP clinical policy states: "Procedural sedation and analgesia is intended to result in a depressed level of consciousness that allows the patient to maintain oxygenation and airway control independently." Patients can progress to each successive stage of sedation to the point of apnea and respiratory arrest. The practitioner's goal is to avoid progressive unconsciousness in the patient, and to remain capable in managing their cardiopulmonary function when necessary.

PROCEDURAL SEDATION & ANALGESIA STAGES

The PSA spectrum involves minimal, moderate, deep, and general anesthesia levels necessitating that the practitioner recognizes the levels of sedation, and be prepared to rescue the next level of sedation if necessary. Several experts have recommended a separate category for dissociative anesthetics such as ketamine because the performance and adverse effect profile differs widely from other forms of sedation. Each degree of sedation increases risk of cardiopulmonary instability with likely need for aggressive intervention.

- **Minimal sedation (anxiolysis):** a drug-induced state during which the patient responds normally to verbal commands. Although cognitive function and physical coordination may be impaired, airway reflexes, and ventilatory and cardiovascular functions are unaffected.

- **Moderate sedation/analgesia (conscious sedation):** a drug-induced depression of consciousness during which the patient responds purposefully to verbal commands, either alone or accompanied by light tactile stimulation. No interventions are required to maintain a patent airway, and spontaneous ventilation is adequate. Cardiovascular function is usually maintained.

- **Deep sedation/analgesia:** a drug-induced depression of consciousness during which the patient cannot be aroused easily but responds purposefully following repeated or painful stimulation. The ability to independently maintain ventilatory function may be impaired. The patient may require assistance in maintaining a patent airway, and spontaneous ventilation may be inadequate. Cardiovascular function is usually maintained.

- **General anesthesia:** a drug-induced loss of consciousness during which the patient cannot be aroused, even by painful stimulation. The ability to maintain ventilatory function independently is often impaired. The patient often requires assistance in maintaining a patent airway, and positive-pressure ventilation may be required because of depressed spontaneous ventilation or drug-induced depression of neuromuscular function. Cardiovascular function may be impaired.

PROCEDURAL SEDATION & ANALGESIA ASSESSMENT

Indications for PSA include pain relief, amnesia, and anxiolysis required for the patient's comfort; therefore, drugs, dosages, depth, and duration of sedation must be considered prior to the initiation of the procedure. PSA requires a presedation assessment, sedation monitoring, and postsedation assessment prior to disposition. In the presedation assessment, history of prior anesthesia/sedation complications should be evaluated along with comorbid conditions and allergies. The American Society of Anesthesiologists (ASA) classifies patient illness severity as categories I, II, III, IV, V, and VI (Table 4–1) using a grading system created in 1941. Each category involves escalating degrees of progressive systemic disease, and is meant to be used for assessment of the illness of the patient prior to surgery. A patient scored as ASA I–II can be reasonably sedated in the emergency department without elevating the risk of sequelae from underlying systemic pathology. When a patient is deemed to be more ill (ASA III-IV), it is often more appropriate to involve anesthesia within the parameters of elective or non–life-threatening scenarios. Category III classifications have shown to be an independent risk factor for adverse outcomes in general anesthesia and pediatric sedation patients. Categories V and VI are usually not applicable within the emergency department setting. The downside to ASA classification is the ambiguity of the category definitions and variable scoring among practitioners.

The patient should be screened for recent illnesses, hospitalizations, birth complications, gastroesophageal reflux disease (GERD), liver or kidney disease, as well as metabolic disorders. Pulmonary diseases such as asthma, cystic fibrosis, pulmonary fibrosis, and tracheomalacia could potentially result in profound hypoxemia. Patient history of supplemental oxygen at

Table 4–1. American Society of Anesthesiologists (ASA) classification.

ASA category I: Normal healthy patient
ASA category II: Patient with mild systemic disease
ASA category III: Patient with severe systemic disease
ASA category IV: Patient with severe systemic disease that is a constant threat to life
ASA category V: Moribund patient who is not expected to survive without the operation
ASA category VI: Declared brain-dead patient whose organs are being removed for donor purposes

home would indicate that ASA category III or IV requires a critical review for the need of emergency department PSA. The pediatric patient with prior history of cardiac surgery (transposition of the great vessels, tetralogy of Fallot, left hypoplastic heart syndrome) requires consultation with an anesthesiologist as well. The patient with GERD may require passive aspiration while sedated, which could result in laryngospasm or aspiration pneumonitis. Food and medication allergies should be documented because egg and soy allergies preclude the option to utilize propofol. Liver disease may indicate a decreased ability to metabolize barbituates and benzodiazepenes potentially prolonging sedation, and methohexital may induce seizure activity in a patient with history of seizure disorder.

Airway assessment is integral in establishing an adequate sedation plan should aggressive maneuvers be necessary. Will the planned procedure involve occluding the airway (oral laceration repairs, GI endoscopy)? Does the patient have a large tongue, an overbite, or micrognathia? Patients with a Mallampati classification less than III, inability to open the mouth greater than 4 cm, a thyromental distance less than 6 cm, history of cervical spinal inflexibility, or history of previous difficult intubation indicate a high risk for intubation failure. If the patient is identified as high risk for airway failure, appropriate precautions should be implemented, and decision to abort the PSA should be considered.

The patient should be assessed for recent oral intake. Patients are at risk for aspiration of gastric contents when they reach deeper levels of sedation, and lose their protective airway reflexes. Although small emergency department studies evaluating pediatric fasting regimens have shown no significant adverse events with known oral intake prior to procedures, ASA guidelines recommend safety parameters of liquids requiring 2 hours, and solids requiring 6 hours prior to procedure. Aspiration under general anesthesia has been estimated to have an incidence of 1:3420 with mortality in 1:125,109 patients with little data to suggest long-term sequelae. General anesthesia is at the end of the sedation spectrum, and often mandates advanced airway manipulation; therefore, aspiration is much more likely. Although no study has demonstrated an elevated risk of aspiration for moderate to deep PSA in the emergency department, it is imperative to consider gastric contents and depth of sedation. A patient presenting with a full stomach would benefit from observation and procedural delay for gastric emptying. Care needs be taken to minimize the likelihood of aspiration and precautions made to manage aspiration should it occur with wall suction, suction catheter, as well as additional personnel should the patient need to be log-rolled into the lateral decubitus position.

MONITORING

When the need for PSA has been confirmed, informed consent should follow, and preparations made for proper monitoring. In the setting of pediatric PSA, the legal guardian should be informed of the risks and benefits, and documented for consent. Patients should have mental status and function documented prior to and following the procedural initiation. Pediatric patients should be placed on a cardiac monitor, pulse oximetry, blood pressure cuff and, if available end-tidal CO_2 ($ETCO_2$). Studies have shown $ETCO_2$ to be more sensitive than pulse oximetry in identification of patients with respiratory depression, although there was no significant difference in outcome. Patients with deep sedation resulting in respiratory depression will demonstrate increase in $ETCO_2$ greater than 10 mm Hg from baseline or greater than 50 mm Hg total before they demonstrate decrease in oxygen saturation. Although the $ETCO_2$ does not differentiate level of sedation, it can accurately detect respiratory depression. While monitoring the patient's sedation course, heart rate, blood pressure, and oxygen saturations should be documented in serial timed intervals.

Airway adjuncts beyond direct laryngoscopy, such as an intubating laryngeal mask airway (LMA), glide scope, light wand, or fiber-optic scope, should remain at the bedside. Supplemental oxygen may need to be delivered via non-rebreather, or nasal trumpet if the patient becomes unexpectedly obtunded. Above all, protection of the patient's airway, and avoidance of respiratory depression is tantamount to a successful sedation.

Hemodynamic stability must be maintained. Many sedative agents and regimens result in vasodilation, and once patients develop a depressed level of consciousness their sympathetic output may also decrease further potentiating bradycardia and decreased mean arterial pressure. Patients with a history of dehydration or acute blood loss anemia should be volume resuscitated prior to PSA. Pressor agents such as norepinephrine, epinephrine, phenylephrine, dopamine, and ephedrine should be available in the event that fluid refractory shock takes place.

Adverse events should be documented with additional descriptions of executed interventions. Standard reporting of adverse events include apnea, oxygen saturation less than 90%, $ETCO_2$ greater than 50, bradycardia, hypotension, and emesis. Continuous cardiac monitoring is important to detect adverse rhythms, and can help determine pain response when the patient develops an increased sinus tachycardia. Additional tools that can prove to be vital during sedations include ACLS medication access, advanced airway equipment, and supplemental oxygen via nasal cannula, non-rebreather, or bag valve mask (Table 4–2).

SEDATION SCALE

A number of sedation scales measure patient levels of comfort, agitation, and sedation in the intensive care unit (ICU), operating room (OR), and emergency department

Table 4–2. Equipment for sedation.

| High flow oxygen |
| Non-rebreather |
| Ambu bag |
| Nasal trumpet |
| Advanced airway equipment |
| Cardiac monitor |
| Blood pressure monitor |
| Pulse oximetry/$ETCO_2$ |
| Reversal agents (naloxone, flumazenil) |
| ACLS medications |
| Defibrillator |
| Suction device with suction catheter |
| IV capabilities |

environments. The scales provide a guide for practitioners to determine depth of sedation and the need for smaller titrations, reversal, or additional medications. Most sedation scales include monitoring agitation which does not directly relate to elective procedural sedation in the emergency department. The Ramsay sedation scale (RSS) has been utilized in studies on emergency department PSA to describe levels of sedation. The RSS is a simple 6-score system with 1 being anxious or restless, and 6 being no response to stimulus (Table 4–3). It has been validated for inter-rater reliability, and simplifies the PSA assessment in the emergency department.

Table 4–3. Ramsay sedation scale.

Score	Responsiveness
1	Patient is anxious and agitated or restless, or both
2	Patient is cooperative, oriented, and tranquil
3	Patient responds to commands only
4	Patient exhibits brisk response to light glabellar tap, or loud auditory stimulus
5	Patient exhibits sluggish response to light glabellar tap, or loud auditory stimulus
6	Patient exhibits no response

SEDATION CONCLUSION & PATIENT DISPOSITION

Care should be taken toward the conclusion of the PSA to limit additional medication administration. Should noxious stimuli cease (distal radius fracture is reduced and splinted) shortly after the last dose, respiratory depression, hypotension, and bradycardia could likely ensue. Depending on the sedative regimen utilized, rapid degradation would mitigate these effects (propofol, dexmedetomidine, etomidate). Long-acting agents such as fentanyl and midazolam can create overt sedation 20–30 minutes beyond the last dose and completion of the emergency department procedure. The patient should respond verbally once sedation has worn off and, after assessment is completed, should return to baseline mental status documented prior to the PSA. Postprocedural emesis may be common following agents such as ketamine; therefore, complete return to baseline is recommended prior to administering oral intake. Studies suggest that a minimum post-PSA observation period of 30 minutes be exercised. Most adverse events such as hemodynamic instability and emesis should have resolved by that time. Upon successful completion of the post-PSA observation period, the patient may be discharged from the emergency department.

AGENTS FOR PROCEDURAL SEDATION & ANALGESIA

The ideal procedural agent for the emergency department patient acts quickly, creates excellent comfort, and resolves soon thereafter with little to no adverse effects. No sedative agent is perfect, but a number of agents exist tailored to each patient encounter (Table 4–4). Analgesia can often be controlled with narcotics, but procedural sedation requires the addition of an amnestic to reach a steady state of comfort. Benzodiazepines are often included with narcotics to facilitate adequate sedation. Ketamine can serve as the sole agent in short-term procedures, whereas midazolam and fentanyl regimens remain the mainstay in a number of emergency departments. Propofol, although a strong agent for moderate to deep sedation, does not satisfy analgesic requirements; however, in multiple studies it is often used solely for the entire PSA.

▶ Fentanyl

Fentanyl is a strong synthetic opiate with potency nearly 100 times that of morphine. Fentanyl lacks amnestic properties, so it is often used in combination with midazolam or propofol. The likelihood of respiratory depression increases greatly when fentanyl is administered with the aforementioned sedatives. It is renally excreted with a half-life of 3.5 hours. Dosing for analgesia is 1-2 mcg/kg IV, but is more optimal if administered as 0.5-2 mcg/kg IV aliquots every 2-3 minutes. Time of onset is 1-2 minutes, and it has a duration of action of 30-45 minutes.

Table 4–4. Sedation and reversal agent dosages.

Agent	Dosage	Onset	Duration
Fentanyl	IV:0.52 mcg/kg Nasal: 1.5-2 mcg/kg	1-2 min 2-5 min	30-45 min 30-60 min
Ketamine	IV: 1-2 mg/kg IM: 3-5 mg/kg	1-2 min 5-10 min	20-60 min 60-120 min
Dexmedetomidine	IV: 1 mcg/kg bolus then 0.5-0.7 mcg/kg/h	15-30 min	240 min
Midazolam	IV: 0.05-0.1 mg/kg (6 mo-5 y) q2-3min prn (max 0.6 mg/kg) 0.025-0.05 mg/kg (6-12 y) q2-3min prn (max 0.4 mg/kg) IM: 1-0.15 mg/kg Nasal: 0.2-0.6 mg/kg	1-5 min 10-15 min 5-10 min	20-60 min 60-120 min 30-60 min
Propofol	IV: 1 mg/kg then 0.5 mg/kg prn IV drip: 5-50 mcg/kg/min	30-60 sec	2-5 min
Etomidate	IV: 0.1-0.2 mg/kg	30-60 sec	3-5 min
Naloxone	IV: 0.01 mg/kg q 2-3 min prn	1-5 min	30-60 min
Flumazenil	IV: 0.01 mg/kg/min to max 0.05 mg/kg	1-5 min	20-75 min

Intranasal fentanyl is dosed 1.5–2 mcg/kg. A number of studies demonstrate efficacy at 2-mcg/kg dosing. Bioavailability is 71% of the IV dose, and typical formulation is 50 mcg/mL. The time of onset is 2–5 minutes. Fentanyl does not induce histamine release, and is less likely to induce hypotension. Fentanyl is also unlikely to cause a cross-reaction allergic response in patients with a known allergy to morphine. Adverse events include bradycardia, hypotension, increased intracranial pressure (ICP), and the potential for chest wall rigidity with high doses.

▶ Ketamine

Ketamine is a dissociative anesthetic which produces analgesic, amnestic, and sedative effects. Ketamine increases endogenous catecholamines by blocking the reuptake pathway facilitating sympathomimetic effects. It maintains protective airway reflexes, and can increase the heart rate and blood pressure as well as intracranial and intraocular pressure (IOP). Patients with head or ocular trauma should be given an alternative agent. Ketamine can cause laryngospasm which may present as persistent cough to complete occlusion with resultant hypoxemia. Recent history of a viral upper respiratory infection (URI), infant younger than 3 months, croup, and stimulation of the posterior pharynx (aggressive suctioning, endoscopy, bronchoscopy) have been demonstrated to increase the likelihood of laryngospasm.

The patient often demonstrates a persistent nystagmus with nonpurposeful movements, but is unable to communicate. Prior to PSA initiation, it may be helpful to describe the phenomenon to friends or family in the room. Drawbacks of ketamine are emergence phenomena and postprocedural emesis. Benzodiazepines have been shown to marginally decrease both effects. Ketamine dosing is 1–2 mg/kg IV with onset within 1–2 minutes, peak levels within 5 minutes, and total duration at 20–60 minutes. Ketamine is administered IM at 3–5 mg/kg with onset in 5–10 minutes, peak levels at 10–15 minutes, and duration of 1–2 hours. Ketamine is a sialagogue, which can produce an increase in tracheobronchial and salivary secretions. An anticholinergic, such as atropine or glycopyrolate, may be given to mitigate the effects. Glycopyrolate can be given at IM/IV at 0.004 mg/kg (usual injection solution is 0.2 mg/mL). Atropine dosing should be 0.01 mg/kg IM/IV with a minimum dose of 0.1 mg and maximum dose of 0.5 mg.

▶ Dexmedetomidine

Dexmedetomidine is a centrally acting α_2-adrenergic agonist with sedating and analgesic effects. Few studies have evaluated the use of dexmedetomidine for PSA in the emergency department; however, a number of studies have demonstrated the safety and efficacy of dexmedetomidine for PSA, surgical interventions, and ICU management. Primary concerns with dexmedetomidine involve its ability to mitigate central sympathetic output. Patients can develop profound bradycardia, sinus arrest, heart block, and hypotension. Patients with a history of cardiovascular disease, heart block, or cardiomyopathy should not be administered dexmedetomidine for PSA. The use of anticholinergics are required to preempt adverse cardiac events.

The standard regimen involves utilizing glycopyrolate at 0.004 mg/kg IV prior to initiation of the PSA. Studies have demonstrated that the preventative measure significantly reduced episodes of bradycardia. The loading does for PSA is 1 mcg/kg bolus over 10 minutes, followed by 0.5–0.7 mcg/kg/hr. The loading dose time should not be less than 10 minutes in order to avoid bradycardia. The patient is capable of participating in painful procedures without developing respiratory depression, and once the PSA is completed, the agent is rapidly metabolized with a short recovery time. The patient should be continuously monitored while on dexmedetomidine.

▶ Midazolam

Midazolam is a benzodiazepine with sedating, anxiolytic, and amnestic effects, but no analgesic effects. It functions through GABA receptors resulting in an influx of chloride, and central nervous system (CNS) depression occurs. It is often used in combination with a narcotic such as fentanyl or a dissociative anesthetic such as ketamine. It is more rapid in onset than diazepam or lorazepam. Midazolam can be given PO, PR, IV, IM, and atomized intranasally. Midazolam has been shown to diminish episodes of postprocedural emesis and emergence reactions with ketamine. Midazolam can cause hypotension and respiratory depression. A patient aged 6 months–5 years should be dosed at 0.05–0.1 mg/kg IV; patient 6–12 years dosed at 0.025 mg-0.05 mg/kg IV. A patient who is administered narcotics simultaneously should have the midazolam dose decreased by 30%. Alternate routes of midazolam and doses include:

- IM: 0.1–0.15 mg/kg
- Oral: 0.25–1 mg/kg
- Intranasal: 0.2–0.6 mg/kg
- Rectal: 0.25–0.5 mg/kg

The pediatric patients requiring gentle anxiolysis for radiologic imaging can receive atomized intranasal midazolam to facilitate the study without the need for parenteral administration. Intranasal midazolam is more effective with atomization versus drip and does tend to burn on administration.

▶ Propofol

Propofol is a nonopioid, nonbarbiturate, sedative hypnotic which is delivered via a lipid emulsion vehicle. Because the emulsion is composed of soy and egg products, patients with these food allergies should not receive this agent. Concentration is 10 mg/mL and is given IV. Propofol does have a tendency to burn on initial IV push. This sensation can be mitigated by pushing 0.5–1.0 mL of lidocine into the peripheral vein. Propofol for PSA is administered as a 1-mg/kg IV loading dose followed by 0.5-mg/kg IV maintenance dose. Propofol drips are initiated at 5–50 mcg/kg/min and titrated to appropriate level of awareness. Risk for respiratory depression and apnea is increased if propofol is given in large, rapid boluses, and significantly more likely if given along with narcotics. Because it is often difficult to titrate correctly the level of sedation with propofol, it is imperative that continuous assessment of the patient's awareness be attained. Should a deeper level of sedation be achieved than warranted, discontinue the agent, observe, and execute rescue maneuvers as needed. Propofol has the benefit of being rapidly metabolized following discontinuation of the PSA or drip, and this enables the practitioner to observe the patient closely for a short period of time until resolution of sedation. Propofol is beneficial in emergent neurologic cases where serial examinations may be necessary to document progression, and it has been shown to decrease ICP. It has been shown to have antiemetic and anticonvulsant properties. Long-term sequelae with propofol are not seen with short-term PSA doses, but include hyperlipidemia, pancreatitis, zinc deficiency, hepatomegaly, rhabdomyolysis, and propofol infusion syndrome. Short-term adverse events include hypotension, hypoxemia, decreased cardiac output, respiratory depression, and apnea.

Etomidate

Etomidate is a short-acting nonbarbiturate hypnotic with GABA-like effects. It has been studied exhaustively in induction of general anesthesia, RSI, and PSA. For PSA, dose is 0.1-0.2 mg/kg IV. Benefits include rapid onset of action, stable hemodynamic effects, and rapid metabolism. Adverse events include laryngospasm, hiccoughs, and myoclonus. Myoclonus can occur in upward of 20-30% of patients which may make the procedure more difficult to complete (shoulder reduction). No long-term sequelae are evidenced from the myoclonus, but the appearance of seizure activity may prompt an unnecessary work up. Etomidate has been shown to blunt response to the adrenocorticotropic hormone (ACTH) stimulation test suggesting an etiology for adrenal suppression; however, studies have not demonstrated a statistically significant difference in outcome with hospitalized patients who received a single dose of etomidate. Greater concern for adrenal suppression is found in patients receiving multiple doses or continuous infusions of etomidate.

REVERSAL AGENTS

Rarely, the physician may need to administer reversal agents in the event that the patient has been deeply sedated to the state of general anesthesia. Although most agents are rapidly metabolized, and no additional medication is necessary, the midazolam and fentanyl regimen could last for 20–30 minutes. Naloxone is given for opiod overdose, and flumazenil is indicated for benzodiazepine overdose. Although naloxone is relatively benign (excluding symptoms of withdrawal), flumazenil can potentially be dangerous in a patient dependent on benzodiazepenes, and may precipitate a refractory seizure.

Naloxone

Naloxone is an opiod antagonist which competes directly with systemic narcotics. It binds all the opiate receptors, but appears to have a higher affinity for the μ receptor. Naloxone may be administered through the endotracheal (ET) tube, IM, IV, IO, or subcutaneously. It is not recommended to administer naloxone via ET tube in newborn infants. Naloxone is dosed at 0.01 mg/kg IV, and it is recommended to give smaller amounts for patients chronically on opiods in order to avoid overt withdrawal. Abrupt reversal in patients chronically administered narcotics may result in seizures, cardiac arrythmias, pulmonary edema, or profound agitation.

Flumazenil

Flumazenil competes directly for the benzodiazepine-binding site on the GABA receptor, thereby reversing some aspects of CNS depression (respiratory depression). Flumazenil does not facilitate the metabolism of benzodiazepenes, and resedation can occur when flumazenil wears off. Flumazil is given IV, undergoes hepatic metabolism, and is excreted renally. The systemic half-life ranges from 20-75 minutes. The pediatric patients is dosed at 0.01 mg/kg up to 0.2 mg IV over 15 seconds. Repeat doses may be given in increments of 0.01 mg/kg up to a maximum dose of 0.05 mg/kg total or 1 mg total. Flumazenil can cause refractory seizures in patients on chronic benzodiazepines. Should a patient develop seizure activity following flumazenil administration, benzodiazepines are likely to be ineffective despite large doses for competitive binding.

American Society of Anesthesiologists: ASA Physical Status Classification System. Park Ridge, IL; 2013. http://www.asahq.org/For-Members/Clinical-Information/ASA-Physical-Status-Classification-System.aspx. Accessed April 24, 2013.

Bahn EL, Holt KR: Procedural sedation and analgesia: A review and new concepts. *Emerg Med Clin N Am.* 2005;23:503 [PMID: 15829394].

Bhatt M, Kennedy RM, Osmond MH, et al: Consensus-based recommendations for standardizing terminology and reporting adverse events for emergency department procedural sedation and analgesia in children. *Ann Emerg Med.* 2009;53:426 [PMID: 19026467].

Borland M, Esson A, Babl F, et al: Procedural sedation in children in the emergency department: A PREDICT study. *Emerg Med Australas.* 2009;21:71 [PMID: 19254316].

Borland M, Jacobs I, King B, et al: A randomized controlled trial comparing intranasal fentanyl to intravenous morphine for managing acute pain in children in the emergency department. *Ann Emerg Medicine.* 2007;49:335 [PMID: 17067720].

Carrasco G: Review: Instruments for monitoring intensive care unit sedation. *Crit Care.* 2000;4:217 [PMID: 11094504].

Deitch K, Miner J, Chudnofsky CR, Dominici P, Latta D: Does end tidal CO_2 monitoring during emergency department procedural sedation and analgesia with propofol decrease the incidence of hypoxic events? A randomized, controlled trial. *Ann Emerg Med.* 2010;55:258 [PMID: 19783324].

Godwin SA, Caro DA, Wolf SJ, et al: American College of Emergency Physicians. Clinical policy: Procedural sedation and analgesia in the emergency department. *Ann Emerg Med.* 2005;45:177 [PMID: 15671976].

Green SM, Krauss B: Barriers to propofol use in emergency medicine. *Ann Emerg Med.* 2008;52:392 [PMID: 18295374].

Hohl C, Sadatsafavi M, Nosyk B, et al: Safety and clinical effectiveness of midazolam versus propofol for procedural sedation in the emergency department: A systematic review. *Acad Emerg Med.* 2009;15:1 [PMID: 18211306].

Klein E, Brown JC, Kobayashi A, et al: A randomized clinical trial comparing oral, aerosolized intranasal, and aerosolized buccal midazolam. *Ann Emerg Med.* 2011;58:323 [PMID: 21689865].

Lamas A, López-Herce J, Sancho L, et al: Assessing sedation in critically ill children by bispectral index, auditory-evoked potentials, and clinical scales. *Intensive Care Med.* 2008;34:2092 [PMID: 18600313].

Lee J, Gonzalez ML, Chuang SK, et al: Comparison of methohexital and propofol use in ambulatory procedures in oral and maxillofacial surgery. *J Oral Maxillofac Surg.* 2008;66:1996 [PMID: 18848094].

Liddo L, D'Angelo A, Nguyen B, et al: Etomidate versus midazolam for procedural sedation in pediatric outpatients: A randomized controlled trial. *Ann Emerg Med.* 2006;48:433 [PMID: 16997680].

McQueen A, Wright RO, Kido MM, et al: Procedural sedation and analgesia outcomes in children after discharge from the emergency department: Ketamine versus fentanyl/midazolam. *Ann Emerg Med.* 2009;54:191 [PMID: 19464072].

Meredith JR, O'Keefe KP, Galwankar S: Pediatric procedural sedation and analgesia. *J Emerg Trauma Shock.* 2008;1:88. [PMID: 19561987].

Miller MA, Levy P, Patel MM: Procedural sedation and analgesia in the emergency department: What are the risks? *Emerg Med N Am.* 2005;23:551 [PMID: 15829397].

Miner J, Biros MH, Heegaard W, et al: Bispectral electroencephalographic analysis of patients undergoing procedural sedation in the emergency department. *Acad Emerg Med.* 2003;10:638 [PMID: 12782525].

Miner J, Danahy M, Moch A, et al: Randomized clinical trial of etomidate versus propofol for procedural sedation in the emergency department. *Ann Emerg Med.* 2007;49:15 [PMID: 16997421].

Messenger D, Murray HE, Dungey PE, et al: Subdissociative-dose ketamine versus fentanyl for analgesia during propofol procedural sedation: A randomized clinical trial. *Acad Emerg Med.* 2008;15:877 [PMID: 18754820].

Newman DH, Azer MM, Pitetti RD, et al: When is a patient safe for discharge after procedural sedation? The timing of adverse effect events in 1367 pediatric procedural sedations. *Ann Emerg Med.* 2003;42:627 [PMID: 14581914].

Newton T, Pop I, Duvall E: Sedation scales and measures—A literature review. *SAAD Dig.* 2013;29:88 [PMID: 23544226].

Riker RR, Shehabi Y, Bokesch PM, et al: Dexmedetomidine vs midazolam for sedation of critically ill patients. *JAMA.* 2009;301:489 [PMID: 19188334].

Roback MG, Bajaj L, Wathen JE, Bothner J: Preprocedural fasting and adverse events in procedural sedation and analgesia in a pediatric emergency department: Are they related? *Ann Emerg Med.* 2004;44:454 [PMID: 15520704].

Roback MG, Wathen JE, Bajaj L, Bothner JP: Adverse events associated with procedural sedation and analgesia in a pediatric emergency department: A comparison of common parenteral drugs. *Acad Emerg Med.* 2005;1:508 [PMID: 15930401].

Saunders M, Adelgais K, Nelson D, et al: Use of intranasal fentanyl for the relief of pediatric orthopedic trauma pain. *Acad Emerg Med.* 2010;17:1155 [PMID: 21175512].

Sivilotti ML, Messenger DW, van Vlymen J, Dungey PE, Murray HE: A comparative evaluation of capnometry versus pulse oximetry during procedural sedation and analgesia on room air. *CJEM.* 2010;12:397 [PMID: 20880431].

Vardy JM, Dignon N, Mukherjee N, et al: Audit of the safety and effectiveness of ketamine for procedural sedation in the emergency department. *Emerg Med J.* 2008;25:579 [PMID: 18723707].

Zed P, Abu-Laban R, Chan WW, Harrison DW: Efficacy, safety and patient satisfaction of propofol for procedural sedation and analgesia in the emergency department: A prospective study. *CJEM.* 2007;9:421 [PMID: 18072987].

Non-Accidental Trauma

Dorian Drigalla, MD, FACEP
C. J. Buckley, MD

IMMEDIATE MANAGEMENT OF LIFE-THREATENING PROBLEMS

As with all patients presenting to the emergency department, the pediatric patient should be evaluated with a timely examination and resuscitated if necessary. A detailed history should be obtained when possible; however, an apparent medical or traumatic life threat must be quickly and adequately addressed.

CHILD MALTREATMENT

Child maltreatment is defined as any behavior toward children that can be viewed as inappropriate or harmful, and consists of four types: physical abuse, neglect, sexual abuse, and emotional abuse. The earliest and best known studies on child maltreatment were conducted in 1946 by John Caffey, a radiologist who recognized the features of non-accidental trauma (NAT) and the psychological entities involved in child maltreatment.

PHYSICAL ABUSE

Physical abuse is broadly defined as an act involving bodily contact intended to cause feelings of intimidation, injury, or other physical suffering or harm. Physical abuse often but not always leaves evidence of a clinically observable injury. The United States Department of Health and Human Services (USDHHS) defines physical abuse as non-accidental physical injury (ranging from minor bruises to severe fractures or death) as a result of punching, beating, kicking, biting, shaking, throwing, stabbing, choking, hitting (with a hand, stick, strap, or other object), burning, or otherwise harming a child, that is inflicted by a parent, caregiver, or other individual who has responsibility for the child. Such damage is deemed maltreatment whether or not the individual planned to harm the child. In the United States, physical forms of

discipline, such as spanking, are common; the clinician must take a careful history to help attempt to discern a history of stated discipline from a pattern consistent with abuse.

NEGLECT

Neglect is more complicated, and it is the most common type of child maltreatment. Neglect is the failure of a caregiver to supply a child's fundamental requirements, and can be divided into four subcategories: physical, medical, educational, and emotional. Physical neglect occurs when a caregiver does not supply necessary supervision, sustenance, or refuge to the child. Medical neglect is the failure to provide essential medical treatment for a child. In the emergency department, the physician often encounters children with multiple medical problems who are especially vulnerable to medical neglect; however, regional or socioeconomic differences may establish variances in cultural values, and therefore different standards of care. Nonetheless, if by a caregiver's refusal to use available resources places a child's well-being in harm's way, corrective action should be considered. It should be noted that if religious beliefs prohibit certain medical interventions, most state laws do not rule this as neglect.

SEXUAL ABUSE

Sexual abuse is defined as the employment, use, persuasion, inducement, enticement, or coercion of a child to engage in, or assist any other person to engage in, any sexually explicit conduct or simulation of such conduct for the purpose of

Acknowledgments The authors would like to extend sincere gratitude to Erica Ward, MD and Sheilah Priori, Forensic Nurse Examiner, McLane Children's Hospital Scott & White, Temple, TX. Your thoughts and experience were great guidance for the work on this chapter. Thank you for all you do to serve the children of our community.

producing a visual depiction of such conduct; or the rape, and in cases of caretaker or interfamilial relationships, statutory rape, molestation, prostitution, or other form of sexual exploitation of children, or incest with children. This topic is covered in greater detail in Chapter 6.

EMOTIONAL ABUSE

Emotional abuse is any action that weakens a child's emotional growth or feelings of self-esteem, such as violent threats, yelling, demeaning language, emotional apathy, or rejection. Without solid substantiation of impairment or mental damage, emotional abuse is extremely difficult to prove. There is a high rate of association between other forms of child maltreatment and emotional abuse.

EPIDEMIOLOGY

Although official reports of child abuse likely understate its true prevalence, a number of studies have demonstrated the pervasive nature of child abuse and neglect. As reported by the USDHHS, the following statistics are specific to 2011, and follow a similar trend of the preceding 5 years.

In the United States, 9.1 per 1,000 children were found to be subjected to maltreatment, most often by a parent, alone or with another individual. Only 13% of the children were abused by someone other than a guardian. Nearly one-half of children were aged 5 years or younger. The highest rate of abuse was for children younger than 1 year, with a victimization rate of 21.2 per 1,000 children. A significant number of abused children will die from their abuse.

In the United States, 1,545 fatalities were reported, at a rate of 2.1 per 100,000 children. Younger children were more likely to die as a result of maltreatment: 81% of fatalities were children younger than 4 years, and 42% were younger than 1 year.

Male and female children are roughly equal to be maltreated. Eighty-eight percent of children reported as maltreated in 2011 fell into three ethnic groups: Hispanic, African American, and white. White children accounted for 44% of maltreatment victims.

The most common type of maltreatment was neglect (78.5%). The second most common was physical abuse followed by sexual abuse.

Risk factors for maltreatment have been identified among child victims. Children with a disability such as mental retardation, emotional disturbance, or chronic medical problems are shown to be at higher risk. Sixteen percent of child abuse victims have a disability, making children with any kind of disability three to four times more likely to be maltreated. Maltreatment can be found in all socioeconomic classes; however, it is predominant in poorer and underprivileged areas. Additional risk factors include domestic violence, parental history of maltreatment, drug and alcohol abuse, and parental psychiatric problems.

HISTORY

When taking the historical assessment of the patient, the following patterns increase suspicion of child abuse. An injury that is not consistent with the reported mechanism should heighten the examiner's concern for potential maltreatment. For example, a 2-year-old child is not likely to fracture a femur by falling from the living room couch. The provider should note injuries inconsistent with the child's physical capabilities, vague explanations of the injuries, delayed presentation, significant changes in the explanation of the injuries, and marked differences in explanations from one witness to another. It is important to assess the affect of the relaying caregiver. It would be abnormal and concerning for the caregiver to appear indifferent toward the injured child.

Gathering information about the child's behavior before, during, and after the injury is important in order to assess the severity and nature of the injury mechanism. Reported deficits in responsiveness should be noted and prompt further investigation. It can be difficult to obtain all the information in a nonaccusatory manner. A caregiver who feels threatened often withholds information for fear of its consequences.

The child's past medical history is important as underlying illness may predispose to the current injury or reveal patterns consistent with abuse. Special attention should be paid to prior trauma or hospitalizations, congenital or genetic conditions, and chronic medical illnesses. Family history can provide useful insight into the child's current state. Screening for family history of bleeding disorders, metabolic disorders, bone disorders, sudden infant death syndrome (SIDS), and genetic disorders help to discriminate between underlying disease and maltreatment. Children with metabolic disorders can appear neglected or malnourished. Pregnancy and birth histories are important, including whether the pregnancy was wanted, whether there was appropriate prenatal care, the presence of postnatal complications, birth trauma, postpartum depression, and where the delivery took place. Injuries during birth are common and more likely if the delivery did not take place in a hospital or under the supervision of health care provider.

There are other less intuitive aspects of the history that are useful when screening pediatric patients for maltreatment. Determination of the family's methods of disciplinary action and the extent of those methods is important. Discipline should not injure the child. The child's baseline temperament can provide insight into stressors that may predispose the child to be maltreated. Fussy children and children with mental disabilities are more likely to be maltreated than those who are easy to care for. The developmental history (language, crawl, walk, fine motor and psychological milestones) provides insight into the child's mental growth and may be delayed in the presence of abuse and neglect. Last, screening for parental or caregiver substance abuse, social and financial stressors, prior child protective services involvement, and domestic violence is helpful to identify risk factors for maltreatment.

PHYSICAL EXAMINATION

The majority of injuries of children presenting to the emergency department are not the result of maltreatment. When examining the pediatric patient, it is important to take into account the history, the nature and mechanism of the injury, and the fact that unusual events do occur in everyday life. There is rarely an injury pattern or finding that is pathognomonic for abuse. However, when examining the child, a thorough, head-to-toe approach is essential in order to minimize missed injuries.

General Assessment

The general assessment of a pediatric patient includes the child's alertness, demeanor, hygiene, and overall interaction with caregiver. The Glasgow coma scale (GCS) is a useful tool if there is suspected compromise in the child's level of alertness. If there is a decrease in mental status, history of trauma, or concern for neurological injury, consider cervical spine immobilization before proceeding with the physical examination. When the child is clinically stable, height and weight are obtained for dosing of medications, if necessary, and to compare with past records if available. Growth failure and inability to gain weight are concerning findings that require further investigation. Figures 5–1, 5–2, and 5–3 show examples of severe growth failure concerning for neglect. It is possible for children to have failure to thrive and, in tandem,

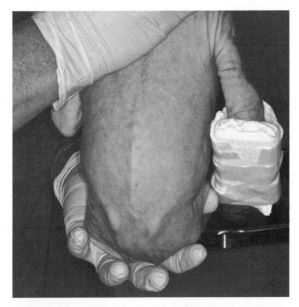

▲ **Figure 5–1.** Example of growth failure concerning for neglect. Note the prominent spinous processes and bony pelvis.

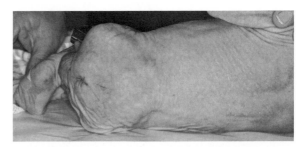

▲ **Figure 5–2.** Example of neglect: Absent gluteal definition reveals lack of muscle and fatty stores.

be abused. Poor hygiene, such as infrequently changed diapers or soiled clothing, may indicate neglect.

Skin Injuries

A thorough physical examination requires fully disrobing the patient so that injuries are not missed. When the examination is complete, rewarm and cover the child in order not to cause discomfort or further injury. The child's skin may reveal injuries, and it is important to document the size, location, and shape of each. An injury's pattern and shape can give clues toward its mechanism and inflicting object. Accidental injuries most commonly occur over bony prominences, so injuries over areas such as the neck, angle of the jaw, ears, scalp, and any posterior aspect of the body are concerning. Not all skin injuries are visible, so palpation for deeper hematomas can be useful. The age of a skin injury can be difficult and occasionally impossible to determine accurately. Lacerations or abrasions in various stages of healing are a nonreassuring finding. Neither visual inspection nor degree of soft tissue swelling will consistently and accurately determine the age of a bruise. Patterned contusions may resemble a looped cord, coat hanger, belt, or other objects and are concerning findings. Figures 5–4, 5–5, 5–6, and 5–7 show examples of skin pattern injuries.

Burns

In burn injuries, take special note of the explanation, number, extent and the distribution of the burns over the body. Scald injuries on the child's upper extremities, torso, neck, or head are more consistent with accidental hot liquid splashes. Inflicted

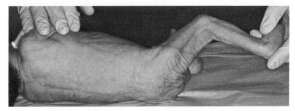

▲ **Figure 5–3.** Clearly evident skeletal structures of the lower extremity with lack of muscular tone or fatty tissue are consistent with neglect.

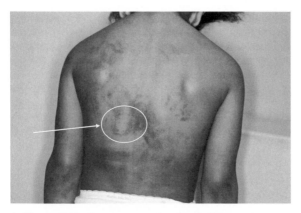

▲ **Figure 5–4.** Pattern contusion (circled) is consistent with a belt buckle.

scald injuries from forced submersion are frequently well demarcated over the buttocks, perineum, or lower extremities and have few splash patterns. Figure 5-8 shows examples of forced submersion burn injury. A stocking and/or glove pattern of burn is concerning for immersion injury. Other patterned burns, such as those from a clothing iron or cigarette, may be clearly demarcated and prompt consideration of abuse; however, accidental injury can also result in a pattern of the hot object.

Head Injuries

Because head injuries are the leading cause of child abuse fatalities, a thorough examination of the head, eyes, ear, nose, and

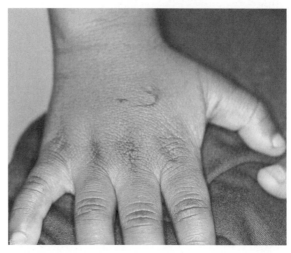

▲ **Figure 5–6.** Pattern contusions are consistent with a loop shape, consistent with the impact of a looped cord.

throat is imperative. Child victims of abuse are more likely to have subdural and subarachnoid bleeds, acute on chronic subdural hematomas, and large retinal hemorrhages compared to children involved in significant accidental trauma. Assessing the skull for deformity or crepitus, hemotympanum, bruising behind the ears (Battle sign), or bruising around the eyes can be useful when evaluating for skull fracture.

The eye examination may be challenging to physicians in care of injured pediatric patients because of patient noncompliance and confounding injury; however, it is a necessary and important aspect to the physical examination. Fundoscopic examination should be performed on all infants when there is concern for abuse. Although small hemorrhages can occur during the birthing process, a finding of retinal hemorrhage is generally concerning if extensive, as 85% of shaken babies will have retinal injury. If an adequate

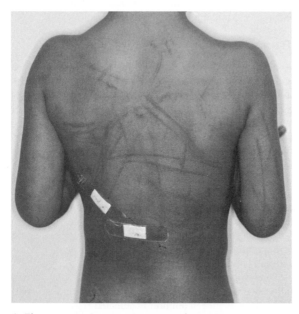

▲ **Figure 5–5.** Pattern contusions, linear in nature, are consistent with being struck by a linear object. Note the central clearing in the pattern of bruising.

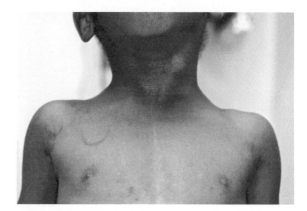

▲ **Figure 5–7.** Example of a loop-shaped pattern contusion of the right anterior chest, consistent with the impact of a looped cord.

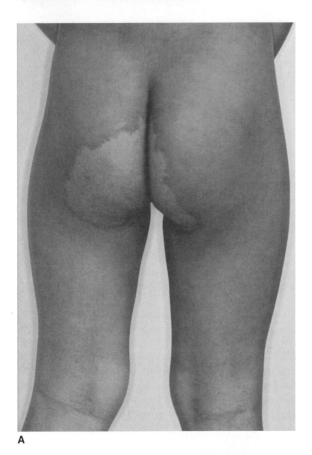

A

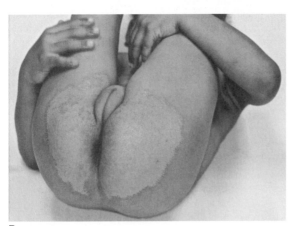

B

▲ **Figures 5–8.** Photographs demonstrate buttock and perineal scald burns consistent with forced submersion.

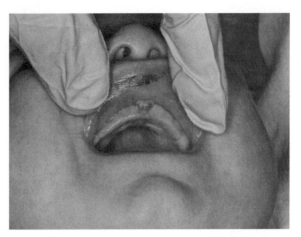

▲ **Figure 5–9.** Frenulum laceration in a 2-month-old bottle-fed child.

fundoscopic examination is unable to be performed, consider consultation with an ophthalmologist. Lastly, assess the pupillary response and extraocular movements if possible. Fixed, dilated pupils are ominous for significant brain injury.

When examining the ears, nose, mouth, and throat of an injured child, look closely. The external ears and lips are common areas for bite injures in maltreated children. The nose is a common site of accidental injury, so nasal injuries are less reliable predictors of NAT. Clues potentially indicating inflicted injury to the mouth of bottle-fed children include inner-lip frenulum lacerations, bruising of the oral mucosa, and bite injuries to the tongue (Figure 5–9).

Truncal Injuries

Accidental injuries to the back, chest, and abdomen are rare, and significant injury to these areas can be severe. In addition to fully disrobing the patient, rolling the patient to examine the back is necessary to minimize missed injuries. Posterior and lateral rib fractures are predictive of inflicted injury and are consistent with a squeeze or crush mechanism. Respiratory distress, splinting, and intractable pain may be signs of rib fracture. Serious cardiac injury resulting from direct blow to chest may include hemopericardium and cardiac contusion. Distended neck veins and cardiovascular collapse can be indicative of hemopericardium or tension pneumothorax, especially if there are diminished breath sounds. Careful auscultation of lung fields prior to palpation is important when assessing for pneumothorax and diaphragmatic rupture, suggested by the presence of bowel sounds in chest.

Solid organ injuries are common both in accidental and inflicted trauma; however, hollow organ injury, like bowel perforation, is more common in inflicted trauma. Physical examination of the pediatric abdomen can be unreliable, but if bruising, guarding, rebound or evidence of significant injury is present, have strong suspicion for solid or hollow organ injury. Children with abdominal injury usually have a delayed presentation and tend to be younger than adolescent age with a higher overall mortality rate. Always inspect the external genitalia for injury or deformity.

Extremity Injuries

Comprehensive examination of the extremities requires a systematic palpation that isolates each joint, hand, and foot to assess for injury. While most extremity injuries are accidental, long bone fractures, spiral fractures, grab marks, and extremity injuries in the nonambulatory child are especially concerning for abuse. In addition to palpation, it is requisite that the neurovascular status of that extremity be assessed, if possible. A large portion of fractures are not clinically detectable on physical examination, thus a negative physical examination should not trump clinical suspicion for injury.

DIFFERENTIAL DIAGNOSIS

The history and physical examination will provide initial insight into the likelihood of abuse, although many findings may be unclear or have potential benign explanations. Laboratory and radiographic evaluation will help clarify the differential diagnosis of other possible explanations of presentation. Bleeding disorders, osteogenesis imperfecta, metabolic and other disorders may be discovered or deemed unlikely through thorough evaluation. The emergency physician should always consider maltreatment when evaluating an injured child (Table 5–1).

DIAGNOSTIC EVALUATION

Diagnostic testing for injury should be completed in the emergency department when possible. Further evaluation for medical conditions or additional injuries may be prompted by initial studies. Admission to the hospital or transfer to an appropriate facility may be necessary for further evaluation.

Laboratory Testing

Toxicology screens, electrolyte evaluation, metabolic screening tests, and other laboratory studies should be ordered as indicated by history and physical examination. The age and condition of the child will be additional guiding factors. The bruised or bleeding child, especially with history of recurrent episodes, should have coagulation studies, a complete blood count, bleeding time, and other hematologic screening tests. Suspected abdominal trauma should prompt consideration for urine analysis, liver and pancreatic enzymes.

Radiographic Evaluation

As in other cases of traumatic injury, the physical examination guides the emergency physician to the choice of initial imaging studies. However, many patients in the setting of abuse present with more subtle history or examination

Table 5–1. Differential diagnosis considerations for suspected physical abuse.

Finding	Possible Causes	Considerations and Tests
Bruising	History of accidental trauma consistent with injury	Mechanism of injury, developmental stage, apparent pattern injuries
	Hematologic or vascular disorders (hemophilia, ITP, DIC, Henoch-Schonlein Purpura, salicylate ingestion, Mongolian spots)	Hematologic screens including CBC, PT, PTT, INR, bleeding time, factor levels
Fractures	History of accidental trauma consistent with injury	Fracture type consistent with mechanism?
	Birth trauma	Further history, chart review, current age of patient
	Skeletal diseases (osteogenesis imperfecta, rickets)	Genetic testing, bone scan, calcium, alkaline phosphatase, phosphorous, vitamin D, parathyroid hormone
Head injury	History of accidental trauma consistent with injury	Consider head CT, MRI
	Hematologic disorders	Coagulation studies, factor levels
	Intracranial vascular anomalies	CTA or MRI/MRA
Altered consciousness	Infection, metabolic, and toxicologic diseases	Medical workup for altered mental status

CBC, complete blood cell count; CT, computed tomography; CTA, computed tomographic angiography; DIC, diffuse intravascular coagulation; INR, international normalized ratio; ITP, idiopathic thrombocytopenic purpura; MRA, magnetic resonance angiography; MRI, magnetic resonance imaging; PT, prothrombin time; PTT, partial thromboplastin time.

findings. Radiographs of the painful, tender, wounded or deformed extremity are indicated. Evidence of injury on initial films, especially in the setting of inconsistent history or examination, should prompt consideration of additional screening imaging, especially in infants and small children. Fractures in multiple stages of healing are particularly concerning for maltreatment.

▶ Skeletal Survey

Given significant clinical suspicion, sources concur that a skeletal survey is indicated for a child 2 years or younger, and is considered for a child upto 5 years of age. The older child rarely presents with occult fracture. Each anatomic area should be independently imaged to assure appropriate radiographic exposure and density, and to maximize clarity of the images. A single "babygram" or series of 2–3 radiographs does not comprise an acceptable substitute. The specified components of a skeletal survey are listed below.

Appendicular Skeleton

Anteroposterior (AP) views of the bilateral humeri, forearms, femurs, lower legs, feet, and posteroanterior (PA) views of the bilateral hands.

Axial Skeleton

Thorax views should include AP, lateral, right and left obliques, including ribs, thoracic spine, and upper lumbar spine. Also included are the pelvis AP view including midlumbar spine, lateral lumbosacral, lateral cervical spine, and skull (frontal and lateral views) radiographs.

▶ Body-Specific Imaging Modalities

Computed tomography (CT) is typically available in the emergency department, and should be considered in the setting of apparent head or body trauma. It may also be used to screen for injury when other diagnostic tests have not explained the patient presentation. Other imaging modalities may prove useful in specific situations.

Evaluation of the Head

Because of the broad range of presentations in the setting of suspected abuse, the emergency physician should consider head injury in all children when suspecting maltreatment. Findings suspicious for a shaken baby range from lethargy to documented retinal hemorrhages. Subdural hemorrhage from this type of acceleration-deceleration injury are believed to result from disrupted bridging veins, and may also be associated with underlying hypoxic brain injury. Alteration in mental status, seizures, inconsolability, and other concerning findings should prompt further evaluation.

In addition to providing excellent evaluation for intracranial injury, modern multislice CT scanners are extremely accurate for assessment of skull fractures. Thus, unenhanced CT of the head is the imaging modality of choice for rapid and sensitive evaluation of pediatric head trauma, and remains preferred over MRI. Specific fracture types occur more predominately in non-accidental injuries to the head; notably multiple fractures, depressed fractures, nonparietal fractures, and fractures widened greater than 3 mm at the suture lines (diastatic fractures). An accidental head injury more commonly results in a single, linear fracture. The most common intracranial finding in NAT is subdural hemorrhage (SDH), and multiple apparent ages of hemorrhage may be seen. Although SDH has been reported as a result of childbirth, asymptomatic term infants tend to show resolution by 4 weeks of age. Subarachnoid hemorrhage, intraventricular hemorrhage, ischemic injury, and cerebral contusions are less frequent findings demonstrated by CT.

If the patient is clinically stable without neurological findings, an initial CT head at acute is sufficient. However, MRI may be more useful in the setting of persistent and concerning neurological findings, as it is more precise at identifying smaller hemorrhages or aged, isodense lesions.

The parent or guardian may insist on obtaining or not obtaining a CT, which may further complicate the emergency department course. Many authorities recommend a head CT for any child with apparent or suspected head trauma, particularly in a child younger than 2 years; however, radiation exposure in children has been an area of increased focus and controversy. A recent prospective study by the Pediatric Emergency Care Applied Research Network (PECARN) has focused on the incidence of injury, with particular regard for the need for acute management or neurosurgical intervention. The resultant guideline may aid clinicians in determining the need to order CT in the setting of pediatric head trauma. In the children younger than 2 years, with normal mental status, absent or frontal-only scalp hematoma, less than 5-second loss of consciousness, nonsevere mechanism, absence of palpable skull fracture, and normal behavior according to parents, the study concluded that urgent management is unwarranted. Similar predictive rules were developed for the child older than 2 years. However, the concern in the emergency department for abuse should prompt serious consideration for evaluation with CT. The emergency physician is charged with assuring a safe medical and social disposition, and CT findings concerning for abuse will be relevant whether or not urgent or surgical intervention is required.

Evaluation of the Body and Extremities

Because the skeletal survey described above increases diagnostic sensitivity toward NAT, it is indicated in the setting of concern for acute or remote injury related to child maltreatment, as well as in head injuries that are suspected or documented by initial single plain films or head CT.

Bone scintigraphy (bone scans) may have higher sensitivity for certain fracture types, such as rib fractures; therefore, the American College of Radiology encourages scintigraphy, either during inpatient evaluation or at follow-up, when significant abuse is suspected but not documented by initial plain radiography. Whole-body MRI has been utilized in adults and children for varying purposes including oncologic evaluation and evaluation for injury when abuse is suspected. Current MRI scanners have low sensitivity in this realm and are not recommended for NAT evaluation.

Imaging of the chest by CT may reveal otherwise occult rib fractures, pneumothorax, cardiac or other injuries. Imaging of the abdomen by CT may reveal viscus or solid organ injury. Liver enzyme elevation, blood in the stool, hematuria, pancreatic enzyme elevation, and abnormal hemoglobin may all be indications for CT imaging when no other explanation seems appropriate.

Pertinent Radiological Findings

1. **Rib fractures** in children suggest severe trauma (Figure 5–10). Young children have particularly flexible ribs, and any acute or healing fracture is concerning for maltreatment. Rib fractures noted in children younger than 1 year are highly concerning. Cardiopulmonary resuscitation (CPR) has not been described as a reliable cause of rib fractures.

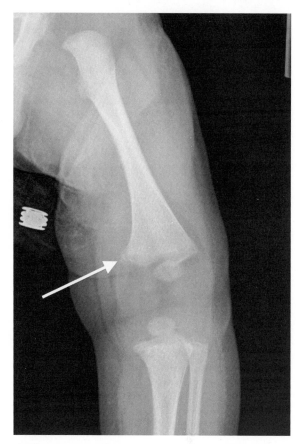

▲ **Figure 5–11.** Classic diaphyseal "corner" fracture of the distal femur (acute).

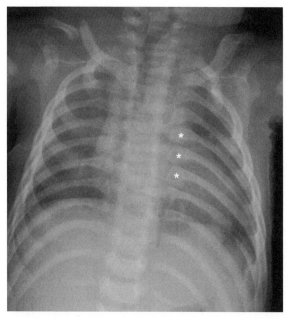

▲ **Figure 5–10.** Left rib fractures suggestive of severe trauma. Asterisks (*) mark areas of callous formation, indicating healing and a subacute time of injury.

2. **Classic metaphyseal lesions** are a concerning fracture type, primarily in the infant. Commonly referred to as corner fractures, or bucket-handle fractures, they result from shearing forces and are angular breaks between the physis and subperiosteal bone collar. The most frequent locations are the distal femur (Figure 5–11), proximal humerus, and both proximal and distal tibia or fibula.

3. **Scapular, spinous process and sternal fractures** should prompt significant concern for abuse (Figure 5–12).

4. Moderate concern should arise when **multiple fractures** are detected, especially when they are **in various stages of healing** (Figure 5–13).

5. Long-bone shaft (diaphyseal) fractures are commonly seen in the emergency department and do not necessarily imply abuse. The likelihood that a diaphyseal fracture resulted from accident increases with patient age. **Nonambulatory infants with long-bone fractures**

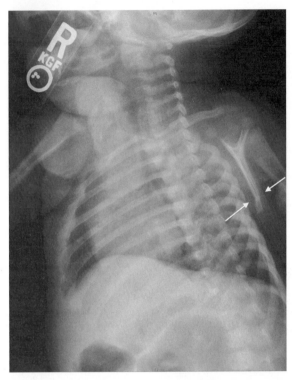

▲ **Figure 5–12.** Scapular fracture. Note the subtle appearance of buckled cortex between the two arrows.

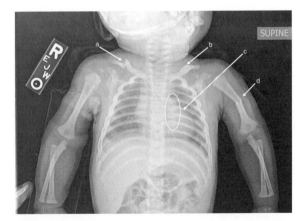

▲ **Figure 5–13.** Fractures in multiple stages of healing: (a), acute right clavicle fracture; (b), healing subacute left clavicle fracture; (c), healing subacute left rib fractures with callous formation; (d), acute left humerus fracture.

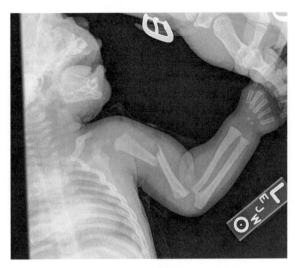

▲ **Figure 5–14.** Left humerus fracture in an infant.

are more concerning, may be seen as result of varying causes, and may appear as spiral, oblique or transverse fractures (Figure 5–14).

6. Linear skull fractures may occur after an accidental 3–4 foot fall, however linear fractures in younger children and all **skull fractures of a complex or depressed nature** are valid indications for consideration of maltreatment.

7. **Pelvic fractures** are typically a result of severe trauma, although reports have described these fractures result from sexual abuse.

8. Determination of the age of a fracture is not an exact science, but most pediatric radiologists can distinguish acute (no sign of healing) from healing fractures.

MANAGEMENT

Documentation

Proof of abuse is not required of the physician in order to report it; however, detailed documentation of the patient encounter is critical. All historical information should be documented clearly in an unbiased fashion. All statements made regarding the injury should be noted, and when multiple explanations or accounts of the history are given, all discussions should include the source.

A detailed physical examination should be documented. The sizes, stage of healing, and exact locations of wounds, abrasions, contusions, and other evidence of injury should be listed. A body diagram tool can be useful in the medical record to document injuries. An example of a body diagram is shown in Figure 5–15. Ideally, permission to photograph

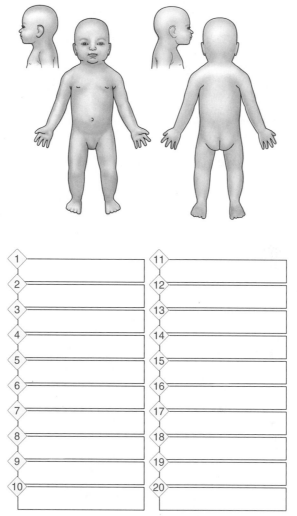

▲ **Figure 5–15.** Body diagram with injury list. Each injury should be diagrammed, and the list used to document size and characteristics of each finding.

injuries should be obtained from the patient's caregiver, and the photographs added to the medical record. All laboratory and radiographic studies should be referenced with regard to noted normal or abnormal findings. Although some findings on examination and in radiographs are thought to be pathognomonic for NAT, the findings should be documented without prejudice. Inconsistencies found within history, examination, and study findings should be specified, as well as the suspicion that neglect or abuse has occurred, if present.

Some facilities have dedicated personnel (Sexual Assault Nurse Examiner [SANE]) or similar program to obtain a comprehensive history and physical examination in the setting of any violent injury or abuse. Many jurisdictions may also authorize or train law enforcement or child protective services professionals to document the case with forensic photography. The emergency physician should be familiar with local resources and standard practices in this area. Many states utilize a formal evidence collection kit for sexual assault examinations.

These issues are discussed in Chapter 6.

When the physician or dedicated personnel collect evidence during the evaluation, it should remain in direct possession of the examiner until sealed and turned over to proper authorities, as the chain of custody for evidence in these situations may have significant legal relevance.

Communication With the Parent or Guardian

The physician caring for the child in the setting of known or suspected abuse should discuss the duty to report once the determination has been made. This communication will frequently be difficult when the parent or guardian present has been involved or is surprised by the information. Typically, authorities recommend reassurance of the caregiver that all testing and evaluation will be in the best interest of the patient.

Legal Aspects and Reporting Abuse

Child abuse and neglect are defined legally at the federal level in the Federal Child Abuse Prevention and Treatment Act (CAPTA) and the CAPTA Reauthorization Act of 2010:

"Any recent act or failure to act on the part of a parent or caretaker which results in death, serious physical or emotional harm, sexual abuse or exploitation" or "An act or failure to act which presents an imminent risk of serious harm." The laws apply primarily to parents or caregivers and usually do not apply to unfamiliar persons or to acquaintances.

Each state has specific definitions for maltreatment, and all states accepting CAPTA funding must meet listed federal standards. Child welfare responsibility is delegated to the state level. All states authorize any person to report known or suspected occurrences of abuse or neglect to child protective services. Mandatory reporting of child abuse varies among states, with a tendency toward mandatory reporting by professions having close or recurrent contact with children. In the United States, physicians in all states are required to report known or suspected abuse. Most states require reporting by social workers, teachers, coaches, child care providers, and law enforcement. Generally, a child is defined as younger than 18 years and is not an emancipated minor.

The ability to place the child on a protective hold in the hospital varies by jurisdiction. The emergency physician should be familiar with local and state statutes regarding their duty to report and time frame required. The emergency physician may be required to submit a sworn statement or to testify in civil or criminal hearings related to the patient care provided.

Disposition

A confirmed safe disposition should be assured in all cases of suspected child maltreatment. An injury requiring surgical management or continuous monitoring should prompt admission. Some cases will involve more minor injuries, or injuries that have already healed. Child protective services may indicate an official position on whether admission to the hospital is required. Temporary custody to a family member or foster care may be provided.

The emergency physician should have confidence in the safe medical and social disposition and confirmed follow-up of the patient. In the event that the medical evaluation is still in progress, a safe discharge plan cannot be formed, or child protective services are unavailable, admission is warranted to complete the workup and to allow the social and legal details to be finalized by appropriate authorities.

Adamsbaum C, Mejean N, Merzoug V, et al: How to explore and report children with suspected non-accidental trauma. *Pediatr Radiol.* 2010;40:932 [PMID: 20432011].

American College of Radiology: ACR-SPR practice guideline for skeletal surveys in children. 2011. Available at http://www.acr.org/~/media/ACR/Documents/PGTS/guidelines/Skeletal_Surveys.pdf. Accessed July 31, 2013.

Guenther E, Olsen C, Keenan H, et al: Randomized prospective study to evaluate child abuse documentation in the emergency department. *Acad Emerg Med.* 2009;16(3):249 [PMID: 19154562].

Hobbs CJ, Bilo RA: Nonaccidental trauma: Clinical aspects and epidemiology of child abuse. *Pediatr Radiol.* 2009;39(5):457 [PMID: 19198825].

Kellogg ND: American Academy of Pediatrics Committee on Child Abuse and Neglect: Evaluation of suspected child physical abuse. *Pediatrics.* 2007;119(6):1232 [PMID: 17545397].

Kemp AM, Dunstan F, Harrison S, et al: Patterns of skeletal fractures in child abuse: Systematic review. *BMJ.* 2008;337:a1518 [PMID: 18832412].

Kuppermann N, Holmes JF, Dayan PS, et al: Identification of children at very low risk of clinically-important brain injuries after head trauma: A prospective cohort study. *Lancet.* 2009;3(374):1160 [PMID: 19758692].

Monuteaux MC, Lee L, Fleegler E: Children injured by violence in the United States: Emergency department utilization, 2000-2008. *Acad Emerg Med.* 2012;19(5):535 [PMID: 22594357].

Rajaram S, Batty R, Rittey CD, et al: Neuroimaging in non-accidental head injury in children: An important element of assessment. *Postgrad Med J.* 2011;87:355 [PMID: 21450760].

Togioka BM, Arnold MA, Bathurst MA, et al: Retinal hemorrhages and shaken baby syndrome: An evidence-based review. *J Emerg Med.* 2009;37(1):98 [PMID: 19081701].

U.S. Department of Health and Human Services–Children's Bureau: Child maltreatment 2011. *U.S. Government Printing Office,* 2011. Also available at http://www.acf.hhs.gov/sites/default/files/cb/cm11.pdf. Accessed July 31, 2013.

U.S. Department of Health and Human Services–Children's Bureau: Definitions of child abuse and neglect. *U.S. Government Printing Office,* 2011. Also available at https://www.childwelfare.gov/systemwide/laws_policies/statutes/define.pdf. Accessed July 31, 2013.

Emergency Department Evaluation of Sexual Abuse

Kathi Makoroff, MD, MEd

Mary Greiner, MD

Brooks Keeshin, MD

▼ OVERVIEW OF SEXUAL ABUSE

DIAGNOSTIC EVALUATION

A patient who has been sexually abused commonly presents to the emergency department for the following:

1. Medical and forensic management of suspected reported acute sexual assault

2. Evaluation after disclosure of sexual abuse

3. Injury or examination finding; for example, bleeding that prompts a differential diagnosis including sexual assault

4. Genital discharge or evidence of sexually transmitted disease (STD)

The history is often the most important part of the diagnosis of sexual abuse. A disclosure of abuse may come during an emergency department physician's history and physical examination. Disclosures should be met with calm and nonjudgmental responses and leading questions should be avoided. The emergency department physician may ask questions about possible sexual assault or abuse if necessary for the medical and forensic evaluation of the patient including

- Nature of the sexual assault and type of contact

- Time interval between assault and arrival at the emergency department

However, forensic interviews should be performed by professionals who are trained in interviewing children for possible sexual abuse. When children with a concern of sexual abuse present to the emergency department, a social worker (in-house or on call) should be notified.

Children who are sexually abused warrant a physical examination; however, the type and urgency of the examination is dictated by the history and temporal relationship to the most recent abusive event. A child who is asymptomatic and discloses a remote history of sexual abuse (>3 days since last contact) may need only a general medical examination in the emergency department, and the genital examination deferred to an outpatient child advocacy center (if available) or to a practitioner trained in child abuse pediatric medicine.

A genital examination is warranted when the child describes genital symptoms (pain, discharge, dysuria, bleeding) or describes sexual abuse involving genital contact that occurred within the last 72 hours. An anxious child will usually cooperate fully with the examination (and evidence collection) if a parent or other support person is present during the examination. Reassurance and distraction techniques are helpful and consultation with a child life specialist (when available) can be useful. Sedation is rarely needed and can be ineffective. An examination should never be forced upon an unwilling child. When an examination is deemed medically necessary; for example, vaginal bleeding without a known source and uncooperative patient, examination under anesthesia should be considered. When a genital examination is performed, a chaperone (hospital personnel) should be present.

A pubertal girl can be examined in the supine position with feet in stirrups. A prepubertal girl should be examined in the supine frog-leg position (hips and knees bent; soles of feet touching). Gentle, even labial traction with gloved hands will allow visualization of the vulva and the hymen (Figures 6–1 and 6–2). Special attention should be given to the hymen, posterior fourchette, and fossa navicularis, the most common sites of injury in a sexually abused patient. In the female patient, a knee-chest position may be required for better visualization of the posterior hymen. Use the clock-face designation when documenting locations around the hymen, with 12 o'clock at the urethra, no matter the positioning of the patient. Adequate lighting is essential. A cotton-swabbed applicator can be used in the postpubescent girl to unfold and examine the edges of the hymen. The prepubescent hymen is sensitive to touch, which should be

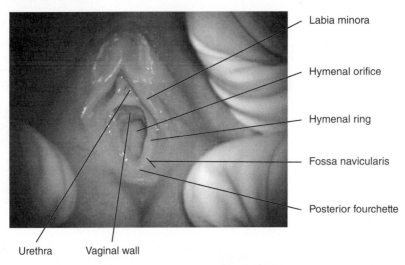

Labia minora

Hymenal orifice

Hymenal ring

Fossa navicularis

Posterior fourchette

Urethra   Vaginal wall

▲ **Figure 6–1.** Labeled anatomy diagram. (Reproduced, with permission, from Dr. Kathi Makoroff.)

avoided if possible. A speculum is never used in the examination of a prepubertal girl. The only time a speculum is used in this age group is during examination under anesthesia.

A male patient can be examined in the supine position, with care to inspect the penis and scrotum in entirety. The anus can be examined in the prone or lateral decubitus position. A colposcope can be used, if available, to magnify the genital and anal areas to look for smaller defects.

Most physical examinations in sexual abuse or assault will be normal. Findings specific for trauma, although not necessarily diagnostic of sexual abuse or assault, include bruising, lacerations, bites, and tears (Figures 6–3 and 6–4). Nonspecific findings include erythema, tenderness, and anal fissures. Signs of a possible sexually transmitted infection (STI), such as discharge or lesions, may be discovered.

Depending on the presentation, the patient may be a candidate for evidence collection. Medical and mental health management and follow-up (as appropriate) are a consideration for the patient.

Before the patient is discharged from the emergency department, it is necessary to

- Assess the emotional state of the patient and family.
- Identify access the alleged perpetrator has to the patient, family, or other individuals in order to ensure a safe discharge plan.

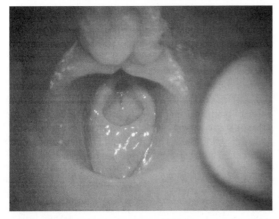

▲ **Figure 6–2.** Labial traction technique showing visualization of the hymen. (Reproduced, with permission, from Dr. Kathi Makoroff.)

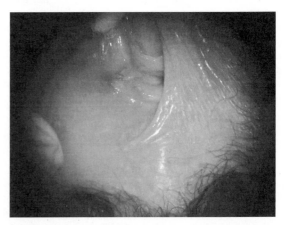

▲ **Figure 6–3.** Acute injury to the female genitalia including a tear to the hymen at the 8-o'clock location. (Reproduced, with permission, from Dr. Kathi Makoroff.)

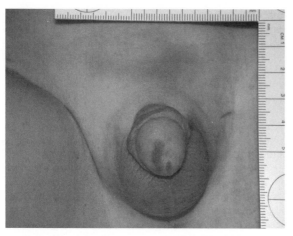

▲ **Figure 6–4.** Injury to the penis in a young boy following acute sexual assault. (Reproduced, with permission, from Dr. Kathi Makoroff.)

ACUTE SEXUAL ASSAULT

Immediate Management of Serious and Life-Threatening Problems

▶ Bleeding

The victim of an acute sexual assault may have genital and/or anal bleeding. The patient who exhibits active genital and/or anal bleeding needs immediate attention and evaluation.

▶ Hemodynamic Stability

Assess the patient's vital signs including pulse, blood pressure for hemodynamic stability and for clinical signs of shock (pale, diaphoretic, delayed cap refill, mental status change).

Treat for Shock, If Present

- Insert two large bore catheters.
- Draw blood for type and cross, a complete blood count, coagulation panel (platelets, prothrombin time [PT], partial thromboplastin time [PTT]), and, in a pubertal or peripubertal female patient, serum pregnancy.
- Begin a rapid infusion of a crystalloid solution and monitor vital signs.
- Infuse cross-matched blood as soon as possible if indicated; if not available, infuse type O blood.
- Continue to monitor vital signs.
- Patient should be monitored in a shock/trauma suite.

Evaluate for Cause of Bleeding

Gynecologic and/or surgical consultation should be obtained immediately.

The patient should have a visual examination to identify the source of bleeding. A prepubertal girl should receive a speculum examination only under anesthesia. The patient may need to go to the operating room for an examination under anesthesia for a complete evaluation.

A pelvic ultrasound may be indicated to look for other causes of bleeding such as pregnancy, ectopic pregnancy, tumor, or trauma.

▶ Suicide & Self-harm

A history of sexual abuse is strongly associated with increased risk of suicidal thinking, as well as suicide and self-harm attempts among older children and adolescents.

A patient evaluated for acute sexual assault should be carefully assessed for current suicidal or self-harm thoughts.

Factors that increase risk for suicide attempts among adolescents include previous suicide attempts, diagnosis of a mood or psychotic disorder (major depressive disorder, bipolar affective disorder), active substance use, history of psychiatric hospitalization, and poor family/social support systems.

A standardized suicide screening protocol should be considered in the emergency department to detect current level of distress and issues related to safety (thoughts of self-harm or suicide) in the sexual assault patient.

Psychiatric consultation should be obtained if there is a question or concern of suicide or self-harm.

▶ Intoxication

Sexual assault can coincide with intentional or covertly administered substance use.

If the patient demonstrates decreased level of consciousness

- Assess airway, ventilation and circulatory status.
- Assess vital signs continuously.
- Send a toxicology screen.
- Begin intravenous hydration.
- Correct electrolyte abnormalities.
- Start specific pharmacologic treatment when available.

Begin the evidence collection of genital/anal examination only when the patient is coherent and can consent or assent to the process and examination.

Diagnostic Evaluation

A child who presents to the emergency room for acute sexual assault should receive a complete physical examination including genital and anal examination, as discussed previously.

Injuries or skin lesions concerning for injuries on the body should be described in detail with the aid of a full body diagram and, when available, photodocumentation.

Evidence collection should be performed if the sexual assault occurred within the last 72 hours (for all boys and prepubertal girls), and can be considered up to 96 hours in pubertal girls if there is potential for the recovery of trace forensic evidence.

A sexual assault evidence collection kit (referred to as a rape kit) includes a checklist, instructions, collection devices, and appropriate labeling and sealing mechanisms to maintain an appropriate chain of custody for evidence collected.

The primary evidence collected are swabs from the mouth, genital, and anal areas, as well as areas reported by the victim that may be sites where bodily fluids (saliva, semen, blood) may have contacted, including skin, fingernails, and pubic hair. When obtaining swabs for evidence, be sure to swab before the patient washes or before the collection of swabs for medical purposes (such as for cultures). The patient should be instructed not to wash, eat/drink, or use the bathroom until swabs have been obtained.

An alternative light source, such as Wood light, as well as direct white light, may be used to identify areas of dried bodily fluids on the skin. These areas should be swabbed.

Patterned injuries on the skin that may be bite marks should be treated as bite marks. The areas should be swabbed to collect DNA and photographed with and without a measuring device (tape measure) in the field of the photograph.

Underwear, as well as any clothing that had potential contact with bodily fluids, should be collected. Clothing should be placed in specially marked paper evidence collection clothing bags.

Testing of a patient for drugs may have clinical and forensic value, and is an important consideration in the evaluation of alleged sexual assault. Testing for drugs should be considered when the patient has difficulty recalling events; reports a period where he/she has a loss of memory; describes intoxication out of proportion to the amount of alcohol or other substance consumed; appears to be intoxicated. Because normal clinical drug screening tests may not detect a number of illicit substances often implicated in drug-facilitated sexual assault, additional testing should be performed as part of the evidence collection process.

A patient with history of sexual assault involving oral, genital, or anal contact warrants testing for STDs and pregnancy (if applicable). When there has been a delay in disclosure, testing performed in the emergency department may be definitive to detect an acquired infection or pregnancy. However, if the sexual assault is recent, testing in the emergency department may be to establish a baseline, and the patient may be required to have follow-up testing performed with the primary care physician or at the local children's advocacy center (≤1–2 weeks if symptoms develop). Testing should be obtained for pregnancy, *Neisseria gonorrhoeae*, *Chlamydia trachomatis*, *Trichomonas vaginalis*, human immunodeficiency virus (HIV), syphilis, hepatitis B virus (HBV), and hepatitis C virus (HCV).

Pregnancy testing should be considered for a postpubertal or peripubertal girl who reports sexual abuse, regardless of type of abuse disclosed. Pregnancy testing should be repeated 2 weeks after acute sexual assault.

Testing for *N. gonorrhoeae* and *C. trachomatis* is performed using nucleic acid amplification test (NAAT) or cultures. When there is a disclosure of genital contact, a "dirty" or nonclean catch urine specimen may be sufficient for NAAT testing. However, if there is a disclosure of anal or oral contact, culture methods are performed (pharyngeal swab for *N. gonorrhoeae* only). If *N. gonorrhoeae* or *C. trachomatis* is positive in a prepubertal child or in a patient who does not give a history of prior sexual contact, repeat testing is necessary for confirmation before the initiation of treatment (see below).

Testing for *T. vaginalis* is performed using a vaginal swab and wet mount using a nonclean catch urine specimen with a Trichomonas antigen test.

Testing for HIV may be performed as a point-of-care testing using an oral swab or blood. Testing at the time of the emergency department visit provides a baseline; follow-up testing at 6 weeks, 3 months, and 6 months is recommended by the Centers for Disease Control and Prevention (CDC).

Blood testing for syphilis, HBV, and HCV should be considered for all genital, oral, or anal disclosures of sexual assault. Follow-up testing should be performed at 6 weeks (syphilis and HBV), 3 months (syphilis and HCV), and 6 months (HCV) or at any time the patient or family notices the appearance of a genital, nonpainful lesion (syphilis) or any symptoms.

Emergency Treatment of Specific Disorders

▶ Pregnancy Prophylaxis

Prophylaxis against pregnancy should be considered for all female pubertal and peripubertal patients who disclose genital-genital or genital-anal (or unknown) contact that occurred in the past 120 hours. A one-dose prophylaxis regimen should be offered in the emergency department. The provider should be familiar with the presumed mechanism(s) of action of the prophylaxis medication in order to counsel the patient and family. If the provider is uncomfortable providing pregnancy prophylaxis for religious or other reasons, an alternate provider should be consulted (Table 6–1).

▶ Sexually Transmitted Infection Prophylaxis

Prophylaxis against *N. gonorrhoeae* or *C. trachomatis* should be considered for pubertal patients who disclose genital-genital

Table 6–1. Prophylaxis after sexual assault.**

	Adolescents or Adults (≥45 kg)*	Children (< 45 kg)*
Pregnancy	Plan B (levonorgestrel 0.75 mg), 2 tabs × 1*	
Chlamydia	Azithromycin 1 g po × 1 or Doxycycline 100 mg po bid × 7 d*	Erythromycin base or Ethylsuccinate, 50 mg/kg/d ÷ 4 doses × 14 days or Azithromycin, 20 mg/kg (maximum 1 g) po × 1
Gonorrhea	Ceftriaxone 250 mg IM × 1 PLUS Azithromycin 1 g po × 1	Ceftriaxone 125 mg IM × 1 PLUS Azithromycin, 20 mg/kg (maximum 1 g) po × 1
Trichomoniasis	Metronidazole 2 g po × 1	Metronidazole 15 mg/kg/d ÷ 3 doses × 7 days; maximum 2 g
Hepatitis	Begin or complete Hepatitis B virus immunization if not fully immunized. If the offender is known to be HBsAg positive, HBIG also should be administered.	Begin or complete Hepatitis B virus immunization if not fully immunized. If the offender is known to be HBsAg positive, HBIG also should be administered.

* Patients who are not pregnant.
**These guidelines reflect current recommendations as of 8/2012.

or genital-anal (or unknown) contact that occurred in the previous 72 hours (see Table 6–1). Prophylaxis is not recommended for a prepubertal patient because of the low incidence of STI in sexually abused prepubertal children and because of the potential forensic importance of the diagnosis of an STI in this age group.

Refer to CDC guidelines for current treatment recommendations.

HIV Postexposure Prophylaxis

When there is a risk of transmission of HIV to a child during sexual assault, HIV postexposure prophylaxis (HIV PEP) should be considered. Risk factors that increase the transmission of HIV include multiple perpetrators, injury at the site of bodily fluid transfer, concurrent STD, and undiagnosed/uncontrolled HIV in perpetrator. Factors about the perpetrator that increase the risk of known or undiagnosed HIV infection include known concurrent STIs, history of drug use, and/or history of incarceration.

HIV PEP should be initiated as soon as possible. Although there is a 72-hour window after sexual assault when the HIV PEP may be initiated, the effectiveness of therapy decreases over the 72-hour time period. It is recommended that a patient who opts for HIV PEP begins a 3-drug antiretroviral regimen with treatment for 28 days. The specific medications to be used should be discussed with a local infectious disease specialist or child abuse specialist. Many emergency departments will stock starter packs of HIV PEP; however, follow-up must be ensured for the remainder of the 28-day course and to check for adverse effects from the medication.

HIV testing should be performed in the emergency department to ensure that the patient does not already have HIV. Testing is repeated at 6 weeks, 3 months, and 6 months.

Mental Health Follow-Up

It is common for a victim of sexual assault to experience emotional distress after the incident. The victim may proceed to have an anxiety disorder, posttraumatic stress disorder, major depressive disorder, or other behavioral/emotional disorder. Provide resources and handouts for each patient and family that detail common emotional responses to sexual assault, how parents can be supportive, and information on signs and symptoms of worsening emotional distress. In addition, supply a list of providers in the area who are experienced in counseling the victim of sexual assault, as well as phone numbers of 24-hour hotlines the sexual abuse survivor can call.

VAGINAL DISCHARGE IN PREPUBERTAL GIRLS

Diagnostic Evaluation

Vaginal discharge in a prepubertal girl can result from infectious agents, sensitivity reaction, foreign body, or a physiologic condition. A number of nonsexually transmitted infections can cause vaginal discharge. However, it is imperative to diagnose correctly an STI (Table 6–2).

The incidence of STIs in sexually abused prepubertal girls is less than 3%, and therefore the positive predictive value of a testing method (culture or NAAT) is greatly reduced. Presumptive treatment for gonorrhea and Chlamydia is not recommended for a prepubertal patient because of the very low

Table 6–2. Causes of vaginal discharge in children.

Nonsexually transmitted organisms
Streptococcus sp.
Staphylococcus sp.
Escherichia coli
Eterococcus
Shigella sp.
Salmonella sp.
Anaerobes (*Clostridium*)
Candida albicans
Gardnerella vaginalis
Sexually transmitted organisms
Neisseria gonorrhoeae
Chlamydia trachomatis
Trichomonas vaginalis
Noninfections
Foreign bodies
Irritation
Poor hygiene
Physiologic

incidence of infection in the patient and because of low risk of ascending infection (infection is a lower-tract disease in prepubertal girls) and the frequent need for confirmatory testing. Because most examination findings in sexually abused prepubertal girls are normal, the discovery of an STI can often be the only forensic evidence.

Cultures for *N. gonorrhea* and *C. trachomatis* are still regarded as the gold standard in prepubertal children because nonculture methods (NAAT) have not yet been rigorously tested in this age group. Nucleic acid amplification tests have replaced culture methods for the detection of *N. gonorrhoeae* and *C. trachomatis* in most laboratories. Regardless of testing method, treatment should not be implemented at the time of testing because of the need for confirmatory testing, if positive.

The presence of an STI in a prepubertal child does not confirm that the child was sexually abused. It is possible that an STI was acquired at birth or by a nonsexual manner such as autoinoculation. Referral and consultation with a child abuse specialist is recommended.

Treatment of Specific Disorders

Refer to CDC guidelines for the most up-to-date treatment recommendations.

A prepubertal girl should be examined in the supine frog-leg position. Gentle, even labial traction with gloved hands will allow better visualization. The patient should be examined for signs of discharge, irritation, injury, lesions, and for the presence of a foreign body in the vagina. The knee-chest position is useful for better visualization into the vagina for foreign body. If visualized, and the patient is cooperative, attempt removal of a foreign body with a steady stream of warm water using a syringe. A speculum is never used in the examination of a prepubertal girl; the only time a speculum is used in this age group is during examination under anesthesia.

VAGINAL BLEEDING IN CHILDREN

Immediate Management of Serious and Life-Threatening Problems

A patient who exhibits active genital bleeding needs immediate attention and evaluation.

▶ Hemodynamic Stability

Assess the patient's vital signs including pulse, blood pressure for hemodynamic stability and for clinical signs of shock (pale, diaphoretic, delayed cap refill, mental status change).

Treatment for Shock, If Present

- Insert two large-bore catheters.
- Draw blood for type and cross, a complete blood count, coagulation panel (platelets, PT, PTT), and (in pubertal or peripubertal patient) serum pregnancy.
- Begin a rapid infusion of a crystalloid solution and monitor vital signs.
- Infuse cross-matched blood as soon as possible if indicated; if not available, O-blood should be infused.
- Continue to monitor vital signs.
- Patient should be monitored in a shock/trauma suite.

▶ Evaluate for Cause of Bleeding

Gynecologic and/or surgical consultation should be obtained immediately.

The patient should have a visual examination to look for the source of bleeding. The source of bleeding should first be determined, whether the source of the bleeding is from the vagina, urethra, or rectum. Prepubertal children should receive a speculum examination only under anesthesia. The patient may need to go to the operating room for an examination under anesthesia for a complete evaluation.

A pelvic ultrasound may be indicated to look for other causes of bleeding such as pregnancy, ectopic pregnancy, tumor, or trauma.

Differential Diagnoses

A differential diagnosis of vaginal bleeding is listed in Table 6–3. It is important to rule out menstruation in peripubertal girls. Signs of pubertal development, symptoms (cramping), and family history of age of menarche can be helpful.

Table 6–3. Causes of vaginal bleeding in children.

Causes in prepubertal children
Trauma
Foreign body
Precocious puberty
Tumor
Nonvaginal bleeding (hematuria, urethral prolapse)
Causes in pubertal children
Trauma
Menses
Hypermenorrhea
Ovarian cyst
Ovarian torsion
Pregnancy
Abortion
Tumor
Coagulopathy
Endocrine abnormality
Menstrual cycle (mittelschmerz)

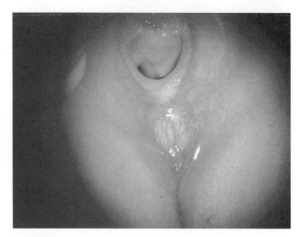

▲ **Figure 6–5.** Failure of midline fusion. (Reproduced, with permission, from Dr. Kathi Makoroff.)

MIMICS

Further Diagnostic Evaluation

▷ Mimics of Anatomy

Failure of Midline Fusion

Perineal failure of midline fusion can occur anywhere along the midline from the labia or scrotum to the anus. Although it appears as a large defect, the finding is congenital and there is no associated pain or bleeding. No treatment is needed, but accurate documentation in the medical record is important (Figures 6–5 and 6–6).

Labial Adhesions

Labial adhesions are common in young children. The etiology is thought to be related to local irritation combined with low levels of estrogen in children. The adhesions can be small and thin (filmy) or very thick and band-like. A small number of children are symptomatic. Adhesions can result in urine retention and "dribbling" in undergarments in a child who is toilet trained. The child can present with a small amount of blood in the underwear if the adhesions are accidentally lysed. There is no known association of labial adhesions and sexual abuse.

Children do not need treatment for asymptomatic labial adhesions, as most will resolve. In a symptomatic patient with evidence of dysuria, urinary retention, or suspected sexual abuse when the genital anatomy needs to be examined, treatment with topical estrogen cream can be used.

Topical estrogen cream should be used sparingly and for a few weeks only. The family should be informed of possible but temporary adverse effects such as breast budding and scan vaginal bleeding. Mechanical separation is painful and not recommended.

▷ Mimics of Trauma

Straddle Injury

Genital injury can result from a fall onto an object. Typically, a straddle injury causes damage to the external genitalia and unilateral bruising, and swelling of labia and periurethral tissues are seen (Figure 6–7). However, occasional penetrating

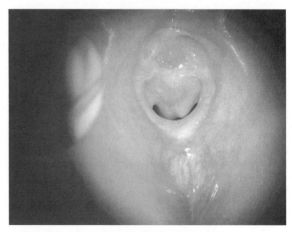

▲ **Figure 6–6.** Failure of midline fusion. (Reproduced, with permission, from Dr. Kathi Makoroff.)

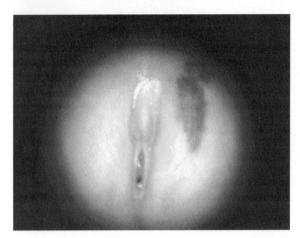

▲ **Figure 6–7.** Straddle injury with injury to the left labia majora. (Reproduced, with permission, from Dr. Kathi Makoroff.)

trauma to the hymen with internal injury is seen. The history and type of object involved in the penetration are needed for documentation. It is imperative to obtain a detailed history of the injury from the child (if developmentally appropriate) separately from the accompanying parent/adult. A number of factors increase concern of possible sexual abuse; including, no history of injury; injury in a child who is non-ambulatory; vaginal or hymenal injury without history of penetrating trauma; history inconsistent with physical findings; and/or additional nongenital trauma.

Treatment is usually symptomatic. If severe injuries occur, surgical repair may be necessary with referral to a pediatric gynecologist or surgeon (see also Immediate Management of Serious and Life-Threatening Problems:Bleeding).

Urethral Prolapse

Urethral prolapse is a condition that only occurs in females and can also occur in school-aged girls. The patient will present with painless bleeding and, on examination, will have what appears as swelling, but is actually the prolapsed portion of the urethra (Figure 6–8). Etiology is unknown but estrogen deficiency may be a risk factor. Additional risk factors include increased intra-abdominal pressure that results from coughing or constipation and anatomic defects. Medical treatment includes sitz bath and topical estrogen cream. Referral to a urologist is indicated, as well as review with the family of indications for emergent return including increased pain or bleeding which are signs of strangulation.

▶ Mimics of Erythema/Bruising

Conditions that mimic erythema are listed in Tables 6–4 and 6–5.

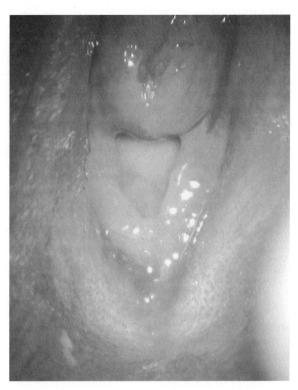

▲ **Figure 6–8.** Urethral prolapse. (Reproduced, with permission, from Dr. Kathi Makoroff.)

Table 6–4. Conditions which mimic genital bruising.

Mongolian spots
Vasculitis
Idiopathic thrombocytopenic purpura (ITP)
Meningococcemia
Erythema multiforme
Dye bleeding from clothing
Henoch-Schonlein purpura (HSP)
Lichen sclerosis
Hemangioma

Table 6–5. Conditions that cause genital erythema in children.

Streptococcal dermatitis
Poor hygiene
Dermatitis
Soap sensitivity
Pinworms
Candida infection (yeast)
Cellulitis

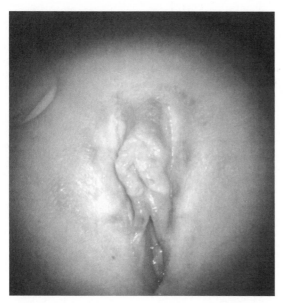

▲ **Figure 6–9.** Lichen sclerosis in a prepuberal female demonstrating hypopigmentation of skin and areas of friability that appear as bruises. (Reproduced, with permission, from Dr. Kathi Makoroff.)

Lichen Sclerosis

Lichen sclerosis is often found in post menopausal women but occasionally in prepubertal girls. Findings include thin hypopigmented easily friable skin in the genital and anal areas that can bleed even without trauma; itching and pain can also occur (Figure 6–9). The exact cause is unknown but thought to involve a genetic susceptibility, autoimmune dysfunction, and state of hypoestrogenism. Treatment consists of high potency corticosteroids and referral to a dermatologist or pediatric gynecologist.

Perianal Streptococcal Disease

Perianal streptococcal dermatitis/disease is an infectious disease caused by group A β-hemolytic streptococci. Signs and symptoms include perianal as well as vulvovaginal or penile erythema, itching, pain, anal fissures, blood-streaked stools, rectal bleeding, anal discharge, and vaginal discharge (Figure 6–10).

A bacterial culture for group A streptococci of the perianal and/or vulvovaginal or penile regions should be obtained by rubbing a dry swab over the affected areas.

Treatment consists of penicillin or amoxicillin. Erythromycin is used in a patient who is penicillin allergic. Treatment is 14–21 days.

Venous Pooling

Venous pooling refers to the purple discoloration of the perianal tissues caused by collection of venous blood in the external

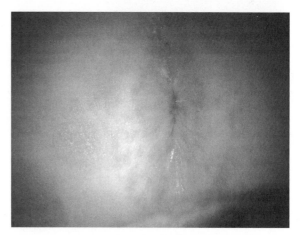

▲ **Figure 6–10.** Perianal streptococcal dermatitis. (Reproduced, with permission, from Dr. Kathi Makoroff.)

hemorrhoidal plexus. Venous blood pools in the plexus when a patient is immobile causing the veins to become distended and visible (Figure 6–11). Pooling can often be eliminated by getting the patient upright and mobile, and reexamining patient immediately after lying down.

Adams JA, Kaplan RA, Starling SP, et al: Guidelines for medical care of children who may have been sexually abused. *J Pediatr Adolesc Gynecol.* 2007;20(3):163-172 [PMID: 17561184].

American Academy of Pediatrics: Sexually transmitted infections in adolescents and children. In: Pickering LK, Baker CJ, Kimberlin DW, Long SS, eds. *Red Book: 2009 Report of the Committee on Infectious Diseases.* 28th ed. Elk Grove Village, IL: American Academy of Pediatrics; 2009.

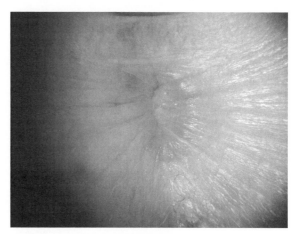

▲ **Figure 6–11.** Venous pooling. (Reproduced, with permission, from Dr. Kathi Makoroff.)

Anveden-Herzberg L, Gaudererx WL: Urethral prolapse: An often misdiagnosed cause of urogenital bleeding in girls. *Pediatr Emerg Care*. 1995;11:212 [PMID: 8532563].

Brent DA, Greenhill LL, Compton S, et al: The Treatment of Adolescent Suicide Attempters study (TASA): Predictors of suicidal events in an open treatment trial. *J Am Acad Child Adolesc Psychiatry*. 2009;48:987 [PMID: 19730274].

Centers for Disease Control and Prevention. *Sexually Transmitted Diseases Treatment Guidelines, 2010*. Atlanta, GA, 2010. Also available at http://www.cdc.gov/std/treatment/2010/sexual-assault.htm. Accessed August 29, 2012.

Davidoff F, Trussell J: Plan B and the politics of doubt. *JAMA*. 2006;296:1775 [PMID: 17032991].

Gavril AR, Kellogg ND, Nair P: Value of follow-up examinations of children and adolescents evaluated for sexual abuse and assault. *Pediatrics*. 2012;129:282 [PMID: 22291113].

Hammerschlag MR: Sexual assault and abuse of children. *Clin Infec Dis*. 2011;53:99 [PMID: 22080264].

Kellogg N: American Academy of Pediatrics, Committee on Child Abuse and Neglect: The evaluation of sexual abuse in children. *Pediatrics*. 2005;116:506 [PMID: 19720674].

Krol A: Perianal streptococcal dermatitis. *Pediatr Dermatol*. 1990;7:97 [PMID: 2359737].

Lang ME, Darwish A, Long AM: Vaginal bleeding in the prepubertal child. *CMAJ*. 2005;172:1289 [PMID: 15883400].

McCann J, Voris J, Simon M, Wells R: Perinal findings in prepubertal children selected for nonabuse: A descriptive study. *Child Abuse Negl*. 1989;13:179 [PMID: 2743179].

Powell JJ, Wojnarowska F: Lichen sclerosis. *Lancet*. 1999;353:1777 [PMID: 10348006].

Cardiac Arrest

Joseph W. Heidenreich, MD, FACEP

J. Scott Wieters, MD

Andrew Morris, DO

▼ PEDIATRIC CARDIAC ARREST

In contrast to cardiopulmonary arrest in adults, most incidences of cardiopulmonary arrest in children are preceded by respiratory failure including hypoxia and hypercarbia. A number of conditions can lead to respiratory failure followed by cardiac arrest, including sepsis, respiratory disease, submersion, trauma, electrolyte and metabolic abnormalities, and sudden infant death syndrome (SIDS). Although the conditions represent the minority of incidences, spontaneous cardiac arrests with initial rhythms of ventricular fibrillation (VF) and ventricular tachycardia (VT) not preceded by any apparent illness also can occur.

Unfortunately, pediatric victims of cardiac arrest have low survival rates. Although survival rates from in-hospital cardiac arrest has increased from 9 to 27% over the past 30 years, no increase has been shown in survival rate from out-of-hospital cardiac arrest with survival stagnating at 6%. Possible reasons for hospital-based increase in survival include rapid recognition of pediatric cardiac arrest, rapid response teams, and availability of pediatric specialists to give immediate care to critically ill children whereas out-of-hospital arrests lack these advantages. Although cardiopulmonary resuscitation (CPR) increases survival rate, fewer than 50% of pediatric cardiac arrest patients receive bystander CPR.

Nothing causes greater concern, fear, and anxiety in a clinician than a major pediatric resuscitation. The successful art of caring for children in cardiac arrest requires a calm and organized team approach. The advent of standardized resuscitation guidelines in the 1980s has aided clinicians in providing the best possible care to critically ill children, and mastery of pediatric advanced life support (PALS) guidelines is important for optimal care of the arresting child. Although PALS is a standard to guide care, resuscitative efforts can go beyond it, including the use of ultrasound, quantitative calorimetric monitoring, and continuous CPR.

Additionally, to optimize outcomes it is vital to recognize signs of shock and respiratory failure early on, before cardiopulmonary arrest occurs. It is also important to have a good understanding of the conditions that can lead up to cardiopulmonary arrest. In many patients, prompt treatment of reversible causes and early resuscitation when indicated will avert impending arrest.

APNEIC/PULSELESS CHILD

Once a child is recognized to be pulseless and/or apneic, PALS algorithms are instituted. A variety of advanced airway management techniques may be used to achieve oxygenation and ventilation. Cardiopulmonary resuscitation should be instituted for all pulseless rhythms or bradycardic infants with aims at circulating blood. Rhythm analysis and electrical stabilization is a priority with a final goal of perfusing oxygenated blood to vital organs, thereby reducing ischemic damage and preserving vital organ function. Actions that are listed in series on PALS algorithms are often performed in parallel by the resuscitating team but directed in a stepwise fashion.

ADJUNCTIVE GUIDES THAT REDUCE ERROR

Adult resuscitation medications have prefilled dosed syringes that reduce medication errors; however, pediatric drugs must be calculated in mg/kg to be dosed correctly. A number of adjuncts exist to aid in reducing errors and reducing the time and cognitive energy involved in calculating doses. Smartphone apps, drug cards, prepackaged weight-based bundles, and **Broselow** tapes are notable adjuncts that aid in error reduction and efficiency of resuscitation. An example of a drug card is shown in Figure 7–1.

The Children's Hospital at SCOTT & WHITE

PRECALCULATED DRUG DOSAGES
Rev. 8/05 Item #D3085-004

Min. (5%) Systolic BP
0-1 mo: 60
1 mo-1yr: 70
1yr: 70 + (2 x age in yr)

ET Tube sizes:
Birth: 3.0-3.5
1yr: 4.0 then ((age/4) +4)

ET tube depth:
3X the correct size tube

AGE	6yr.	7yr.	8yr.	9yr.	10yr.	11yr.	12yr.	13yr.	14yr.	15yr.	16yr.	Adult
WEIGHT (kg)	20	22	25	28	34	36	40	45	50	57	62	70
EPI (1;10,000) IV Dose												
ml's at 0.1 ml/kg	2	2.2	2.5	2.8	3.4	3.6	4	4.5	5	5 to 10	5 to 10	5 to 10
EPI (1;1,000) ETT Dose												
ml's at 0.1 ml/kg	2	2.2	2.5	2.8	3.4	3.6	4	4.5	5	5	5	5
ATROPINE mg's at 0.02 mg/kg (max = 1 mg)	0.4	0.44	0.5	0.5	0.5	0.5	0.5	0.5	1	1	1	1
ml's of 0.1 mg/ml	4	4.4	5	5	5	5	5	5	10	10	10	10
ml's of 0.4 mg/ml	1	1.1	1.25	1.25	1.25	1.25	1.25	1.25	2.5	2.5	2.5	2.5
CALCIUM 10 mg/kg Elemental Ca++ (100 mg/ml) ml's of Ca++ Gluconate (100 mg/kg)	10	10	10	10	10	10	10	10	10	10	10	10
ml's of Ca++ Chloride (20 mg/kg)	4	4.4	5	5.6	6.8	7.2	8	9	10	10	10	10
ADENOSINE mg's at 0.1 mg/kg (max = 12 mg)(3 mg/ml)	2	2.2	2.5	2.8	3.4	3.6	4	4.5	5	5.7	6	6
ml's of 1st dose (0.1 mg/kg)	0.7	0.7	0.8	0.9	1.1	1.2	1.3	1.5	1.7	1.9	2	2
ml's of 2nd dose (0.1 mg/kg)	1.3	1.5	1.7	1.9	2.3	2.4	2.7	3	3.3	3.8	4	4
SODIUM BICARBONATE mEq's at 1 mEq/kg	20	22	25	28	34	36	40	45	50	50	50	50
ml's of 1 mEq/ml	20	22	25	28	34	36	40	45	50	50	50	50
ml's of PediVial (0.5 mEq/ml)	40	44	50	56	68	72	80	90	100	100	100	100
NARCAN mg's at 0.1 mg/kg	2	2	2	2	2	2	2 to 4	2 to 4	2 to 4	2 to 4	2 to 4	2 to 4
ml's at 1 mg/ml	2	2	2	2	2	2	2 to 4	2 to 4	2 to 4	2 to 4	2 to 4	2 to 4
GLUCOSE ml's of D25 at 0.5 gm/kg	40	44	50	56	68	72	80	90	100	100	100	100
ml's of D50 at 0.5 gm/kg	20	22	25	28	34	36	40	45	50	50	50	50
DEFIBRILLATION Joules at 2 Joules/kg	40	44	50	56	68	72	80	90	100	100	100	100
Joules at 4 Joules/kg	80	88	100	112	136	144	160	180	200	200	200	200
CARDIOVERSION Joules at 0.5 Joules/kg	10	11	13	14	17	18	20	23	25	29	31	35
Joules at 1 Joules/kg	20	22	25	28	34	36	40	45	50	57	62	70
EPI/*PGE/NOREPI/TERB (1 mg/100 ml concentration) Rate in ml/hr for: *0.05 mcg/kg/min	6	6.7	7.5	8.5	10	11	12.5	13.5	15	17	18.5	21
*0.1 mcg/kg/min	12	13	15	17	20	22	24	27	30	34	37	42
0.17 mcg/kg/min	20	22	26	29	35	37	41	46	51	58	63	71
0.34 mcg/kg/min	41	45	51	57	69	73	82	92	102	116	126	143
0.51 mcg/kg/min	61	67	77	86	104	110	122	138	153	174	190	214
DOPAMINE/DOBUTAMINE (80 mg/100 ml Concentration) Rate in ml/hr for: 6.66 mcg/kg/min	10	11	12.5	14	17	18	20	22.5	25	28.5	31	35
13.32 mcg/kg/min	20	22	25	28	34	36	40	45	50	57	62	70
20 mcg/kg/min	30	33	37.5	42	51	54	60	67.5	75	85.5	93	105
LIDOCAINE mg's at 1 mg/kg (max = 100 mg)	20	22	25	28	34	36	40	45	50	57	62	70
ml's of 1% (10 mg/ml)	2	2	3	3	3	4	4	5	5	6	6	7
ml's of 2% (20 mg/ml)	1	1	1	1	2	2	2	2	3	3	3	4
LIDOCAINE DRIP (400 mg/100 ml concentration) Rate in ml/hr for: 20 mcg/kg/min	6	7	8	8	10	11	12	14	15	17	19	21
40 mcg/ kg/min	12	13	15	17	20	22	24	27	30	34	37	42
AMIODARONE mg at 5 mg/kg (50 mg/ml)	100	110	125	140	170	180	200	225	250	285	300	300
ml's for V tach (max 3 ml's)	2	2.2	2.5	2.8	3	3	3	3	3	3	3	3
ml's for V fib (max 6 ml's)	2	2.2	2.5	2.8	3.4	3.6	4	4.5	5	5.7	6	6
AMIODARONE DRIP (450 mg/250 ml D5W glass btl.) Rate in ml/hr for: 15 mg/kg/day	6.9	7.6	8.7	9.7	11.8	12.5	13.9	15.6	17.4	19.8	21.8	24.3

▲ **Figure 7–1.** Precalculated drug dose card.

PRECALCULATED DRUG DOSAGES
Rev. 8/05 Item #D3085-004

The Children's Hospital at SCOTT & WHITE

Min. (5%) Systolic BP
0-1 mo: 60
1 mo-1yr: 70
1yr: 70 + (2 x age in yr)

ET Tube size
Birth: 3.0-3.5
1yr: 4.0 then ((age/4) +4)

ET tube depth:
3X the correct size tube

AGE	B	1mo.	2mo.	4mo.	6mo.	8mo.	10mo.	12mo.	2yr.	3yr.	4yr.	5yr.
WEIGHT (kg)	3	4	5	6	7	9	10	15	12	14	16	18
EPI (1;10,000)												
IV Dose												
ml's at 0.1 ml/kg	0.3	0.4	0.5	0.6	0.7	0.9	1	1	1.2	1.4	1.6	1.8
EPI (1;1,000)												
ETT Dose												
ml's at 0.1 ml/kg	0.3	0.4	0.5	0.6	0.7	0.9	1	1	1.2	1.4	1.6	1.8
ATROPINE												
mg's at 0.02 mg/kg (max = 1 mg)	N/A	0.1	0.1	0.12	0.14	0.18	0.2	0.2	0.24	0.28	0.32	0.36
ml's of 0.1 mg/ml	N/A	1	1	1.2	1.4	1.8	2	2	2.4	2.8	3.2	3.6
ml's of 0.4 mg/ml	N/A	0.25	0.25	0.3	0.35	0.45	0.5	0.5	0.6	0.7	0.8	0.9
CALCIUM												
10 mg/kg Elemental Ca++ (100 mg/ml)												
ml's of Ca++ Gluconate (100 mg/kg)	3	4	5	6	7	9	10	10	10	10	10	10
ml's of Ca++ Chloride (20 mg/kg)	0.6	0.8	1	1.2	1.4	1.8	2	2	2.4	2.8	3.2	3.6
ADENOSINE												
mg's at 0.1 mg/kg (max = 12 mg)(3 mg/ml)	0.3	0.4	0.5	0.6	0.7	0.9	1	1	1.2	1.4	1.6	1.8
ml's of 1st dose (0.1 mg/kg)	0.1	0.1	0.2	0.2	0.2	0.3	0.3	0.3	0.4	0.5	0.5	0.6
ml's of 2nd dose (0.1 mg/kg)	0.2	0.3	0.4	0.4	0.4	0.6	0.6	0.6	0.8	1	1	1.2
SODIUM BICARBONATE												
mEq's at 1 mEq/kg	3	4	5	6	7	9	10	10	12	14	16	18
ml's of 1 mEq/ml	3	4	5	6	7	9	10	10	12	14	16	18
ml's of PediVial (0.5 mEq/ml)	6	8	10	12	14	18	20	20	24	28	32	36
NARCAN												
mg's at 0.1 mg/kg	0.3	0.4	0.5	0.6	0.7	0.9	1	1	1.2	1.4	1.6	1.8
ml's at 1 mg/ml	0.3	0.4	0.5	0.6	0.7	0.9	1	1	1.2	1.4	1.6	1.8
GLUCOSE												
ml's of D25 at 0.5 gm/kg	6	8	10	12	14	18	20	20	24	28	32	36
ml's of D50 at 0.5 gm/kg	3	4	5	6	7	9	10	10	12	14	16	18
DEFIBRILLATION												
Joules at 2 Joules/kg	6	8	10	12	14	18	20	20	24	28	32	36
Joules at 4 Joules/kg	12	16	20	24	28	36	40	40	48	56	64	72
CARDIOVERSION												
Joules at 0.5 Joules/kg	2	2	3	3	4	5	5	5	6	7	8	9
Joules at 1 Joules/kg	3	4	5	6	7	9	10	10	12	14	16	18
EPI*/PGE/NOREPI/TERB												
(1 mg/100 ml concentration)												
Rate in ml/hr for:												
*0.05 mcg/kg/min	1	1.2	1.5	1.8	2.1	2.7	3	3	3.6	4.2	4.8	5.4
*0.1 mcg/kg/min	1.8	2.4	3	3.6	4.2	5.4	6	6	7.2	8.4	9.6	10.2
0.17 mcg/kg/min	3.1	4.1	5.1	6.1	7.1	9.2	10.2	10.2	12.2	14.3	16.3	18.4
0.34 mcg/kg/min	6.1	8.2	10.2	12.2	14.3	18.4	20.4	20.4	24.5	28.6	32.6	36.7
0.51 mcg/kg/min	9.2	12.2	15.3	18.4	21.4	27.5	30.6	30.6	36.7	42.8	49	55.1
DOPAMINE/DOBUTAMINE												
(80 mg/100 ml Concentration)												
Rate in ml/hr for:												
6.66 mcg/kg/min	1.5	2	2.5	3	3.5	4.5	5	5	6	7	8	9
13.32 mcg/kg/min	3	4	5	6	7	9	10	10	12	14	16	18
20 mcg/kg/min	4.5	6	7.5	9	10.5	13.5	15	15	18	21	24	27
LIDOCAINE												
mg's at 1 mg/kg (max = 100 mg)	3	4	5	6	7	9	10	10	12	14	16	18
ml's of 1% (10 mg/ml)	0.3	0.4	0.5	0.6	0.7	0.9	1	1	1.2	1.4	1.6	1.8
ml's of 2% (20 mg/ml)	0.15	0.2	0.25	0.3	0.35	0.45	0.5	0.5	0.6	0.7	0.8	0.9
LIDOCAINE DRIP												
(400 mg/100 ml concentration)												
Rate in ml/hr for:												
20 mcg/kg/min	0.9	1.2	1.5	1.8	2.1	2.7	3	3	3.6	4.2	4.8	5.4
40 mcg/ kg/min	1.8	2.4	3	3.6	4.2	5.4	6	6	7.2	8.4	9.6	10.8
AMIODARONE												
mg at 5 mg/kg (50 mg/ml)	15	20	25	30	35	45	50	50	60	70	80	90
ml's for V tach (max 3 ml's)	0.3	0.4	0.5	0.6	0.7	0.9	1	1	1.2	1.4	1.6	1.8
ml's for V fib (max 6 ml's)	0.3	0.4	0.5	0.6	0.7	0.9	1	1	1.2	1.4	1.6	1.8
AMIODARONE DRIP												
(450 mg/250 ml D_5W glass btl.)												
Rate in ml/hr for:												
15 mg/kg/day	1	1.4	1.7	2.1	2.4	3.1	3.5	3.5	4.2	4.9	5.6	6.3

▲ **Figure 7–1.** (*Continued*)

Atkins DL, Everson-Stewart S, Sears GK, et al: Epidemiology and outcomes from out-of-hospital cardiac arrest in children: The resuscitation outcomes consortium epistry–cardiac arrest. *Circulation.* 2009;119:1484 [PMID: 19273724].

Rodriguez-Nunez A, Lopez-Herce J, Garcia C, et al: Pediatric defibrillation after cardiac arrest: initial response and outcome. *Crit Care.* 2006;10:R113 [PMID: 16882339].

Young KD, Gausche-Hill M, McClung CD, et al: A prospective, population based study of the epidemiology and outcome of out of hospital pediatric cardiopulmonary arrest. *Pediatrics.* 2004;114:157 [PMID: 15231922].

CARDIOPULMONARY RESUSCITATION

BASIC LIFE SUPPORT/ PEDIATRIC ADVANCED LIFE SUPPORT

In the American Heart Association (AHA) most recent iteration of PALS, the ubiquitous ABC (airway, breathing, circulation) of cardiopulmonary resuscitation has been changed to CAB (circulation, breathing, airway) for adults and children. The change from ABC to CAB marks a significant paradigm shift in cardiac arrest care that prioritizes early high-quality chest compressions and prompt defibrillation over airway management and rescue breathing. Although most data supporting this change in emphasis is from adult literature, the decision was made to apply the new mnemonic to children as well in order to simplify training. However, as discussed previously, most instances of cardiac arrest in children are precipitated by respiratory arrest and in children airway and breathing deserve much more attention than in adults.

Witnessed out-of-hospital cardiac arrest should begin with a check for responsiveness and normal breathing, followed by chest compressions if a pulse is absent. A pulse check should not delay chest compressions by more than 10 seconds. Studies show that even health care providers may have difficulty correctly identifying a pulse; therefore, if there is uncertainty and the patient shows signs of poor perfusion, CPR should be initiated immediately. If a pulse is present but is less than 60 beats/min and the patient is showing signs of poor perfusion, chest compressions should be initiated as if there were no pulse. If two rescuers are available, one should alert emergency medical services (EMS) immediately; however, if a second rescuer is not available and there is no way to call for help immediately, the single rescuer should administer 2 minutes of CPR prior to leaving the patient's side to call EMS. A high percentage of pediatric arrest patients respond very well to early CPR.

High-quality chest compressions, early defibrillation, and treating reversible causes have been shown to improve survival from cardiac arrest. In 2010 the recommended compression rate was revised from 100 to *at least* 100 reflecting data showing that a rate greater than 100 results in better outcomes than a rate less than 100. Also, the recommended compression depth was revised to *at least* one-third of diameter of the chest or *at least* 1.5 in for infants, and *at least* 2 in for children. The revisions were based on adult data showing that as little as 5 mm of increased compression depth results in measurable improvement in survival from cardiac arrest. Additionally, incomplete recoil should be avoided and interruptions in chest compressions should be minimized. The role of compressor should be rotated every 2 minutes if possible.

With a single rescuer the compression-to-ventilation ratio is 30:2, whereas with two rescuers the ventilation ratio is 15:2. If an advanced airway is placed, chest compressions and ventilations should be asynchronous with a compression rate of at least 100 and a ventilation rate of 8 to 10 (one breath every 6-8 seconds). In newborns, the recommended chest compression-to-ventilation ratio is 3:1.

Hands-only or compression-only CPR is an alternative to standard basic life support (BLS) CPR according to current PALS guidelines. The data supporting hands-only CPR come predominantly from adult studies where most arrests are cardiac in origin. Hands-only CPR has several advantages over traditional CPR and results in survival rates equal to or better than standard CPR for cardiogenic arrest. Bystanders are more likely to perform hands-only CPR because there is no need for mouth-to-mouth contact and it is an easy skill to master. Hands-only CPR will deliver significantly more chest compressions with fewer interruptions. Patients most likely to benefit from hands-only CPR have maximally oxygenated blood at the time of arrest. It is important to note, however, that in asphyxial arrest hands-only CPR has comparable outcomes to no CPR. Hands-only CPR, therefore, must be applied judiciously in the pediatric out-of-hospital population and likely has no role in the hospital setting.

DEFIBRILLATION/CARDIOVERSION

Management of dysrhythmias in pediatric patients differs greatly from management of dysrhythmias in adult patients. Primary cardiac arrest in the pediatric population is relatively rare but usually results from a secondary insult such as hypoxia, trauma, sepsis, or overdose. Most children will undergo a pattern of bradycardia that leads to pulseless electrical activity (PEA) or asystole. Therefore, when concerns of cardiac dysrhythmias develop, children tend to respond better to addressing the primary insult rather than cardiac-directed treatments. Children can have sinus rhythms in excess of 220/min and rates lower than this range should be assumed to be compensating for illness rather than exhibiting a primary dysrhythmia. With that said, it is difficult to discern sinus tachycardia from a poorly perfusing dysrhythmia. Cardioversion should be considered in a child with abnormal perfusion and abnormal cardiac rhythm with a synchronized cardioversion at 2 J/kg. If a second shock is required, the dose should be increased to 4 J/kg. Lethal dysrhythmias such as ventricular tachycardia, ventricular fibrillation, PEA, and asystole should be treated according to PALS algorithms.

AUTOMATIC EXTERNAL DEFIBRILLATOR

A number of types of automatic external defibrillator (AED) are available to deliver attenuated doses of energy to pediatric patients. The AEDs, if available, are recommended for use in a child younger than 8 years, and strongly recommended for an infant (< 1 year). If an AED with ability to attenuate energy dose for children is not available, it is considered safe and effective to use a standard adult AED on a child older than 1 year. An adult AED may be used for an infant if no other AED is available; however, there is little data on safety for this age group.

AIRWAY

A physician's knowledge of when a pediatric patient needs an adjunct or advanced airway is one of the most critical skills of pediatric resuscitation. Because most incidences of cardiac arrest in children are preceded by respiratory arrest, management of airway and breathing deserves special attention. The astute physician must watch closely for signs of respiratory decline. Respiratory failure is characterized by inadequate oxygenation, ventilation, or both. Signs of impending respiratory failure include increased respiratory rate and effort with signs of distress (nasal flaring, retractions, grunting), decreased respiratory rate and effort particularly with accompanying lethargy, or persistent cyanosis with abnormal breathing.

AIRWAY ADJUNCTS

Nasopharyngeal and oropharyngeal airways are excellent adjuncts that can help maintain airway patency by displacing the soft palate or the tongue from the pharyngeal air passages. An oropharyngeal airway is used only in a patient with an absent gag reflex; whereas a nasopharyngeal airway can be used in all patients. To function properly, the device must be appropriately sized. An oropharyngeal airway should reach from the corner of the mouth to the angle of the jaw, whereas a nasopharyngeal airway should reach from the nare to the tragus when held up against the face. The devices are particularly useful during bag-mask ventilations and can improve airflow in an otherwise difficult-to-bag patient.

ADVANCED AIRWAY

A comprehensive review of pediatric airway adjuncts as well as endotracheal (ET) intubation are mentioned in Chapter 9.

BREATHING

During CPR it is acceptable to give 100% oxygen; however, newer guidelines stress that pre- and postarrest oxygen levels should be titrated to an oxyhemoglobin saturation of 94% or greater in pre- and postarrest periods. Administering excessive oxygen is not necessary and may even be harmful.

Bag-mask ventilation is a critical skill in the resuscitation of a crashing pediatric patient. Not only is bag-mask ventilation usually a bridge to mechanical ventilation, but it may be the only type of ventilation needed in the resuscitation. Bag-mask ventilation is a skill that requires training and practice to maintain, and is arguably the most difficult skill in pediatric resuscitation. It is important to choose a properly sized mask, maintain an open airway, ensure a tight seal between the mask and the face, and assess for the effectiveness of each ventilation.

Excessive force, volume, and frequency of ventilation are a common problem during pediatric cardiac arrest and can reduce the likelihood of a successful outcome. Most importantly, hyperventilation increases intrathoracic pressure, impedes venous return, and decreases cardiac output during CPR. This leads to decreased cardiac and cerebral blood flow and increased mortality. Additionally, hyperventilation can induce air trapping and barotrauma as well stomach insufflation, regurgitation, and aspiration. To avoid entry of air into the stomach, cricoid pressure may be applied during bag-mask ventilations. Immediately following ET intubation, a nasogastric (NG) tube should be passed to relieve gastric insufflation which can impair resuscitative efforts.

Current CPR guidelines recommend that after every 30 compressions, two ventilations should be delivered over 1 second each for single rescuer CPR. For two-rescuer CPR two rescue breaths should follow every 15 compressions. The rescuer should deliver enough volume to see a visible chest rise but not more. If an advanced airway is in place, the respiratory rate during CPR should be 8 to 10 or one breath every 6 to 8 seconds. If there is a perfusing cardiac rhythm but the patient is apneic, the ventilation rate should be 12 to 20 or one breath every 3 to 5 seconds.

End-tidal CO_2 ($ETCO_2$) monitoring is now formally recommended both during and after arrest for assessment of appropriate ventilation/tube placement as well as assessment of chest-compression efficiency and detection of return of spontaneous circulation (ROSC). During CPR, $ETCO_2$ levels are loosely correlated with the quality of chest compression with effective compressions. When ROSC occurs a sudden, dramatic increase in $ETCO_2$ will be observed.

The following caveats are important to remember when interpreting the $ETCO_2$. The presence of a capnography waveform confirms that an endotracheal tube is in the airway but does not rule out right mainstem intubation. Occasionally bolus epinephrine can transiently reduce pulmonary blood flow hence decreasing $ETCO_2$. Severe asthma and pulmonary edema can markedly reduce $ETCO_2$ sometimes below detectable limits. Also a large glottic air leak can result in artificially low $ETCO_2$.

CIRCULATION

ASSESSMENT

The first component of assessment of the circulatory status of the pediatric patient is the "clinical gestalt" or "doorway impression" of the health care provider. Important information can be gathered by the patient's level of activity, muscle tone, appearance, and the context of presentation. The presence of a pulse should be assessed for no more than 10 seconds. In children, carotid or femoral artery palpation are the most reliable noninvasive methods to assess the pulse. In infants, brachial artery palpation or chest auscultation are preferred. If no adequate pulse is detected within 10 seconds, CPR should be initiated.

The presence of a pulse alone does not preclude the need for chest compressions as inadequate pulse rates will not achieve effective end-organ perfusion. Initiate chest compressions if the pulse rate is less than 60 per minute with signs of poor perfusion. Skin temperature and color and capillary refill (normal < 2 seconds) can be used as adjunct methods of assessing perfusion status but may be influenced by environmental status such as ambient temperature. In the hospital setting, the health care provider will often have the benefit of cardiac monitors and other advanced methods of monitoring circulatory status. Care must be taken to avoid "treating the monitor" as a good electrocardiographic tracing may not necessarily correspond to adequate end-organ perfusion, for example, the patient with PEA.

INTRAVENOUS ACCESS

Vascular access is an essential component of the effective pediatric resuscitation effort. Although support of airway, breathing, and circulation should not be delayed by attempts to establish vascular access, it is imperative to secure a reliable means to administer medication and fluids to the patient as well as to obtain blood samples for laboratory studies.

Peripheral venous cannulation is often the initial method by which vascular access is attempted and it is acceptable if it can be established quickly. Common sites of cannulation in the pediatric patient include the dorsum of the hand or foot, the forearm, or in neonates, the scalp. Current guidelines recommend that health care providers limit the time attempting peripheral venous cannulation and instead obtain intraosseous (IO) access. IO catheters can be placed rapidly and safely and used both for medication administration and for obtaining blood samples (including type and cross-matching or blood gas analysis). Medications should be administered at the same doses as those used with IV access and followed with normal saline flushes.

Pediatric providers should be skilled in the placement of the IO line. In addition to the Jamshidi IO needle, which is placed manually and has historically been used in pediatric cardiac arrest, there are several commercially available IO devices including the EZ-IO which have been shown to reduce the placement time and reduce complications related to IO placement. Central venous cannulation is not recommended as the initial method of vascular access during the resuscitative effort as it requires both special training and time to be safely obtained. Placement of a central line may be useful in the postresuscitation period for ongoing administration of vasoactive medications.

LETHAL DYSRHYTHMIAS

When following PALS algorithms, the physician should carefully consider reversible causes of cardiac arrest. Formerly, these reversible causes were emphasized for PEA and asystole but are now emphasized during cardiac arrest with any rhythm. Reversible causes can be recalled using the mnemonic, 5Hs and 5Ts (hypoxia, hypovolemia, hydrogen ion [acidosis], hypo/hyperkalemia, hypoglycemia, hypothermia, toxins, tamponade, myocardial thrombosis, pulmonary thrombosis, and tension pneumothorax). Special care addressing oxygenation, breathing, and shock will be most beneficial. In neonatal patients, ductal-dependent lesions should be considered in the differential and prostaglandin E (PGE) may have a role in resuscitation. Often, ultrasound/Doppler will detect pulses not able to be palpated in the central area. The physician should use adjunctive ultrasound to detect cardiac activity and correlate with electrical monitoring to guide resuscitation. Ultrasound will be able to detect pericardial effusion and tension pneumothorax or hemoperitoneum as well, which are potentially reversible causes of pulseless electrical activity (PEA) and asystole.

PULSELESS VENTRICULAR TACHYCARDIA/VENTRICULAR FIBRILLATION

Recognition of wide complex tachycardia can be difficult in a tachycardic patient. QRS width greater than 0.09 millisecond are considered wide complex in children younger than 4 years, and greater than 0.1 millisecond in children 4 years and older. Defibrillation should be delivered as soon as possible for ventricular tachycardia (VT) without a pulse or ventricular fibrillation (VFib). Biphasic defibrillation of pulseless ventricular tachycardia and ventricular fibrillation should be at 2 J/kg to maximum of 10 J/kg (or adult maximum 200 J). Primary dysrhythmias will usually respond better to defibrillation than dysrhythmias that develop as a secondary cause of illness. Pads can be placed in anterior-posterior or axillary-sternal positions. Pediatric pads and pediatric AEDs are preferred, however, adult AEDs are not harmful in children older than 1 year with studies showing that adult AEDs are 96% sensitive and 100% specific at recognizing VFib and VT. Older monophasic defibrillators can be used to defibrillate at 2 J/kg and subsequent shocks at 4 J/kg. It should be noted that conversion rates are as low as 20% with monophasic shocks at 2 J/kg.

In contrast to PALS recommendations, many recommend that CPR should not be interrupted during defibrillation. Studies and experience have failed to show significant transmission of energy from defibrillation to the person performing chest compression. Interruptions serve only to preclude circulation of high-quality CPR. The physician may use a small towel or rubber mat to aid in reducing concerns about provider injury from defibrillation.

NEONATAL CONSIDERATIONS

Neonatal resuscitation skills are not employed daily in the emergency department, but are a set of skills that should be revisited periodically. As with any resuscitation or procedure, preparation is paramount. Emergency physicians and staff should be aware of the type and location of equipment needed for adequate resuscitation, including general knowledge of the type of team available to respond.

INITIAL RESUSCITATION

Neonates should be expeditiously dried and warmed as they are prone to hypothermia, a condition which requires more oxygen consumption on their part. The goal for initial temperature is 36.5°C (97.7°F) axillary. Immediately after delivery warm towels or blankets may be used, but a radiant heat source is preferred, such as the type used in standard delivery rooms. Remember to preheat the warming mechanism. Premature infants may be wrapped in plastic wrap to further prevent heat loss. All ventilatory interventions should include warm humidification. The room should be warmed if at all possible to 26°C (~78°F).

AIRWAY/BREATHING

Ventilation is the cornerstone of neonatal resuscitation and should be reassessed regularly during resuscitation. The newborn's mouth and nares should be suctioned shortly after birth with a bulb syringe. Be cognizant of the color of the suctioned fluid (meconium). Suctioning not only clears the newborn's airway, but also provides necessary stimulation. Meconium-stained fluid may herald the need for more aggressive ventilation measures.

Care must be taken when using supplemental oxygen in this age group, specifically the preterm infant. Pulse oximetry is a valuable tool for assessment of adequate oxygenation of the newborn. Supplemental oxygen should be titrated such that the Spo_2 is 85-95%. Remember that the Spo_2 levels will not rise to this level until 10 minutes after delivery. If there is not a response of increased heart rate (< 100 beats min) after 90 seconds, the Fio_2 may be increased. Positive-pressure ventilation is indicated if there is no improvement in the heart rate or if there if the infant remains apneic. This should ideally be applied with a bag or other device capable of providing positive end-expiratory pressure. CPAP should only be employed only to infants who are breathing spontaneously.

Selection of proper equipment is important when intubation is necessary. A Miller or other straight blade is preferred for optimal airway visualization. The majority of term infants can be intubated with a size 1 blade, while smaller or premature neonates may require a size 0 blade. The ET tube should be inserted to just past the vocal cords. It may also be beneficial to apply positive end-expiratory pressure (PEEP) through the ventilator.

CARDIOPULMONARY RESUSCITATION AND MEDICATIONS

Chest compressions are indicated for infants with a heart rate that remains less than 60 beats/min despite adequate ventilation. Compressions should be performed at a 3:1 ratio to positive-pressure ventilations, for a total of 90 compressions and 30 breaths in 1 minute. After a heart rate of 60 beats/min or greater is achieved, CPR should be discontinued.

If the heart rate remains below 60 despite adequate ventilation and compressions, epinephrine is indicated. The recommended dose is 0.01-0.03 mg/kg (0.1-0.3 mL of the 1:10,000 solution) IV. This dose may be tripled if given via ET tube. Reassess the patient's heart rate and ventilation frequently.

Volume expansion is provided with an initial 10 mL/kg bolus of isotonic fluid (normal saline or lactated Ringer solution). If blood loss is suspected, then type O-negative packed red blood cells should be transfused. Optimally, transfused blood should be cross-matched against the mother. Routine administration of naloxone for volume expansion is no longer recommended.

POSTRESUSCITATION MEASURES

After initial resuscitation, assess the newborn's airway, breathing, and circulation once more, as well their fluid and electrolyte status. Treat this expectantly, paying special attention to serum glucose levels. Treat hypoglycemia promptly and aggressively with dextrose. The neonate should then be admitted to the nearest accepting neonatal intensive care unit (NICU).

Berg M, Schexnayder S, Chameides M, et al: Part 13: Pediatric Basic Life Support: 2010 American Heart Association Guidelines for Cardiopulmonary Resuscitation and Emergency Cardiovascular Care. *Circulation.* 2010;122:S862 [PMID: 20956229].

Berg MD, Samson RA, Meyer RJ, et al: Pediatric defibrillation doses often fail to terminate prolonged out-of-hospital ventricular fibrillation in children. *Resuscitation.* 2005;67:63 [PMID: 16199288].

Chameides L, Samson RA, Schexnayder SM, et al: *Pediatric Advanced Life Support Provider Manual.* Dallas: American Heart Association; 2011.

Edson DP, Abella BS, Kramer-Johansen J, et al: Effects of compression depth and pre-shock pauses predict defibrillation failure during cardiac arrest. *Resuscitation.* 2006;71:137 [PMID: 16982127].

Hoke RS, Heinroth K, Trappe HJ, et al: Is external defibrillation an electric threat for bystanders? *Resuscitation.* 2009;80:395 [PMID: 19211180].

International Liaison Committee on Resuscitation: 2005 International consensus on cardiopulmonary resuscitation and emergency cardiovascular care science with treatment recommendations. Part 7: Neonatal resuscitation. *Resuscitation.* 2005;67:293 [PMID: 16324993].

Kattwinkel J, Bloom RS, American Academy of Pediatrics: *Textbook of Neonatal Resuscitation.* Dallas: American Academy of Pediatrics; 2011.

Kattwinkel J, Perlman J, Aziz K, et al: Part 15: Neonatal resuscitation: 2010 American Heart association guidelines for cardiopulmonary resuscitation and emergency cardiovascular care. *Circulation.* 2010;122:S909 [PMID: 20956231].

Kitamura T, Iwami T, Kawamura T, et al: Conventional and chestcompression-only cardiopulmonary resuscitation by bystanders for children who have out-of-hospital cardiac arrests: A prospective, nationwide, population-based cohort study. *Lancet.* 2010;375:1347 [PMID: 20202679].

Kleinman M, Chareides L, Schexnayder S, et al: Part 14: Pediatric basic life support: 2010 American Heart Association guidelines for cardiopulmonary resuscitation and emergency cardiovascular care. *Circulation.* 2010;122:S876 [PMID: 20956230].

Kligman RM, Stanton B, Geme J, et al: *Nelson Textbook* of *Pediatrics: Expert Consult Premium Edition.* Philadelphia, PA.: Saunders; 2011.

Loyd MS, HeekeB, Walter PF, et al: An analysis of electrical current glow through rescuers in direct contact with patients during biphasic external defibrillation. *Circulation.* 2008;117:2510 [PMID:18458166].

Noori S, Wlodaver A, Gottipati V, et al: Transitional changes in cardiac and cerebral hemodynamics in term neonates at birth. *J Pediatr.* 2012;160:943 [PMID: 22244465].

Perlman JM, Wyllie J, Kattwinkel J, et al: Neonatal resuscitation: 2010 international consensus on cardiopulmonary resuscitation and emergency cardiovascular care science with treatment recommendations. *Pediatrics.* 2010;126:e1319 [PMID:20956431].

Tibballs J, Carter B, Kiraly NJ, et al: External and internal biphasic direct current shock doses for pediatric ventricular fibrillation and pulseless ventricular tachycardia. *Pediatr Crit Care Med.* 2011;12:14 [PMID: 20308928].

Tibballs J, Russell P: Reliability of pulse palpation by healthcare personnel to diagnose pediatric cardiac arrest. *Resuscitation.* 2009;80:61 [PMID: 18992985].

Watkinson M: Temperature control of premature infants in the delivery room. *Clin Perinatol.* 2006;33:43 [PMID:16533632].

PHARMACOLOGIC MANAGEMENT

Medication doses for the pediatric patient are weight dependent and as such, the most recent reliable weight measurement should be used. In the setting of cardiac arrest such measurements are often unavailable and the use of length-based adjuncts (such as a Broselow tape) is an acceptable alternative. Despite the fact that most adjuncts indicate precalculated dosages based on ideal body weight, data is lacking on the safety of adjusting precalculated doses for obese children. Although several of the medications used in the PALS protocols can be given via the endotracheal tube in 2.5 times the IV dose, ET dosing of medications is discouraged in favor of using IV as a first choice, and IO as a second choice. Only as a last resort with inability to establish an IO should drugs be given endotracheally. Table 7–1 lists the common medications with doses that are used in pediatric resuscitation.

SELECTED MEDICATIONS

Adenosine

Adenosine is an endogenous nucleoside with very short half-life. This drug causes a short-lived AV node blockade which makes this drug the first-line therapy for SVT or PSVT. Administration should be via rapid IV push followed by saline flush with careful cardiac monitoring. Adenosine may cause a brief asystolic period. If the initial dose of 0.1 mg/kg (6 mg maximum) does not resolve the SVT or PSVT, it may be repeated by up to two additional doses of 0.2 mg/kg (12 mg maximum).

Amiodarone

Amiodarone is a potassium channel blocker (class III anti-antiarrhythmic) with some Na channel blocker, beta-blocker and calcium channel blocker effects. Amiodarone slows AV conduction and prolongs the AV refractory period. It also widens the QRS complex and prolongs the QT interval. It is indicated for the treatment of VF or pulseless VT as a rapid bolus of 5 mg/kg (maximum single dose of 300 mg) for up to 15 mg/kg total. It is also indicated in the treatment of VT with pulses and as a second-line agent for the treatment of SVT if adenosine fails. In these patients it should be administered as a slow infusion over 20 to 60 minutes under cardiac and blood pressure monitoring as QT prolongation and hypotension may develop.

Atropine

Atropine is a parasympatholytic useful in the treatment of symptomatic bradycardias. Atropine accelerates sinoatrial pacemaker rhythm and shortens AV conduction. Avoid use in high grade heart blocks (Mobitz type II or third-degree heart blocks). Administer 0.02 mg/kg IV or IO (minimum single of dose 0.1 mg to avoid paradoxical bradycardia, maximum single dose 0.5 mg). Repeat once if needed. Atropine can also be given via ET tube if IV or IO access is unavailable. In this patient give 2 to 2.5 the usual dose. Atropine is no longer indicated for children with PEA or asystole.

Calcium

Available as calcium chloride or calcium gluconate, calcium administration is recommended in the setting of

Table 7–1. Drugs commonly used in pediatric arrest.

Drug	Indications	Dose
Adenosine	SVT	0.1 mg/kg rapid push. May repeat with up to 2 additional doses of 0.2 mg/kg (max 12 mg/dose)
Albumin	Shock, burns, trauma	0.5-1.0 g/kg IV/IO rapid infusion
Albuterol	Asthma, hyperkalemia	2.5-5.0 mg neb q20 min as needed or 0.5 mg/kg/h continuous (max 20 mg)
Amiodarone	VF, pulseless VT	5 mg/kg IV/IO bolus (max 300 mg per single dose). May repeat to daily max of 15 mg/kg.
	Stable VT and SVT	5 mg/kg IV/IO over 20-60 min. Repeat to daily max of 15 mg/kg
Atropine	Symptomatic bradycardia	0.02 mg/kg IV/IO. May repeat once, max dose 1 mg child, 3 mg adolescent
	Organophosphate poisoning	< 12 years 0.02-0.05 mg/kg IV/IO repeated q30 min until reversal. > 12 y 2 mg IV/IO then 1-2 mg IV/IO until reversal
Calcium chloride	Hypocalcemia, CCB overdose, hyperkalemia, hypermagnesemia	20 mg/kg IV or IO slow push during arrest as needed (max dose 2 g)
Diphenhydramine	Anaphylactic shock	1-2 mg/kg IV/IO/IM q4-6h (max 50 mg)
Epinephrine	Pulseless arrest, symptomatic bradycardia	In arrest 0.01 mg/kg IV/IO (1:10,000 concentration) max dose of 1 mg.
	Hypotensive shock	0.1-1.0 mcg/kg/min IV/IO
	Anaphylaxis	0.01 mg/kg 1:1000 IM q15 min (max dose 0.3 mg). If hypotensive, give 0.01 mg/kg 1:10,000 IV/IO q3-5 (max dose 1 mg)
Etomidate	Rapid sequence intubation	0.2-0.4 mg/kg IV/IO over 30 sec
Glucose (dextrose)	Hypoglycemia	0.5-1.0 g/kg IV/IO. May be necrotic if extravasation occurs
Hydrocortisone	Adrenal insufficiency	2 mg/kg IV (max 100 mg)
Lidocaine	VFib, pulseless VT, stable VT	1 mg/kg IV or IO bolus. 20-50 mcg/min IV or IO infusion
Magnesium sulfate	Hypomagnesemia, torsade de pointes	25-mg/kg IV or IO slowly over 10-20 min (max dose 2 g)
Milrinone	Myocardial dysfunction with increased SVR/PVR	Load 50 mcg/kg IV/IO over 10-60 min, then 0.75 mcg/kg /min infusion
Naloxone	Opioid toxicity	1-5 mcg/kg IV/IO—partial reversal 0.1 mg/kg (max 2 mg)—total reversal
Procainamide	Afib, atrial flutter, SVT, or VT (with good perfusion)	15 mg/kg IV or IO over 30-60 min
Sodium bicarbonate	Severe metabolic acidosis, hyperkalemia	1 mEq/kg IV/IO slow bolus
	Tricyclic antidepressant overdose	1-2 mEq/kg IV/IO bolus until serum pH is > 7.45 followed by infusion to maintain alkalotic pH
Terbutaline	Status asthmaticus, hyperkalemia	0.1-10 mcg/kg/min IV/IO, may give 10 mcg/kg SQ until IV started
Vasopressin	Cardiac arrest	0.4-1 unit/kg bolus to replace 1st or 2nd dose of epinephrine (max 40 units)
	Catecholamine-resistant hypotension	0.2-2 milliunits/kg/min continuous infusion

documented hyperkalemia or hypermagnesemia or in incidences of calcium channel blocker overdose or documented hypocalcemia. Calcium may be irritating to the peripheral vessels and as such a central line should be used if available. Dosing will vary according to formulation and concentration with calcium chloride delivering approximately three times as much elemental calcium as calcium gluconate.

Epinephrine

Epinephrine is an α- and β-adrenergic agonist indicated for the treatment of all pulseless rhythms. It may be repeated every 3-5 minutes as needed and may be given via ET tube as described in Table 7–1.

Glucose

A carbohydrate, glucose is essential in the treatment of hypoglycemia. It is available as dextrose in different concentrations (D50, D25, and D10). It should be administered carefully since its hyperosmolar nature means it may cause necrosis of surrounding tissue if extravasation occurs.

Lidocaine

Lidocaine is a class IB anti-arrhythmic that decreases automaticity of pacemaker cells. Its use is indicated in the treatment of ventricular arrhythmias. Monitor for signs of toxicity which include cardiovascular depression, diminished cardiac output, and seizures. After successful treatment of dysrhythmia with a bolus, an infusion should be administered as described in Table 7–1.

Magnesium Sulfate

Magnesium is indicated in the treatment of polymorphic VT (torsades des pointes) or in incidences of documented hypomagnesemia. It should be given slowly at 25 mg/kg (max dose of 2 g) IV or IO over 10-20 minutes as rapid administration may cause hypotension. Monitor the patient for signs of toxicity which include QT prolongation and decreased deep tendon reflexes.

Procainamide

Procainamide is a class IA antiarrhythmic which increases the refractory period in both the atria and ventricles. It may be used on the treatment of atrial fibrillation or atrial flutter even though evidence of benefit in pediatric resuscitation efforts is lacking. Avoid concurrent administration with other drugs that prolong QT interval. It should be infused slowly over 30-60 minutes. Infusion should be discontinued if signs of toxicity are observed.

Berg M, Schexnayder S, Chameides M, et al: Part 13: Pediatric Basic Life Support: 2010 American Heart Association Guidelines for Cardiopulmonary Resuscitation and Emergency Cardiovascular Care. *Circulation.* 2010;122:S862 [PMID: 20956229].

Chameides L, Samson RA, Schexnayder SM, et al: *Pediatric Advanced Life Support Provider Manual.* Dallas: American Heart Association; 2011.

Kleinman M, Chareides L, Schexnayder S, et al: Part 14: Pediatric basic life support: 2010 American Heart Association guidelines for cardiopulmonary resuscitation and emergency cardiovascular care. *Circulation.* 2010;122:S876 [PMID: 20956230].

Kliegman RM, Stanton B, Geme J, et al: *Nelson Textbook of Pediatrics: Expert Consult Premium Edition.* Philadelphia, PA.: Saunders; 2011.

POSTRESUSCITATION CARE

Postresuscitation care of the pediatric cardiac arrest patient deserves special mention. Recent improvements in survival of arrest victims comes, in part, because of postresuscitation measures in addition to high-quality CPR, and current PALS guidelines include a dedicated algorithm for postcardiac arrest care.

The priority immediately after obtaining ROSC is to optimize ventilation and oxygenation. Titrate O_2 to an oxygen saturation of 94-99%. Additionally, if advanced airway management has not yet been obtained, it is now considered. Waveform capnography helps ensure adequate ventilation and should be now considered.

The circulatory system should be addressed for any signs of persistent hypotension or shock. The most common reversible causes (5Hs and 5Ts) should be reviewed, but remember that this list is not exhaustive. Fluid boluses of 10-20 mL/kg should be given as needed to support the circulatory system. If fluid alone does not resolve hypotension, consider inotropic or vasopressor support. Norepinephrine, dopamine, or epinephrine are indicated for hypotensive shock, whereas milrinone, dobutamine, ephedrine, or dopamine are preferred in normotensive shock.

Therapeutic hypothermia has been shown to clearly improve outcomes for comatose survivors of cardiac arrest in adult populations. Although there is likely a subset of pediatric patient who would benefit from therapeutic hypothermia such as those whose initial insult was a primary cardiac dysrhythmia, data supporting this practice in children has been mixed. The PALS postresuscitation guidelines recommend that therapeutic hypothermia should be "considered" for pediatric comatose survivors of cardiac arrest.

Finally, intensive monitoring for agitation, seizures, hypoglycemia, electrolyte, and other laboratory abnormalities is essential, and patients should be promptly transferred to the pediatric intensive care unit (PICU) or nearest tertiary care center for critical care monitoring.

FAMILY PRESENCE DURING RESUSCITATION

The resuscitation process can be psychologically and emotionally troubling for family members as well as providers. Many developments have been made in this area over the last few decades. While perceptions of this concept differ much research has been done in this area. Some providers fear family will interrupt. However, research has shown that when families have a dedicated personnel attending to them (usually chaplain or nurse), they are not disruptive. Further concerns of increased litigation have been disproven in studies even when mistakes were made.

Family presence during resuscitation (FPDR) is gaining more and more acceptance. Many studies have shown benefits from FPDR to include allowing the family to see the seriousness of their loved one's condition, dispels wonders if "everything was done," reduces guilt, encourages closure, and overall facilitates the bereavement process. Benefits to the providers are that FPDR encourages professionalism, dignity, and makes the process of delivering news of death easier. As a result of the research findings, many organizations have developed position statements on the subject. Associations and organizations that endorse FPDR include American College of Emergency Physicians (ACEP), American Academy of Pediatrics (AAP), American Heart Association (AHA), and American College of Critical Care Medicine.

FPDR should be offered during resuscitation. Dedicated staff should be responsible for explaining and caring for the family present. When done appropriately, benefits will be gained by the provider team as well as family.

TERMINATION OF RESUSCITATION

There are no ridged well-established predictors of outcome to guide termination of efforts of resuscitation. Many authors would suggest concepts such as prolonged down time, unwitnessed collapse, increasing doses of epinephrine, and age, as well as total length of CPR as poorer predictors of good outcomes. Bystander CPR, witnessed arrest, and hypothermic temperatures are better prognostic indicators. Termination of efforts should be considered after the patient has been ventilated with oxygen, volume-resuscitated, electrical dysrhythmias addressed, and reversible causes of PEA and asystole have been addressed. Family present during resuscitation should not be forced to make the decision to terminate efforts. As the leader of the resuscitation, the physician should take all data and circumstances in account to make the difficult but final decision to terminate efforts.

POST DEATH CARE

There is probably no more traumatic or painful experience than the death of a person's child. Parents should be allowed to grieve the loss of their child. Encouraging parents to hold their children and be with them can be powerful adjuncts to aid in the grieving process. Providers should be available to address questions of family members and offer condolences. Chaplains and child life specialists play an important role and should be included in the grieving process at parental discretion. Provider teams also have emotional and psychological effects that require addressing. Both formal and informal debriefing sessions can be powerful tools to maintain the provider team morale, cohesiveness, and maintain job satisfaction.

American Academy of Pediatrics & American College of Emergency Physicians, O'Malley P, et al: Patient and family centered care and the role of the emergency physician providing care to a child in the emergency department. *Pediatrics.* 2006;118:2242-2244 [PMID: 17079599].

American Academy of Pediatrics, Committee on Pediatric Emergency Medicine, American College of Emergency Physicians: Joint policy statement: Guidelines for care of children in the emergency department. *Pediatrics.* 2009;124:1233 [PMID: 19770172].

Berg MD, Samson RA, Meyer RJ, et al: Pediatric defibrillation doses often fail to terminate prolonged out-of-hospital ventricular fibrillation in children. *Resuscitation.* 2005;67:63 [PMID: 16199288].

Davidson JE, Powers K, Hedayat KM, et al: Clinical practice guidelines for support of the family in the patient-centered intensive care unit: American College of Critical Care Medicine Task Force 2004-2005. *Crit Care Med.* 2007;35:605 [PMID: 17205007].

Doherty DR, Parshuram CS, Gaboury I, et al: Hypothermia therapy after pediatric cardiac arrest. *Circulation.* 2009;119:1492 [PMID: 19273725].

Hanson C, Strawser D: Family presence during cardiopulmonary resuscitation: Foote Hospital emergency department's nine-year perspective. *J Emerg Nurs.* 1992;18:104 [PMID: 1573794].

Sudden Infant Death Syndrome and Apparent Life-Threatening Events

Brandon Pace, MD

Brian Hawkins, MD

OVERVIEW OF CLINICAL CONDITIONS

Sudden infant death syndrome (SIDS), apparent life-threatening event (ATLE), and infantile apnea are three clinical conditions that have specific definitions. The first, ALTE is defined as a collection of symptoms that is frightening to the observer which may include color change, apnea, change in muscle tone, and/or choking or gagging. The second, SIDS is a diagnosis rather than a collection of symptoms and is defined as a sudden unexpected infant death for which there is no explanation. In order to make the diagnosis of SIDS, there must be a complete autopsy, review of the medical and family history, and death scene investigation that excludes predisposing environmental factors and does not result in a clear explanation for the infant's death. The third, infantile apnea is defined by the American Academy of Pediatrics (AAP) as "an unexplained episode of cessation of breathing for 20 seconds or longer, or a shorter respiratory pause associated with bradycardia, cyanosis, pallor, and/or marked hypotonia."

ALTE should not be considered as a "near-miss SIDS." There is insufficient evidence to suggest that ALTE precedes SIDS. Current literature indicates that ALTE, SIDS, and apnea are unrelated; instead, ALTE is a multifaceted all-encompassing term with the inclusion of apnea as one of the symptoms which may be perceived as life threatening by an observer. The literature has not reached consensus on components of the standard workup for an ALTE. This is in contrast to SIDS where a consensus has been reached that in order to make the diagnosis, a complete autopsy, review of the medical and family history, and death scene investigation that excludes predisposing environmental factors should be performed. Both ATLE and SIDS are similar in that the differential for the cause of each is vast and a definitive cause may never be found in each case.

SUDDEN INFANT DEATH SYNDROME

▶ Evaluation

 ESSENTIALS OF DIAGNOSIS

▶ In order to make the diagnosis of SIDS, there must be a complete autopsy, review of the medical and family history, and death scene investigation that excludes predisposing environmental factors and does not result in a clear explanation for the infant's death.

▶ General Considerations

The definition of SIDS has evolved as our understanding of the syndrome has changed due to research and clinical experience. The National Institute of Health (NIH) originally defined SIDS as "sudden death of an infant or young child, which is unexpected by history, and in which a thorough postmortem examination fails to demonstrate an adequate cause." Further research indicated that environmental conditions can play a role in SIDS such as trauma, hyper/hypothermia, and asphyxia. The definition of SIDS has been updated to include review of the medical and family history and a death scene investigation in addition to an autopsy. It is only after a complete review of the patient's and family's medical records, death scene investigation, and autopsy resulting in no clear explanation for the infant's death is the term SIDS used.

▶ Epidemiology

A number of factors have been previously associated with SIDS including preterm infants, socioeconomically disadvantaged families, nonwhite ethnicity, unwed status of the mother, use of illicit substances by the mother, and maternal age younger than 20 years. Infants sleeping in the same bed as parents and infants sleeping alone in the prone position have been correlated with SIDS. Paternal and maternal smoking is a strong risk factor for SIDS. In some studies there is a 2- to 5-fold increased risk with maternal smoking.

As a result of the updated definition of SIDS, the incidence has declined. A factor that has led to a decline in the incidence of suffocation (formerly classified as SIDS) is the Back to Sleep campaign which began in 1994 and advocated for infants to sleep in the supine position rather than the prone position. This campaign was initiated after studies in the 1980s and 1990s indicated that infants who slept in the supine position were at the lowest risk for SIDS. Following this campaign, the rate of prone sleeping in infants decreased and a resultant decline in SIDS was also appreciated with an overall decrease in the rate of SIDS by 58% since 1992.

The majority of SIDS deaths occur in males and most commonly in infants aged 2-4 months. Very few deaths occur in infants younger than 1 month and older than 8 months.

▶ Presentation

The hallmark presentation for SIDS includes an infant who is found dead after having been put to bed by the caretaker. Although there is no evidence that an infant who presents to the emergency department with an ALTE will subsequently suffer from SIDS, it has been reported that infants had presented with vomiting, diarrhea, and/or lethargy in the weeks before death.

Cases characteristic with SIDS include those where the infant died between 2 and 4 months of age, the peak incidence for SIDS, and the infant was found to be normal during intermittent checks after being put to bed, but was then found to be dead at a subsequent check. Cases that are uncharacteristic of SIDS include those where there was a prolonged amount of time between when the infant was last found to normal and when the infant was found dead; and infants who die older than 6 months of age.

▶ Differential Diagnosis

The differential diagnosis for SIDS is broad and includes metabolic derangements, cardiac channelopathies, infections, unsafe sleeping positions and/or conditions, and trauma such as child abuse.

Inborn errors of metabolism may be the cause of death in a SIDS infant. Specifically there have been cases of reported disorders of fatty acid metabolism contributing to infant death. Medium-chain acyl-CoA dehydrogenase deficiency (MCADD) is the most common fatty acid metabolism disorder. In this disorder the infant is unable to oxidize fatty acids when glucose is unavailable and may result in a metabolic crisis and sudden death.

Cardiac channelopathies account for 10-15% of SIDS cases. Long QT syndromes are related to sodium channel abnormalities and potassium channel abnormalities that increase risk of sudden death. The majority of the abnormalities are secondary to genetic mutations in those specific channels. Infants with cardiac sodium channel mutation are at increased risk of sudden death during sleep whereas those with potassium channel mutation are at increased risk of sudden death during periods of sympathetic nervous system stimulation.

Genetic mutations that affect the immune system make an infant more susceptible to infection that results in sudden death. Previous studies have looked at the possibility of a correlation between deletion of a specific gene and a trivial infection shortly before death of the infant. There have also been studies looking at the possibility of abnormal interleukin genotypes and how this may result in an abnormal immune response to infection in infants resulting in sudden death.

Unsafe sleeping conditions and/or positions may result in a sudden unexpected infant death. Couch or sofa sleeping is an example of unsafe sleeping conditions given the possibility of the infant slipping in-between couch cushions and suffocating. Memory foam is especially dangerous for infants due to the risk of its molding to the shape of the infant and occluding the airway. Prone sleeping has been indicated in up to 50% of sudden unexpected death cases in previous studies. An infant sleeping in the same bed with another individual, places the infant at a greater risk for sudden death due to the risk of suffocation. A previous study performed by the National Institute of Child Health and Human Development and Consumer Product Safety Commission showed that an infant sleeping with an individual in an adult bed had a risk of death of 25.5/100,000 versus sleeping alone in a crib of 0.63/100,000.

Based on 2006 data from the AAP, the incidence of intentional infant suffocation is between 1% and 5%. It can be nearly impossible to discriminate intentional suffocation from accidental suffocation on examination or autopsy. Review of the history may be helpful to identify elements that suggest foul play, such as, repeated episodes of cyanosis, apnea, or ALTEs while supervised by the same caretaker, unexpected deaths in one or more siblings, and simultaneous death of twins. As stated, it is only after a complete review of the patient's and family's medical records, death scene investigation, and autopsy resulting in no clear explanation for the infant's death that the term SIDS may be used. Because autopsy in the case of child abuse may reveal occult injuries and result in cause of death, these cases do not fall under the category of SIDS.

SUMMARY

SIDS is defined as the unexplained death of an infant younger than 1 year after a complete review of the patient's and family's medical records, death scene investigation, and autopsy resulting in no clear explanation for the infant's death. If medical history were to reveal a recent infection, medical history of a cardiac malformation, sleeping prone or signs of trauma on autopsy, then by definition these cases are not SIDS. Factors which are associated with SIDS include preterm status, socioeconomically disadvantaged families, nonwhite ethnicity, unwed status, use of illicit substances by the mother, maternal and paternal smoking, maternal age younger than 20 years, parents sleeping in the same bed as the infant, and infants sleeping alone in the prone position. The hallmark presentation for SIDS includes an infant who is found dead after having been put to bed by the caretaker despite normal checks intermittently. The differential diagnosis for SIDS includes metabolic derangements, cardiac channelopathies, infections, unsafe sleeping positions, and child abuse.

APPARENT LIFE-THREATENING EVENT

 ESSENTIALS OF DIAGNOSIS

▶ An ALTE should best be considered a description of concerning symptoms rather than a diagnosis.

▶ The differential diagnosis should remain broad with careful attention made to the history and physical examination.

▶ There is no standardized approach to the emergency department evaluation of an ALTE.

General Considerations

An apparent life-threatening event (ALTE) is a description of a group of specific symptoms rather than a definitive diagnosis. An ALTE is defined as "an episode that is frightening to the observer and that is characterized by some combination of apnea, color change, marked change in muscle tone, choking, or gagging." The causes are broad and diverse, and 50% of evaluations determine a definitive cause.

An ALTE accounts for fewer than 1% of all emergency department visits and there is no gender preference. It remains a concerning problem because of the frightening nature of the presentation as contained in the definition, as well as the difficulty in obtaining a definitive diagnosis.

Initial Management

If the patient appears acutely ill or distressed, those issues must be addressed quickly and the patient resuscitated according to standard advanced cardiac life support (ACLS) protocols. A typical airway, breathing, circulation approach is needed.

Differential Diagnosis

Three diagnoses comprise 50% of diagnoses in which a final diagnosis is made. The diagnoses are gastroesophageal reflux, seizure, and lower respiratory tract infection. Nonaccidental trauma must be considered in the differential as it may be difficult to diagnose. There are a large number of potential causes to be maintained in the differential. For example, one study showed a potential for ALTE events related to the positioning of infants in a car safety seat. Table 8–1 lists causes of ALTE.

Table 8–1. Causes of apparent life-threatening events.

Cause	Description
Accidental smothering	Occurred while sleeping In prone position Had soft objects near face
Seizure	Loss of consciousness Deviation of eyes Convulsion Hyper- or hypotonia
Apnea of infancy	Exclusion of other causes Absence of breathing > 20 sec
Metabolic (inborn error)	Family history of metabolic disorder Seizure activity Frequent illnesses Dysmorphism
Cardiac	Feeding difficulties Diaphoresis Central cyanosis
Infections (meningitis, sepsis, UTI)	Fever or hypothermia Lethargy
Medications	Lethargy History of medication use
GERD	Pulling up the legs during ALTE Association with feeding
Intussusception	Blood in stool and lethargy
Volvulus	Bilious vomiting Distended abdomen
Respiratory infection	Cough Coryza Wheezing
Airway abnormality	Stridor and feeding difficulties
Foreign body	History of ingestion Stridor
Nonaccidental trauma	Blood in mouth or nose Sibling with SIDS Delayed presentation

Risk factors for ALTE include preterm infants due to their immature physiology, as well as healthy-term infants during the first 2 hours after birth.

Home monitoring has not been shown to prevent ALTE or SIDS; however, it is currently recommended for preterm infants at high risk of apnea, bradycardia, and hypoxia, as well as infants who are technologically dependent such as being on a home ventilator, and infants who have medical conditions associated with breathing issues that would benefit from home monitoring.

Despite the frequent association, there is no evidence that ALTE is a precursor to SIDS. Risk factors for ALTE and SIDS are different, and the epidemiology reveals distinctly different patient populations.

▶ Evaluation

When evaluating an infant with an ALTE, it is very important to obtain an accurate description of the event. We must be able to discern true apnea (> 30 seconds) versus periodic breathing. It is important to determine if the episode spontaneously resolved or required stimulation for resolution. Determination of central cyanosis versus acrocyanosis is also vitally important. A careful physical examination with attention to neurologic and cardiovascular abnormalities is required. Important historical factors for ALTE are listed in the following box. Important physical examination findings are listed in Table 8–2.

The diagnostic evaluation of ALTE events is controversial with some authorities recommending baseline screening tests for all ALTE patients, but the evidence behind a baseline set of recommendations remains underwhelming. A recent study documented a wide variation in how emergency physicians evaluate ALTE events in the emergency department. For most tests used in the evaluation of ALTE, the likelihood of positive test is low and the importance of testing is minor when compared with the importance of a good clinical history and physical examination. Most would agree that there is no standard workup for ALTE. Diagnostic tests include EEG, neuroimaging, serum metabolic studies, toxicology screens, and investigative studies for gastric reflux. Patients who have seizures caused by ALTE often have a normal EEG and neuroimaging. Therefore, the diagnoses must be made clinically. Table 8–3 lists tests and considerations for diagnosis of ALTE.

▶ Disposition

Because of a high risk of recurrent episodes (12% in first 24 hours), most would recommend an observation admission for most episodes of ALTE. Studies are underway to aid in determination of a predictive model to help identify patients that require admission. Some authorities state that discharge may be reasonable if it was the first episode of ALTE, no history of prematurity, no significant past medical history, well appearing with stable vital signs, and if the

Table 8–2. Physical examination considerations for infant with apparent life-threatening event.

Type of examination	Considerations
Level of Consciousness Vital signs Head circumference	Is infant arousable, irritable?
Examination of the head	Look for signs of trauma. Fontanelle size and fullness.
Tympanic membrane examination	Look for asymmetry; hemotympanum.
Pupillary examination Eye examination	Look for conjunctival and retinal hemorrhage.
Nasopharynx examination	Look for signs of congestion, presence of refluxed meals, blood (abuse).
Neck examination	Listen for tracheomalacia/laryngomalacia.
Lung examination	Assess work of breathing and abnormal lung sounds (stridor, wheezes, crackles, rhonchi).
Cardiac examination	Pay particular attention to cardiac auscultation (rhythm, murmur) and perfusion (capillary refill, pulses).
Abdominal examination	Look for distention or signs of an acute abdomen.
Musculoskeletal examination	Evaluate for signs of trauma.
Skin examination	Look for bruising or rash.
Neurologic examination	Evaluate for muscle tone (hyper- or hypotonicity), movement, reflexes.
Body-type examination	Evaluate for dysmorphic features.

episode is brief and self-resolving with a high likelihood of a nonprogressive cause such as gastric reflux. One study indicated high-risk patients as being younger than 1 month and having multiple events. If a patient is discharged, resources for basic life support should be made available to caregivers.

SUMMARY OF APPARENT LIFE-THREATENING EVENT AND SUDDEN INFANT DEATH SYNDROME

The ALTE is defined as an episode that is frightening to the observer and that is characterized by some combination of apnea, color change, marked change in muscle tone, choking,

Important historical factors for ALTE.

Presence or absence of apnea (with particular attention for obstructive vs central apnea)

Color change and distribution (acrocyanosis vs central cyanosis)

Change in muscle tone and distribution

Rhythmic shaking and distribution

Presence of choking, gagging, coughing, or vomiting

Duration of the episode

Association with feeding

Feeding difficulties (aversion, choking, diaphoresis, fatigue)

Eye deviation and abnormal eye movements

Level of consciousness

Fever

Coryza and upper respiratory symptoms

History of trauma

Appearance prior to ALTE

Location and sleep position at time of ALTE

Requirement of resuscitation

Medications (also medications taken by mother if breastfeeding)

Past medical history

Family history of ALTS, SIDS

Table 8–3. Diagnostic testing for apparent life-threatening events.

Test	Considerations
EEG	Difficult to obtain in the emergency department Poor sensitivity for diagnosing epilepsy Possibly for recurrent ALTE
Neuroimaging (CT/MRI/US)	Not indicated for all patients as a routine study Radiation risk with CT Perform in cases suspicious for abuse (will also need retinal examination and skeletal survey)
Serum laboratory studies	May detect electrolyte abnormality (hyponatremia) or be useful in detecting an inborn error. Choices include CBC with differential, electrolytes, ammonia, lactate, pyruvate, CRP (C-reactive protein), urinalysis
Toxicological studies	Many authorities would recommend a urine toxicology screen A recent study showed 8.4% of infants with an ALTE tested positive for a medication that could cause apnea
Investigations for gastric reflux	Most authorities suggest testing (UGI, pH probe) if the patient has reported frequent reflux or if the event was preceded by feeding or gastric contents noted in the mouth or nose at the time of the ALTE
CSF studies	Low likelihood of giving contributory information unless clinical diagnosis of meningitis is considered
Echocardiogram	Low yield unless history is suggestive of cardiac problem
Nasopharyngeal swabs (RSV, pertussis)	Order if clinical suspicion

or gagging. The ALTE is not a diagnosis but is designated as a group of symptoms. The three most symptoms of an ALTE include those associated with gastroesophageal reflux disease, seizure disorders, and lower respiratory tract infections. Risks factors for ALTE include preterm infants and healthy-term infants during the first 2 hours after birth. There is wide variability in the workup of ALTEs and there is no standard workup; rather, a detailed history and physical are essential in each case of ALTE in search of a cause. In most cases admission is recommended given that previous studies have found that 12% of patients may have a recurrent episode within 24 hours. If a patient is discharged home, basic life support resources should be made available to the patient's caretakers.

There is insufficient evidence to suggest that ALTE precedes SIDS; therefore, ALTE should not be considered as a "near-miss SIDS." SIDS is considered a definite diagnosis in contrast to ALTE which is a group of symptoms. SIDS is defined as the unexplained death of an infant younger than 1 year after a complete review of the patient's and family's medical records, death scene investigation, and autopsy resulting in no clear explanation for the infant's death. In order to reach the diagnosis of SIDS, the physician must review the patient's and family's medical records, perform a death scene investigation and autopsy for all cases where SIDS is considered. The hallmark presentation for SIDS includes an infant who is found dead after having been put to bed by the caretaker despite normal checks intermittently. Risk factors for SIDS include preterm status, socioeconomically disadvantaged families, nonwhite ethnicity, maternal unwed status, use of illicit substances by the mother, maternal and paternal smoking, maternal age younger than 20 years, parents' sleeping in the same bed as the infant, and infant sleeping alone in the prone position.

Berkowitz C: Advances in pediatrics sudden infant death syndrome, sudden unexpected death, and apparent life-threatening events. *Adv Pediatr.* 2012;59:183-208 [PMID: 22789579].

Bonkowsky JL, Guenther E, Srivastava R, Filloux FM. Seizures in children following an apparent life-threatening event. *J Child Neurol.* 2009;24:709-713 [PMID: 19289698].

Brand DA, Altman RL, Purtill K, Edwards KS. Yield of diagnostic testing in infants who have had an apparent life-threatening event. *Pediatr.* 2005;115:885-893 [PMID: 15805360].

Chu A, Hageman JR. Apparent life threatening events in infancy. *Pediatr Ann.* 2013;42:78-83 [PMID: 23379411].

Claudius I, Keens T. Do all infants with apparent life-threatening events need to be admitted? *Pediatr.* 2007;119:679-683 [PMID: 17403838].

Dewolfe CC: Apparent life-threatening event: A review. *Pediatr Clin North Am.* 2005; 52;1127-1146 [PMID: 16009260].

Edner A, Katz-Salamon M, Lagercrantz H, Reicson M, Milerad J: Heart rate variability in infants with apparent life-threatening events. *Acta Paediatr.* 2000;89:1326-1329 [PMID: 11106044].

Fu LY, Moon RY. Apparent life-threatening events: An update. *Pediatr Rev.* 2012;33:361-368 [PMID: 22855928].

Genizi J, Pillar G, Ravid S, Shahar E. Apparent life-threatening events: Neurological correlates and the mandatory work-up. *J Child Neurol.* 2008;231305-1307 [PMID: 18645202].

Grylack LJ, Williams AD: Apparent life-threatening events in presumed healthy neonates during the first three days of life. *Pediatr.*1996;97:349-351 [PMID: 8604268].

Kundra M, Duffy E, Thomas R, Mahajan PV. Management of apparent life-threatening event: A survey of emergency physicians practice. *Clin Pediatr.* 2012:51:130-133 [PMID: 21903620].

Okada K, Motoko M, Honma S, Wakabayashi Y, Sugihara S, Osawa M: Discharge diagnoses in infants with apparent life-threatening event. *Pediatr Int.* 2003;45:560-563 [PMID: 14521532].

Pitetti RD, Maffei F, Chan K, Hickey R, Berger R, Pierce MC: Prevalence of retinal hemorrhages and child abuse in children who present with an apparent life-threatening event. *Pediatr.* 2002;Sept:557.

Pitetti RD, Whitman E, Zaylor A. Accidental and nonaccidental poisonings as a cause of apparent life-threatening events in infants. 2008;122:e359-362 [PMID: 18676522].

Tonkin SL, Vogel SA, Bennet L, Gunn AJ. Apparently life threatening events in infant safety seats. *BMJ.* 2006;333:1205-1206 [PMID: 17158387].

Wong LCH., Behr ER: Sudden unexplained death in infants and children: The role of undiagnosed inherited cardiac conditions. *Europace.* 2014;Feb 28 (Epub ahead of print) [PMID: 24585884].

Compromised Airway

Andrew L. Juergens II, MD
Jenny Glover, MS
Manoj P. Reddy, BS

ANATOMIC CONSIDERATIONS OF THE PEDIATRIC PATIENT

Endotracheal intubation of children may be more difficult compared with intubation of adults because of anatomical differences. A number of differences are illustrated in Figure 9–1. Children have a small mouth aperture with a hyomental distance of 1.5 cm or less in a newborn or infant and 3 cm or less in a child. Children also have impaired head and neck mobility, especially a child with Down syndrome or juvenile rheumatoid arthritis.

Children have airways that are cephalad compared with adults. Children have a larynx that is closer to the C3 spinal level, whereas the larynx in adults is at the C4 level. The higher position of the larynx in a child causes the tongue to be located higher in the airway and at a more acute angle to the larynx. This causes the larynx to appear anterior in the airway. Moreover, the larynx can be partially shielded by the hyoid superiorly.

Because children naturally have larger occiputs in comparison with their bodies, intubation of pediatric patients on backboards or other firm surfaces is often difficult. A large occiput requires the physician to position a pediatric patient differently. If the head is flexed, it may cause a collapse of the upper airway. The neck must be extended or kept in a neutral position to maintain a patent airway. Proper patient position can be achieved by using blankets or towels to support the body.

The narrowest portion of the airway in a child is at the level of the cricoid membrane, compared with the level of the vocal cords in an adult. Conventional teaching is that cuffed tubes should not be used in a child younger than 8 years. Appropriately sized uncuffed tubes seal well at the cricoid ring where the airway is the narrowest. Uncuffed tubes are preferred because cuffed tubes increase the risk of ischemic damage to the tracheal mucosa from compression between the cuff and cricoid ring. However, the design of

modern endotracheal tube (ETT) has improved and this may be less of a risk than previously thought, and many practitioners use cuffed tubes in small children. ETT cuffs now are designed to be high volume and low pressure, thus producing a seal at a lower pressure. Several studies have shown no increase in postextubation stridor or reintubation rates when cuffed tubes were used in controlled settings with frequent cuff pressure monitoring. Cuffed tubes may provide some protection from aspiration. Potential benefits of ETT cuffs include facilitating ventilation with higher pressures, more consistent ventilation, and decreased need to exchange inappropriately sized tubes.

Children may have proportionally larger tongues, tonsils, and adenoids compared with adults. A large tongue is a common cause of airway obstruction, especially in children who are seizing, postictal, or obtunded. The physician should be cautious when placing a nasal airway in young infants because large adenoids and tonsils can be traumatized during insertion. This can result in bleeding.

The pediatric airway is smaller than the adult airway in all dimensions, including the diameter. Because the area of a circle is proportional to the square of the radius, a very small change in the radius will result in a dramatic change in the airway. This concept is explained in Poiseuille law of resistance, which states that resistance is inversely proportional to the radius to the power of 4 ($R \propto 1/r^4$). Based on this equation, the physician should note that pediatric patients have a lower tolerance to airway edema or obstruction (Figure 9–2).

SIGNS OF RESPIRATORY DISTRESS

When a child presents to the emergency department, parents should be asked if the child has had symptoms of noisy breathing (during exercise, at rest, when feeding), previous surgeries or intubations, neck pain, fever, recent respiratory infections, birth trauma, or congenital anomalies. On physical

Respiratory Rate

The child's respiratory rate should be determined upon arrival at the emergency department, before disturbing the child. Infants frequently have periodic breathing, so it is important to count respirations over a full minute and frequently reassess respiratory rate. The appropriate respiratory rate varies across age. Oxygen saturation should also be measured in the pediatric patient.

Accessory Muscle Use

Several visual cues indicate that a pediatric patient is in respiratory distress. The physician must pay attention to the use of accessory muscles of respiration. Retractions are a commonly seen sign of respiratory distress, in which skin and soft tissues are drawn inward during inspiration. Retractions can occur in the substernal, intercostal, supraclavicular, and suprasternal areas. The child should be undressed for a complete assessment.

Nasal flaring is a form of accessory muscle use and represents nostril widening during respiratory distress. Nasal flaring is an attempt to decrease airway resistance. Infants who have severe respiratory distress are also noted to bob their heads frequently. This occurs as a result of the neck muscles being used to increase respiratory pressure.

Infants have a lower percentage of type 1 or slow-twitch skeletal muscle fibers in the intercostal muscles and diaphragm, which are less prone to fatigue. Moreover, infants have lower stores of glycogen and fat in the respiratory muscles. These differences predispose infants to respiratory muscle fatigue. Also, the young infant preferentially breathes through the nose; in cases of oral breathing, an infant must use soft palate muscles to maintain an open oral airway—expending further energy.

Color Change

A key symptom of respiratory distress is cyanosis, mottling, or other color change. Cyanosis can present at any age in childhood and may be intermittent or persistent. Central cyanosis typically involves the lips, tongue, and mucous membranes, whereas peripheral cyanosis involves the fingers and toes. Pseudocyanosis is a bluish tinge to the skin or mucous membranes that is not associated with hypoxemia or peripheral vasoconstriction.

The physician's ability to recognize cyanosis depends on several factors, including skin tone, room lighting, the level of deoxygenated hemoglobin, the total hemoglobin concentration, and the general state of perfusion. Checking the patient's pulse oximetry will discriminate cyanotic from pseudocyanotic states, although the accuracy of oximetry is influenced by alterations in pH levels, hemoglobin levels, arterial carbon dioxide tension, peripheral perfusion, and movement artifact. Measuring the oxygen tension from arterial blood is the most valid reflection of arterial oxygenation status.

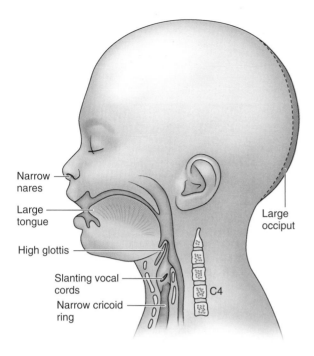

▲ **Figure 9–1.** Anatomical difference in pediatric airways.

examination, the physician assesses respiratory rate and accessory muscle use, including nasal flaring. Stridor, cough, and voice changes are several of the most frequently signs of respiratory distress.

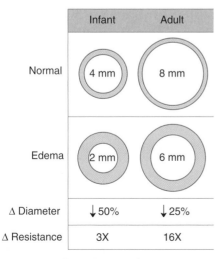

	Infant	Adult
Normal	4 mm	8 mm
Edema	2 mm	6 mm
Δ Diameter	↓50%	↓25%
Δ Resistance	3X	16X

▲ **Figure 9–2.** Effect of airway diameter on resistance in pediatric versus adult airways.

Cyanosis can result from several disease processes. Pulmonary and cardiovascular issues must be considered. Cyanosis produced as a result of a primary respiratory disorder can be caused by respiratory distress, pneumonia, chronic lung disease, pulmonary malformation, and other causes of lung dysfunction. The physician should evaluate the patient for signs of respiratory distress, apnea, or clubbing. In the presence of a significant murmur, cardiomegaly, or hepatomegaly, cyanosis is most likely cardiac in origin. Tests that may confirm the cause of the cyanosis include a chest radiograph, an electrocardiogram, an arterial blood gas, and assessment for clinical change after supplemental oxygen is initiated.

Breath and Airway Sounds

Audible and auscultated respiratory sounds can provide clues to the cause of respiratory distress. Expiratory wheezing is a common sign of respiratory distress. The high-pitched sound is made during attempts at exhalation against an intrathoracic airway obstruction, which can be caused by asthma, a mass or vascular structure compressing the airway, or a foreign object in the airway. A history of an unexplained cough can be suggestive of a foreign body in the larynx, trachea, or bronchi. Wheezing can occur in inspiratory and expiratory phases with severe obstruction. Wheezing is generally heard only with a stethoscope, but in severe cases, it can be heard without one.

Inspiratory stridor is a high-pitched sound caused by turbulent airflow across an extrathoracic airway obstruction. Causes of stridor include croup, retropharyngeal abscesses, and foreign bodies in the upper airway. Changes in the quality of voice or cry can be an indication of the cause of respiratory distress.

A muffled voice may indicate a retropharyngeal or peritonsillar abscess. Snoring noises may indicate partial airway obstruction from the tongue falling back to the posterior oropharynx and is often seen in seizing patients. Gurgling sounds can indicate that there is blood or secretions in the airway.

Another sign of respiratory distress is grunting, the sound produced when an infant exhales against a partially closed glottis which increases end-expiratory pressure. Grunting occurs frequently in patients who have pneumonia, pulmonary edema, and bronchiolitis.

However, it is important to note that once a child is in severe respiratory distress, many signs of respiratory distress diminish. The disappearance of retractions or slowing of respiratory rate can be a sign of fatigue and impending respiratory arrest.

Liess BD, Scheidt TD, Templer JW: The difficult airway. *Otolaryngol Clin North Am.* 2008;41(3):567 [PMID:18435999].

Ondik MP, Kimatian S, Carr MM: Management of the difficult airway in the pediatric patient. *Operative Techniques Otolaryngol.* 2007;18(2):121.

Porepa W, Benson L, Manson DE, et al: True blue: A puzzling case of persistent cyanosis in a young child. *CMAJ.* 2009;180(7):734. [PMID: 19332754].

Santillanes G, Gausche-Hill M: Pediatric airway management. *Emerg Med Clin North Am.* 2008;26(4):961 [PMID: 19059095].

DETERMINING CAUSE OF RESPIRATORY DISTRESS

The causes of respiratory distress in pediatric patients can be broadly divided into upper and lower airway conditions.

Conditions that can cause upper respiratory distress in children include croup, epiglottis, bacterial tracheitis, peritonsillar or retropharyngeal abscess, and foreign bodies. Less common conditions include vocal cord edema or dysfunction, tumors, or vascular structure impinging on the airway.

Special care must be taken in the general approach to the pediatric patient with upper airway pathology. In severe cases the patient may present in a tripod position, attempting to maximize airflow. The child may not be able to handle his or her own secretions. If intubation becomes necessary, the swollen tissues or foreign body causing airway obstruction may pose a particular challenge. Upper airway obstruction may be exacerbated by the child's crying and becoming upset. With the child in severe distress from an upper airway issue, the most prudent course of action is often to have airway equipment ready at the bedside to use if needed, but to avoid distressing the child as much as possible. The child should be escorted to the operating room as soon as possible where the airway may be secured in a more controlled environment with specialist care.

Conditions that can affect the lower airway of children and cause respiratory symptoms include asthma, pneumonia, congestive heart failure, acute respiratory distress syndrome, and neonatal lung disease. See also Chapter 12.

Choi J, Lee GL: Common pediatric respiratory emergencies. *Emerg Med Clin North Am.* 2012;30(2):529 [PMID: 22487117].

Chung S, Forete V, Campisi P: A review of pediatric foreign body ingestion and management. *Clin Ped Emerg Med.* 2010;11(3):225.

Liess BD, Scheidt TD, Templer JW: The difficult airway. *Otolaryngol Clin North Am.* 2008;41(3):567 [PMID:18435999].

TREATMENTS

The presenting clinical scenario will guide specific treatment and airway management. Noninvasive and invasive approaches are discussed below.

NONINVASIVE MODALITIES

Simple airway management maneuvers can ensure an open pathway between the patient's lungs and mouth cavity. The child has a relatively large tongue in comparison with adults.

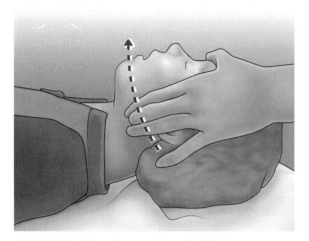

▲ **Figure 9–3.** The jaw thrust technique.

The tongue is a common cause of airway obstruction in the unconscious child. Several techniques are available to open the airway to alleviate such issues.

Jaw Thrust

The jaw thrust maneuver acts to open the airway by lifting the mandible to alleviate any pressure the tongue or epiglottis may have on the posterior pharynx. To perform this maneuver, the operator stands cephalad to the supine patient, positions thumbs on each side of the patient's maxilla and lifts the jaw by pushing anteriorly with fingers on the angle of the mandible (Figure 9–3). The jaw thrust is preferred to the chin lift in patients where spinal injury is suspected.

Chin Lift

If an injury to the cervical spine is not suspected, the chin lift maneuver may be used. The chin lift maneuver accomplishes the same intended goals as the jaw thrust technique. With the patient in the supine position, the operator places one hand on the patient's forehead and the other hand at the point of the chin. The forehead is pushed down while lifting anteriorly and superiorly on the chin to tilt the head back.

Suction Catheter

The suction catheter can be a vital component in effective removal of secretions in airway management. The removal of obstructions in the mouth and pharynx can clear the opening and remove any barriers to clear channeled breathing.

Oropharyngeal Airway

An oropharyngeal airway (OPA) is a useful adjunct that can help ventilate an unconscious pediatric patient. An OPA is generally less tolerated than a nasopharyngeal airway due to the risk of sudden vomiting and laryngospasm, as well as stimulation of the gag reflex. Sizing of an OPA is measured by gauging the distance between the corners of the mouth and the angle of the mandible. An OPA is inserted with the tip facing the roof of the mouth before inverting it 180 degrees. The end opposite to the tip of the curvature is placed between the patient's teeth to prevent biting.

Nasopharyngeal Airway

A nasopharyngeal airway (NPA) should be avoided if skull base trauma is suspected in a patient, due to the risk of infection or penetration in the anterior cranial fossa. The appropriate NPA length is measured from the patient's nose to the external auditory meatus. The size of the NPA can be approximated by comparing the diameter of the tube with the patient's little finger. A correctly sized NPA will separate the soft palate from the pharynx and avoid irritating stimulus to the gag or cough reflex. An NPA is inserted by first lubricating the tip and then visually confirming its placement in the back of the mouth upon placement as shown in Figure 9–4.

Oxygen Administration

Supplemental oxygen can be effective therapy in pediatric patients that display respiratory conditions and hypoxemia. Excessive oxygen administration can have negative effects on patients, whereas insufficient oxygen therapy (hypoxia) can lead to tissue damage.

▶ Nasal Cannula

The nasal cannula is a proven and effective measure in administering oxygen in patients with mild to moderate hypoxia. Children generally tolerate nasal cannula administration at levels less than 4 liters per minute, with lower rates typically given to infants and smaller children. Cooling and drying of the airways can cause discomfort to the patient. High-flow nasal cannula (HFNC) has proven to be useful in some instances of respiratory distress in children and neonates, if used with caution.

▶ Simple Oxygen Mask

Simple oxygen masks are widely used for patients with hypoxemia. The masks tend to be diluted by room air and can result in unpredictable oxygen concentrations, particularly when the mask is loose fitting.

▶ Non-rebreather Oxygen Mask

A non-rebreather oxygen mask uses a reservoir bag where oxygen enters between breaths. The mask has the potential

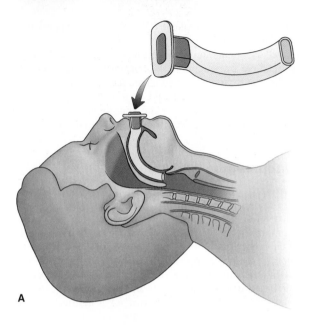

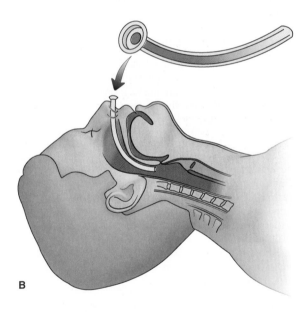

▲ Figure 9–4. Important basic airway devices to relieve upper airway obstruction from collapsed pharyngeal tissues. A. Oral airway. B. Nasal airway. (Adapted, with permission, from Stone CK, Humphries RL: *Current Diagnosis and Treatment Emergency Medicine,* 7th ed. McGraw-Hill, 2011. Copyright © McGraw-Hill Education LLC.)

to provide oxygen concentration levels (FiO_2) close to 100%. This type of oxygen mask has a valve that prevents room air from entering the mask and may be useful for patients requiring a high FiO_2.

▶ Bag-valve-mask

A bag-valve-mask (BVM) is used to oxygenate and ventilate patients by providing positive pressure ventilation (PPV). The technique is often implemented before intubation. A BVM is applied over the nose and mouth of the patient to form an airtight seal across the face without encroaching on the eyes or chin. The BVM operator stabilizes the seal by pressing down on the mask with the thumb and index finger in the shape of the letter *C*. The remaining three fingers subsequently form the shape of the letter *E* beneath the patient's chin. This is known as the **E-C method.** The bag may be squeezed with the operator's free hand or with the help from another provider. The two-person technique has been shown to administer mean tidal volumes in children and infants more effectively than the one-person method. The size of the bag and rate of inflation is dependent on patient's age and condition. Confirmation of proper technique can be made by visualizing chest rise. Improper inflation of a BVM can lead to gastric distention that may further complicate the patient's respiratory problem.

Flow-inflating bags require the use of an external flow source in order to inflate. From a patient's perspective, the flow-inflating bag may be easier to breathe through compared with the self-inflating bag. A flow-inflating bag gives stronger tactile feedback to the operator, and it is easier to tell if a good seal is being made between the mask and patient. However, the self-inflating bag is easier to use with fewer technical difficulties than the flow-inflating bag, including not being dependent on a constant, pressurized source of oxygen in order to function.

Nebulized Treatment

Nebulized treatments are commonly used for emergency department patients, inpatients, and small children who cannot properly control their breathing enough to use an inhaler. Pharmacologic intervention via nebulizer can be effective treatment for certain obstructive airway diseases in pediatric patients. Nebulized medications such as albuterol and other β-agonists act directly at $β_2$-adrenergic receptors to dilate the bronchioles.

▶ β₂-Agonists

Albuterol is a selective $β_2$-receptor agonist used to limit bronchospasms by relaxing lower airway muscles. Albuterol is first-line therapy for acute asthma due to its high $β_2$-adrenergic selectivity and minimal toxicity.

Dosing of albuterol (nebulized) by age:

- < 2 years (off-label): 0.2-0.6 mg/kg/day divided every 4 to 6 hours nebulized
- 2-12 years > 15 kg: 0.63-2.5 mg every 6 to 8 hours nebulized
- Serum potassium levels should be monitored closely in patients who receive continuous albuterol

Levalbuterol is the R-enantomer of albuterol, and may be more specific to the β_2-receptor than racemic albuterol, which would result in fewer side effects. However, clinical trials demonstrate no clear advantage of levalbuterol over albuterol.

▶ Epinephrine

Epinephrine acts as a nonselective agonist of all adrenergic receptors. A primary use in emergent pediatric situations is in the treatment of croup or upper airway obstruction. A 2.25% solution of nebulized racemic epinephrine has been shown to significantly reduce the symptoms of patients with croup. Nebulized epinephrine has also been described as treatment for bronchiolitis and asthma. However, albuterol remains the first-line choice for treatment in children with asthma. Use of nebulized medication for bronchiolitis is no more effective than nebulized saline.

Dosing of 2.25% racemic epinephrine solution for asthma and croup by age:

- < 4 years 0.05 mL/kg nebulized (diluted to 3 mL with NS); no more than every 12 hours; maximum 0.5 mL/dose
- > 4 years 0.5 mL nebulized every 3 to 4 hours as needed

▶ Humidified Oxygen

Humidified oxygen can be used in the treatment of croup. Its theoretical mechanism of action includes decreasing airway edema and loosening and moistening secretions. It may be effective in acute exacerbations of bronchial asthma when used as an adjunct with nebulized albuterol. Humidifying oxygen can help reduce mucous membrane drying and discomfort for those on oxygen therapy.

▶ Heliox

Heliox is a gas composed of various mixtures of helium and oxygen. The composition of heliox allows for its density to be less than that of air and therefore provides a reduction in the resistance of flow. Heliox has been studied in patients with asthma, acute bronchiolitis, and bronchopulmonary dysplasia. Its use has been particularly successful in upper respiratory obstructions. Controversy still remains on the use of heliox as a first-line therapy in asthma and bronchiolitis. In patients with moderate to severe croup, heliox has been shown to be effective in symptom improvement. Heliox can be administered in a number of ways including nebulizers, non-rebreather reservoir masks, and mechanical ventilators. Possible disadvantages and risks include cost, risk of anoxia, hypothermia, high-delivery volume to lungs, and inaccurate administration of oxygen when utilizing heliox in the emergent setting.

Noninvasive Positive Pressure Ventilation

Noninvasive positive pressure ventilation (NIPP) is an effective means of stabilizing breathing in a patient in order to avoid intubation or surgical intervention. Continuous positive airway pressure (CPAP) and bilevel positive airway pressure (BiPAP) are two methods that are considered NIPPV. The two methods have been used as first-line therapy in patients requiring primary ventilatory support or to help wean patients from invasive ventilation. The NIPPV measures may also be used to bridge the gap before more invasive procedures are implemented. Indications for use of NIPPV include respiratory fatigue, asthma, bronchiolitis, pneumonia, and obstructive sleep apnea.

▶ Continuous Positive Airway Pressure

Continuous positive airway pressure (CPAP) facilitates ventilation by keeping a patient's airway open to allow for supplemental oxygen to flow to the lungs. Depending upon the age of the patient, CPAP can be placed with either a facemask or nasal prongs. Pressure settings generally start at 5 cm H_2O and increase in smaller increments before reaching a level that is comfortable for the patient and clinically effective, usually without surpassing a recommended maximum of 15 cm H_2O.

▶ Bilevel Positive Airway Pressure

Bilevel positive airway pressure (BiPAP) can provide preset inspiratory (IPAP) and expiratory (EPAP) pressure levels that can react to a patient's breathing accordingly. BiPAP may be preferred at times over CPAP because of its ability to provide additional aid in inspiration and ventilation. Settings generally used for a BiPAP are as follows:

- IPAP: 10-12 cm H_2O
- EPAP: 5-7 cm H_2O

Bingham RM, Proctor LT: Airway management. *Pediatr Clin North Am.* 2008;55(4):873.

Bjornson C, Russell KF, Vandermeer B, et al: Nebulized epinephrine for croup in children. *Cochrane Database Syst Rev.* 2011;Feb 16:2011 [PMID: 21328284].

Davidovic L, LaCovey D, Pitetti RD: Comparison of 1- versus 2-person bag-valve-mask techniques for manikin ventilation of infants and children. *Ann Emerg Med.* 2005;46(1):37 [PMID: 15988424].

Eastwood GM, O'Connell B, Considine J: Oxygen delivery to patients after cardiac surgery: A medical record audit. *Crit Care Resusc.* 2009;11(4):238 [PMID: 20001870].

Garcia Figueruelo A, Urbano Villaescusa J, Botran Prieto M: Use of high-flow nasal cannula for non-invasive ventilation in children. *An Pediatr* (Barc). 2011;75(3):182 [PMID: 21511547].

Hostetler M: Use of noninvasive positive-pressure ventilation in the emergency department. *Emerg Med Clin North Am.* 2008;26(4):929 [PMID: 19059092].

Kim IK, Corcoran T: Recent developments in heliox therapy for asthma and bronchiolitis. *Clin Pedi Emerg Med.* 2009;10(10):68.

Kleinman ME, Chameides L, Schexnayder SM, et al: 2010 American Heart Association Guidelines for Cardiopulmonary Resuscitation and Emergency Cardiovascular Care. *Circulation.* 2010;122(3):S876 [PMID: 20956230].

Krebs SE, Flood RG, Peter JR et al: Evaluation of a high-dose continuous albuterol protocol for treatment of pediatric asthma in the emergency department. *Pediatr Emerg Care.* 2013;29(2):191 [PMID: 23364383].

Martinón-Torres F: Noninvasive ventilation with helium-oxygen in children. *J Crit Care.* 2012;27(2):220.e1 [PMID: 21958976].

Navaratnarajah J, Black AE: Assessment and management of the predicted difficult airway in babies and children. *Anaesth Intensive Care Med.* 2012;13(5):226.

Nibhanipudi K, Hassen GW, Smith A: Beneficial effects of warmed humidified oxygen combined with nebulized albuterol and ipratropium in pediatric patients with acute exacerbation of asthma in winter months. *J Emerg Med.* 2009;37(4):446 [PMID: 19062230].

O'Driscoll BR, Howard LS, Davison AG: BTS guideline for emergency oxygen use in adult patients. *Thorax.* 2008;63(Suppl 6) vi1[PMID 18838559].

Rechner JA, Loach VJ, Ali MT, et al: A comparison of the laryngeal mask airway with facemask and oropharyngeal airway for manual ventilation by critical care nurses in children. *Anaesthesia.* 2007;62(8):790 [PMID: 17635426].

Simşek-Kiper Po, Kiper N, Hascelik G, et al: Emergency room management of acute bronchiolitis: A randomized trial of nebulized epinephrine. *Turk J Pediatr.* 2011;53(6):651 [PMID: 22389988].

Skierven HO, Hunderi JO, Brügmann-Pieper SK, et al: Racemic adrenaline and inhalation strategies in acute bronchiolitis. *N Engl J Med.* 2013;368(24):2286 [PMID: 23758233].

Spentzas T, Minarik M, Patters AB, et al: Children with respiratory distress treated with high-flow nasal cannula. *J Intensive Care Med.* 2009;24(5):323 [PMID: 19703816].

Stafford RA, Benger JR, Nolan J: Self-inflating bag or Mapleson C breathing system for emergency pre-oxygenation? *Emerg Med J.* 2009;25(3):153 [PMID: 18299363].

INVASIVE MODALITIES

ENDOTRACHEAL INTUBATION

Endotracheal intubation in airway management is the placement of an endotracheal tube (ETT) in a patient's trachea to maintain an open airway.

Indications for Intubation

▶ **Neonates**

Cardiopulmonary Instability

Distress may include atypical vital signs, respiratory distress, low blood pressure, low heart rate, and low O_2 saturation, as well as other atypical findings in the patient. Intubation can help provide oxygenation and alleviate the neonate from the work of breathing. Less stress will be placed on the patient and allow for improved management of cardiorespiratory symptoms.

Meconium

Meconium is one of the first stools produced by a newborn infant after birth. It is made up of ingested intestinal epithelial cells, bile acids, digestive enzymes, lanugo hair, and amniotic fluid. Respiratory problems can occur as a result of meconium aspiration syndrome (MAS) when infants pass stool into the amniotic fluid prior to birth. Current protocol recommends intubation for MAS when the newborn infant presents as nonvigorous, defined as either poor muscle tone, HR < 100 beats/min, or a poor respiratory effort.

Prematurity With Respiratory Distress

Respiratory distress in infants may be caused by an insufficiency in the production of surfactant. When noninvasive measures prove ineffective, a physician can utilize tracheal intubation to provide adequate ventilation.

▶ **Infants and Children**

Respiratory Failure

See Cause of Respiratory Distress discussed previously, and Chapter 12.

Airway Compromise

Airway obstruction that is caused by a foreign body, or swelling, or by an injury to the trachea, larynx, or bronchi may be treated by tracheal intubation. Bypassing the blockage with an ETT allows the patient to maintain an open airway and preserve normal respiration.

Transport to a Higher Level of Care

Controversy exists on the necessity of intubation prior to transfer to higher level of care in patients in whom there is a danger of airway decompensation. Community physicians may not express the same level of comfort and self-confidence in performing advanced procedures in pediatric patients as their receiving hospital counterparts. If a child is in danger of losing his or her airway, the transferring physician must weigh the benefits and risks of deferring intubation. A child who decompensates during transport may have a worse outcome if intubation is required in an out-of-hospital setting. However, specially trained critical care transport providers demonstrate a high rate of successful intubation.

Grading Scales

Visual grading scales have been utilized to aid the physician in assessment of a patient's predicted difficulty with endotracheal intubation. Studies have questioned the specificity of such grading systems. The classifications may not be as applicable to small children due to patient's cooperation with examination and anatomical variation.

▶ Mallampati Classification

The Mallampati score is a grading scale that applies a 1-4 numerical annotation: 1 is a patient who is relatively easy to intubate, and 4 is a patient who is very difficult to intubate. Numerical values are assigned by assessing a patient's oral cavity preprocedure (Figure 9–5).

▶ Cormack-Lehane System

The Cormack-Lehane system categorizes the difficulty of intubation by the visibility of specific anatomical features upon laryngoscopy (Figure 9–6).

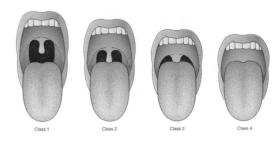

Class 1   Class 2   Class 3   Class 4

▲ **Figure 9–5.** Mallampati classifications.
Class 1: visualize faucial pillars, soft palate, and uvula
Class 2: visualize faucial pillars and soft palate
Class 3: visualize hard and soft palates
Class 4: visualize hard palate only

Equipment
▶ Endotracheal Tube

An argument has been made for the use of an uncuffed endotracheal tube (ETT) for intubation of children younger than 8 years. However, the advantages of a cuffed ETT include a possibly better seal, lower gas leak, and a decreased chance of recurrent laryngoscopy. The recommended cuff inflation pressure is less than 20 cm H_2O.

Sizing:

The traditional teaching of using a patient's fifth finger to gauge the size of the ETT may result in tube sizes that are 1-2 mm larger than necessary. Age formulas given below are preferred over finger estimations, however the latter is clinically acceptable when no other means are available.

- Cuffed: ETT size (mm ID) = (age in years ÷ 4) + 3
- Uncuffed: ETT size (mm ID) = (age in years ÷ 4) + 4

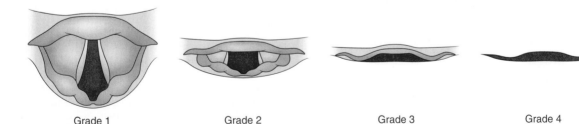

Grade 1   Grade 2   Grade 3   Grade 4

▲ **Figure 9–6.** Cormack-Lehane Classification.
Grade 1: view the entire laryngeal aperture
Grade 2: view parts of the laryngeal aperture or the arytenoids
Grade 3: view only the epiglottis
Grade 4: view of only the soft palate

Broselow Tape

The Broselow tape is a color-coded system used by health care professionals to determine appropriate medication doses and equipment sizes based on a pediatric patient's height and weight. The Broselow tape is a means to determine the correct ETT size for a pediatric patient in the absence of age-related information in emergent situations.

Bag-valve-mask

A bag-valve-mask is a noninvasive means of providing oxygen to a patient during preparation for intubation, as discussed previously in the Bag-valve-mask section.

Suction

Suction is used during intubation to remove apparent secretions that can potentially hinder the procedure.

Laryngoscope Blade: Miller vs MacIntosh

A laryngoscope blade is used during endotracheal intubation to allow the physician to view the larynx directly. The blades come in variable sizes and shapes with the most common the Miller (straight) and the Macintosh (curved). The difference in intubation success with the blades can be attributed to the proper technique relative to the blade used, as well as the choice of correct size.

The Miller blade is placed posterior to the epiglottis and directly lifts the epiglottis. This is the preferred blade for infants and young children, who may have a "floppy" epiglottis. The Miller blade is generally used for children years and older, but if necessary the Miller blade can be used for children of any age. A Miller 0 blade should be used only in premature infants and average-sized newborns. A Miller 1 blade is appropriate for most infants beyond the immediate newborn period.

The Macintosh blade slips in the vallecula (space between the epiglottis and the tongue) and indirectly lifts the epiglottis. The Macintosh curved blade is used primarily in older children and adults.

The size of the laryngoscope blade is estimated using the distance between the upper incisor teeth and the angle of the mandible. In children younger than 8 years, studies have shown that blades that measured within 1 cm of this anatomical distance had better first attempt results.

Stylet

A stylet is a device used to assist and guide in the placement of an ETT during the intubation of patient. The stylet is placed in the ETT tube and removed only after the tube has been placed successfully for intubation. It is essential to leave enough distance between the end of the stylet and the end of the ETT to avoid injury to the airway.

Preparation

Preoxygenation

Preoxygenation with a 100% oxygen source in a spontaneously breathing patient allows for "nitrogen washout" and provides an oxygen reservoir for patients while they are apneic during an intubation procedure. Studies have shown that preoxygenation greater than the customary 3-4 minutes has little to no benefit.

Current recommendations indicate the use of a non-rebreather facemask to provide preoxygenation. Noninvasive ventilation by means of CPAP may be a more effective means of preoxygenation in critically ill patients.

Positioning

The "sniffing" position is recommended for a patient in preparation for intubation. The position provides adequate visualization of the glottis opening. It is achieved by moving the head forward and slightly extending the atlanto-occipital joint (Figure 9–7).

Rapid Sequence Induction

Rapid sequence induction (RSI) is the preferred method of intubation in patients with no known increased risk of complication. The RSI consists of prompt administration of an induction agent and neuromuscular blocking agent. The combination of the two drugs causes immediate paralysis and sedation in a patient and results in ideal tracheal intubation conditions (Table 9–1). Studies have shown efficacy and safety of RSI in pediatric patients.

Pretreatment

The procedure of RSI and intubation can cause undesirable physiologic changes. Pretreatment is used to help blunt the negative effects. Pretreatment medications should be given 3-5 minutes prior to RSI.

Atropine

The use of atropine as a pretreatment for intubation in pediatric intubation is controversial. Atropine has traditionally been used in tracheal intubation to depress the heightened vagal response (bradycardia) of pediatric patients. However, some studies have shown an increase in tachycardia and cardiac arrhythmia in patients who were administered atropine as pretreatment for intubation.

Neuroprotective Induction

Patients who require intubation and have sustained head trauma or are otherwise at risk for increased intracranial pressure (ICP) may benefit from pretreatment measures designed to lower ICP. Classically, lidocaine and fentanyl

Correct

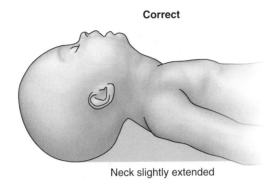

Neck slightly extended

Incorrect

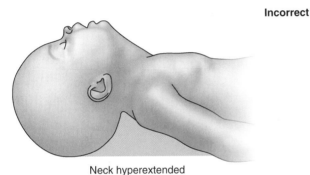

Neck hyperextended

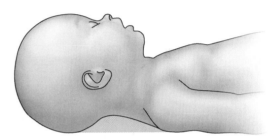

Neck underextended

▲ **Figure 9–7.** The sniffing position.

have been used. Lidocaine is believed to decrease the cough reflex and prevent elevation in ICP. Fentanyl is an opioid analgesic that can blunt the sympathetic response to intubation. A defasiculating dose of rocuronium or vecuronium may also be given at 1/10th the standard paralytic dose to prevent fasiculations and subsequent elevation in ICP.

▶ Sedation Agents

Etomidate

The use of etomidate in RSI remains controversial. Studies have shown that the use of etomidate can result in adrenal suppression and therefore have the potential to cause complications in children with septic shock. It is unclear if such complications will occur after administration of a single dose. Other studies support the efficacy of etomidate as a sedation treatment for RSI in children. Etomidate is still a widely used induction agent due to its relative hemodynamic stability.

Benzodiazepines

Of the benzodiazepines, midazolam is the most commonly used for induction. Midazolam has the potential to cause

respiratory depression and may have some undesirable hemodynamic effects. Benzodiazepines can be reversed with flumazenil, however this may reduce the seizure threshold.

Barbiturates

Thiopental is a drug capable of induction of sedation for RSI. Thiopental has been used in patients with elevated ICP who are hemodynamically stable. The adverse effects of thiopental include histamine release, myocardial depression, venodilation, and hypotension.

Propofol

Propofol is a powerful sedative/hypnotic, and may depress pharyngeal and laryngeal muscle tone to allow for ease of tracheal intubation. The use of propofol can cause hypotension and myocardial depression. Propofol does not have strong analgesic properties, and may cause pain upon infusion.

Ketamine

Ketamine is an *N*-methyl-D-aspartate (NMDA) receptor antagonist that has a wide range of effects including

Table 9–1. Drug dosages.

	Dosage	Comments	Onset	Duration
Pretreatment				
Atropine	.02 mg/kg IV IV/IO: .04-.06 mg	Minimum dose: 0.1 mg Maximum dose: Child: 0.5 mg Maximum dose: Adult: 1 mg	2-4 min	4 h
Neuroprotective				
Fentanyl	2-3 mcg/kg IV		30-60 sec	30-45 min
Lidocaine	1-1.5 mg/kg IV		45-90 sec	120 min
Sedation				
Etomidate	0.3 mg/kg IV		30-60 sec	3-5 min
Midazolam	0.1-0.3 mg/kg IV	Benzodiazepine	60-90 sec	15-30 min
Thiopental	3-5 mg/kg IV	Barbiturate of choice	< 30 sec	5-10 min
Propofol	2-3 mg/kg IV		15-45 sec	3-10 min
Ketamine	1-2 mg/kg IV		30-60 sec	5-10 min
Paralysis				
Succinylcholine	0.3-2 mg/kg IV	Depolarizing agent	45 sec	4-6 min
Rocuronium	0.6-1.2 mg/kg IV	Nondepolarizing	< 1 min	30-60 min
Vecuronium	0.08-0.1 mg/kg IV	Nondepolarizing	2 min	45-65 min

analgesia and anesthesia. Ketamine is one of the few RSI induction agents that will also cause analgesia in addition to its sedative effects. The adverse side effects of ketamine include possible increased heart rate and blood pressure, and this drug should be used with caution in patients who are hypertensive.

Neuromuscular Blocking Agents (Paralytics)

Succinylcholine

Succinylcholine is a depolarizing agent and recommended by many sources for neuromuscular block in RSI. Although succinylcholine is the most widely used medication for paralysis, it is not without adverse effects. Succinylcholine can potentially cause hyperkalemia, muscle fasiculations, and increased intraocular pressure. The potential for hyperkalemia restricts the use of succinylcholine for patients with malignant hyperthermia, hyperkalemia, recent burn or severe infection, denervating injuries, acute lateral sclerosis (ALS), or multiple sclerosis. In young children, the administration of succinylcholine in undiagnosed myopathies may leave patients at risk of hyperkalemia.

Despite its drawbacks, it has a faster onset of action and far shorter duration of effect than the nondepolarizing agents. This can be advantageous in a patient in whom there is a risk of failed intubation, especially if that patient is otherwise spontaneously breathing, or would be difficult to ventilate by other means if paralyzed for an extended period.

Rocuronium

Rocuronium is part of a class of agents known as short-acting nondepolarizing neuromuscular blockers. Rocuronium exhibits less danger for hyperkalemia than succinylcholine. However, it has a longer time of onset and duration of effect. A physician may elect to give higher doses to shorten the onset of paralysis, however the duration of effect will also be lengthened.

Vecuronium

Vecuronium is a nondepolarizing medication that acts similarly to rocuronium. Vecuronium also has a relatively longer onset and duration of action compared with succinylcholine.

Direct Laryngoscopy

▶ Technique

Direct laryngoscopy can be used to assist in the visualization of the larynx for endotracheal intubation. Before intubation, all equipment, including suction, light bulbs on laryngoscope blades, and cuffs on ETT should be checked. The patient is placed in as ideal a position as possible (see Figure 9-7). The patient is given pretreatment and rapid sequence medications as indicated. The laryngoscope blade is held in the left hand. The right hand is used to part the lips and teeth. The laryngoscope blade is inserted along the right side of the mouth, sweeping the tongue to the left. Using the laryngoscope, the jaw, tongue, and epiglottis are lifted upward, taking care not to rock the laryngoscope backward and leverage against the upper teeth or maxilla. The vocal cords are visualized, and the appropriate ETT is inserted between them. The ETT is inserted to an appropriate depth, an initial estimation of which can be made by taking the diameter of the tube (in mm) and multiplying by 3. This will give an initial depth in centimeter. However, the position of the tube must be verified.

▶ Tube Placement Verification Methods

The verification of ETT placement is a critical step in the intubation procedure. The possibility of misplacement can lead to hypoxic brain injury and death in a pediatric patient. It is important to note that no single verification method is 100% reliable and sensitive. Multiple methods should be considered and utilized in a patient to confirm the proper execution of endotracheal intubation. Verification should be repeated in patients who are moved or transported.

Direct Visualization

Visualization of the ETT passing through the vocal cords provides strong evidence of proper placement. However, difficult intubations under emergent conditions can limit and prohibit direct visualization.

Auscultation

Auscultation of equal breath sounds in the lungs can indicate proper ETT placement. The juxtaposition of the esophagus to the trachea in a pediatric patient can create sounds that may mask an esophageal intubation. During BVM-induced ventilation, breaths auscultated over the patient's bilateral axillae are reassuring; however, breaths heard over the stomach indicate improper placement of the tube.

Chest Rise

The rising and falling of a child's chest may indicate proper ETT placement, however esophageal ventilation has also been shown to produce a similar chest rise.

Water Vapor

Condensation seen in the ETT may be seen with tracheal placement. This method is considered unreliable because of the occurrence of water vapor in misplaced esophageal tubes.

Esophageal Intubation Detectors

Esophageal intubation detectors (EIDs) are more reliable than auscultation or chest rise for patients that are in cardiac arrest or are hypotensive. Self-inflating bulbs can be placed on an ETT and will inflate rapidly if correct placement is made. The absence of inflation or inflation taking longer than 5 seconds will indicate the necessity for ETT reassessment. Self-inflating bulbs are not recommended for children younger than 5 years or who weigh less than 20 kg.

End-Tidal CO_2

A colorimetric device can be placed on an ETT to identify the presence of exhaled carbon dioxide. Patients who have been successfully intubated will exhale enough carbon dioxide to cause a color change from purple to yellow. In patients receiving humidified gas, the colorimetric device can be rendered useless within 15 minutes. The device contains paper that changes color in an acidic environment. Several conditions can cause difficulties in using a colorimetric device, such as the endotracheal administration of epinephrine, status asthmaticus, large glottic air leak, and acidic contamination.

Capnography is the detection of end-tidal CO_2 on a breath-to-breath basis using measurements made by infrared spectrometry. Strong constant waveforms indicate proper tracheal intubation. There is a danger of false positives in patients who are bag-valve-mask ventilated and have had ETT placement in the pharynx. In the prehospital setting, capnography has been found to be more reliable than auscultation in the verification of ETT placement. However, end-tidal CO_2 detection as a whole is less accurate in patients who are in cardiac arrest.

Chest X-ray

Intubation is considered successful if the tip of the ETT is between 2 and 6 cm above the carina, subject to variation with patient size. Verification of placement in the trachea can be made via a chest x-ray (CXR) to rule out placement in the esophagus. Chest radiographs are taken traditionally from anteroposterior view with the patient in the supine position and the head midline. Chest radiography is often discouraged as sole confirmation of correct ETT placement in an emergent setting because of the amount of time necessary to complete the procedure.

▶ Possible Complications

The most common complications of endotracheal intubation include esophageal intubation, aspiration, dental trauma, laceration to the oral airway, and hypoxia. Esophageal intubation increases the risk of gastric inflation and oxygen deprivation in the patient. Hypoxia can lead to tissue and cerebral damage, bradycardia, arrhythmia, and death. Proper tube placement verification methods identify most improperly placed ETTs.

▶ Alternative Methods to Secure the Airway

Laryngeal Mask Airway

A laryngeal mask airway (LMA) can be a successful alternative in patients who are difficult to intubate. It should be considered in situations where bag-mask ventilation and intubation are difficult or not possible. An LMA is usually placed in a patient's pharynx and is subsequently easier to manage in an emergent setting. A balloon cuff is inflated to create a seal to establish a clear airway. A higher rate of complication has been noted in children compared with adults in the clinical setting. However, LMA is preferred over endotracheal intubation when a skilled practitioner is unavailable for endotracheal intubation. Relative contraindications for LMAs include unsedated patients and children with clear gag reflexes.

An LMA can also be used as a channel to assist in the tracheal intubation of a patient. Intubating laryngeal mask airways (ILMAs) provide specific features that can assist during intubation. An ILMA allows for larger ETT, a removable circuit connector, and the ability to lift the epiglottis. An ETT may be channeled through an LMA or ILMA to facilitate access to the trachea.

Trans-tracheal Techniques

Cricothyrotomy (also called cricothyroidotomy) is an emergency procedure used to create a patent airway between the cricoid and thyroid cartilage. It is generally indicated in conditions where intubation or ventilation is contraindicated or cannot be performed. Cricothyrotomy may be performed on patients who are expected to have a difficult airway as determined by preprocedure tests. Serious complications of cricothyrotomy make it the "last ditch effort" in oxygenating a patient in acute distress. It has few absolute contraindications beyond that of accessibility and/or identification of the cricothyroid membrane. Two different methods of cricothyrotomy are available for short-term emergent use: surgical and needle.

Indications for cricothyrotomy include

- Failure to intubate
- Failure to ventilate
- Airway obstruction
- Hemorrhage to the nasopharyngeal airway
- Cervical spinal injury preventing traditional ventilation/intubation

Surgical Cricothyrotomy

Surgical cricothyrotomy is indicated for patients older than 12 years who meet the criteria for emergent ventilation as listed above. It allows for ventilation and oxygenation. Identification of the cricothyroid membrane is the first step in the procedure. A midline incision should be made on the cricothyroid membrane while avoiding the branches from the inferior thyroid and anterior jugular veins. The incision should be deep enough to gently enter the tracheal space. A tracheal hook may be used to maintain the tract to the trachea. The tracheostomy tube is then placed through the membrane. Care must be given not to insert the tube too far, because it can easily pass the carina and into a main bronchus. There are a number of commercially produced cricothyrotomy kits.

Tube size will be smaller than that used for orotracheal intubation to allow for the diminished cricothryroid space. A 6.0 ETT is often used in adult-sized patients. For smaller pediatric patients, a 4.5-5.5 ETT may be used. The ETT should be cuffed. The cuff allows some flexibility in tube selection if a slightly smaller size is chosen, but the largest size that can easily and safely be passed will allow for improved airway resistance and pulmonary toilet.

Needle Jet Cricothyrotomy

Needle jet cricothyrotomy is the preferred method used in patients younger than 12 years. A needle jet cricothryotomy is very similar to the surgical technique except for the use of a needle to puncture and gain access to the trachea. A syringe with approximately 1-2 mL of saline solution is mounted on a large bore (14-16 gauge) IV catheter with needle. The cricothyroid membrane is punctured, and angled at a 45-degree angle, pointed inferiorly. The needle is advanced while withdrawing with the syringe. Once the trachea is reached, air will be aspirated into the syringe. The catheter may be slid over the needle into the trachea. Many commercially available IV catheters have relatively flimsy plastic walls, and care must be taken not to kink them. Alternatively, if a kit is used, a small incision is then made to create a larger opening. A guide wire is fed through the needle and the needle is withdrawn. A dilator and subsequently a catheter are placed over the wire.

Once the catheter is secured, it must be attached directly to wall oxygen (not through a regulator) via tubing with a release valve. Alternatively a hole may be cut into the tubing small enough for a thumb to occlude which may serve as a pressure release valve. The patient should receive 1 second of jetted, pressurized 100% oxygen for every 4 seconds of pressure release. The patient is not effectively ventilated during this time. This is a temporizing measure only to allow for other definitive airway management techniques to be initiated.

Complications of cricothyrotomy are numerous and serious, including

- Incision displacement
- Needle displacement

- Hemorrhage
- Obstruction
- Aspiration
- Incorrect placement leading to hypoxia
- Tracheal and laryngeal trauma
- Pneumothorax

▶ Postintubation Care

Ventilator Settings

Multiple modes of ventilation are available for postintubation care in the pediatric patient. Ventilator management is an extensive topic, covered briefly below.

Volume controlled ventilation (VCV) uses a set volume as the marker for cycling the ventilator. The ventilator functions by delivering constant volumes of inhalation to the patient. Improperly managed VCV may result in excessive pressure, especially under conditions of decreased compliance and may result in ventilator induced lung injury.

Care must be taken, especially in small children, if VCV is used. The volumes used in such patients are small. When the volume of the tubing and the rest of the circuit is added, the margin of error in many ventilators may not be within sufficient limits to avoid barotrauma.

Pressure controlled ventilation (PCV) delivers pressure to the patient as the driving force for ventilation. The volume that a patient receives is a function of the pressure administered, as well as other factors such as lung compliance.

Studies suggest some advantages of PCV over VCV. Airway pressures can be better controlled in patients who receive PCV over VCV, resulting in less lung injury.

Sedation

Sedation after intubation is necessary when the duration of action of paralytic drugs outlasts the induction medication. A study of short-acting etomidate and rocuronium or vecuronium in pediatric patients showed that patients experienced inadequate sedative effects in the presence of paralysis. Emergency physicians should be aware of drug duration during RSI to avoid having a paralyzed patient who is not appropriately sedated. This is particularly apparent when using the longer lasting paralytics such as rocuronium or vecuronium.

Postintubation sedation also helps with patient comfort and ability to tolerate the ventilator. It can help reduce airway pressures and be beneficial for hemodynamics. Commonly used emergency department sedation regimens include intravenous (IV) continuous drips of fentanyl, versed, propofol, and ketamine.

Suction

Suction catheters are used in postintubation care to prevent aspiration. It is important to have a suction catheter available to remove any secretions in the oral cavity, pharynx, or trachea. Installed and portable suction units provide varying vacuum forces and must be adjusted before use. Recommended maximum tracheal suction force is between 80 and 120 mm Hg in children. Suction catheters that are used via the ETT should not be inserted farther than the ETT to avoid tracheal trauma.

Achen B, Terblanche OC, Finucane BT: View of the larynx obtained using the Miller blade and paraglossal approach, compared to that with the Macintosh blade. *Anaesth Intensive Care.* 2008;36(5):717 [PMID: 18853593].

den Brinker M, Hokken-Koelega AC, Hazelzet JA, et al: One single dose of etomidate negatively influences adrenocortical performance for at least 24h in children with meningococcal sepsis. *Intensive Care Med.* 2008;34(1):163 [PMID: 17710382].

Escobedo M: Moving from experience to evidence: Changes in US neonatal resuscitation program based on International Liaison Committee on Resuscitation review. *J Perinatol.* 2008;28:S35 [PMID: 18446175].

Holm-Knudsen RJ, Rasmussen LS, Charabi B, et al: Emergency airway access in children: Transtracheal cannulas and tracheotomy assessed in a porcine model. *Paediatr Anaesth.* 2012;22(12):1159 [PMID 23134162].

Katos MG, Goldenberg D: Emergency cricothyrotomy. *Operative Techniques Otolaryngol.* 2007;18(2):110.

Kendrick DB, Monroe KW, Bernard DW, et al: Sedation after intubation using etomidate and a long-acting neuromuscular blocker. *Pediatr Emerg Care.* 2009;25(6):393 [PMID: 19458564].

Kleinman ME, Chameides L, Schexnayder, SM, et al: 2010 American Heart Association Guidelines for Cardiopulmonary Resuscitation and Emergency Cardiovascular Care. *Circulation.* 2010;122(3):S876 [PMID: 20956230].

Krage R, van Rijn C, van Groeningen D, Loer, SA, et al: Cormack-Lehane classification revisited. *Br J Anaesth.* 2010;105(2):220 [PMID: 20554633].

Le Cong M: Flying doctor emergency airway registry: A 3-year, prospective, observational study of endotracheal intubation by the Queensland section of the Royal Flying Doctor Service of Australia. *Emerg Med J.* 2012;29(3):249 [PMID: 20844099].

Mallampati S, Gatt S, Gugino L, et al: A clinical sign to predict difficult tracheal intubation: A prospective study. *Can Anaesth Soc J.* 1985;32(4):429 [PMID 4027773].

Mort TC, Waberski BH, Clive J: Extending the preoxygenation period from 4 to 8 mins in critically ill patients undergoing emergency intubation. *Crit Care Med.* 2009;37(1):68 [PMID: 19050620].

Nishisaki A, Marwaha N, Kasinathan V, et al: Airway management in pediatric patients at referring hospitals compared to a receiving tertiary pediatric ICU. *Resuscitation.* 2011;82(4):386 [PMID: 21227561].

Perry JJ, Lee JS, Sillberg VA, et al: Rocuronium versus succinylcholine for rapid sequence induction intubation. *Cochrane Database Syst Rev.* 2008;(2)Apr 16. [PMID: 18425883].

Rudraraju P, Eisen LA: Confirmation of endotracheal tube position: A narrative review. *J Intensive Care Med.* 2009;24(5):283 [PMID: 19654121].

Scherzer D, Leder M, Tobias JD: Pro-con debate: etomidate or ketamine for rapid sequence intubation in pediatric patients. *J Pediatr Pharmacol Ther*. 2012;17(2):142 [PMID: 23118665].

Sprung CL, Annane D, Keh D, et al: Hydrocortisone therapy for patients with septic shock. *N Engl J Med*. 2008;358:111 [PMID: 18184957].

Weiss M, Dullenkopf A, Fischer JE, et al: Prospective randomized controlled multi-centre trial of cuffed or uncuffed endotracheal tubes in small children. *Br J Anaesth*. 2009;103(6):867 [PMID: 19887533].

Wong DT, McGuire GP: Endotracheal intubation through a laryngeal mask/supraglottic airway. *Can J Anaesth*. 2007;54(6):489 [PMID: 17541083].

Zuckerbraun NP, Pitetti RD, Herr SM, et al: Use of etomidate as an induction agent for rapid sequence intubation in a pediatric emergency department. *Acad Emerg Med*. 2006;13(6):602.

Shock

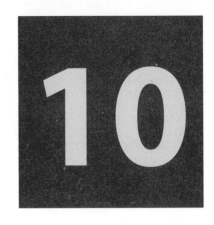

Subhankar Bandyopadhyay, MD
Irma Ugalde, MD

Any condition that results in inadequate tissue oxygen delivery triggers an autonomic response in human body to maintain homeostasis. A cellular response to decreased oxygen delivery activates cascades of physiologic compensatory mechanisms to maintain normal functions. Therefore, in a state of shock, inadequate oxygen delivery fails to meet cellular metabolic demands and results in global tissue hypoperfusion and metabolic acidosis. Cellular response to decreased oxygen delivery causes adenosine triphosophate (ATP) depletion, energy-dependent ion pump dysfunction, and loss of cell membrane integrity. These events lead to systemic lactic acidosis with overpowering of various compensatory mechanisms that progress to multiple organ failure and ultimately death.

Clinically, shock is a complex syndrome associated with acute disruption of macro-and microcirculation resulting from disruption of blood flow. Hypotension may present in shock, but shock may not be diagnosed by virtue of hypotension alone. In the pediatric patient, presence of hypotension is regarded as a sign of decompensated shock.

PATHOPHYSIOLOGY

FAILURE IN MACROCIRCULATION

Blood (fluid) is pumped from the heart (pump), carried in the vessels (pipe), and delivered to the tissues. Therefore, inadequate perfusion may result from malfunction of the pump; that is, decreased cardiac output (CO) from inadequate preload, poor contractility, and excessive afterload. These result in decreased stroke volume (SV). Because CO is a function of SV and heart rate (HR), diminished HR may also cause decrease in tissue perfusion. Stroke volume is the difference between end-diastolic volume (EDV) and end systolic volume (ESV), as expressed in the following equation.

$$\text{Cardiac output (CO)} = \text{stroke volume (SV)} \times \text{heart rate (HR)}$$

and

$$\text{Stroke volume} = \text{end-diastolic volume (EDV)} - \text{end-systolic volume (ESV);}$$

therefore

$$CO = EDV - ESV \times HR.$$

End-diastolic volume is largely dependent on preload, whereas ESV reflects afterload. The parameter that best relates to SV and can be measured is ejection fraction (EF), the fraction of blood that is ejected by the left ventricle during the contraction or ejection phase of the cardiac cycle (systole). Normal range of EF is 55-70%. Increasing EDV with volume resuscitation and decreasing ESV by increasing myocardial contractility or decreasing afterload, will increase SV and hence the cardiac output.

Inadequate fluid volume causes a state of hypovolemia, decreased EDV, and decreased tissue perfusion. Increased HR (tachycardia) and increased vasodilatation with a decrease in systemic vascular resistance (SVR) may be an initial compensatory mechanism during early stages of shock to restore cardiac output, as expressed in the following equation.

$$\text{Blood pressure (BP)} = \text{cardiac output (CO)} \times \text{systemic vascular resistance (SVR);}$$

therefore

$$CO = BP/SVR.$$

However, cardiac output decreases eventually and hypotension ensues because of decrease in preload. Changes that occur in a state of shock are loss of preload volume or EDV, increased heart rate, vasodilatation and decreased systemic vascular resistance (SVR), and loss of myocardial contractility (increased ESV). As EDV and SV decrease, this along with decreased SVR (hypotension) results in heart failure.

Malfunction in the normal circulatory state leads to inadequate end organ perfusion and dysfunction. Hence, poor peripheral perfusion (delayed capillary refill time), decreased urinary output, and altered mental status, are components of clinical vignette of shock.

NORMAL OXYGEN DELIVERY & FAILURE IN MICROCIRCULATION

Normal cellular function and survival is dependent upon continuous supply of oxygen. Inspired oxygen moves across the alveolar capillary membrane into blood and transported to the tissues for sustenance of aerobic cellular metabolism. Any disruption in the circulatory circuit results in decreased oxygen delivery to the tissues (failure in microcirculation) and converts the normal aerobic metabolic pathway to anaerobic metabolism resulting in metabolic lactic acidosis. Tissue oxygen extraction is maximal and reflected in decreased mixed venous oxygen saturation, as expressed in the following equation.

Oxygen delivery (DO_2)

$DO_2 = CO \times CaO_2$

- CaO_2 = arterial oxygen content
- $CaO_2 = (Hgb \times SaO_2 \times 1.34) + (0.003 \times PaO_2)$

Oxygen consumption (VO_2)

$VO_2 = CO \times Hgb \times 13.8 \times (SaO_2 - SvO_2)$

SaO_2 = Arterial oxygen saturation

SvO_2 = Venous oxygen saturation

TYPES OF SHOCK

HYPOVOLEMIC SHOCK

Hypovolemia, which is decreased circulatory blood volume, is the most common type of shock in children. Acute decrease in circulating intravascular volume either by the loss of fluids and electrolytes (gastroenteritis, burns) or by the loss of blood (trauma), activates the vasomotor center in the medulla in the midbrain through arterial baroreceptors. This is in turn results in sympathetic outflow to the heart, blood vessels, adrenal medulla, and juxtaglomerular cells in kidneys. This results in an increase in circulating catecholamines and angiotensin II, along with the increase in autonomic reflexes, increase heart rate, myocardial contractility and ejection fraction (cardiac output), vasoconstriction in skin and visceral organs (peripheral vascular resistance). If there is delay in resuscitation with adequate fluids or blood (if hemorrhage continues), these compensatory mechanisms fail resulting in multi-organ dysfunction and death.

DISTRIBUTIVE SHOCK

Unequal distribution of blood, due to vasodilatation and pooling in the peripheral vascular bed, is the cause of a distributive shock. The most common cause of distributive shock in children is sepsis. Other common causes are anaphylaxis, neurogenic or spinal cord injuries, and certain drug toxicities.

▶ Anaphylactic Shock

Anaphylactic shock results as a systemic immune response to an allergen. Both immunoglobulin E (IgE)- and non–IgE-mediated responses can cause mast cell degranulation resulting in histamine release. Histamine is the primary mediator of anaphylactic response and causes relaxation of vascular smooth muscle, constriction of bronchial smooth muscle, alters cardiac output, and causes leakage of plasma through the transcapillary membrane. The other potent mediator of anaphylactic shock is platelet-activating factor (PAF), which is a coronary vasoconstrictor, peripheral vasodilator, and a negative inotrope.

▶ Neurogenic Shock

Disruption of the sympathetic efferent fibers resulting from a spinal cord injury is the usual cause of a neurogenic shock. This is a selective sympathetic outflow disruption keeping the vagal outflow intact. Hypotension with bradycardia are the most consistent clinical features of neurogenic shock.

▶ Septic Shock

Sepsis is a systemic inflammatory response syndrome (SIRS) in the presence of suspected or proven infection. SIRS in the pediatric population is defined by the presence of at least two of the four criteria.

1. One criterion must be abnormal temperature (> 38.5°C or < 36°C).

2. Tachycardia defined as > 2 standard deviation (SD) above normal for age **or** for children < 1 year, bradycardia persisting > 30 minutes (Table 10–1).

3. Mean respiratory rate > 2 SD for age; or in mechanical ventilation, without any evidence of neuromuscular disease or general anesthesia.

4. Abnormal leukocyte count for age (leukocytosis or leucopenia) without any evidence of being induced by chemotherapy.

Systemic inflammatory response syndrome was originally described in adults, but the definition was subsequently modified for children. Elevated heart rate or respiratory rate alone is not sufficient to diagnose SIRS in the pediatric population. Septic shock in children can be divided into early and late clinical stages. In early septic shock, cardiac output is normal, or

Table 10–1. Normal values for pulse and mean arterial pressure–central venous pressure (mm Hg) by age.

	Term Newborn	≤ 1 y	≤ 2 y	≤ 7 y	≤ 15 y
Pulse (bpm)	120-180	120-180	120-160	100-140	90-140
Mean arterial pressure–central venous pressure (mm Hg)	> 55	> 60	> 65	> 65	> 65

increased, blood pressure is normal or there may be widened pulse pressure due to reduction in peripheral vascular resistance. The patient usually presents with an intact sensorium, tachycardia, bounding pulses, and warm extremities. Late septic shock consists of signs and symptoms of hemodynamic instability consistent with decompensated shock such as, altered sensorium, hypotension, tachycardia, feeble peripheral pulses, and cool extremities.

CARDIOGENIC SHOCK

Cardiogenic shock is caused by decrease in cardiac output with primary dysfunction within the heart. Low cardiac output in this scenario is usually from decreased cardiac contractility. Decreased cardiac output that is unable to meet tissue demands of the nutrients and oxygen, progressively leads to cardiac failure. Myocardial infarction is the most common cause of cardiogenic shock in adults, whereas the following that directly damage the myocardium are primary causes of cardiogenic shock in children.

- Dysrhythmias (supraventicular and ventricular tachycardias)
- Cardiomyopathies: Hpoxia, infections, viral myocarditis, connective tissue disease, metabolic, toxins
- Congenital heart disease
- Post cardiac surgery
- Trauma

Signs and symptoms of either left (thready peripheral pulses, pulmonary edema, weak peripheral pulses) or right (jugular venous distention, hepatomegaly) ventricular failure usually present in cardiogenic shock.

OBSTRUCTIVE SHOCK

A mechanical obstruction causing impedance to effective cardiac outflow and thus causing decreased cardiac output to occur is a cause of obstructive shock. Critical aortic stenosis, interrupted aortic arch, pericardial tamponade, and tension pneumothorax, can cause mechanical obstruction of the heart and its outflow tracts, and thus decrease the cardiac output. Pulmonary embolism, although it can cause obstruction of flow through the pulmonary artery and thus a cause of obstructive shock, is also categorized as a cause of cardiogenic shock.

CLINICAL PRESENTATION & RECOGNITION OF SHOCK

COMPENSATED SHOCK

The earliest sign of a compensated shock regardless of its etiology is likely unexplained tachycardia without other signs. Regardless of the primary cause, shock occurs due to diminished effective intravascular volume or hypovolemia. Hypovolemia is either absolute or relative. Absolute hypovolemia occurs due to loss of fluids and electrolytes (vomiting, diarrhea), blood loss (trauma), third spacing of fluids (peritonitis, ascites). Relative hypovolemia exists when there is intravascular space without adequate intravascular fluid. This occurs due to decreased intravascular resistance such as seen with sepsis, anaphylaxis, drug intoxications, and spinal cord injuries. Early signs of shock include tachycardia, tachypnea, and normal or slightly delayed capillary refill time. As effective intravascular volume decreases, tachycardia occurs to maintain cardiac output while compensating for the stroke volume. Endogenous catecholamines initially increase myocardial contractility and peripheral vascular resistance. In early septic shock, however, there is peripheral cutaneous vasodilatation causing increased peripheral blood flow along with increased cardiac output characterized by bounding pulses (warm shock).

UNCOMPENSATED SHOCK

Uncompensated shock occurs when physiologic compensatory mechanisms fail. Tachycardia and tachypnea become progressively severe. Decreased intravascular volume causes tissue ischemia and acidosis, and tachypnea, a hallmark of a compensatory mechanism of metabolic acidosis, leads to a reduction in PCO_2 blood level. Vasoconstrictions occur in both splanchnic and cutaneous blood vessels leading to various signs and symptoms. Oliguria occurs because of decreased renal blood flow, gastric motility decreases due to decreased blood flow in the abdominal blood vessels. Finally, sensorium is altered due to lack of blood flow and oxygenation in the brain. Multiple organ dysfunction syndrome (MODS) is one end of spectrum of septic shock. Released vasoactive substances in the blood lead to endothelial cell damage along the capillary walls with capillary leaks in end organs resulting in MODS. This process in the lungs leads to acute respiratory distress syndrome (ARDS) and respiratory failure.

Keet C: Recognition and management of food-induced anaphylaxis. *Pediatr Clin North Am.* 2011;58(2):377 [PMID: 21453808].

Mack E: Neurogenic Shock. *Open Pediatr Med J.* 2013;7 (Suppl: M4)16.

Soar J, Pumphrey R, Cant A, et al: Emergency treatment of anaphylactic reactions: Guidelines for healthcare providers. *Resuscitation.* 2008;77(2):157 [PMID: 18358585].

MANAGEMENT

The goal of therapy for all forms of shock is to restore adequate oxygen and nutrients to the cells of vital organs to meet metabolic demands. To meet this goal, airway, breathing, and circulation (ABC) need to be addressed rapidly.

Providing an intact airway and effective ventilation must be present or quickly established. Applying a non-rebreather (oxygen at 100% FiO_2) may be the first step. Almost simultaneously intravascular access as well as laboratory studies must be obtained on all patients. Aggressive fluid resuscitation is started with a rapid bolus of 20 mL/kg of crystalloid 0.9% sodium chloride or ringer's lactate with subsequent boluses determined by the examination and suspected continued shock. The exception is treatment of cardiogenic shock. See Cardiogenic Shock section below.

Each intervention must be followed by reassessment of the patient. This is facilitated with continuous monitoring of hemodynamic status with cardiac telemetry, oximetry, and frequent or continuous assessment of vitals including heart rate, blood pressure, and respirations. Once resuscitation has been initiated, a targeted history and clinical evaluation to ascertain the cause of shock is performed. Specific shock reversal measures are then tailored to specific shock states.

HYPOVOLEMIC SHOCK

Aggressive fluid administration is the hallmark of therapy for hypovolemic shock presuming an intact airway. This is best accomplished by placing two large bore intravenous (IV) lines since repeated normal saline boluses of 20 mL/kg may be indicated. Intraosseous or central venous access should be considered without significant delay if IV access is not successful. Fluids are given by push or rapid infusion device (pressure bag) while observing for signs of fluid overload (the development of increased work of breathing, rales, gallop rhythm, or hepatomegaly). In the absence of these clinical findings, repeated fluid boluses to as much as 200 mL/kg may be required during resuscitation. Children commonly require 40-60 mL/kg in the first hour.

In the setting of trauma, the first-line fluid is still IV crystalloid which should be administered as 20 mL/kg over 5-10 min using two large bore IV sites. A second 20 mL/kg bolus may be repeated. If vital signs do not improve, blood is the next choice of fluids. Other than blood, colloids do not offer a mortality benefit compared to crystalloids. It is important to remember that in an anemic patient, the adjunct of 100% oxygen administration is essential because dissolved oxygen will make up a large portion of the oxygen content. Rapid evaluation in a systematic, organized, and efficient manner is critical in recognizing sites of bleeding that may benefit from prompt surgical correction or readily reversible causes of shock such as cardiac tamponade or tension pneumothorax. See Section III, trauma chapters. The standard of care currently focuses on control of the hemorrhage, careful monitoring of hemodynamics, and use of fluids to maintain tissue perfusion until operative control is available.

CARDIOGENIC SHOCK

Fluid resuscitation must be approached with caution in children with cardiogenic shock. These children require small fluid boluses of 5–10 mL/kg if hypovolemia is a contributing factor to their depressed cardiac function. This is followed by immediate reassessment of the patient. Inotropic therapy is initiated early with dobutamine being an ideal agent with its characteristic β_1-agonist inotropic properties and β_2 effects of afterload reduction. Dopamine at lower doses can also be used. Phosphodiesterase inhibitors like milrinone can be administered although onset of action is not immediate. Monitoring for hypotension during the loading dose is important or a maintenance infusion without a loading dose is another option. Steady state is not reached for at least 6 hours following infusion of a maintenance dose. Pharmacologic or electrical conversion may be needed for tachyarrhythmias while chronotropic agents or pacemaker may be needed for bradyarrhythmias resulting in hemodynamic instability. Consultation with cardiologist is important to help guide resuscitation efforts.

DISTRIBUTIVE SHOCK

1. Neurogenic Shock

When hemorrhage is ruled out in the setting of trauma and spinal shock is suspected (hypotension with bradycardia), agents with α_1-agonist properties are needed to oppose the underlying peripheral vasodilation. Phenylephrine is a good choice. Alternatively, norepinephrine and high-dose dopamine have both β_1- and α_1-action, providing cardiac inotropy.

2. Septic Shock

The 2009 updated 2007 critical care guidelines for septic shock stress that infants and children, in comparison with adults, require proportionally larger fluid volumes, inotrope and vasodilator therapies, hydrocortisone for adrenal insufficiency, and ECMO for refractory septic shock.

Sepsis guidelines for infants and children

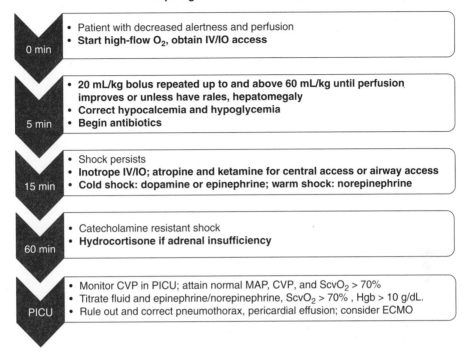

0 min
- Patient with decreased alertness and perfusion
- **Start high-flow O₂, obtain IV/IO access**

5 min
- **20 mL/kg bolus repeated up to and above 60 mL/kg until perfusion improves or unless have rales, hepatomegaly**
- **Correct hypocalcemia and hypoglycemia**
- **Begin antibiotics**

15 min
- Shock persists
- **Inotrope IV/IO; atropine and ketamine for central access or airway access**
- **Cold shock: dopamine or epinephrine; warm shock: norepinephrine**

60 min
- Catecholamine resistant shock
- **Hydrocortisone if adrenal insufficiency**

PICU
- Monitor CVP in PICU; attain normal MAP, CVP, and ScvO₂ > 70%
- Titrate fluid and epinephrine/norepinephrine, ScvO₂ > 70% , Hgb > 10 g/dL.
- Rule out and correct pneumothorax, pericardial effusion; consider ECMO

▲ **Figure 10–1.** Algorithm for time sensitive, goal-directed stepwise management of hemodynamic support in infants and children. (Adapted, with permission, from Brierley J, Carcillo JA, Choong K, et al: Clinical practice parameters for hemodynamic support of pediatric and neonatal septic shock: 2007 update from the American College of Critical Care Medicine. *Crit Care Med* 2009;37(2):666.)

The major recommendation in the update is the earlier use of inotrope support through peripheral access until central access is attained (Figures 10–1 and 10–2).

Airway and breathing are stabilized initially with high-flow oxygen delivery per pediatric advanced life support (PALS) guidelines. Intubation and mechanical ventilation are warranted if there is increased work of breathing, hypoventilation, or declining mental status. Intubation may help in patients requiring large volumes of fluid resuscitation and inotropes as it can decrease oxygen requirements. This is because up to 40% of cardiac output maybe required for work of breathing. Ketamine with atropine has been advocated for use as an induction agent. And etomidate is not recommended secondary to evidence of adrenal suppression in adults with its use.

Fluid infusion is begun with boluses of 20 mL/kg of crystalloid or colloid over 5-10 minutes in rapid succession with clinical endpoints being threshold heart rates, normal blood pressure, and capillary refill less than 2 seconds. With continued reassessment of the patient after each intervention for any signs of congestive heart failure (rales, gallops,

hepatomegaly or jugular venous distension), up to 60 mL/kg of fluid can be given in the first 15 minutes. Rapid fluid administration can be achieved with an inflatable pressure bag, maintained at 300 mm Hg, or manual pushing of fluids. Traditional IV pumps or IV fluids by gravity (wide open) are unacceptable. If shock reversal has still not occurred, vasoactive agents can be started while simultaneously continuing fluid resuscitation. Dopamine is the drug of choice for shock unresponsive to fluids in the setting of low systemic vascular resistance. At medium doses (5-10 mcg/kg/min), dopamine can increase cardiac output by acting like an inotrope and at higher doses (> 10 mcg/kg/min) it increases systemic vascular resistance by acting like a vasopressor. If shock persists, it is important to discriminate between cold and warm shock. For cold shock, epinephrine is recommended; for warm shock, norepinephrine.

While obtaining IV access, blood work is sent which should include, glucose, lactate and ionized calcium, and efforts should be made to correct these. Within the first hour of treatment, antibiotics should be started after obtaining blood, urine, or other tissue cultures when time allows. Stress

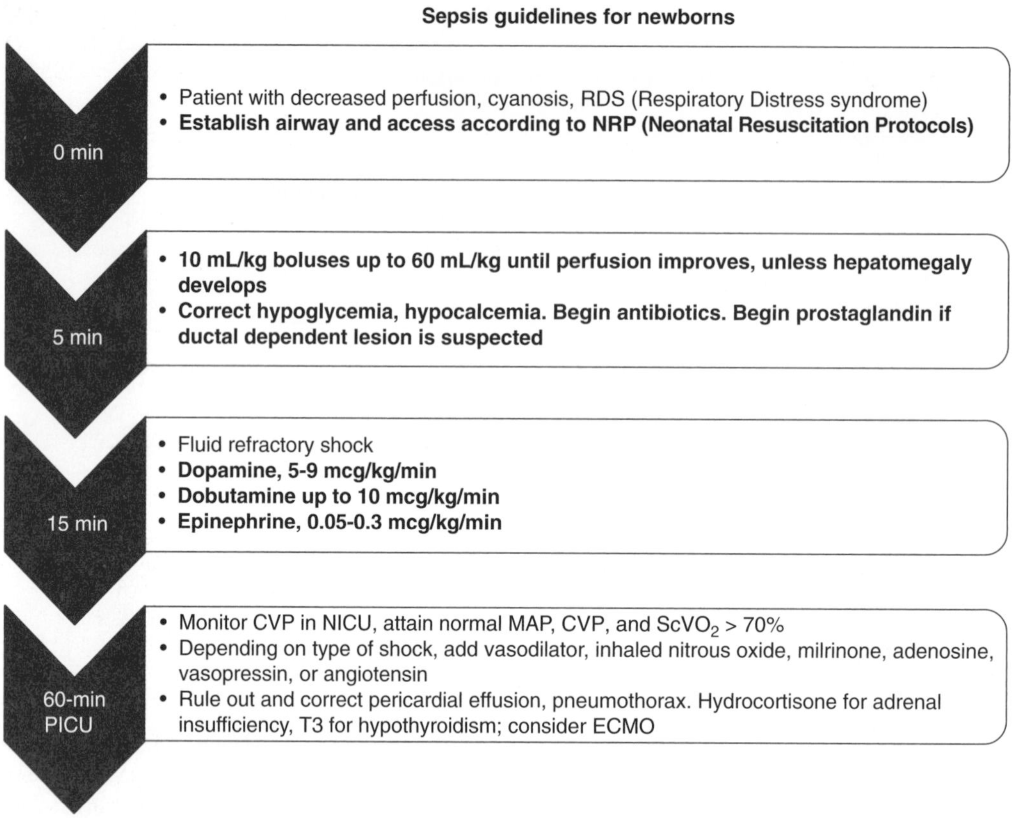

Sepsis guidelines for newborns

0 min
- Patient with decreased perfusion, cyanosis, RDS (Respiratory Distress syndrome)
- **Establish airway and access according to NRP (Neonatal Resuscitation Protocols)**

5 min
- **10 mL/kg boluses up to 60 mL/kg until perfusion improves, unless hepatomegaly develops**
- **Correct hypoglycemia, hypocalcemia. Begin antibiotics. Begin prostaglandin if ductal dependent lesion is suspected**

15 min
- Fluid refractory shock
- **Dopamine, 5-9 mcg/kg/min**
- **Dobutamine up to 10 mcg/kg/min**
- **Epinephrine, 0.05-0.3 mcg/kg/min**

60-min PICU
- Monitor CVP in NICU, attain normal MAP, CVP, and $ScVO_2 > 70\%$
- Depending on type of shock, add vasodilator, inhaled nitrous oxide, milrinone, adenosine, vasopressin, or angiotensin
- Rule out and correct pericardial effusion, pneumothorax. Hydrocortisone for adrenal insufficiency, T3 for hypothyroidism; consider ECMO

▲ **Figure 10–2.** Algorithm for time sensitive, goal-directed stepwise management of hemodynamic support in neonates. (Adapted, with permission, from Brierley J, Carcillo JA, Choong K, et al: Clinical practice parameters for hemodynamic support of pediatric and neonatal septic shock: 2007 update from the American College of Critical Care Medicine. *Crit Care Med* 2009;37(2):666.)

dose steroids (hydrocortisone at 2.5 mg/kg) may be given to children with known adrenal disorders or those receiving chronic steroids who remain in shock despite norepinephrine or epinephrine. Therapeutic endpoints are capillary refill less than 2 seconds, threshold HR and normal pulses without a differential between central and peripheral pulses, urine output greater than 1 mL/kg/h, and normal mental status. Extracorporeal membrane oxygenation (ECMO) may be an important therapy for refractory septic shock.

3. Anaphylaxis

Epinephrine is the mainstay of treatment for anaphylactic reactions and delays in administration are associated with worse outcomes. Cardiovascular collapse requires IV saline fluid boluses, starting at 20 mL/kg, in concert with the epinephrine. The recommended doses are listed in Table 10–2. Ventricular arrhythmias, angina, myocardial infarction, pulmonary edema, hypertensive emergency, and intracranial hemorrhage are rare side effects of epinephrine administration and are more commonly associated with intravenous administration. Adjuncts to therapy such as antihistamines, inhaled adrenergic agonists, corticosteroids and H_1 and H_2 blockers do not reverse the life-threatening symptoms that are characteristic of anaphylaxis, but are recommended.

▶ Special Population

The Neonate in Shock

When shock is recognized, airway and breathing must be stabilized by assuring patency and ventilation and oxygenation. IV or intraosseous access must be secured rapidly. However, unlike most shock, high volumes of fluid input may be associated with higher pulmonary, cardiac, gastrointestinal, and CNS morbidity in premature infants. Thus a term neonate (not in cardiogenic shock) may receive a 20-mL/kg bolus of crystalloid while a preterm neonate

Table 10–2. Medication dosing in treatments for shock.

Hypovolemic shock	Restore volume, start with crystalloid 20 mL/kg until patient's perfusion improves or until signs of volume overload appear (rales, hepatomegaly). Blood products used early in cases of trauma and known or suspected blood loss. Hemorrhage control in an important adjunct.
Cardiogenic shock	Smaller boluses (5-10 mL/kg) with careful evaluation of patient's response to fluid. Early inotropy is used. Dopamine at doses < 10 mcg/kg/min or dobutamine 1-20 mcg/kg/min. Milrinone may be used on consultation with cardiology. Begin with a loading dose of 50-75 mcg/kg, with maintenance infusion doses of 0.5-0.75 mcg/kg/min. Monitor for hypotension during loading dose or consider maintenance infusion without loading dose.
Anaphylactic shock	IM epinephrine 0.01 mg/kg to a maximum of 0.3 mg in children, given as a 1:1000 solution (1 mg/1 mL). IV infusions for persistent hypotension, 0.1-1 mcg/kg/min. Fluids, corticosteroids (dose 1-2 mg/k methylprednisolone), antihistamines are adjuncts to care.
Neurogenic shock	Phenylephrine (1 mcg/kg IV and titrate; 0.01 mcg/kg/min drip), with α_1-agonist properties, is a good choice but may cause reflex bradycardia so must be used with caution. An alternative is norepinephrine (0.5-2 mcg/kg/min) with α_1- and β_1-agonist properties. Epinephrine (0.5-2 mcg/kg/min) or vasopressin (0.5 mU/kg/h) can be used for refractory cases.
Septic shock	See Figures 10–1 and 10–2.

should start out with a 10-mL/kg bolus and both should be carefully reexamined after each intervention. If the source of hypovolemia is hemorrhage, whole or reconstituted blood is more appropriate than crystalloid. Colloid infusion in the perinatal period may impair long-term lung function.

In the setting of acidosis, shock, and hypoxemia, increased pulmonary artery pressure can lead to persistent pulmonary hypertension of the neonate. This may improve with inhaled nitric oxide with greatest effects seen at 20 ppm. Furthermore, the infant who presents with heart failure from congenital obstructive left heart syndromes will require the administration of prostaglandin E (PGE) to maintain a patent ductus arteriosus. The typical start dose in this life-saving intervention is 0.05-0.1 mcg/kg/min, but it can be titrated up to effect to a maximum of 0.4 mcg/kg/min. Effects can be seen within 15 minutes. Because apnea can be an adverse reaction of PGE infusion, these infants should be intubated.

Neonates respond to vascular agents differently than do older children and adults. Although dopamine can be used as the first-line agent, it may be less effective as the myocardial norepinephrine stores are immature and become rapidly depleted. A combination of dopamine at low dosage (8 g/kg/min) and dobutamine ($\geq$ 10 g/kg/min) is initially recommended. If the patient does not adequately respond to these interventions, then epinephrine (0.05-0.3 g/kg/min) can be infused to restore normal blood pressure and perfusion. For management of septic shock in newborns, see Figure 10–2.

Alderson P, Bunn F, Lefebvre C, et al: Human albumin solution for resuscitation and volume expansion in critically ill patients. *Cochrane Database Syst Rev.* 2004;(4):CD001208.

Arnal LE, Stein F: Pediatric septic shock: Why has mortality decreased? The utility of goal-directed therapy. *Semin Pediatr Infect Dis.* 2003;14(2):165 [PMID: 12881803].

Brierley J, Carcillo JA, Choong K, et al: Clinical practice parameters for hemodynamic support of pediatric and neonatal septic shock: 2007 update from the American College of Critical Care Medicine. *Crit Care Med.* 2009;37(2):666 [PMID: 19325359].

de Oliveira CF: Early goal-directed therapy in treatment of pediatric septic shock. *Shock.* 2010;34 (Suppl 1):44 [PMID: 20523274].

Jackson WL, Jr: Should we use etomidate as an induction agent for endotracheal intubation in patients with septic shock?: A critical appraisal. *Chest.* 2005;127(3):1031 [PMID: 15764790].

Roberts I, Alderson P, Bunn F, Chinnock P, Ker K, Schierhout G: Colloids versus crystalloids for fluid resuscitation in critically ill patients. *Cochrane Database Syst Rev.* 2004;(4):CD000567.

Schweer L: Pediatric trauma resuscitation: Initial fluid management. *J Infus Nurs.* 2008;31(2):104 [PMID: 18344770].

Simpson JN, Teach SJ: Pediatric rapid fluid resuscitation. *Curr Opinion Pediatr.* 2011;23(3):286 [PMID: 21508842].

Stoner MJ, Goodman DG, Cohen DM, Fernandez SA, Hall MW: Rapid fluid resuscitation in pediatrics: Testing the American College of Critical Care Medicine guideline. *Ann Emerg Med.* 2007;50(5):601 [PMID: 17764783].

Cyanosis

Taylor Ratcliff, MD, EMT-P

Brett Trullender, MS, PT, MS IV

LeeAnne Feher, MS III

GENERAL CONSIDERATIONS

Neonatal and pediatric cyanosis is a common complaint seen in the emergency department. The incidence of pediatric cyanosis declines with age; however, the severity of the underlying cause can become more ominous. Accordingly, it is important to categorize and understand various etiologies of cyanosis as they relate to age and presentation in order to stratify risk and severity. This chapter will differentiate peripheral cyanosis from central cyanosis and the benign and pathologic causes and treatment of each.

Cyanosis is visually perceived as blue or purple discoloration in body tissues resulting from abnormalities of hemoglobin and oxygen saturation in the capillary beds within those tissues. Primarily, desaturated hemoglobin gives the characteristic appearance of cyanosis. Any factor that decreases the overall oxygen saturation of hemoglobin in the arterial blood (loading) or increases the oxygen consumption from hemoglobin in peripheral tissues (unloading) can cause cyanosis. Accordingly, hypoxia or other causes of decreased oxygen exchange at the pulmonary capillary level will cause systemic or central cyanosis.

Central cyanosis becomes visible to the human eye when desaturated hemoglobin reaches 5 g/dL, which roughly corresponds to an oxygen saturation of approximately 85%. The saturation of hemoglobin and oxygen saturations causing peripheral cyanosis are more variable. A number of factors other than central causes contribute to peripheral cyanosis, ranging from normal physiologic events to life-threatening causes. Most factors relate to changes in arterial flow such as vasomotor tone, perfusion, and temperature changes.

Although uncommon in the emergency department, the most common type of cyanosis is commonly called acrocyanosis, or cyanosis of the hands, feet, and perioral area. The nonscientific term refers to peripheral cyanosis most common in newborns during the first minutes of life.

Neonates are born with a high degree of intrinsic peripheral vascular resistance and vasomotor instability. Normally, with rewarming, suctioning, and oxygenation, acrocyanosis remains confined to the periphery and lasts several minutes only. Cyanosis is included in the APGAR scoring system for newborns (Figures 11–1 and 11–2). In some infants, acrocyanosis may persist longer or become central cyanosis which may become pathologic.

Well infants may present to the emergency department with peripheral cyanosis. Parents may be concerned about peripheral cyanosis associated with bath time, feedings and sometimes, tantrums. In infants, vasomotor changes associated with temperature, feeding, and agitation or crying can produce transient peripheral cyanosis. Central cyanosis is not typically seen in these patients and should prompt investigation for more serious causes such as "Tet spells" occurring with tetralogy of Fallot. Central cyanosis is considered pathologic until proven otherwise.

Additionally, parents or caretakers may bring in young children with concerns about livedo, commonly referred to as "mottling." Livedo (l. reticularis) is a lace-like pattern of purple discoloration frequently mistaken for cyanosis. In most patients, the cause is benign and due to sluggish venous flow. However livedo in the presence of an ill child or other skin findings such as purpura, ulceration, or skin or mucosal lesions should promote further investigation. Persistent livedo not linked to an environmental cause may suggest vasculitis or thrombotic disease.

PHYSICAL EXAMINATION FINDINGS

Diagnosis of cyanosis is uncomplicated and commonly made by physical examination alone. Exposed skin should be examined for the aforementioned signs, bluish or purple tinged or discolored skin. Peripheral cyanosis generally will be confined to the hands, feet and, occasionally, areas with

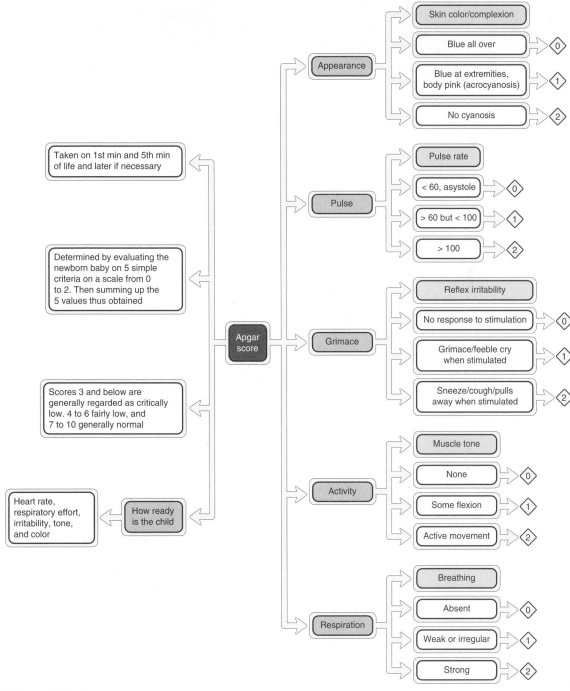

▲ **Figure 11–1.** Apgar score.
- Taken at first and fifth minutes of life (and as needed)
- Sum of A, P, G, A, and R, each scaled 0-2

- Scores
  ≤ 3 = critical low
  4-6 = low
  7-10 = generally normal

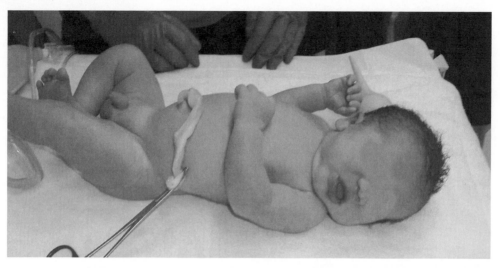

▲ **Figure 11–2.** Cyanosis. (Reprinted with permission from Charles Goldberg, MD, University of California, San Diego School of Medicine.)

terminal capillary beds such as the ears, nose, and the perioral area. Clinicians testing, and laboratory will often check perfusion as well using capillary refill by quickly blanching and then releasing capillary beds, most refilling to normal color in less than 2 seconds. Peripherally in the nail beds and distal tissues, measurement of capillary refill is confounded by temperature, vasomotor tone, and other factors that can give false results. Capillary refill in central areas, for example, over the chest or forehead, is more reliable and subject to less error. Of note, cyanosis becomes imperceptible with the human eye after hemoglobin levels fall below 5 mg/dL making physical examination in severely anemic patients difficult.

DIFFERENTIAL DIAGNOSIS

Cardiac, hematologic, pulmonary, trauma, and environmental exposure are known etiologies of cyanosis in children. The age of the child should be taken into account when considering the differential for cyanosis. Neonates can have age-specific signs and symptoms for their accompanying illness and considerations vary with advancing age. Older children may have a differential diagnosis similar to that of adults to include other cardiac causes.

Cardiac Causes of Cyanosis

Because cardiac output and oxygen extraction rates are defining factors in the physiology of cyanosis, a cardiac abnormality or congenital cardiac defect can cause varying degrees and instances of cyanosis. Clinically relevant cardiac factors are discussed in Chapter 35.

Hematologic Causes of Cyanosis

Cyanosis in children can result from anemia and hemoglobin abnormalities such as methemoglobinemia (see Chapter 40).

▶ Anemia

Anemia is a decrease in red blood cell mass or blood hemoglobin concentration. This reduction decreases the effective hemoglobin and oxygen carrying capacity of the blood. Pallor caused by anemia can usually be appreciated when the hemoglobin concentration is below 8-9 g/dL. The hemoglobin concentration in the blood can be lowered by three basic mechanisms: decreased erythrocyte production, increased erythrocyte destruction (eg, hemolysis), and blood loss.

Anemia can also be classified by the size or morphology of the red blood cell. These classifications include microcytic, normocytic, and macrocytic. Normal hemoglobin and hematocrit values for children 6-12 years of age are approximately 13.5 g/dL and 40%, respectively.

In evaluation of a young patient for anemia, it is important to take a thorough history that may expose genetic or long-standing causes of anemia, episodes of blood loss, or signs of hemolysis. Signs of hemolysis include changes in urine color, scleral icterus, and jaundice. Questions regarding recent or chronic infections should be asked, as well as recent travel to regions with endemic diseases (eg, malaria). Potential drug or toxin exposure should also be considered.

Methemoglobinemia

Methemoglobinemia is a cause of cyanosis. Methemoglobin is an altered state of hemoglobin in which the ferrous (Fe^{2+}) iron components of heme are converted to an oxidized ferric (Fe^{3+}) state. Causes can be endogenous or exogenous, classically associated with genetic causes such as glucose-6-phospate deficiency (G6PD), and medications such as local anesthetics, sulfonamides, and dapsone. Methemoglobinemia should be suspected in patients with cyanosis and normal arterial pO_2, partial pressure of arterial oxygen (PaO_2). Similarly, standard pulse oximetry may be inaccurate in the presence of methemoglobinemia. If the oxygen saturation as measured by standard pulse oximetry is significantly different from that measured by arterial blood gas, the presence of methemoglobinemia should be suspected.

Pulmonary Causes of Cyanosis

Pulmonary causes of cyanosis in children are thought to be the most common cause of central cyanosis. The respiratory causes are variable but include anything that inhibits oxygen from reaching the alveoli or disrupts diffusion of oxygen across the alveolar membrane. Patient history and clinical examination should point the physician to suspect the clinical cause, whether infection, intrinsic lung disease, or upper or lower airway problem.

Infection may be bacterial or viral and include pneumonia, empyema, or viral processes such as respiratory syncytial virus (RSV) bronchiolitis. These infections may cause exacerbation of intrinsic lung disease such as asthma or cystic fibrosis. Upper airway disturbance may be associated with croup, epiglottitis, or bacterial tracheitis although the clinician should also consider foreign body and inhalation injury. Physical findings of airway obstruction may include stridor, voice changes, drooling, sternal retractions, and prolonged inspiratory time.

Pulmonary edema can be due to cardiogenic or noncardiogenic etiology. Pulmonary edema reduces diffusion of oxygen across the alveoli into the pulmonary capillaries. Cardiogenic pulmonary edema typically is the result of left heart failure, but in children it can be associated with a myriad of congenital heart lesions. Ischemic heart disease is uncommon in children; however, myocarditis and various cardiomyopathies can produce heart failure. Causes of noncardiogenic pulmonary edema include illness-induced acute respiratory distress syndrome (ARDS), pneumonitis from near-drowning, and chemical exposure. History, physical examination, and chest radiography help the clinician determine a correct differential diagnosis (see Chapter 12).

Traumatic Causes of Cyanosis

Trauma is a consideration in the differential diagnosis of cyanosis. Whether due to impaired oxygenation, circulatory compromise or both, the traumatized pediatric patient may be cyanotic. Suspect pneumothorax or other intrathoracic injury in the cyanotic child presenting after traumatic injury, particularly when the mechanism suggests the possibility of chest trauma, or visual clues of chest wall trauma are observed.

Pneumothorax can be classified as spontaneous or traumatic, and simple versus tension. Tension pneumothorax is a true emergency, resulting in a marked impairment of ventilation and venous return. Findings may include abnormal chest wall movement, chest pain, abnormal breath sounds, subcutaneous emphysema, and late findings that include tracheal deviation and/or jugular venous distention. Vital signs may reflect rapidly worsening hypotension, tachycardia, and hypoxia. Tension pneumothorax should be treated immediately with needle decompression and/or tube thoracostomy. The treatment of traumatic pneumothorax is addressed in Chapter 25.

Environmental Causes of Cyanosis

Cyanosis in children can result from environmental causes. Common environmental considerations include cold exposure (hypothermia), poisoning, and inhalation injuries. The specific cause is often identified by careful history-taking from family members or caregivers (see Chapters 45 and 46).

EVALUATION OF PEDIATRIC & NEONATAL CYANOSIS

Initial investigation should focus on common age-based considerations and be guided by the clinical history. Patients may have a history of pulmonary infection, cardiac abnormality, or other likely cause or exposure. Physical examination, directed bedside testing, and laboratory evaluation will guide the clinician in unclear cases.

Pulse Oximetry

Pulse oximetry is a valuable bedside tool, is rapidly deployable, and gives instant information. Pulse oximetry readings can be taken in all four limbs to assist in identification of vascular abnormalities such as coarctation of the aorta and anomalous great vessels. However, misinformation can be provided by pulse oximetry. Methemoglobinemia and carbon monoxide poisoning are two clinical conditions in which pulse oximetry data and physical examination can be erroneous. Specialized multispectrum co-oximeters should be utilized for such cases as they can differentiate between regular, methemoglobin, and hemoglobin saturated with carbon monoxide. In most cases of concern, an arterial blood gas measurement should also be obtained to evaluate peripheral blood PaO_2.

Hyperoxia Test

In most cases of pediatric cyanosis, supplemental oxygen will increase oxygen diffusion tension in the lungs and increase PaO_2, resulting in improvements in peripheral oxygenation and reduction of cyanotic appearance. A select group of patients with arteriovenous shunting may not improve with oxygenation, and in fact, may worsen. For these patients, the hyperoxia test may prove beneficial.

The hyperoxia test is considered the gold standard to discriminate pulmonary conditions and hemoglobinopathies from cardiac conditions. As the patient is breathing room air, an arterial blood gas measurement is acquired from the right radial artery. Another measurement is obtained after the patient inspires 100% oxygen for 10 minutes. As an alternative to arterial blood gas values, pulse oximetry measurements can be used comparing room air to 100% oxygen. In patients without cardiopulmonary shunting, the PaO_2 should rise above 150 mm Hg after providing 100% oxygen, which predicts the absence of a cardiac shunt. In patients with cardiopulmonary shunting, the PaO_2 will not exceed 150 mm Hg, and/or minimal changes in pulse oximetry values will be noted after administration of 100% oxygen.

As mentioned above, some hemoglobinopathies, such as methemoglobinemia, may produce different patterns such as a PaO_2 greater than 200 mm Hg with a low pulse oximetry reading after hyperoxia. It is important to note that the hyperoxia test cannot function alone to exclude all forms of congenital heart disease, as left-sided obstructions may not follow this pattern of findings.

TREATMENT

Initial management of the pediatric patient presenting with cyanosis is centered on normal pediatric critical care measures. Immediate severity assessment and rapid identification and correction of any life threat are warranted. Specific attention to airway patency and correction of inadequate breathing are the initial priorities. Standard measures should be initiated, including peripheral IV access, laboratory evaluation, and vital sign monitoring including noninvasive blood pressure (NIBP) and SaO_2. A 12-lead electrocardiogram should be obtained.

Once the airway, breathing, circulation (ABC) and initial critical care steps are managed, high-concentration supplemental oxygen is the most common primary intervention. Administration of supplemental oxygen may worsen the patient's hemodynamic status and demonstrates no improvement in oxygenation, especially in the neonate. In these patients, a ductal dependent lesion should be suspected and supplemental oxygen should be restricted. If available, emergent cardiology consultation should be sought. If unavailable or in the presence of significant hemodynamic compromise, prostaglandin E_1 (PGE_1) therapy should be initiated (see Chapter 35).

Aside from identifying concerns about hyperoxia and ductal lesions, further determination of the etiology is critical. A specific consideration is persistent pulmonary hypertension. In select patients, high pulmonary vascular tone persists after birth, known as persistent pulmonary hypertension of the newborn (PPHN). The syndrome stresses right heart circulation and prohibits effective pulmonary circulation and oxygen exchange. In the neonate with PPHN, the result is a persistently open ductus arteriosus, causing an effective shunt. Treatment includes increasing FiO_2 and effective alveolar ventilation to maximize oxygenation. The patient likely will need intubation, sedation, and mechanical ventilation to maximize alveolar conditions. Inotropic agents may be used to support right heart function in the interim, followed by targeted medical therapy to dilate the pulmonary vasculature. Medications are directed at endothelial signaling cascades that produce pulmonary vasodilation. Nitric oxide (NO) has been the inhaled medication of choice but has limited availability and is contraindicated in other types of congenital heart disease that may not have been excluded. Sildenafil is not FDA approved for use in the pediatric population but is the subject of ongoing research. In older children, appropriate management of underlying disease that may contribute to persistent pulmonary hypertension should be considered, from obstructive sleep apnea to metabolic pathology, but will likely require workup outside the emergency department setting.

DISPOSITION

Ensuring a safe disposition and appropriate follow-up is a main priority of the emergency physician. The pediatric patient presenting with central cyanosis and concerning features on examination should routinely be admitted for workup and treatment. It is also likely that a cyanotic patient with a chronic cause such as asthma should be admitted unless markedly improved, because the initial clinical condition was likely severe in order to produce cyanosis. The patient with known reversible causes such as known Tet spells or other causes may be able to return home with close follow-up. Similarly, the well-appearing patient with a benign cause such as acrocyanosis or livedo with a clear explanation can likely be discharged home.

REFERENCES

Dolbec K, Mick NW: Congenital Heart Disease. *Emerg Med Clin North Am*. 2011;29(4):811-27 [PMID: 22040709].

Fouzas S, Priftis KN, Anthracopoulos MB: Pulse oximetry in pediatric practice. *Pediatrics*. 2011;128(4):740-52 [PMID: 21930554].

Jopling J, Henry E, Wiedmeier SE, et al: Reference ranges for hematocrit and blood hemoglobin concentration during the neonatal period: Data from a multihospital health care system. *Pediatrics*. 2009;123(2):e333-7 [PMID: 19171584].

Konduri GG, Kim UO: Advances in the diagnosis and management of persistent pulmonary hypertension of the newborn. *Pediatr Clin North Am*. 2009;56(3):579-600 [PMID: 19501693].

Kurklinsky, AK, Miller, VM, Rooke, TW: Acrocyanosis: The Flying Dutchman. *Vasc Med*. 2011;16(4):288-301 [PMID: 21427140].

Scott JA, Wonodi C, Moïsi JC, et al: The definition of pneumonia, the assessment of severity, and clinical standardization in the Pneumonia Etiology Research for Child Health Study. *Clin Infect Dis*. 2012;54(Suppl 2):S109-16 [PMID: 22403224].

Steinhorn, RH: Evaluation and management of the cyanotic neonate. *Clin Pediatr Emerg Med*. 2008;9(3):169-175 [PMID: 19727322].

Yap SH, Anania N, Alboliras ET, et al: Reversed differential cyanosis in the newborn: A clinical finding in the supra-cardiac total anomalous pulmonary venous connection. *Pediatr Cardiol*. 2009;30(3):359-62 [PMID: 18923862].

Zhang L, Mendoza-Sassi R, Santos JC, et al: Accuracy of symptoms and signs in predicting hypoxemia among young children with acute respiratory infection: A meta-analysis. *Int J Tuberc Lung Dis*. 2011;15(3):317-25 [PMID: 21333097].

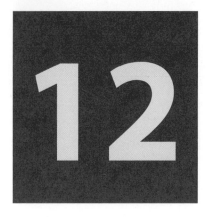

Respiratory Distress

Dominic Lucia, MD

Anthony James, MD

ASSESS SEVERITY AND GIVE IMMEDIATE NECESSARY CARE

The pediatric patient presenting in respiratory distress can represent a challenge to the emergency department physician. Respiratory failure is a common cause of cardiac arrest of the pediatric patient and hence the patient in respiratory distress should be of the highest priority in the emergency department.

The patient should receive, in parallel, an evaluation and immediate therapy. Maintaining an adequate airway and breathing should be the initial primary consideration. Respiratory evaluation begins with the general appearance of the patient. The patient should have a visible abdomen, chest wall, neck, and abdomen. Infants and toddlers often compensate their respiratory efforts with signs such as nasal flaring, clavicular and/or sternal retractions. A decline in mental status is a critical component of advanced respiratory distress and pending respiratory failure.

Immediate oxygen supplementation should occur during initial assessment and continue in patients with severe respiratory distress. A rapidly performed and focused physical examination of the oropharynx, neck, lungs, heart, chest, and extremities should be done in parallel with getting the child on cardiovascular monitoring and obtaining a focused history. A chest x-ray should be obtained as soon as possible as it can provide immediate valuable diagnostic information. Caution should be used that the acquisition of a chest x-ray does not delay immediate life saving care or remove the child from an environment of close monitoring.

ASSESS ADEQUACY OF OXYGENATION

Mental Status

In a child, mental status can be of utmost important in the initial evaluation of oxygenation. Hypoxia can manifest as a variety of behavioral changes that include persistent sleepiness, fussiness, and irritability. More advanced and concerning behaviors associated with hypoxia are inconsolability, restlessness, overt agitation, confusion, lethargy, and reduced response to painful stimuli. The emergency department physician must be cautious not to attribute these signs and symptoms to normal infant or child behaviors in the setting of possible hypoxia.

Pulse Oximetry

Bedside pulse oximetry is a useful tool for rapid feedback that measures percent saturation of oxygen in capillary blood. It can be particularly useful during procedural sedation or endotracheal intubation because of the real-time delivery of physiological information. The information should be considered as part of the ventilation assessment because it does not measure PCO_2 and does not account for initial hypoventilation. It can be a challenge to obtain a consistent waveform in an uncooperative child or in a child who is in subsequent cardiopulmonary collapse with poor peripheral perfusion. Mental status paired with respiratory status of the child should therefore be used as oxygenation assessment until objective data may be obtained.

Arterial Blood Gas

Similar information regarding arterial oxygenation can be taken from an arterial blood gas (ABG) compared with pulse oximetry. The ABG adds essential information about the effectiveness of ventilation in the form of pH, pO_2, and PCO_2. A more complete picture of the patient's physiologic status provides an initial baseline for later management. Obtaining the ABG should not delay immediate treatment based on real-time evaluation of the respiratory distress patient.

SEVERE UPPER AIRWAY OBSTRUCTION

▶ Clinical Findings

If the child does not present with overt apnea, the diagnosis of upper airway obstruction can usually be obtained based on overt stridorous respirations as well as significant respiratory effort. The range of clinical findings in a child with upper airway obstruction may be initially as subtle as anxiousness and parental reports of unusual breathing to the frightening presentation of stridor along with suprasternal and or supraclavicular retractions. The child may not be able to cry or speak. Because of the mobile infant's and toddler's propensity for oral exploration, the risk for inhalation of foreign bodies should be high on the differential. Viral illness or seasonality may make croup the likely reason for the stridor. Physical clues such as visible neck swelling or mass may be present. Swollen lips and tongue may result from upper airway obstruction. Laryngoscopy may be required to determine the true cause of the obstruction, but as discussed below the child should be approached with extreme caution.

▶ Treatment

Discretion should be used in the clinical treatment of the conscious child with presentation of upper airway compromise and/or stridor. In cases such as epiglottitis, supraglottic swelling, or precarious airway foreign body, examination of the child in distress can worsen the clinical status very quickly. (See Chapter 9 for approach to the child in respiratory distress.)

In patients with upper edema or swelling from infection or allergic reaction, treatment is directed at reducing the airway swelling. Therapy of cooling and vasoconstriction of affected tissue while treating the cause is the goal. Epinephrine by inhalation, intramuscular, or parenteral route is the most effective and rapid medication to reverse edema of the upper airway from a variety of causes. Epinephrine is usually well tolerated in children and should be given without delay via chosen route in a normally healthy child with signs of upper airway edema.

Acute obstructing or partially obstructing foreign bodies should be attempted to be visualized and extracted with appropriate sized nonview-obstructing forceps (McGill) in the child who is deteriorating (Figure 12–1). If the child is stable, extraction in the more controlled environment of the operating room (OR) by subspecialists and anesthesiology should be considered. Liquids and particulate matter obstructing the upper airway should be suctioned out using an appropriate-sized rigid blunt-tipped suction device. Moldable foreign bodies such as hot dog pieces or latex balloons may require Heimlich maneuver. The physician most skilled in airway management should care for the patient. The use of adjuncts such as fiberoptic laryngoscopy or video-assist laryngoscopy can be a critical resource in the removal of foreign body from the pediatric airway. If less invasive methods fail, immediate use of jet needle ventilation or cricothyroidotomy may be required, but are generally avoided in children younger than 10 years.

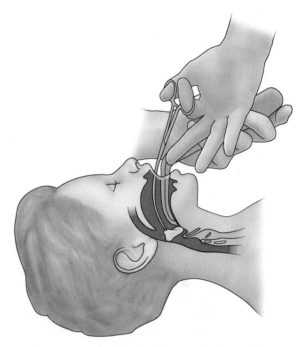

▲ **Figure 12–1.** Foreign body removal with McGill forceps.

▶ Disposition

The pediatric patient with an uncomplicated foreign body removal with no loss of consciousness and complete recovery to baseline may be observed in the emergency department for a period of time prior to discharge with specific return precautions. Most patients with lingering symptoms require admission for observation. Children who experienced any level of hypoxia, instrumentation, or epinephrine treatment should be highly considered for a period of inpatient observation. Children with possible liquid or material aspiration should also be observed. Disposition directly to the OR may be required for a patient requiring sedation and airway exploration by pediatric anesthesiologists and otolaryngology surgical subspecialists.

ALTERED MENTAL STATUS WITH SHALLOW BREATHING

▶ Clinical Findings

Altered mental status presenting in a child with respiratory distress is a diagnostic dilemma because one condition may be the cause of the other. Initial actions should be aimed at evaluation and treatment of the airway and breathing. Hypoxia in a child may progress and manifest mental status findings such as sleepiness, irritability, agitation, confusion, and/or lethargy. Obvious respiratory distress may cause profound labored breathing with the aforementioned obvious clinical symptoms of inspiratory retractions and nasal flaring.

The unique diagnostic challenge is the child with hypoxia who presents with subtle tachypnea and shallow respirations from causes such as occult trauma, shock, or metabolic derangements such as diabetic ketoacidosis (DKA). With a pediatric patient presenting with altered mentation, the determination of oxygenation status and bedside blood glucose should occur in the initial minutes of patient assessment. Altered mentation with loss of airway protective reflexes (gag reflex) are indications for immediate intubation.

▶ Treatment

When determination has been made that protection of the airway is required for a patient with altered mentation, ventilatory support should be initiated while preparing for intubation. High-flow (10-15 L/min) supplemental oxygen via non-rebreather is a bridging measure to intubation in the partially conscious patient who will not tolerate positive pressure ventilation (PPV). Adequate PPV via bag-valve-mask (BVM) should be initiated immediately in the patient who tolerates it. Positive pressure ventilation via BVM is often considered the most important skill in treatment of the pediatric patient in respiratory distress (see Chapter 9).

Endotracheal intubation provides a definitive airway by prevention of aspiration as well as facilitating effective respiratory support by BVM and eventual ventilator. If there is uncertainty regarding intubation of the patient with altered metal status, err on the side of intubation. After the airway is determined to be secure, evaluation and treatment for causes of altered mentation may be conducted via appropriate management.

▶ Disposition

The pediatric patient with altered mentation and respiratory distress should be admitted to a high-level care unit for further diagnostics and treatment.

TENSION PNEUMOTHORAX

▶ Clinical Findings

Tension pneumothorax is caused by an accumulation of air in the chest cavity outside the lung parenchyma. It is typically the result of trauma, though rarely develops spontaneously. The underlying etiology is a tear in the lung tissue allowing air to escape into the pleural space causing an increase in the positive pressure in the chest cavity on the affected side. The patient may complain of chest pain and will likely present in respiratory distress. Examination may reveal hyperresonance on chest wall percussion and poor chest wall movement on the affected side. Tachycardia, tachypnea, and hypoxia are expected findings as well as hypotension due to venous blood flow obstruction to the

heart. Radiographic findings include hyperexpansion of the affected side of the chest and shift of mediastinal contents away from the affected side.

▶ Treatment

Treatment should not be delayed for chest x-ray if clinical examination findings suggest tension pneumothorax. Immediate needle decompression should be performed on the affected side followed by tube thoracostomy. Tube sizes vary by age and size of the child; an 18 French tube is appropriate for most children, a 10-12 French appropriate for a newborn or infant. Improvement in blood pressure, hypoxia, tachycardia, and tachypnea should follow treatment as the positive pressure in the chest cavity is relieved. (See Chapter 3 for specifics of procedure.)

▶ Disposition

Hospitalization is indicated for management of the thoracostomy tube and further workup of underlying trauma or pathology.

SEVERE ASTHMA

▶ Clinical Findings

The most common cause for respiratory distress in the pediatric patient is an acute asthma exacerbation. The most important aspect of acute distress from an asthma event is the initial physical appearance of the child. Examination of the child with the chest and abdomen exposed is of utmost clinical importance. Findings such as respiratory status, color, and mentation can provide rapid guidance in severity and treatment. Other common findings are tachypnea, tachycardia, chest hyperexpansion, inspiratory retractions, and nasal flaring. In a child with a history of asthma, diffuse wheezing on auscultation or the more serious "quiet chest" can be a rapid examination finding that confirms suspicion of an asthma exacerbation, as well as a focused history. The child's ability to speak along a range from silence to full sentences can be a useful finding to determine the severity of the particular event. For children with inability to speak full sentences (if verbal at baseline), pulse oximetry less than 92%, declining mental status, or quiet chest, immediate treatment cannot be understated. Important focused points include history of asthma, related number of clinic or emergency department visits, hospitalizations, intubations, and current, past, and home treatment.

▶ Treatment

Oxygen

Oxygen should be given immediately. The modality of delivery depends on the severity of illness and method the child tolerates best. If tolerated, initial nasal cannula of 1-3 L/min is a good starting point unless the child is in extremis. If the child does not tolerate nasal cannula, blow-by oxygen delivery may suffice in milder cases. If escalation of oxygenation is needed, consider an appropriate-sized non-rebreather mask. If further therapy is needed because the child is not improving or is worsening, escalation to noninvasive ventilation should occur if this is an option in your facility.

The importance of noninvasive ventilation in the treatment of acute asthma exacerbations cannot be overstated. If time, equipment, and circumstances allow, noninvasive ventilation should occur prior to the decision to intubate. The decision to intubate an asthmatic child should not be made lightly. Mental status and respiratory effort serve as the initial guidepost for this decision point.

β-Adrenergic Sympathomimetic Bronchodilators

Bronchodilator medication should be given in aerosol form in the initial phase. It can be given in concert with oxygen supplementation. Consider addition of ipratropium bromide to the initial aerosol dose as this has been shown to reduce the need for hospitalization in the pediatric asthma patient. Continuous nebulizer treatments are generally used in the severe asthmatic. Parenteral therapy with epinephrine does not offer increased effectiveness over inhaled β-agonists. If the patient lacks adequate tidal volume to deliver the inhalation medication, intramuscular administration of epinephrine 1:1000 concentration at a dosage of 0.01 mL/kg up to 0.3 mL can be considered. Monitoring should be used on all patients receiving this therapy as tachycardia is the most common side effect.

Corticosteroids

Giving steroids early in the course of an asthma exacerbation has shown many benefits. The oral route has been shown to have similar efficacy to parenteral routes and may allow the physician to get them "on board" sooner that awaiting IV access in a child. The initial dose of 1-2 mg/kg of prednisone or a dose of dexamethasone at 0.6 mg/kg has shown to have similar benefit. Although inhaled corticosteroids have a role in the maintenance of medication regimen, it is not currently indicated at the time of an acute exacerbation.

Magnesium Sulfate

Intravenous magnesium has a potential bronchodilating effect and should be considered to treat moderate to severe asthma exacerbation. It should be reserved for patients who do not experience a significant response to initial therapy of inhaled β-agonist and ipratropium. A generally recognized dose of 50 mg/kg IV is given over a 20-minute period. Use caution with repeated dosing as the effects of magnesium toxicity include loss of deep tendon reflexes and eventual respiratory depression or cardiac arrest.

Invasive Mechanical Ventilation

Intubation may be required in the decompensating asthmatic patient. If this decision is made, it is important to remember a few basic principles. Ketamine is an excellent sedative choice due to its bronchodilating properties. The patient may not improve rapidly as the initial issue of lower airway obstruction is still present. Air trapping and breath stacking may occur due to the prolonged exploratory phase. To prevent these problems, the inspiratory time to exploratory ratio should be initially set at 1:3 and adjusted based on clinical findings.

Other Considerations

Consider rehydration with isotonic crystalloid in the patient with acute asthma. A patient often presents with some level of dehydration due to poor oral intake and insensate losses associated with tachypnea. Alternative therapies include Heliox inhalation and ketamine infusion.

▶ Disposition

Hospitalization should be considered if near or complete resolution of symptoms associated with the exacerbation has not occurred after three albuterol treatments and steroids. The level of care (floor vs pediatric intensive care unit [PICU]) required depends on the real-time clinical evaluation of the child after treatment in the emergency department. Caution should be used in rapid home disposition after improvement of a child who presented in distress. Relapse of asthma exacerbation is not uncommon; therefore, a period of observation in the emergency department, proper discharge plan, medications, return precautions, and follow-up instructions should be in place prior to discharge of patient. Further management of the distressed patient is discussed in Chapter 34.

Berg MD, Schexnayder SM, Chameides L, et al: Pediatric life support: 2010 American Heart Association guidelines for cardiopulmonary resuscitation and emergency cardiovascular care. *Circulation.* 2010;122:S876-908 [PMID: 20956230].

Browne LR, Gorelick MH: Asthma and pneumonia. *Pediatr Clin North Am.* 2010;57:1347-1356 [PMID: 21111121].

Carroll CL, Schramm CM: Noninvasive positive pressure ventilation for the treatment of status asthmaticus in children. *Ann Allergy Asthma Immunol.* 2006;96:454-459 [PMID:16597080].

Choi J, Lee GL: Common pediatric respiratory emergencies. *Emerg Med Clin North Am.* 2012;30:529-563 [PMID: 22487117].

Donoghue AJ, Nadkarni V, Berg RA, et al: Out-of-hospital pediatric cardiac arrest: An epidemiologic review and assessment of current knowledge. *Ann Emerg Med.* 2005;46:512 [PMID: 16308066].

Dotson K, Dallman M, Bowman CM, et al: Ipratropium bromide for acute asthma exacerbations in the emergency setting: A literature review of the evidence. *Pediatr Emerg Care.* 2009;25:687-692 [PMID: 19834421].

Fidkowski CW, Zheng H, Firth PG: The anesthetic considerations of tracheobronchial foreign bodies in children: A literature review of 12,979 cases. *Anesth Analg.* 2010;111:1016-1025 [PMID: 20802055].

Iramain R, Lopez-Herce J, Coronel J, et al: Inhaled salbutamol plus ipratropium in moderate and severe asthma crises in children. *J Asthma.* 2011;48:298-303 [PMID: 21332430].

Mayordomo-Collunga J, Medina A, Rey C, et al: Non-invasive ventilation in pediatric status asthmaticus: A prospective observational study. *Pediatr Pulmonol.* 2011;46:949-955 [PMID: 21520437].

Walker DM: Update on epinephrine (adrenaline) for pediatric emergencies. *Curr Opin Pediatr.* 2009;21:313-319 [PMID: 19444115].

Wang XF, Hong JG: Management of severe asthma exacerbation in children. *World J Pediatr.* 2011;7:293-301 [PMID: 22015722].

Zur KB, Litman RS: Pediatric airway foreign body retrieval: surgical and anesthetic perspectives. *Paediatr Anaesth.* 2009'19(Supp1):109-117 [PMID: 19572850].

EMERGENCY TREATMENT OF SPECIFIC DISORDERS

PULMONARY COLLAPSE

Pulmonary collapse may not always elicit physical examination findings. The severity of the collapse will be manifested in the degree of patient's respiratory distress. Physical examination and chest radiography will detect underlying pathology and guide the emergency physician toward the correct treatment. Management of specific causes of pulmonary collapse is addressed below.

Pneumothorax

▶ Clinical Findings

Patients with a spontaneous pneumothorax may present with chest pain, tachypnea, and tachycardia. The findings of respiratory distress may be accompanied by physical examination findings of hyper-resonance on chest wall percussion and decreased breath sounds on the affected side. Spontaneous pneumothorax consists of two categories: primary and secondary. Primary spontaneous pneumothorax occurs in the absence of any underlying lung disease, whereas secondary spontaneous pneumothorax is caused by known underlying lung disease such as cystic fibrosis or asthma. Chest x-ray (Figure 12–2) is diagnostic and will guide the treatment.

▶ Treatment

Treatment of primary spontaneous pneumothorax depends on the size of the pneumothorax and symptomatology. Small pneumothoraces, less than 10-20%, or apical pneumothoraces in children with minimal symptoms, may be treated conservatively with supplemental oxygen. The recurrence rate among patients treated conservatively with supplemental oxygen only is 50%. Small pneumothoraces with significant symptoms may be treated with manual aspiration via thoracentesis, with or without placement of a catheter connected to a Heimlich valve. Tube thoracostomy is indicated for large pneumothoraces.

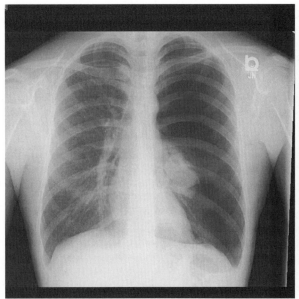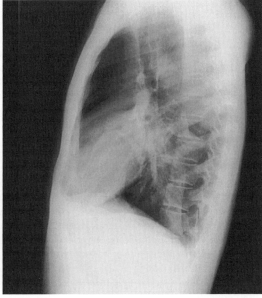

▲ **Figure 12–2.** Pneumothorax demonstrated on chest x-ray.

Disposition

Admission is indicated for supplemental oxygen and observation. Some patients may require video-assisted thoracoscopic surgery (VATS) to relieve persistent or recurrent pneumothoraces.

Hydrothorax/Hemothorax

Clinical Findings

Accumulation of fluid in the pleural space will lead to pulmonary collapse. The degree of respiratory distress is dependent on the volume of fluid in the chest cavity. Physical examination findings may include dullness to percussion and diminished breath sounds on auscultation. Chest radiography is diagnostic. (See Chapter 25.)

Treatment

Acute respiratory distress due to hydrothorax is uncommon in the pediatric population. If the dyspnea is of acute onset and the etiology felt to be the hydrothorax, drainage is indicated. A small-gauge catheter can be inserted for drainage of low-viscosity fluids. If the fluid is particularly viscous, insertion of a thoracostomy tube is indicated. A sample of the fluid removed should be sent to the laboratory for analysis (cell count, glucose, pH, protein, lactate dehydrogenase [LDH], specific gravity), culture, and cytologic studies.

Respiratory distress from hemothorax is almost always the result of trauma. Hemothorax may be the result of rib fractures, tears in the lung parenchymal, or cardiac and vascular injuries. Tube thoracostomy is indicated for drainage. Chest computed tomography (CT) is warranted to identify the source of the hemothorax and guide patient management, which may include surgical exploration.

Disposition

The patient should be admitted to the hospital for further workup and management of drainage catheters or thoracostomy tubes.

Atelectasis

Clinical Findings

Collapse of the alveoli that is not caused by hydrothorax, hemothorax, or pneumothorax is known as atelectasis. The most common cause of atelectasis is shallow inspiration. This may be caused by conditions such as pneumonia, pre-existing neuromuscular disorders that cause difficulty with chest wall expansion, or prolonged immobility from chronic disease states.

Treatment

Degree of dyspnea or respiratory distress depends upon the severity of the atelectasis. Supplemental oxygen and respiratory support is warranted. Positive pressure ventilation may be indicated for severe cases and can include Bilevel positive airway pressure (BiPAP) or intubation with mechanical ventilation. Positive pressure will open the alveoli and should improve the patient's respiratory status.

Disposition

Hospitalization is indicated for all patients with atelectasis, unless the severity is mild and does not result in hypoxia.

LOSS OF FUNCTIONAL LUNG PARENCHYMA

Respiratory distress may be due to conditions that cause a decrease in the functionality of the lung parenchyma. Physical examination findings include inspiratory crackles, dullness to chest wall percussion, and auscultory changes such as egophany. Chest radiography will reveal infiltrates or consolidations and is diagnostic. Conditions causing a decrease in the functionality of the lung parenchyma in children include pulmonary edema, pneumonia, bronchopulmonary dysplasia, and aspiration.

Pulmonary Edema

Clinical Findings

Pulmonary edema in children usually results from underlying cardiac abnormalities, most of which are congenital in nature. Changes in the cardiac function curve (Frank Starling curve) due to underlying congenital cardiopulmonary abnormalities can result in pulmonary edema. As pulmonary edema worsens, the lung tissue becomes less compliant and results in tachypnea and hypoxia. Physical examination findings may reveal crackles and decreased breath sounds on auscultation. Tachypnea, tachycardia, and hypoxia progress in relation to the severity of the pulmonary edema. In children, peripheral edema may or may not be present, depending on the chronicity of the pulmonary edema. Cardiomegaly and prominent pulmonary vasculature on chest x-ray are diagnostic (Figure 12–3).

Treatment

Initial treatment should begin with supplemental oxygen. If this therapy fails, BiPAP may be used to avoid endotracheal intubation in the appropriate clinical setting. If the child is not able to protect the airway or is combative, endotracheal intubation should be performed.

Disposition

Hospitalization is indicated for a child with pulmonary edema unless the severity of symptoms is very mild, there is no hypoxia, and the etiology is from a known cardiopulmonary abnormality. Pulmonary edema in a child with no known cardiopulmonary abnormality mandates hospitalization.

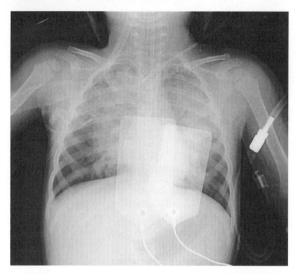

▲ **Figure 12–3.** Pulmonary edema demonstrated on chest x-ray.

Pneumonia

▷ **Clinical Findings**

Fever and cough are symptoms consistently seen in children with pneumonia. Additional symptoms may include wheezing, tachypnea, chest pain, and hypoxia. Physical examination findings may reveal wheezing and rales on auscultation, and overlying areas of consolidation can produce egophany and dullness to percussion. Chest x-ray is diagnostic (Figure 12–4).

▷ **Treatment**

Supplemental oxygen should be administered to support respiratory status. Bronchodilator therapy can be effective when wheezing and hypoxia are present. Parenteral antibiotics should be considered in the child who is not tolerating oral intake with the choice of agent guided by age. General recommendations for children older than 2 years are ceftriaxone at 50 mg IV and atypical coverage with azithromycin (initial dose 10 mg/kg on the first day). Evaluate the child's volume status and administer IV fluids as indicated. (See Chapter 34 for a detailed discussion of pneumonia.)

▷ **Disposition**

In children younger than 5 years, pneumonia is a leading cause of death. Mild cases with no signs of hypoxia in an otherwise well-appearing child can be treated with oral antibiotics and follow-up with a primary care physician. In all other cases, admission for IV antibiotics and respiratory therapy is indicated.

Bronchopulmonary Dysplasia

▷ **Clinical Findings**

Children with bronchopulmonary dysplasia may present with tachypnea, tachycardia, retractions, hypoxia, hypercapnia,

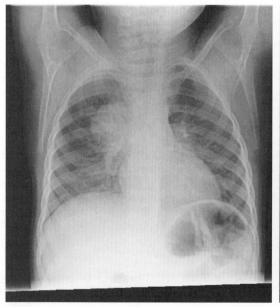
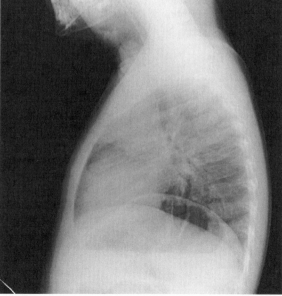

▲ **Figure 12–4.** Pneumonia demonstrated on chest x-ray.

wheezing, and other findings consistent with an acute exacerbation of the underlying lung disease. They may clinically appear like a child suffering from asthma, but their history is significant for prematurity, low birth weight, and/or history of mechanical ventilation at birth. Chest x-ray findings include hyperexpansion and atelectasis, as well as the possibility of superimposed pneumonia or pulmonary edema.

▶ Treatment

Treatment should include respiratory support as indicated with supplemental oxygen and bronchodilator therapy. More aggressive management is indicated if the child's respiratory status deteriorates, and includes BiPAP and possible intubation with mechanical ventilation. Intravenous corticosteroids, diuretics (in cases of fluid overload), and inhaled nitric oxide are of benefit. If concomitant pneumonia is present, intravenous antibiotics should be initiated.

▶ Disposition

Children with bronchopulmonary dysplasia frequently have other significant comorbidities and should be strongly considered for admission to the hospital for further care.

Aspiration

▶ Clinical Findings

Aspiration of food, fluids, or vomitus may present with respiratory distress of varying degrees. Aspiration of foreign bodies is discussed later in this chapter. Be suspicious for aspiration in the child with altered mental status that presents with respiratory distress. The findings of vomitus on clothing or the mouth can confirm the physician's suspicions. The clinical picture may be similar to pneumonia with tachypnea, tachycardia, and hypoxia present. Chest radiography may reveal infiltrates or a consolidation depending on when the aspiration occurred.

▶ Treatment

Supportive care with supplemental oxygen should be initiated. The mouth should be suctioned and cleared of debris. For more severe cases, endotracheal intubation may be required. Bronchoscopy can be beneficial to clear the large particulate matter. As the clinical findings may mimic pneumonia, especially on chest x-ray, broad spectrum antibiotics are typically initiated.

▶ Disposition

All patients should be hospitalized as pulmonary status can deteriorate due to progressive inflammation from the initial insult to the lung parenchyma.

Bhandari A, Bhandari V: Pitfalls, problems, and progress in bronchopulmonary dysplasia. *Pediatrics*. 2009;123:1562-1573 [PMID: 19482769].

Browne LR, Gorelick MH: Asthma and pneumonia. *Pediatr Clin North Am*. 2010;57:1347-1356 [PMID: 21111121].

Choi J, Lee GL: Common pediatric respiratory emergencies. *Emerg Med Clin North Am*. 2012;30:529-563 [PMID: 22487117].

de Benedictis FM, Carnielli VP, de Benedictis D: Aspiration lung disease. *Pediatr Clin North Am*. 2009;56:173-190 [PMID:19135587].

Don M, Canciani M, Korppi M: Community-acquired pneumonia in children: What's old? What's new? *Acta Paediatr*. 2010;99:1602-1608 [PMID: 20573146].

Lee LP, Lai MH, Chiu WK, et al. Management of primary spontaneous pneumothorax in Chinese children. *Hong Kong Med J*. 2010;16:94-100 [PMID: 20354242].

Lynch T, Bialy L, Kellner JD, et al: A systematic review on the diagnosis of pediatric bacterial pneumonia: When gold is bronze. *PLoS One*. 2010;5:e11989 [PMID: 20700510].

Robinson PD, Cooper P, Ranganathan SC: Evidence-based management of paediatric primary spontaneous pneumothorax. *Paediatr Respir Rev*. 2009;10:110-117 [PMID: 19651381].

Seguier-Lipszyc E, Elizur A, Klin B, et al: Management of primary spontaneous pneumothorax in children. *Clin Pediatr (Phila)*. 2011;50:797-802 [PMID: 21482575].

Shah S, Sharieff GQ: Pediatric respiratory infections. *Emerg Med Clin North Am*. 2007;25:961-979 [PMID: 17950132].

AIRWAY DISEASE

AIRWAY OBSTRUCTION

Obstruction of a child's airway results in dyspnea and may progress to severe respiratory distress. Physical examination may reveal a child with wheezing or stridor, tachypnea, tripodding, intercostal and substernal retractions, and choking. Multiple etiologies can result in obstruction of the upper airway and include foreign bodies, epiglottis, croup, tonsillar hypertrophy, retropharyngeal abscess, anaphylaxis, bacterial tracheitis, and congenital anomalies.

Identification of the underlying cause and timely management of obstruction relief are critical. Chest x-ray and lateral x-rays of the soft tissues of the neck can aid in identification of foreign bodies if they are radiopaque. Children can aspirate small objects such as nuts, coins, beads, and toys with resultant obstruction in multiple sites along the trachea and bronchial tree. Chest x-ray with a dedicated expiratory view will reveal a unilateral hyperexpansion on the affected side if the foreign body is lodged in the bronchus.

Foreign Body

Asphyxiation from inhaled foreign bodies is a leading cause of accidental death in young children. The foreign body must be removed to relieve the obstruction. The timing and location of the removal is dependent upon the severity of the child's symptoms. Children in acute respiratory distress mandate evaluation of the airway and, if visible, removal of the object via direct visualization. If the object cannot be visualized and respiratory failure is imminent, endotracheal intubation is warranted. If the object causing the obstruction prevents endotracheal intubation and cannot be removed, emergent crichothyrotomy may be required. Fiberoptic laryngoscopy, if available, can assist with removal. For the child who is not in respiratory distress, removal with rigid bronchoscopy under general anesthesia is the gold standard as well as the safest route. (See also Chapter 33.)

Anatomic

Anatomic causes for airway obstruction include epiglottitis, croup, tonsillar hypertrophy, retropharyngeal abscess, and laryngeal edema.

Epiglottitis should be managed carefully as any attempts to visualize or manipulate the airway can result in worsening symptoms. Children with this condition are now rarely seen due to vaccination against *Haemophilus influenza*. Children with epiglottitis should be evaluated in the OR by an anesthesiologist and a surgeon should tracheostomy be required.

Croup results in swelling of the larynx and trachea. It is identified by a barking cough and stridor. The classic "steeple sign" is visible on anteroposterior (A-P) view radiograph of the neck. Treatment includes supplemental oxygen as needed, single-dose steroids, and nebulized epinephrine for moderate to severe cases.

Tonsillar hypertrophy is a common pediatric finding. Children with this condition are often noted to be snore while sleeping and may even have intermittent episodes of brief apnea while asleep. Acute inflammation of the tonsils, such as in cases of tonsillitis, may result in an anatomic obstruction to the upper airway. Treatment should include supplemental oxygen as needed, single-dose steroid, and antibiotics for acute tonsillitis. These children should be referred to an ear, nose, and throat (ENT) surgeon for evaluation of elective tonsillectomy. Severe hypertrophy causing acute respiratory distress should be managed with endotracheal intubation.

Retropharyngeal abscesses can also cause an anatomic upper airway obstruction. Supplemental oxygen should be administered in addition to IV antibiotics. Surgical incision and drainage is necessary. For cases of imminent respiratory compromise, endotracheal intubation is required.

Congenital Upper Airway Abnormalities

▶ Clinical Findings

Common congenital upper airway abnormalities include laryngomalacia, vocal cord dysfunction/paralysis, and subglottic stenosis. Other causes include obstructive sleep apnea, tumors, vascular anomalies, micrognathia, retrognathia, cleft palate, and a number of rare conditions.

Clinical presentation may range from minor to severe respiratory distress depending upon the underlying etiology. As congenital abnormalities are structural in nature, mild airway irritation or trauma may lead to significant swelling and subsequent respiratory distress. Patients may present with stridor, tachypnea, retractions, hypoxia, and tachycardia.

▶ Treatment

Supplemental oxygen should be initiated. Use of PPV with BiPAP may be helpful in some patients, depending on the underlying etiology. Should endotracheal intubation be required, the emergency department physician should be familiar with, and have at his or her disposal, difficult airway adjuncts to assist with intubation. The physician should investigate other potential causes for the child's acute respiratory distress, such as infections, trauma, or exacerbations of other comorbid conditions and treat accordingly.

▶ Disposition

Discharge or admission depends on the severity of the patient's condition and the etiology of the acute event. Any concern for potential deterioration of the child's respiratory status warrants hospital admission.

Anaphylaxis

▶ Clinical Findings

Anaphylaxis is caused by the rapid release of inflammatory mediators in response to a specific trigger, most commonly food, medicines, or insect stings/bites in children. This is a potentially life-threatening condition that requires immediate action by the emergency physician. The child may present with tachypnea, tachycardia, swelling (localized or diffuse), hives, wheezing, stridor, and itching.

▶ Treatment

Epinephrine (0.01 mg/kg) as intramuscular injection (repeated every 5-20 minutes up to three doses as indicated) is the first line of treatment. Other treatments include nebulized bronchodilators, antihistamines (diphenhydramine), and corticosteroids. Severe anaphylaxis may result in hypotension, so monitor and treat with fluid resuscitation as needed. Manage the child's respiratory status with supplemental oxygen as needed and be prepared for more advanced respiratory support (BiPAP or endotracheal intubation) if respiratory status deteriorates.

▶ Disposition

Patients with very mild symptoms should be observed after treatment for a minimum of 4 hours and discharged home if stable. All other patients require admission.

Bacterial Tracheitis

Clinical Findings

Children will present with symptoms that can include a cough (barking cough similar to croup), stridor, tachypnea, retractions, tachycardia, sore throat, and fever. Patients with bacterial tracheitis will not respond to the standard treatment for croup and typically appear more ill. The inflammatory process in the larynx, trachea, and bronchi results in the formation of a mucopurulent membrane. The membrane can dislodge that results in airway obstruction. Radiography of the neck may reveal a "steeple sign" similar to croup, or an irregular border of the upper airway.

Treatment

Provide supplemental oxygen and assess respiratory status. If endotracheal intubation is indicated, use a slightly smaller endotracheal tube (ETT) to accommodate for the swelling of the airway and to minimize potential trauma. Intravenous antibiotics should be initiated and should include a third-generation cephalosporin or clindamycin. Toxic appearing children should be given vancomycin.

Disposition

All patients with bacterial tracheitis require hospital admission.

Bronchiolitis

Clinical Findings

Bronchiolitis is a unique pediatric clinical presentation occurring most commonly in children aged 6 months to 2 years. Strong consideration of this diagnosis should be applied to a child younger than 2 years who presents with rhinorrhea, wheezing, and tachypnea especially in the winter and early spring months. Respiratory syncytial virus (RSV), rhinovirus, adenovirus, human metapneumovirus, influenza, and parainfluenza virus have been named as culprits in this disease entity with RSV being the most common. The pathology of the disease is caused from the edema, inflammation, and epithelial necrosis and sloughing into the infant-sized bronchioles. Hypoxia may occur from the variable obstruction that is resultant from these factors. The course of bronchiolitis can be variable and prolonged with the child experiencing more than one episode of illness within the same season. Diagnostic studies are not always required as bronchiolitis is a clinical diagnosis. Recent studies have shown there to be a higher rate of concomitant urinary tract infections and/or acute otitis media in infants younger than 3 months with RSV.

A typical CXR in an infant with uncomplicated bronchiolitis reveals a variable combination of hyperinflation, peribronchial cuffing, and possible atelectasis. Chest x-ray is not indicated as routine workup in the current American Academy of Pediatrics (AAP) guidelines for bronchiolitis. Viral panels may reveal the culprit for the specific episode of bronchiolitis, but have rare effect on the actual clinical management.

Treatment

Treatment of bronchiolitis is based on supportive care. Nasal suctioning can be an initial and simple treatment that may clinically improve the infant significantly due to their obligate nasal breathing. Hydration status of the child should be considered as this can be an issue in bronchiolitis due to the insensate losses from tachypnea and poor feeding due to respiratory effort.

The AAP practice guidelines recommend supplemental oxygen if the SpO_2 is less that 90%. Oxygen may be delivered by nasal cannula or blow-by oxygen if better tolerated. Inhaled bronchodilator therapy has not been shown to have a significant benefit to be standard therapy. Many clinical practitioners do a trial dosage of β-adrenergic agonist. Subsequent dosing should be performed only if the initial dosage provided a clear benefit. Albuterol has the advantage of possible home usage upon discharge as opposed to other inhaled therapies that may be trialled in bronchiolitis that include racemic epinephrine or hypertonic saline. Corticosteroids and antibiotics do not have a role in standard therapy unless other disease entities that require these treatments exist. As with asthma, intubation should be considered last resort in a child with bronchiolitis. Many of the complications that occur with the intubated asthmatic can occur with the intubated bronchiolitic including air trapping and barotrauma.

Disposition

Clinical status of the bronchiolitic child should be the basis of disposition. Young age and comorbid conditions are the most useful predictors of severity. Factors such as oxygen requirement to keep SpO_2 above 90%, or inability to feed and stay hydrated indicate a need for admission. Another consideration should be the ability of the caretaker to return for acute therapy if the child should worsen at home.

Before a patient with bronchiolitis is discharged home, the caretaker should have education, including suctioning instructions, possible bronchodialator therapy, hydration instructions, and explicit return instructions. Infants younger than 3 months should be considered for admission. If there is an infant history of apnea with the illness course, admission should occur. The decision to admit to the hospital floor versus PICU should be based on each institution's ability to care for the patient. A patient with significant respiratory distress or ventilatory support requirements (noninvasive or intubation) should be monitored in the PICU.

OTHER CONDITIONS

Pertussis

▶ Clinical Findings

Pertussis is a bacterial respiratory infection that is extremely contagious via droplet contact to respiratory epithelium. Incidence has been increasing with several localized endemic outbreaks occurring in the United States. The classic clinical presentation occurs in sequence: catarrhal, paroxysmal, and convalescent phases. The symptoms associated with each phase are listed in Table 12–1. Pertussis should be high on the differential in a patient with persistent cough without other signs of overt illness such as lung sounds, fever, sore throat, or flu-like symptoms. A common presentation may be an afebrile adolescent with persistent cough longer than 1 week. Another presentation may be a nontoxic toddler who has a rapid prolonged coughing spell with posttussive emesis. Children may exhibit evidence of prolonged episodes of increased intrathoracic pressure from the coughing with upper body petechiae or subconjunctival hemorrhage. Young infants may be a more challenging diagnosis. History of cyanosis, apnea, and a prolonged worsening convalescent phase may be present. A significant leukocytosis may be present usually in the catarrhal stage.

▶ Treatment

Treatment is generally aimed at supportive care with special caution to avoid stimuli that may trigger a cough, including allergens, cold temperatures, and vigorous physical activity. Antihistamines and corticosteroids are not of significant clinical value. Antibiotic treatment can be used presumptively based on clinical findings. The benefits of antibiotic treatment include reduction in disease severity, symptoms, and potential transmission. Macrolides are the generally recommended class of antibiotics with azithromycin being the most commonly prescribed due to safety profile and simplicity of dosing.

▶ Disposition

If treatment is not provided at point of care, close follow-up with laboratory results should occur. Household contacts should be treated if a positive test occurs in a symptomatic patient. Immunity is not obtained from natural disease and immunization does not confer lifelong immunity. The decision to hospitalize the patient is based on clinical picture including severity of illness, comorbid conditions, age, hydration status, history of apnea or cyanosis. If hospitalization is required, the child should be placed on isolation within the institution until diagnosis is confirmed or denied.

Pulmonary Embolism

▶ Clinical Finding

Pulmonary embolism (PE) in children often occurs with major risk factors. Risk factors include hematologic disorders (sickle cell disease, leukemias, inherited thrombophilias), neoplasms, trauma, congenital heart disease, or presence of central venous lines. Most cases occur in adolescents and risk factors, similar to adults, such as oral contraceptive use, smoking, pregnancy, and abortion, should be considered when suspecting PE.

Historical findings of unexplained dyspnea, pleuritic chest pain, cough (with or without hemoptysis), tachypnea, fever, extremity pain, or swelling can be elicited in PE. Because of the strong correlation with central venous lines, upper extremity deep vein thrombosis (DVT) should be a consideration in the pediatric population with history or presence of central line.

Physical examination of the patient with PE may reveal tachycardia, tachypnea, increased work of breathing, abnormal lung sounds, or cyanosis. Physical findings of DVT, which has a strong incidence of subsequent pulmonary embolism, include extremity swelling, tenderness, erythema, warmth, and venous distension. There are no clinical prediction rules currently specific to the pediatric population. Laboratory findings such as D-dimer are often not as useful in children because many children with PE already have a high pretest probability. Imaging diagnostic modalities for PE include chest x-ray (CXR), ventilation perfusion scan, pulmonary angiography, and CT pulmonary angiography. The choice of imaging should be made in concert with radiology colleagues as each study has varying specificity and sensitivity in varying age and body habitus for detection of PE.

▶ Treatment

With DVT and high suspicion or when diagnostics detect a PE, treatment should not be delayed. If possible, treatment

Table 12–1. Symptoms for the clinical phases of pertussis.

Catarrhal Phase (7–14 d)	URI type symptoms Low-grade fever Rhinorrhea Intermittent dry irritating cough
Paroxysmal phase (2–4 wk)	Persistent paroxysms of coughing Possible characteristic "whoop" at end of cough Child is infectious during this phase until resolution of treatment
Convalescent phase (1–6 wk)	Symptoms gradually decrease Infants cough may worsen during this period

should be in cooperation with a pediatric hematologist. Consultation should not delay treatment of the child. Air, breathing, and circulation (ABC) should be the initial priority.

After the patient's airway is deemed stable, medical therapy should ensue. General recommendations are divided by age. The unfractionated heparin IV loading dose from neonate to adolescent is 70-75 units/kg.

- Infants < 1 year, initial IV infusion rate starts at 28 units/kg/h.
- Children 1-16 years, IV infusion rate of 20 units/kg/h with a maximum of 1650 units per hour.
- Adolescents > 16 years, IV infusion rate of 15 units/kg/h with a maximum of 1650 units per hour. Low molecular weight heparin via subcutaneous (SC) route reaches therapeutic range more quickly.
- Child ≥ 2 months initial dosing is 1 mg/kg SC twice daily.
- Infants < 2 months dosing should be increased to 1.6 mg/kg SC twice daily.

▶ Disposition

Patients with equivocal imaging or studies, but evidence by history or physical examination should be considered for treatment and hospital admission in a monitored setting. Patients with a diagnosis of new DVT or PE should be admitted. The pediatric intensive care setting should be strongly considered for children with confirmed PE.

Psychogenic Hyperventilation

▶ Clinical Findings

Adolescents are most likely to present with hyperventilation in the emergency department. Although a diagnosis of exclusion, it can be made based on past episodes and some subtle but useful physical examination findings. The adolescent subset of patients often presents with history of acute dyspnea and anxiety that may have been preceded by stressful personal events. If the patient is hyperventilatory to the point of tetany, it is strongly in favor of the diagnosis. Patients also report light headedness (cerebral vasoconstriction), and perioral and/or limb paresthesias. The dyspnea may improve with exercise. The patient often times can be calmed enough to speak clearly and halt the very loud breathing pattern. Normal pulse oximetry on room air and lower lung sounds that are clear can be helpful physical examination findings. Screening laboratories reveal only a low arterial PCO_2, normal or high PO_2, and an elevated pH. Organic etiology should be considered, but often patients can be diagnosed in the emergency department. After calming and reassurance, the patient will often completely resolve in the emergency department.

▶ Treatment

No specific treatment is required. Reassurance may help in the medical environment. In older adolescent patients with symptomatic hypocapnea (perioral tingling, carpopedal spasm, tetany) or marked respiratory alkalosis (pH > 7.55), breathing into a patient-held air-tight bag may help alleviate the hypocapnic symptoms.

▶ Disposition

The patient should not be sent home with continued symptoms. If symptoms resolve, outpatient follow-up with a pediatrican or pediatric pulmonologist may be helpful for complete workup and reassurance.

REFERENCES

Bettitol S, Wang K, Thompson MJ, et al: Symptomatic treatment of the cough in whooping cough. *Cochrane Database Syst Rev.* 2012;5:CD003257 [PMID: 22592689].

Bjornson CL, Johnson DW: Croup. *Lancet.* 2008;371:329-39 [PMID: 18295000].

Bordley WC, Viswanathan M, King VJ, et al: Diagnosis and testing in bronchiolitis: A systematic review. *Arch Pediatr Adolesc Med.* 2004;158:119-26 [PMID: 14757603].

Cherry J: Clinical practice. Croup. *N Engl J Med.* 2008;358:384-91 [PMID: 18216359].

Choi J, Lee GL: Common pediatric respiratory emergencies. *Emerg Med Clin North Am.* 2012;30:529-63 [PMID: 22487117].

Daniel SJ: The upper airway: Congenital malformations. *Paediatr Respir Rev.* 2006;7:S260-3 [PMID: 16798587].

Fidkowski CW, Zheng H, Firth PG: The anesthetic considerations of tracheobronchial foreign bodies in children: A literature review of 12,979 cases. *Anesth Analg.* 2010;111:1016-25 [PMID: 20802055].

Healy F, Hanna BD, Zinman R: Pulmonary complications of congenital heart disease. *Paediatr Respir Rev.* 2012;13:10-5 [PMID: 22208788].

Muraro A, Roberts G, Clark A, et al: EAACI task force on anaphylaxis in children. The management of anaphylaxis in childhood: position paper of the European academy of allergology and clinical immunology. *Allergy.* 2007;62:857-71 [PMID: 17590200].

Parasuraman S, Goldhaber S: Venous thromboembolism in children. *Circulation.* 2006;113:e12-6 [PMID: 16418440].

Shah S, Sharieff GQ: Pediatric respiratory infections. *Emerg Med Clin North Am.* 2007;25:961-79 [PMID: 17950132].

Simons FE: Anaphylaxis. *J Allergy Clin Immunol.* 2010;125:S161-81 [PMID: 20176258].

Steinhorn RH: Neonatal pulmonary hypertension. *Pediatr Crit Care Med.* 2010;11:S79-84 [PMID: 20216169].

Walker DM: Update on epinephrine (adrenaline) for pediatric emergencies. *Curr Opin Pediatr.* 2009;21:313-9 [PMID: 19444115].

Zur KB, Litman RS: Pediatric airway foreign body retrieval: Surgical and anesthetic perspectives. *Paediatr Anaesth.* 2009;19(Suppl 1):109-17 [PMID: 19572850].

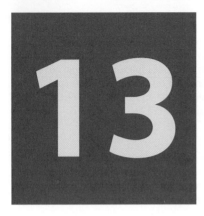

Submersion Injuries

Sameer Desai, MD

Mary Wardrop, MD

Thomas Cunningham, MS IV

SUBMERSION INJURIES

The World Health Organization (WHO) estimates the annual incidence of death by drowning to be approximately 500,000 a year worldwide; and in males aged 5-14 years, the leading cause of death worldwide. The pediatric population is most at risk for drowning events. Submersion injuries are the second leading cause of death from unintentional injuries in children aged 1-18 years, and leading cause of accidental death in children aged 1-4 years. For 2009, the Centers for Disease Control and Prevention (CDC) reported 983 fatal and 5,624 nonfatal injuries due to unintentional drowning or submersion injuries in the pediatric population.

EPIDEMIOLOGY

Age distribution of drowning incidents in the pediatric population follows a bimodal distribution. The first and larger peak occurs among children aged 1-4 years who are inadequately supervised in swimming pools, bathtubs, buckets, and other bodies of water. The second age peak occurs among adolescent males, which has been attributed to higher risk-taking behavior, overestimating of swimming abilities, use of alcohol and/or illicit drugs, and greater exposure to bodies of water. There exists a higher drowning rate in African American and Native American children. Drowning is much more common during the summer months when swimming pools, beaches, and other bodies of water are more frequented, particularly during daylight hours and on weekends. There are special populations at increased risk for drowning, specifically patients with epilepsy, children with developmental delay, and individuals with long QT syndrome or other cardiac arrhythmias.

DEFINITION

Historically, there has been considerable confusion due to the varied terminology used to describe drowning symptoms. In 2002, the World Congress on Drowning met and established the official Utstein style which standardized the medical discourse currently used. The following terms have been abandoned in medical discourse: dry versus wet drowning; active versus silent drowning; secondary drowning; near-drowned. The Utstein style defines drowning as "a process resulting in primary respiratory impairment from submersion/immersion in a liquid medium." Implicit in this definition is that a liquid/air interface is present at the entrance of the victim's airway, preventing the victim from breathing air.

PATHOPHYSIOLOGY

The drowning process begins when the victim's airway lies below the surface of liquid, usually water, at which time the victim voluntarily holds his or her breath. The breath-holding period is followed by an involuntary period of laryngospasm secondary to the presence of liquid in the oropharynx or larynx. The lack of ventilation and oxygenation results in hypoxia and ultimately death if the process is not reversed. The majority of submersion injuries involve aspiration of liquid. The distinction between freshwater and saltwater drowning historically was significant due to concerns that the tonicity of water could cause major electrolyte disturbances, and influenced past treatment and management protocols. It is now recognized that this distinction has no bearing on the treatment of victims. Aspiration of more than 11 mL/kg of body weight must occur before blood volume changes occur, and 22 mL/kg must be aspirated before electrolyte abnormalities take place. The majority of submersion injuries involve aspiration of a small quantity of water secondary to associated laryngospasm. It is unusual for drowning victims to aspirate more than 3-4 mL/kg. Aspiration of 1-2 mL/kg of liquid medium can destroy pulmonary surfactant, resulting in decreased lung compliance, atelectasis, significant intrapulmonic shunting and V-Q mismatch, and pulmonary edema. This ultimately develops into acute respiratory distress syndrome (ARDS). When a patient is successfully resuscitated, studies have shown the lungs are capable of full recovery with no long-term pulmonary complications from the drowning and aspiration event, although reports of airway hyper-responsiveness have been reported.

Loss of consciousness during a drowning incident is a direct result of cerebral hypoxia. The areas of the brain most susceptible to injury are watershed regions at the end of vascular beds, in particular the hippocampus, insular cortex, and basal ganglia. When hypoxia continues, global ischemia and neurologic damage ensues. This results in posthypoxic encephalopathy and an increase in intracranial pressure (ICP). The rise in ICP and its persistence over time reflects the severity of neurologic injury. Prolonged elevation of ICP is a poor prognostic indicator. It has been well documented that patients who suffer submersion injuries in very cold or icy water have a better chance of neurologic recovery, although complete neurologic recovery is reported in warm water submersion injuries. If the patient is able to be cooled rapidly it slows overall metabolism and has a protective effect on neuronal tissue. This is especially true if the patient is able to oxygenate while the cooling is taking place and when hypoxia does not set in until the patient has already cooled. The neurologic damage following a drowning incident is the limiting factor in recovery and functionality for patients successfully resuscitated. The best prediction of final neurologic outcome is found via repeat neurologic examinations during the first 24-72 hours of therapy.

Patients resuscitated will not have long-term cardiac damage. If the drowning victim suffers prolonged asphyxiation, the resultant hypoxia will ultimately lead to cardiac arrest. By the time severe myocardial damage sets in, the patient will have sustained severe neurologic injury that is not survivable. There is a well-known association between drowning and primary cardiac events. The act of swimming and the breath-holding involved can precipitate lethal arrhythmias, especially in patients with previously undiagnosed prolonged QT syndrome.

EMERGENCY DEPARTMENT MANAGEMENT

Resuscitation should be performed following current advanced cardiac life support (ACLS) guidelines, with the exception that the traditional airway, breathing, and circulation (ABC) pattern of resuscitation should be used as opposed to the circulation, airway, and breathing (CAB) sequence given the hypoxic causation of arrest. Time to initiation of cardiopulmonary resuscitation (CPR) plays a key role in the success and neurologic outcome of drowning victims. Patients should be immobilized and C-collar placed until definitive determination as to mechanism of injury. Many drowning victims have traumatic injuries in addition to their submersion injury. If the drowning is precipitated by medical conditions (eg, seizures, ingestions), treatment decisions must be adjusted to appropriately evaluate the situation.

It is important in the initial assessment to obtain a baseline temperature as many drowning victims are submerged in cold water and suffer from hypothermia. If the patient is hypothermic, immediate rewarming should be undertaken. External rewarming can be performed with warm blankets, Bair Hugger, heat lamps, increased ambient air temperature, and warm IV fluid bags applied to groin and axillae. Methods of internal rewarming include warm IV fluids, bladder irrigation with warm saline, and administration of warmed humidified oxygen. Some patients may appear lifeless until their core temperature has been sufficiently warmed. Hypothermic patients should be actively warmed to a temperature of 32-34°C (89.6-93°F). Recent data suggests that hypothermia has a neuroprotective effect and may improve neurologic outcome, although definitive studies of this practice after submersion injuries in the pediatric population are still lacking. Given the success of therapeutic hypothermia in postcardiac arrest patients, a number of institutions currently perform therapeutic hypothermia on drowning patients who suffer cardiac arrest. In the past, hyperventilation, barbiturate coma, aggressive diuresis, and neuromuscular blockage were used in an effort to improve neurologic outcomes. However, studies have shown these measures do not improve outcomes and should not be used.

Patients who present to the emergency department with a Glasgow coma scale (GCS) of 14 or 15 and oxygen saturations at or above 95% on room air can be classified as low risk for complications. These patients require a 4- to 6-hour period of observation in the emergency department. Studies have shown that patients with clinical sequelae from submersion injuries will become symptomatic within this time frame. Patients require serial pulmonary examinations and continuous pulse oximetry. Laboratory studies and chest radiography are not required or indicated in this low-risk subset. It is common for the patient to initially have a normal chest radiograph despite lung injury, and physical examination findings will precede any radiographic abnormalities. Basic laboratory testing and blood gas studies are unnecessary if the patient is breathing independently and maintaining oxygen saturations on room air.

Patients who have suffered insult from drowning injuries will begin to show symptoms such as rales, rhonchi, wheeze, stridor, increased work of breathing, or decreased oxygen saturations. Symptomatic patients with respiratory findings on physical examination, inability to maintain oxygen saturation at or above 95% on room air, or any other abnormal findings require an in-depth evaluation and admission to a monitored bed. The main focus from a respiratory standpoint is to prevent further hypoxia while the patient is recovering from the drowning incident. Patients unable to maintain their oxygen saturations at or above 95% on room air require respiratory support with supplemental oxygen. Oxygen saturations at or below 90% or PaO_2 less than 60 on high flow oxygen indicate the need for positive airway pressure. Continuous positive airway pressure (CPAP) can be used to accomplish this. However, the danger of gastric distention and vomiting with aspiration is a consideration as drowning patients have frequently ingested water, which puts them at higher risk. If the patient is unable to maintain saturations with non-invasive ventilation strategies, or develops a $PaCO_2$ greater than 50, intubation is recommended for further support with positive pressure ventilation. High levels of positive end-expiratory pressure (PEEP) may be necessary to recruit fluid-filled areas of lung parenchyma. This must be balanced with the risk of developing lung barotrauma from high peak pressures. Also, PEEP can increase intrathoracic pressures and compromise cardiac return and output which can in turn decrease overall cerebral perfusion. There is no established PaO_2 goal to guide resuscitation. Treatment management must be aimed at prevention of any further hypoxia while the patient is recovering from their injury to optimize neurologic outcome. For critical patients needing frequent arterial blood gas (ABG) monitoring, placement of an arterial line to facilitate these blood draws is reasonable. Administration of prophylactic antibiotic to treat for possible aspiration is still a controversial option, although current studies do not support this practice.

Key steps in management and discharge of emergency department pediatric patients are listed in the following two boxes.

Initial emergency department management of submersion injury.

1. Assess airway, intubate if significant hypoxia or altered mental status using RSI.
2. If not intubated, oxygen via NC, mask, or CPAP.
3. Consider trauma, immobilize C-spine if any concern of injury, including if unknown mechanism.
4. IVF with NS or LR, use warm fluids if hypothermic.
5. If signs of bronchospasm, may try β-agonists.
6. Observe for lung injury.
7. Imaging as needed.

Criteria for patient to be safely discharged home.

- Asymptomatic for observation period of 4-6 h
- Maintain oxygen saturations ≥ 95% on room air
- Patient does not require respiratory support at any time
- GCS 14- GCS 15
- No findings on serial pulmonic physical examination

PROGNOSIS

Extensive studies have been conducted to classify the long-term neurologic outcome of drowning injuries. The efforts have focused on how to predict prognosis upon arrival at the emergency department, and thereby guide resuscitation efforts in the emergency department. There is no classification system to date that predicts which patients will have a poor neurologic outcome. Current systems have misclassified patients as poor outcome when they subsequently had full recovery. It is accepted that prolonged cardiopulmonary arrest, fixed and dilated pupils, and a GCS 3 are indicators of poor neurologic outcome. Likewise, there have been reported cases of complete recovery of patients after cold water submersions, with these same poor prognostic criteria, although this does not appear to be the norm. The question of how aggressively to resuscitate these patients on arrival to emergency department is still up for debate. Ultimately the decision to resuscitate lies with the treating physician.

REFERENCES

American Academy of Pediatrics Committee on Injury, Violence, and Poison Prevention: Prevention of drowning. *Pediatrics.* 2010;126(1):253-262. Epub 2010 May 24 [PMID 20498167].

Bowman SM, Aitken ME, Robbins JM, Baker SP: Trends in US pediatric drowning hospitalizations, 1993-2008. *Pediatrics.* 2012;129(2):275-81. Epub 2012 Jan 16 [PMID: 22250031].

Centers for Disease Control, National Center for Injury and Prevention Control: WISQARS. Available at http://www.cdc.gov/injury/wisqars/. Accessed August 28, 2012.

Dean R, Mulligan J: Management of water incidents: Drowning and hypothermia. *Nurs Stand.* 2009;24(7):35-9 [PMID: 19927557].

Kawati R, Covaciu L, Rubertsson S: Hypothermia after drowning in paediatric patients. *Resuscitation.* 2009;80(11):1325-6. Epub 2009 Aug 26 [PMID: 19713025].

Kenny D, Martin R: Drowning and sudden cardiac death. *Arch Dis Child.* 2011;96(1):5-8. Epub 2010 Jun 28 [PMID: 20584851].

Layon AJ, Modell JH: Drowning: Update 2009. *Anesthesiology.* 2009;110(6):1390-401 [PMID: 19417599].

Szpilman D, Bierens J, Handley A, Orlowski J: *Drowning. N Engl J Med.* 2012;366(22):2102-2110 [PMID: 22646632].

Torres SF, Rodríguez M, Iolster T, et al: [Near drowning in a pediatric population: epidemiology and prognosis]. *Arch Argent Pediatr.* 2009;107(3):234-40 [PMID: 19543632].

Vanden Hoek TL, Morrison LJ, Shuster M, et al: Part 12: cardiac arrest in special situations: 2010 American Heart Association Guidelines for Cardiopulmonary Resuscitation and Emergency Cardiovascular Care. *Circulation.* 2010;122(18 Suppl 3):S829 [PMID: 20956228].

Weiss J: American Academy of Pediatrics Committee on Injury, Violence, and Poison Prevention. Prevention of drowning. *Pediatrics.* 2010;126(1):e253-62. Epub 2010 May 24 [PMID: 20498167].

Wester TE, Cherry AD, Pollock NW, et al: Effects of head and body cooling on hemodynamics during immersed prone exercise at 1 ATA. *J Appl Physiol.* 2009;106(2):691-700. Epub 2008 Nov 20 [PMID: 19023017].

World Health Organization: Media Centre Fact Sheet, Drowning. Available at http://www.who.int/mediacentre/factsheets/fs347/en/. Accessed August 28, 2012.

Youn CS, Choi SP, Yim HW, Park KN: Out-of-hospital cardiac arrest due to drowning: An Utstein style report of 10 years of experience from St. Mary's Hospital. *Resuscitation.* 2009;80(7):778-83. Epub 2009 May 13 [PMID: 19443097].

Fever

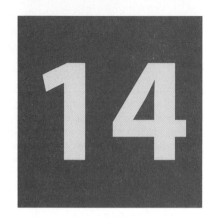

Charles Tad Stiles, MD, FACEP

GENERAL CONSIDERATIONS

Fever constitutes approximately 20% of visits to emergency departments nationwide. It is also the most common pediatric emergency concern. Fever is defined as body temperature greater than 38°C (100.4°F). Fever is induced by exogenous pyrogens from invading organisms and by endogenous pyrogens that are released by immune mediating cells to fight infectious pathogens. The pyrogens cause the body's central "thermostat" in the hypothalamus to reset.

The majority of children presenting with fever will have benign causes and self-limited illness. The child's parent may overtreat a fever or the physician may prescribe antibacterial therapy for a viral illness. Body temperature elevations alarm parents and caretakers, and may result in the child's being brought for evaluation before a clinical syndrome can manifest itself. Fever can make a child uncomfortable, which can cause dehydration from insensible water loss.

The method of temperature measurement should be rectal in a child younger than 2 years as it is the most reliable means in this age group where detecting a fever is imperative. Oral temperatures are typically 1°C (1.8°F) lower and axillary 2°C (3.6°F) lower than rectal but should not be converted or substituted when a rectal measurement is indicated. Axillary temperatures are never appropriate in the emergency department. Tympanic and temporal thermometry are attractive as a less invasive technique but both are well studied to have demonstrated somewhat poor sensitivity for fever detection in pediatric patients.

Research regarding maternal tactile fever detection has shown the child's mother to be accurate slightly greater than 50% of the time. This bears clinical consideration whereas nonvalidated fever is a not an uncommon complaint of emergency department pediatric illness. Excessive swaddling, environmental temperature, operator technique, digital versus mercury thermometer, type of device used,

and consumption of liquids prior to oral measurements can affect measured temperatures.

Although most pediatric fever is caused by viral pathogens, the identification of cause of the fever as an invasive organism and/or a serious bacterial infection (SBI) is imperative to prevent morbidity or death in children. The younger the patient the less reliable the physical examination; infants younger than 3 months must be approached with utmost caution using appropriate clinical guidelines as serious bacterial illness is prevalent in that age group. However, all children younger than 3 years merit thorough evaluation.

ACUTE FEVER FROM BIRTH TO 29 DAYS

General Considerations

Neonates are at high risk for SBI, the incidence of which is approximately 15-20%. Their immune systems are not fully developed, and clinical signs and findings are unreliable. The most common etiology of fever is viral, but group B streptococci, *Escherichia coli*, and *Listeria monocytogenes* are the most common causes of SBI.

Premature rupture of maternal membranes at delivery can be causative of early-onset neonatal sepsis, from days 1 to 8 of life, is usually caused by group B streptococci. Late-onset neonatal sepsis, 8 days and older, is usually caused by Gram-negative enteric organisms and sometimes coagulase-negative *Staphylococcus*. Always investigate the maternal status of herpes simplex virus (HSV) and group B streptococci prophylaxis, prior or active infection, and/or treatment.

Urinary tract infection (UTI) in neonates may not be detectable on initial microscopic examination, and culture only may confirm the diagnosis when the organism is isolated.

Clinical Findings

Important clinical findings that suggest SBI may be subtle or difficult to detect in the neonate and their absence should never be relied upon. Signs in addition to actual or reported fever (≥100.4°F) include hypothermia (≤95°F), poor feeding, cough, vomiting, diarrhea, breathing difficulty, lethargy, or excessive crying. Physical findings may include poor arousability, irritability (crying more when picked up due to meningeal irritation), a bulging fontanelle, respiratory distress such as nasal flaring, grunting, retractions, tender tense abdomen, and vasculitic rashes such as petechiae and/or purpura which are always ominous. Cellulitis of the abdominal wall may be due to omphalitis, an inflammation of the umbilical cord which can cause sepsis. Neonates with HSV infections may present with seizures, focal neurologic findings, elevated liver function tests, or lethargy, with or without characteristic HSV-1 (cold sore) mucous membrane lesions, and/or rhinorrhea.

▶ Evaluation & Treatment

Figure 14–1 outlines the evaluation and treatment for neonates with fever. It cannot be overemphasized that neonates with fever should be assumed to be septic due to the unreliability of clinical findings and the neonate's underdeveloped immune system. Attention to airway, breathing, and circulation (ABC) is paramount, and fluid maintenance and resuscitation should be initiated as necessary. Lumbar puncture should be performed.

Laboratory studies and interventions include complete blood cell count (CBC) with blood culture, urinalysis and urine culture, chest x-ray, examination of cerebrospinal fluid (CSF) for white blood cell count (WBC), glucose, protein, Gram stain and culture, and stool culture if diarrhea

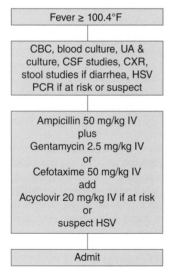

▲ **Figure 14–1.** Evaluation and treatment guideline for infants aged ≤ 28 days.

is present. Consider viral testing of CSF for HSV when suspected. Seasonal testing for other viral illnesses (influenza, enterovirus) yields information but should not change overall management for hospital admission and antibacterial therapy.

Antibiotic choices are targeted to cover group B streptococci, *Escherichia coli*, and *Listeria monocytogenes* which include ampicillin 50 mg/kg combined with either cefotaxime 50 mg/kg (if meningitis suspected or confirmed) or gentamycin 2.5 mg/kg. Data show that survival in neonatal sepsis may be increased with empiric use of gentamycin over cefotaxime. Ceftriaxone use in this age group is discouraged because neonates cannot metabolize and/or excrete it well, especially with preexisting hyperbilirubinemia.

▶ Disposition

All patients in this age group should be admitted for IV antibiotic therapy for treatment of SBI.

ACUTE FEVER IN INFANTS AGED 29-90 DAYS

▶ General Considerations

The reliability of the clinical assessment improves with the age of the child in this group. The risk of SBI in infants aged 60-80 days decreases from approximately 12% until risk approaches that in older children. Pneumococcus and influenza virus type B are prevalent pathogens in this age group although the latter continues to decrease in surveillance studies.

Infants with an obvious viral syndrome such as bronchiolitis, croup, or viral stomatitis have a lower risk for concomitant SBI with the exception of urinary tract infection. This holds true for infants who test positive for influenza. Several observation tools and clinical assessment criteria have been described for assessment of infants with SBI, but most have a only a moderate positive predictive value despite their demonstrated high sensitivity.

▶ Clinical Findings

In addition to clinical findings discussed above for the neonatal age group, an irritable fussy infant, or one who refuses to feed with a fever can be harboring a serious bacterial infection. Classic nuchal rigidity is found in approximately 25% of patients in this age group. Poor muscle tone, poor skin perfusion, weak cry, minimal response to painful procedures, and overall lethargy suggest sepsis. On the other hand, infants older than 30 days who have nasal congestion, coughing, and sneezing with an overall good clinical appearance with a fever likely manifest a viral upper respiratory infection (URI).

Evaluation & Treatment

Figure 14–2 outlines evaluation and treatment for infants aged 29 days to 3 months. In this age group the septic evaluation may be tailored. A chest x-ray may not be necessary in a child who is well-appearing and does not exhibit tachypnea, tachycardia, wheezing, a cough, or other respiratory symptoms. A urinalysis should always be obtained noting that UTIs may not present with pyuria, and a urine culture should be obtained and followed up. A CBC and blood culture should be obtained, and admission is recommended for SBI if the WBC is greater than 15,000, although the recommendations come from the prepneumococcal and pre-HIB vaccine era. A lumbar puncture may not be necessary if the infant aged 60-90 days is clearly not toxic; however, it should be performed in the 29- to 60-day-old infant.

Disposition

Well-appearing infants in this age group may be managed as outpatients if their workup is normal. If the decision is made to discharge the patient, the caregivers must be responsible and reliable. Assured clinical follow-up must be arranged and available within 24 hours. A third-generation cephalosporin (ceftriaxone) may be used as empiric antibiotic therapy for occult bacteremia if the child is discharged, but if this antimicrobial modality is used, a lumbar puncture should then be performed. Patients should be admitted who are ill-appearing, have abnormal workup, or have unreliable care giver.

ACUTE FEVER AGE 3 TO 36 MONTHS

General Considerations

Most causes of infection in this age group are viral. Day care attendance and immunization status should be strongly considered in the evaluation. The older and more verbal the child makes the physical assessment more reliable. Fever without a source (FWS) is clinical instance of a child in whom the history, physical and laboratory/radiological investigations are unable to reveal a source of the temperature elevation, but when this occurs it is less of a concern for serious infection in the well-appearing immunized infant and toddler.

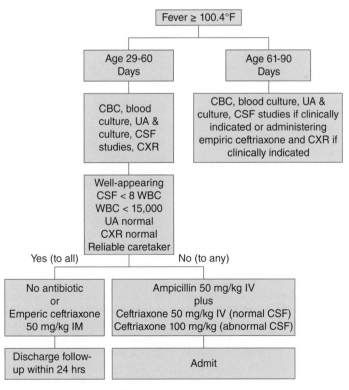

▲ **Figure14–2.** Evaluation and treatment guideline for infants aged 29-90 days.

An important clinical consideration for investigations (with the exception of urinalysis) and empiric antimicrobial therapy in children with FWS is whether they have had at least three of the pneumococcal and HIB vaccinations which are given at approximately 6 months of age. The heptavalent pneumococcal vaccine has markedly decreased the incidence of SBI from this organism in this age group, and newer more polyvalent vaccines are in development that may cover more than a dozen strains. The *H. influenza* vaccine has been highly effective in decreasing infections from this organism.

Skin infections from group A β-hemolytic *Strepococcus* (GAS) and *S. aureus* (especially community-acquired methicillin resistant) are more common. If bacteremia occurs in this age group, many will be from *S. pneumoniae* with overall favorable outcomes, even in children not treated with antimicrobials. Causes of fever such as autoimmune disease (discussed below), Kawasaki, osteomyelitis, atypical infections, and/or zoonoses, oropharyngeal including odontogenic infections, malignancy/leukemia, and appendicitis are included in the differential diagnosis. Children in this age group may complain of headache with fever, and it is not unusual to have them present to the emergency department on oral antibiotic therapy for a presumed otitis or sinusitis. In these children, the classic signs of meningeal irritation may not be present due to partially treated meningitis.

Clinical Findings

The overall appearance of the child is more helpful in this age group because well-appearing patients are less likely to harbor an SBI. Head, ears, eyes, nose, and throat (HEENT) examination may reveal otitis or pharyngitis with minimal concerns. Otitis media alone is a rare cause of the fever when fever results from an overlying associated viral URI. Rhinorrhea or nasal congestion with active coughing and sneezing that accompany a viral URI is often the hallmark of the diagnosis as cause of a fever.

Neck and facial masses may be odontogenic infections or lymphadenopathy (LAN), whereas the latter is usually associated with streptococcus pharyngitis. Massive cervical LAN may be seen with mononucleosis or leukemia.

Lungs may have rhonchi, rales and/or wheezes, and the presence or absence of retractions and/or accessory muscle use should be noted. Palpation of the abdomen is important to document for the presence of absence of tenderness as well as masses, liver, or splenic enlargement. Palpation of the extremities or observation of the child walking is important for the consideration of soft tissue, bone, or joint infections.

The presence of types of rashes can be either diagnostic or confounding but the presence of morbilliform or migrating nonspecific maculopapular rashes are seen frequently with viral illness, whereas characteristic rashes can be seen with rubella, fifth disease, and other viral xanthems. The nonspecific rash of Kawasaki can involve the palms and soles, and characteristically is associated with a strawberry tongue, cheilosis of the lips, and an exudative conjunctivitis.

Evaluation & Treatment

Following attention to ABCs, the overall clinical appearance of the child is a reliable indicator as to whether an evaluation for sepsis is necessary. Obtaining CBC and blood culture are necessary only in ill children or those with a suspected bacterial focus such as pneumonia or significant abscess or soft tissue infection. Routine blood cultures are simply not indicated for this age group in vaccinated, well-appearing children.

Chest x-ray is indicated if respiratory symptoms do not appear to be viral, when tachypnea or tachycardia are present, and with first-time wheezing episodes. Urinalysis and urine culture should be obtained if UTI is suspected, especially if no other source for fever is found in high-risk groups such as uncircumcised males.

CSF studies would be indicated in children with altered mental status that does not improve with resuscitative measures, children with headache or neck pain, and or stiffness especially if the child is on oral antibiotic therapy, as partially treated meningitis can be clinically misleading. Upper respiratory tract viral antigen testing should be obtained if it will prognosticate outcome or change management, as with RSV or influenza. An abscess drainage or joint fluid obtained should be cultured for sensitivities of the organism in order to tailor antimicrobial therapy.

The major cause for fever in this age group is viral; therefore, strong consideration of this should weigh in regarding the treatment of otitis, sinusitis, and other URIs with antimicrobial therapy.

Disposition

Close follow-up is necessary for children upon discharge from the emergency department because illness can progress and bacterial superinfections with viral URIs can occur. Ill-appearing children or those identified with a serious infection from the evaluation should be admitted.

ACUTE FEVER IN THE OLDER CHILD

General Considerations

With the exception of children with developmental delay or impaired communication, older pediatric patients will be able to localize their symptoms and give more reliable history. When the examiner is able to approach the child in a nonthreatening manner, the reward is not infrequently a presumed diagnosis at the bedside. The risk of bacteremia in this age group is less than 1%, and meningitis can frequently be suspected clinically. However, UTIs still occur in children, especially those with congenital urologic abnormalities or spina bifida.

Children with cerebral palsy, impaired airway reflexes or swallowing, or with significant gastroesophageal reflux are at risk for aspiration pneumonia. Day care centers and schools transmit a number of infections among children. Additionally, nonimmunized or underimmunized children may harbor illness outside the "herd immunity" benefit of their environment. Adolescents may manifest systemic symptoms of a sexually transmitted pathogen. Most infections will be determined to be viral based upon a reliable clinical assessment.

▶ Clinical Findings

Because they are verbal, children in this age group are able to localize their symptoms for bacterial causes of the fever, and the general malaise associated with viral infections will be apparent. Clinical findings for children aged 3-36 months apply to older children (discussed previously). Abdominal and neurological examination will be more reliable as age and development progress. The sinuses become more developed with age and an intranasal examination and palpation of the sinuses should be done on older children with fever. Inspection of the skin and perineum should be done, and palpation of the joints and regional lymph nodes should not be overlooked.

Mononucleosis syndromes may have characteristic anterior and posterior cervical adenopathy, exudative pharyngitis, hepatosplenomegaly, and telltale rash. Adolescent patients with sexually transmitted infection (STI) may have pustular rashes, arthritis, urethritis or cervicitis; however, patients with primary HIV may have only flu-like presentation with diffuse lymphadenopathy. Skin abscesses and cellulitis are more common with community-acquired MRSA causing the majority of skin abscesses, and M-protein–producing streptococcus strains are becoming a major pathogen in cellulitis.

▶ Evaluation & Treatment

Attention to ABCs is the priority, with consideration of sepsis in ill-appearing children prompting adequate and prompt resuscitation and appropriate empiric antibiotic therapy. In well-appearing children who are fully vaccinated, blood cultures are not necessary as bacteremia should not be a major concern. As for the possibility of UTI, the algorithms and current recommendations in regards to risk should be followed, including urine culture. Viral antigen testing and management in this age group of children is the same as for infants 3-36 months (discussed above) because the positive and negative predictive values of rapid influenza testing deceases with age; therefore, the practitioner should be cautious about foregoing a lumbar puncture for the sake of a positive influenza screen.

Rapid streptococcus screen laboratory testing of the throat is likely to yield a true positive as a bacterial cause of fever and pharyngitis in the absence of viral symptoms; however, the resource can be overutilized if the clinician does not consider the Centor criteria in decision making. Blood cultures should be obtained in patients with complicated bacterial pneumonia and cellulitis as well as suspected bacteremia. A CSF should be obtained for a clinically significant headache with fever, in all children who are taking antibiotics and an alternative HEENT infection cannot be identified. It is not unusual for a child with fever and vague abdominal pain to harbor lower lobe pneumonia, thus a chest x-ray should be considered in cases of upper quadrant pain or tenderness.

Aspiration and drainage of inflamed joints, abscesses, and infected wounds for culture and sensitivity should be undertaken. Sexually active adolescent patients with referable symptoms should have skin pustules opened for Gram stain and culture, and urethral and cervical specimens sent for genitourinary symptoms, groin lymphadenopathy, or lower abdominal pain with fever. Testing for HIV disease should be done either in the emergency department or by referring the patient to their primary care physician or local health department, if STD is suspected.

Consider noninfectious causes of fever when prolonged or unusual fever patterns occur, especially with marked constitutional symptoms, lymphadenopathy, joint involvement, and other uncommon manifestations. Ultimately viral syndromes and fever can be managed expectantly and treated symptomatically as in other age groups.

Any unclear source of fever or fever associated with abdominal symptoms after appropriate CT, magnetic resonance imaging (MRI), or ultrasound imaging should have close follow-up with instructions to return to the emergency department if symptoms worsen or have not significantly improved as expected, and symptoms reviewed with caregivers.

▶ Disposition

Most children in this age group can be discharged from the emergency department. Ill-appearing patients or those identified with a serious infection from the evaluation should be admitted.

FEVER OF UNKNOWN ORIGIN

▶ General Considerations

Fever of unknown origin in children most often is eventually determined to be an unusual or atypical presentation of a more common entity. The practical definition is fever of at least 8 days in duration without apparent source from an adequate history, physical examination, appropriate ancillary laboratory, and/or radiologic imaging as either outpatient or inpatient. The common causes are infections, neoplasms, or connective tissue disease. The source of reported fever should be considered, as a malfunctioning electronic thermometer or factitious fever can prompt a litany of resource-consuming diagnostic studies.

The pattern of fever is important. Fluctuating or spiking fever can be seen with lymphomas, endocarditis, sarcoidosis, tuberculosis, occult abscesses, or juvenile idiopathic arthritis (JIA; formerly juvenile rheumatoid arthritis). Patients may be fever-free between pyrexic episodes with malaria, other bloodborne cancers, and rat-bite fever. Hereditary dysautonomic syndromes may cause isolated fever episodes over a period of weeks or months. Travel history is important for consideration of malaria, dengue, or other arthropod-associated or hemorrhagic fever viruses, hepatitis, Rocky Mountain spotted fever (RMSF), or typhus. Camping, dense wood exposure, or tick bites suggest RMSF or Lyme disease.

Food consumption must be reviewed with consideration for hepatitis, brucellosis, and salmonella. Contact with animals or possession of pets is important with consideration for parvovirus (dogs), pasteurella or bartonella (dog or cat bite/scratch), salmonella (captive bred reptiles), toxoplasmosis (cat excrement), recently pregnant cats or cattle (Q fever), or skinned animals while hunting (tularemia). Consideration of HIV infection should be included and the environmental or exposure risk examined.

▶ Clinical Findings

The child with sinusitis may not be diagnosed if one is not looking for physical examination findings such as purulent drainage from the posterior nose to the throat accompanied by sinus tenderness. Conjunctivitis may be associated with Kawasaki or leptospirosis, whereas uveitis may develop in various autoimmune conditions.

Oropharyngeal or tonsillar exudates associated with an assumed resistant streptococcus infection may be seen with mononucleosis or Epstein-Barr virus (EBV). Regional lymphadenopathy can occur in lymphoma, EBV, cytomegalovirus (CMV), or catscratch disease (CSD), whereas diffuse lymphadenopathy may be appreciated in leukemia or HIV disease. A new or pathological murmur suggests endocarditis. Hepatosplenomegaly is often present in EBV, whereas splenic enlargement may be seen in salmonella infection. A palpable abdominal mass with fever and hematuria suggests a Wilm tumor of the kidney. Periodic fevers with aphthous stomatitis, pharyngitis, and adenitis (PFAPA syndrome) is considered when fever-free episodes occur over months and sometimes years with the characteristic clinical findings in its eponym.

Characteristic rashes include pupura as seen in vasculitic or platelet-related illness, or petechiae in rickettsial illness, endocarditis, and other systemic infections or endothelial processes. The typical rash of RMSF appears petechial and begins on the wrists and ankles to spread centrally, whereas chickenpox lesions are pustular and vesicular and usually appear on the scalp or hairline before becoming generalized. Diffuse deep-colored macular rashes may be seen with serum sickness and are accompanied by joint swelling; however, if these occur after amoxicillin use for a pharyngitis the physician should consider undiagnosed EBV rather than a drug reaction if the arthritis component is not present.

Acute rheumatic fever (ARF) can be diagnosed with multiple joint arthritis, cardiac findings, chorea, and or characteristic skin findings of erythema marginatum or subcutaneous nodules in the setting of recent GAS infection. Eschars or pustules may develop at the inoculation site for tularemia or CSD. A salmon-colored macular rash is associated with JIA. Palpation of the muscles is important to detect a deep soft tissue abscess, and bone tenderness may be seen in osteomyelitis and malignancies.

▶ Evaluation & Treatment

Laboratory studies should be ordered by considering the history, physical examination, demographics, and exposures of the child with an ongoing unknown origin fever. The CBC should include a smear for consideration of hematologic malignancy and malaria. High neutrophil counts are associated with infection. A number of authorities recommend erythocyte sedimentation rate (ESR) test and C-reactive protein (CRP) test as these are generally indicated as markers of inflammation. If the indices are normal a factitious cause for fever remains in the differential. Despite their lack of specificity, markedly high levels of CRP and especially ESR suggest autoimmune disease or malignancy.

Several sets of blood cultures should be obtained over time in a 12- to 24-hour period when suspecting occult abscesses or endocarditis. Urinalysis and urine culture should be done, and repeated if equivocal results occur. Chest x-ray should be included in the evaluation, and sinus imaging, preferably limited CT, should be considered with persisting upper respiratory symptoms with or without headache. If significant headache is present with fever, lumbar puncture should be performed, especially in a child who is already on antibiotic therapy. If focal neurological findings are noted with any CSF pleocytosis, tuberculosis (TB), fungal studies, and HSV PCR/culture should be ordered on the fluid obtained.

Liver enzyme abnormalities may be seen with CMV or EBV. Testing for HIV should be considered in children evaluated for FUO. Specific serologies may be sent for JIA, lupus, EBV, CMV, toxoplasmosis, tularemia, brucellosis, leptospirosis, CSD, and rickettsial illnesses. If intra-abdominal abscess is considered, ultrasound imaging is preferred to CT as the first study.

▶ Disposition

Children with FUO can be discharged from the emergency department with close follow-up. Patients should be admitted for treatment or further evaluation if they are ill-appearing or a serious infection has been diagnosed from the emergency department.

FEVER IN THE IMMUNE COMPROMISED CHILD

Children with fever and malignancy are a potential medical emergency and their absolute neutrophil count should be evaluated, blood, urine, and other appropriate cultures obtained, and the hematologist/oncologist consulted for definitive care (see Chapter 40).

Immune deficiency syndromes may require gamma globulin or other immune-modulating therapy in consultation with the appropriate specialist. Sickle cell patients are usually functionally asplenic by 10 years of age, and antimicrobial therapy selected should cover encapsulated organisms. The treatment choice holds for children who have undergone splenectomy. Children with connective tissue diseases, idiopathic thrombocytopenic purpura (ITP), or other illnesses taking chronic steroids should be considered to be functionally immune suppressed with their fever. The child with HIV and fever should be managed in close consultation with an infectious disease specialist. Pediatric patients with indwelling lines or devices should have the sites cultured where possible with line sepsis or device infection considered as a possible source of the fever. Consider tapping ventricular drainage devices or shunts for a sample of CSF to check for bacterial infection, using strict sterile technique in consultation with a neurosurgeon.

FEVER MANAGEMENT

Discomfort associated with fever can be distressing for a child due to the release of endogenous and exogenous pyrogens that cause myalgia and overall body discomfort, particularly in some viral infections. As discussed previously, recalibration of the hypothalamic set point to induce fever is an important mechanism by which the body blocks metabolism and replication of an invasive organism. Proven therapies for fever reduction include acetaminophen and ibuprofen. It is commonplace for children to have been underdosed with these antipyretics upon initial presentation to the emergency department, as the package recommended dosing regimens are based upon age and not weight. In addition, for safety reasons, the packaging indicates a lower dosage than expected body weight within each age group. Because of the association with Reye syndrome, aspirin and aspirin products should never be given to febrile children.

Fever phobia is a common phenomenon among care takers of children as well as medical and hospital personnel regarding the danger of fever. Frequently unjustified fears about fever range from seizures to brain damage, in addition to the legitimate fear of possibility of an SBI being present. Individuals unrealistically expect a child's body temperature to normalize with antipyretic therapy. Ancillary emergency department personnel may believe it is necessary for a child's temperature to be markedly improved prior to discharge. Chills and shivering may be misinterpreted by observers to be seizure activity. Parents may utilize cool baths or more unconventional means such as bathing with rubbing alcohol. These measures may actually induce more shivering and paradoxically raise body temperature while alcohol vapors may induce toxicity or hypoglycemia.

An important component of the disposition and parental education for the febrile child includes appropriate and safe use of antipyretic medications. The optimal dosing regimen for acetaminophen is 10-15 mg/kg orally every 4 to 6 hours as needed. Rectal doses may be administered safely up to 30 mg/kg on the same schedule. A notable caution about acetaminophen is that it is available in two different concentrations: 160 mg/5 mL and as a 100 mg/mL dropper for infants. The latter is being phased out by pharmaceutical companies for safety reasons, as the potential for dosing confusion exists.

Ibuprofen may be given at 5-10 mg/kg every 6 to 8 hours as needed for children older than 6 months. It is commonplace for parents to use an "alternating" regimen between acetaminophen and ibuprofen, although no data shows that this method is substantially more effective than using either agent alone. For extreme malaise or myalgias with fever there is no harm in taking both drugs together at appropriate intervals (acetaminophen every 4 hours and ibuprofen every 8 hours) as long as care is taken not to confuse dosing. Although data show fever may be lowered earlier with ibuprofen which has a longer duration of action than acetaminophen, there is no overall difference in effectiveness. Ibuprofen has been reported to cause renal toxicity in patients with marked volume depletion, and it can also be difficult to tolerate for children with gastritis and vomiting. There is potential for liver toxicity to develop if acetaminophen is overdosed. A useful patient education and safety tool is to offer parents a premarked syringe to take home after demonstrating how to dose and administer the drugs with it.

Children with unrelenting high fever greater than 103°F (39.4°C) should be reevaluated for progressive or new infection, and a child with a body temperature greater than 105.8°F (41.0°C) should be treated as hyperpyrexia as a medical emergency with appropriate cooling measures.

American College of Emergency Physicians Clinical Policies Committee: Clinical policy for children younger than three years presenting to the emergency department with fever. *Ann Emerg Med.* 2003;42:530-545 [PMID:14520324].

Bilavsky E, Shouval DS, Yarden-Bilavshy H, et al: A prospective study of the risk for serious bacterial infections in hospitalized febrile infants with or without bronchiolitis. *Pediatr Infect Dis J.* 2008;27:269-270 [PMID: 18277919].

Clark RH, Bloom BT, Spitzer AR, et al: Empiric use of ampicillin and cefotaxime, compared with ampicillin and gentamycin, for neonates at risk for sepsis is associated with an increased risk for neonatal death. *Pediatrics.* 2006;117:67-74 [PMID: 16396862].

Claudius I: An evidence-based review of neonatal emergencies. *Pediatr Emerg Med Pract.* 2010;7:8.

Crocetti, M, Moghbeli N, Serwint J: Fever phobia revisited: Have parental misconceptions about fever changed in 20 years? *Pediatrics.* 2001;107:1241-6 [PMID: 11389237].

Hurt TL, Kim T, Washke D, el al: The things kids bring home from abroad: Evaluating the returning child traveler with fever. *Pediatr Emerg Med Pract.* 2005;2:11.

Ingarfield SL, Celenza A, Jacobs IG, Riley TV: Outcomes in patients with an emergency department diagnosis of fever of unknown origin. *Emerg Med Australas.* 2007;19:105-12 [PMID: 17448095].

Krief WI, Levine DA, Platt SL, et al: Influenza virus infection and the risk of serious bacterial infections in young febrile infants. *Pediatrics.* 2009;124:30-9 [PMID: 19564280].

National Center for Biotechnology Information: Evidence Report/ Technology Assessment, No. 205: Diagnosis and Management of Febrile Infants (0-3 Months). Rockville, MD: 2012. Available at http://www.ncbi.nlm.nih.gov/books/NBK92690/pdf/TOC. pdf. Accessed May 5, 2013.

Pierce CA, Voss B: Efficacy and safety of ibuprofen and acetaminophen in children and adults: A meta-analysis and qualitative review. *Ann Pharmacother.* 2010;44:489-506 [PMID: 20150507].

Vergnano S, Sharland M, Kazembe P, et al: Neonatal sepsis: An international perspective. *Arch Dis Child Fetal Neonatal Ed.* 2005;90:F220-4 [PMID: 15846011].

Abdominal Pain

Ryan P. Morrissey, MD

Emily A. Porter, MD

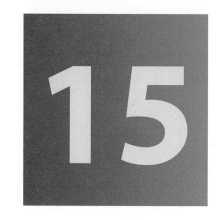

EVALUATION OF THE PEDIATRIC PATIENT WITH ABDOMINAL PAIN

HISTORY

A detailed history should be performed only after the practitioner has evaluated and stabilized the patient, and established that no life-threatening conditions are present. A meticulous history is crucial in guiding the practitioner in the management of abdominal pain including laboratory and radiographic evaluations, differential diagnosis, necessity for specialist consultation, and disposition. Depending on the age of the child, obtaining a detailed history of abdominal pain can be challenging. In younger children, parents often perceive that their child's abdomen hurts based on facial expression or body movements such as writhing or drawing up the knees. Localization of pain may prove difficult based on history alone. Key features of history include presence, duration, and location of pain; presence or absence of fever; feeding and bowel habits; last oral intake; frequency and character of stools and vomitus; presence of blood in stools or vomitus; urinary symptoms; menstrual history; vaginal discharge/bleeding; respiratory symptoms; travel history, and changes in weight.

Special attention should be paid to significant past medical history including history of prematurity, congenital anomalies, inborn errors of metabolism, sickle cell disease, necrotizing enterocolitis, cystic fibrosis, and intussusception. A thorough review of systems is mandatory as abdominal pain is often a symptom of disorders originating in other organ systems such as ear, nose, and throat (ENT [pharyngitis]), genitourinary(GU [UTI, ectopic pregnancy, hernia]), vascular (Henoch-Schönlein purpura), and pulmonary (lower lobe pneumonia). The discriminating practitioner keeps in mind an age-appropriate differential during the history as common causes of abdominal pain vary significantly in the pediatric population, especially among infants.

The differential diagnosis of common causes of acute abdominal pain is listed in Table 15–1.

Age

Age-specific causes of abdominal pain help determine the differential diagnosis, as many causes occur primarily during infancy, the toddler years, or after further development. For example, appendicitis is exceedingly rare in children younger than 2 years and malrotation is extremely uncommon in children older than 2 years. Necrotizing enterocolitis can present with very few symptoms before overt sepsis, but knowing that a neonate was born at 29 weeks' gestation and is presenting with apparent abdominal pain 3 weeks later will aid the practitioner in early diagnosis.

Gender

There are several conditions that tend to occur with greater frequency in either males or females, which can help the clinician further narrow the differential diagnosis. In addition to the more complex differential diagnosis for females of reproductive age, there are other disease processes when gender makes a diagnosis more or less likely in the pediatric patient with abdominal pain. Both intussusception and pyloric stenosis occur more than twice as frequently in males. Females have three to four times the incidence of urinary tract infections (UTIs) as uncircumcised males.

Anorexia, Nausea, & Vomiting

While common, the presence or absence of anorexia, nausea, and vomiting does not rule out surgical causes of abdominal pain in children. A key distinguishing factor in the pediatric patient is the presence of bilious emesis, usually indicative of a surgical emergency such as obstruction, intussusception, malrotation with or without midgut volvulus, or incarcerated

Table 15–1. Differential diagnosis of acute abdominal pain.

Disease	Characteristics of Pain	Epidemiology	Associated Symptoms	Physical Examination	Laboratory and Radiographic Evaluation
Appendicitis +/− perforation	Periumbilical gradually localized to RLQ becoming acute and persistent	Peaks in adolescence (due to maximal lymphoid hyperplasia) & rare < 2 y; often presents with peritonitis or sepsis due to delayed diagnosis in young children; perforation: (90% < 3 y, < 15% adolescents)	Fever, vomiting, diarrhea, diffuse pain, distention, right hip complaints, lethargy, or irritability	Fever, RLQ, or periumbilical tenderness	Leukocytosis not sensitive; abdominal ultrasound (sensitivity, 80–92%; specificity, 86–98%; appendix not visualized in 10% with appendicitis); abdominal CT (sensitivity, 87–100% and highest with both oral and colonic contrast; specificity 83–97%)
Intussusception	Colicky, severe, and intermittent. Child may draw legs up to abdomen and kick legs in air. Child appears calm and relieved between attacks.	Peak at 10 mo; rare < 3 mo; 2–4 times more common in males	Intermittent pain, fever, vomiting, poor feeding, lethargy, bloody or mucous stools	"Dance sign" or "sausage" in RLQ; abdominal mass	Barium or water-soluble enema gold standard for diagnosis and therapy; US (sensitivity, 95–98%; specificity 88–94%) as adjunct to monitor therapeutic effect
Malrotation/ midgut volvulus	Vague, diffuse, or nonexistent	75% diagnosed by 1 y; Peak at < 1 mo (50%)	Feeding intolerance, bilious emesis, abdominal pain, peritonitis and shock	Normal abdominal examination in 50% of patients due to proximal obstruction; distention; peritoneal signs; signs of shock	Upper GI is gold standard, revealing taper/beak of contrast and malpositioned ligament of Treitz; plain films may reveal SBO, LBO, or nothing
Pyloric stenosis	Intermittent, diffuse, vague, or nonexistent	Peaks at 3–5 wk; Males 2–5 times more common (especially firstborn or with family history)	Postprandial projectile nonbilious emesis; dehydration	May reveal palpable "olive-sized" mass at RUQ (90% specific, < 50% sensitive) or increased LUQ peristalsis	Hypochloremic metabolic alkalosis, hypokalemia, hyponatremia, paradoxical aciduria; US or UGI is gold standard (both > 90% sensitive and specific)
Incarcerated hernia	Intermittent at first; then steady in unilateral groin	Inguinal hernia ranges from 3–5% in term; 7–30% preterm; familial; 90% of inguinal hernias occur in males; 6:1 male to female ratio of incarcerated inguinal hernia; R 60%, L 30%, 10% bilateral. Highest risk of incarceration is 1st y of life, hence most congenital hernias repaired	Painful, swollen bulge under the skin, usually worse with crying or straining; anorexia, nausea, vomiting, and fever	Tender inguinal bulge cannot be reduced; worse when child crying; dusky overlying skin. Reduction of nonincarcerated hernia easier with analgesics and/or sedation	Testicular ultrasound helpful to rule out testicular torsion but should not delay immediate surgical consultation
Necrotizing enterocolitis	Diffuse, vague, or nonexistent	Neonates—equal gender term infants < 7 d; premature infants < 21 d	Distention; poor feeding; vomiting; diarrhea; lethargy; apnea; gross blood in stool (25%)	Increased abdominal girth, visible intestinal loops, decreased bowel sounds, palpable mass, abdominal wall erythema	KUB shows pneumatosis intestinalis in 50–75%; delayed gastric emptying

(Continued)

Table 15–1. Differential diagnosis of acute abdominal pain. (*Continued*)

Disease	Characteristics of Pain	Epidemiology	Associated Symptoms	Physical Examination	Laboratory and Radiographic Evaluation
Hepatitis	RUQ, vague, or nonexistent	HBV and HCV can be transmitted in utero; 70-80% are HAV	Headache, anorexia, malaise, abdominal discomfort, nausea, vomiting	Hepatomegaly, sometimes tender; icterus, jaundice; ascites, varices, or splenomegaly	Serum AST, ALT, alkaline phosphatase, GGT, bilirubin, and albumin; coagulation studies; lactic acid; consider viral serology
Pancreatitis	Epigastric—radiates to back; post prandial; rapid onset; continuous; severe	Mostly idiopathic or congenital; sometimes medications, hypertriglyceridemia, cholelithiasis, or trauma	Nausea; vomiting; diarrhea; sometimes fever or lethargy	Epigastric tenderness; ecchymosis at epigastrium or flank; severe cases may present with sepsis	Serum lipase, amylase, electrolytes, and CRP; CBC; ultrasound for cholelithiasis and pancreatic edema; CT with PO and IV contrast may help to evaluate pseudocyst
Cystitis & pyelonephritis	Suprapubic or generalized abdominal pain; sometimes flank or back pain	Account for 5-14% of pediatric emergency department visits; prevalence highest for females < 2 y and males < 1 y; uncircumcised males 6-20 times risk vs circumcised; females < 12 mo 3-4 times risk	Vomiting; poor feeding; fussiness; dysuria, frequency, or new incontinence; fever (2-12%) more likely in younger patients	Suprapubic tenderness; fever; costovertebral angle tenderness	Clean catch or catheterized urinalysis; consider urine culture
Renal colic	Costovertebral or lower quadrant along course of ureter	10 times less common than in adults; 20-40% incidentally found; associated with family history, congenital diseases and metabolic derangements	Asymptomatic; generalized pain; hematuria; recurrent UTI; vomiting; constipation; enuresis	Abdominal examination usually normal; generalized tenderness	Urinalysis; serum creatinine; renal/abdominal ultrasound adequate primary imaging modality; CT more sensitive and specific (may require contrast to evaluate obstruction or radiolucent stones)
Ovarian torsion	Unilateral	Females; 25% have normal ovaries	Unilateral lower abdominal pain (maybe intermittent); nausea, vomiting;	Adnexal mass palpable 20-40%	Ultrasound diagnostic (Doppler); may be false negative if study done during period of detorsion; US or CT may show ovarian cyst/mass or pelvic free fluid; laparoscopy diagnostic
Ectopic pregnancy	Unilateral early; may become diffuse after rupture	Females; sudden onset of sharp pain with rupture	Nausea, vomiting, abdominal pain, vaginal bleeding; frequently asymptomatic	Adnexal tenderness +/– palpable mass	Ultrasound showing extrauterine pregnancy +/– pelvic free fluid; positive pregnancy test
Testicular torsion	Unilateral in scrotum or groin; may wax and wane	Males; rarely before puberty; 12% bilateral	Testicular, inguinal, lower abdominal, or flank pain; nausea, vomiting	Tender, "high-riding" testis with horizontal lie; epididymis indistinguishable from testis; absent cremasteric reflex; ipsilateral leg flexed at hip and knee;	Ultrasound diagnostic (Doppler); may be false negative if study done during period of detorsion; surgical exploration definitively diagnostic

inguinal hernia. Bilious emesis typically requires emergent surgical consultation.

Fever & Rigors

Fever is a common presenting symptom for which parents seek emergency treatment of their child. It is also commonly associated with many causes of abdominal pain, mostly infectious. In cases of delayed diagnosis, especially with nonverbal children, fever or sepsis may be the presenting symptom in the absence of any known abdominal pain. Systemic inflammatory signs such as fever and rigors, when observed in patients with abdominal pain, suggest either an extrabdominal/systemic disease with abdominal manifestations or abdominal pathology that has progressed to become systemic. The combination of vital signs, physical examination, including a detailed abdominal examination, and a review of symptoms should help differentiate these two possibilities.

Character of Stool

▶ Diarrhea, Constipation, & Obstipation

It is important to ask about the frequency and characteristics of stool in the pediatric patient as details can hint toward causes of abdominal pain. Diarrhea in the setting of abdominal pain suggests an infectious or allergic process. It is of special consequence in younger children as they may dehydrate much more quickly than adults. The parents and clinician should focus on signs of dehydration and attempt rehydration via oral, intravenous, or the emerging dermoclysis method. Constipation is a common cause of functional abdominal pain in children, particularly if it is chronic. New onset constipation combined with abdominal pain or nausea and vomiting is more suggestive of an obstructive process. Beware the patient with diarrhea and a history of constipation and laxative use, as there is likely encopresis with ongoing fecal impaction.

▶ Hematochezia & Melena

Hematochezia is associated with conditions such as constipation with hemorrhoids, anal fissure, and lower gastrointestinal (GI) bleeding. In children, this may be in the form of Meckel diverticulum which can also serve as a lead point for intussusception. Melena is generally from upper GI bleeding, but in breast-fed infants, it can also be from swallowed maternal blood or a nasopharyngeal source such as epistaxis. The classic "currant jelly" stool in intussusception is a late and somewhat ominous finding as it suggests bowel necrosis.

PHYSICAL EXAMINATION

The abdominal examination in younger children can be quite difficult resulting from pain and trust issues, thus requiring the utilization of more nontraditional methods than with adults. Distraction is especially helpful as are serial examinations.

When possible, examine the younger child's abdomen while he or she is being held by the parent. Assess peritoneal signs by secondary methods such as having the child skip, hop, climb, or play. Engage the child or parent in palpation of the abdomen by having him or her place a hand on the abdomen with the practitioner's on top, which can also reduce ticklish sensation. Close examination of the overall appearance (lethargic versus playful, hydration status, toxic appearance) of the child may be as helpful as the abdominal examination itself.

A thorough general physical examination is required in addition to a focused abdominal examination to exclude extra-abdominal causes of abdominal pain such as pharyngitis and pneumonia. When appropriate, a pelvic examination should be performed.

Inspection

Evaluate for scars, feeding tubes, ostomies, distention, ecchymosis, erythema, jaundice, abnormal vasculature, peristalsis, and protruding masses.

Auscultation

With the bell of the stethoscope, listen in all four quadrants and midline for peristaltic sounds. High-pitched sounds are indicative of partial obstruction.

Percussion

Normal percussion should elicit dullness in the right upper quadrant (RUQ) over the liver, hollow note over the stomach in the left upper quadrant (LUQ), and a flat percussion note elsewhere. Splenic enlargement produces dullness in the LUQ over the lower ribs. Bladder enlargement produces dullness in the suprapubic area. Rebound is pain elicited by percussion remote to the immediate site of examination and is suggestive of peritoneal inflammation.

Palpation

Relaxation of the abdominal musculature is necessary for diagnostic abdominal palpation. This can often be best achieved in sheepish children while in their parent's arms. Distractive conversation may aid in relaxation of some children. Always begin with light palpation and palpate the area of maximal tenderness last. Watch the child's face for evidence of discomfort as you palpate. In ticklish children, deep palpation may be accomplished with pressure from the stethoscope or have the older child place his or her fingers on top of the examiner's and follow the motions. The examiner should also assess for hepatosplenomegaly. Note palpable feces. Rectal examination, both external and internal, should be done when indicated to assess for fissures, skin tags, presence of fecal impaction, and presence of gross and occult blood.

Special Signs

▷ Obturator Sign

While supine, the patient flexes the right thigh to 90 degrees and then gently rotates internally and externally. Pelvic pain indicates an inflamed muscle and raises the possibility of appendicitis.

▷ Iliopsoas Sign

While supine, the patient with extended knee flexes thigh against the resistance of the examiner's hand. If painful, it indicates an inflammatory process involving the psoas muscle.

▷ Rovsing Sign

Positive when palpation of the left lower quadrant (LLQ) causes increased pain in the right lower quadrant (RLQ) and is suggestive of appendicitis.

LABORATORY EXAMINATION

Blood Count

Similar to fever and rigors, leukocytosis and thrombocytosis are neither specific nor sensitive for a surgical abdomen, nor does their absence rule out serious pathology, especially in children with immunie compromise. Likewise, leukopenia may be a presenting sign of sepsis in the presence of other SIRS criteria. Polycythemia vera, although rare in children, is consistent with severe dehydration. Anemia in the absence of trauma should alert the practitioner to an underlying hematologic sequestration or an anemic process such as infectious mononucleosis or sickle cell anemia.

Serum Amylase & Lipase

Elevated amylase and lipase in the presence of epigastric pain suggest pancreatitis. Their degree of elevation is not predictive of the severity of pancreatitis. Serum lipase is more specific for pancreatitis as it is found only in the pancreas, while measurement of the less-specific amylase has become less common.

Hepatic Function Tests

Elevated hepatic function tests including transaminases and bilirubin in the setting of abdominal pain suggest hepatocellular dysfunction, and confirmatory viral serology should follow. Elevated alkaline phosphatase and gamma-glutamyl transferase (GGT) with or without hyperbilirubinemia is more indicative of a cholestatic process, usually idiopathic or medication induced.

Urine

Urine should be sent for urinalysis and microscopy in order to rule out cystitis or pyelonephritis. In the febrile child or child with history of UTIs, urine should also be sent for culture and sensitivities. Leukocyte esterase has fairly good sensitivity and specificity (both 80-90%) for UTIs. Conversely, nitrites are insensitive (49%) but highly specific (98%) for UTIs. Urine should be collected in a sterile fashion from a urinary catheter when indicated. In addition to cystitis, hematuria can be associated with poststreptococcal glomerulonephritis or renal colic, although red blood cells can be absent in the latter in cases of obstruction.

Serum Electrolytes & Renal Function Tests

Although the results of a basic chemistry panel may indicate varied metabolic derangements, in the setting of abdominal pain the focus is an objective assessment of volume status, and can refute, confirm, or emphasize findings on physical examination. Findings consistent with dehydration include hypobicarbonatemia and an elevated BUN-to-creatinine ratio.

Pregnancy Test & Polymerase Chain Reaction for Chlamydia/Gonorrhea

A pregnancy test should be ordered in all perimenarchal and postmenarchal females. A positive pregnancy test in the presence of abdominal pain is an ectopic pregnancy until proven otherwise. A quantitative beta-human chorionic gonadotrophin of 1500 IU/L defines the discriminatory zone for visualizing an intrauterine pregnancy with an intercavitary ultrasound probe, whereas 5000 IU/L is the value consistent with transabdominal visualization. For patients in whom pelvic infection is suspected but who lack specific physical examination findings, the results of polymerase chain reaction (PCR) for gonorrhea and chlamydia can increase clinical accuracy.

Fecal Occult Blood Testing of Stool

Testing for the presence of occult blood in stool is helpful in certain gastrointestinal bleeding disorders and intussusception. It may also be positive in severe constipation due to internal hemorrhoids or anal fissures.

RADIOLOGIC EXAMINATION

When history is lacking, radiologic examination may be especially helpful in diagnosis of abdominal disease, and in some cases, even therapeutic. In recent years, there has been a trend toward minimizing the amount of radiation exposure from radiographic studies in emergency departments, especially for pediatric patients. In general, start with plain abdominal radiographs to assess for free air, constipation, obstruction, foreign bodies and stones. A chest radiograph may reveal lower lobe pneumonia. Abdominal ultrasonography is often practical when diagnosing appendicitis, cholelithiasis, pancreatitis, pyloric stenosis, intussusception, obstructive renal colic, and in evaluation of the liver. Pelvic ultrasound will evaluate for ovarian cysts, ovarian torsion, and ectopic pregnancy. Scrotal ultrasound assesses for testicular torsion and inguinal hernia. Air enema studies with or without contrast can sequentially diagnose and treat intussusception. Upper GI studies can diagnose malrotation and pyloric stenosis.

Abdominal computed tomography (CT) (ideally with enteric, rectal, and intravenous [IV] contrast) can diagnose appendicitis, pancreatitis, and obstruction, among others. Noncontrast abdominal CT can reveal ureterolithiasis. Compared with other common radiographic modalities, CT exposes patients to much more ionizing radiation. Given the stochastic risk for neoplasm, conservative guidelines for risk reduction include limiting scans to the anatomy of interest, limiting multiphase studies, scaling radiation dose to patient size, and appropriate use of alternative modalities such as ultrasound when possible.

ADDITIONAL MEASURES FOR THE MANAGEMENT OF ABDOMINAL PAIN

Serial Examination & Evaluation

When opting to minimize radiation, repeated or serial abdominal examinations (ideally by the same clinician) are useful in tracking progression of disease and can aid decisions regarding the acquisition of a radiographic study and the patient's disposition. This is especially true when the diagnosis is uncertain based on history and initial physical examination alone. The practitioner should inquire as to the progression of symptoms, need for analgesia, change in vital signs, and repeat the abdominal examination. Successful serial examinations can avoid unnecessary radiation or surgeries without the risk of delayed diagnosis. If patients remain unimproved after a period of hours, the prudent clinician may admit for observation and/or seek surgical consultation. If the patient is discharged home, the guardian should always be given both verbal and written precautions for return to the hospital.

Nutrition

In general, a patient presenting with abdominal pain should be made *nil per os* (nothing by mouth [NPO]) until it is determined that the pain is nonsurgical in nature or until an oral challenge is necessary. In the setting of ongoing losses or prolonged withholding of oral intake, start appropriate weight-based maintenance intravenous fluids.

Analgesia

Traditionally, analgesia was withheld in the setting of abdominal pain to avoid masking the degree of discomfort prior to deciding the need for surgical intervention. However, especially in the pediatric patient, analgesia may aid in a more accurate physical examination with a relaxed patient and improve the overall experience for the family. A recent study revealed no delay in diagnosis after administration of 0.05-0.1 mg/kg IV morphine sulfate.

Emesis Control & Nasogastric Suctioning

Children may often complain of abdominal pain due to emesis. In the vomiting patient, begin with parenteral or orally dissolving antiemetics. A nasogastric catheter and suctioning may be necessary in refractory cases or in the setting of obstruction.

Antimicrobials

Antimicrobials should be reserved for abdominal pain with at least a tentative diagnosis unless there are overt signs of sepsis such as high fever, rigors, and hemodynamic instability. In some cases, surgical consultants may ask that perioperative antimicrobials be given in the emergency department. However, administering antimicrobials in undifferentiated abdominal pain can lead to complications due to subclinical progression and delayed diagnosis or abscess formation.

Surgical Consultation

Early surgical consultation is helpful in cases of pediatric abdominal pain, especially in efforts to minimize radiation exposure. Some surgeons will operate based on history and physical examination alone, and early consultation can thus prevent undesirable sequelae. It is also helpful in establishing a baseline for serial examinations in the case of admission for observation of undifferentiated abdominal pain. In cases of apparent surgical emergency, a surgical subspecialist should be consulted as soon as possible, even before confirmatory studies have been performed.

Chawla S, Seth D, Mahajan P, et al: Upper gastrointestinal bleeding in children. *Clin Pediatr.* 2007;46(1):16-21 [PMID: 17164504].

Holtz LR, Neill MA, Tarr PI: Acute bloody diarrhea: A medical emergency for patients of all ages. *Gastroenterology.* 2009;136(6):1887-1898 [PMID: 19457417].

Marin JR, Alpern ER: Abdominal pain in children. *Emerg Med Clin North Am.* 2011;29(2):401, ix-x [PMID: 21515185].

McCollough M, Sharieff GQ: Abdominal pain in children. *Pediatr Clin North Am.* 2006;53(1):107-137, vi [PMID: 16487787].

Ross A, LeLeiko NS: Acute abdominal pain. *Pediatr Rev.* 2010; 31(4):135-144 [PMID: 20360407].

Sharwood LN, Babl FE: The efficacy and effect of opioid analgesia in undifferentiated abdominal pain in children: A review of four studies. *Paediatr Anaesth.* 2009;19(5):445-451 [PMID: 19453578].

Sivit CJ: Contemporary imaging in abdominal emergencies. *Pediatr Radiol.* 2008;38(4):S675-8 [PMID: 18810420].

MANAGEMENT OF SPECIFIC DISORDERS

Gastrointestinal (Chapter 36), renal and genitourinary (Chapter 38), and gynecologic (Chapter 39) disorders are discussed in detail in the chapters listed in parentheses.

INTESTINAL DISORDERS

Acute Appendicitis

▶ **Clinical Findings**

Appendicitis peaks in adolescence and is rare in children younger than 2 years. It generally manifests itself as gradual onset of pain that eventually localizes to the right lower quadrant and becomes persistent. It maybe accompanied by anorexia or fever. Absence or presence of leukocytosis is of little help with diagnosis. It is generally diagnosed by ultrasound or contrast CT.

▶ **Treatment & Disposition**

Appendicitis warrants a surgical consultation, analgesics, occasionally antimicrobials based on consultant's preferences, and admission for surgery.

Intussusception

▶ **Clinical Findings**

Intussusception usually presents as colicky, severe, and intermittent pain in a child younger than 1 year and is more common in males. The child may kick legs in the air during attacks, and then be calm. Intussusception can also present with lethargy as the main symptom. Occasionally, a palpable mass is present in the RLQ. It can be diagnosed with barium or water-soluble enema or ultrasound.

▶ **Treatment & Disposition**

Diagnostic enema is often therapeutic, but intussusception may recur and can be monitored with serial ultrasounds. Admit refractory patients or those with dehydration, sepsis, or signs of perforation or other complication.

Malrotation With Midgut Volvulus

▶ **Clinical Findings**

Infants with malrotation with or without midgut volvulus generally present within the first year of life (one-half present in the first month) with the hallmark sign of bilious emesis, feeding intolerance, abdominal pain, or in severe cases, peritonitis and shock. One-half of patients have a normal abdominal examination while others have peritoneal signs, distention, or shock. Upper GI study reveals a taper/beak of contrast and malpositioned ligament of Treitz.

▶ **Treatment & Disposition**

Because it is a true surgical emergency, children should receive *nil per os* and be admitted with emergent surgical consultation. Appropriate resuscitation should begin in the emergency department.

Pyloric Stenosis

▶ **Clinical Findings**

Patients with pyloric stenosis are more frequently males, often firstborn, with a peak between 3-5 weeks of life. Parents often report postprandial projectile vomiting that is not bilious and may be associated with intermittent abdominal pain, generally relieved by emesis. Patients may present with severe dehydration from ongoing losses despite normal intake. The classic palpable "olive" has a low sensitivity but is highly specific. Laboratory testing may reveal hypochloremic metabolic alkalosis, but this finding is not always present early in the course of illness. Ultrasound and upper GI have similar sensitivities and specificities for diagnosis.

▶ **Treatment & Disposition**

In dehydrated children, immediate treatment includes correction of fluid loss, electrolytes, and acid-base imbalance with a crystalloid bolus. Children should be made *nil per os* and a surgeon consulted for admission.

Incarcerated Hernia

▶ **Clinical Findings**

Incarcerated hernias typically present in males in the first year of life, especially preterm males with a family history. They are usually inguinal and can be bilateral. Parents notice a painful, swollen bulge under the skin that is worse with crying, and the practitioner is unable to reduce the bulge despite appropriate analgesia and sedation. There may be associated anorexia, nausea, vomiting, and fever. Testicular ultrasound is helpful to rule out torsion.

▶ **Treatment & Disposition**

Incarcerated hernias are a surgical emergency requiring immediate surgical consultation for repair to avoid progression of bowel necrosis. Patients should be given appropriate parenteral analgesics and made *nil per os* in preparation for surgery.

Necrotizing Enterocolitis

▶ **Clinical Findings**

Necrotizing enterocolitis is an illness of neonates, especially those born prematurely, and has a variable presentation from little to no abdominal pain to vague and diffuse pain accompanied by distention, poor feeding, vomiting, diarrhea, lethargy, and bloody stools. Examination also varies depending on degree of illness and accompanying intestinal air but can reveal large abdominal girth with abdominal wall erythema and decreased bowel sounds. Abdominal radiograph usually shows pneumatosis cystoides intestinalis.

▶ **Treatment & Disposition**

Begin emergent resuscitation with IV fluids, nasogastric decompression, make the infant *nil per os*, and begin immediate broad-spectrum antimicrobials. Necrotizing enterocolitis is a true surgical emergency and early surgical consultation is crucial to avoiding further bowel damage. These patients should be admitted to a pediatric intensive care unit which may require transfer to another facility. Be prepared to administer blood, vasopressors, and intubate patients as rapid deterioration and sepsis may occur.

Lampi B, Levin TL, Berdon WE, et al: Malrotation and midgut volvulus: A historical review and current controversies in diagnosis and management. *Pediatr Radiol.* 2009;39(4):359-366 [PMID: 19241073].

Neu J, Walker WA: Necrotizing enterocolitis. *N Engl J Med.* 2011;364(3):255-264 [PMID: 21247316].

Pandya S, Heiss K: Pyloric stenosis in pediatric surgery: An evidence-based review. *Surg Clin North Am.* 2012;92(3):527-539, vii-viii [PMID: 22595707].

Pepper VK, Stanfill AB, Pearl RH: Diagnosis and management of pediatric appendicitis, intussusception, and Meckel diverticulum. *Surg Clin North Am.* 2012;92(3):505-526, vii [PMID: 22595706].

HEPATOBILIARY DISORDERS

Hepatitis

▶ **Clinical Findings**

Acute hepatitis presents with flu-like symptoms including headache, anorexia, malaise, abdominal discomfort and pain in the RUQ, nausea, and vomiting. Physical examination may include hepatomegaly and tenderness, icterus, jaundice, ascites, varices, or splenomegaly. Liver function tests are elevated as may be coagulation profile and lactic acid.

▶ **Treatment & Disposition**

Treatment of hepatitis is mostly supportive as there are only investigational antivirals for hepatitis A, the most common form of hepatitis in children. Hospitalization is indicated for patient with significant dehydration due to vomiting or those with fulminant hepatitis, as indicated by very high serum bilirubin, prolonged prothrombin time, low serum albumin, and hypoglycemia.

Pancreatitis

▶ **Clinical Findings**

Pancreatitis typically presents with severe and unrelenting epigastric pain, sometimes with radiation to the back. It can be associated with nausea, vomiting, fever, or lethargy. In addition to epigastric tenderness, ecchymosis of the epigastrium or flank is sometimes present in cases of hemorrhagic conversion. Serum lipase and amylase are elevated to at least three times the normal limit. Ultrasound may reveal cholelithiasis or pancreatic edema, and CT may show pancreatic inflammation or pseudocyst.

▶ **Treatment & Disposition**

Patients should be made *nil per* os and admitted for IV hydration and parenteral analgesics.

Bai HX, Lowe ME, Husain SZ: What have we learned about acute pancreatitis in children? *J Pediatr Gastroenterol Nutr.* 2011;52(3):262-270 [PMID: 21336157].

Devictor D, Tissieres P, Afanetti M, et al: Acute liver failure in children. *Clin Res Hepatol Gastroenterol.* 2011;35(6-7):430-437 [PMID: 21531191].

OTHER DISORDERS CAUSING ABDOMINAL PAIN

Cystitis & Pyelonephritis

▶ **Clinical Findings**

Urinary tract infections are a common finding in the pediatric emergency patient and occur mostly in children younger than 2 years unless there is a history of predisposition, occurring most frequently in females followed by uncircumcised males. Simple cystitis often presents with suprapubic or generalized abdominal pain, whereas pyelonephritis may additionally present with flank or back pain and fever. The infections are diagnosed on clinical complaints in the setting of positive leukocyte esterase, nitrite, or bacteriuria on a urinalysis or a sufficient number of bacterial colony-forming units on a urine culture.

▶ **Treatment & Disposition**

Treat with age- and community-appropriate antimicrobials (usually oral) taking into account local resistance. Children with complicated recurrent urinary tract infections or refractory symptoms or signs of sepsis should be admitted for parenteral antimicrobials and urologic consultation.

Renal Colic

▶ **Clinical Findings**

Renal colic presents with severe and intermittent pain in the costovertebral area or along the course of the ureter in a lower quadrant. Additional symptoms vary from urinary frequency or enuresis to hematuria and vomiting. Patients usually have a normal abdominal examination. Stones can sometimes be seen on renal or abdominal ultrasound which can evaluate for obstruction. Computed tomography is more sensitive and specific than ultrasound, but has the downside of radiation.

Treatment & Disposition

Most renal colic can be managed outpatient with appropriate analgesia and urology referral. In the setting of fever, pyelonephritis, renal function impairment or for larger stones, urology consultation and admission are appropriate.

Ovarian Torsion

Clinical Findings

Ovarian torsion presents with unilateral pain (often intermittent as ovary torses and detorses) in a female, often with an ovarian cyst larger than 5 cm. Nausea and vomiting may be associated. Occasionally an adnexal mass may be palpated. Doppler reveals decreased arterial flow to the ovary and ultrasound may reveal a corresponding ovarian cyst.

Treatment & Disposition

Ovarian torsion is a gynecological emergency requiring admission for immediate laparoscopy to avoid ovarian necrosis.

Ectopic Pregnancy

Clinical Findings

Ectopic pregnancy, in the case of rupture, typically presents as a sudden onset of sharp unilateral pain that may become diffuse. There is often amenorrhea with new onset vaginal bleeding and other signs of pregnancy. Women are occasionally asymptomatic. Adnexal tenderness and mass may be present. It can be diagnosed on ultrasound with direct visualization of the extrauterine pregnancy and free fluid in the pelvis, or lack of intrauterine pregnancy with an established beta-human chorionic gonadotropin that is within the discriminatory zone.

Treatment & Disposition

Patients with ectopic pregnancies may opt for methotrexate under close observation of a gynecologist in the correct clinical setting. In the case of advanced gestational age or rupture, admission and laparoscopy are necessary.

Testicular Torsion

Clinical Findings

Testicular torsion presents with pain in the unilateral scrotum or groin that may wax and wane. It is usually at or after puberty and can be bilateral. The testis is "high-riding" with a horizontal lie and an absent cremasteric reflex. Doppler will show a lack of arterial blood flow to the testicle but can be falsely negative during periods of detorsion.

Treatment & Disposition

In cases of torsion, urologic consult for immediate surgical visualization and repair is warranted, even if the Doppler is nondiagnostic in the appropriate clinical setting.

REFERENCES

Baldisserotto M: Scrotal emergencies. *Pediatr Radiol.* 2009;39(5):516-521 [PMID: 19189096].

McGrath NA, Howell JM, Davis JE: Pediatric genitourinary emergencies. *Emerg Med Clin North Am.* 2011;29(3):655-666 [PMID: 21782080].

McKay CP: Renal stone disease. *Pediatr Rev.* 2010;31(5):179-188 [PMID: 20435709].

Pecile P, Miorin E, Romanello C, et al: Age-related renal parenchymal lesions in children with first febrile urinary tract infections. *Pediatrics.* 2009;124(1):23-29 [PMID: 19564279].

Shaikh N, Monroe NE, Lopez J, et al: Does this child have a urinary tract infection? *JAMA.* 2007;298(24):2895-2904 [PMID: 18159059].

Vichnin M: Ectopic pregnancy in adolescents. *Curr Opin Obstetr Gynecol.* 2008;20(5):475-478 [PMID: 18797271].

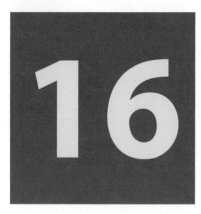

16

Vomiting and Diarrhea

Corinne L. Bria, MD

Constance M. McAneney, MD, MS

VOMITING

Vomiting is the act of disgorging the contents of the stomach through the mouth. It can be a symptom of something as benign as infant overfeeding to as serious and intestinal obstruction (Table 16–1). In the approach to the vomiting pediatric patient, the physician should consider four basic classifications: age, associated symptoms, degree of illness, and etiologies outside the GI tract that can cause vomiting.

As with all pediatric patients the general approach begins with a complete history and precise physical examination (Table 16–2). History should include the age of the patient as well as the onset (duration of illness, relation to feeding, time of day), quantity (number of times), and character of emesis (color, forcefulness, presence of blood, food contents, mucus). Additional history includes travel, ingestions (food and drug), antibiotic use, day care outbreaks, chronic illness, and immunocompetency of the patient. Associated gastrointestinal (GI) symptoms such as fever, abdominal pain, diarrhea, anorexia, and flatulence should be elicited. Signs and symptoms suggestive of etiologies outside the GI tract should be obtained such as headache, neck stiffness, clumsiness, blurred vision, sore throat, rash, cough, chest pain, increased work of breathing, dysuria, urinary frequency, flank pain, vagina discharge, and amenorrhea.

During the physical examination, the overall general appearance should be noted assessing the degree of illness, including responsiveness, mental status, irritability, and vital signs. A head-to-toe examination should be performed making special note of hydration status (mucous membranes, tears, skin turgor, heart rate, pulses, capillary refill, weight), and the abdominal examination (distension; presence, location, and quality of pain; mass; presence of bowel sounds). Note any neurologic, metabolic, cardiac, infectious, gynecologic, renal, and toxic etiologies for vomiting.

The broad differential for the symptom of vomiting makes a prescribed diagnostic set of laboratory tests and radiographs impossible. History, physical, patient's age, and degree of toxicity should guide the workup.

NEONATES (< 3 MONTHS)

A careful birth and perinatal history should be obtained. Onset and duration, quality and color of emesis, associated GI symptoms, and review of systems should be noted (Table 16–3).

Gastrointestinal Obstruction

▶ **Clinical Findings**

Vomiting early in life may be indicative of GI congenital anomalies and a sign of obstruction. Bilious vomiting is a hallmark finding for intestinal obstruction such as malrotation with or without volvulus, meconium ileus, intestinal atresia, incarcerated hernia, or Hirschsprung disease (aganglionic segment of colon). Generally these obstructive processes have accompanying abdominal pain (drawing legs up with pain), poor feeding, and abdominal distension or rigidity. Incarcerated hernia can present with a swollen scrotum or inguinal area. Emesis due to esophageal atresia will not be bilious. Generally esophageal atresia presents very early in the nursery with poor feeding and immediate vomiting. In addition to poor feeding, vomiting and abdominal distension, in the neonate, Hirschsprung disease presents when no meconium has been passed and no stool is present in the rectum on examination. Other clinical features of intestinal obstruction in the neonate include lethargy, dehydration, and poor perfusion. Neonates may show signs of compensated or uncompensated shock quickly in their illness.

Pyloric stenosis, gastric outlet obstruction, generally presents in infants aged 3-6 weeks. It is rare in infants

Table 16–1. Life-threatening causes of vomiting.

Neonates (birth-3 mo)

Obstruction: Malrotation, volvulus, Hirschsprung disease, esophageal atresia, pyloric stenosis

Infections: Necrotizing enterocolitis, peritonitis, meningitis, sepsis, gastroenteritis with dehydration

Nongastrointestinal causes: Hydrocephalus, brain tumor, intracranial hematoma, inborn errors of metabolism

Infants and toddlers (3 mo-3 yr)

Obstruction: Volvulus, intussusception, incarcerated hernia, Hirschsprung disease

Infections: Meningitis, sepsis, gastroenteritis with dehydration

Nongastrointestinal causes: Hydrocephalus, brain tumor, intracranial hematoma, cranial abscess, renal tubular acidosis, renal obstruction, hemolytic uremic syndrome, toxins (drugs, lead, iron), myocarditis

Older child and adolescent (3 yr-18 yr)

Obstruction: Volvulus, intussusception

Infections: Meningitis, sepsis, appendicitis

Nongastrointestinal: Brain tumor, intracranial hematoma, uremia, diabetic ketoacidosis, toxins (drugs, lead, iron)

Table 16–2. Evaluation of acute vomiting and diarrhea.

History

Present illness: Time of onset, duration and nature of symptoms, associated symptoms (fevers, abdominal pain, myalgias, cephalgia, anorexia, neurological symptoms)

Travel: International or domestic, backpacking, new water supplies

Exposures: Community outbreaks, day care exposure, hospitalization, institutionalization

Ingestion: Mushrooms, plant products, herbal preparations, seafood, 24-h food history

Toxins: Medications, recreational drugs, recent antibiotic use, exposure to heavy metals, pesticides, carbon monoxide

Radiation therapy or chemotherapy

Medical and surgical history: Endocrine disorders, HIV, malignancies, gastrointestinal bleeds, abdominal surgeries

Sexual contacts

Physical examination

General appearance: Patient's overall health, toxic appearance, jaundice, or evidence of volume depletion

Complete set of vital signs: Blood pressure, heart rate, respiratory rate, pulse oximetry, rectal temperature

Abdominal examination: Focal tenderness, signs of peritoneal inflammation, pain out of proportion to the examination, distended abdomen

Rectal examination: Fecal impaction, melena, hematochezia, occult blood

Laboratory and diagnostic studies

Fecal cell count: Limited clinical utility because fecal erythrocytes and leukocytes are associated with dysentery and noninfectious processes

Stool cultures: In patients who appear toxic, patients who are immunocompromised, and those with chronic diarrhea

Stool for ova and parasites: In patients with chronic diarrhea, those with history of international travel, HIV-infected patients, and day care exposures

C. difficile toxin: Consider if recent antibiotic use. No indication for testing in children < 1 yr

Giardia antigen: Consider in HIV-infected patients, in patients with history of travel to developing countries, in those with a history of backpacking, and in day care exposures

Complete blood count, blood urea nitrogen, creatinine, glucose, lipase, liver function test, and blood cultures as indicated

Urinalysis: Urinalysis and a urine pregnancy test if indicated

Radiographic evaluation: Consider an acute abdominal series in suspected bowel obstruction; abdominal CT scan or ultrasound as indicated

older than 3 months. The history obtained reveals gradual increasing nonbilious emesis that progresses to projectile vomiting, soon after or during a feed. The infant usually continues to be hungry, has no abdominal pain or distension, and a small olive-like mass may be palpated in the right upper quadrant (RUQ), which is best palpated after vomiting has occurred. A peristaltic wave, moving from the left upper quadrant (LUQ) to the RUQ, may be observed. These infants are usually well appearing unless they have progressed to dehydration.

▶ **Treatment**

When a neonate shows signs of intestinal obstruction a surgical consult is warranted immediately. In ill-appearing infants, initiate intravenous (IV) fluids of normal saline (NS); obtain CBC, electrolytes, and glucose. Flat and upright or lateral decubitus x-rays of the abdomen are necessary. Free air is indicative of an intestinal perforation, air-fluid levels are indicative of obstruction, dilated proximal colon with paucity of gas in the pelvis is indicative of Hirschsprung disease, and gaseous distension of the stomach and proximal duodenum (double bubble) is indicative of duodenal atresia. An upper gastrointestinal (UGI) series that shows the duodenojejunal junction in an abnormal location (right side of spine) is suspicious for malrotation. Barium enema which demonstrates a mobile cecum located midline, in the RUQ or on the left side of the abdomen can confirm malrotation. Surgery is indicated for most neonatal intestinal obstruction.

Prognosis is based on the amount of bowel necrosis and bowel loss, presence of peritonitis, presence of perforation, presence of other life-threatening congenital anomalies, and general underlying condition of the neonate at the time of surgery.

Table 16–3. Common causes of vomiting.

Neonates (birth-3 mo)

Gastroesophageal reflux
Obstruction: Esophageal/intestinal atresia, pyloric stenosis
Infections: Gastroenteritis, necrotizing enterocolitis, meningitis, sepsis

Infants and toddlers (3 mo-3 yr)

Gastroesophageal reflux
Obstruction: Intussusception, incarcerated hernia
Infections: Gastroenteritis, otitis media, urinary tract infection, meningitis, sepsis
Nongastrointestinal causes: Toxins, post-tussive

Older child and adolescent (3-18 yr)

Obstruction: Volvulus, intussusception, incarcerated hernia
Infections: Appendicitis, gastroenteritis, meningitis, urinary tract infection
Nongastrointestinal causes: Diabetic ketoacidosis, toxins, post-tussive emesis, pregnancy

If pyloric stenosis is suspected, then an ultrasound or UGI series should be performed. Ultrasound has become the study of choice but is operator dependent. The ultrasound will show a thickened pylorus (> 3 mm) with a long canal (> 15 mm). Some centers are more comfortable with UGI series. If pyloric stenosis has been identified or the patient is dehydrated, electrolytes should be obtained. Hypokalemic hypochloremic metabolic alkalosis is often present and will need to be corrected prior to the definitive surgical pylorotomy.

Infections

Clinical Findings

Other serious causes of vomiting in the neonate are infectious in etiology. The neonate may be hypothermic, normothermic, or febrile. If diarrhea is present, gastroenteritis may be the cause. Abdominal pain or distension is not typically present with acute gastroenteritis (AGE). Although generally not life threatening, AGE may become life threatening in the neonate if caused by bacterial infection or with the development of dehydration or hypoglycemia. Hematemesis or melena should alert the health care provider to more serious gastroenteritis or to broaden the differential diagnosis. Necrotizing enterocolitis (NEC) can present with vomiting, feeding intolerance, abdominal distension, erythema, and tenderness, and bloody stools. The exact pathogenesis of NEC is thought to be due to previous intestinal ischemia, infection, and immunologic immaturity of the intestine. NEC generally occurs in premature infants, but up to 10% of NEC occurs in full-term infants. Presentation occurs within the first few weeks of life.

Infectious etiologies of vomiting outside the GI tract need to be considered. Altered mental status, bulging fontanel,

poor feeding, poor capillary refill, in addition to vomiting, could be indicative of meningitis and/or sepsis. Urinary tract infections (UTIs) may present with just vomiting, with or without fever, and should be considered in the differential diagnoses. The neonate could appear otherwise well.

Treatment

Assess the neonate's general appearance. Vital signs should be noted. If viral gastroenteritis is suspected in a well appearing, well-hydrated infant, with good urine output, and still feeding, observation and trial of oral feeding in the emergency department is appropriate. Immediate resuscitative measures should be initiated in any ill-appearing infant with the following symptoms: abdominal distension, pain, bloody stools, irritability, somnolence, poor capillary refill, tachycardia for age, tachypnea for age, fever, apnea, or bulging fontanel. Intravenous catheter placement with a NS bolus, complete blood count (CBC), blood culture, catheterized urinalysis and urine culture, renal panel, point of care capillary gas, and glucose should be a priority after assessing and managing airway and breathing. Antibiotics should be given. Antibiotic choice is usually broad and based on what in particular you are treating. Generally ampicillin plus an aminoglycoside are first-line drugs. Strongly consider acyclovir in the neonate in which meningitis is suspected. A lumbar puncture should be performed on any neonate with a fever or suspected to have meningitis. Abdominal x-ray in NEC classically shows pneumatosis cystoides intestinalis (bubble or soap-suds-like appearance of gas in the intestinal wall).

Nongastrointestinal Causes of Vomiting

Clinical Findings

Vomiting can be indicative of central nervous system pathology. The most common etiologies in the neonatal age group are due increased intracranial pressure (ICP). Hydrocephalus, a mass lesion, and subdural or epidural hematoma can cause increased ICP. Cerebral edema from meningitis or diffuse axonal loss of gray-white matter (nonaccidental trauma) may also be the reason for increased ICP. Kernicterus can be a cause for vomiting in neonates but is rarely seen in developed countries.

Inborn errors of metabolism, specifically amino acidemias, organic acidemias, carbohydrate metabolism disorders can present with vomiting, but generally the infant will have a constellation of symptoms including lethargy, seizures, hypo- or hypertonia, tachypnea/hyperpnea, failure to thrive (FTT), and possibly hepatomegaly. Metabolic disorders should be suspected as the cause for vomiting when the neonate is ill appearing, symptoms present with change in diet, family history of mental retardation and/or parental consanguinity.

Treatment

Airway, breathing, and circulation (ABC) are attended to first with IV catheter placement and a bolus of NS. It is important to get a CBC and blood culture as stated above because sepsis or an infectious process is always in the differential for the ill newborn. Electrolytes and glucose are important as well as a point of care capillary gas, if available, to help determine the acid-base status. Patients with hypoglycemia and acidosis should have an ammonia level and liver function tests obtained. Hypoglycemia should be treated immediately with 5-10 mL/kg of $D_{10}W$. Obtain a repeat glucose to ensure that the glucose has corrected.

Patients with vomiting and symptoms of neurological derangement (bulging fontanel, seizures, lethargy, sluggishly reacting pupils, retinal hemorrhages) require resuscitation with intubation to secure the airway, head CT scan to rule out intracranial process (ICP) and lumbar puncture. Infants who are this ill would need to have antibiotics started until the etiology is determined.

Colletti JE, Brown KM, Sharieff GQ, Barata IA, Ishimine P: ACEP Pediatric Emergency Medicine Committee. The management of children with gastroenteritis and dehydration in the emergency department. *J Emerg Med.* 2010;38(5):686-698 [PMID: 19345549].

Freedman SB, Ali S, Oleszczuk M, Gouin S, Hartling L: Treatment of acute gastroenteritis in children: An overview of systematic reviews of interventions commonly used in developed countries. *Evid Based Child Health.* 2013;8(4):1123-1137 [PMID: 23877938].

Gastroesophageal Reflux

Clinical Findings

The most common cause for vomiting in the neonate is gastroesophageal reflux disease (GERD), which is the regurgitation of esophageal or stomach contents usually resulting from lower esophageal sphincter dysfunction. The neonates have a normal birth and perinatal history. They appear normal on examination, gaining at least 5 ounces per week after they regained their birth weight in the first week of life. They are generally hungry. In infants GERD resolves by 1 year of age and is usually a benign condition. Rarely, GERD can become more severe causing FTT, aspiration pneumonia, chronic cough, apnea, esophagitis and irritability, wheezing, and even an acute life-threatening event (ALTE). As the infant becomes more upright and solids are added to the diet, GERD usually improves. By 1 year of age, 95% of GERD in infants is resolved.

Treatment

Gastroesophageal reflux is a clinical diagnosis in normal infants who are growing and thriving and usually require no therapy. In neonates with no change in weight, continuing to thrive and pain free, therapy consists of leaving the infant in an upright position after feeds and offering smaller amounts of thickened feeds more often. If the neonate is in pain or has frequent emesis, arching, or difficulty gaining weight, medical intervention may be warranted. Histamine antagonist (ranitidine) may be started but there is limited data available for its safety in infants younger than 44 weeks corrected for prematurity. In very low-birth-weight infants, studies demonstrate an increase in the incidence of NEC, mortality, and infections of those receiving ranitidine. In nonpremature or very low-birth-weight infants, ranitidine (2 mg/kg/dose three times per day) and proton pump inhibitors (PPIs) (omeprazole 0.7-1 mg/kg/day in one dose or lansoprazole 0.2 mg/kg/day in one dose) may relieve symptoms of esophagitis and help improve pain. But note, they do not resolve the vomiting. Prokinetic drugs are not used as routinely as in the past. Cisapride may cause severe cardiac arrhythmias in children and has been recalled for pediatric use. Metoclopramide has shown limited efficacy with adverse effects (dystonic reactions, agitation).

Infants with symptoms of GERD refractory to conservative treatment may warrant an esophageal pH probe. A gastroesophageal scintiscan or upper GI scan can elicit delayed gastric emptying and any anatomic reasons for the delay. The tests can be performed as an outpatient and arranged through the patient's primary care provider.

Admission should be considered in a neonate with cyanotic color (an ALTE) change due to presumed GERD. A period of observation on monitors will determine the severity of GERD, the need for therapy, and eliminate other causes of cyanosis other than GERD.

Guillet R, Stoll BJ, Cotten CM, et al. Association of H2-blocker therapy and higher incidence of necrotizing enterocolitis in very low birth weight infants. National Institute of Child Health and Human Development Neonatal Research Network. *Pediatrics.* 2006;117(2):e137-42 [PMID: 23877938].

Terrin G, Passariello A, De Curtis M, Manguso F, Salvia G, Lega L, et al. Ranitidine is associated with infections, necrotizing enterocolitis, and fatal outcome in newborns. *Pediatrics.* 2012;129(1):e40-5 [PMID: 22157140].

OLDER INFANTS (3 MONTHS-3 YEARS)

Older infants and toddlers have similar general reasons for vomiting.

Gastrointestinal Obstruction

Clinical Findings

Intussusception is the most frequent cause of obstruction in the older infant and child that occurs from 6 months to 3 years of age (60% < 1 year; 90% < 2 years). The most common form involves the ileocecal junction when the proximal segment telescopes into the distal segment causing venous and lymphatic congestion and edema. The obstruction can lead to ischemia, perforation, and peritonitis. Intermittent colicky abdominal pain (drawing up of legs) and vomiting are the hallmark signs. The emesis is initially nonbilious but can progress to bilious if it goes undiagnosed. The infant can have periods that are pain free but eventually can progress to lethargic periods between the episodes of abdominal pain. If the condition continues, bloody stools may develop, classically described as currant jelly stools. The absence of currant jelly stools does not rule out intussusception. On examination, the infant may have a palpable sausage mass in the right side.

Incarcerated hernias, volvulus, and Hirschsprung disease are causes of obstruction in this age group. Incarcerated hernias present with groin swelling, pain, as well as vomiting. Volvulus generally presents with bilious vomiting, abdominal distention, and pain. Patients generally appear ill. Patients with Hirschsprung disease usually have a history of not having a normal stool without some form of rectal stimulation. On rectal examination they will have no stool in the rectal vault. Meckel diverticulum (omphalomesenteric duct remnant) can cause recurrent intussusception or volvulus and therefore obstruction should be considered as an etiology in vomiting patients who have had previously diagnosed asymptomatic Meckel diverticulum that has not been resected. Volvulus is diagnosed with UGI or barium enema.

Treatment

If the patient is ill appearing or in compensated shock attention to the ABC is primary. Administer NS bolus of 20 mL/kg (repeat if necessary). Complete blood count, electrolytes, glucose, and a point of care glucose and capillary gas should be obtained for ill-appearing patients. Surgical consultation should be obtained immediately. In older infants who present with vomiting, intermittent abdominal pain with lethargy, or heme positive stools, evaluate for intussusception. Most infants and children who present with intussusception are not ill appearing, but look uncomfortable if you observe them during their episodes of abdominal pain. Two radiographs of the abdomen (anteroposterior [AP] and upright or lateral decubitus views) should be obtained to look for air fluid levels, free air, paucity of air in the RLQ, or mass effect. Abdominal x-ray is not a definitive test and cannot rule out intussusception, but will direct the physician to notify the surgeon if there are signs of perforation. Ultrasound is used to diagnose intussusception, but is operator dependent. Air enema can diagnose and reduce intussusception. Up to 90% are reduced via air enema. After successful reduction by air enema, the patient should be observed for signs of perforation or reoccurrence. Laparotomy is indicated in failed reduction via enema, perforation, and in patients who present in shock.

As with neonates, older infants with signs of intestinal obstruction (bilious vomiting, abdominal distension, abdominal pain) should have immediate consultation with the surgeon. Initiate fluid resuscitation and laboratory analysis as previously described. Remember that infants and children will maintain their blood pressure despite being in shock.

Mandeville K, Chien M, Willyerd FA, Mandell G, Hostetler MA, Bulloch B: Intussusception: Clinical presentations and imaging characteristics. *Pediatr Emerg Care.* 2012;28(9):842-844 [PMID: 22929138].

Infections

Clinical Findings

The most common infectious etiology of vomiting in this age group is viral gastroenteritis. Viral gastroenteritis usually is paired with diarrhea but commonly begins with vomiting as the first presenting sign. Symptoms include possible fever, crampy abdominal pain, and depending on the duration and severity of the illness, dehydration. Bacterial gastroenteritis can occur (*Salmonella, Shigella*) but diarrhea is a prominent feature. Consider nongastrointestinal infectious causes as an etiology for vomiting. Meningitis, encephalitis, or sepsis can cause vomiting in the older infant with history of fever, decreased activity, altered mental status, poor feeding, and poor capillary refill. Meningismus may not be present in the older infant or young child. Otitis media, UTI, pneumonia, hepatitis, and viral myocarditis can present with vomiting. Careful attention should be paid to tachycardia in the older febrile infant who does not improve with antipyretics and a decrease in fever. A thorough cardiac examination, with attention to the presence of murmurs or gallops, hepatomegaly, or presence of wheezing or rales, should be performed, as the differential diagnoses would include myocarditis.

Treatment

Evaluate the general appearance, mucous membranes, presence of tears, and to determine capillary refill greater than 2 seconds. It has been shown that these four factors predict dehydration. If resuscitative efforts are indicated (> 10% dehydration), they should be performed immediately. Generally, older infants and children with viral gastroenteritis do not require any intervention. Serum electrolytes are not routinely recommended unless the patient exhibits altered mental status, moderate to severe dehydration, clinical signs of hypokalemia, hypoglycemia, or hyponatremia, infants less than 6 months of age, or suspicious presentations. Older infants and children with mild to moderate dehydration can be orally rehydrated. If 6-9% dehydrated by clinical estimation, then begin oral rehydration at 100 mL/kg over

3-4 hours. If 3-5% dehydrated, begin oral rehydration at 50 mL/kg over 3-4 hours. Remember to replace ongoing losses. The oral rehydration solution is ideally a solution containing sodium, potassium, chloride, and carbohydrates (Pedialyte, Rehydralyte, Infalyte, World Health Organization solution). Sports beverages and apple juice are not recommended as solutions because of their high carbohydrate content and low electrolyte content. Antiemetics are traditionally not recommended (sedation effects, dystonic reactions), but there is evidence that ondansetron (IV: 0.15-0.3 mg/kg/dose; PO: 8-15 kg give 2 mg/dose, > 15-30 kg give 4 mg/dose, > 30 kg give 8 mg/dose) is effective in reducing the rate of vomiting, increasing the effectiveness of oral rehydration, decreasing the need for IV hydration, and decreasing admissions with less adverse side effects.

If oral rehydration is contraindicated (rare), fails, or is not accepted by the parents, IV therapy can be instituted in the emergency department. Serum electrolytes are not routinely indicated. A bolus of 20 mL/kg of NS or Ringer lactate can be given. After the bolus, if the patient's heart rate is down and the patient has urinated, an oral challenge should be given. The use of ondansetron may improve the chances that the patient will not need admission. If the patient has not urinated or hydration status has not improved, a second bolus of NS 20 mL/kg is indicated. Criteria for admission include the following:

- Greater than 5% dehydration *and* inability to tolerate oral fluids
- Serious underlying illness (sepsis, UTI, inborn errors of metabolism, diabetic ketoacidosis [DKA])
- Bilious emesis
- Poor social situation

The younger the patient the more conservative the health care provider should be and may wish to consider admission.

If vomiting is present with diarrhea longer than the usual 2-6 days of viral gastroenteritis or bloody diarrhea is prominent, consider bacterial gastroenteritis. Stool culture may be indicated in these patients.

For vomiting caused by other infections etiologies, directed care is indicated. Meningitis, encephalitis, or sepsis requires IV placement, CBC, blood culture, electrolytes, glucose, and fluid resuscitation. Broad spectrum antibiotics are indicated. A lumbar puncture should be obtained if the patient is stable; however, antibiotics should not be delayed if the lumbar puncture is not able to be obtained immediately.

Otitis media, UTI, pneumonia should be worked up appropriately and treated. If myocarditis is suspected (tachycardia despite defervesce, new murmur, gallop, hepatomegaly, rales) a chest x-ray and electrocardiogram (ECG) are indicated. If cardiolmegaly is present or signs of myocarditis on ECG, a pediatric cardiologist should be consulted. An echocardiogram is indicated with admission.

Nongastrointestinal Causes of Vomiting

▶ Clinical Findings

Noninfectious extragastrointestinal causes of vomiting are important to consider. In the older infant and child, central nervous system etiologies are uncommon but can be devastating if missed. Brain tumors, hydrocephalus, hematomas (non-accidental or accidental trauma), and abscesses, can cause increased ICP and vomiting. The increased ICP may cause sutures to split, increasing head circumference and bulging fontanel if the patient is younger than 6-9 months. Papilledema may be present. Lethargy or irritability may be the presenting symptom. A patient in this age group cannot complain about the presence of a headache. Cushing triad (hypertension, bradycardia, and respiratory depression) is indicative of brain stem herniation, requiring intubation, resuscitation, and investigation.

Inborn errors of metabolism can still present after the first 3 months of life. Their presentations involve vomiting, lethargy, possible seizures, hypo- or hypertonia, tachypnea/hyperpnea, FTT, and possible hepatomegaly. Obtain history concerning symptoms are related to change in diet, fasting, or family history of metabolic disorders or developmental delay.

Renal disorders such as renal tubular acidosis or renal failure are possible. Although these disease processes tend to occur in older children, renal failure secondary to hemolytic uremic syndrome (HUS) can affect this age group. Infants are usually ill appearing and may have a history of hematuria, polyuria, anuria, edema, and hypertension.

Because of their exploring nature, toddlers are at risk for ingestions. Vomiting can be the primary symptom. Consider lead poisoning in patients with pica. These patients can also exhibit abdominal pain. Developmental delay is a later sign. Careful examination of the toddler for signs of toxin with special attention to vital signs and mental status should be performed. Common ingestions that cause vomiting are salicylates, theophylline, alcohol, hydrocarbons, lead, iron, and digoxin.

▶ Treatment

Noninfectious extragastrointestinal etiologies for vomiting require a focused workup and treatment. Serum electrolytes as well as a point of care capillary gas and glucose, if available, are important to help determine acid-base status and electrolyte etiology for the symptoms. Ammonia level and liver function tests should be included if the patient has hypoglycemia. Hyperglycemia in the setting of severe dehydration and vomiting may be evidence of diabetic ketoacidosis. Hypoglycemia should be treated immediately with 2-4 mL/kg $D_{25}W$. Intravenous fluids containing dextrose should be instituted after the patient has received initial bolus. Consultation with a specialist in metabolic and genetic disorders is warranted.

In the infant with signs of increased ICP or altered mental status, attention to the ABC is first. After the patient is deemed stable, a CT scan of the head is necessary. Appropriate subspecialty consultations should be obtained or transfer to a tertiary care center for definitive care should be initiated.

Vomiting secondary to toxin ingestion requires a focused evaluation.

OLDER CHILDREN & ADOLESCENTS

Vomiting caused by obstruction, infection, and nongastrointestinal causes continues throughout the pediatric age group. NEC, pyloric stenosis, intestinal atresias, and meconium ileus do not occur in older children (> 3 years). Although it occurs throughout life, GERD does not generally cause vomiting in children older than 1 year. Intussusception is rare in children older than 5 years and occurs usually secondary to a mass as a lead point. Metabolic disorders and Hirschsprung disease have usually been diagnosed by the first year. The older pediatric patient is able to provide a history of symptoms (headache, specific areas that are in pain) and thus specific reasons for vomiting may be elicited. Gastroenteritis affects all ages and the general principles of assessing hydration status, rehydrating with oral rehydration solution if indicated, and determination of patient disposition are the same.

Gastrointestinal Obstruction

Obstruction as an etiology can occur throughout life. Volvulus continues to occur and should be considered when a patient presents with colicky abdominal pain, bilious vomiting, and abdominal distension. A patient who has had previous surgery has the possibility of postoperative adhesions and may present with the same symptoms. The treatment is the same with stabilization as the cornerstone and surgical consultation for definitive care (see Older Infants above).

Infection

▶ **Clinical Findings**

Vomiting as sign of infection in the older children is similar to children in other age groups. One disease entity more common in the children older than 2 years is appendicitis. Although appendicitis has been seen at all ages, in children younger than 2 years, it is usually diagnosed late, after perforation, because of the nonspecific symptoms. In school-aged children, the abdominal pain usually begins periumbilically and migrates to the RLQ. Anorexia is followed by vomiting. Fever can develop and is usually low grade. Diarrhea is not a symptom, but its presence does not rule out appendicitis. The child may complain of increased pain with movement, walking, jumping, coughing, or being in a moving vehicle.

As the inflammation progresses, the child may exhibit rebound tenderness and referred pain on examination. Younger children have more vague complaints on examination and a quicker progression of symptoms. The signs and symptoms of appendicitis vary widely and the diagnosis can be difficult to make. Ovarian torsion, sexually transmitted infection (STI), tubo-ovarian abscess, gastroenteritis, and UTI should be in the differential diagnosis.

▶ **Treatment**

When an older child presents with vomiting, anorexia, periumbilical or RLQ abdominal pain, low-grade fever, pain with movement, appendicitis is suspected. A CBC should show an elevated white blood cell (WBC) count. A WBC greater than 10,000 with an absolute neutrophil count (ANC) greater than 6750 puts a patient at increased risk of appendicitis. Electrolytes are not necessary unless the patient exhibits signs of dehydration. Both CT scan and ultrasound are radiographic modalities that can aid in the diagnosis. Ultrasound has the advantage of no radiation, lower cost, and better modality for assessing the presence of flow to the ovary in female patients. It is slightly less sensitive than CT scan when the appendix is visualized (sensitivity 97.5%). Ultrasound is operator dependent and in institutions where pediatric ultrasound expertise is not present, CT scan of the abdomen is the study of choice. If perforation is suspected, CT scan is the study of choice. Intravenous NS bolus followed by maintenance fluids are indicated if the older child is dehydrated. Surgical removal of the appendix is usually performed; however, in a patient with perforation, the surgeon may prefer to treat with antibiotics and postpone the appendectomy.

Bundy DG, Byerley JS, Liles EA, Perrin EM, Katznelson J, Rice HE: Does this child have appendicitis? *JAMA*. 2007;298(4):438-451 [PMID: 17652298].

Mittal MK, Dayan PS, Macias CG, et al; Pediatric Emergency Medicine Collaborative Research Committee of the American Academy of Pediatrics. Performance of ultrasound in the diagnosis of appendicitis in children in a multicenter cohort. *Acad Emerg Med*. 2013;20(7):697-702 [PMID: 23859583].

Nongastrointestinal Causes of Vomiting

▶ **Clinical Findings**

As with children in other age groups metabolic abnormalities cause vomiting. Inborn errors of metabolism (previously diagnosed), uremia, and adrenal insufficiency can present in this age group. Diabetes more commonly presents in this age group. Polydipsia, polyuria, and polyphagia with weight loss are the classic presenting symptoms, but if the child has progressed vomiting may be the chief complaint. First, the presentation of diabetes can be missed and attributed to gastroenteritis. The child may have fruity smelling breath, hyperpnea, altered mental status, and appear more dehydrated than expected.

The differential diagnosis for vomiting in the adolescent age group must include pregnancy. According to the Youth Risk Behavior Survey, 33% of high school freshman, 44% of sophomores, 53% of juniors, and 63% of seniors in this country have had vaginal sexual intercourse. Historic factors may be denied and physical symptoms may be subtle.

Cyclic vomiting is an entity that presents initially between 3 and 5 years of age and is distinguished by numerous episodes of vomiting interspersed with well periods. It may have a prodrome of fever, nausea, headache, or lethargy. Etiology includes altered intestinal motility or abdominal migraine. It is a diagnosis of exclusion after other causes of vomiting have been considered and the patient has undergone testing including metabolic studies, UGI series, endoscopy, and MRI of the brain. The diagnosis is not generally made in the emergency department.

▶ **Treatment**

When a nongastrointestinal etiology for vomiting is suspected in a child in this age group, the workup is based on clinical suspicion. Because the older child is better at communicating, the investigation can be focused. If diabetic ketoacidosis is suspected, then serum glucose, electrolytes, point of care capillary gas (to determine pH), and urinalysis are indicated. Treatment includes correcting dehydration, hyperglycemia, and acidosis and preventing hypokalemia (Chapter 42). Cerebral edema, exhibited by a change in mental status, is a life-threatening complication of diabetic ketoacidosis in the pediatric population. Therefore, monitoring of the mental status and neurologic examination is important.

A pregnancy test should be performed on all females who are postmenarchal. If the test is positive, treatment of the vomiting with an antiemetic such as ondansetron may relieve symptoms. Referral to appropriate primary care is a necessity.

Yen S, Martin S: Contraception for adolescents. *Pediatr Ann.* 2013;42(2):21-25 [PMID: 23379400].

DIARRHEA

In pediatric patients, the term diarrhea refers to the softening of stools without necessarily the inclusion of an increased number of stools. Any change in the pattern of stooling in a pediatric patient should raise suspicion for diarrhea. Although diarrhea can accompany common pediatric illness such as acute viral gastroenteritis, diarrhea may be a symptom of a life-threatening illness (Table 16–4).

Table 16–4. Common causes of diarrhea.

Infections: Viral enteritis, parasitic enteritis, bacterial enteritis
Parenteral diarrhea
Dietary disturbances
Antibiotic use
Irritable bowel syndrome
Inflammatory bowel disease

INFECTIOUS DIARRHEA

Viruses

Rotavirus, caliciviruses (Norwalk and Sapporo viruses), enteroviruses, adenoviruses, and astroviruses.

Parasites

Giardia lamblia, Entamoeba histolytica, and *Cryptosporidia.*

▶ **Clinical Findings**

Viruses and parasites are two sources of infectious diarrhea, which cause soft or watery stools that may be malodorous in nature. Pediatric patients may have an increased frequency of stooling and abdominal pain may accompany the diarrhea. Most patients with viral causes of diarrhea have fever and the stools are nonbloody. Most patients with parasitic causes of diarrhea have diarrhea for 1 week or more, and had exposure to contaminated water such as at a lake or stream, or attend a day care center where outbreaks occur.

When obtaining a history, it is important to ascertain the patient's intake and output during the course of the illness. Specific questions about volume of intake and output, for example, the number of wet diapers during the course of the illness and the number, frequency, and size of stools help to estimate fluid balance.

Viral and parasitic causes of diarrhea may lead to dehydration as evidenced by change in mental status (lethargy), vital sign abnormalities (tachycardia, hypotension), and weight loss. In addition, examination of the mucous membranes and skin turgor are useful in gauging dehydration. The abdominal examination usually reveals a soft, nondistended abdomen that the patient may perceive as uncomfortable but the examination does not elicit localized or rebound tenderness.

▶ **Treatment**

Table 16–5 lists differential diagnostic features of common pediatric diarrhea. Viral and parasitic causes of diarrhea require supportive care with oral or IV rehydration depending on the degree of dehydration and careful monitoring of intake and output. Symptoms usually remit in 2-5 days. Oral

Table 16–5. Differential diagnostic features of common pediatric diarrhea.

Cause	Mode of transmission	Incubation	Comments	Therapy
Salmonella sp.	Contaminated food or water (eggs, poultry, milk). Animals or pets (turtles, chickens, lizards). Group gatherings.	8–72 h	Very common. Fever, abdominal pain, headache, myalgia, diarrhea with little vomiting. Risk of sepsis in the young, or the compromised (sickle cell disease, diabetes, HIV, the asplenic). Rare fecal RBCs; common WBCs.	Antimicrobial therapy usually not indicated for patients with either asymptomatic infection or uncomplicated (noninvasive) gastroenteritis Treat infection in those with severe illness or sepsis, the immunocompromised, or the hospitalized. If antimicrobial therapy is initiated in patients with gastroenteritis, amoxicillin or trimethoprim-sulfamethoxazole is recommended for susceptible strains. Alternative: azithromycin or ceftriaxone for resistant strain. Floroquinolones not approved for children < 18 yr.
Shigella sp.	Fecal–oral, person-to-person transmission, or contaminated food. Day care and institutions. Poor sanitation. Highly contagious.	1–3 d	Very common. Children 1–5 yr, institutionalized patients. Fever, headache, abdominal pain, myalgia, diarrhea with little vomiting. Febrile seizures and a toxic appearance may prompt lumbar puncture. Diarrhea may begin during the procedure. Fecal RBCs common; sheets of WBCs.	Treat infection in those with severe dysentery, sepsis, or institutional outbreaks. Treat with ampicillin or trimethoprim-sulfamethoxazole for 5 d. Resistant strains: treat with parenteral azithromycin for 3 d, ceftriaxone for 5 d, or a fluoroquinolone (such as ciprofloxacin if > 18 yr) for 3 d should be administered. Oral cephalosporins are not useful for treatment. Floroquinolones not approved for children < 18 yr.
Campylobacter sp.	Unchlorinated water, contaminated food (unprocessed milk, poultry). Animals or pets. Natural water supplies in the national parks.	1–7 d	Very common. Backpacker diarrhea, summer months, children and young adults. Fever, headache, abdominal pain, myalgias for several days followed by diarrhea with little vomiting. May mimic appendicitis. Fecal RBCs and WBCs common.	Treat infection in those who are compromised or appear toxic. Azithromycin and erythromycin shorten duration of illness and prevent relapse when given. Treatment with azithromycin (10 mg/kg/d for 3–5 d) or erythromycin (40 mg/kg/d in 4 divided doses for 5 d). Fluoroquinolone, such as ciprofloxacin, may be effective, but resistance to ciprofloxacin is common. Floroquinolones not approved for children < 18 yr.
Yersinia enterocolitica	Contaminated food or water (pork, milk). Fecal-oral, person-to-person transmission. Wild and domestic animals.	1–5 d	Children and young adults. Anorexia, low-grade fever, RLQ abdominal pain, and vomiting may precede diarrhea and mimic appendicitis. Bacteremia may occur in children < 1 y or others with conditions such as excessive iron storage (ie, use of defeoroxime in sickle cell disease/beta-thalessemia), and immunosupressive states. Fecal RBCs and WBCs common. (Iron overload situations substantially increases the pathogenicity of enterocolitica)	Treat infection in severely ill patients. Usually self-limiting. Treat with trimethoprim-sulfamethoxazole, aminoglycosides, or cefotaxime. May use tetracycline or doxycycline (for children ≥ 8 yr); fluoroquinolones (for patients ≥18 yr). Usually resistant to first-generation cephalosporins and most penicillin.
Enterohemorrhagic E. coli 0157:H7	Contaminated food or water; raw undercooked meats, hamburger; fecal-oral, person-to-person transmission; institutions, day care.	3–8 d	Children and the elderly; fever, abdominal pain, vomiting, grossly bloody diarrhea; may mimic gastrointestinal bleed or mesenteric ischemia; hemolytic uremic syndrome (common cause of renal failure in children) occurs in 5%, 5–20 d postinfection; fecal RBCs and WBCs common	Supportive care; antibiotics not recommended.

Organism	Source	Incubation	Clinical Features	Treatment
Aeromonas hydrophilia	Contaminated water.	1-5 d	More common in the immunocompromised; more severe in children; cause of 10-15% of cases of pediatric diarrhea; diarrhea, vomiting, and abdominal cramps with or without fever; chronic infection may mimic inflammatory bowel disease; fecal RBCs and WBCs common.	Treat with trimethoprim-sulfamethoxazole. May use tetracycline (children ≥ 8 yr; Fluoroquinolones (patients ≥ 18 yr;
Strongyloides stercoralis	Soils with fecal contamination. Warm climates, poor sanitation, institutions.	Wk-mo	Fever, abdominal pain, vomiting, diarrhea, and sepsis in the immunocompromised; the compromised may develop cutaneous, pulmonary, or central nervous system symptoms.	Ivermectin 200 mcg/kg/d x 2 d. Alternative : abendazole 400 mcg/kg/d x 7 d
Clostridium difficile (antibiotic associated)	Recent antibiotic use. Clindamycin, penicillins, and cephalosporins are most commonly implicated.	1-12 wk	Fever, abdominal pain, diarrhea, rarely vomiting; may cause significant illness especially in the compromised; fecal RBCs and WBCs common. Intestinal colonization rates in healthy infants can be as high as 50% but usually < 5% in children > 5 yr and adults.	Discontinue associated antibiotics; Metronidazole (30 mg/kg/d in 4 divided doses, maximum 2 g/d) is drug of choice for initial treatment of children and adolescents with mild to moderate diarrhea and for first relapse. or vancomycin, 40 mg/kg/d, orally, in 4 divided doses, to a maximum daily dose not to exceed 2 g) Therapy x 10 d
Entamoeba histolytica (amebic dysentery)	Contaminated food or water. Poor sanitation, institutions. Travel to developing countries.	1-12 wk	Patients with acute amebic dysentery present with abrupt onset of fever, abdominal pain, tenesmus, and bloody diarrhea; vomiting is rare; chronic dysentery causes malaise, weight loss, bloating, and blood-streaked diarrhea; may develop an hepatic abscess; fecal RBCs and WBCs common.	Metronidazole, 35-50 mg/kg/d orally 3 times a day x 10 days followed by iodoquinol 30-40 mg/kg/d (max 2 g) orally 3 times a day x 20 days.
Giardia intestinalis (formerly *Giardia lamblia*)	Infected directly from an infected person or through ingestion of fecally contaminated water or food.	1-3 wk	Acute watery diarrhea, abdominal pain, or protracted intermittent, often debilitating disease characterized passage of foul-smelling stools associated with flatulence, abdominal distention, and anorexia. Malabsorption with significant weight loss, failure to thrive, and anemia.	Metronidazole 15 mg/kg/d orally 3 times a day x 7 days
Cryptosporidia	Ocysts are excreted in feces and transmitted via fecal-oral route. Extensive waterborne disease outbreaks have been associated with contamination of drinking water and recreational water.	3-14 d	Nonbloody, watery diarrhea, abdominal cramps, fatigue, fever, vomiting, anorexia, weight loss. Usually lasts 6-14 d. In immunocompromised chronic, severe diarrhea, which can lead to malnutrition and weight loss.	Nitazoxanide: 1-3 yr: 100 mg PO bid x 3 d 4-11 yr: 200 mg PO bid x 3 d > 12 yr: 500 mg PO bid x 3 d

(Adapted with permission from Stone CK, Humphries RL: *Current Diagnosis and Treatment Emergency Medicine*, 7th ed. Copyright © The McGraw-Hill Companies, 2011. Chapter 36. Gastrointestinal Emergencies.Empiric Management and Disposition of Patients with Infectious Gastroenteritis. Empiric Chemotherapy.)

rehydration solutions contain both glucose and electrolytes and reintroduction of feedings should occur early in the illness. If a patient is estimated to be 5-10% dehydrated, a basic metabolic panel, looking specifically at the electrolytes and blood urea nitrogen (BUN), should be obtained. The study reveals the degree of acidosis and whether the patient is hypo- or hypernatremic. A bedside glucose level will determine whether the patient is hypoglycemic. For patients who require IV rehydration, a 20 mL/kg bolus of NS should be initiated. Following this intervention, the patient should be reassessed and if improved, the patient can undergo a trial of oral fluids. If the patient is more severely dehydrated, more than one NS bolus is required and then IV fluids with dextrose at a maintenance rate or higher to maintain hydration in light of the diarrhea. Examination of the stools specifically for ova and parasites may confirm identification of the infectious agent as certain forms of diarrhea may be a public health concern (*Cryptosporidia* outbreaks).

Most pediatric patients with viral and parasitic causes of diarrhea can tolerate oral fluids and thus can undergo oral rehydration at home. Admission should be considered in pediatric patients who have developed 5-10% dehydration with continued diarrhea or who are hypo- or hypernatremic. It is important to note that infants and young children do not have the same reserve as older children and may demonstrate dehydration more quickly and with more subtle historical features than older children.

Antidiarrheal medications should not be used in children with gastroenteritis. In recent years probiotics (members of the *Lactobacillus bifidobacterium* genera that alter the microflora of the host) have been studied and used in children with gastroenteritis. An American Academy of Pediatrics Committee on Nutrition report stated that there is evidence in otherwise healthy infants and young children to support the use of probiotics early in the course of gastroenteritis. Studies show that probiotics reduces the duration of diarrhea caused by viral gastroenteritis by 1 day. There is not conclusive evidence to show that probiotics are efficacious in prevention of diarrhea.

Bacteria

Salmonella, Shigella, Yersinia, Campylobacter, pathogenic *Escherichia coli, Aeromonas hydrophila, Vibrio* spp., *Clostridium difficile,* tuberculosis.

▶ Clinical Findings

Bacteria serve as a source of infectious diarrhea. In comparison with viral and parasitic causes of diarrhea, the two hallmark features of bacterial causes of diarrhea are abdominal cramping and hematochezia or bloody stools. Given the infectious nature of this type of diarrhea, fever is often found in patients.

When obtaining a history, it is important to ask about exposure to raw or undercooked eggs or chicken (*Salmonella*), public swimming pools (*Shigella*), unpasteurized apple cider (*Campylobacter*), undercooked red meat such as hamburgers (pathogenic *Escherichia coli*), or shellfish (*Vibrio* spp.).

Hemolytic uremic syndrome (HUS) is a serious sequela of shiga-toxin *E. coli* (STEC). Enteric infection *E. coli* O157:H7 is the STEC serotype most commonly associated with HUS. Microangiopathic hemolytic anemia, thrombocytopenia, and acute renal insufficiency/failure may be seen on laboratory analysis. HUS occurs in up to 15% of shiga-toxin *E. coli*-infected children. It typically develops 7 days (≥ 3 weeks) after onset of diarrhea. Greater than 50% of children require dialysis, and 3-5% die. Neurologic complications (seizures, coma, stroke) have been reported.

Clostridium difficile is the most common cause of antimicrobial-associated diarrhea and is a common health care–associated pathogen. Clinical symptoms include asymptomatic colonization, watery diarrhea, bloody diarrhea, fever, and abdominal pain. Pseudomembranous colitis generally is characterized by diarrhea with mucus in feces, abdominal cramps and pain, fever, and systemic toxicity. Colonization by toxin-producing strains without symptoms occurs in children younger than 5 years and is common in infants younger than 1 year. The most common testing method used today for *C. difficile* toxins is the commercially available enzyme immunoassay (EIA), which detects toxins A and/or B. Molecular assays using nucleic acid amplification tests (NAATs) are also available. The American Academy of Pediatrics Policy Statement on testing recommends the following: testing for *C. difficile* colonization or toxin should be performed only in children with diarrhea who meet the clinical and age-related criteria listed in the following recommendations. Testing in infants (< 12 months) is complicated by a high rate of asymptomatic colonization. Testing should be limited to infants with Hirschsprung disease or other severe motility disorders or in an outbreak situation. Alternative etiologies should be sought even in those with a positive test result for *C. difficile*.

It is important to ascertain the patient's intake and output during the course of the illness. Specific questions about volume of intake and output, for example, the number of wet diapers during the course of the illness and the number, frequency, and size of stools help to estimate fluid balance. In most patients, the blood in the stool will appear as a small quantity specifically as drops on the surface of the stool. Bacterial causes of diarrhea may lead to dehydration as evidenced by vital sign abnormalities specifically tachycardia, hypotension, and decrease in weight. In addition, examination of the mucous membranes and skin turgor are useful in gauging dehydration.

Treatment

Bacterial causes of diarrhea require supportive care with oral or IV rehydration depending on the degree of dehydration and careful monitoring of intake and output. Oral rehydration solutions contain both glucose and electrolytes, and reintroduction of feedings should occur early in the illness. If a patient is estimated to be 5-10% dehydrated, a metabolic panel should be obtained. The panel evaluates possible hypoglycemia, hypo- or hypernatremia, elevated BUN or creatinine. A CBC, blood smear may reveal anemia or thrombocytopenia if HUS is suspected. For patients who require IV rehydration, a 20 mL/kg bolus of NS should be initiated. Following this intervention, the patient should be reassessed and, if improved, can undergo a trial of oral fluids. In more severe dehydration, the patient may require more than one NS bolus and then IV fluids with dextrose at a maintenance rate or higher to maintain hydration in light of the diarrhea.

In the febrile pediatric patient with bloody diarrhea, a stool culture may help to determine the infectious agent; however, in most patients, antibiotic therapy is not indicated even with a positive stool culture. Testing for *C. difficile* is discussed above.

Antibiotic therapy is indicated in shigellosis as the antibiotics shorten the course of the illness and the duration of excretion of the organisms in the stool. Table 16–5 lists treatment options for specific etiologies of diarrhea.

Most pediatric patients with bacterial causes of diarrhea can undergo oral rehydration at home. Families frequently require reassurance that bloody stools are not an ominous sign. Admission should be considered in pediatric patients who are mildly to moderately dehydrated with continued diarrhea. It is important to note that infants and young children do not have the same reserve as older children and may demonstrate dehydration more quickly and with more subtle historical features than older children.

American Academy of Pediatrics. *Red Book: 2012 Report of the Committee on Infectious Diseases.* Section 4: Antimicrobial Agents and Related Therapy. Drugs for parasitic infections, 29th ed. Pickering LK, ed. Elk Grove Village, IL: American Academy of Pediatrics; 2012: 848-868.

Schutze GE, Willoughby RE; Committee on Infectious Diseases; American Academy of Pediatrics: Clostridium difficile infection in infants and children. *Pediatrics.* 2013;131:196-200 [PMID: 23277317].

Stutman HR: Salmonella, shigella, and campylobacter: Common bacterial causes of infectious diarrhea. *Pediatric Ann.* 1994;23(10):538-543 [PMID: 7838603].

Inflammatory Bowel Disease

Clinical Findings

Inflammatory bowel disease (IBD) includes both ulcerative colitis and Crohn disease. Clinical features of both disorders include diarrhea, GI blood and protein loss, abdominal pain, fever, anemia, weight loss, and growth failure. Extraintestinal manifestations (arthritis, uveitis, erythema nodosum, chronic hepatitis, and sclerosing cholangitis) are more common in Crohn disease. A typical presentation to the emergency department includes severe abdominal pain and diarrhea with or without occult blood in the stool. Abdominal examination may reveal tenderness, guarding, and/or rebound tenderness. Perianal disease (fissures, skin tags, fistulae, and abscesses) may precede the intestinal manifestations of Crohn disease by several years.

Treatment

If a patient has known IBD, initial emergency department management involves an assessment of the severity of GI symptoms and systemic toxicity.

Mild Disease

Mild disease consists of the following:

- Fewer than six stools passed daily
- Absence of systemic signs.

Moderate Disease

Severe disease consists of the following:

- More than six stools passed daily
- Fever (temperature > 38°C or 100.4°F)
- Hypoalbuminemia (serum protein concentration < 3.2 g/dL)
- Anemia (hemoglobin concentration < 10 g/dL)

Severe Disease

Severe disease consists of the following:

- More than six stools passed daily
- Marked abdominal cramping and tenderness
- Fever
- Significant anemia
- Leukocytosis (WBC count > 15,000)
- Hypoalbuminemia (3 mg/dL)
- Toxic megacolon

In patients with known or suspected IBD, laboratory studies including a CBC with differential, basic metabolic panel, serum albumin, liver function tests, erythrocyte sedimentation rate (ESR), and C-reactive protein level are indicated. Abdominal radiographs are helpful in establishing the diagnosis of toxic megacolon, bowel obstruction, or perforation. Stool examination for occult blood, fecal leukocytes, and culture of infectious agents is important.

The patient with suspected or known IBD can be discharged from the emergency department when the patient presents with mild manifestations of disease *and* the patient's laboratory and radiographic studies do not reveal significant abnormality *and* follow-up with a gastroenterologist has been arranged.

In patients with moderate to severe disease, initial management is supportive with IV rehydration with NS followed by maintenance IV fluids with dextrose. Admission of these patients may be necessary to initiate or modify specific therapy, such as corticosteroids or immunosuppressive medications. Consultation with a gastroenterologist is recommended.

PARENTERAL DIARRHEA

▶ Clinical Findings

Pediatric patients can develop diarrhea without an infectious or inflammatory etiology. Acute otitis media can cause diarrhea in infants and young children. The patients may have fever associated with acute otitis media and may develop dehydration from the diarrhea.

▶ Treatment

In this case, treatment of the acute otitis media will lead to the resolution of the diarrhea. Patients are safe for discharge from the emergency department as long as they can maintain hydration despite diarrhea. Dehydrated patients may require admission to the hospital for IV rehydration and strict monitoring of intake and output.

Dietary Disturbances

▶ Clinical Findings

Dietary disturbances such as overfeeding and sugary drink intake such as apple juice may lead to diarrhea in infants and young children. Patients are afebrile and thriving despite the diarrhea. Historical features including specific questions regarding frequency and volume of feeds or sugary drinks and appearance of a large infant or young child may indicate that overfeeding or increased intake of sugary drinks as the cause of the diarrhea. Patients usually do not demonstrate significant dehydration; however, the softening in the stool, or the change in pattern of stooling raises concerns in the parent which prompts the emergency department visit.

▶ Treatment

It is important to identify dietary disturbances as the cause of the diarrhea so that appropriate guidance can be provided to the parents. Decreasing the volume of feeds and limiting the volume of sugary drinks will cause remittance of the diarrhea. Unless moderately to severely dehydrated due to the diarrhea, the patient can be discharged home with modified feeding instructions. It is important to have the patient follow-up with pediatrician to reinforce the anticipatory guidance and to follow up the patient's diarrhea.

Thomas DW, Greer FR: American Academy of Pediatrics Committee on Nutrition; American Academy of Pediatrics Section on Gastroenterology, Hepatology, and Nutrition. *Pediatrics.* 2010;126(6):1217-31 [PMID: 21115585].

Irritable Bowel Syndrome

▶ Clinical Findings

Irritable bowel syndrome (IBS) differs from IBD in that the anatomy of the bowel in IBS is not abnormal. IBS is characterized by abdominal pain, fullness, and bloating present at least 3 days a month for the past 3 months. The symptoms of IBS are usually reduced after a bowel movement or occur when there is a change in the frequency of bowel movements. Patients with IBS may vacillate between constipation and diarrhea though most patients have a tendency to be either constipated or have diarrhea.

▶ Treatment

Treatment of IBS is directed at relieving symptoms and includes lifestyle changes such as increased sleep or exercise, dietary changes such as decreased caffeine, and certain medications such as anticholinergic medications to control intestinal muscle spasms. While IBS is a lifelong disorder, it does not lead to permanent damage of the intestines and rarely leads to admission to the hospital.

Aloi M, D'Arcangelo G, Pofi F, et al.: Presenting features and disease course of pediatric ulcerative colitis. *J Crohns Colitis.* 2013;7(11):e509-e515 [PMID: 23583691].

Suares, NC, Ford AC: Diagnosis and treatment of irritable bowel syndrome. *Discov Med.* 2011;11(60):425-33 [PMID: 21616041].

Fluids and Electrolyte Balance

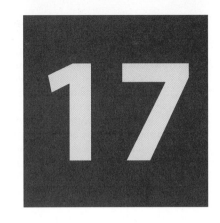

Jon Jaffe, MD

Richard Whitworth, MD

The management of fluid and electrolyte balance in children is an ever-present challenge in the practice of emergency medicine. The varying size of patients coupled with their dependency on others to provide alimentation, both during healthy times and illness, add to the challenge. The ambient environment and multiple organ systems, including the skin, alimentary tract, lungs, kidneys, heart, vasculature, and muscles, joined by multiple endocrine systems create the balance. Although most patients are in the emergency department for short periods of time, the diagnosis of the fluid and electrolyte status needs to have a wider scope. There are formulas for calculating the proper amounts of fluids and solute for patients, but the calculations have to be modified over time. The fluid status of a patient needs to be reassessed on a regular basis regardless of the calculations.

DISORDERS OF VOLUME

GENERAL CONSIDERATIONS

Intravascular volume is crucial to homeostasis and survival. The pediatric population is a great deal more sensitive to derangements in volume than their adult counterparts. The volume status of a child is determined largely in part on the sodium concentration which is regulated by the kidney's ability to alter the amount of sodium reabsorbed along the nephron. The kidneys have a remarkable ability to vary the amount of sodium resorption and thus regulate volume status. However, the renal system's ability to compensate can be overcome by extreme volume loss, markedly decreased intake, volume redistribution, or disease in the kidney itself.

VOLUME DEPLETION

▶ Clinical Findings

History and physical examination contribute significantly to the evaluation and the treatment of children with presumed volume depletion. Important historical elements involve the presence of gastrointestinal (GI) symptoms which are among the most common conditions requiring fluid therapy. Other conditions resulting in volume depletion are poor intake, sepsis, burns, cystic fibrosis, and conditions of the kidney or regulating hormones.

Knowing the severity or quantity of volume depletion is helpful in directing therapy as well as the urgency and duration of therapy. Dehydration is classified into < 5%, 5-10%, and > 10%. For many years a variety of physical findings and scales (collections of findings) have been proposed. None of these is as good as accurate weights.

Look for the presence of dry mucous membranes, absence of tears, tachycardia at rest, capillary refill greater than 3 seconds, abnormal respiratory pattern, and hypotension. In the absence of a documented baseline weight, which is generally not available to the emergency department physician, the patient with a history of poor intake and extra loss may be considered to be hydrated to less than 5% dehydrated. The presence of one or more of these signs would put the patient in the 5-10% range of dehydration. The patient who demonstrates all the signs is profoundly ill and in shock. Ultrasound measuring the ratio of the aorta and inferior vena cava has shown promise in assessing the degree of dehydration.

▶ Treatment

Treatment of the volume-depleted child is dictated by the degree of dehydration, and is typically accomplished in two phases: primary and secondary. Primary replacement is often directed by the emergency department physician, and secondary replacement occurs in the inpatient setting after initial stabilization. In moderate to severe dehydration, emergent replacement of circulating volume with isotonic crystalloid solution is required. The child should be given repeated 20 mL/kg boluses of normal saline (NS) IV or (IO). Repeat administration is indicated based on reassessment and the patient's responsiveness to the fluids. In the primary replacement stage, there is no indication for hypotonic or hypertonic solutions as the goal of therapy is improvement of circulating volume and thus tissue perfusion. Volume expansion with tonic solutions can cause rapid shifts in serum sodium and osmolality resulting in devastating neurologic consequences.

After correction of severe depletion and stabilization, the second stage of replacement therapy begins. The goal of this stage is to continue the volume restoration, correction of electrolyte derangements, as well as providing adequate maintenance fluids. Secondary correction depends upon sodium concentration. In the eunatremic patient correction can continue with NS. However, in the hyponatremic and hypernatremic children volume replacement is not as simple and requires calculation of total body water (TBW), sodium excess or deficit, and the sodium concentration of the fluids.

▶ Disposition

Patients with mild dehydration who respond to hydration can be treated as outpatients with attention to the underlying cause. Patients with moderate or severe dehydration should be hospitalized.

VOLUME OVERLOAD

▶ Clinical Findings

Excessive volume is a rare problem in healthy children due to the kidney's regulation of volume balance via the excretion and resorption of sodium. Children with underlying renal disorders are susceptible to the effects of decreased sodium excretion. Similarly, children with cardiovascular disorders can manifest increased intravascular volume in an attempt to improve perfusion resulting in congestive heart failure (CHF).

Increased volume without underlying renal or cardiovascular disorders can be seen in the presence of water intoxication. Historical clues include lethargy, neurological symptoms, in the setting of increased free water intake. The result is dilutional hyponatremia which will be evident on an electrolyte panel.

▶ Treatment

Treatment of volume overload in the child with chronic health conditions is best managed with specialist consultation. Diuresis and possibly dialysis may be indicated. In the setting of water intoxication hyponatremia, fluid restriction is the treatment of choice.

▶ Disposition

Most children with volume overload, regardless of the underlying etiology, should be considered for admission.

Chen L, Hsiao A, Langhan M, et al: Use of bedside ultrasound to assess degree of dehydration in children with gastroenteritis. *Acad Emerg Med.* 2010;17:1042-1047 [PMID: 21040104].

Colletti JE, Brown KM, Sharieff GQ, et al: The management of children with gastroenteritis and dehydration in the emergency department. *J Emerg Med.* 2010;38:686-698 [PMID: 19345549].

Freedman SB, Adler M, Seshadri R, et al: Oral ondansetron for gastroenteritis in a pediatric emergency department. *N Engl J Med.* 2006;354:1698-1705 [PMID: 16625009].

Friedman JN, Goldman RD, Srivastava R, et al: Development of aclinical dehydration scale for use in children between 1 and 36 months of age. *J Pediatr.* 2004;145:201-207 [PMID: 15289767].

Simpson JN, Teach SJ: Pediatric rapid fluid resuscitation. *Curr Opin Pediatr.* 2011;23:286-292 [PMID: 21508842].

Johnston BC, Shamseer L, da Costa BR, et al: Measurement issues in trials of pediatric acute diarrheal diseases: A systematic review. *Pediatrics.* 2010;126:e222-e231 [PMID: 20566617].

Kinlin LM, Freedman SB: Evaluation of a clinical dehydration scale in children requiring intravenous rehydration. *Pediatrics.* 2012;129:e1211-1219 [PMID: 22529270].

Saba TG, Fairbairn J, Houghton F, et al: A randomized controlled trial of isotonic versus hypotonic maintenance intravenous fluids in hospitalized children. *BMC Pediatr.* 2011;11:82 [PMID: 21943218].

DISORDER OF SODIUM

GENERAL CONSIDERATIONS

Sodium is the most abundant cation in the extracellular fluid (ECF) and therefore the primary determinant of osmolality. By means of a variety of hormonal mechanisms, the kidney regulates volume status via the excretion and resorption of sodium and therefore alteration in sodium concentration can be accompanied by swings in volume and vice versa. Treatment of sodium disorders is based on several factors including severity of symptoms, chronicity, and the patient's volume status. Treatment decisions are based upon these factors in hopes to prevent the potentially devastating neurologic sequelae from sodium correction.

Hypernatremia is sodium concentration greater than 145 mEq/L. Simply put, hypernatremia is water deficit for total body sodium and develops by water loss and less commonly excessive sodium intake or administration. Each category can be further subdivided and the differential can be extensive (Table 17–1).

Table 17–1. Causes of hypernatremia.

Water loss	Sodium Intake
Gastrointestinal	Improperly mixed formula
Increased insensible losses	Iatrogenic
Renal loss (diabetes insipidus)	Abuse
Decreased intake	

Clinical Findings

A thorough nutrition and feeding history must be obtained as well as history of any potential sources of volume loss, including, but not limited to, GI losses and chronic conditions such as diabetes insipidus. The emergency department physician must have a high index of suspicion for sodium disorders in children and infants because they are dependent upon others for fluids and nutrition. In addition, infants are prone to increased insensible losses and the kidneys' ability to concentrate are not fully developed thus providing additional sources of water loss.

The dominant signs and symptoms of infantile and childhood hypernatremia are dehydration and generalized neurological complaints. The neurological complaints may be subtle consisting of irritability, lethargy, weakness, and restlessness. The parents of infants may report a high-pitched cry and the physician may witness hyperpnea. Neurological symptoms progress as a result of water loss from brain cells in response to increased osmolarity. The most devastating impact of hypernatremia is intracranial hemorrhage. The increase in extracellular sodium concentration drives free water from brain cells causing dehydration and shrinkage of the brain. As the brain moves away from the skull meninges, vascular structures are disrupted.

Elevated serum sodium confirms the diagnosis and if the apparent cause is not clear from the history or physical examination, further workup is required to determine the etiology of free water loss. Urine studies are useful to determine whether the loss is primarily renal pathology or results from an extrarenal mechanism. Inappropriately dilute urine indicates a renal pathology such as diabetes insipidus. In contrast, hypernatremia from an extrarenal cause should have urine osmolality greater than 1000 mOsm/kg.

Treatment

The treatment of hypernatremia depends upon chronicity and volume status. In the severely volume-depleted and hypernatremic child, the priority is the restoration of intravascular volume and should be achieved with repeated 20 mL/kg boluses of NS until improvement of vital signs. After stabilization is achieved, the emergency department physician must initiate correction based on rate of development. As hypernatremia develops, the brain produces idiogenic osmoles to combat the osmotic effects of increased ECF osmolarity. The process occurs over time and therefore is most prominent when the hypernatremia develops slowly. When hypernatremia is corrected rapidly, the idiogenic osmoles create an osmotic gradient causing the movement of water from the ECF into the brain causing cerebral edema. When the onset is unknown or known to be chronic, the goal of correction is to decrease the sodium no greater than 0.5 mEq/L/hr or 12 mEq/L/day and TBW corrected over 48-72 hours. Several equations exist for correction, each of which relies on the correction of water deficit which in turn

Table 17–2. Equations for correction of hypernatremia.

Calculate TBW = weight (kg) × 0.6 (child) or 0.8 (infant)
Calculate TBW deficit = {[Na−140] / 145} × TBW
Calculate replacement volume for desired fluid = volume = TBW deficit × {1/(1-[fluid Na/154])}
Calculate rate of infusion to correct over 48-72 hours = volume of desired fluid in mL/hr

will correct sodium. Acute severe hypernatremia is usually a product of sodium excess, not free water loss, and can be corrected more rapidly; however, it may be impossible for correction with hypotonic solution. Sodium concentrations greater than 180 may require peritoneal dialysis. Equations that are used to correct hypernatremia are listed in Table 17–2. Sodium concentration contained in typical fluids are listed in Table 17–3.

Disposition

Children with significant hypernatremia, regardless of the etiology, should be hospitalized.

Hyponatremia

Hyponatremia is sodium concentration less than 135 mEq/L. In contrast to hypernatremia, the diagnosis and treatment of hyponatremia is much more complex. Whereas hypernatremia is associated with some element of volume depletion and hyperosmolality, hyponatremia can be found in hypo-, hyper-, and euvolemic states, as well as in all spectrums of osmolality. The same factors that guide treatment of hypernatremia, chronicity, severity of symptoms, and volume status, are integral to the emergent management of hyponatremia.

The manifestations of hyponatremia are more a product of a decreased serum osmolality and the osmotic effect on the brain. Fluid is driven into brain as a result of the osmotic gradient between brain cells and the ECF causing cerebral edema. Compensation mechanisms explain chronic hyponatremia; however, if the sodium derangement develops quickly, there is no time for compensation and symptoms progress rapidly.

Table 17–3. Sodium concentrations of common intravenous fluids.

NS (0.9%)-154 mEq/L
½ NS (0.45%)-77 mEq/L
0.2%-34 mEq/L
D5W-0 mEq/L

Clinical Findings

Patients present with a constellation of vague neurologic complaints from headache, emesis, and loss of appetite that ultimately progress to seizure and coma. The astute clinician can identify and correct the problem before it progresses to that point but like most other diagnoses a high index of suspicion is required. Interview of parents for a detailed feeding history and history of recent or ongoing GI illnesses is mandatory. Review of medications for potential causes of syndrome of inappropriate antidiuretic hormone (SIADH) can assist in making the diagnosis.

The emergency department physician must ascertain the volume status of the patient as well as the chronicity of symptoms. Measurement of serum sodium makes the diagnosis. Factors that can cause pseudohyponatremias are hyperglycemia, hyperproteinemia, and hyperlipidemia. Testing should be done to exclude these spurious causes. In hyponatremia of uncertain etiology, urine osmolality and urine sodium can be helpful.

Treatment

The severity of symptoms and the chronicity of symptoms will dictate initial management. Rapid correction of indolent hyponatremia can have devastating delayed neurological consequences. Central pontine myelinosis has been associated with rapid correction of sodium and may present 4-5 days after correction. In light of this, the sodium should be corrected by no greater than 8 mEq/L/day. Regardless of the fluid status in the setting of severe symptoms (seizure and coma), rapid partial correction with 3% saline may be necessary. Small aliquots of 1-2 mL/kg of 3% NS can be used until the seizure resolves. Emergent management of hypovolemic hyponatremia resuscitation begins with the treatment of severe neurological symptoms and replacement of intravascular volume and can occur in parallel if necessary. Nonemergent sodium correction is achieved by means of water restriction or parenteral fluid administration and is dependent upon intravascular volume status. Equations useful to correct hyponatremia are listed in Table 17–4.

Table 17–4. Equations for correcting hyponatremia.

Calculate TBW = weight (kg) × 0.6 (child) or 0.8 (infant)
Change in serum sodium per 1 L of fluid = (infusate Na − serum sodium) / (TBW +1)
Volume required = (serum sodium − desired sodium) / change in Na per L infusate
Calculate hours of infusion required for change in sodium correction rate (0.3 to 0.5 mEq/L) = (serum sodium − goal sodium) / 0.3
Calculate rate of infusion = volume required/hours to correct

Disposition

Severity and chronicity of symptoms will guide the disposition. Hospitalization will be required for most patients.

El-Bayoumi MA, Abdelkader AM, El-Assmy NM, et al: Normal saline is safe initial rehydration fluid in children with diarrhea-related hypernatremia. *Eur J Pediatr.* 2012;17:383-388 [PMID: 21909623].

Moritz ML, Ayus JC: New aspects in the pathogenesis, prevention, and treatment of hyponatremic encephalopathy in children. *Pediatr Nephrol.* 2010;25:1225-1238 [PMID: 19894066].

Moritz ML, del Rio M, Crooke GA, et al: Acute peritoneal dialysis as both cause and treatment of hypernatremia in an infant. *Pediatr Nephrol.* 2001;16:697-700 [PMID: 11511979].

DISORDERS OF POTASSIUM

GENERAL CONSIDERATIONS

Potassium (Na) is regulated by the kidney and the hormone aldosterone has the most profound effect on potassium regulation. Serum potassium levels (not necessarily total body potassium) is also altered by pH, circulating catecholamine, and insulin as these hormones stimulate the cell to either take up potassium or release it into the ECF. Potassium is the primary intracellular cation, and it is the intracellular concentration that is responsible for the membrane potential of cells. Therefore, variations in potassium will alter the contractility and responsiveness of nervous and muscular tissues.

Hyperkalemia

The upper limit of normal potassium varies by age with the level in neonates and young infants greater than 6.5 mEq/L, and in infants and children greater than 5.5 mEq/L. Hyperkalemia is a true electrolyte emergency due to the potential for lethal arrhythmias. There are four primary causes of hyperkalemia: increased intake, cellular shifts, decreased excretion, and factitious. The disorders and primary causes are detailed in Table 17–5.

Clinical Findings

Complaints associated with hyperkalemia are often mild and nonspecific and related to the underlying pathology not the electrolyte disturbance. Historical elements of particular interest are past medical history, medications, and previous episodes. Electrocardiography (ECG) and cardiac monitoring are of utmost importance when hyperkalemia is discovered or suspected. Hyperkalemia history and further diagnostic testing may help tease out the underlying cause but all attention should be focused on immediate stabilization. Supplementary testing can be obtained to assist the inpatient team but are not of primary concern in the

Table 17–5. Causes of hyperkalemia.

Increased Intake	Cellular Shift	Decreased Excretion	Factitious
Blood transfusion	Acidosis	Renal failure	Hemolyzed sample
Potassium containing IVF	Rhabdomyolysis	Adrenal disease	Leukocytosis
Oral supplementation	Tumor lysis	Renal tubular disease	
	Hemolysis		
	GI bleeding		

emergent setting. Tests for hyperkalemia include urine electrolytes, urine osmolality, plasma osmolality, and aldosterone.

As serum potassium reaches approximately 6 mEq/L, tall narrowed based peaked T waves may be present. As potassium climbs, the P-R interval prolongs and then eventually flattening of the P wave. If uncorrected, the QRS will widen and progress to a sine wave followed by ventricular fibrillation arrest and asystole. The ECG changes seen with increasing potassium concentrations are shown in Figure 17–1.

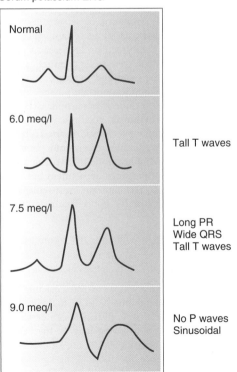

Serum potassium EKG

Normal

6.0 meq/l — Tall T waves

7.5 meq/l — Long PR / Wide QRS / Tall T waves

9.0 meq/l — No P waves / Sinusoidal

▲ **Figure 17–1.** Typical ECG findings with elevated potassium concentration.

Treatment

Treatment of hyperkalemia is warranted if for a serum potassium greater than 6 mEq/L with ECG changes or a serum potassium greater than 7 mEq/L with or without ECG changes. Emergent treatment can be divided into three sequential steps: cardiac stabilization, temporization, and elimination.

Cardiac stabilization is achieved by means of IV calcium. Two options exist: calcium chloride and calcium gluconate. Although calcium chloride contains approximately three times the elemental calcium, it must be given via central line and therefore calcium gluconate is a more rapidly available option. Dose of calcium gluconate is 60-100 mg/kg repeated in 10 minutes if no response in QRS duration.

Temporization is achieved by taking advantage of the ability of cells to store potassium and thus decrease serum levels. It is important to note that total body potassium has not changed but excess potassium is temporarily stored in the cells. Several methods for temporization are available. Insulin causes potassium uptake in cells and must be administered concomitantly with dextrose solutions to prevent hypoglycemia. A β_2-agonist such as albuterol will promote cellular uptake of potassium. Sodium bicarbonate can cause transient shift in cellular potassium uptake by raising the pH driving potassium into cells. Of all the temporizing measures, sodium bicarbonate has the most variable results.

Elimination is the final step in emergent treatment and is usually accomplished by exchange resins. Other options for potassium elimination are loop diuretics and, in severe refractory potassium elevations, emergent hemodialysis.

Disposition

Children with hyperkalemia require admission for monitoring and treatment of the underlying cause.

Hypokalemia

Hypokalemia is serum potassium less than 3.5 mEq/L. In the pediatric patient, hypokalemia is a usually a product of GI loss (diarrhea) or renal loss (renal tubular acidosis). Regardless of the mechanism, the effects of hypokalemia can have a profound effect on cardiac, skeletal, and smooth muscles.

▶ **Clinical Findings**

The child with hypokalemia may present with a myriad of complaints. As a result of the effects on cardiac, skeletal, and smooth muscles, the patient may complain of or exhibit muscle cramps, weakness, and possibly paralysis. When hypokalemia is discovered, an ECG should be obtained as well as serum magnesium and phosphate levels. Characteristic ECG findings include flattened T waves, S-T segment depression and, occasionally, a U wave between the T wave and P wave. As with hyperkalemia, recognition and correction of hypokalemia are priorities in the emergency department. After stabilization, additional testing to confirm the underlying diagnosis may be initiated, such as blood gas, urine potassium, urine osmolality, and serum osmolality.

▶ **Treatment**

Goals of treatment are to replace potassium at a safe rate and to stop ongoing potassium loss. For mild decreases in potassium, oral replacement may be sufficient and the oral dose of potassium is 0.5-2 mEq/kg every 12 hours. Severely symptomatic or potassium-depleted patients may require IV potassium. Intravenous potassium should always be given in a monitored setting and delivered by a pump at 0.5 mEq/kg over 1-2 hours. Replace magnesium concurrently. Caution should be taken when correcting hypokalemia in patients with renal disease as they have a decreased ability to regulate excrete the excess potassium.

▶ **Disposition**

Consider admission for the child with hypokalemia for monitoring, replacement, and treatment of the underlying cause.

Ingram TC, Olsson JM: In brief: Hypokalemia. *Pediatr Rev.* 2008;29:e50-e51 [PMID: 18765467].

Mahoney BA, Smith WA, Lo DS, et al: Emergency interventions for hyperkalemia. *Cochrane Database Syst Rev.* 2005;18:CD003235 [PMID: 15846652].

DISORDERS OF CALCIUM

GENERAL CONSIDERATIONS

Approximately 99% of total body calcium is found in skeletal tissue. The remaining 1% is distributed among the intracellular and extracellular compartments (ECF) and is vital for cell function and survival. Fluctuations in calcium can have a variety of manifestations that include GI, psychiatric, neurological, and cardiac effects. Within the ECF, calcium exists

Table 17–6. Causes of calcium disorders.

Hypercalcemia	Hypocalcemia
Hypoparathyroidism	Hyperparathyroidism
Maternal hypoparathyroidism	Vitamin D intoxication
Vitamin D deficiency	Exogenous calcium administration
Hyperphosphatemia	Diuretics
Ingestions (ethylene glycol)	Malignancy

either bound to proteins and ions or free. It is the free or "ionized" calcium that is physiologically active. The percentage of bound calcium is dependent upon several factors, the two most notable are albumin level and the pH. Table 17–6 lists the most common causes for calcium derangements.

Hypocalcemia

▶ **Clinical Findings**

Similar to electrolyte abnormalities, manifestations of hypocalcemia are dependent upon chronicity. Mild hypocalcemia may present as paraesthesias of face and hands and progress to the more severe symptoms of seizure, laryngospasam, and tetany. A Chvostek (facial nerve tapping causing facial muscles to twitch or contract) or Trousseau sign (inflating a blood pressure cuff above systolic pressure causing spasm of the muscles of the hand and forearm) may be present. Significant cardiac complications are possible in the setting of hypokalemia and include hypotension, CHF, prolonged Q-T, and other dysrhythmias.

Upon diagnosis of hypocalcemia, ionized calcium should be ordered as well as albumin, magnesium, phosphate, renal profile, and parathyroid hormone (PTH). The tests may not prove useful in the emergency department but will identify the underlying cause. The clinician must remember to correct the serum calcium for the albumin level, using the equation

$$[0.8 \times (4 - \text{patient's albumin})] + \text{serum calcium}$$

▶ **Treatment**

In severe hypocalcemia with a corrected calcium of less than 7.5 or significant symptoms or ECG findings, IV replacement is necessary. Calcium gluconate can be given peripherally and the emergent setting may be the better option. Calcium gluconate is given 50-100 mg/kg over 3-5 minutes for cardiac disturbance and 100-200 mg/kg over 5-10 minutes for severe neurological disturbance. Doses are repeated until symptoms resolve. Oral replacement is an option for less severe hypocalcemia. Magnesium should be corrected concomitantly with hypocalcemia. In patients with severe hypophosphatemia, aggressive calcium replacement may result in the precipitation of calcium and phosphate in the tissues.

▶ Disposition

Patients requiring IV replacement should be hospitalized for monitoring and treatment of the underlying cause.

Hypercalcemia

▶ Clinical Findings

Presenting signs and symptoms will depend upon the severity and the chronicity of the elevated calcium level. Mild elevations (< 12 mg/dL) may be asymptomatic and as levels increase symptoms develop and the child may present with complaints of anorexia, irritability, and abdominal pain. If hypercalcemia is severe, presentation may include weakness, seizure, and coma. When hypercalcemia is profound, dehydration and signs and symptoms of hypovolemia may present.

Once hypercalcemia is suspected or confirmed, treatment should begin as well as investigation to identify underlying cause. Laboratory workup includes a basic metabolic panel, ionized calcium, magnesium, phosphorus, albumin, and assessment of acid-base status. A parathyroid hormone level should be obtained, although, in most cases, results will not be available during the acute phase of treatment. However, the results may be vitally important to the follow-up or inpatient providers.

▶ Treatment

Mild (> 12 mg/dL) and moderate (< 14 mg/dL) hypercalcemia may not require emergent treatment, instead investigation to identify the underlying cause. Symptomatic or severe (> 14 mg/dL) hyercalcemia requires treatment. Initial management is aimed at fluid resuscitation. Once adequate circulating volume is restored, calcium excretion can be promoted with loop diuretics. Alternative treatments include calcitonin, bisphosphonates, and hemodialysis. Consultation with a pediatric nephrologist is warranted prior to initiating these therapies.

▶ Disposition

Children with symptoms or those with moderate and severe hypercalcemia should be admitted for monitoring and treatment.

Lietman SA, Germain-Lee EL, Levine MA: Hypercalcemia in children and adolescents. *Curr Opin Pediatr.* 2010;22:508-515 [PMID: 20601885].

Shaw N: A practical approach to hypocalcaemia in children. *Endocr Dev.* 2009;16:73-92 [PMID: 19494662].

Table 17–7. Maintenance of fluid requirements by weight.

Weight (mass)	Fluid/day
< 10 kg	100 mL/kg
11-20 kg	1000 mL + 50 mL/kg
> 21 kg	1500 mL + 20 mL/kg

INTRAVENOUS MAINTENANCE THERAPY

GENERAL CONSIDERATIONS

Maintenance fluids for children are commonly based on the weight (mass) of the patient. Formulas used are based on caloric expenditure and body surface area and are not linear. The formulae are for parenteral therapy only and are listed in Table 17–7. The fluid calculations are often coupled with deficit fluid therapy as needed.

Sodium and potassium requirements are related to the maintenance formulae.

- Sodium ~ 2-3 mEq/100 mL of fluid administered per day
- Potassium ~ 2 mEq/100 mL of fluid administered per day

The 10-kg child would receive 1 L of fluid. In that would be 30 mEq sodium and approximately 20 mEq potassium. Commonly this is administered in a hypotonic solution of D5½ NS and D5¼ NS in infants younger than 6 weeks. Although controversy exists regarding use of hypotonic solutions in perioperative patients for a prolonged period causing iatrogenic hyponatremia, the 12-hour window for emergency resuscitation and fluid administration remains incontrovertible. Thus, D5½ NS remains the standard.

Moritz ML, Ayus JC: Improving intravenous fluid therapy in children with gastroenteritis. *Pediatr Nephrol.* 2010;25:1383-1384 [PMID: 20309584].

Mortiz ML, Ayus JC: Inravenous fluid management for the acutely ill child. *Curr Opin Pediatr.* 2011;23:186-193 [PMID: 21415832].

DEFICIT FLUID THERAPY

GENERAL CONSIDERATIONS

Deficit therapy is more clearly weight based because rapid weight loss is invariably equivalent to water loss. Replacement can be estimated based on weight and the estimated percentage of dehydration (weight loss) based on physical findings. Fluid deficit is calculated using the following equation.

$$\text{Fluid deficit (mL)} = \text{weight (kg)} \times \% \text{ dehydration} \times 10$$

In a practical situation, some of the deficits are replaced with recussitative therapy and should be included in the total calculation. For example, in a 10-kg infant with 10 % dehydration, the fluid deficit equals 1000 mL. If the patient is given a 20-mL/kg fluid bolus, the deficit equals 800 mL of water. However, maintenance fluid should be calculated and administered. The volume of maintenance fluid for the example is 1000 mL (100 mL/kg × 10 kg). As a result, ongoing therapy would be 1800 mL over the next 24 hours by administering D5½ NS at 75 mL/hr for 24 hours. From a pure fluid standpoint, this is adequate maintenance and deficit therapy. However, there remains a significant caloric deficit. For the emergency department physician, the goal is to normalize vital signs and then give patient a small amount of salt water and sugar, with the hope of early return to normal alimentation.

Disposition

Patients who have fluid deficits of 5% or greater should be admitted.

Moritz ML, Ayus JC: Improving intravenous fluid therapy in children with gastroenteritis. *Pediatr Nephrol.* 2010;25:1383-1384 [PMID: 20309584].

Mortiz ML, Ayus JC: Inravenous fluid management for the acutely ill child. *Curr Opin Pediatr.* 2011;23:186-193 [PMID: 21415832].

Simpson JN, Teach SJ: Pediatric rapid fluid resuscitation. *Curr Opin Pediatr.* 2011;23:286-292 [PMID: 21508842].

HYDRATION TECHNIQUES

GENERAL CONSIDERATIONS

There are various techniques for hydration. They vary because of location, availability of resources, and cultural norms. The emergency department physician should be acquainted with all.

Oral Rehydration

Oral rehydration is the preferred route for the World Health Organization (WHO) and many centers in the United States. Oral rehydrating solutions are designed to provide volume, mineral, and carbohydrate support without osmotic taxation soft drinks or juices can bring with them. Oral hydration cannot be used in the presence of an ileus; therefore, bowel sounds must be present to begin therapy. Administer slowly with a syringe or teaspoon and replace ongoing losses, stool, and urine using diaper weight. Nasogastric tube rehydration can be used effectively even in the presence of vomiting. Dosage is typically 50-100 mL/kg of oral rehydrating solution over 4 hours.

Intraosseous Infusion

Intraosseous infusion is frequently used in the prehospital setting or in the setting of a patient in extremis. It has the advantage of being a rapid and safe way to administer fluids and drugs. Similar to venous access, irritative drugs and fluids need to be considered carefully to avoid complication.

Subcutaneous Infusion

Infusion of fluids into the subcutaneous tissue is an old technique to treat the mild to moderately dehydrated patient. Currently it is that has been augmented by recombinant haluronidase. The enzyme loosens the subcutaneous space and makes it more receptive to volume. It is helpful to augment oral rehydration as well as to improve the intravascular compartment to make venous access easier. Inject 150 units of recombinant hyaluronidase prior to subcutaneous fluid administration. Typically the injection is done with 24-gauge catheter placed into the subcutaneous space on the patient's back between the scapulae or in the anterior thigh. The hyaluronidase can facilitate absorption of 1000 mL or greater of solution at a rate and volume that does not exceed the intravenous infusion.

Mortiz ML, Ayus JC: Intravenous fluid management for the acutely ill child. *Curr Opin Pediatr.* 2011;23:186-93 [PMID: 21415832].

Rouhani S, Meloney L, Ahn R, et al: Alternative rehydration methods: A systematic review and lessons for resource-limited care. *Pediatrics.* 2011;127:e748-57 [PMID: 21321023].

Simpson JN, Teach SJ: Pediatric rapid fluid resuscitation. *Curr Opin Pediatr.* 2011;23:286-92 [PMID: 21508842].

Spandorfer PR: Subcutaneous rehydration: Updating a traditional technique. *Pediatr Emerg Care.* 2011;27:230-6 [PMID: 21378529].

Syncope

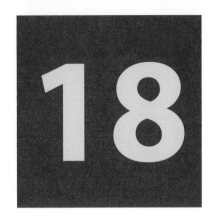

18

Brit Anderson, MD

Seema Bhatt, MD, MS

Although vasodepressor syncope is the most common cause of syncope in older children and adolescents, cardiac causes are the most concerning and life threatening in this group. Approximately 2–6% of all cases of pediatric syncope can be attributed to the heart. The rare, yet life-threatening causes of syncope must be discriminated from more benign etiologies. History, physical examination findings, and electrocardiograph (ECG) findings can be used by the emergency medical practitioner to screen for patients who may be at risk for cardiac pathology. Historical "red flags" include syncope with exertion and a positive family history (Table 18–1). Cardiac causes of syncope can be divided into structural, functional, and primary electrical categories. Table 18–2 lists ECG findings associated with specific cardiac abnormalities.

STRUCTURAL HEART DISEASE

Structural heart disease includes a wide range of pathologies defined by an alteration in the physical architecture of the heart. History of syncope with exertion and anginal chest pain are concerning for structural heart disease. Mechanisms by which structural heart disease can cause syncope include arrhythmias and outflow obstruction. Structural abnormalities include hypertrophic cardiomyopathy, anomalous coronary arteries, and congenital heart conditions that have undergone repair.

Hypertrophic Cardiomyopathy

▶ Clinical Findings

Hypertrophic cardiomyopathy (HCM) is characterized by asymmetric hypertrophy of the left ventricle. It is the most common genetic cardiovascular disease with an autosomal dominant pattern of inheritance. It is caused by a mutation in one of several genes, which accounts for the heterogeneity of clinical presentation.

HCM can lead to outflow obstruction or arrhythmias. The rate of sudden death is approximately 1 in 200,000, most commonly occurring during exercise.

A careful history and physical examination are important if there is concern for HCM, with close attention to family history. Patients with HCM present with chest pain, dizziness, or syncope on exertion. Because a high percentage of pediatric patients do not have outflow obstruction, a murmur is not always found on physical examination. Classically, a systolic murmur with HCM will increase with decreased venous return to the heart (Valsalva or standing), and will decrease with increased return to the heart (sitting). An ECG should be carefully read for axis deviation, left ventricular hypertrophy, and ST-wave abnormalities. An echocardiogram is diagnostic and should be done if HCM is suspected.

▶ Treatment

All patients suspected of having HCM or who have a concerning history, physical examination, or ECG findings should be followed by a cardiologist and should refrain from physical exertion. Screening of family members is often indicated. Treatment depends upon the patient because of the heterogeneity of the disease. Treatment includes beta blockers, calcium channel blockers, and implantable defibrillators.

▶ Disposition

Patients who present to the emergency department with findings concerning for HCM should be evaluated by a cardiologist. Patients should abstain from physical activity until evaluation is complete. Patients with signs of heart failure or who are unstable should be admitted for further management.

Table 18–1. Historical findings for syncope.

- History of heart disease
- Syncope during exercise or exertion
- Absence of prodromal symptoms
- History of chest pain, palpitations, difficulty breathing
- Family history
  - Sudden death
  - Pacemaker placement
  - Car accidents/drowning
  - Dysrhythmia
  - SIDS
  - Deafness

Table 18–2. ECG findings associated with specific cardiac abnormalities.

Disease	ECG findings
Hypertrophic cardiomyopathy	LAE LVH Axis deviation Abnormal ST-segments Q waves in lateral leads TWI
Aortic stenosis	LVH LV strain
Vascular anomalies	ST/T wave changes Q waves Strain/infarction
Myocarditis	Sinus tachycardia ST and T wave changes Q waves BBB Wide QRS
Dilated cardiomyopathy	Sinus tachycardia ST/T wave changes Q waves Dysrhythmias
Long QT syndrome	QTc > 450 msec
Brugada syndrome	ST elevation in right, precordial leads
Wolff-Parkinson-White syndrome	Short PR interval Delta wave SVT (usually narrow complex tachycardia with absent or polymorphic P waves)
Catecholaminergic polymorphic ventricular tachycardia	Resting: Normal or sinus bradycardia, U wave

LAE, left atrial enlargement; LVH, left ventricular hypertrophy; TWI, T-wave inversions; LV, left ventricular; BBB, bundle branch block.

Anomalous Right or Left Coronary Artery From the Opposite Aortic Sinus

▶ Clinical Presentation

Anomalous right or left coronary artery from the opposite aortic sinus can lead to myocardial ischemia and ventricular dysrhythmias when exercising. During exercise it is hypothesized that the anomalous coronary artery may be kinked or compressed by the expanding aorta. A history of syncope during exercise is particularly concerning for HCM. Unfortunately, diagnosis challenging as physical examination and ECG may be normal. Echocardiography, computed tomography (CT), or magnetic resonance imaging (MRI) may be utilized to delineate the abnormal origin of the coronary arteries.

▶ Treatment

Treatment is surgical and includes coronary artery reimplantation and unroofing procedures.

▶ Disposition

If a child has syncope during exercise, a careful evaluation must be done to rule out anomalous coronary arteries. Disposition is made in conjunction with a pediatric cardiologist so that the evaluation can be completed in a safe and timely manner. Patients should be restricted from physical activity.

Anomalous Left Coronary Artery From the Pulmonary Artery

▶ Clinical Presentation

Anomalous origin of left coronary artery from pulmonary artery (ALCAPA) can lead to syncope or sudden death. As pulmonary pressures fall after birth, perfusion to the anomalous left coronary artery falls leading to myocardial ischemia. Myocardial steal syndrome can occur if collaterals between the left and right coronaries develop. The direction of blood flow reverses and drains from the left coronary artery into the pulmonary artery (aorta to right coronary to left coronary to pulmonary artery). In addition to ischemia, fibrosis, dilation, or aneurysms of the left ventricle can occur. Patients may have associated mitral valve insufficiency. History includes symptoms of heart failure, episodic chest pain, and symptoms with exertion. Physical examination can reveal a gallop or murmur from mitral insufficiency. Cardiomegaly may be seen on chest x-ray. Findings of myocardial infarctions or ischemia may be present on ECG (ST- and T-wave changes, Q waves). Diagnosis can be difficult. Echocardiography, exercise testing, CT, MR, or coronary angiography may be indicated.

Treatment

Treatment depends upon the clinical presentation and includes surgical repair of the primary problem. Patients may need medical management for consequences of ALCAPA (myocardial ischemia).

Disposition

Patients with history concerning for ALCAPA warrant echocardiography and cardiology consultation. Disposition should be made in conjunction with a pediatric cardiologist.

Leong SW, Bordes AJ, Henry J, et al: Anomalous left coronary artery from the pulmonary artery: A case report and review of the literature. *Int J Cardiol.* 2009;133:132-134 [PMID: 18279981].

OTHER STRUCTURAL HEART DISEASES

Patients with repaired congenital heart disease or prosthetic heart disease who present with syncope warrant special attention. Acquired coronary lesions can lead to syncope as well and include Kawasaki disease (KD), atherosclerosis, and drug abuse. Patients with KD may have coronary artery aneurysms, stenosis, or occlusions which persist after the acute phase of illness and can lead to serious morbidity and mortality. Other structural heart diseases which can lead to syncope include cardiac masses, atrial septal defect (ASD), arrhythmogenic right ventricular dysplasia, and primary or secondary pulmonary hypertension.

FUNCTIONAL HEART DISEASE

Functional heart disease is a disorder primarily affecting cardiac myocyte function and cell architecture. Myocarditis, dilated cardiomyopathy, and pericarditis with effusion are functional cardiac diseases which can lead to syncope. Syncope is likely caused by a secondary arrhythmia.

Myocarditis

Clinical Presentation

Myocarditis is inflammation, necrosis, or myocytolysis of the myocardium which can lead to heart failure, arrhythmias, or sudden death. The most common cause of myocarditis is a viral infection, although inflammatory, toxic, and other etiologies exist. Clinical presentation depends on the age and etiology and is varied. Symptoms can range from a mild flu-like illness to chest pain, heart failure, hemodynamic instability, or death. Fever and persistent tachycardia can suggest the diagnosis. Chest x-ray reveals an enlarged heart and pulmonary edema. Findings from ECG include sinus tachycardia, reduced QRS voltage, and ST-segment and T-wave abnormalities. Arrhythmias may be present as well. Echocardiography is significant for poor ventricular function. The gold standard for diagnosis is myocardial biopsy.

Treatment

Treatment depends on the etiology of myocarditis and the condition of the patient. The patient should have careful cardiac monitoring. Supportive care is important. Treatment for arrhythmias and heart failure may be warranted. Therapies such as intravenous immunoglobulin (IVIG) and immunosuppression are controversial.

Disposition

Although a number of patients with myocarditis improve spontaneously, some patients become very ill and require escalation of care. Cardiology and cardiothoracic surgery consultations may be necessary. Patients with myocarditis should be observed closely, and if a fulminant course is suspected, the patient should be transferred to a tertiary care facility.

Sagar S, Liu PP, Cooper LT, Jr: Myocarditis. *Lancet.* 2012;379: 738-747 [PMID: 22185868].

Dilated Cardiomyopathy

Clinical Presentation

Left ventricular dilation (although the right ventricle may be involved) can be caused by several etiologies. In the child it is often idiopathic, but myocarditis and neuromuscular disorders are other etiologies. A genetic cause may be present in some patients and can be inherited in an autosomal dominant fashion. Pediatric patients can have systolic and diastolic dysfunction in addition to arrhythmias. All age groups can be affected and clinical presentations vary. Onset is often insidious and symptoms include respiratory distress and abdominal pain. ECG can reveal atrial enlargement, left or right ventricular hypertrophy, and T-wave abnormalities. Chest x-ray is significant for cardiomegaly and may have pulmonary congestion or edema. Echocardiography is diagnostic.

Treatment

If dilated cardiomyopathy is suspected in a child, a cardiologist should be consulted. Management depends on etiology. Medical therapy for heart failure can be successful although heart transplantation is occasionally necessary.

Disposition

Disposition of the child with or suspected of having dilated cardiomyopathy is made in conjunction with a cardiologist based on the clinical condition of the child.

Black KD, Seslar SP, Woodward GA: Cardiogenic causes of pediatric syncope. *Clin Pediatr Emerg Med.* 2011;12(4):266-277; http://www.sciencedirect.com/science/article/pii/S1522840111000620.

Carabello BA, Paulus WJ: Aortic Stenosis. *Lancet.* 2009;373:956-966 [PMID: 19232707].

Cooper LT: Myocarditis. *N Engl J Med.* 2009;360:1526-38 [PMID: 19357408].

Jefferies JL, Towbin JA: Dilated cardiomyopathy. *Lancet.* 2010;375 (9716):752-762 [PMID: 20189027].

Walsh KE, Sanders LK, Ross JC: A-9-year old boy with exertional syncope. *J Emerg Med.* 2012;43(5):e319-e324 [PMID:22445680].

Washington R: Syncope and sudden death in the athlete. *Clin Pediatr Emerg Med.* 2007; 8(1): 54-58.

PRIMARY ELECTRICAL HEART DISEASE

Primary electrical heart disease is the disturbance of normal cardiac activity without a structural or functional abnormality. Long QT syndrome, Brugada syndrome, Wolff-Parkinson-White (WPW) syndrome, heart block, and ventricular tachycardia are included in this category.

Long QT Syndrome

▶ Clinical Presentation

Long QT syndrome (LQTS) is an ion channelopathy. There is interference with ventricular repolarization which predisposes to unstable arrhythmias. Syncope or sudden death results from arrhythmias such as torsade de pointes or ventricular fibrillation. Estimated prevalence in the general population in the United States is 1 in 5000. There are several etiologies including congenital and acquired. Congenital LQTS is a heterogeneous disorder resulting from mutations in one of three genes and can be categorized as LQT1, LQT2, and LQT3. Presentations differ among the types: LQT1 tends to be triggered by emotional or physical stress, and LQT2 is classically triggered by loud noises. Long QT can be associated with specific genetic syndromes: Romano-Ward with autosomal dominant inheritance and Jervell and Lange-Nielsen syndrome with deafness and autosomal recessive transmission. LQTS can be acquired through electrolyte disturbances (hypocalcemia), hypothyroidism, or medications (antiarrhythmic agents, tricyclic antidepressants, antipsychotics, antibiotics, antifungals, and antihistamines).

It is essential to obtain a careful family history of arrhythmia or sudden death because long QT can be inherited. Syncope with LQTS is precipitous. Patients do not usually report prodromal symptoms. Diagnosis is made on ECG (Figure 18–1). Bazet formula is used to calculate the corrected QT interval (QTc) when an ECG is obtained.

$$QTc = QT / \sqrt{RR}$$

Upper limit of normal for QTc depends upon sex and age. Echocardiography is normal. Genetic testing for mutations is available and may be appropriate in patients with family history of sudden death or ECG findings.

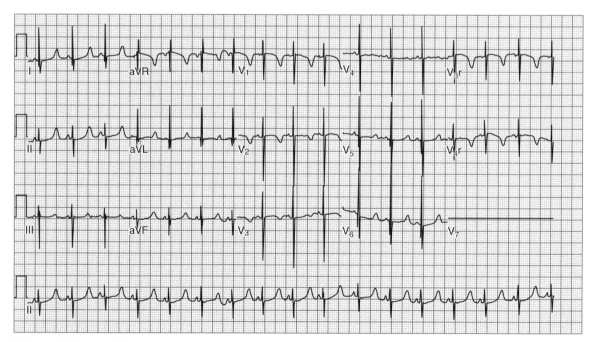

▲ **Figure 18–1.** Long QT.

Treatment

Treatment depends upon etiology and includes β blockade and implantable cardioverter defibrillator (ICD) placement. Patients with LQTS should abstain from competitive sports and medications known to prolong the QT interval.

Disposition

Children and adolescents with syncope and prolonged QTc should be evaluated in the emergency department by a cardiologist. It is appropriate to refer a patient with borderline prolonged QTc as outpatient to a cardiologist. Physical activity must be restricted until the patient is evaluated.

Roden DM: Long-QT syndrome. *N Engl J Med.* 2008;358(2): 169-176 [PMID: 18184962].

Brugada Syndrome

Clinical Presentation

Brugada syndrome is a channelopathy predisposing to arrhythmias. The syndrome can present with syncope or sudden death. Patients have a mutation in the SCN5A channel, a sodium channel, but they have a structurally normal heart. It is an inherited disorder, likely autosomal dominant. Diagnosis is made by finding ST-segment elevation in the right precordial leads on ECG (Figure 18–2). Patients who present with syncope appear be at high risk for sudden death.

Treatment

The mainstay of treatment in patients who present with syncope is ICD placement.

Disposition

Patients suspected of having Brugada syndrome who present with syncope should be evaluated by a cardiologist in the emergency department as they are at risk for sudden death.

Probst V, Veltmann L, Eckardt PG, et al: Long-term prognosis of patients diagnosed with Brugada syndrome: Results from the FINGER Brugada syndrome registry. *Circulation.* 2010;121:635-643 [PMID: 20100972].

Supraventricular Tachycardia

Clinical Presentation

Supraventricular tachycardia (SVT) is a tachyarrhythmia that requires atrial or AV nodal tissue for conductance. Tachycardia can occur through several mechanisms, one of which is an accessory pathway (see Wolff-Parkinson-White Syndrome discussed below). Clinical presentations of SVT include palpitations, chest pain, difficulty breathing, and syncope. Young children will have a heart rate greater than 220 beats per minute, whereas older children have a heart rate greater than 180 beats per minute. Rapid onset and rapid termination discriminate SVT from sinus tachycardia.

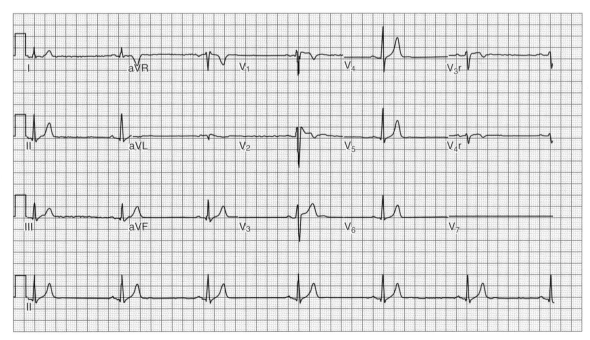

▲ **Figure 18–2.** Brugada syndrome; note the abnormal QRS in the right precordial leads.

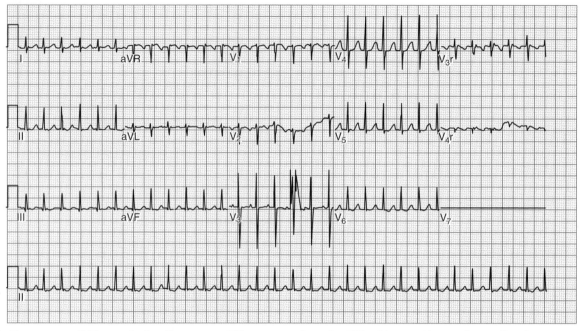

▲ **Figure 18–3.** SVT; note the fast (heart rate ~170) narrow and regular QRS, without evidence of preceding P waves.

Findings of ECG can include a narrow complex tachycardia without beat-to-beat variability and an absent or polymorphic P wave (Figure 18–3). Patients with SVT and an accessory pathway or bundle branch block can present with a wide-complex tachycardia.

▶ Treatment

Treatment for SVT in the acute setting varies depending on hemodynamic stability of the patient. If unstable, cardioversion is the mainstay of treatment. In the stable patient, vagal maneuvers, adenosine, or other medications can be attempted. Wide complex tachycardia should be treated as ventricular tachycardia unless it is known to be SVT. Long-term therapy depends upon the etiology and includes medical therapy (β blockers) and ablation.

▶ Disposition

SVT associated with syncope or preexcitation should be referred to an electrophysiologist.

Wolff-Parkinson-White Syndrome

▶ Clinical Presentation

Wolff-Parkinson-White (WPW) syndrome is characterized by an accessory pathway from the atrium to the ventricle bypassing the AV node (Figure 18–4). It results in earlier activation of the ventricle. Syncope occurs when there is rapid conduction from the atrium which can deteriorate into ventricular fibrillation. In contrast to LQTS and Brugada syndrome, most patients with WPW report heart palpitations from SVT.

▶ Treatment

Catheter ablation of the accessory pathway can be curative. In stable patients, vagal maneuvers and adenosine are recommended, synchronized cardioversion for unstable patients.

▶ Disposition

Patients with SVT should be referred to an electrophysiologist for ablation of the accessory pathway.

Catecholaminergic Polymorphic Ventricular Tachycardia

▶ Clinical Presentation

Catecholaminergic polymorphic ventricular tachycardia (CPVT) is an inherited arrhythmia which is characterized by polymorphic ventricular tachycardia during physical or emotional stress. Symptoms usually present in childhood and include dizziness, palpitations, and syncope during times of stress. There is often a family history of similar symptoms. Diagnosis is made by exercise stress test or Holter monitoring. Polymorphic tachycardia or premature ventricular

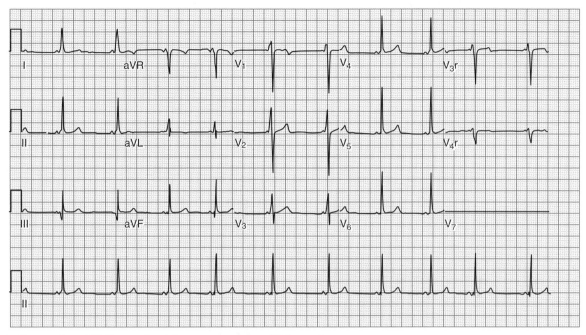

▲ **Figure 18–4.** WPW; note the delta waves and short PR interval.

contractions (PVCs) can be seen as heart rate increases. Resting ECG is typically normal as is echocardiography. Untreated patients have a high mortality rate.

▶ Treatment

Treatment options include β blockers and ICD placement.

▶ Disposition

Patients suspected of having CPVT should be referred to a cardiologist. Physical activity should be restricted until evaluation is complete.

Ylanen K, Poutanen T, Hiippala A, et al: Catecholaminergic polymorphic ventricular tachycardia. *Eur J Pediatr.* 2010;169: 535-542 [PMID: 20143088].

Atrioventricular Block

▶ Clinical Presentation

Atrioventricular (AV) block can be a cause of syncope in children and adolescents. Type II second-degree block is the sudden, intermittent failure of conduction from the atria to the ventricles without a gradual lengthening of the PR interval seen on ECG. Third-degree, or complete heart block, is the complete absence of conduction from atria to the ventricles. Atrioventricular block can be congenital, for example,

if structural anomalies are present or in the case of neonatal lupus. Acquired heart block can be due to many conditions including history of cardiac surgery or myocarditis. Patients can present with syncope due to poor cardiac output.

▶ Treatment

Patients who have syncopal episodes caused by second- or third-degree heart block are candidates for pacemaker placement.

▶ Disposition

Patients should be evaluated by a cardiologist as pacemaker placement may be indicated.

Sick Sinus Syndrome

▶ Clinical Presentation

Sick sinus syndrome (SSS) is complex disease involving the sinus node, which can lead to bradycardia and occasionally intermittent tachycardia. The mechanism of SSS is unclear and likely multifactorial. Potential causes of SSS are intrinsic problems in the sinus node, defects in conduction from the node to the rest of the atria, and abnormal autonomic influences. Clinical presentation varies and range from asymptomatic bradycardia to dizziness, syncope, and signs of heart failure. It can present after heart surgery.

Treatment

Treatment depends on the stability of the patient. A number of patients can be observed, whereas symptomatic patients may require pacing.

Disposition

Patients who are symptomatic (present with syncope) should be evaluated by a cardiologist immediately.

Anderson JB, Benson DW: Genetics of sick sinus syndrome. *Card Electrophysiol Clin.* 2010;2:499-507 [PMID: 21499520].

Hanash CR, Crosson JE: Emergency diagnosis and management of pediatric arrhythmias. *J Emerg Trauma Shock.* 2010;3:251-260 [PMID: 20936909].

EMERGENCY TREATMENT OF SPECIFIC DISORDERS

DEFINITION AND CAUSES OF SYNCOPE:

Syncope is defined as an abrupt loss of consciousness associated with a loss of postural tone. Episodes are typically brief and resolve spontaneously. It is a common emergency department presenting complaint during childhood and adolescence.

Causes of syncope can be classified into general categories: autonomic, cardiac, metabolic, and conditions that mimic syncope. The etiology is most often benign although there are rare, life-threatening causes of syncope that should not be missed. Life-threatening causes are typically cardiac in nature. Table 18-3 lists causes of syncope.

EPIDEMIOLOGY

True incidence of syncope in the pediatric population is unknown as many people do not seek medical care. However, pediatric syncope is commonly encountered in the emergency department. In fact, it accounts for approximately 1% of patient visits to emergency department in the United States. It has been reported that syncope is more common in the adolescent age group with a peak between 15 and 19 years of age. Females are affected more often than males.

HISTORY

A careful history can help identify true syncope as well as point to those at high risk for life-threatening causes of syncope (cardiac disease). Description of what happened prior to the syncopal event as well as during the event are important to elicit from the patient as well as witnesses. A history should be obtained including details about what the patient was doing when syncope occurred (standing, exercise), the position the patient was in before syncope,

Table 18–3. Causes of syncope.

Autonomic
- Vasovagal syncope
- Situational syncope (includes breath-holding spells)
- Orthostatic hypotension
- Postural orthostatic tachycardia syndrome (POTS)
- Carotid sinus hypersensitivity
- Pregnancy

Cardiogenic
- Structural
  - Hypertrophic cardiomyopathy
  - Aortic stenosis
  - Pulmonary hypertension
  - Anomalous coronary vessel
  - Kawasaki disease
  - Cardiac mass
  - Other unrepaired or repaired congenital heart disease
- Functional
  - Dilated cardiomyopathy
  - Myocarditis
  - Pericarditis with effusion
- Primary electrical
  - Long-QT syndrome
  - Brugada syndrome
  - AV block
  - Supraventricular tachycardia/ Wolff-Parkinson-White syndrome
  - Ventricular tachycardia
  - Arrhythmogenic right ventricular dysplasia

Metabolic
- Electrolyte disorder
- Carbon monoxide exposure

duration of loss of consciousness, prodromal symptoms (dizziness, diaphoresis, nausea, and vision changes), chest pain or heart palpitations, presence or absence of seizure activity. Syncope occurring during physical exertion may be a red flag pointing to an underlying cardiac etiology. Injuries may be sustained by falling when consciousness is lost. Any significant past medical history including new medications, use of illicit drugs, or family history especially of cardiac etiology should be elicited.

PHYSICAL EXAMINATION

Complete examination should be performed including vital signs (at rest and orthostatic), with special attention to neurological and cardiac examination.

DIAGNOSTIC EVALUATION

Further evaluation should be tailored to history and physical examination findings. It has been found that extensive testing in routine patients with syncope is expensive and ineffective. At minimum an ECG should be obtained on each child presenting with a syncopal episode to screen for cardiac disease. Laboratory studies that may be useful include glucose level, hematocrit, urine pregnancy test, and urine toxicology screen. If concern for neurologic insult or seizure, consider neuroimaging or electroencephalogram (EEG), respectively.

Anderson JB, Czosek RJ, Cnota J, et al: Pediatric syncope: National Hospital Ambulatory Medical Care Survey Results. *J Emerg Med.* 2012;43 (4):575-583. [PMID: 22406025].

Task Force for the Diagnosis and Management of Syncope, European Society of Cardiology, European Heart Rhythm Association: Guidelines for the diagnosis and management of syncope (version 2009). *Eur Heart J.* 2009;30:2631-2671 [PMID: 19713422].

Vasovagal Syncope

Clinical Presentation

Vasovagal syncope is the most common cause of syncope in children, accounting for one-half of all emergency department syncope-related visits. Patients tend to have complaints of prodromal symptoms immediately before loss of consciousness which include dizziness, diaphoresis, warm sensation, light-headedness, nausea, and vision changes. Loss of consciousness follows, which typically lasts several seconds. Witnesses may report that the patient appears pale and sweaty. There can be seizure-like activity after loss of consciousness, usually one to two jerking movements, caused by cerebral hypoperfusion. Recovery is spontaneous, but it may take several minutes before sweating, nausea, and other symptoms resolve.

Common triggers for vasovagal syncope include prolonged standing, warm temperatures, stress, fear, pain, or the sight of blood. Presence of these triggers is suggestive of vasovagal syncope. The mechanism of vasovagal syncope is complex, but involves decreased vascular tone and cardiac output due to a strong vagal stimulus.

Workup in the emergency department, as with all complaints of syncope, includes a careful history, physical examination, pregnancy test if needed, and ECG. If this is consistent with vasovagal syncope, no further diagnostic evaluation is necessary.

Treatment

Patients with vasovagal syncope should be reassured in the emergency department. Methods for aborting a syncopal episode can be discussed including the importance of recognizing presyncopal symptoms, lying down, getting a drink, and avoidance of known triggers. Patients should be advised to drink plenty of fluids and eat healthy, regular meals.

Disposition

Patients with history and physical examination consistent with vasovagal syncope who have normal ECG in the emergency department can be discharged to home. They should seek care with their primary doctor as needed.

Situational Syncope

Clinical Presentation

Situational syncope is a reflex syncope triggered by specific situations. Triggers include micturition, defecation, coughing, sneezing, diving, hair-combing, and even swallowing. Stimuli tend to cause recurrent episodes of syncope in susceptible patients. Patients may experience presyncopal symptoms including dizziness, diaphoresis, nausea, and vision changes followed by loss of consciousness. Patients regain consciousness within seconds but may continue to have symptoms for several minutes.

Treatment

Avoidance of known triggers, if possible is advised. Patients should drink plenty of fluids.

Disposition

Patients with a clinical presentation and emergency department evaluation consistent with situational syncope can be discharged to home. For recurrent syncope or triggers which cannot be avoided, consultation with a cardiologist may be beneficial.

Breath-holding Spells

Clinical Presentation

Breath-holding spells occur in children between 6 and 24 months of age, which can be frightening events for parents. A breath-holding spell is usually triggered by an emotion such as fear, pain, or anger. The child holds his/her breath, often turns pale or cyanotic, and loses consciousness. The event ends spontaneously as the child takes a breath.

Treatment

Breath-holding spells are benign events that do not usually require treatment.

Disposition

Children can be discharged to home with parents with reassurance.

Whitehouse WP: Breath holding spells. *J Pediatr Neurol.* 2010;8: 49-50. doi 10.3233/JPN-2010-0353.

Orthostatic Hypotension

Clinical Presentation

Orthostatic hypotension is the failure of normal compensatory mechanisms to maintain adequate cardiac output during postural changes (supine-to-standing position) and can result in syncope. Patients may experience vision changes, light-headedness, dizziness, and weakness when changing position. Dehydration, blood loss, pregnancy, or medications may be responsible. Diagnosis is made by obtaining orthostatic vital signs. A pregnancy test should be done in females. If there is concern for blood loss, additional testing is indicated.

Treatment

If dehydration is the likely cause of orthostatic hypotension, hydration, either IV or orally, is the treatment. If blood loss is suspected, attention should be paid to fluid resuscitation (crystalloid, blood products), stabilization of blood pressure, as well as identification and treatment of source of bleeding. The patient's medication list should be screened for medications that could contribute to orthostatic hypotension.

Disposition

Disposition with orthostatic hypotension depends upon the underlying etiology. Patients with dehydration can be discharged if the clinician is confident that patient can maintain hydration at home. If a patient is pregnant, obstetrical care should be arranged. If the patient is unstable because of blood loss or extreme hypovolemia, disposition depends upon the clinical picture.

Postural Orthostatic Tachycardia Syndrome

Clinical Presentation

Postural orthostatic tachycardia syndrome (POTS) symptoms are induced by postural changes. Symptoms are accompanied by tachycardia, in adults defined as at least 30 beats per minute increase over baseline, without hypotension. Patients may experience syncope, fatigue, heart palpitations, exercise intolerance, and general malaise. The syndrome tends to present in adolescents, typically after a prolonged period of inactivity, such as illness or injury.

Treatment

Acute POTS symptoms improve with sitting. First-line treatment includes aerobic exercise, strengthening exercises, increased fluid and salt intake. Patients may require medication to control symptoms.

Disposition

Patients with POTS can be discharged to home from the emergency department.

Johnson JN, Mack KJ, Kuntz NL: Postural orthostatic tachycardia syndrome: A clinical review. *Pediatr Neurol.* 2010;42:77-85 [PMID: 20117742].

Pregnancy

Syncope can occur during pregnancy, therefore all females of childbearing age who present with the complaint of syncope should have a urine pregnancy test. Syncope can be a normal occurrence during pregnancy, but could signal a more serious process including ectopic pregnancy or pulmonary embolism. If there is concern for these processes in a pregnant patient, appropriate workup should be conducted.

Treatment

In most patients, syncope during pregnancy does not require treatment. It is important to advise pregnant women to drink plenty of fluids and avoid triggers that may cause syncope.

Disposition

Obstetric care should be arranged for pregnant adolescents. If there is concern for a process such as ectopic pregnancy, transfer to a facility which can appropriately manage this condition is important.

Carbon Monoxide Poisoning

Clinical Findings

Severe carbon monoxide poisoning can lead to syncope. Common sources of carbon monoxide include engine exhaust and furnaces in disrepair. Headache, dizziness, and confusion result from mild exposures, although syncope or even death occurs with more serious exposure. Exposure causes hypoxia as carbon monoxide has a much higher affinity for hemoglobin than oxygen. Arterial or venous blood gas should be obtained with co-oximetry for diagnosis (see Chapter 46, Poisonings).

Treatment

Patients who have been exposed to carbon monoxide should be placed on a non-rebreather ventilator with 100% oxygen. Hyperbaric oxygen is controversial in the treatment of carbon monoxide poisoning. It is not clear which patients should receive hyperbaric oxygen although the practitioners may consider loss of consciousness as an indication.

Weaver LK: Clinical practice: Carbon monoxide poisoning. *N Engl J Med.* 2009;360:1217-1225 [PMID: 19297574].

Hypoglycemia

► Clinical Findings

Hypoglycemia can be a cause of syncope in the insulin-dependent child with diabetes. Preceding symptoms include weakness, hunger, diaphoresis, agitation, and confusion. Diagnosis is made by low glucose blood levels.

► Treatment

Treatment includes oral or IV dextrose containing fluids or solids.

► Disposition

The patient can be discharged to home when glucose level has returned to normal and the patient is back to baseline mental status.

Fischer JW, Cho CS: Pediatric syncope: Cases from the emergency department. *Emerg Med Clin North Am.* 2010;28:501-516 [PMID: 20709241].

Goble MM, Benitez C, Baumgardner M, et al: ED management of pediatric syncope: Searching for a rationale. *Am J Emerg Med.* 2008;26:66-70 [PMID: 18082784].

MISCELLANEOUS CONDITIONS

CONDITIONS THAT MIMIC SYNCOPE

In the differential of true syncope there are conditions that mimic syncope. Included are seizures, migraines, and specific psychiatric disorders. History is key in making an accurate diagnosis.

Patients with seizures often describe a premonition before the seizure which differs from the prodromal symptoms of syncope. Supine position before the event is more suggestive of seizure than syncope. Jerking of the extremities is seen before the loss of conscious in a seizure, and incontinence or cyanosis can be reported. A seizure typically lasts longer than a syncopal episode. Patients often have a postictal period which is not experienced after true syncope. However, it can be difficult to discriminate a syncopal event from a seizure based on clinical presentation alone. Often the patient has returned to baseline health upon presentation. Further complicating the history is that children who have syncope can have seizure-like activity while unconscious due to cerebral hypoperfusion. If there is a concern for epileptic activity, referral to a neurologist is recommended in order to obtain an EEG.

Migraines can present with loss of consciousness but typically have associated headache and nausea.

Hyperventilation and pseudosyncope are events which can be confused with syncope but have a psychiatric etiology. The two events are common in adolescent females and are triggered by extreme emotional stress. Hyperventilation is characterized by deep breathing and may be accompanied by chest pain, anxiety, tingling of the extremities, and occasionally loss of consciousness. Pseudosyncope is often a prolonged, emotional event which may be in front of an audience. The patient with pseudosyncope rarely sustains injury on the fall and often is able to describe the entire event. These patients lack the hemodynamic or autonomic changes associated with causes of true syncope. If the history is suggestive of these events rather than syncope, referral to a psychiatrist may be warranted.

Thijs RD, Bloem BR, van Dijk JG: Falls, faints, fits and funny turns. *J Neurol.* 2009;256:155-167 [PMID: 19271109].

Yilmaz S, Gokben S, Levent E, et al: Syncope or seizure? The diagnostic value of synchronous tilt testing and video-EEG monitoring in children with transient loss of consciousness. *Epilepsy Behav.* 2012;24:93-96 [PMID: 22459868].

Coma

James E. Morris, MD, MPH

Blake D. Hatfield, MSIV

IMMEDIATE MANAGEMENT OF LIFE-THREATENING PROBLEMS

GENERAL CONSIDERATIONS

Coma is defined as the total absence of arousal, and awareness of the self and surroundings that last at least 1 hour. Coma is characterized by the absence of sleep-wake cycles and unarousable unresponsiveness, which are associated with injury or functional disruption of the ascending reticular activating system in the brainstem or bilateral cortical structures. Comatose patients demonstrate no eye opening, age-appropriate speech/vocalizations, or normal spontaneous movements. Movement elicited by painful stimuli (if present) is abnormal or reflexive rather than purposeful. Although definitive discrimination of coma from other pathological states associated with decreased consciousness such as delirium, vegetative state, and brain death should be attempted, but it may be difficult in the emergency setting. Terms such as obtundation, stupor, and lethargy are imprecise and there is variability among physicians in their use. A specific description of the patient's level of consciousness or the stimuli to which the patient arouses is preferable.

INITIAL MANAGEMENT

The initial management of the comatose patient presenting to the emergency department should proceed similar to that for any critically ill patient. Patients who do not respond to empiric therapy for coma should have immediate assessment and support of airway, breathing, and circulation (ABC) before efforts to diagnose or address specific causes of coma are undertaken. Empiric therapy, referred to as the "coma cocktail," consists of intravenous (IV) naloxone and dextrose (Table 19–1). Naloxone (IV 0.1 mg/kg in neonates and children < 5 yr; 2 mg in children > 5 yr) rapidly reverses coma

and respiratory depression secondary to narcotic overdose but has a short half-life and multiple doses or continuous infusion may be required. Dextrose (0.5 g/kg) reverses coma secondary to hypoglycemia and is indicated if rapid testing of blood glucose is unavailable. Agents, such as flumazenil, are rarely given empirically as they may precipitate seizures that are then refractory to benzodiazepines. Flumazenil may be indicated in iatrogenic coma secondary to excess benzodiazepine administration, such as following procedural sedation.

Coma that persists following the administration of naloxone and dextrose should prompt consideration of definitive management of airway and breathing. Intravenous access should be obtained and blood pressure (especially hypotension) managed aggressively. Focused physical examination, including a complete set of vital signs, should be obtained to evaluate for potential precipitating exposures such as trauma or evidence of drug use as well as to avoid missing complicating factors such as hypo- or hyperthermia and hypoxia. Maintain cervical spine immobilization if there is suspicion or evidence of trauma. Additional history obtained from friends, relatives, teachers, or emergency medical services (EMS) personnel is imperative.

NEUROLOGICAL ASSESSMENT

After immediate threats to life have been addressed, a structured neurological assessment including level of consciousness, cranial nerve examination, and sensorimotor examination should be conducted as soon as possible. Structural lesions are more likely to produce lateralizing deficits and a rostrocaudal progression of brainstem dysfunction, whereas involuntary movements are suggestive of a metabolic cause of coma. Pediatric Glasgow coma scale (GCS) has been shown to be prognostic in many different types of coma. Both total and component (eye, verbal, motor) scores should be documented (Table 19–2).

Table 19-1. Pediatric coma cocktail.

Agent	Neonate (0-3 mo)	Infant (3-12 mo)	Child < 5 yrs or < 20 kg	Child > 5 yrs or > 20 kg
Naloxone	TB > 0.1 mg/kg IV/IO/IM	0.1 mg/kg IV/IO/IM	0.1 mg/kg IV/IO/IM	2 mg/kg IV/IO/IM
Dextrose	0.5 g/kg of D10	0.5 g/kg of D10 or D25	0.5 g/kg of D25 or D50	0.5 g/kg of D25 or D50

A careful cranial nerve examination (especially pupillary response) may help determine the level of brainstem dysfunction (Table 19-3). Lesions rostral to the midbrain usually result in normal pupillary function and eye movements. Pupillary abnormalities (especially unilateral) may be an early indicator of herniation, and pupillary function should be assessed frequently when increased intracranial pressure (ICP) is a concern. Symmetrically reactive pupils that are usually large or small are suggestive of drug ingestions.

Motor examination should focus on the presence of spontaneous and elicited movements and whether they are reflexive, involuntary, or purposeful. Purposeful movements such as localization require some degree of cortical processing, whereas reflexes are stereotypical responses that occur in the absence of cortical input and typically disappear in sequence (Table 19-4). Structural lesions caudal to the midbrain are characterized by extension of both upper and lower extremities (decerebrate posturing), whereas lesions rostral to the midbrain are characterized by flexion of the upper extremities and extension of the lower extremities (decorticate posturing). Decerebrate and decorticate posturing often presents with intermittent and asymmetric patterns that should not be mistaken for seizures.

INCREASED INTRACRANIAL PRESSURE & HERNIATION

Increased intracranial pressure (ICP) usually results from a space-occupying lesion such as a hematoma or tumor; however, ICP may also result from cerebral edema secondary to trauma, infection, or severe metabolic derangements such as aggressive treatment of diabetic ketoacidosis. The Monro-Kellie principle conceptualizes the relationship of intracranial contents; that is, the volume within the skull is fixed and normally contains three components: brain, blood, and cerebrospinal fluid (CSF). Increase in the amount of one component (cerebral edema, hematoma, or hydrocephalus), or the addition of components (tumor) results in increased ICP, which can be visible in neonates and infants from a displaced fontanelle. Using the Monro-Kellie principle, treatment is aimed at reducing the volume of components or expanding the volume available by means of surgical decompression. The goal of treatment is to keep cerebral perfusion pressure (CPP) (CPP = mean arterial pressure [MAP] - ICP), between 30 and 40 mm Hg for premature neonates, approximately 40 mm Hg in neonates and infants, and between 50 and 60 mm Hg in children older than 2 years.

Table 19-2. Pediatric Glasgow coma scale.

Category	Score	Child < 5 yr	Child > 5 yr
Eye opening	4	Spontaneously	Spontaneously
	3	To voice	To voice
	2	To pain	To pain
	1	No response	No response
Verbal responsiveness	5	Age-appropriate speech/vocalizations	Oriented
	4	Less than usual ability; irritable cry	Confused
	3	Cries to pain	Inappropriate words
	2	Moans to pain	Incomprehensible
	1	No response	No response to pain
Motor responsiveness	6	Normal spontaneous movements	Follows commands
	5	Localizes to supraocular pain (> 9 mo)	Localizes to pain
	4	Withdraws from nailbed pressure	Withdraws from pain
	3	Flexion to supraocular pain	Decorticate posturing
	2	Extension to supraocular pain	Decerebrate posturing
	1	No response	No response

Table 19–3. Brainstem reflexes.

Reflex	Examination Technique	Normal Response	Brainstem Location
Pupils	Response to light	Direct and consensual restriction	Midbrain
Oculocephalic	Turn head from side to side	Eyes move conjugately in direction opposite to head	Pons
Vestibulo-oculocephalic	Irrigate external auditory canal with cold water	Nystagmus with fast component away from stimulus	Pons
Corneal reflex	Stimulation of cornea	Eyelid closure	Pons
Cough reflex	Stimulation of carina	Cough	Medulla
Gag reflex	Stimulation of soft palate	Symmetric elevation of soft palate	Medulla

Herniation syndromes result from increased ICP and lead to brainstem compression manifested by arterial hypertension, bradycardia, and respiratory irregularities (Cushing triad). Herniation may be uncal, central, or cerebellar (Table 19–5). Initial emergency department management of herniation consists of prompt recognition and aggressive resuscitation. Avoidance of hypoxia and hypotension is essential and other adverse systemic factors such as hyperglycemia and fever should be addressed. Cerebral venous outflow should be promoted by elevation of the patient's head to 30 degrees, and adequate sedation and analgesia provided to minimize cerebral metabolic activity. Seizure prophylaxis should be considered, particularly when paralytics have been given. When available, further treatment should be guided by ICP monitoring. When ICP monitoring is unavailable, slight hyperventilation to a $PaCO_2$ of 30-35 mm Hg should be initiated (excessive or prolonged hyperventilation has been associated with a negative prognosis), followed by mannitol (0.25-0.5 g/kg IV every 4-6 hours) or hypertonic saline (2 mL/kg of 3% solution IV). If the ICP remains high and craniectomy is not indicated or not available, barbiturates may be used to decrease cerebral metabolism and thus cerebral blood flow. Barbiturate therapy is most effective in patients with preserved autoregulatory response, and should only be considered after patients have not responded to other treatments. Corticosteroids in the setting of trauma have not demonstrated decrease in cerebral edema, but may be indicated in nontraumatic pathologies (brain tumor).

Fouad H, Haron M, Halawa EF, et al: Nontraumatic coma in a tertiary pediatric emergency department in Egypt: Etiology and outcome. *J Child Neurol.* 2011;26(2):136-141 [PMID: 20606061].

Ghosh A, Wilde EA, Hunter JV, et al: The relation between Glasgow Coma Scale score and later cerebral atrophy in paediatric traumatic brain injury. *Brain Inj.* 2009;23:228-233 [PMID: 19205959].

Jindal A, Singhi SC, Singhi P: Non-traumatic coma and altered mental status. *Indian J Pediatr.* 2012;79:367-375 [PMID: 21870145].

Pitfield AF, Carroll AB, Kissoon N: Emergency management of increased intracranial pressure. *Pediatr Emerg Care.* 2012;28:200-204 [PMID: 22307193].

Seshia SS, Bingham WT, Kirkham FJ, et al: Nontraumatic coma in children and adolescents: Diagnosis and management. *Neurol Clin.* 2011;29:1007-1043 [PMID: 22032671].

Table 19–4. Neurological landmarks and reflexes.

Reflex	Description	Age of Disappearance
Parachute	Outstretched arms as if breaking a fall, seen before infant can walk	~ 6 mo
Moro	Infant's face looks startled, and arms move abduct with palms pointing up	3-4 mo
Tonicneck	When infant's face is tilted to one side, arm on that side reaches away from body, and contralateral arm is flexed with clenched fist	~ 6 mo
Palmar grasp	When a finger is placed in infant's hand, it causes a grasping action	4-5 mo
Plantar grasp	Infant flexes its toes in response to plantar stimulus	9-12 mo
Babinski	Infant extends its toes in response to plantar stimulus	2 yr
Stepping	Infant makes stepping action with both feet on a surface and with its body supported	4-5 mo

Table 19–5. Signs of increased intracranial pressure and herniation syndromes.

Sign	Mechanism	Type of Herniation
Coma	Compression of midbrain tegmentum	Uncal, central
Pupillary dilation	Compression of ipsilateral third nerve	Uncal
Miosis	Compression of midbrain	Central
Lateral gaze palsy	Stretching of CNVI	Central
Hemiparesis	Compression of contralateral cerebral peduncle	Uncal
Decerebrate posturing	Compression of midbrain	Central, uncal
Hypertension, bradycardia	Compression of medulla	Central, uncal, cerebellar
Abnormal breathing	Compression of pons or medulla	Central, uncal, cerebellar

▼ FURTHER EVALUATION OF THE COMATOSE PATIENT

HISTORY

The number of disorders that produce coma is vast (Table 19–6). History should be obtained from available sources, including friends, teachers, police, and EMS personnel. Crucial points include the following:

- Recent head trauma, even seemingly trivial
- Drug use or potential exposure
- Past medical history, including history of seizures, diabetes, liver or metabolic diseases, or other neurological disease
- Precomatose activity and behavior (headache, confusion, vomiting)
- Sudden versus gradual onset of coma
- Individuals who have similar symptoms
- Concern for non-accidental trauma (NAT)
- Accidental overdose or poisoning including potential exposure to family members' prescription medications

PHYSICAL EXAMINATION

In addition to a focused neurological examination, physical examination should focus on evidence of other threats to life such as hypovolemia and systemic trauma. Trauma elsewhere on the body is presumptive evidence of head trauma in the comatose patient.

Table 19–6. Etiology of coma and altered consciousness.

Primary cerebral disorders
Bilateral or diffuse hemispheric disorders
  Traumatic brain injury
  NAT
  Ischemic
  Hemorrhagic (subarachnoid hemorrhage, intraventricular hemorrhage)
  Hypoxic-ischemic encephalopathy
  Cerebral venous thrombosis
  Malignancy
  Meningitis/encephalitis
  Generalized or complex partial seizures; status epilepticus
  Hypertensive encephalopathy
  Posterior reversible encephalopathy syndrome
  Acute disseminated encephalomyelitis
  Hydrocephalus
Unilateral hemispheric disorders (with displacement of midline structures)
  Traumatic (contusions, SDH, epidural hematoma)
  Large hemispheric ischemic stroke
  Primary intracerebral hemorrhage
  Cerebral abscess
  Brain tumor
Brain stem disorders (pons, midbrain)
  Hemorrhage, infarction, tumor, trauma
  Central pontine myelinolysis
  Compression from cerebellar infarct, hematoma, abscess, tumor

Systemic derangements causing coma
Toxic
  Medication overdose/adverse effects
  Drugs of abuse
  Exposures (carbon monoxide, heavy metals)
Metabolic
  Systemic inflammatory response syndrome/sepsis
  Hypoxia
  Hypercapnia
  Hypothermia
  Hypoglycemia
  Hyperglycemic crises (DKA, NHHS)
  Hypo- or hypernatremia
  Hypercalcemia
  Hepatic failure
  Renal failure
  Reye syndrome
  Wernicke encephalopathy
Endocrine
  Panhypopituitarism
  Adrenal insufficiency
  Hypo- or hyperthyroidism

IMAGING

Noncontrast head CT is an integral part of the workup for coma that is not obviously related to hypoglycemia, overdose, or other metabolic cause, and should be strongly considered in a patient who remains comatose after dextrose and naloxone. Magnetic resonance imaging (MRI), magnetic resonance spectroscopy, electroencephalography (EEG), and testing such as evoked potentials are studies that may be obtained in the intensive care unit (ICU) to determine the etiology of coma but have limited utility in the emergency department. Magnetic resonance spectroscopy can be useful in detecting hypoxic-ischemic encephalopathies, inborn errors of metabolism, and acute encephalopathy with biphasic seizures and late reduced diffusion (AESD). Use of EEG is helpful diagnostically and for determining prognosis in the setting of coma, particularly when there is concern for nonconvulsive status epilepticus. Bedside ultrasonography of the optic nerve sheath may reveal increased ICP, a potential contributor to the cause of coma.

LABORATORY EVALUATION

Rapid determination of blood glucose levels is the most important initial laboratory study in the comatose patient. Electrolytes, LFTs, CBC, UA, urine-serum toxicology screens, thyroid function studies, BUN/Cr, and ABG or VBG should be obtained early in the evaluation of coma. Lumbar puncture and CSF analysis should be performed if not contraindicated (mass lesions or other evidence of increased ICP) in patients for whom the cause of coma is unclear or in whom an infectious cause is suspected. Electrocardiogram (ECG) should be obtained and cardiac monitoring instituted to eliminate cardiac arrhythmias or toxic ingestions as a contributing factor. In intubated patients receiving paralytics or in those for whom nonconvulsive status epilepticus is a consideration, obtain an EEG as soon as practical.

Colbert CA, Holshouser BA, Aaen GS, et al: Value of cerebral microhemorrhages detected with susceptibility-weighted MR Imaging for prediction of long-term outcome in children with nonaccidental trauma. *Radiology.* 2010;256:898-905 [PMID: 20720073].

Jindal A, Singhi SC, Singhi P: Non-traumatic coma and altered mental status. *Indian J Pediatr.* 2012;79:367-375 [PMID: 21870145].

Seshia SS, Bingham WT, Kirkham FJ, et al: Nontraumatic coma in children and adolescents: Diagnosis and management. *Neurol Clin.* 2011;29:1007-1043 [PMID: 22032671].

▼ EMERGENCY TREATMENT OF SPECIFIC DISORDERS CAUSING COMA

STRUCTURAL LESIONS

INTRACEREBRAL HEMORRHAGE

General Considerations

Intracerebral hemorrhage (ICH) can be classified as primary (unrelated to congential or acquired lesions) or secondary (related to vascular malformations, tumors, or other lesions). Primary ICH is rare in children, with the vast majority of primary ICH related to hypertension and amyloid angiopathy, which occurs in characteristic areas of the brain: deep white matter, basal ganglia, thalamus, cerebellum, and pons. Secondary ICH is more variable in location and is considered the most common type of ICH to occur in pediatric patients. This consists of arteriovenous malformations, hematologic abnormalities, and brain tumors. Rapid deterioration (within the first 6 hours of presentation) is most commonly related to early hematoma growth. Cytotoxic and vasogenic edema surrounding the hemorrhage may result in ischemia and are likely responsible for delayed deterioration (see Chapter 37).

Idiopathic thrombocytopenia purpura (ITP) may cause ICH or complicate other types of ICH. According to published cases between 1954 and 1998, 72% of patients with ITP had developed ICH within 6 months of diagnosis, and a majority of patients presented with platelet counts less than 10,000/μL ITP with ICH produced a 55% mortality rate. Children with hemophilia are also at increased risk of spontaneous ICH. Up to 12% of patients with hemophilia will develop ICH, most commonly between 6 months and 2 years of age. Sickle cell patients receiving corticosteroids, nonsteroidal anti-inflammatory drugs (NSAIDs), or transfusions within the past 14 days, and patients with premorbid hypertension can be at an increased risk for ICH.

▶ Clinical Findings

The clinical features of a patient's presentation are related to the size and location of the hemorrhage (Table 19-7). Headache is universally present in awake patients and may accompany other signs of increased ICP. Patients with large areas of hemorrhage often show signs of herniation and may be comatose on arrival. Seizures occur in 10% of all ICH but in 50% of patients with lobar hemorrhage. Most patients are hypertensive on presentation, even if previously normotensive.

▶ Treatment & Disposition

The diagnostic study of choice is CT scan. Care is primarily supportive and aimed at reducing ICP and controlling

Table 19-7. Primary idiopathic cortical hyperostosis syndromes.

Location	Findings
Basal ganglia	Contralateral motor deficits, gaze paresis, aphasia
Thalamus	Contralateral sensory loss
Cerebellum	Nausea, vomiting, ataxia, nystagmus, AMS, ipsilateral gaze/facial palsy
Pons	Coma, pinpoint pupils, autonomic instability, quadriplegia, altered respiratory patterns

blood pressure, although consensus on optimal management is lacking. Aggressive blood pressure control using IV labetalol or nicardipine should be considered. A lower MAP may result in decreased hematoma growth and improved outcomes; however, care must be taken to ensure that age-appropriate CPPs are maintained. Hemorrhages in characteristic areas may not require further diagnostic evaluation and are rarely amenable to surgery. Younger patients with no clear source of hemorrhage should be considered for cerebral angiography and possible surgery. Symptomatic cerebellar hemorrhage requires surgery. All patients should be admitted for further care.

SUBDURAL HEMATOMA

▶ General Considerations

The possibility of subdural hematoma (SDH) must be considered in a comatose patient. Trauma is the most common cause of SDH in older children, and shaken baby syndrome (SBS) is the most common cause in neonates and infants. Patients may present without a history of or external evidence of trauma. Neonates and infants presenting to the emergency department with SDH must be considered as potential abuse victims (see Chapter 23).

▶ Clinical Findings

Subdural hematomas have a highly variable presentation. Symptoms and signs of SDH are nonspecific, nonlocalizing, or absent and may be either stable or rapidly progressive. SDH is often bilateral and may be associated with underlying cerebral contusion. Hemiparesis, when present, is contralateral to the lesion in approximately 60% of patients; ipsilateral pupillary dilation occurs in approximately 75% of patients. Diagnostic study of choice is CT scan, which typically reveals hyperdense extra-axial crescent-shaped collection of blood, which rarely crosses the falx or tentorium but which otherwise is not constrained by sutures. Subacute (> than 10-14 days) lesions may appear as isodense on CT.

▶ Treatment & Disposition

Immediate hospitalization and emergent neurosurgical consultation should be obtained. Rapid decline of mental status or other neurological deficit suggests increase in hematoma size and may warrant intubation and aggressive treatment for increased ICP as discussed above. Steroids have not been shown to be of benefit in ICP management.

EPIDURAL HEMATOMA

▶ General Considerations

Epidural hematoma (EDH) is a collection of blood between the periosteal layer of the dura and the inner table of the skull that happens almost exclusively in the setting of trauma. Commonly, EDH occurs in the temporoparietal region secondary to laceration of the middle meningeal artery. In children, EDH in the frontoparietal region is more common than in adults because of the larger frontoparietal to temporo-occipital ratio. Although uncommon, occipital EDH may result from a dural sinus laceration and is frequently rapidly progressive. It may extend beneath the tentorium resulting in apnea. Arterial EDH occurs more frequently in older children, whereas venous EDH slightly more frequently in younger children (see Chapter 23).

▶ Clinical Findings

Symptoms of EDH progress rapidly. Classic presentation of head trauma followed by brief loss of consciousness, return to alertness, then worsening headache, and vomiting with subsequent coma (lucid interval or "talk and die" phenomenon) is seen in 20% of patients. Diagnostic study of choice is CT scan, which reveals a hyperdense lenticular (biconvex) collection of blood that usually does not cross suture lines, which discriminates it from SDH. However, a retrospective study on EDH in children demonstrated that 11% of EDH crossed suture lines. Ipsilateral pupillary dilation and contralateral hemiparesis are ominous findings suggestive of impending herniation.

▶ Treatment & Disposition

Immediate neurosurgical consultation should be obtained. If a neurosurgeon or CT confirmation of the diagnosis is unavailable and the patient is actively herniating, a burr hole performed ipsilateral to the area of trauma (or to the dilated pupil if external trauma is not apparent) may be lifesaving. Care is otherwise supportive and aimed at decreasing ICP. Patients presenting with small EDH not causing herniation or neurological deficits may be considered for conservative management in consultation with a neurosurgeon. Approximately 50% of neonates with EDH can be treated without surgery.

BRAIN TUMOR

▶ General Considerations

Coma is an uncommon symptom of primary or metastatic tumors in the central nervous system (CNS), but may arise from tumor-induced seizures or increased ICP secondary to acute bleeding into a tumor. Mass lesions leading to herniation syndromes provide a constellation of symptoms that require immediate management as discussed in the section, Increased Intracranial Pressure and Herniation, earlier in this chapter.

▶ Clinical Findings

Patients typically have a history of headache, focal weakness, and altered or depressed consciousness lasting several days to weeks. Headache presentation is commonly worse in the morning followed by a decline in symptoms within 2 hours of awakening. Symptoms may worsen with increases in intrathoracic pressure (exercise, coughing, or position changes). Common focal weaknesses include gradual loss of movement or feeling in upper or lower limbs, ataxia, speech difficulties, visual abnormalities, and hearing loss. Dizziness or other posterior circulation signs may also be present. Depressed consciousness may present with increased sleep, difficulty reasoning, behavioral changes, and memory loss. Papilledema, absent red reflex, positive Babinski reflex, and separated sutures are possible physical examination findings. Noncontrast CT, followed by contrast-enhanced if needed, is the initial diagnostic study of choice, followed by MRI, and possibly EEG.

▶ Treatment & Disposition

Glucocorticoids and osmotic agents (dexamethasone and mannitol, respectively) are remarkably effective at reducing surrounding edema and should be initiated early. Administration of anticonvulsants should be considered to prevent or reduce seizures. Neurosurgical consultation should be obtained. Hospitalization for supportive care and further evaluation is indicated.

BRAIN ABSCESS

▶ General Considerations

Brain abscess should be considered in immunocompromised patients who exhibit a change in mentation. Etiologically, local invasion from organisms that cause sinusitis and otitis media and hematogenous seeding from dental infections is more common among immunocompetent patients.

▶ Clinical Findings

Progression to coma can occur over days or, rarely, hours. Often the usual signs of infection are absent. In particular, fever and leukocytosis may not be present even in confirmed cases. Temperature is normal in 50% of patients, and the white blood cell count (WBC) is less than 10,000/mL in greater than 25% of patients. Blood cultures (preferably 2 before antibiotic administration) should be obtained although 30% of patients may have positive results. Elevated erythrocyte sedimentation rate and C-reactive protein may be present. Noncontrast CT, followed by contrast-enhanced CT if needed, may reveal large abscesses; however, MRI has higher sensitivity. Lumbar puncture is contraindicated secondary to a space-occupying lesion.

▶ Treatment & Disposition

Initiate antibiotic therapy early when clinical suspicion of CNS infection is high, prior to imaging if possible. Antibiotic choice should cover anaerobes as well as aerobes, and coverage for fungal or other organisms may be indicated depending on patient history. Empiric therapy in combination with vancomycin, metronidazole, and a third- or fourth-generation cephalosporin is indicated. Use of corticosteroids for increased ICP secondary to brain abscess should be reserved for patients in which edema causes major neurological deficits. Steroids decrease antibiotic penetration to the abscess, and alter capsule formation, which can cause rupturing into the cerebral ventricles or subdural space. Neurosurgical consultation and hospitalization are necessary, although many surgeons defer intervention initially.

Frazier JL, Ahn ES, Jallo GI: Management of brain abscesses in children. *Neurosurg Focus.* 2008;24:E8 [PMID: 18518753].
Huisman TA, Tschirch FT: Epidural hematoma in children: Do cranial sutures act as a barrier? *J Neuroradiol.* 2009;36:93-97 [PMID: 18701165].
Jordan LC, Hillis AE: Hemorrhagic stroke in children. *Pediatr Neurol.* 2007;36:73-80 [PMID: 17275656].
Piatt JH: Intracranial suppuration complicating sinusitis among children: An epidemiological and clinical study. *J Neurosurg Pediatr.* 2011;7:567-574 [PMID: 21631191].

▼ METABOLIC CAUSES OF COMA

GENERAL CONSIDERATIONS

Metabolic encephalopathies are characterized by a period of intoxication, toxic delirium, or agitation, after which the patient gradually becomes drowsy and finally comatose. Headache is not an initial symptom of metabolic encephalopathy except in meningitis, or poisoning caused by organophosphate compounds or carbon monoxide. Neurological examination typically fails to reveal focal hemispheric lesions (hemiparesis, hemisensory loss, aphasia) before loss of consciousness. Neurological findings are usually symmetric except in patients with hepatic encephalopathy and hypoglycemic coma, which may be accompanied by focal signs that lateralize or alternate sides. Asterixis may be present. The hallmark of metabolic encephalopathy is reactive pupils (a midbrain function) in the presence of impaired function of the lower brain stem (hypoventilation, loss of extraocular movements), an anatomically inconsistent set of abnormalities.

HYPOGLYCEMIA

▶ General Considerations

Unlike other organs, the brain relies almost entirely on glucose to supply its energy requirements. Abrupt hypoglycemia interferes rapidly with brain metabolism and produces symptoms quickly. The occurrence of hypoglycemia is most common in neonates followed by toddlers and infants, and rarely older children. Persistent hyperinsulinemic hypoglycemia of infancy (PHHI) is the most common cause of hypoglycemia in neonates, and insulin treatment for type 1 diabetes is the most common cause of hypoglycemia in infants and children (see Chapter 42).

▶ Clinical Findings

Symptoms of hypoglycemia are likely to occur in neonates when blood sugar is less than 40-45 mg/dL, and in older children when blood sugar is less than 60-65 mg/dL. Signs and symptoms include tachycardia, sweating, blurred vision, cyanosis, apnea, poor feeding, and anxiety. Symptoms may warn the patient of impending hypoglycemia, but may be absent in patients with diabetic autonomic neuropathy or (more commonly) go unreported in preverbal children. Common neurological abnormalities are delirium, seizures, focal signs that alternate sides, and coma. Hypoglycemic coma may be tolerated for 60-90 minutes, but when flaccidity with hyporeflexia has been reached, glucose administration within 15 minutes is essential to avoid irreversible damage.

▶ Treatment & Disposition

If possible, confirm hypoglycemia by analysis of drawn blood before treatment with bolus of dextrose solution. IV dose is dependent on weight/age/condition (see Table 19–2). Give an additional dose of dextrose solution as needed or begin dextrose infusion for patients who do not respond to initial treatment or who respond and relapse. Other therapies such as glucagon or octreotide typically have little role in routine cases of hypoglycemia but may be considered in specific cases such as overdose.

Awake patients should be fed and then observed for 1-2 hours after glucose supplementation has been discontinued to ensure that hypoglycemia does not recur before they are discharged from the hospital. Refractory or recurrent hypoglycemia may require hospitalization, especially if hypoglycemia recurs despite aggressive treatment or in the event of long-acting insulin or oral hypoglycemic agent overdose.

DRUG OVERDOSE

Drug overdose is one of the most common causes of coma in patients presenting to the emergency department. Drugs may be implicated, including alcohol, opiates, sedative-hypnotics, antiepileptics, and cyclic antidepressants. Management of drug overdose is discussed in Chapter 46.

ALCOHOL INTOXICATION

Alcohol poisoning in children can arise from ingestion of ethanol, isopropyl alcohol, or methanol. Common household products containing alcohol (mouthwash) can be a cause of intoxication in children presenting to the emergency department. Alcohol intoxication produces a metabolic encephalopathy similar to that produced by sedative-hypnotic drugs, although nystagmus during wakefulness and early impairment of lateral eye movements are not as common. Peripheral vasodilation is a prominent manifestation and produces tachycardia, hypotension, and hypothermia. Symptoms include nausea, vomiting, confusion, seizures, cyanotic or pale skin, slow breathing, and unconsciousness.

Signs of intoxication occur when blood alcohol levels reach 50-75 mg/dL with absolute ethanol (95-99%) in young children, and coma commonly occurs when levels reach 125-200 mg/dL. Because alcohol has significant osmotic pressure (100 mg/dL = 22.4 mOsm), alcohol intoxication is a cause of hyperosmolality.

Patients should be observed until improvement has occurred with normal orientation and judgment, and satisfactory coordination. Hospitalize patients who have abnormalities that require hospitalization (metabolic abnormalities or other underlying conditions) or in whom the exposure suggests neglect or an unsafe disposition. Management of alcohol intoxication is discussed in Chapter 46.

NARCOTIC OVERDOSE

Hypoventilation and pinpoint pupils are the cardinal features present in narcotic overdose, as well as absent extraocular movements in response to the doll's eye maneuver. Pinpoint pupils are associated with disorders that must be ruled out, such as use of miotic eye drops, pontine hemorrhage, Argyll-Robertson pupils from syphilis (congenital or acquired), and organophosphate insecticide poisoning.

Narcotic intoxication is confirmed by rapid pupillary dilation and awakening after administration of a narcotic antagonist such as naloxone (see Table 19–1). Patients who have overdosed on a specific narcotic (propoxyphene) may not respond to initial dosing and may require twice the recommended amount. The duration of action of naloxone varies with the dose and route of administration and repeat doses or a continuous infusion may be necessary following intoxication with a long-acting narcotic (methadone).

Opioids such as methadone, hydrocodone, and fentanyl patches have proven fatal in children from accidental exposure. Clinical presentation is variable depending on the amount of opioid ingested and time of exposure, but commonly includes decreased respiration and mentation. Fentanyl patches in particular may deliver very high doses to young children who chew on them. Of the 26 reported cases of fentanyl toxicity since 1997, most children were younger than 2 years. There were 10 deaths and 12 hospitalizations.

Hospitalization is indicated for patients who do not recover completely in the emergency department or who have taken long-acting narcotics. Treatment of drug overdose and poisoning is discussed in Chapter 46.

GAMMA-HYDROXYBUTYRATE

Gamma-hydroxybutyrate is a CNS depressant and can induce coma. Known as the "date rape drug," it is frequently used at parties although in younger children exposure may be more difficult to determine. Detection of the drug is difficult, because most is eliminated through the lungs. Treatment is primarily supportive and may involve endotracheal intubation. Some patients require hospitalization for prolonged supportive care.

DRUGS THAT CAUSE STATUS EPILEPTICUS

Ingestion of drugs that can cause status epilepticus leading to coma should be considered. Theophylline, tricyclic antidepressants (TCAs), amphetamines, cocaine, phenylpropanolamine, ephedra, and heroin in high doses can cause seizure. Tricyclic antidepressants are a class of drugs used to treat depression, as prophylaxis for migraine, and some chronic pain disorders. Their narrow therapeutic index increases the probability of overdose. Although infrequently used in the pediatric patients, unintentional exposure to a family member's medication is possible. Most pediatric patients receive a therapeutic dose between 5-10 mg/kg/day. Adverse effects usually occur greater than 20 mg/kg/day with altered mental status and cardiovascular toxicity commonly appearing in presentation. Airway control and cardiac monitoring should be considered early in management. Seizures or arrhythmias associated with TCA ingestion may be refractory to commonly used agents and treatment with sodium bicarbonate or hypertonic saline indicated (Chapter 46).

HYPONATREMIA

Hyponatremia may present with delirium, seizures, vomiting, bradycardia, circulatory collapse, and respiratory depression, or coma. Hyponatremia may cause neurological symptoms when serum sodium levels are less than 120 mEq/L, and symptoms are common with levels less than 110 mEq/L. When the serum sodium level falls rapidly, symptoms occur at higher serum sodium levels (Chapter 17).

▶ Treatment & Disposition

Hypertonic saline solution is a common treatment for hyponatremia in the setting of refractory seizures or coma. Conventional therapies such as fluid restriction, demeclocycline, lithium carbonate, or urea for hyponatremia can be toxic and take a number of days to reach maximal effect. Recently AVP-receptor antagonists (conivaptan, lixivaptan, and tolvaptan) are proving beneficial in raising serum sodium levels. Hospitalization is mandatory in symptomatic patients or in newly diagnosed hyponatremia with serum sodium levels less than 125 mEq/L.

HYPOTHERMIA & HYPERTHERMIA

▶ Clinical Findings

Hypothermia and hyperthermia are associated with symmetric neurological dysfunction that may progress to coma. Comatose patients must have rectal temperature taken with an extended range thermometer if the standard thermometer fails to register.

Internal body temperature less than 26°C (78.8°F) uniformly causes coma; hypothermia with core temperature greater than 32°C (89.6°F) does not typically cause coma. Body temperatures of 26°C-32°C (78.8°F-89.6°F) are associated with varying degrees of decreased consciousness. Pupillary reaction will be sluggish below 32°C (89.6°F) and lost below 26.5°C (80°F). Internal body temperatures above 41°C-42°C (105.8°F-107.6°F) are associated with coma and may also rapidly cause permanent brain damage. Seizures are common, especially in children.

▶ Treatment & Disposition

Hospitalization is mandatory for patients with altered mental status or other neurological deficits. Diagnostic and treatment measures for hypothermia and hyperthermia are discussed in Chapter 45.

MENINGITIS

▶ Clinical Findings

Classic triad of fever, neck stiffness, and altered mental status is poorly sensitive for bacterial meningitis. Clinicians should have a low threshold for performing lumbar puncture to confirm suspected cases of meningitis. Patients with bacterial meningitis typically have a CSF pleocytosis, and a CSF glucose level less than 40 mg/dL or less than 60% of serum glucose levels, which are consistent with bacterial infection. Patients with viral or other infectious causes may have a pleocytosis but typically have normal CSF glucose levels. However, a patient with altered mental status, seizure, focal neurological deficit, or evidence of increased ICP should undergo neuroimaging prior to lumbar puncture to minimize risk of herniation. See Chapter 41 for additional information about meningitis.

▶ Treatment & Disposition

Intiate antibiotic therapy immediately based on clinical findings, prior to obtaining imaging. Do not delay administration of antibiotics to obtain imaging or CSF studies. Current recommendations for neonates are ampicillin plus gentamycin or cefotaxime. Recommendations for infants are vancomycin and ampicillin plus ceftriaxone. Children 3 months and older should be administered cefotaxime or ceftriaxone, plus vancomycin. Dexamethasone given with antibiotics may be

Table 19–8. Treatment for meningitis.

Antibiotic	Neonate (< 1 mo)	Infants (1-3 mo)	Children > 3 mo
Ampicillin	50-100 mg/kg every 6 h	50-100 mg/kg every 6 h	
Gentamycin	2.5 mg/kg every 8 h		
Cefotaxime	50 mg/kg every 6-8 h		75 mg/kg every 6-8 h, up to 12 g daily max
Vancomycin		15 mg/kg every 6 h	15 mg/kg every 6 h, up to 1 g max per dose
Ceftriaxone		50 mg/kg every 12 h	50 mg/kg every 12 h, up to 4 g daily max
Rifampicin			10 mg/kg every 12 h, up to 600 mg daily max

considered in older children (see Table 19–8). Hospitalization is indicated for all patients with meningitis who present in coma or in whom bacterial meningitis cannot be excluded. Acyclovir should be administered to patients for whom there is a clinical suspicion of herpes simplex virus encephalitis. Pediatric patients of the postneonatal age should receive a dosage of 10 mg/kg at 3 times per day, for 21 days. Neonatal administration has not been correlated with favorable outcomes compared with untreated patients (67% vs. 69%).

INBORN ERRORS OF METABOLISM THAT CAUSE COMA

General Considerations

Inborn errors of metabolism (IEM) is a broad category of metabolic disorders with some leading to altered mental status in children that are undiagnosed at birth. Neonates receive a heel-stick for laboratory testing to identify and potentially decrease the progression of the conditions, although many clinically significant disorders are not diagnosed at the time of birth. Notable IEMs leading to coma include maple syrup urine disorder, fatty acid oxidation disorders, urea cycle disorders, and nonketotic hyperglycinemia.

Clinical Findings

Children with IEMs can have symptoms consistent with other causes of coma (nausea, vomiting, feeding difficulties), which are challenging to identify in the differential diagnosis. Distinguishing features for IEMs (urine with a maple syrup smell) and blood analysis become vital in initiating early treatment. Adequate history should be taken to give the clinician possible causes of coma, particularly information relevant to IEM.

Treatment & Disposition

Immediate management of ABC should be achieved. Hypoglycemia is a common complicating presentation of several IEMs and may result in worse outcomes and thus should be avoided. In children with known disorders, parents may be knowledgeable regarding their child's condition or may be able to provide the contact information for the specialist who follows their child. Admission for further management and consultation with metabolic disorders specialists is indicated.

REYE SYNDROME

General Considerations

Reye syndrome is a rare, but potentially life-threatening condition that causes cerebral and hepatic edema. The syndrome has been strongly linked with the use of salicylates following a viral illness (chickenpox, influenza virus, herpes simplex virus). Children with fatty oxidation disorders are at an increased risk of developing Reye syndrome.

Clinical Findings

Patients usually have cerebral edema and fatty deposits in the liver that cause degeneration. Symptoms are progressive and typically begin 3-5 days after viral infection. Children younger than 2 years initially present with diarrhea and tachypnea. Older children initially exhibit continuous vomiting and unusual sleepiness. As the syndrome progresses, patients can show irritability, confusion, decerebrate posturing, paralysis (arms and legs), staring, seizures and convulsions, decreased consciousness, and coma. Laboratory evaluations can reveal decreased glucose, and increased acidity and ammonia levels. Testing for Reye syndrome is nonspecific, but typically includes CT, lumbar puncture, and liver biopsy to help determine diagnosis.

Treatment & Disposition

Diuretics should be considered to decrease ICP. Administration of IV glucose and antiepileptic medications are indicated. Platelets, plasma, and vitamin K should be given as well as medications to prevent bleeding resulting from liver pathology as indicated.

Crawford, JR: Advances in pediatric neurovirology. *Curr Neurol Neurosci Rep.* 2010;10:147-154 [PMID: 20425240].

Faustino EV, Hirshberg EL, Bogue CW: Hypoglycemia in critically ill children. *J Diabetes Sci Technol.* 2012;6:48-67 [PMID: 22401322].

Gosalakkal JA, Kamoji V: Reye syndrome and Reye-like syndrome. *Pediatr Neurol.* 2008;39:198-200 [PMID: 18725066].

Kim KS: Acute bacterial meningitis in infants and children. *Lancet Infect Dis.* 2010;10:32-42 [PMID: 20129147].

Kraut JA, Kurtz I: Toxic alcohol ingestions: Clinical features, diagnosis, and management. *Clin J Am Soc Nephrol.* 2008;3:208 [PMID: 18045860].

Kwon KT, Tsai VW: Metabolic emergencies. *Emerg Med Clin North Am.* 2007;25:1041-1060 [PMID: 17950135].

Munger MA: New agents for managing hyponatremia in hospitalized patients. *Am J Health Syst Pharm.* 2007;64(3):253-265 [PMID: 17244874].

Thompson C, Kneen R, Riordan A, et al: Encephalitis in children. *Arch Dis Child.* 2012;97:150-161 [PMID: 21715390].

OTHER DISORDERS CAUSING COMA

NON-ACCIDENTAL TRAUMA

General Considerations

Non-accidental trauma (NAT) resulting in coma usually occurs in neonates and infants as a result of angular acceleration-deceleration forces that tear cortical veins draining to the dural venous sinuses. Patients presenting to the emergency department with the triad of SDH, retinal hemorrhage, and encephalopathy should be considered as potential abuse victims of NAT, referred to as SBS (Chapter 5).

Clinical Findings

The triad of NAT may present with or without noticeable external evidence of head trauma. Other symptoms are vomiting, irritability, seizure, and coma. Noncontrast head CT is the initial diagnostic study of choice. Radiographic studies have indicated that SDHs appearing as heterogenous/mixed-density scans on noncontrast CT are indicative of repetitive injuries. Interhemispheric SDH is thought to be another sign of NAT in children. Many cases of non-accidental head trauma may initially have relatively normal CTs or evidence of diffuse axonal injury.

Treatment & Disposition

Neurological consultation with possible evacuation of any resultant hematoma is indicated. Diuretics and anticonvulsants in consultation with neurosurgery may be used to alleviate cerebral edema. Immediate hospitalization is required.

SEIZURE

General Considerations

Nonconvulsive status epilepticus should be considered in any patient with no other apparent cause of coma, especially in those with a history of seizure disorder. Prolonged postictal coma of several hours followed by several days of confusion may occur after status epilepticus, in patients with brain damage (eg, multiple cerebral infarctions, head trauma, encephalitis, or mental retardation) and in patients with metabolic encephalopathy that alters consciousness and induces seizures (eg, hyponatremia, hyperglycemia).

Clinical Findings

The neurological examination is usually nonfocal, although Babinski sign may be transiently present. Uncommonly, there may be focal abnormalities (Todd paralysis) referable anatomically to the focus of seizure activity in the brain. Generalized, tonic-clonic seizures are the most common type of childhood seizures exhibiting rapid onset, pale skin, miosis, eye deviations, bladder and bowel incontinence, and muscle rigidity.

Physical examination may elicit evidence of a recent seizure, such as trauma to the tongue from biting or incontinence. Rapid resolution of coma in a patient with a witnessed seizure or known seizure disorder should suggest the diagnosis of the postictal state as the cause of coma. Coma that is first thought to be postictal but fails to improve should prompt an investigation for underlying processes contributing to mental status depression, including metabolic encephalopathy, underlying diffuse brain damage, encephalitis, and structural lesion. Appropriate investigations include measurements of serum electrolytes (particularly sodium and calcium), CT scan, and lumbar puncture.

Treatment & Disposition

Treatment depends on underlying cause of the seizure, but IV lorazepam (0.5-0.1 mg/kg, ≥ 2 mg) is the first choice for most causes. Phenytoin, fosphenytoin, or levetiracetam are the next-line agents when repetitive seizures are suspected. Be alert for metabolic causes and treat them appropriately. Immediate hospitalization is required for children with status epilepticus, prolonged postictal coma, and for seizures due to metabolic causes that are not quickly correctable (Chapter 20).

CRITERIA FOR BRAIN DEATH

Brain death is a clinical diagnosis supported by the loss of neurological function of the brain and brain stem, with concurrent irreversible coma (known etiology), and apnea. Before accurate neurological and apnea testing is conducted to confirm diagnosis, the patient must meet certain criteria.

- Clinical or neuroimaging evidence of catastrophic CNS event compatible with clinical diagnosis of brain death
- Exclusion or correction of medical conditions that may confound clinical assessment, such as
  - Shock or hypotension relative to patient's age
  - Acid-base disorders
  - Severe electrolyte disorders
  - Endocrinopathies
  - Drug intoxication/poisoning
  - Core temperature < 35ºC (95ºF)

If the patient meets the following criteria, two examinations with an intermittent observation period are performed by different physicians. The observation period for neonates (37 weeks-30 days) is 24 hours, with infants and children (> 30 days) 12 hours. If patient testing remains unchanged, a diagnosis of brain death can be made.

- Coma (unresponsiveness): No cerebral motor response to pain
- Absence of brain-stem reflexes (all of the following)
- No pupillary response to light
- No oculocephalic reflex (doll's eyes maneuver)
- No response to cold water calorics
- No corneal reflexes
- No jaw reflex
- No grimacing to painful stimulus
- No gag reflex
- No cough response to tracheal/bronchial stimulation
- Apnea > 15 minutes with Pco_2 > 60 mm Hg

Ancillary testing may be used when complicating factors are present such as severe facial trauma, preexisting pupillary abnormalities, or toxic drug levels. Ancillary tests result in findings that are consistent with brain death, but are not diagnostic. The standard ancillary tests include four-vessel cerebral angiography, EEG, and radionuclide technetium-99m-hexamethlypropyleneamine brain scan. In some patients tests may aid in the diagnosis, but in others may confuse the picture. Repeat ancillary testing after a 24-hour observation period. Ancillary tests such as transcranial Doppler, somatosensory evoked potential, CT angiography, and MRI angiography have not been adequately studied and are not currently recommended in children. Documentation of diagnosis of brain death should include the cause and irreversibility of the condition, absence of brain-stem reflexes, absence of motor response to pain, formal apnea test results, and justification for and results of any confirmatory tests. The initial and repeat examinations should be included.

Colbert CA, Holshouser BA, Aaen GS, et al: Value of cerebral microhemorrhages detected with susceptibility-weighted MR Imaging for prediction of long-term outcome in children with nonaccidental trauma. *Radiology.* 2010;256:898-905 [PMID:20720073].

Gill JR, Goldfeder LB, Armbrustmacher V, et al: Fatal head injury in children younger than 2 years in New York City and an overview of the shaken baby syndrome. *Arch Pathol Lab Med.* 2009;133:619-27 [PMID: 19391663].

Nakagawa TA, Ashwal S, Mathur M, et al: Clinical report—guidelines for the determination of brain death in infants and children: An update of the 1987 task force recommendations. *Pediatrics.* 2011;128:e720-40 [PMID: 21873704].

Sharieff GQ, Hendry PL: Afebrile pediatric seizures. *Emerg Med Clin North Am.* 2011;29:95-108 [PMID: 21109106].

Squier W: The "Shaken Baby" syndrome: Pathology and mechanisms. *Acta Neuropathol.* 2011;122:519-42 [PMID: 21947257].

Thompson C, Kneen R, Riordan A, et al: Encephalitis in children. *Arch Dis Child.* 2012;97:150-61 [PMID: 21715390].

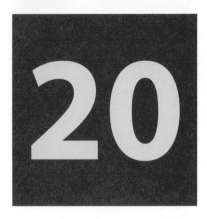

Status Epilepticus

C. Keith Stone, MD, FACEP

▼ CONVULSIVE STATUS EPILEPTICUS

GENERAL CONSIDERATIONS

A seizure that lasts longer than 5 minutes, or multiple seizure episodes with no intervening periods of consciousness is the current accepted definition of status epilepticus. Observe carefully for seizure activity in the patient in coma. Signs of convulsive status epilepticus (CSE) may be subtle (deviation of head or eyes; repetitive jerking of fingers, hands, or one side of the face).

PROTECT THE AIRWAY

Use a nasopharyngeal airway. Administer 100% oxygen by nasal cannula or non-rebreathing face mask and monitor with pulse oximetry. Be prepared for possible endotracheal intubation if anticonvulsants therapy fails to terminate the seizure or causes respiratory depression after seizure termination (see Chapter 9).

INSERT AN INTRAVENOUS CATHETER

Obtain blood specimens for glucose, electrolytes, magnesium, and phosphate determinations; hepatic and renal function tests; and complete blood count; as well as additional tubes of blood for possible toxicology screen or measurement of anticonvulsant levels if the patient is known or suspected to be on these medications. Consider blood and urine cultures as needed based on the presentation.

RULE OUT HYPOGLYCEMIA

Obtain bedside glucose and administer 2.5 mL/kg of 10% dextrose solution if the patient is hypoglycemic. If an intravenous (IV) line cannot be established, hypoglycemia can be treated with glucagon, given intramuscularly or subcutaneously at a dose of 0.03 mg/kg, maximum of 1 mg.

PHARMACOLOGICAL TREATMENT PROTOCOL

First-line Agent

▶ Benzodiazepines

Administer lorazepam, 0.1 mg/kg IV (max dose 5 mg) over 1 minute. Repeat lorazepam dose in 5 minutes if the seizure has not terminated. Diazepam 0.2 mg/kg is an alternative. The two drugs have been shown to be equally effective as first-line choices. Lorazepam has a longer duration of action compared with diazepam. Because of this property, lorazepam is currently considered the drug of choice. If venous access cannot be obtained, midazolam, 0.2 mg/kg, can be administered by several routes: intramuscularly, intranasal, or buccal. Alternatively, diazepam can be given rectally 0.2-0.5 mg/kg (Figure 20–1).

Second-line Agents

▶ Phenytoin or Fosphenytoin

If the seizure persists after two adequate doses of benzodiazepine, administer phenytoin or fosphenytoin as the second-line anticonvulsant drug. Infusion of phenytoin at rapid rates can precipitate cardiac arrhythmias and hypotension. These unwanted side effects can be avoided by the use of fosphenytoin (a prodrug of phenytoin) which can be given faster than phenytoin. Fosphenytoin dosage is expressed as phenytoin equivalent (PE). The dose is 25-30 mg PE/kg IV at a rate up to 150 PE/min. Administer phenytoin 25-30 mg/kg by IV infusion at a maximum rate of 50 mg/min.

Third-line Agents

There is no consensus on the definition for refractory status epilepticus (RSE). Recent literature is supporting a definition of RSE to be any seizure that continues for

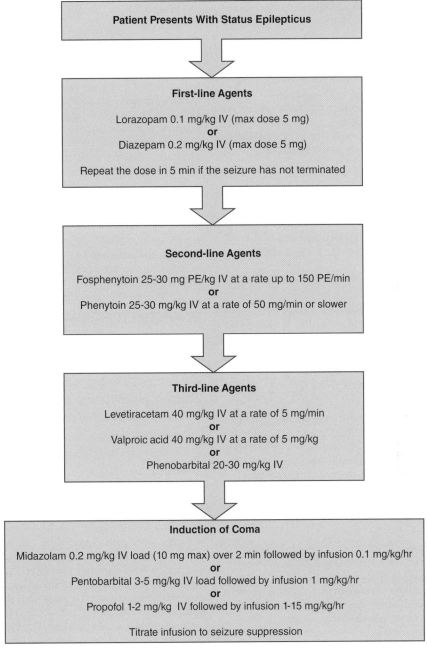

Figure 20–1. Pharmacological treatment for status epilepticus.

60 minutes after the administration of both first- and second-line agents. Consider administration of one of the following anticonvulsant drugs for patients with RSE (levetiracetam, valproic acid, phenobarbital). Intubation may be required with the administration of these drugs. Continuous electroencephalography (EEG) monitoring should be considered if it is readily available while using these drugs in patients with RSE. If seizure activity persists for 5 minutes after

completion of administration of a third-line agent, consider administration of an additional third-line agent, or proceed to induction of coma.

Levetiracetam

Levetiracetam has shown to be effective in termination of RSE. Administer a dose of 40 mg/kg IV at a rate of 5 mg/kg/min. The drug has attractive features for RSE with almost no drug interactions, rare allergic reactions, and minimal respiratory and cardiovascular effects with IV dosing. In addition, it is safe in patients with metabolic and liver disease.

Valproic Acid

Valproic acid is reported to be effective in termination of RSE. Administer a dose of 40 mg/kg IV at a rate of 5 mg/kg/min. Advantages of the drug are excellent safety profile and ease of administration. It is contraindicated in patients with metabolic and liver disease and in patients with thrombocytopenia.

Phenobarbital

Administer phenobarbital at a dose of 20-30 mg/kg. Common complications with phenobarbital at this dose include hypotension and respiratory depression. Endotracheal intubation is often necessary. Patients with hemodynamic instability should not receive this drug.

Induction of Coma

Failure to terminate seizure activity after administration of a third-line agent is the indication for general anesthetics to induce coma. The selection of agent should be based on availability, physician familiarity with the drugs, and side effects. Consultation with a neurologist and continuous EEG monitoring are indicated. Endotracheal intubation will typically be required.

Midazolam

Administer midazolam in a loading dose of 0.2 mg/kg (10 mg max) given over 2 minutes followed by an infusion of 0.1 mg/kg/hr. If seizure activity persists, administer a second bolus dose of 0.2 mg/kg and continue the infusion. If the seizure is not terminated, administer a third bolus and increase infusion to 0.2 mg/kg/hr. Side effects are minimal, and hypotension is rare. There seems to be increased risk of seizure recurrence with midazolam compared with other agents.

Pentobarbital

Administer pentobarbital at a loading dose of 3-5 mg/kg followed by infusion of 1 mg/kg/hr titrated to burst suppression on EEG with maximum infusion dose of 10 mg/kg/hr. Hypotension and myocardial depression are prominent side effects.

Propofol

Evidence exists that propofol is superior to midazolam and the shorter-acting barbiturates to terminate RSE. Administer propofol at a dose of 1-2 mg/kg load followed by infusion of 1-15 mg/kg/hr. Propofol infusion syndrome in children is well described and limits use of the drug for RSE. Clinical features are acute refractory bradycardia leading to asystole with at least one of the following: hyperlipidemia, rhabdomyolysis, metabolic acidosis, or fatty infiltration of the liver. It is strongly associated with prolonged use greater than 48 hours and dose greater than 4 mg/kg/hr.

MAINTAIN VENTILATION

Patients in status epilepticus or those given anticonvulsant medications that are strong respiratory depressants often require endotracheal intubation to protect the airway and maintain adequate ventilation. Monitor pulse oximetry and blood gas measurements to follow the adequacy of oxygenation and ventilation.

COMPUTED TOMOGRAPHY SCAN

Noncontrast head computed tomography (CT) scan should not be performed routinely for patients with status epilepticus. After termination of the seizure and stabilization, the following should undergo CT scan.

- Patients presenting with partial seizures
- Patients with a focal neurological examination
- Patients suspected to have intracranial hypertension
- Patients with a head injury
- Neonates and infants

LUMBAR PUNCTURE

Lumbar puncture should not be performed routinely on a patient with status epilepticus. The decision should be driven based on the clinical presentation. Perform lumbar puncture if fever is greater than 38.5°C (101.2°F) or nuchal rigidity is present. Muscle activity of status epilepticus may produce transient fever. Neonates that present with status epilepticus should have a lumbar puncture. Status epilepticus may produce a mild transient cerebrospinal fluid pleocytosis in up to 20% of patients.

DISPOSITION

Patients with CSE should be admitted to the hospital. Admission to intensive care unit (ICU) is required for patients who received large doses of antiepileptic agents, and those requiring continuous EEG and respiratory monitoring or support.

Abend NS, Gutierrez-Colina AM, Dlugos DJ: Medical treatment of pediatric status epilepticus. *Semin Pediatr Neurol.* 2010;17:169-75 [PMID: 20727486].

Kam PC, Cardone D: Propofol infusion syndrome. *Anaesthesia.* 2007;62:690–701 [PMID: 17567345].

Owens J: Medical management of refractory status epilepticus. *Semin Pediatr Neurol.* 2010;17:176-81 [PMID: 20727487].

Penas JJ, Molins A, Salas Puig J: Status epilepticus evidence and controversy. *Neurologist.* 2007;13:S62-S73 [PMID: 18090953].

Shah AM, Vashi A, Jagoda A: Review article: Convulsive and nonconvulsive status epilepticus: An emergency medicine perspective. *Emerg Med Australas.* 2009;21:352-66 [PMID: 19840084].

Shearer P, Riviello J: Generalized convulsive status epilepticus in adults and children: Treatment guidelines and protocols. *Emerg Med Clin N Am.* 2011;29:51-64 [PMID: 21109102].

▼ NONCONVULSIVE STATUS EPILEPTICUS

GENERAL CONSIDERATIONS

Nonconvulsive status epilepticus (NCSE) presents in a diverse manner, is difficult to diagnose, and frequently has a prolonged delay before definitive diagnosis can be made. Although there is no standard definition for NCSE, prolonged seizure activity longer than 30 minutes with no major motor manifestations and altered behavior or cognition are definitive. Controversy exists regarding EEG findings to diagnose NCSE and how aggressive the physician should be in treating the condition especially in patients in coma or who are critically ill. There are many types of NCSE recognized: absence NCSE, complex partial NCSE, and NCSE in coma. Classification by clinical findings alone is problematic but unnecessary in the emergency setting.

CLINICAL FINDINGS

Clinical picture of NCSE is diverse (Table 20–1). The hallmark is behavioral or cognitive alteration. Patients presenting with a prolonged postictal state after a convulsive seizure, altered patients with subtle motor manifestation such as twitching and blinking, those with fluctuating mental status, and patients with no definite cause of altered mental status, especially those with history of seizure, should raise a high index of suspicion for NCSE.

EVALUATION

Key to an accurate diagnosis lies in obtaining results from an EEG in patients suspected of having NCSE. This can be challenging as EEGs are not readily available for emergency department patients. In patients with a strong suspicion of NCSE, the risk of delay in definitive diagnosis must be measured and transfer to a facility with EEG capabilities should be considered. Consultation with a neurologist is mandatory.

Table 20–1. Clinical findings in nonconvulsive status epilepticus.

Altered mentation
Slow mentation
Disorientation
Confusion
Slow responses
Psychosis
Unresponsiveness
Delusions
Paranoia
Hallucinations
Catatonia
Motor manifestations
Positioning
Flexion or extension of extremities
Head deviation
Cyclonic jerks
Twitches
Other findings
Automatisms
Eye twitching
Eye deviation
Verbal perseveration
Aphasia
Speech arrest
Disorganized speech

TREATMENT

NCSE has traditionally been considered a benign condition because of the absence of systemic sequelae of CSE, such as hyperthermia, metabolic acidosis, and respiratory compromise. However, recent evidence indicates that NCSE be considered an emergency condition with treatment initiated in a timely manner. Treatment for NCSE mirrors treatment for CSE with benzodiazepines as first-line treatment, followed by second-line agents (fosphenytoin or phenytoin) and third-line agents (levetiracetam, valproic acid, phenobarbital). Dosing guidelines are outlined above.

DISPOSITION

Patients with suspected NCSE or those with a definitive diagnosis should be admitted to the hospital in consultation with a neurologist.

Chang AK, Shinnar S: Nonconvulsive status epilepticus. *Emerg Med Clin N Am.* 2011;29:65-72 [PMID:21109103].

Galimi R: Nonconvulsive status epilepticus in pediatric populations: Diagnosis and management. *Minerva Pediatr.* 2012;64: 347-55 [PMID: 22555329].

Shah AM, Vashi A, Jagoda A: Review article: Convulsive and nonconvulsive status epilepticus: An emergency medicine perspective. *Emerg Med Australas.* 2009;21:352-66 [PMID:19840084].

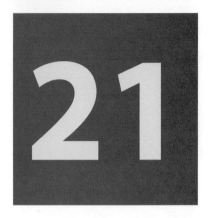

Headache

C. Keith Stone, MD, FACEP

Sophia A. Koen, MD

IMMEDIATE EVALUATION AND MANAGEMENT OF HEADACHE CAUSED BY LIFE-THREATENING CONDITIONS

ACUTE BACTERIAL MENINGITIS

▶ General Considerations

Meningitis is a life-threatening infectious disease affecting the central nervous system (CNS). Bacteria that are pathogenic to humans can produce meningitis. However, a fairly small number of pathogens (group B streptococci, *Escherichia coli*, *Listeria monocytogenes*, *Haemophilus influenzae* type b, *S pneumoniae*, and *Neisseria meningitides*) account for most incidences in neonates and children. Despite antibiotic treatment, mortality is significant and some survivors will have permanent neurological sequelae. Survival depends on prompt diagnosis and antibiotic treatment (see Chapter 41).

▶ Signs and Symptoms

Signs and symptoms of meningitis are age dependent. Symptoms may be nonspecific, subtle, or even absent. Older children often present with complaint of headache. Additional symptoms include fever, photophobia, nausea and vomiting, confusion, lethargy, and irritability. Physical findings include nuchal rigidity, Kernig sign (flexing the hip while extending the knee to elicit pain in the back and legs), Brudzinski sign (passive flexion of the neck causing flexion of the hips), focal neurological findings, and increased intracranial pressure (ICP). On presentation, signs of meningeal irritation are present in 75% of children with acute bacterial meningitis.

▶ Laboratory Findings

Perform lumbar puncture (LP) in a patient in which the clinical picture is suspicious for meningitis. In the absence of papilledema and focal neurological findings, computed tomography (CT) scan before LP is not indicated. Gram staining of cerebrospinal fluid (CSF) will allow presumptive identification of bacterial agent in most patients and can guide antimicrobial therapy. Bacterial meningitis is a likely diagnosis if total CSF leukocytes are more than 1000, CSF glucose is less than 10 mg/dL, and CSF protein is greater than 100 mg/dL.

▶ Treatment

Antimicrobial Therapy

If bacterial meningitis is suspected, begin administration of appropriate empiric antibiotics immediately based on age and suspected organism (see Chapter 41). Administer the first dose as soon as LP has been performed. If LP must be delayed for CT scan, obtain two blood samples for culture and begin appropriate antimicrobials. CSF culture may be negative in patients who receive antibiotic treatment before CSF has been obtained.

Corticosteroids

Studies have failed to demonstrate the usefulness of corticosteroids in patients with bacterial meningitis. However, evidence suggests a potential benefit and no prominent negative effects. National Institute for Health and Clinical Excellence (NICE) guidelines for children and young persons aged up to 16 years recommend dexamethasone 0.15 mg/kg, to a maximum dose of 10 mg, four times a day for 4 days for suspected or confirmed bacterial meningitis. Corticosteroids should not be given to children younger than 3 months. If dexamethasone was not given before or with the first dose of antibiotics, but the indication was met, the first dose should be given within 4 hours of starting antibiotics. Dexamethasone should not be started more than 12 hours after initiating antibiotic therapy.

Disposition

Immediate hospitalization is indicated for all patients.

HERPES SIMPLEX ENCEPHALITIS

General Considerations

Herpes simplex encephalitis (HSE) is an infectious disease of the CNS in which rapid diagnosis and treatment is paramount to avoid significant mortality. Without acyclovir treatment, HSE has mortality rate of 70%. With the use of herpes polymerase chain reaction (PCR) testing, clinical presentation and disease progression in children is more varied. This variation may result in a delay in acyclovir administration with major implications on morbidity and mortality.

Signs and Symptoms

Classic signs of HSE include fever, altered level of consciousness, disturbances in behavior, and neurological symptoms and signs that include seizures and focal motor deficits. Signs of meningeal irritation include headache, neck stiffness, vomiting, and photosensitivity.

Laboratory Findings

Perform LP in patients in which the clinical picture is suspicious for HSE. In the absence of papilledema and focal neurological findings, CT scan before LP is not indicated. If CT scan is done, children with HSE often demonstrate changes in the frontal temporal regions with loss of the normal gyral pattern. The CSF findings of children with HSE characteristically show increase in number of leukocytes(< 1000) with a predominance of lymphocytes, an increased protein (< 100 mg/dL), and a normal glucose. Studies of CSF PCR should be obtained as PCR is the gold standard for diagnosis of HSE. Sensitivity and specificity are 96% and 99%, respectively in studies that include all age groups of patients. However, case reports and studies have demonstrated a significant number of false-negative PCR studies in children with sensitivity of 70-75%, particularly in the early stages of the disease.

Treatment

Acyclovir is the agent of choice in children with HSE. The current recommended dose is 15 mg/kg every 8 hours for 15 days. There is evidence that indicates early relapse may occur and as a result some authors recommend a dose of 20 mg/kg every 8 hours for 21 days.

Disposition

Immediate hospitalization is indicated for all patients.

SUBARACHNOID HEMORRHAGE

General Considerations

Subarachnoid hemorrhage (SAH) is a medical emergency with most resulting from ruptured aneurysms. A small number result from trauma, infection, or dissection. Intracranial aneurysms in children are rare and account for less than 5% of patients of all ages with aneurysms. Most aneurysms in children are symptomatic and there is male predominance. In comparison with adults, the location in the cerebral circulation of aneurysms differs in children with an approximately threefold increased incidence for posterior circulation lesions.

Clinical Findings

Signs and symptoms of SAH include headache and focal neurological deficits (40%), increased ICP (20%), and seizures. When headache is the primary complaint, history classically is a severe, sudden severe headache. In the absence of family history of migraine, SAH should be considered.

Imaging & Laboratory Findings

A CT scan should be performed as the first diagnostic study when SAH is suspected. Lumbar puncture should be performed if CT scan does not demonstrate blood but suspicion for SAH remains high. Spinal fluid demonstrating xanthochromia is diagnostic. However, it takes 12 hours after the bleeding for spinal fluid to become xanthochromic, and it will remain xanthochromic for approximately 2 weeks. Blood in the CSF may be due to SAH or a traumatic LP. Cerebral angiography is the gold standard for detection of aneurysms; however, MR angiography (MRA) and CT angiography (CTA) are improving as diagnostic imaging techniques. In critically ill patients, CTA is easier to perform than MRA.

Treatment & Disposition

Treatment is determined by the location and etiology of the SAH. Aneurysm type and location will dictate the treatment as endovascular coiling or surgical clipping. Neurosurgical consultation and intensive care unit (ICU) admission is required for all patients.

Berardi A, Lugli L, Rossi C, et al: Neonatal bacterial meningitis. *Minerva Pediatr.* 2010;62:51-54 [PMID: 21089719].

De Tiege X, Rozenberg F, Heron B: The spectrum of herpes simplex encephalitis in children. *Eur J Paediatr Neurol.* 2008;12: 72-81 [PMID: 17870623].

Do corticosteroids improve outcome in meningitis. *Drug Ther Bull.* 2010;48:116-120 [PMID: 20926448].

Kim KS: Acute bacterial meningitis in infants and children. *Lancet Infect Dis.* 2010;10:32-42 [PMID: 20129147].

Krings T, Geibprasert S, terBrugge KG: Pathomechanisms and treatment of pediatric aneurysms. *Childs Nerv Syst.* 2010;26:1309-1318 [PMID: 20033187].

Regelsberger J, Heese O, Martens T, et al: Intracranial aneurysms in childhood: Report of 8 cases and review of the literature. *Cent Eur Neurosurg.* 2009;70:79-85 [PMID: 19711260].

Thompson C, Kneen R, Riordan A, et al: Encephalitis in children. *Arch Dis Child.* 2012;97:150-161 [PMID: 21715390].

MANAGEMENT OF SPECIFIC DISORDERS CAUSING PRIMARY HEADACHE

MIGRAINE

General Considerations

Migraine headache is a primary brain disorder in which neural events result in vasodilation of blood vessels that causes pain and further nerve activation. Migraines are extremely common in childhood and adolescence. The reported prevalence increases as children age. Migraine is reported in 3% of preschool children, 4-11% of elementary school-aged children, and 8-23% of high school–aged children. There is prevalence of migraine in boys before puberty and in girls after puberty. A family history of migraine is commonly present.

Clinical Findings

Pediatric migraine headache is classified by the International Headache Society (IHS) in three categories: migraine without aura, migraine with aura, and childhood periodic syndromes which are precursors of migraine.

In migraine without aura, pain is throbbing or pulsing, unilateral, and of moderate or severe intensity. Symptoms may include nausea and vomiting, photophobia, and phonophobia. Also included are pallor, change in personality, or change in appetite or thirst. The prodrome may occur several hours prior to headache onset. Continuing pain may cause cervical muscle contraction, leading to an erroneous diagnosis of tension headaches.

Migraine with aura is preceded by progressive neurological symptoms (the aura) with subsequent complete recovery. Most common auras are visual disturbances and are termed ophthalmic aura. They include hemianopic field defects, scotomas, and scintillations that enlarge and spread peripherally. Other auras include sensory symptoms, which may include numbness or tingling of the face, lips, or fingers. It is rare for children to have motor or speech deficits. As the aura fades, vasodilation occurs producing the headache that has identical characteristics as migraine without aura.

In childhood periodic syndromes that are precursors of migraine, children may present with cyclical vomiting, abdominal symptoms, benign vertigo symptoms, and have a family history of migraine headaches.

Migraine attacks can be precipitated by certain foods such as tyramine-containing cheeses, meats with nitrite preservatives, chocolate containing phenylethylamine, and monosodium glutamate (a flavor enhancer). Fasting, emotion, menses, drugs, and sunlight may also trigger attacks.

Treatment

Analgesics

Over-the-counter medications that include acetaminophen and ibuprofen are safe and effective in treating pediatric patients with migraine headaches mild to severe in nature. Ibuprofen 7.5-10 mg/kg or acetaminophen 15 mg/kg are often effective first-line agents. In addition, ketorolac 0.5 mg/kg IV or IM is effective but has a high incidence of headache recurrence. Opiates should be avoided because they can exacerbate gastrointestinal symptoms and have a high abuse potential.

Dopamine Antagonists (Antiemetics)

Dopamine antagonists have been shown to be effective in aborting acute migraine headaches. Prochlorperazine and metoclopramide are most widely used. Prochlorperazine dosing is 0.15 mg/kg IV. Side effects include hypotension and akathisia. Metoclopramide is also effective and should be dosed 0.1-0.2 mg/kg.

Triptans

Triptans have an advantage of being selective pharmacological agents for the treatment of migraine headaches. These compounds are serotonin 5-HT receptor agonists. All these drugs have been found to be effective in aborting acute migraine headache; however, most are not approved for use in children. Almotriptan is approved for adolescents (12-17 years), but is available only in oral form at a dose of 6.25-12.5 mg. Rizatriptan 5-10 mg oral dissolving tablets is approved and found to have good efficacy for children 6 years and older. Other considerations are sumatriptan nasal spray 5-20 mg (approved for children > 12 years) and zolmitriptan 5 mg intranasal for adolescents (off-label use in children).

Ergot Derivatives

Ergot preparations have been widely used in the past for acute treatment of migraine headaches and can be effective in children. Because of the effectiveness of dopamine antagonists and triptans, ergot preparations should be abandoned for abortive therapy in the emergency department.

Prophylactic Drugs

Prophylactic therapy may be useful in prevention of migraine headaches, but it should not be initiated in the emergency department. Patients should be referred to a neurologist for the evaluation of preventive treatment.

Biobehavioral Therapy

In addition to pharmacological therapy, biobehavioral therapy is important for management of migraines which include discussion with patient about healthy lifestyle, such as a well-balanced diet, not skipping meals, regular exercise, and good sleep hygiene. Behavioral counseling and coping techniques should be considered for the patient suffering from recurrent or disabling headaches; therefore, a referral from the emergency room should be considered for these patients.

▶ Disposition

Referral to a neurologist or primary care physician is indicated. Hospitalization (other than a brief stay in the emergency department for parenteral medication) is rarely needed.

CLUSTER HEADACHE

▶ Clinical Findings

Cluster headache is a syndrome of distinct attacks of severe, unilateral headache with ipsilateral cranial autonomic symptoms. Autonomic symptoms include ptosis, lacrimation, miosis, conjunctival injection, eyelid edema, nasal congestion, and rhinorrhea. Cluster headache is rare in children and the presentation of the disease in children is similar to adults and distinct from migraine. The prevalence in childhood is 0.1% and is more common in boys.

Pain caused by cluster headache occurs in distribution of the trigeminal nerve and most commonly in the ocular, frontal, and temporal areas. There are two types of cluster headache: episodic and chronic. In episodic cluster headaches, headache may last from 7 days to 1 year separated by pain-free episodes that can last 1 month. Chronic cluster headaches occur for longer than 1 year without remission or remission lasting less than 1 month.

▶ Treatment

Standard treatment for acute attacks is oxygen (7 L/min for 15 minutes) delivered by face mask. Sumatriptan is administered subcutaneously or intranasally, although it is off-label use for children younger than 12 years and there are no studies for effectiveness in children. Verapamil has been found to be effective as preventative treatment in adults with no studies in the pediatric population. Treatment with medications such as ibuprofen and codeine has largely proved ineffective. Prednisone 2 mg/kg may be an effective treatment in children.

▶ Disposition

Because of the severity, reoccurrence, and chronicity of attacks, consultation with neurologist or referral should be considered. Hospitalization is rarely indicated.

TENSION HEADACHE

▶ Clinical Findings

Tension headache most commonly presents as constant pressure. Location is typically bilateral. Most tension headaches are described as mild to moderate pain but severe pain can be present. There are usually no associated symptoms such as nausea, vomiting, and photophobia. Pain is constant and nonthrobbing and persists for hours or entire day. Neurological examinations should be normal.

▶ Treatment

Treatment approach for tension headaches in the emergency department is nonsteroidal anti-inflammatory drugs for abortive treatment of tension headache. Referral for prophylactic treatment or nonpharmacological treatment should be considered.

▶ Disposition

Referral to neurologist may be necessary if simple measures are not successful. Hospitalization is not indicated.

Eilandand LS, Hunt MO: The use of triptans for pediatric migraines. *Paediatr Drugs.* 2010;12:379-389 [PMID: 21028917].

Lewis DW: Pediatric migraine. *Neurol Clin.* 2009;27:481-501 [PMID: 19289227].

Majumdar A, Ahmed MA, Benton S: Cluster headache in children. Experience from a specialist headache clinic. *Eur J Paediatr Neurol.* 2009;13: 524-529 [PMID: 19109043].

Mariani R, Capuano A, Torriero R et al: Cluster headache in childhood: Case series from a pediatric headache center. *J Child Neurol.* 2014;29:62-65 [PMID: 23307881].

O'Brien HL, Kabbouche MA, Hershey AD: Treating pediatric migraine: An expert opinion. *Expert Opinion Pharmacotherapy.* 2012;13:959-966 [PMID: 22500646].

Ozge A, Termine C, Antonaci F, et al: Overview of diagnosis and management of paediatric headache. Part 1: Diagnosis. *J Headache Pain.* 2011;12:13-23 [PMID: 21359874].

▼ MANAGEMENT OF SPECIFIC DISORDERS CAUSING SECONDARY HEADACHE

POSTCONCUSSION SYNDROME

Children and adolescents who have mild traumatic brain injury (concussion) typically recover from acute symptoms within several weeks. However, some patients may experience continued symptoms for weeks or months and present to the emergency department with a constellation of postconcussive symptoms termed postconcussive syndrome (PCS).

Clinical Findings

Clinical signs and symptoms of PCS include headache (72-93%), nausea, photophobia, phonophobia, vision changes, and dizziness. In addition, there may be emotional disturbances (irritability, anxiety, depression) or cognitive impairment (loss of concentration, slow processing, attention deficit).

Treatment & Disposition

The role of CT scan for PCS is limited if the patient did not undergo imaging at the time of the acute traumatic event. The character of the headache dictates the treatment of PCS. Pharmacologic treatments for migraine and tension headache are appropriate for PCS and are dictated by the patient's symptoms. Physical and cognitive rest (elimination of computers, video games, television) is the most important treatment. Hospitalization is typically not indicated for PCS.

INTRACRANIAL MASS

Clinical Findings

Headaches caused by brain tumors are a common concern to parents despite the statistically small number of children with headaches caused by tumors. Children with an intracranial mass lesion typically present with signs and symptoms of acute or chronic elevated ICP. Elevation in ICP may increase from days to months dependent on the location and rate of the tumor growth. Classic presentation is headache that occurs daily and is exacerbated by Valsalva pressure or lying supine. Vomiting is typically present with a history of vomiting that occurs either during the night or in early morning. An acute, rapid elevation of ICP can lead to an altered level of consciousness. Physical examination findings of elevated ICP include papilledema, pallor of the optic disc, and vision disturbances.

Imaging

Patients with signs and symptoms consistent with an elevated ICP or alteration in mental status should undergo neuroimaging in the emergency department. Initial study is noncontrast head CT, with the exception of infants with open fontanel. In these infants, ultrasound avoids radiation exposure and is more useful for the investigation of a rapid increase in head circumference. The definitive test for a suspicious lesion on CT is high-quality MRI with and without contrast.

Treatment & Disposition

Children with acute hydrocephalus often require emergent treatment. Neurologic or neurosurgical consultation is indicated. Cushing triad (elevated blood pressure, bradycardia, and irregular respiration) is an emergency that requires aggressive treatment aimed at lowering ICP. Treatment includes dexamethasone, mannitol, or hyperventilation. Shunt procedures are often needed to stabilize patients. Children who are stable can be managed using dexamethasone until definitive treatment can be started. Hospitalization is indicated for all patients.

IDIOPATHIC INTRACRANIAL HYPERTENSION (PSEUDOTUMOR CEREBRI)

Clinical Findings

Idiopathic intracranial hypertension is a syndrome characterized by papilledema, increased ICP (with normal CSF), and nonspecific brain imaging study demonstrating normal or small-sized ventricles. The syndrome is typically seen in obese women but with the rise in childhood obesity, it is becoming more prevalent in children and adolescents.

Diffuse headache is almost always a presenting symptom. Pain is usually present upon awakening or while in the recumbent position. Symptoms may include vomiting, changes in vision, and sixth nerve palsy impairment, with reports of horizontal diplopia and pulsatile tinnitus. Young children may be difficult to diagnose with symptoms of irritability, listlessness, dizziness, somnolence, back and neck pain. Older children show symptoms similar to adults. They may have concerns of diplopia and blurred vision or transient visual obscuration which occur in more than 60% of patients. Moderate to severe papilledema is seen in greater than 40% of affected persons. Diagnosis is made when the patient has symptoms of increased ICP, no localizing symptoms, nonspecific or normal imaging study, and elevated CSF pressures (> 180 mm of H_2O in child < 8 years; > 200 mm of H_2O in child $\geq$ 8 years) with otherwise normal CSF findings. The course in idiopathic cases is generally self-limited over several months, but visual loss may occur. Discrimination of pseudotumor cerebri from space-occupying intracerebral mass lesions is critical and can be identified by CT scan.

Treatment & Disposition

Hospitalization is indicated for evaluation and treatment of patients with newly diagnosed idiopathic intracranial hypertension in the emergency department. Acetazolamide 15-25 mg/kg/day is first-line treatment. Furosemide 0.3-0.6 mg/kg/day combined with potassium has been used as second-line treatment. Topiramate 1.5-3 mg/kg/day in two divided doses, with maximum dose of 200 mg/day may be used. For children with visual concerns, IV methylprednisolone 15 mg/kg can be used. Serial LPs may provide temporary relief only and are uncomfortable for the patient; however, they may be indicated if visual loss is severe, progressive, or unresponsive to medications. Surgical maneuvers, including lumbar-peritoneal shunting or optic nerve sheath decompression, may be required. Patients who present to the emergency department with diagnosis of pseudotumor cerebri should receive treatment in consultation with the patient's neurologist, neurosurgeon, or ophthalmologist.

ACUTE SINUSITIS

▶ Clinical Finding

Sinusitis is usually preceded by a viral upper respiratory infection (URI). When symptoms persist for 7-10 days, diagnosis of sinusitis should be considered. Symptoms include headache, facial pressure, nasal congestion, nasal discharge, maxillary dental pain, and cough. Younger children rarely have facial pressure, but can be irritable and may vomit from gagging on secretions. Symptoms seen less frequently include fever, malaise, fatigue, bad breath, and sore throat.

Physical findings are typically not helpful in discrimination of viral URI from sinusitis. Facial tenderness on palpation or percussion is often absent in young children and unreliable in older children. Purulent drainage seen on examination of the nasal cavity can be a reliable finding for sinusitis but is difficult to perform in very young children. If periorbital edema is present, sinusitis involving the ethmoid sinus should be considered.

▶ Imaging

Plain-film radiographs of the sinuses are typically not needed to diagnose sinusitis. Clinical suspicion based on history and examination findings suffice in most patients to make the diagnosis and begin treatment. Although CT scans of the sinuses can show great detail of the paranasal sinuses to include air fluid levels and mucosal thickening, they are recommended only to confirm diagnosis of chronic sinusitis.

▶ Treatment & Disposition

Sinusitis will resolve without antibiotic treatment in more than one-half of patients. However, antibiotics are recommended to shorten the clinical course. Guidelines from the American Academy of Pediatrics recommend amoxicillin for uncomplicated mild to moderate sinusitis. The dose is 45-90 mg/kg/day in two divided doses. Alternative treatment for patients with penicillin allergy includes second-generation cephalosporins, clarithromycin, or azithromycin. Risk factors for amoxicillin-resistant sinusitis are attendance at day care, antimicrobial therapy in the past 3 months, and age younger than 2 years. These patients as well as with those with severe symptoms should be given high-dose amoxicillin-clavulanate 80-90 mg/kg/day amoxicillin with 6.4 mg/kg/day clavulanate in two divided doses. Nasal or oral steroids may be adjunctive therapy but efficacy is controversial. Patients can be discharged to follow up with pediatrician. Hospitalization is not indicated.

Blume HK, Lucas S, Bell KR: Subacute concussion-related symptoms in youth. *Phys Med Rehabil Clin N Am.* 2011;22:665-681 [PMID: 22050942].

Fleming AJ, Chi SN: Brain tumors in children. *Curr Probl Pediatr Adolesc Health Care.* 2012;42:80-103 [PMID: 22433905].

Ko MW, Liu GT: Pediatric idiopathic intracranial hypertension (pseudotumor cerebri). *Horm Res Paediatr.* 2010;74:381-389 [PMID: 20962512].

Mercille G, Ospina LH: Pediatric idiopathic intracranial hypertension: A review. *Pediatr Rev.* 2007;28:e77-86 [PMID: 17974701].

Tan R, Spector S: Pediatric sinusitis. *Curr Allergy Asthma Rep.* 2007;7:421-426 [PMID: 17986371].

Approach to the Multiple Trauma Patient

Heather Kleczewski, MD
Susan M. Scott, MD

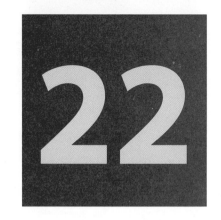

OVERVIEW

As reported by the Advanced Trauma Life Support Course (2010), "Injury mortality and morbidity surpass all major diseases in children and young adults, making it the most serious health care problem in this population."

Injury is the number 1 cause of death and long-term disability in the children older than 1 year (Table 22–1). It is estimated that for one child's death from an injury, 34 children are admitted to the hospital for treatment of a nonfatal injury, and 1000 children are seen in the emergency department and discharged home following evaluation for an injury. Data from the Centers for Disease Control and Prevention (CDC) confirm that injury, both intentional and unintentional, accounts for more than one-half of pediatric deaths per year.

Indications

Unintentional injury is the leading mechanism of injury followed by homicide and suicide (Table 22–2).

Mechanism rate of occurrence varies by locale. The most frequent unintentional injury event is motor vehicle-related, followed by drowning, fire/burns, and poisonings. Deaths following accidents on motorized land vehicles such as ATVs are increasing. Blunt trauma is the major mechanism of injury in children with penetrating trauma accounting for 10-20% of injury events. The injured child dies from head injury, with and without other major trauma, accounting for greater than 80% of fatalities.

Anatomic Characteristics in Children

Children have distinct physiological and anatomic characteristics that put them at risk for injury. Characteristics include varying body sizes and shapes with anterior placement of internal organs. Infants and young children have a large head-to-body ratio as well as a pliable developing skeleton with active growth centers. In addition, their large body surface area predisposes them to hypothermia and insensible fluid loss. During evaluation and management of the injured child, these characteristics can present a challenge to the provider. Centers caring for the pediatric trauma victim must have available age- and size-appropriate equipment as well as methods to ensure correct dosing of medications because of the varying sizes and weights of trauma victims.

Evaluation

Major and multisystem trauma victims require a concise, systematic, and thorough evaluation utilizing a multidisciplinary approach at, ideally, a designated trauma center. The American College of Surgeons developed the Advanced Trauma Life Support (ATLS) guidelines to standardize evaluation of trauma patients. The approach focuses on rapid identification and stabilization of life-threatening injuries. A series of steps and reevaluation guide the practitioner from initial stabilization through transfer for definitive care of the injuries sustained.

PRIMARY SURVEY

Initial evaluation of the pediatric trauma patient is the primary survey. The primary survey is divided into airway, breathing, and circulation (ABC). The goal of the survey is to identify and treat life-threatening injuries rapidly before proceeding to the next step in the primary survey. It also allows for reevaluation of ABC if the child becomes unstable at any point during the evaluation.

AIRWAY

In children, cardiac arrest is often due to a respiratory cause. It may begin with hypoxemia, hypercapnia, and acidosis progressing to bradycardia and hypotension that precede a cardiac arrest.

Table 22–1. Ten leading causes of death, the United States 2007, all races, both sexes.

Rank	< 1	1-4	5-9	10-14	15-24
1	Congenital anomalies 5,785	Unintentional injury 1,588	Unintentional injury 965	Unintentional injury 1,229	Unintentional injury 15,897
2	Short gestation 4,857	Congenital anomalies 546	Malignant neoplasms 480	Malignant neoplasms 479	Homicide 5,551
3	SIDS 2,453	Homicide 398	Congenital anomalies 196	Homicide 213	Suicide 4,140
4	Maternal pregnancy comp 1,769	Malignant neoplasms 364	Homicide 133	Suicide 180	Malignant neoplasms 1,653
5	Unintentional injury 1,285	Heart disease 173	Heart disease 110	Congenital anomalies 178	Heart disease 1,084

Data Source: National Center for Health Statistics (NCHS), National Vital Statistics System. Produced by: Office of Statistics and Programming, National Center for Injury Prevention and Control, CDC using WISQARS™.

EVALUATION

The initial step of the primary survey is to assess the patency of the airway and ability of the child to maintain his or her airway.

In infants and toddlers, the patency of the airway can be assessed by observing the patient for crying. In older children, eliciting a verbal response to questions can be used to determine patency of the airway. If the child is unable to respond appropriately and in a timely manner because of suspected head injury, facial injury, or declining mental status, the airway should be secured prior to proceeding to the next step in the primary survey.

Anatomic Differences in Child's Airway

Special attention must be paid to several anatomic differences in the airway of children in comparison with adults. The child's tongue is disproportionately large in comparison to the oropharynx. This puts the child at greater risk for upper airway obstruction by the tongue. The airway of infants and toddlers is also positioned anterior and has a larger, floppy epiglottis in comparison with older children and adults, which can make endotracheal intubation difficult.

EMERGENCY AIRWAY INTERVENTIONS

Airway Maneuvers

A number of maneuvers can be used to open a child's airway. The chin-tilt maneuver includes the operator's placing the fingers of one hand under the child's mandible, while the thumb applies gentle downward pressure to the upper lip. The jaw-thrust method uses two hands, one on each side, to gently place upward pressure on the angles of the mandible.

Table 22–2. Ten leading causes of unintentional injury deaths, the United States 2007, all races, both sexes.

Rank	< 1	1-4	5-9	10-14	15-24
1	Unintentional suffocation 959	Unintentional drowning 458	Unintentional motor vehicle traffic 456	Unintentional MV Traffic 696	Unintentional MV Traffic 10,272
2	Unintentional motor vehicle traffic 122	Unintentional motor vehicle traffic 428	Unintentional fire/burn 136	Unintentional drowning 102	Unintentional Poisoning 3,159
3	Unintentional drowning 57	Unintentional fire/burn 204	Unintentional drowning 122	Unintentional other land transport 80	Unintentional Drowning 630
4	Unintentional fire/burn 39	Unintentional suffocation 149	Unintentional suffocation 42	Unintentional fire/burn 78	Unintentional Other Land Transport 310
5	Unintentional fall 24	Unintentional pedestrian, other 124	Unintentional other land transport 40	Unintentional poisoning 69	Unintentional Fall 233

Data Source: National Center for Health Statistics (NCHS), National Vital Statistics System. Produced by: Office of Statistics and Programming, National Center for Injury Prevention and Control, CDC using WISQARS™.

Each maneuver elevates the tongue to prevent occlusion of the airway, while preventing hyperextension of the neck.

Noninvasive Airways

Oropharyngeal airway and nasopharyngeal airway can be used as adjuncts to improve patency of the child's airway.

Oropharyngeal Airway

Oropharyngeal airway (OPA) is used in unconscious patients to relieve airway obstruction that is caused by the tongue. An OPA is never used in conscious patients because of the risk for vomiting and aspiration associated with eliciting the gag reflex. The OPA is placed by depressing the tongue with a tongue blade or with the OPA with its tip pointing to the roof of the mouth. The OPA is then placed with the curvature of the airway following the curvature of the tongue. Special care must be taken to ensure that the OPA does not cause gagging or vomiting.

Nasopharyngeal Airway

Nasopharyngeal airway (NPA) can be used in conscious patients without suspected facial or nasal injuries to open the airway. Appropriate size of NPA is determined by measurement of the distance between the nare and the external auditory meatus. The NPA is lubricated and gently placed in an unobstructed nare. It is advanced slowly with the curvature of the airway following the curvature of the nasopharynx. The NPA can become obstructed by secretions and should be suctioned frequently.

Intubation

Indications

Children with a Glasgow coma scale (GCS) less than 8, large volumes of secretions, blood, vomitus in the airway, or difficulty ventilating with bag-valve-mask (BVM) require placement of a definitive airway. Endotracheal intubation will maintain the patency of the airway and protect the airway in patients meeting the criteria. It is important to obtain a brief history regarding past intubations and preexisting cardiac, neurological, genetic, and respiratory conditions that could cause the child to have a difficult airway.

Equipment

It is important to gather all necessary supplies, such as functioning laryngoscope with blades, suction, and devices for checking tube placement, prior to beginning the procedure. Preparation ensures minimal interruptions and enhances patient safety (see Box: Supplies Required for Endotracheal Intubation).

Size of the endotracheal tube (ETT) is selected based on the actual or estimated age of the child. A cuffed ETT may

---

Supplies required for endotracheal intubation
Self-inflating or anesthesia bag
Appropriately fitting face mask
Blankets for shoulder roll
Suction
Laryngoscope
Laryngoscope blades
Endotracheal tubes
Stylet
Nasograstric or orogastric tube
Colorimeter
End-tidal CO$_2$ monitor alternative airways (LMA)

---

be used in all children following the neonatal period. The formula commonly used is shown in the following equation.

$$\text{Cuff size (mm)} = 4 + (\text{age}/4)$$

Weight-based measuring tapes can be used to determine appropriate tube size and often the products have recommended sizes per unit of weight printed on them. A tube one-half size smaller should be available if resistance is met during intubation.

Rapid Sequence Intubation

In children with significantly depressed mental status or patients in extremis, induction medications may not be required for intubation. In the semiconscious patient, rapid sequence intubation (RSI) medications are used to provide sedation and paralysis. Medication choices are often guided by the clinical picture of the patient (Table 22–3). The presence of hypotension, bradycardia, or suspected head injury impacts the medications chosen for RSI.

Immediately prior to intubation, the patient should be preoxygenated with 100% oxygen. This provides the patient with an oxygen reserve, which allows the patient to tolerate interruptions in oxygenation during intubation. The functional residual capacity of children is less than adults, which shortens the amount of time a child can go without oxygenation. During intubation, the oxygen saturation of the patient should be closely monitored. If at any time the oxygen saturation begins to rapidly decline and between intubation attempts, the patient should again be preoxygenated with 100% oxygen to replenish the reserve.

Airway Confirmation

Following intubation, it is important to check ETT placement using several methods. Auscultation for breath sounds over both lung fields and absence of breath

Table 22-3. Rapid sequence intubation medications and their indications and contraindications.

Medication	Dosing	Indication	Contraindications/cautions
Atropine	0.02 mg/kg Minimum dose: 0.1 mg Maximum dose: 0.5 mg	Bradycardia Premedication in children < 1 yr Use of succinylcholine	Tachycardia Inhibits pupillary light reflex
Etomidate	0.5 mg/kg	Hypotension Suspected head injury	Produces myoclonus Transient adrenal suppression
Fentanyl	2-4 mcg/kg	Sepsis Concern for adrenal suppression	Hypotension
Lidocaine	1 mg/kg	Elevated intracranial pressure	Must be given several minutes prior to intubation
Propofol	2 mg/kg	Rapid onset paralysis	Very short duration of action
Rocuronium	1 mg/kg	Paralysis	Masks seizure activity duration 5-20 min
Succinylcholine	1-2 mg/kg	Rapid onset paralysis	Bradycardia Hyperkalemia in patients with renal failure or myopathies Malignant hyperthermia
Versed	0.1-0.3 mg/kg	Sedation	Hypotension

sounds of the stomach is one method. Use of an end-tidal CO_2 colorimeter, observation of color change, and looking for mist within the ETT are other methods. Presence of an end-tidal CO_2 tracing, if available, is also useful. Chest x-ray should be performed rapidly after intubation to verify ETT placement and to determine depth. If the patient's oxygen saturation declines, the patient becomes difficult to ventilate, or if there are other significant respiratory changes, it is advised to remove the ETT and bag-valve mask the patient and reattempt endotracheal intubation. Laryngeal mask airway (LMA) can be placed in the event of a difficult airway. This, however, is not a definitive airway but rather a temporizing measure until an ETT is able to be placed.

CERVICAL SPINE IMMOBILIZATION

Indications

In addition to assessment of the airway, it is important to protect the cervical spine of the patient. Because of the large size of their heads in proportion to their bodies, infants and toddlers are at increased risk of cervical spine injury. A cervical spine collar (C-spine collar) and manual holding of the patient's head in a neutral position should be used on children with any risk factors for cervical spine injury. Risk factors include mechanism with rapid deceleration, direct injury to the head or neck, multiple injuries, altered mental status, complaints of neck pain, weakness, numbness, or neurologic deficits on examination.

BREATHING

ASSESSMENT

Assessment of breathing is the second step in the primary survey, which includes assessment of the adequacy of oxygenation and ventilation. In addition to physical examination, pulse oximetry is useful in determination of oxygenation of the patient. Examination includes observation of adequacy of spontaneous respiration, auscultation of the lung fields, and inspection of the neck and chest. Inspection of the neck and chest includes feeling for the position of the trachea and palpation for subcutaneous emphysema, inspection for distended neck veins, identification of penetrating injury, and observation of asynchronous movement of the chest wall.

The most important injuries to identify during assessment of breathing are tension pneumothorax, open pneumothorax, hemothorax, and flail chest.

TENSION PNEUMOTHORAX

Tension pneumothorax results from injury that causes air to build up in the pleural space. Due to a "one-way valve" effect, the trapped air shifts the mediastinum away from the site of the air build up. The increased pressure within the pleural space can compress and impair venous return to the heart, which manifest as tachycardia and hypotension. Physical findings of tension pneumothorax include tracheal deviation away from the side of air build-up, decreased or absent breath sounds over the affected side, hyperresonance of the affected side, and distension of the neck veins.

Tension pneumothorax must be rapidly decompressed to improve oxygenation, ventilation, and circulation. A large-bore angiocath or spinal needle should be inserted into the second to third intercostal space at the midclavicular line on the affected side. A rush of air will be heard once the needle is within the pleural space. Often times, an improvement in vital signs and ease of BVM will also be observed. Following decompression, a chest tube must be placed to prevent reaccumulation of the tension pneumothorax.

OPEN PNEUMOTHORAX

Open pneumothorax is caused by a chest wall defect that allows air into the pleural space. Small open chest wounds act as a one-way valve that prevents air escape to the pleural cavity creating a tension pneumothorax. In larger open pneumothoraces, the chest wall defect creates equilibrium between in the intrathoracic and atmospheric pressure, allowing air to enter the pleural space when the intrathoracic pressure decreases during inspiration rather than entering the lung through the bronchi. These wounds are referred to as "sucking" chest wounds. On physical examination, penetrating wounds to the thorax associated with decreased or absent breath sounds on the affected side are observed. Vital sign changes, such as tachycardia, tachypnea, and hypoxia can be observed.

If an open pneumothorax is detected, the wound should be immediately covered with an occlusive dressing. Petroleum-coated gauze should be placed over the wound and secured on three sides. This allows for air to exit the chest cavity, but prevents air from entering the chest cavity. A chest tube should be placed on the affected side. The chest tube should not be placed through the chest wall defect, and the defect should not be closed in the emergency department. Following chest tube placement, the wound should be fully occluded. Often, large chest wall defects will require surgical closure in the operating room.

HEMOTHORAX

Hemothorax is caused by accumulation of blood within the chest causing compression of the lung. The patient will present with signs of shock due to blood loss and impaired ventilation and oxygenation. On physical examination, the patient will have decreased breath sounds and dullness to percussion over the affected lung. The patient must be aggressively fluid resuscitated, and a chest tube must be placed to drain the collection of blood.

CARDIAC TAMPONADE

Cardiac tamponade can impair circulation. Cardiac tamponade is the accumulation of blood within the pericardial sac. It is often secondary to penetrating trauma, which is uncommon in children. Beck triad is the presence of distended neck veins, hypotension, and muffled heart tones in cardiac tamponade. In patients with significant volume loss, distended neck veins may not be present. Emergent pericardiocentesis must be performed. Bedside ultrasonography can be used as an adjuvant to physical examination for detection of a pericardial effusion. Pericardiocentesis is a temporizing measure to improve circulation, but not a cure. The patient will require thoracotomy and exploration for isolation and repair of the source of bleeding.

FLAIL CHEST

Flail chest is an injury that can impair breathing. Flail chest occurs when multiple consecutive ribs are fractured creating a segment of the chest wall that no longer has bony continuity. Underlying pulmonary contusions are a common associated injury. Flail chest is uncommon in younger pediatric patients because of decreased calcification and increased pliability of the ribs, but is seen in older children and adolescents.

Flail chest and pulmonary contusions affect respiration in two ways. First, due to pain, the patient often exhibits splinting and shallow breathing which lead to inadequate oxygenation and ventilation. Secondly, the underlying pulmonary contusion, an area of the lung that will have decreased oxygen exchange capabilities, leads to hypoxia.

On physical examination, the flail segment will show paradoxical movement during the respiratory cycle. The broken ribs can also be felt on palpation. Chest x-rays can be useful in visualizing broken ribs. However, x-rays do not adequately identify bone and cartilage separation.

Treatment of flail chest includes aggressive pain control to allow the patient to take deep breaths. Pain control can be achieved using intravenous narcotics and local anesthesia. Patients might benefit from intercostal nerve blocks or epidural anesthesia. Fluids should be used judiciously to prevent accumulation of pulmonary edema in the underlying pulmonary contusions. Aggressive pain control and appropriate fluid management can prevent intubation of patients with flail chest.

CIRCULATION

ASSESSMENT

The third step of the primary survey is assessment of circulation. During this step, it is important to identify sources of hemorrhage and sources of nonhemorrhagic shock.

PHYSIOLOGIC CHARACTERISTICS OF CHILDREN

In children, tachycardia will be the only vital sign change associated with acute hemorrhage due to an increased physiologic reserve. In children, it is important to determine if tachycardia is a function of anxiety or if it is due to shock. Blood pressure can remain normal or slightly decreased due to vasoconstriction and tachycardia. Children require a loss 30-45% of their blood volume prior to a decrease in systolic blood pressure. Hypotension is a late finding and often occurs shortly before circulatory collapse.

Circulatory status is assessed by first looking at the patient's vital signs. Vital signs should be assessed for hypotension, narrowing or widening of pulse pressure, and tachycardia. The lower limit of normal systolic blood pressure can be determined using the formula of 70 mm Hg plus the child's age in years times two. On physical examination, capillary refill, peripheral pulses, temperature of the skin, mottling of the skin, changes in mental status, bruising, and lacerations should be noted. Common sites for blood loss in children include bleeding lacerations, the thigh, the abdomen and pelvis, the cranium in children with open sutures, and the chest.

FLUID RESUSCITATION

Initial management of hemorrhagic shock includes stopping the source of active bleeding. Actively bleeding lacerations should be sutured or a pressure dressing should be put in place. Two peripheral intravenous (IV) lines of the largest gauge possible should be placed. Initial fluid resuscitation can be given in 20 mL/kg boluses of warmed isotonic fluids administered as quickly as possible. If the patient continues to have tachycardia or hypotension following 40-60 mL/kg of isotonic fluids, O negative, warmed packed red blood cells (PRBCs) can be given in 10 mL/kg aliquots. Vital signs should be closely monitored for changes during fluid resuscitation. Signs of successful fluid resuscitation include return of heart rate and blood pressure to normal values, improved mental status, warming of the extremities, improvement in capillary refill, and improvement in skin color.

DISABILITY

GLASGOW COMA SCALE IN INFANTS AND ADULTS

Disability is the fourth step of the primary survey. Disability includes assessment for severe head injury. The Glasgow coma scale (GCS) can be applied to children that are verbal. A modified scale can be used in preverbal children (Table 22–4). Head trauma is categorized as minor, moderate, or severe based on the GCS score of the patient. Minor head trauma is defined as a GCS score of 13-15. Moderate head trauma is defined as a score of 9-12 and severe head trauma is a GCS score of 8 or less. GCS scores of less than 8 often require endotracheal intubation for airway protection. The

Table 22–4. Modified Glasgow coma scale for pediatrics.

	Child	Infant	Score
Eye opening	Spontaneous	Spontaneous	4
	To speech	To speech	3
	To pain	To pain	2
	No response	No response	1
Verbal	Oriented	Coos and babbles	5
	Confused	Irritable cry	4
	Inappropriate	Cries to pain	3
	Incomprehensible	Moans to pain	2
	No response	No response	1
Motor	Obeys commands	Spontaneous, purposeful	6
	Localizes pain	Withdraws to touch	5
	Withdraws to pain	Withdraws to pain	4
	Flexion to pain	Flexion posture	3
	Extension to pain	Extension posture	2
	No response	No response	6

severity of the GCS score does not always correlate with intracranial findings on computed tomography (CT) scan.

PHYSICAL SIGNS AND FINDINGS IN INTRACRANIAL PRESSURE

Head injury can be accompanied by increased intracranial pressure (ICP). Cushing triad of hypertension, bradycardia, and agonal respirations is indicative of increased ICP and impending uncal herniation. The pupils should be checked for dilation and reactivity. Dilated and nonreactive pupils are also signs of impending herniation.

TREATMENT

Children with signs of increased ICP and impending herniation require immediate intervention and consultation with a neurosurgeon. Several temporizing measures can be performed prior to emergent neurosurgical intervention. Mannitol (0.5-1 g/kg IV infusion) or 3% hypertonic saline (2-3 mL/kg IV infusion) can be given acutely to patients with symptomatic increases in ICP. Mannitol creates an osmostic diuresis, which can worsen the volume status of patients who are already dehydrated. Intubated patients can be hyperventilated for short periods of time to a $PaCO_2$ of 30 mm Hg as a rescue therapy in acutely decompensating patients. End-tidal capnography is useful in guiding brief periods of hyperventilation. Prolonged hyperventilation has not been shown to be of benefit in patients with head injury. These temporizing measures should not delay definitive care by a neurosurgeon.

EXPOSURE AND ENVIRONMENT

REMOVAL OF CLOTHING AND LOG ROLLING

The final step of the primary survey is exposure and environment. All pediatric trauma patients should have all their clothing removed to properly assess for injuries. The patient should also be log rolled while maintaining cervical spine precautions to adequately assess the spine and back for injury.

The perineum should be assessed for bleeding or bruising. The urethral meatus should be visualized to determine the presence of blood. The presence of blood can be associated with urethral or bladder injury that would require further evaluation. If blood is present at the urethral meatus, a Foley catheter should not be placed until the integrity of the urethra and bladder has been assessed.

A rectal examination should be done in all pediatric trauma patients to assess for rectal tone and rectal injury. In males, the position of the prostate should be noted. A high-riding prostate is indicative of urethral injury.

Risk of Hypothermia

Following exposure and examination, the child should be covered with warmed blankets. Infants and toddlers have higher body surface area to body volume ratio making them most susceptible to hypothermia. As a child gets older, this ratio decreases.

Normothermia should be maintained in the trauma patient. Fevers should be treated with antipyretics to decrease the body's metabolic rate. In addition to warmed blankets, warmed IV fluids can be used to maintain normothermia.

With any acute change in patient status, the primary survey should be repeated starting with airway to reassess for life-threatening emergencies. Once the patient is stable, the secondary survey and any adjuvants can be completed.

SECONDARY SURVEY

Following stabilization and assessment for life-threatening injuries, a more detailed physical examination and a brief history should be performed.

HEAD-TO-TOE EXAMINATION

Physical examination of the multiple trauma patients should be conducted in a head-to-toe fashion to assess for non–life-threatening injuries.

The head should be assessed for lacerations, bony instability, and hematomas. The eyes should be assessed for hemorrhage, lacerations, and the presence of contact lens. The ears should be evaluated for the presence of cerebral spinal fluid otorrhea, hemotympanum, and Battle sign, which are signs of skull fractures. The nose should be assessed for bleeding, CSF drainage, and septal hematomas. Septal hematomas require emergent drainage and packing to prevent cartilage damage. The oropharynx should also be assessed for lacerations and dental injuries. The facial bones should be palpated for fractures.

Careful examination of the neck while maintaining cervical spine precautions should be performed. The paraspinal muscles should be palpated for spasm and the vertebrae should be palpated for tenderness and step-offs. Range of motion of the neck should not be attempted until concern for cervical spine fractures is eliminated.

The chest should be examined for hematomas, lacerations, subcutaneous emphysema, and fractures that were not identified on the primary survey. It is also important to auscultate breath sounds to reexamine for pneumothorax. In intubated patients, breath sounds should be auscultated to ensure equal ventilation of lungs.

The abdomen should be palpated for tenderness, guarding, or peritoneal signs, which are indicative of solid organ or hollow viscous injury. Close attention should be paid to the presence of bruising. Bruising in a seatbelt distribution can be associated with solid organ injury. Bruising that occurs in a patterned distribution can be indicative of nonaccidental trauma.

The arms and legs should be assessed for range of motion and presence of bony deformities. A thorough neurologic examination should also be performed at this time.

HISTORY

A member of the trauma team should also be gathering a focused history from the emergency medical service providers and parents if they are available. The mnemonic AMPLE is useful for quickly gathering pertinent information that can enhance the patient care.

A: Allergies

M: Medications

P: Past medical history

L: Last meal

E: Events leading up to and following the injury

LABORATORY STUDIES

Following thorough physical examination and obtaining a brief history, laboratory studies and imaging can be used to further delineate the child's injuries. If studies cannot be safely obtained, planning for transfer to definitive care should also occur at this time.

Chest, pelvis, and cervical spine x-rays can be obtained quickly to examine for injuries not apparent on physical examination. Chest x-ray is useful in identification of pneumothorax, pulmonary contusion, and ETT placement in intubated patients. If a pelvic fracture is identified, a pelvic binder or sheet tied tightly around the pelvis should be placed. Pelvic fractures in children cause increased blood loss in comparison with adults. Binders help to tamponade bleeding resulting from a fracture. Pelvis x-rays can be deferred if the patient is cooperative, has no distracting injuries, and no pain with palpation of the pelvis.

Because of the large amount of radiation delivered by the CT scan, cervical spine x-rays are the preferred methods of imaging in pediatric patients. For thorough evaluation of the cervical spine, a minimum of an anterior-posterior and lateral cervical series should be performed. In older and cooperative children, an odontoid view can be obtained.

In children with abdominal tenderness, guarding, or seatbelt distribution bruising, a CT scan of abdomen and pelvis can be obtained to assess for solid organ and hollow viscous injury. The patient should be stabilized prior to going to the CT scanner. Unstable patients should receive prompt evaluation and treatment prior to being scanned. Additional imaging should not delay transfer of a patient to a facility that can provide definitive care.

LABORATORY STUDIES AND IMAGING

Laboratory studies can be used as an adjuvant to physical examination. Hemoglobin and hematocrit are useful in determining the degree of blood loss in a trauma patient. The hematocrit also guides the need for transfusion. Aspartate aminotransferase (AST), alanine aminotransferase (ALT), amylase, and lipase can be used to screen for solid organ injury. The presence of elevated laboratory markers should prompt CT evaluation for abdominal trauma. Urinalysis should be done to assess for kidney and urethral injury. The presence of large blood on bedside testing or greater than 40 red blood cells on microscopy should prompt further imaging with CT scan or retrograde urethrogram to assess for urethral, bladder, and kidney injury. In children with injuries requiring an operation, clotting studies and type and crossing the patient are useful.

Focused assessment sonography in trauma (FAST) is increasingly being used in pediatric trauma. It can identify small amounts of abdominal free fluid in pediatric trauma patients, which may be insignificant. However, large amounts of abdominal fluid is abnormal and may require further imaging with CT.

NASOGASTRIC TUBE, OROGASTRIC TUBE & FOLEY CATHETER

In children receiving continuous positive airway pressure or BVM ventilation, a nasogastric tube or orogastric tube might be required to decompress the stomach. Nasogastric tube should be placed in patients who are awake or with a gag reflex. Orogastric tube can be placed in intubated patients. Prior to placing a nasogastric tube, it is important to assess for facial bone fractures. Placement of a nasogastric tube in patients with facial bone fractures can cause additional injury. Urinary output is a sensitive indicator of volume status and renal perfusion. A urinary catheter may be placed once urethral injury has been excluded.

Following the initial evaluation, resuscitation, and stabilization, the provider must assure ongoing monitoring of the patient with frequent reassessments as well as the appropriate disposition of the patient. Consideration for transfer to a designated trauma center should be considered for any patient with unstable vital signs, GCS of less than 12, or any injury requiring subspecialty evaluation.

American College of Surgeons Committee on Trauma: *Advanced Trauma Life Support for Doctors*, 8th ed. Chicago, IL: American College of Surgeons; 2008.

Kleinman ME, et al: Pediatric advanced life support: 2010 American Heart Association Guidelines for Cardiopulmonary Resuscitation and Emergency Cardiovascular Care. *Circulation*. 2010;122:S876 [PMID: 20956230].

Kortbeek JB, et al: *Advanced Trauma Life Support*, 8th ed. The evidence for change. *J Trauma*. 2008;64:1638 [PMID: 18545134].

Head Trauma

Jakob Kissel, MD
Julia Martin, MD, FACEP

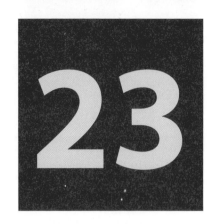

IMMEDIATE MANAGEMENT OF SERIOUS & LIFE-THREATENING PROBLEMS

CERVICAL SPINE IMMOBILIZATION

Pediatric patients with blunt force trauma to the head should be assumed to have cervical spine injury until proven otherwise and thus should be managed with full immobilization during transport and initial evaluation. An important consideration is the use of an appropriately fitting cervical collar. Improper fitting can lead to poor immobilization of the cervical spine, and in some patients can obstruct the airway if it rides up over the chin and mouth. Additionally, the pediatric patient should be secured to a rigid backboard, with blocks for the head and towel rolls or other bulky buffers along the lateral aspect of the child to prevent side-to-side slippage.

AIRWAY

Transient respiratory arrest and hypoxia may occur, which can lead to secondary brain injury. Hypoxia must be avoided at all costs and maintenance of an oxygen saturation of greater than 98% is preferred. Therefore, early endotracheal intubation should be performed for Glasgow coma scale (GCS) scores of 3-8 (see below and Figure 23-1), or for any patient with a decompensating level of consciousness and inability to protect the airway. On arrival to the emergency department, the patient should be provided 100% oxygen via a non-rebreather mask, and bag-valve-mask (BVM) with 100% oxygen can be used as well for apneic or bradypneic patients as a temporizing measure to a definitive airway.

BREATHING

Once a definitive airway is established, or the patient is stable enough to maintain airway, blood gas measurements should be obtained. Gas measurements are important because, in addition to hypoxemia, hypo- and hypercarbia can lead to secondary brain injury. Hypocarbia leads to decreased cerebral perfusion and hypercarbia is associated with increased morbidity and mortality, so in general it is best to keep the pCO2 at about 35 mm Hg. In the rare case that there are incontrovertible signs of imminent or concurrent transtentorial herniation, such as a unilaterally blown pupil or acute neurological deterioration, hyperventilation with resultant permissive hypocarbia may be employed briefly until more definitive neurosurgical intervention is possible.

CIRCULATION

Hypotension in the setting of trauma is most likely a marker of severe blood loss, indicating Class III or IV shock. In pediatric patients, it is more ominous because children usually can compensate for hypovolemia farther into the disease process than adults. Hypotension in the brain-injured patient leads to secondary brain injury, and is therefore to be avoided. The mortality for patients with severe brain injury is more than double that of patients who do not have hypotension. The presence of hypoxia in addition to hypotension is associated with a mortality of approximately 75%. A single occurrence of hypotension and hypoxia is associated with a 150% increase in mortality. Fluid bolus with normal saline or lactated Ringer solution at 20 mL/kg twice a day is an appropriate initial intervention and hypotonic or glucose containing solutions should be avoided. However, neurogenic shock from spinal cord injury, cardiac tamponade, and tension pneumothorax are possible etiologies for hypotension.

Cushing triad (hypertension, bradycardia and widened pulse pressure) heralds a marked increase in intracranial pressure (ICP). Children may present with tachycardia rather than bradycardia. Intracranial hypertension may be managed with mannitol 0.5-1 g/kg, or 3% hypertonic saline (5 mL/kg) in the hypotensive patient. Although there is no consensus about the benefit of these interventions, consultation with a neurosurgeon is advised in these cases.

If normotension is unobtainable despite aggressive fluid resuscitation, and a focused assessment with sonography for trauma (FAST) examination is positive, the patient should go emergently to the operating room (OR) for a laparotomy. Neurological examination and computed tomography (CT) head scan can be deferred until the source of hypotension is identified and reversed.

DISABILITY

The GCS can be used in pediatric head trauma patients, with some adjustments made for preverbal children (Table 23–1). The GCS score is important to establish upon arrival of the patient in the emergency department, before sedatives, paralytics, or analgesics are administered, as it separates patients into mild brain injury (GCS 13-15), moderate brain injury (GCS 9-12), and severe brain injury (GCS 3-8). The most sensitive aspect of the GCS is the motor score. If the patient's motor score is variable, or one side is more responsive, the overall best motor score is a more accurate prognostic indicator than the worst score. Stimulation can be provided by nailbed pressure or pinching the trapezius muscle. A pupillary examination should be performed. Pupil response and GCS constitue a limited neurologic examination, which is appropriate in the setting of trauma. In pediatric patients, drugs, alcohol, and other intoxicants taken accidentally or on purpose can confound the neurologic examination.

EXPOSURE

Pediatric patient's body must be fully exposed and examined, including the back. Logroll precautions are taken in the setting of head trauma until the cervical spine is cleared. Cover the patient with warm blankets. Administer warmed fluids if needed, as children are more sensitive than adults to temperature fluctuations because of their increased surface area-to-volume ratio. The room should also be kept warm.

Avoid hyperthermia as well as hypothermia, as both conditions can lead to secondary brain injury.

OTHER ISSUES

SEIZURES

Posttraumatic seizures may occur in the brain-injured child. Early-onset seizures are more common and less worrisome than delayed-onset seizures, as the latter may represent increasing ICP. Acute seizures should be treated with lorazepam, fosphenytoin, and phenobarbital as needed. The evidence for prophylactic treatment with antiepileptics is currently a level III recommendation and guidelines indicate that prophylaxis with phenytoin be considered to reduce posttraumatic seizures in pediatric patients with severe traumatic brain injury (TBI). Realize that the postictal period may confound the neurologic examination, as will the treatment with sedatives or antiepileptic drugs, or long-acting paralytics in the patient with rapid sequence intubation (RSI). Use short- or intermediate-acting paralytics (authors prefer succinyl choline to rocuronium) if RSI is indicated.

COMBATIVENESS

Aggressive behavior and combativeness are ominous signs in the head-injured child that may signal a more serious brain injury or herald imminent neurologic decline. Confirm that organic causes of altered mental status have been investigated and treated accordingly, including hypoxemia, hypoglycemia, and hypotension. Additionally, a combative patient is more likely to injure her- or himself further and worsen a head injury or cervical spine injury. Therefore, the physician should have a low threshold to intubate a combative patient. Intoxication and pain can cause the patient to become more combative. Make every attempt to obtain an adequate neurologic examination, with best GCS and pupillary function

Table 23–1. Pediatric Glasgow coma scale.

	Eyes	Verbal	Motor
1.	Not open eyes	No verbal response	No motor response
2.	Opens eyes in response to painful stimuli	Inconsolable, agitated, moans to pain	Abnormal extension to pain
3.	Opens eyes in response to speech	Inconsistently inconsolable, cries to painful stimulus	Abnormal flexion to pain for an infant
4.	Opens eyes spontaneously	Cries but consolable, inappropriate interactions	Infant withdraws from painful stimulus
5.	N/A	Smiles, orients to sounds, follows objects, interacts, coos, babbles	Infant withdraws from touch
6.	N/A	N/A	Infant moves spontaneously or purposefully; normal

before RSI. Furthermore, short-acting paralytics such as succinylcholine should be used where appropriate and available, as the neurosurgical consultants will want to perform more extensive neurologic examination as soon as possible.

PAIN CONTROL

After initial evaluation, control the pediatric patient's pain with narcotics and sedatives as needed for adequate control. Fentanyl at 1 mcg/kg is a good first-choice agent because it tends to have less effect on blood pressure than longer-acting narcotics. Also, in the intubated patient, adequate sedation is important to avoid rapid fluctuations in blood pressure. Consider propofol, or fentanyl and midazolam. However, it is important to be aware that an analgesic will counteract some native sympathetic stimulation, which may be an important pillar supporting the patient's blood pressure; therefore, titrate an analgesic carefully

Kochanek PM, Carney N, Adelson PD, et al: Guidelines for the acute medical management of severe traumatic brain injury in infants, children and adolescents, 2nd ed. *Pediatr Crit Care Med.* 2012;13(1) [PMID: 22217782].

▼ FURTHER DIAGNOSTIC EVALUATION EMERGENCY TREATMENT OF SPECIFIC DISORDERS

CONCUSSION/CLOSED HEAD INJURY

Trauma is the leading cause of death among children, and TBI accounts for almost half a million emergency room visits per year by children aged 0-14 years. Of these visits, about 75% are nonserious, mild TBI, or concussions. A concussion is a closed head injury that results in metabolic insults, rather than gross structural changes. The most important method for determining intracranial abnormalities in pediatric patients with head injuries is a CT head scan. However, most scans will be negative, and CT head scan is not without risk. Besides the monetary cost and the cost in time and emergency department length of stay, the radiation dose to the developing brain is nontrivial. Estimates are as high as 1 in 2000 neonates who undergo CT head scan will ultimately die from cancer caused by the radiation exposure of the scan. Although this ballpark estimate is based on a number of variables, the risk from CT scan radiation is real, and must be weighed by physicians when deciding which patients need imaging, and those that can be safely observed. To this end, a number of prediction algorithms have been developed and tested that help identify, from history and examination, the patient in the low-risk pool and the patient who needs a CT head scan, in order to minimize this potentially harmful and costly test. The most current of the decision trees is Pediatric Emergency Care Applied Research Network (PECARN)

Table 23–2. Low-risk criteria for infants and children, obviating need of computed tomography head scan.

Age	< 2 yr	> 2 yr
Low-risk criteria	Normal mental status No scalp hematoma except frontal Loss of consciousness < 5 s Nonsevere mechanism* No palpable skull fracture Normal behavior per parents	Normal mental status No loss of consciousness No vomiting Nonsevere mechanism* No signs of basilar skull fracture No severe headache
Sensitivity	100%	96.80%
NPV	100%	99.95%

*Severe mechanism: motor vehicle collision with ejection, rollover, or fatality of another passenger; pedestrian or bicyclist without helmet versus motor vehicle; fall > 2 mo (age ≥ 2 years) or > 1 mo (age < 2 years); head struck by high-impact object.
Data from Kuppermann N et al: Identification of children at very low risk of clinically-important brain injuries after head trauma. *Lancet.* 2009;374:1160.

Low-Risk Criteria for Infants and Children with Minor Head Injury. Children are divided into two age groups (< 2 y and ≥ 2 y) and, when all low-risk criteria are met, the negative predictive value reaches nearly 100% in both groups (Table 23–2). These children require observation in the emergency department.

▶ Clinical Findings

Concussion is a trauma-induced alteration in mental status that may or may not involve loss of consciousness.

▶ Treatment

Treatment for concussion is supportive, and may include acetaminophen for headache, low-stimulation environment including dimmed lights and quiet room. There are many guidelines for athletes' return to practice/competition. In general, these guidelines are conservative and recommend athletes do not return to practice or competition until they have been free of symptoms for a period of time. The major concern is that if the athlete suffers another concussive injury before fully recovered from the first insult, severe neurologic decompensation (and even death) termed, second impact syndrome, can occur.

▶ Disposition

For patients who suffer a concussion, a period of observation in the emergency department of 4-6 hours postinjury is appropriate, followed by close monitoring by a responsible adult for the following 24 hours. A detailed set of written instructions including symptoms to watch for and return to the emergency department for reevaluation must be given to the caregiver. Symptoms include steadily worsening headache, uncontrolled nausea/vomiting, late-onset seizures, and altered mental status. Provide reassurance that the child may sleep if it is naptime or bedtime, and that headache may persist for several days despite treatment with acetaminophen. Close follow-up with a primary care physician should be arranged, and for significant concussions, consideration should be given to neuropsychiatric testing to establish a baseline from which to gauge recovery. Symptoms, such as amnesia surrounding the injury, short-term memory loss, and mental sluggishness may persist for weeks to months in patients with serious concussions. Return to circumstances where the patient may suffer further head injury, such as competition or full-contact sports, should be delayed for as long as even minor symptoms persist, and the patient should follow up with a primary care physician or concussion specialist for clearance to return to play.

Brenner DJ: Estimating cancer risks from pediatric CT: Going from the qualitative to the quantitative. *Pediatr Radiol.* 2002;32(4):228-231 [PMID: 11956700].

Chodick G, Ronckers CM, Shalev V, Ron E: Excess lifetime cancer mortality risk attributable to radiation exposure from computed tomography examinations in children. *Israel Med Assoc J.* 2007;9(8):584-587 [PMID: 17877063].

Faul M XL, Wald MM, Coronado VG: Traumatic brain injury in the United States: Emergency department visits, hospitalizations and deaths 2002–2006. *In: Centers for Disease Control and Prevention NCfIPaC,* ed. Atlanta, GA; 2010.

Kuppermann N, Holmes JF, Dayan PS, et al: Identification of children at very low risk of clinically-important brain injuries after head trauma: A prospective cohort study. *Lancet.* 2009;374(9696):1160-1170 [PMID: 19758692].

Schunk JE, Schutzman SA: Pediatric head injury. *Am Acad Pediatr.* 2012;33(9):398-411 [PMID: 22942365].

Schutzman SA, Barnes P, Duhaime AC, et al: Evaluation and management of children younger than two years old with apparently minor head trauma: Proposed guidelines. *Pediatrics.* 2001;107(5):983-993 [PMID: 11331675].

Smith-Bindman R, Lipson J, Marcus R, et al: Radiation dose associated with common computed tomography examinations and the associated lifetime attributable risk of cancer. *Arch Intern Med.* 2009;169(22):2078-2086 [PMID: 20008690].

SCALP HEMATOMA

► Clinical Findings

A hematoma may be an isolated soft tissue injury, or may overlie or indicate more serious injury. As the sinuses have not fully aerated in young children, the frontal bones are stronger and hematoma on the forehead is less likely to be associated with intracranial or cranial injury. Nonfrontal boggy hematoma increases the likelihood of intracranial injury, and the CT head scan should be obtained in children younger than 2 years.

► Treatment

After examination for bogginess or underlying depressed skull fracture, ice and gentle compression may be applied with a towel over the hematoma to reduce edema. Avoid direct application of ice to skin as this may cause tissue damage from frostbite. The closed head injury observation and guidelines previously discussed should be followed.

► Disposition

Patients with scalp hematomas may be discharged to responsible, reliable adult caregivers with ability to closely follow up with primary care physician. Give instructions to apply cold compresses for comfort, avoid direct contact with ice or prolonged application, and may take acetaminophen for pain and discomfort.

SCALP LACERATIONS

► Clinical Findings

Lacerations result from either blunt or penetrating trauma—there is scant subcutaneous padding on the scalp and therefore blunt trauma pinches the skin between the object and the skull and can result in significant lacerations. The scalp is a highly vascular region and will bleed profusely. It can bleed enough to cause hypovolemic shock, and thus active bleeding should be controlled quickly. Prehospital estimates of blood loss from scalp lacerations are important but are frequently over- and underestimated, and so must be evaluated with caution and correlated with the patient's examination. Bleeding may need to be controlled with cautery, sutures, or Raney clips before an examination of the laceration and any more major, underlying trauma. Note the length, depth, layers of tissue involved (dermis, superficial fascia, galea aponeurosis, pericranium), and the condition of the wound edges. Once bleeding is controlled, the CT head scan should be obtained to look for structural intracranial abnormalities if indicated (altered mental status).

► Treatment

Sedation may be required for preparation, exploration, and repair of scalp lacerations in pediatric patients. Topical, local, or regional anesthesia may be employed. Lidocaine with epinephrine is often used to help control bleeding and oozing. Irrigate copiously with high pressure to reduce contamination and lower the risk of infection, although the vascularity of the scalp protects it against infection. Do not shave the scalp as this increases the risk of wound infection. Pull hair away from wound and mat it down with ointment to visualize the laceration. Explore the wound for foreign bodies. If the galea is involved, it may be closed with simple absorbable interrupted sutures. Close the skin with staples or simple interrupted sutures, either nonabsorbable or rapidly absorbable, and leave long tails to facilitate nonabsorbable suture removal. Consider a pressure dressing for deep lacerations to avoid hematoma formation.

Disposition

Patients with scalp lacerations can be discharged with routine wound care instructions: rinse area but avoid scrubbing or soaking, remove pressure dressing after 24 hours, and no need for continued dressing or antibiotic ointment. Consider concussion precautions as well. Sutures or staples should be removed in 10 days, with an interval wound check if necessary.

SKULL FRACTURES: CLOSED/OPEN/ DEPRESSED/BASILAR

Clinical Findings

Skull fractures are identified in 2-20% of pediatric head trauma patients (Figure 23–1A, 1B). All patients with a suspected skull fracture should undergo CT head scan after bleeding from an associated scalp laceration is controlled,

and the wound is explored as described above. Overlying nonfrontal scalp hematoma, especially in children younger than 2 years may be the only sign of a closed skull fracture, and these children should undergo CT head scan. A closed skull fracture that is depressed more than one thickness of skull is often lifted surgically. Investigate carefully any scalp lacerations for evidence of underlying fracture, foreign body, deformity, or skull fragments or brain parenchyma. Basilar skull fracture may be associated with Battle sign (mastoid ecchymosis), raccoon eyes (periorbital ecchymosis), or CSF otorrhea or rhinorrhea, and is a significant risk factor for intracranial injury.

Treatment

The literature is unclear on the proper treatment of any open fracture, fracture of the sinuses, or fracture associated with pneumocephalus or CSF leak regarding the administration of IV antibiotics to avoid meningitis. CSF leaks can be difficult to detect, and therefore a sample may need to be sent to the laboratory for confirmation. Elevate the head of the bed to 30 degrees, and arrange for consultation with a pediatric neurosurgeon.

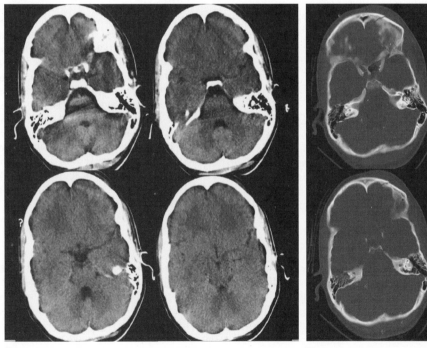

A   B

▲ **Figure 23–1A, B.** A 15-year-old boy involved in MVC with signs of left facial trauma and altered mental status. (**A**) Noncontrast CT with brain windows. A small amount of pneumocephalus is noted in top-left image in the left frontal area. (**B**) Noncontrast CT with bone windows more clearly demonstrating a slightly displaced skull fracture through the left supraorbital area. Also noted is frontal scalp hematoma.

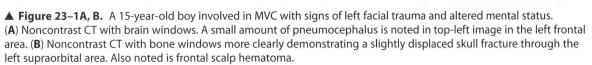

Disposition

Pediatric patients with skull fractures should be admitted to the neurosurgical service, with the possible exception of closed, nondisplaced fractures without any underlying intracranial injuries. Pediatric patients with skull fractures need close follow-up to ensure proper healing. Unique to children is the complication of leptomeningeal cysts or "growing fractures" in which the fracture line does not close normally but continues to separate as the child's head grows. For the patient with closed fractures, after consultation with a neurosurgeon, if there is no concern for non-accidental trauma and the parents are responsible and have reliable transportation, the patient may be discharged to home with close follow-up. Detailed instructions to return to the emergency department for any signs of infection, altered mental status, worsening headache, seizures, uncontrolled nausea/vomiting, or other symptoms concerning to the family must be reviewed with caregivers.

CEREBRAL CONTUSIONS

Clinical Findings

Cerebral contusions occur after significant mechanism, so it is important to get a detailed history if possible. They can be caused by direct force transmission, often to the frontal cortex, or by contra-coup forces opposite the site of impact. Usually they will show up on CT head scan, and are associated with intraparenchymal and subarachnoid hemorrhages. Significant edema may occur.

Treatment

Initial treatment of cerebral contusions involves avoiding secondary injury by providing good emergency care, adequate but not overly aggressive resuscitation, oxygenation, and quality supportive care. Patients are at increased risk for delayed intraparenchymal hemorrhage and their coagulation status should be monitored and corrected if necessary with platelets, fresh frozen plasma, or specific factors if indicated. Emegent consultation with a neurosurgeon should be arranged.

Disposition

Patients need to be admitted and monitored closely for evolution of concerning symptoms. Intracranial pressure monitoring may be required if signs of elevated ICP such as coma and GCS less than nine develop.

DIFFUSE AXONAL INJURY

Clinical Findings

Diffuse axonal injury is caused by the shearing forces of deceleration on the neurons of the brain. It is caused by blunt trauma, often motor vehicle crash (MVC), but also shaken baby syndrome (SBS). Cerebral edema may develop rapidly. There is often no abnormality on CT scan, but punctate lesions at the gray-white junction may sometimes be seen.

Treatment

Document the best GCS and brief neurological examination. The physician should have a very low threshold for intubation of these patients, as cerebral edema and resultant decline in ability to protect airway may develop rapidly. Early consultation with a neurosurgeon is advised. Maintain blood pressure and oxygenation status to avoid secondary injury. With signs of herniation, hypertonic saline (3% at 5 mL/kg) or mannitol (0.25-1 g/kg IV bolus) may stabilize the cerebral edema.

Disposition

Admit cerebral contusion patients to the neurosurgical and/or pediatric intensive care unit for close observation.

EPIDURAL HEMATOMA

Clinical Findings

Classic presentation of epidural hematoma is blunt force trauma to the lateral aspect of the head with immediate altered mental state, followed by a lucid interval, and then rapid neurological decline and death. Epidural hematoma is caused most often by disruption of the middle meningeal artery after a blow to the temporal or temporoparietal area, usually with depressed skull fracture, and resultant collection of blood between the skull and the dura mater. It has also been reported to occur with damage to the venous sinuses and adjacent collection of blood in the same space. Diagnosis is by noncontrast CT scan (Figure 23–2), where a biconvex hematoma will be evident at the margin of the brain. Unlike subdural hematoma, epidurals cannot cross suture lines, as the blood is outside the dura and therefore is contained by the adhesion of suture to cranium.

Treatment

It is important to stabilize, scan, and diagnose patients because the underlying brain parenchyma is often uninjured, and full recovery can be expected after neurosurgical evacuation. However, because of the often high pressure accumulation of blood, herniation leading to irreversible damage and death can occur within a few hours following injury.

Disposition

Consultation with a neurosurgeon and craniotomy with epidural hematoma evacuation should be arranged as soon as possible after diagnosis.

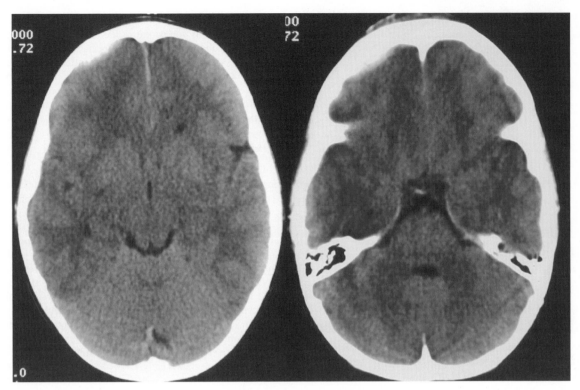

▲ **Figure 23–2.** A pediatric patient with a subtle small epidural hematoma in the right frontal area. Using lower dose pediatric imaging protocols, occasionally epidural hematomas are difficult to visualize on noncontrast CT using brain windows so consider others looking on bone windows as well.

SUBDURAL HEMATOMA

▶ Clinical Findings

Resulting from tearing of the bridging veins between the cranium and the brain parenchyma, subdural hematomas collect deep to the dura mater. On CT scan, they show up as crescent-shaped collections of blood that follow the inner contour of the skull (Figure 23–3). Acute subdural hematomas appear hyperdense, but subacute and chronic hematomas may be isodense or hypodense because the hemoglobin in the blood has been reabsorbed, and these may be difficult to appreciate. Children younger than 2 years are at increased risk of subdural hematoma because of the fragility of their bridging veins and because there is more room in the calvarium for the brain to move during trauma. Subdural hematoma, especially bilaterally, should prompt consideration of non-accidental trauma, often from shaking (SBS).

▶ Treatment

Depending on the neurologic status of the patient, these injuries can either be evacuated or observed. Consultation with a pediatric neurosurgeon is important. If the child has no, or minor, neurologic deficits, the body can often reabsorb these hematomas without surgery.

▶ Disposition

Admit patients for observation or surgery.

TRAUMATIC SUBARACHNOID HEMORRHAGE

▶ Clinical Findings

Most common finding in patients with GCS score less than 13 is traumatic subarachnoid hemorrhage, which results from tearing of the subarachnoid vessels and presents with blood in the CSF. Patients often complain of headache, photophobia, and meningismus. Usually, this injury can be picked up on CT head scan, but scans performed at 6-8 hours postinjury may be more sensitive. Subarachnoid hemorrhage is associated with a steep increase in mortality, especially when it is early onset or combined with severe range GCS 3-8.

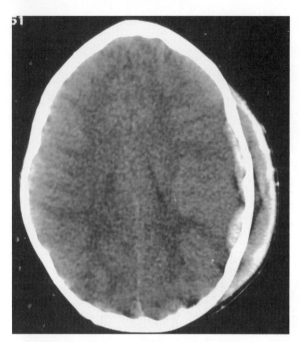

▲ **Figure 23–3.** A pediatric patient with a left parietal subdural hemorrhage with associated scalp hematoma overlying the intracranial hemorrhage.

▶ **Treatment**

Obtain a thorough history and a complete physical examination because patients have the potential to decline rapidly. Consultation with a neurosurgeon is advised.

▶ **Disposition**

Admit patients for close observation and possible repeat CT scans or neurosurgical intervention.

MISCELLANEOUS (Special Cases/Populations, Other Misfit Items)

NON-ACCIDENTAL TRAUMA

Intentional injury to a child from a parent, guardian, or acquaintance is considered child abuse. If abuse goes unrecognized, it is likely to escalate and, on subsequent occasion, may result in the child's death. Of child fatalities from non-accidental trauma (NAT), 66% in children younger than 5 years is from abusive head trauma, and children younger than 1 year make up the vast majority of these deaths. The physician must suspect abuse if the history from the parent/caregiver does not coincide with the physical examination (infant < 6 months "rolled off" table, long bone injury in a child too young to walk), a prolonged interval elapses

between injury and presentation for medical care, history given differs from one parent to the other, or in instances of multiple subdural hematomas, especially without a concomitant skull fracture. Head injuries often result from shaking a child. Maintain a low threshold of suspicion, and alert social services to any instances of potential abuse. Remember, these children are at risk for death if discharged into the same circumstances.

COAGULOPATHY

Children with hemophilia, other bleeding dyscrasias, those on anticoagulant medications who present with a head injury represent a very low percentage of the head-injured patient population. However, they do present special challenges. Obviously, these children are at increased risk for intracranial hemorrhage, with continued expansion of hematoma and resultant increase in ICP. At this time, no specific guidelines exist for management of these patients. Self-reported physician management for children with hemophilia and head trauma is diverse, but includes a lower threshold for CT scan and prophylactic factor transfusion, with a higher percentage admitted for observation and continued factor transfusion. Until further research defines best practices, it is prudent to err on the side of caution and involve pediatric hematology consultants early.

DISCHARGE CRITERIA

Most pediatric head trauma is nonserious. Patients can be evaluated, observed, and safely discharged to home. Asymptomatic infants and children who are at least 4 hours postinjury can safely be discharged to reliable caregivers without imaging. Children younger than 2 years with intermediate risk for intracranial hemorrhage or skull fracture can either be observed for 4-6 hours and discharged if stable or improving, or CT head scan may be obtained and the child discharged if normal. The risk of delayed deterioration after a normal CT head scan is near zero. Parents/caregivers should be counseled on postconcussive syndrome and what to watch for in their child, and a child with concussion should be followed up by either primary care physician or a specialized concussion clinic for neuropsychiatric baseline testing. A child with an intracranial injury should be admitted to the hospital, as well as a child who shows signs of even mild deterioration during their emergency department stay.

Klevens J, Leeb RT: Child maltreatment fatalities in children under 5: Findings from the National Violence Death Reporting System. *Child Abuse Negl.* 2010;34(4):262-266 [PMID: 20304491].

Witmer CM, Manno CS, Butler RB, Raffini LJ: The clinical management of hemophilia and head trauma: A survey of current clinical practice among pediatric hematology/oncology physicians. *Pediatr Blood Cancer.* 2009;53:406-410 [PMID: 19489052].

Maxillofacial & Neck Trauma

Stephen McConnell, MD
Dorian Drigalla, MD, FACEP

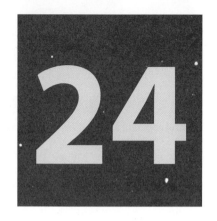

IMMEDIATE MANAGEMENT OF LIFE-THREATENING CONDITIONS

Evaluation of the pediatric patient with maxillofacial and neck trauma begins with the primary trauma assessment. Depending on the injuries present, airway management may be difficult due to distortion of normal landmarks or blood present in the path of visualization. It is often difficult to determine the severity of an injury by external examination alone, and complete evaluation may require the use of advanced imaging techniques or consultation with a trauma surgeon.

The complexity and intricacies of the structures of these regions require a thorough examination. Airway management may be difficult in patients with traumatic injuries to the face or neck, and the airway should be secured whenever compromise is present or felt to be imminent.

A number of imaging modalities may be employed to evaluate potential injuries. Computed tomography (CT) scans are commonly used in the emergency department to evaluate for traumatic injuries. Magnetic resonance imaging (MRI) and swallow studies may be used to identify or exclude injury. The emergency department physician should maintain diligence in identifying the patient who may be a victim of non-accidental trauma.

AIRWAY MANAGEMENT

Continuous monitoring of the airway is crucial. A thorough evaluation of the airway should be made while maintaining cervical spine immobilization with a cervical collar. Patients may initially display little to no external evidence of tracheal injury.

LARYNGEAL & TRACHEAL INJURIES

Monitor for changes in phonation, presence of subcutaneous emphysema, development or worsening of edema, expanding hematoma, as well as deviation of the trachea from its midline position. These signs all suggest a potential laryngeal injury and possibly worsening airway compromise.

Tracheal injuries are suggested by mediastinal air on chest radiograph, development of subcutaneous emphysema, or development of a simple or tension pneumothorax.

Endotracheal intubation should be attempted to secure the airway when laryngeal or tracheal injury is suggested. Simultaneous preparation for surgical airway is advised. Cricothyroidotomy or tracheostomy may be necessary if intubation fails.

FACIAL & NECK INJURIES

Traumatic injuries to the face or jaw may present with airway obstruction resulting from the displacement of tissue, or from a significant amount of bleeding, which prevents the patient from being able to ventilate or oxygenate effectively. Perform a jaw thrust maneuver when injuries allow, and utilize suctioning to clear blood or secretions that may be complicating ventilation. Neck injuries may include damage to the cervical spinal cord with a reduction in effective spontaneous respirations. In these patients, endotracheal intubation or other airway management should be performed, while maintaining cervical spine alignment. Rapid sequence induction followed by orotracheal intubation is the preferred method for securing an airway. Consider avoidance of paralytics if facial deformity is likely to prevent successful bag-valve-mask ventilation during the procedure. Airway adjuncts may be employed to perform this procedure successfully (see Chapter 9). Be prepared to perform a surgical airway for patients with laryngeal or tracheal injuries, as passage of endotracheal tube (ETT) through the injured area may not be successful.

BREATHING

Monitor breathing continuously to maintain acceptable oxygenation and ventilation. Arterial blood gas analysis will guide appropriate oxygen administration. Concomitant pneumothorax should be treated appropriately (see Chapter 3). Frequent reassessment and management of secretions should be maintained. Place an orogastric or nasogastric tube to decompress the stomach.

CIRCULATION

Control apparent hemorrhage when vascular injury is apparent. An expanding hematoma, carotid bruit, absence of the carotid pulse, and worsening oxygenation are indicators of potential vascular injury. Do not remove foreign bodies or explore open wounds in the emergency department, as worsening hemorrhage may result.

Direct pressure to hemorrhaging facial or neck wounds is recommended. Do not apply circumferential pressure (tourniquet) to the neck, as it likely will cause vascular or airway compromise. If a bleeding vessel can be clearly seen and direct pressure fails to control hemorrhage, consider a controlling figure-of-eight stitch or direct clamping with hemostats, using caution to avoid adjacent structures.

Closely monitor heart rate and blood pressure. Treat apparent hemorrhagic shock as described in Chapter 10. Aggressive administration of intravenous fluids, blood products, and vasopressors may be required. Consider spinal shock in patients with hypotension and bradycardia, and initiate supportive measures.

DISABILITY

In the presence of facial or soft tissue neck trauma, strong suspicion of intracranial or cervical spine injury is warranted. Evaluation for related or adjacent trauma is indicated. Prompt consultation of a neurosurgeon or spine surgeon is indicated when these injuries are identified.

Chapman VM, Fenton LZ, Gao D, et al: Facial fractures in children: Unique patterns of injury observed by computed tomography. *J Comput Assist Tomogr.* 2009;33(1):70-72 [PMID: 19188788].

Dufresene CR, Manson PN: Pediatric craniofacial trauma: Challenging pediatric cases–Craniofacial trauma. *Craniomaxillofac Trauma Reconstr.* 2011;4(2):73-84 [PMID: 22655118].

Hopper RA, Salemy S, Sze RW: Diagnosis of midface fractures with CT: What the surgeon needs to know. *Radiographics.* 2006;26(3):783-793 [PMID: 16702454].

Imahara SD, Hopper RA, Wang J, et al: Patterns and outcomes of pediatric facial fractures in the United States: A survey of the National Trauma Data Bank. *J Am Coll Surg.* 2009;207(5): 710-716 [PMID: 18954784].

NECK TRAUMA

Life-threatening injuries to the structures of the neck require prompt intervention. Laryngeal, tracheal, esophageal, vascular, and spinal injuries are possible when evidence of penetrating or blunt trauma is present. Spinal cord injuries and thrombosis of the common or internal carotid artery comprise 50% of the mortality associated with blunt or penetrating neck injuries. Early airway management is appropriate, and a judicious search for underlying injury is warranted.

PENETRATING NECK INJURIES

▶ Clinical Findings

Penetrating injuries are most commonly caused by gunshot or stab wounds. Airway and esophageal injuries are rare. Direct airway injuries may present with hoarseness, cough, or shortness of breath. Subcutaneous emphysema may be present. Indirect involvement of the airway (such as an expanding hematoma) may cause stridor, tachypnea, dysphonia, or cyanosis.

Esophageal injuries present with dysphagia and/or odynophagia, as well as drooling and hematemesis. Clinical signs are not always present, and a high degree of clinical suspicion should be coupled with a thorough diagnostic evaluation when mechanism suggests this possibility.

The neck is divided into three zones, based on anatomic landmarks (Figure 24–1). Zone I extends from the thoracic

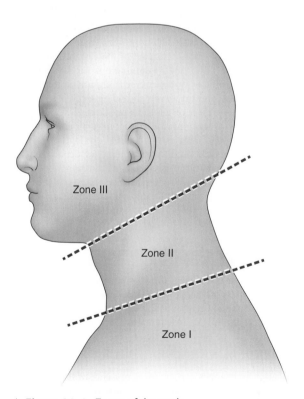

▲ **Figure 24–1.** Zones of the neck.

outlet to the inferior aspect of the cricoid cartilage. Zone II spans from the cricoid cartilage to the angle of the mandible. Zone III extends from the angle of the mandible to the base of the skull.

Potentially damaged structures are delineated by the zone of the neck involved. Zone I injuries may involve major thoracic or neck structures such as the subclavian vessels, pleura, trachea, or esophagus. Damage to these structures in this location may require surgical exploration. Proximal control of the vessels in this region may necessitate a thoracotomy. Evaluation of zone I injuries frequently requires advanced imaging including angiography, as well as swallow studies to exclude injury to the esophagus.

Zone II injuries are often noticed on physical examination. The presence of an expanding hematoma or bruit may signify vascular injury, whereas stridor or phonation changes may signify tracheal or laryngeal injury. Historically, penetrating trauma to zone II would lead to surgical exploration. Currently, it is more common to observe hemodynamically stable patients with the assistance of advanced imaging that is now readily available.

Injuries to zone III have a high rate of vascular injury. These injuries are often challenging to manage surgically because of the difficulty in obtaining distal control. Angiography is often needed and interventional radiology may be required.

▶ **Treatment**

Unstable patients may be defined as those in hemorrhagic shock, as well as those with an expanding neck hematoma, unstable airway that cannot be secured, or apparent stroke with central nervous system (CNS) signs. The unstable patient with a penetrating neck injury requires surgical exploration. The airway should be secured when possible, and prompt surgical consultation sought.

Stable patient should have a physical examination followed by a chest and soft-tissue neck radiograph. The patient with a normal examination and normal radiographs may be clinically observed for developing signs or symptoms. The patient with an abnormal examination or initial x-ray requires further diagnostic studies. Conventional angiography or CT scan is warranted to assess for vascular injury. Suspicion of airway or esophageal injury warrants esophagoscopy and laryngoscopy/bronchoscopy. A contrast-enhanced swallow study will increase sensitivity in evaluation for airway or esophageal injury.

▶ **Disposition**

Unstable patients require operative exploration. Patients with a zone I, II, or III injury and positive angiographic findings of vascular injury should undergo surgical exploration. Patients noted to have injury during esophageal or laryngeal endoscopy require surgical evaluation and exploration.

Stable patients with a suspicious mechanism for underlying injury, but no evidence of injury on examination, or during procedural or radiographic evaluation should be clinically observed in the inpatient setting.

BLUNT TRAUMA NECK INJURIES

▶ **Clinical Findings**

Motor vehicle collisions are the most common source of blunt neck injury. The seatbelt, dashboard, or other object may directly traumatize the anterior neck. Strangulation is another source of injury, usually evident by clinical signs such as subconjunctival hemorrhages, facial petechiae, or direct ligature markings. The injury, termed "clothesline" may occur during sports, martial arts, and while riding recreational vehicles.

Laryngeal fracture above the glottis presents with subcutaneous emphysema in the neck, dysphagia, hoarseness, worsening airway obstruction, and occasionally thyroid cartilage deformity. Injury below the glottis typically presents with hemoptysis and persistent air leak from the endotracheal tube.

Blunt esophageal injuries may be suggested by bloody gastric tube aspirate, or crepitus in the superficial neck tissues. No initial signs of injury may be noted, and the mechanism of the injury should prompt consideration of advanced imaging.

▶ **Treatment**

Approach to the patient with blunt trauma follows a similar course as that of penetrating trauma: evaluate and stabilize the airway as needed, then pursue advanced imaging to evaluate damage to the great vessels and other deep space tissues. Esophageal evaluation with a water-soluble swallow study may also be indicated.

The unstable patient should have the cervical spine immobilized, airway secured, and be evaluated further for likely causes. Hemorrhagic shock should be treated with blood products. Assessment for signs of vascular injury begins with a focused examination. A carotid bruit, expanding hematoma, pulsatile bleeding or hematoma, or pulse deficit indicate likely vascular injury. Hypotension, stable hematomas, and CNS ischemic signs also point to vascular injury. These patients should undergo CT angiography of the head and neck to assess for vascular integrity. A number of centers prefer conventional four-vessel cerebral angiography to assess the vertebral and carotid arteries.

Stable patients should have a thorough physical examination including careful neurological assessment, as well as neck and chest radiographs. Abnormal findings indicate need for CT angiography. The CT studies will also evaluate the nonvascular structures of the neck. Normal studies in clinically symptomatic patients should be followed by endoscopic evaluation of the airway and/or esophagus.

▶ Disposition

Patients with diagnosed vascular, airway, or esophageal injury require surgical consultation. Interventional radiology may benefit patients with vascular injury or cerebrovascular compromise. Patients with no hard findings of injury during diagnostic studies may still be observed in the inpatient setting when clinical suspicion for occult injury exists.

Rathlev NK, Medzon R, Bracken ME: Evaluation and management of neck trauma. *Emerg Med Clin North Am.* 2007;25(3): 679-694 [PMID 17826212].

Tisherman SA, Bokhari F, Collier B, et al: Clinical practice guideline: Penetrating zone II neck trauma. *J Trauma.* 2008;64(5):1392-1405 [PMID: 18469667].

MAXILLOFACIAL SOFT TISSUE TRAUMA

Pediatric patients may present to the emergency department with various injuries to the musculoskeletal structures of the face and neck. Many patients are capable of being managed entirely in the emergency department and do not require specialty consultants or admission. Soft tissue injuries of the face and neck are two common conditions for which patients may seek medical care. Discussion of soft tissue injuries and wound care is discussed in Chapter 31.

Detailed history and physical examination is necessary for proper management. Identification of the mechanism injury and assessment for the presence of foreign body may help dictate care. Timely closure of a wound may lead to better outcomes, including reduction in scar formation and likelihood of infection. Thorough irrigation and cleansing of the wound is especially important. Deep soft tissue injuries to the face or neck may require in-depth evaluation to exclude damage to nerves, blood vessels, muscular structures, or the salivary glands and ducts.

NERVE INJURY

Nerve supply to the face is large, including the facial, trigeminal, auditory, lingual, and hypoglossal nerves. Test the branches of the facial nerve and observe for facial asymmetry. Observe movement of the forehead and eyelids, as well as smiling. Assess for sensation and taste. Assess hearing as well as tongue movement.

PAROTID GLAND INJURY

Consider parotid gland injury when the wound implies likely injury. Probe Stensen's duct from inside the mouth and observe for pass-through into the wound. If a parotid gland injury is left untreated, a salivary fistula may develop and be difficult or impossible to repair. Consult a maxillofacial specialist in this setting.

EYE INJURY

Carefully evaluate the eyes and visual acuity (see Chapter 32). A slit lamp examination with fluorescein staining is indicated for assessment of globe injury. Eyelid lacerations pose a risk of improper healing without specialized repair. Complete ocular examination to exclude underlying fracture of the orbital wall or damage to the globe is indicated. Complete through-and-through lacerations, those that involve the eyelid margin or canalicular system, or those where the overall function of the eyelid is distorted, should be managed by a plastic surgeon or ophthalmologist.

ANIMAL BITES

Animal bites are a specific injury to the soft tissue that requires attention. Evaluate the neurovascular status as well as both the immunization status of the patient and the animal. Animal bite wounds should not be closed unless loss of function will result. Many clinicians loosely approximate animal wounds for better cosmetic healing. All bite wounds should be thoroughly cleansed and irrigated.

TISSUE AVULSION

Tissue avulsion is an injury that may be seen in the pediatric patient. Care should be taken to evaluate and cleanse the wound fully, and determine if specialist consultation is indicated. Patients with extensive injury may require exploration and intervention in the operating room; specifically, avulsions that involve structures near the eye, nose, ear, or mouth. Avulsions with significant tissue loss should be managed by a specialist.

NASAL INJURY

Inspect the bilateral nares for apparent septal hematoma, ongoing epistaxis, or obstruction. Thorough examination is required to identify the presence of a septal hematoma, which appears as an erythematous or violaceous bulge on the septum. An adjacent fracture is likely in the presence of hematoma (Figure 24–2). A nasal septal hematoma should be emergently drained, preferably by a specialist. Drainage can be performed in the emergency department by an experienced clinician. Early evacuation of the hematoma is recommended to prevent the formation of an abscess or septal perforation. Rarely, intracranial spread of bacteria may occur.

Observe for the possibility of cerebrospinal fluid (CSF) leakage, which points to communicating intracranial injury and likely underlying fracture. Cartilaginous injury requires specialized repair to ensure proper cosmetic result, especially in the growing pediatric patient.

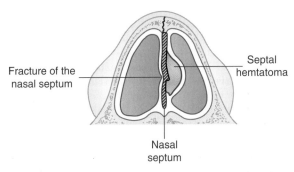

Fracture of the nasal septum

Septal hemtatoma

Nasal septum

▲ **Figure 24–2.** Nasal septal hematoma. (Reproduced, with permission, from Reichman EF, Simon RR: *Emergency Medicine Procedures*. McGraw-Hill, 2004. Copyright © McGraw-Hill Education LLC.)

EAR INJURY

Auricle lacerations and auricle hematomas require specific attention (see Auricle Lacerations). These findings should prompt evaluation for hemotympanum, as well as postauricular hematoma (Battle sign) and CSF otorrhea. Any of these three findings suggests associated fracture or intracranial injury, and should prompt further diagnostic evaluation and specialist consultation.

Hogg NJ, Horswell BB: Soft tissue pediatric facial trauma: A review. *J Can Dent Assoc.* 2006;72(6):549-552 [PMID: 16884647].
Singh G, Mohammad S, Pal US, et al: Pediatric facial injuries: It's management. *Natl J Maxillofac Surg.* 2011;2(2):156-162 [PMID: 22639504].

MAXILLOFACIAL FRACTURES

MANDIBLE FRACTURES

▷ Clinical Findings

Pediatric patients rarely encounter injury to the mandible, although this injury is more common than fractures to the midface. This is likely due to the unsupported structure of the mandible. Most injuries are caused by blunt trauma from falls or motor vehicle accidents. Some suggest that the mandible is at extra risk due to the presence of permanent tooth buds, which may lead to a relative thinning of the bone as well as the curvature of the mandible. Mandible injuries are usually accompanied by injury to the tooth, described in the Dental Injuries section of this chapter. The frequency of mandibular fractures increases with age in the pediatric population. The astute clinician will suspect mandibular injury in a patient with pain, swelling, asymmetry, trismus, malocclusion, or the presence of sublingual ecchymosis. Patients may also have damage to the inferior alveolar nerve producing loss of

sensation along the mandible to the midline of the lower lip. A laceration should be evaluated to exclude an open fracture. Any finding suggestive of mandibular fracture should prompt suspicion of associated facial or intracranial injury.

▷ Treatment

Assess and stabilize the patient's airway and breathing first. CT scan of the mandible alone or in conjunction with maxillofacial views is considered the imaging modality of choice. Dedicated views of these structures will help determine the extent of the injury and may help the specialist plan appropriate treatment options. The most common mandibular fracture in the pediatric patient is "greenstick" fracture (Figure 24–3). This occurs when one cortex wall is broken and the other cortex wall is bent. Pediatric patients have a high healing rate of the periosteum, which leads to faster healing.

Confirmed mandible fracture should be considered open, given the adjacent teeth, and broad-spectrum antibiotics are typically recommended. Consultation with an oral surgeon or maxillofacial surgeon is indicated.

▷ Disposition

Management of a greenstick fracture without displacement or malocclusion is conservative.

Reduction of a mandibular fracture does pose a challenge and should be performed by an oral or maxillofacial surgeon. Closed reduction with splinting is preferred in most patients with mandibular fracture. Open reduction may need to be

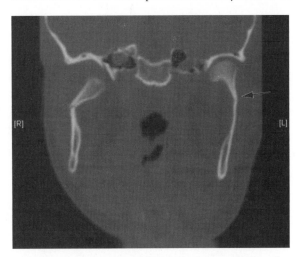

▲ **Figure 24–3.** Greenstick fracture of the mandible: The CT demonstrates bilateral mandibular condylar fractures in a 12-year-old. The left fracture (*arrow*) is an incomplete (greenstick) fracture. (Reproduced, with permission, from Shah BR, Lucchesi M (eds): *Atlas of Pediatric Emergency Medicine*, 2nd ed. McGraw-Hill, 2013. Copyright © McGraw-Hill Education LLC.)

performed in some patients, and with recent advances in materials, complications are fewer.

John B, John RR, Stalin A, et al: Management of mandibular body fractures in pediatric patients: A case report and review of the literature. *Contemp Clin Dent.* 2010;1(4):291-296 [PMID: 22114443].

Laster Z, Muska EA, Nagler R: Pediatric mandibular fractures: Introduction of a novel therapeutic modality. *J Trauma.* 2008;64(1):225-229 [PMID: 18188125].

DENTAL INJURIES

▶ Clinical Findings

Patients who sustain fractures to the midface or mandible often have associated dental injury. The incidence is higher in the anterior teeth, and is common in younger children learning to mobilize and with less developed coordination. Regaining occlusion is important in caring for the patient with dental injury, as well as identifying any potential underlying fracture.

Patients may present to the emergency department after isolated trauma results in damage to one or more of the primary or secondary teeth. Damage may range from a small crack or chip to complete avulsion. Understanding how to manage the pediatric patient is critical. Treatment of dental injuries is focused primarily on survival of the secondary tooth. Damage to a primary tooth is not critical, as it will normally be replaced by the emergence of the secondary tooth. Figure 24–4 diagrams the anatomy of a tooth.

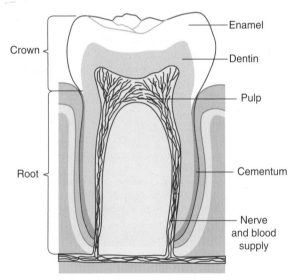

▲ **Figure 24–4.** Tooth anatomy in cross-section. (Reproduced with permission from Stone CK, Humphries RL: *Current Diagnosis & Treatment Emergency Medicine,* 7th ed. New York: McGraw-Hill, 2011. Copyright © McGraw-Hill Education LLC.)

▶ Treatment

Dental fractures through the enamel are usually managed as an outpatient with dental referral. However, damage that goes through to the dentin or pulp should be addressed in the emergency department. Untreated, these injuries may result in necrosis or infection and timely management is indicated.

Ellis classification is commonly used to describe the dental layers involved in the fracture. Ellis I fractures involve the enamel, whereas Ellis II and Ellis III fractures involve the dentin and pulp, respectively (Figure 24–5).

Dental Fractures and Temporary Seals

A fractured tooth warrants a temporary seal placed in the emergency department. Prior to attempting temporary seal of the tooth, provide adequate analgesia as the exposed pulp and dentin are very sensitive. Consider performing a nerve block or providing systemic analgesics. Several commercially available preparations may be placed over the fractured tooth to seal it, with calcium hydroxide being one of the more common applications. Apply the mixture over

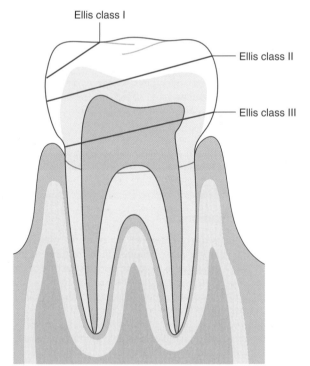

▲ **Figure 24–5.** Ellis classification of dental fractures. (Reproduced with permission from Stone CK, Humphries RL: *Current Diagnosis & Treatment Emergency Medicine,* 7th ed. New York: McGraw-Hill, 2011. Copyright © McGraw-Hill Education LLC.)

the fractured tooth and allow to dry, forming a seal over the fracture site.

Replacement of a Tooth Avulsion

Dental avulsion, displacement of a tooth from its normal anatomical position, may also occur. The first step in managing the patient is locating the missing tooth. Avulsed teeth pose an aspiration hazard to the patient. Attempts at reimplanting an avulsed tooth should be made with a secondary tooth only. Time is critical in replacing a secondary tooth as the periodontal ligament may become necrotic. Scrubbing the avulsed tooth may damage the periodontal ligament and is not recommended. Placing the avulsed tooth in a container of milk may help slow the death of the cells associated with the periodontal ligament.

Attempting to replace the avulsed tooth is usually painful. Provide the patient with sufficient analgesia or anesthesia. If the buccal evaluation reveals significant trauma, attempting to replace the avulsed tooth should not occur. Gently suction the socket to remove any blood clot and gently irrigate the area with saline. Blood clot that remains in the dental socket may inhibit anatomic alignment of the tooth. It is important not to damage the periodontal ligament that is lining the socket. Gently, and with firm pressure, insert the tooth into the socket in anatomic alignment. The tooth will need to be splinted in place, typically with temporary adhesive and a short section of wire.

Alveolar Ridge Fracture

On occasion dental trauma may be associated with a fracture of the alveolar ridge, the section of the maxilla or mandible where the teeth normally reside. This is more common when multiple teeth are displaced or undergo luxation. These injuries may be noted on physical examination as a section of teeth, or an individual tooth that is misaligned and partially mobile. If the section is mobile and poses an aspiration risk, splinting should be performed in the emergency department before disposition.

▶ Disposition

Most patients with dental injuries with appropriate hemostasis can be discharged home. After placement of a temporary seal over a fractured tooth, follow-up with a dentist for definitive care is indicated. Reassessment after secondary tooth avulsion and emergency department replacement is urgent and definitive dental follow-up care should be arranged. Repair of alveolar ridge fractures should be done by an oral surgeon or dentist as soon as possible, preferably within the first 24 hours after injury. Definitive care with a dentist or oral surgeon should be arranged prior to discharge.

Iso-Kungas P, Törnwall J, Suominen AL, et al: Dental Injuries in pediatric patients with facial fractures are frequent and severe. *J Oral Maxillofac Surg.* 2012;70(2):396-400 [PMID: 22260909].

Lieger O, Zix J, Kruse A, et al: Dental injuries in association with facial fractures. *J Oral Maxillofac Surg.* 2009;67(8):1680-1684 [PMID: 19615582].

MAXILLARY (LE FORT) FRACTURES

Midface fractures in the young pediatric patient are rare. Some authors have hypothesized that this finding is due to the elasticity of the skeletal structure as well as the midface being less prominent than in the adult. In addition, the pediatric patient younger than 5 years does not have a well-aerated sinus system, likely adding to the protection of the midface. Midface fractures in children younger than 5 years are reported to be fewer than 1% of fractures and are primarily caused by blunt trauma.

As the pediatric patient enters adolescence, the skeletal structure develops to resemble that of an adult and the sinus cavities become aerated. This is believed to play a role in the increase of sinus fractures in adolescent patient population. The presence of a facial fracture following blunt trauma, primarily from motor vehicle collisions, is associated with a higher injury severity score and longer hospital stay in patients requiring admission.

The Le Fort classification system is classically used to describe typical patterns of injury to the maxilla. Three different types are described, and all involve the pterygoid plate. The fracture may be unilateral or bilateral. The classification system is useful when discussing a patient's injuries with a specialist. Le Fort fractures are associated with a significant mechanism of injury, and require a broader consideration of associated injuries, particularly to the brain and cervical spine.

Le Fort I fractures are roughly horizontal in nature, across the maxilla above the dental structures and teeth. These fractures communicate with the nasal opening(s) inferiorly. These fractures lie below the zygomaticomaxillary complex (ZMC) junction. Essentially, the upper jaw and teeth are disassociated from the upper midface.

Le Fort II fractures involve the maxilla as in a Le Fort I fracture, but extend superiorly and through the zygomaticomaxillary buttress, including the orbital floor and inferior rim. They may involve the medial orbital wall and nasal septum and have a pyramidal shape. The nasal region and maxilla are separated from the other facial bones.

Le Fort III fractures includes the entire zygomatic arch, across the orbit(s), and through the nasal and ethmoid bones. These fractures are referred to as craniofacial disjunctions, as the maxilla, zygoma, and naso-orbital-ethmoid complex are divided from the cranium. Figure 24-6 demonstrates the different appearances of Le Fort fractures.

▶ Clinical Findings

Patients with Le Fort fractures usually present with obvious apparent facial trauma. Swelling, ecchymosis, mobility, and

Anterior views

Lateral views

A

B

C

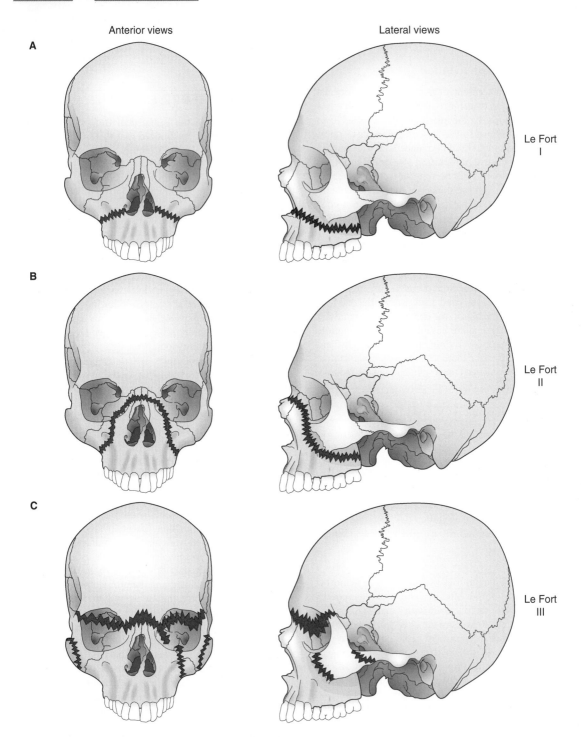

Le Fort
I

Le Fort
II

Le Fort
III

▲ **Figure 24–6.** Le Fort fracture classification system. (Reproduced with permission from Stone CK, Humphries RL: *Current Diagnosis & Treatment Emergency Medicine,* 7th ed. New York: McGraw-Hill, 2011. Copyright © McGraw-Hill Education LLC.)

deformity vary according to underlying injury. Malocclusion is commonly reported. In a Le Fort I fracture, the patient may have a swollen upper lip and grating sensation when the hard palate is palpated. If the fracture is bilateral, the maxilla may feel unstable to the examiner.

A Le Fort II fracture may have worse deformity, including a widening of the intercanthal space. Infraorbital ecchymosis is likely. Mobility of the maxilla and hard palate will be notable mobile on examination.

A Le Fort III fracture will reveal more significant and complete facial mobility when manipulated. Significant swelling and ecchymosis are usually present, as well as elongation and flattening of the facial appearance.

Assess the face on each side for orbital entrapment, nerve deficits, and mobility. Examine the patient carefully for associated injuries.

▶ Treatment

Most fractures to the maxilla and zygoma are identified on a dedicated maxillofacial CT scan. As these injuries result primarily from blunt trauma, a thorough evaluation of the patient is indicated. Head and cervical spine CT scans are usually indicated. Involve a facial surgeon early when a Le Fort fracture is identified.

Le Fort I and II fractures are rarely associated with airway complications. A Le Fort III fracture may have airway involvement due to edema and dissection of expanding hematomas. Consider securing the airway early, but avoid use of nasotracheal or nasogastric tubes.

▶ Disposition

The facial surgeon should determine the disposition of patients with a Le Fort fracture. Cosmetic and functional damages are usually surgically repaired. Most patients are admitted for observation, if surgical repair is not immediately planned.

Gentile MA, Tellington AJ, Burke WJ, et al: Management of midface maxillofacial trauma. *Atlas Oral Maxillofac Surg Clin N Am*. 2013;21(1):69-95 [PMID: 23498333].

ZYGOMATICOMAXILLARY COMPLEX FRACTURE

The zygomaticomaxillary complex (ZMC) is composed of the lateral and inferior orbital rims, as well as the ZMC buttress and zygomatic arch. The fracture lines are through the inferior rim, zygomatic-temporal junction, and zygomatic-frontal suture (Figure 24–7). The fracture through the three areas is commonly termed, "tripod fracture." Because of the involvement of two sides of the orbit, injury in this area has potentially significant impact on the integrity of the orbit, intraorbital structures, and eye.

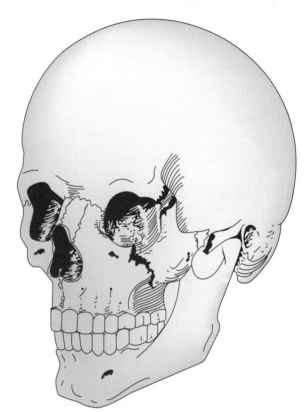

▲ **Figure 24–7.** Tripod (zygomaticomaxillary complex) fracture. (Reproduced with permission from Stone CK, Humphries RL: *Current Diagnosis & Treatment Emergency Medicine*, 7th ed. New York: McGraw-Hill, 2011. Copyright © McGraw-Hill Education LLC.)

▶ Clinical Findings

Dramatic swelling, pain, and local ecchymosis are common in a ZMC fracture. Subconjunctival hemorrhage and a malpositioned globe point to this injury. Diplopia on examination is possible. The infraorbital nerve may be damaged causing decreased sensation. Palpable emphysema and step-offs may be noted on careful examination. A majority of paresthesias noted on examination may become permanent, and careful documentation of sensory loss is warranted.

▶ Treatment

A CT scan of the maxillofacial structures and orbits is warranted. Fractures and soft tissues, including the globe, extraocular muscles, and nerves can be seen with modern scans. Three-dimensional reconstruction images, when available, offer a clearer picture of the damage. Evaluation by a specialist is indicated when diagnosis is confirmed. Early surgical fixation is indicated with displaced fracture fragments or extraocular muscle entrapment.

Disposition

Consultation with a maxillofacial surgeon should both be arranged in the emergency department for patients with a ZMC fracture. An ophthalmologist should be consulted, especially if intraorbital complications such as ruptured glove or retrobulbar hematoma occur. Most patients should be admitted if immediate surgical repair is not planned.

Gaziri DA, Omizollo G, Luchi GH, et al: Assessment for treatment of tripod fractures of the zygoma with microcompressive screws. *J Oral Maxillofac Surg.* 2012;70(6):e378-388 [PMID: 22608820].

ORBITAL FRACTURES

Orbital fractures present with various symptoms dependent on the fracture, associated swelling and displacement. Associated injuries range from simple contusion, to adjacent laceration, to globe injury. Most orbital fractures are the result of physical assault or motor vehicle collision.

Clinical Findings

At minimum, examination should test visual acuity, as well as presence of visual field deficit or diplopia throughout all extraocular movements. Pupillary response and integrity of the globe should be assessed. Palpate the orbital rim for deformity, and observe for enophthalmos and exophthalmos.

As the pediatric patient becomes the adolescent patient, injury patterns resemble those in adults. However, in the younger pediatric patient, injuries that are sustained may differ from adults. The orbital roof is more likely to be fractured in the younger pediatric patient because of the relatively large size of the cranium and absence of pneumatization of the sinuses. There is a strong association of orbital roof fractures with intracranial abnormality and frontobasal fractures.

Treatment

Apparent injury to the globe should prompt noncompressing coverage of the eye and emergent ophthalmologic consultation. Additional orbital wall injuries may occur in the pediatric patient. Fractures of the medial or inferior orbital wall may occur as the patient enters adolescence because of the pneumatization of the sinuses. Both orbital floor and medial wall fractures may lead to ocular-muscle entrapment. Detailed physical examination will allow for these fractures to be suspected prior to imaging. A slit lamp examination with fluorescein staining will help evaluate for globe injury.

The positive presence of a Seidel sign (fluorescein flowing at the site of injury) indicates a penetrating globe wound.

CT imaging is indicated for suspected orbital wall injuries. Complete maxillofacial and head CT scans are usually performed, but some hospitals have dedicated orbital CT protocols with greater precision. Evaluation for entrapment of extraocular muscles, in addition to assessment for fractures and globe injury, may require coronal and sagittal images.

Disposition

Pupillary defect, apparent entrapment, or open globe injury are indications for emergency ophthalmologic consultation. All orbital fractures should be discussed in consultation with an ophthalmologist to form a plan of care.

Most pediatric patients with diagnosed orbital fractures are admitted for observation and detailed examination. Nondisplaced, closed orbital roof fractures are usually managed nonoperatively in children. However, thorough ophthalmic evaluation may be required to exclude ocular injury. This may prove difficult in younger children, who often require examination under sedation. If a specialist is unavailable, or examination cannot be reliably performed, transfer of the patient to a trauma center is recommended. Isolated and nondisplaced fractures with no evidence of entrapment rarely require surgical intervention. However, evaluation for concomitant traumatic injury is prudent.

Gerbino G, Roccia F, Bianchi FA, et al: Surgical management of orbital trapdoor fracture in a pediatric population. *J Oral Maxillofac Surg.* 2010;68(6)1310-1316 [PMID: 20381939].

Joshi S, Kassira W, Thaller SR: Overview of pediatric orbital fractures. *J Craniofac Surg.* 2011;22(4):1330-1332 [PMID: 21772188].

Nowinski D, Di Rocco F, Roujeau T, et al: Complex pediatric orbital fractures combined with traumatic brain injury: Treatment and follow-up. *J Craniofac Surg.* 2010;21(4): 1054-1059 [PMID: 20613557].

Thiagarajah C, Kersten RC: Medial wall fracture: An update. *Craniomaxillofac Trauma Reconstr.* 2009;2(3):135-139 [PMID: 22110807].

NASAL FRACTURES

Clinical Findings

Patients with nasal fractures commonly present after anterior-posterior directed blunt trauma to the face. Injury may be either isolated or in conjunction with other midface injuries. Unilateral or bilateral epistaxis, nose pain, nasal septal deviation and hematoma, nasal deformity, and septal mucosal injury are likely clinical findings associated with a nasal fracture.

Treatment

Nasal fractures may exist in combination with other injuries to the midface. Simple nasal injuries do not require imaging to diagnose. However, associated adjacent injuries should be excluded when the mechanism or examination suggests additional injury. Primarily caused by blunt trauma, naso-orbito-ethmoid fractures may result from significant force (Figure 24–8). The literature suggests that these types of injuries may account for up to 15% of pediatric facial fractures. The affected area is usually significantly swollen, and may have ipsilateral increased lacrimation and loss of structural nasal support. A CT scan of the maxillofacial structures will reliably confirm or exclude such fractures.

With all nasal injuries, the clinician should evaluate the patient for evidence of other traumatic findings. It is important to stabilize the patient's airway as some fractures may result in a significant amount of epistaxis or airway compromise. Avoid insertion of objects (nasotracheal or nasogastric tubes) into the nose until a complete evaluation of the extent of the injury can be obtained. Control epistaxis with nasal packing, if underlying penetrating injury has been excluded. A nasal septal hematoma should be drained prior to disposition, unless immediate (same day) follow-up is available. Follow-up should be confirmed prior to disposition.

Disposition

Isolated nasoseptal injuries are primarily managed by a facial surgeon. Depending on the patient's age at the time of the injury, one of the concerns is long-term skeletal development of the nose and midface if the reduction is not performed properly. Most patients with a significantly displaced fracture will require a repeat surgical procedure. Simple, minimally displaced nasal fractures include follow-up on an urgent basis with an otolaryngologist or plastic surgeon; Most authors recommend antibiotic prophylaxis in consideration of the usual nasal colonization with bacteria. Appropriate analgesics should be prescribed.

Significant overlying wounds (open fractures) and nasal deformities warrant consultation in the emergency department. A patient with a naso-orbito-ethmoid fracture should be evaluated by a specialist in the emergency department, or transferred to a facility which has specialist availability.

Desrosiers AE, Thaller SR: Pediatric nasal fractures: Evaluation and management. *J Craniofac Surg.* 2011;22(4):1327-1329 [PMID: 21772190].

Liau JY, Woodlief J, van Aalst JA: Pediatric nasoorbitoethmoid fractures. *J Craniofac Surg.* 2011;22(5):1834-1838 [PMID: 21959446].

Nguyen M, Koshy JC, Hollier LH Jr: Pearls of nasoorbitoethmoid trauma management. *Semin Plast Surg.* 2010;24(4):383-388 [PMID: 22550462].

Umana AN, Offiong ME, Francis P, et al: Nasal septal hematoma: Using tubular nasal packs to achieve immediate nasal breathing after drainage. *Int J Med Science.* 2011;3(7):233-235.

Wright RJ, Murakami CS, Ambro BT: Pediatric nasal injuries and management. *Facial Plast Surg.* 2011;27(5):483-490 [PMID: 22028012].

FRONTAL SINUS FRACTURES

Frontal sinus fractures result from significant force, most commonly motor vehicle collisions. Fracture is to the frontal bone, and therefore considered a skull fracture. The sinus begins forming in children between 1 and 2 years of age, and typically completes development by 12 years of age. Associated intracranial and facial injuries should be expected, and a thorough evaluation is required. Neurologic injury is likely. The anterior table of the sinus lies just beneath the skin, whereas the posterior table is behind the sinus and adjacent to the brain. Frontal sinus fractures typically involve the anterior table, with more significant injuries also involving the posterior table. Posterior table fractures are considered open fractures and a CSF leak may result. The inferior aspect of the sinuses is formed by the bilateral superior orbital rims.

Clinical Findings

Apparent swelling to the forehead in the setting of a significant mechanism of injury should prompt concern for frontal sinus fracture. Crepitus over the sinus may be present. Adjacent injuries to the orbits, scalp, and midface may also be present. Many patients have underlying neurologic

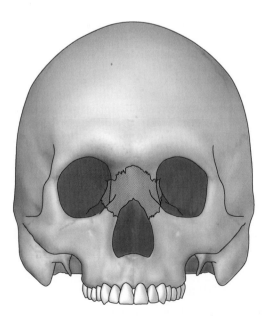

▲ **Figure 24–8.** Nasoorbitoethmoid fracture.

or intracranial injury from the force of injury, and a detailed neurologic examination may not be possible.

Treatment

A CT scan of the head and maxillofacial structures will confirm frontal sinus fractures. The cervical spine should also be imaged for injury. Displacement of the anterior table correlates with cosmetic deformity and need for surgical correction. The greater the displacement of the posterior table, the more likely associated intracranial injury has occurred. Rhinorrhea should be considered a CSF leak until excluded. Ocular injuries may result if the frontal sinus fracture involves the superior orbital rim. Severe frontal sinus fractures may also extend into the temporal bone, with additional signs of injury.

Disposition

Significantly deformed anterior table fractures, as well as all posterior table fractures, indicate need for surgical correction. CSF rhinorrhea and open fractures are also surgical indications. A facial surgeon should be consulted on all frontal sinus fractures, and a neurosurgeon consulted in patients with posterior table fractures or with associated intracranial injury. Isolated nondisplaced frontal sinus fractures may be discharged if the specialist deems outpatient management appropriate. Pediatric patients with frontal sinus fractures are admitted for close observation and surgical repair as needed.

Boswell KA: Management of facial fractures. *Emerg Med Clin N Am.* 2013;31(2):539-551 [PMID: 23601488].

TEMPORAL BONE FRACTURES

The majority of basilar skull fractures include associated or extension of fracture in the temporal bone. The temporal bone surrounds and encompasses several delicate structures, including the cochlea, vestibule, internal carotid artery, jugular vein, and facial nerve canal. Significant head injury may limit clinical examination.

Clinical Findings

Awake patients may complain of facial nerve deficit, dizziness, hearing loss, or fluid leakage from the ear. Evaluate the patient's hearing and facial nerve function when possible. Examine the ear canal and tympanic membrane, paying close attention for hemotympanum, or any leakage of CSF or blood from the canal. Postauricular hematoma (Battle sign) or periorbital ecchymosis (often bilateral, "raccoon eyes") may be present.

Treatment

CT scans of the head and maxillofacial structures are warranted. Fractures may be longitudinal along the temporal bone's long axis, or transverse to this axis. Transverse fractures cause more severe injuries compared with longitudinal. Significant force is usually associated with these fractures, and other injuries should be suspected in accordance with the mechanism. Cervical spine precautions should be followed. Do not manipulate or pack the auditory canal, as open injury can cause direct contamination to the inner ear, with spread to the cerebrospinal fluid, meninges, and brain.

Disposition

Patients with temporal bone fractures should be admitted. A maxillofacial or ear, nose, and throat (ENT) surgeon should be consulted for evaluation. Temporary and long-term hearing complications may result. A neurosurgeon should be consulted for associated intracranial injuries.

EAR INJURIES

AURICULAR HEMATOMA

Clinical Findings

Direct blunt trauma to the ear, including injuries sustained in contact sporting events, is the main cause of auricular hematomas. Separation of the perichondrium from the cartilage on the auricle, as well as small vessel damage leads to hematoma formation. Hematomas gradually enlarge to maximal size fairly rapidly, and are readily apparent on physical examination.

Treatment

Auricular hematomas should be evacuated in the emergency department. If the hematoma is not sufficiently drained, complications such as infection, perichondritis, and necrosis may occur. Replacement of a hematoma by fibrous tissue is known as "cauliflower ear."

Draining an auricular hematoma is not challenging. Providing adequate analgesia throughout the procedure may require the use of an auricular block. Patient cooperation is crucial throughout the procedure. Some clinicians prefer to use an 18-gauge needle attached to a syringe to drain the hematoma. This may not be sufficient if clot has already formed, and a larger incision with a scalpel may be required. The scalpel incision should be parallel to the helix. The use of small hemostats may be required to break up the clot. Firm pressure is required to achieve hemostasis. Placement of a pressure dressing is then indicated. Bolstering the auricle on both sides with cotton rolls that are sutured in place will provide enough pressure.

Disposition

Isolated auricular hematoma injuries may be discharged home after hematoma drainage. The patient should be evaluated in 24 hours by a otolaryngologist to look for reaccumulation, and to direct further management.

AURICLE LACERATIONS

▶ Clinical Findings

Auricle lacerations may overlie the surface, penetrate through the auricle, or extend through its outer margin. Careful cleansing of the wound will allow for a complete evaluation to determine the extent and depth of injury. If the mechanism of injury includes blunt trauma such as a motor vehicle collision, the presence of an auricle laceration should prompt consideration of underlying skull or intracranial injury.

▶ Treatment

Repairing most auricle lacerations may be performed in the emergency department. Evaluation for tissue loss is important as loss of any cartilaginous structure will likely lead to a permanent defect. An auricle block may be necessary to provide sufficient analgesia.

If the cartilage is minimally involved, approximate the wound margins together. On occasion, absorbable suture may be required. The overlying skin should be closed to ensure that no cartilage is exposed. Exposed cartilage may lead to chondritis or deformities. If there is not enough skin and soft tissue to cover the cartilage or the cartilage defect is severe, consider specialist consultation.

▶ Disposition

Lacerations managed by the emergency physician should have prompt follow-up with otolaryngologist or plastic surgeon to ensure appropriate healing. Surgical consultation in the emergency department is appropriate for near-amputation of the auricle, deep or complex wounds.

Greywoode JD, Pribitkin EA, Krein H, et al: Management of auricular hematoma and the cauliflower ear. *Facial Plast Surg.* 2010;26(6):451-455 [PMID: 21086231].

Lavasani L, Leventhal D, Constantinides M, et al: Management of acute soft tissue injury to the auricle. *Facial Plast Surg.* 2010;26(6):445-450 [PMID: 21086230].

OTOLOGIC DISORDERS FOLLOWING HEAD TRAUMA

▶ Clinical Findings

Complications following temporal bone fractures are common, but fortunately, many are not associated with high mortality rates. The most common concern following temporal bone injury is hearing loss, which may be a result of sensory-neural, conductive, or mixed hearing loss.

Sensory-neural hearing loss may be the result of damage to the cochlea or the auditory nerve. This hearing loss

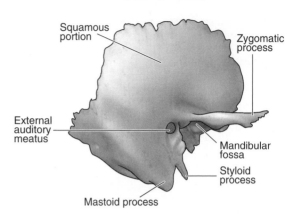

▲ **Figure 24–9.** Temporal bone diagram.

may be seen in patients who do not sustain a fracture to the temporal bone. Individuals with low-frequency hearing loss regain more function than those with high-frequency hearing loss.

Conductive hearing loss occurs when there is a structural change in sound transmission. Although the cochlea and nerves are functioning appropriately, a change in the external auditory canal, tympanic membrane, or the ossicles may result in a conductive hearing loss. Two of the more common causes of conductive hearing loss are tympanic membrane rupture and hemotympanum. If either is the cause of the hearing loss, recovery is usually good. However, the clinician should consider ossicle displacement if recovery doesn't occur, or if there is no evidence of the two findings on physical examination. Correcting conductive hearing loss may require surgical intervention, specifically in the patient with displaced ossicles.

Other otologic findings that may suggest damage to the temporal bone include deafness, tinnitus, vertigo, facial nerve palsy, cerebrospinal fluid otorrhea, and hemotympanum. If any of these symptoms are found on physical examination, the clinician should be concerned for possible temporal bone fracture. Figure 24–9 illustrates the structures of the temporal bone.

▶ Treatment and Disposition

Treat acute temporal bone fractures as described earlier in this chapter (Temporal Bone Fractures). Urgent otolaryngologist consultation should be obtained in the setting of hemotympanum. Consultation in the emergency department or follow-up with an otolaryngologist is indicated for traumatic hearing loss after head injury.

Johnson F, Semaan MT, Megerian CA: Temporal bone fracture: Evaluation and management in the modern area. *Otolaryngol Clin North Am.* 2008;41(3):597-618 [PMID: 18436001].

Chest Trauma

Jo-Ann O. Nesiama, MD, MS

Craig J. Huang, MD

▼ OVERVIEW

Trauma is the leading cause of childhood morbidity and mortality in the United States, accounting for greater than 7.5 million emergency department visits annually. Chest trauma is the second leading cause of mortality in pediatric trauma patients and is often encountered in the setting of multisystem trauma, usually caused by high-energy impact incidents such as motor vehicle collisions. Blunt-chest injuries account for greater than 80% of pediatric chest trauma and often require a longer hospital length of stay compared with penetrating chest injuries.

PATHOPHYSIOLOGY

The following anatomic and pathophysiologic features of children differentiate chest trauma in children from those in adults:

- Increased chest wall compliancy due to pliability of cartilage allows the chest to absorb energy and dissipate it to the internal organs without necessarily resulting in rib fractures.
- Increased incidence of traumatic asphyxia and commotio cordis because of increased chest wall compliancy.
- A larger blood volume relative to body weight can result in a higher incidence of hypovolemia and shock despite smaller amounts of blood loss.
- Relatively smaller body mass index results in greater energy of forces dispersed over a smaller area.
- A more mobile mediastinum increases the incidence of intrathoracic injuries such as pneumothorax, hemothorax, which can lead to cardiovascular compromise.

IMMEDIATE MANAGEMENT OF LIFE-THREATENING PROBLEMS

ESTABLISH AIRWAY, BREATHING, & CIRCULATION

Priorities for trauma patients are to establish a definitive airway, manage breathing and then circulation. Causes of airway compromise, which can occur at any level from the pharynx to the trachea, as well as disorders of ventilation/oxygenation in the pediatric chest trauma patient include

- Direct interruption or injury of the respiratory tract
- Impairment in gas exchange from hypoventilation secondary to pain or neurological injury
- Injuries to the chest wall, pleura, and lung parenchyma (atelectasis, contusions, hemothorax, or pneumothorax)

PAIN CONTROL

Adequate pain control is important to ensure maximal comfort, resulting in improved chest wall movement and expansion to optimize oxygen exchange and ventilation. Parenteral narcotics (morphine, fentanyl) are used for this goal, and may require multiple doses.

IMMEDIATE MANAGEMENT OF LIFE-THREATENING INJURIES

Life-threatening injuries should be identified on the primary survey, and require immediate action without definitive diagnostic testing, as these measures are often lifesaving.

TENSION PNEUMOTHORAX

Tension pneumothorax occurs when air accumulates in the intrapleural space (Figure 25–1). It is often seen with injury to the lung parenchyma or bronchus, as air flows unidirectionally into the pleural space. Air flows in during inspiration and is unable to escape during expiration. The accumulated air can lead to lung collapse on the affected side and shift of the mediastinal contents to the contralateral side. A large tension pneumothorax can decrease venous return to the heart, with subsequent cardiovascular collapse.

▶ Diagnosis

Tension pneumothorax is a clinical diagnosis with patients presenting with signs and symptoms that include severe respiratory distress with tachypnea and hypoxia, or decreased or absent breath sounds on the affected side. Distension of neck veins on the affected side may be seen, but this finding is not consistently present. Tracheal deviation may be evident on chest radiographs, if obtained. Bedside ultrasonography can accurately diagnose a pneumothorax (see Chapter 2).

▶ Treatment

When tension pneumothorax is suspected in a patient with either respiratory or cardiovascular compromise, rapid decompression should be instituted before chest radiographs

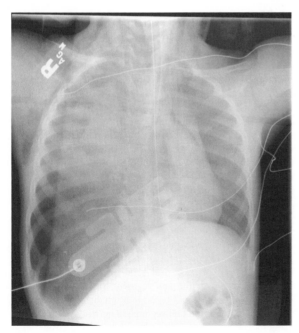

▲ **Figure 25–1.** Right-sided tension pneumothorax with massive displacement of mediastinal structures to the left.

are obtained. Rapid decompression, using a large-bore needle placed in the second intercostal space, will convert a tension pneumothorax to a simple pneumothorax and provide immediate relief of symptoms. The needle should remain in place until a chest tube has been placed, usually along the midaxillary line in the fifth intercostal space.

Two conditions that mimic tension pneumothorax in children are intubation of the right main stem bronchus, leading to collapse of the left lung; and massive gastric distension that can elevate the left hemidiaphragm diaphragm, reducing ventilation in the left lung.

Brook OR, Beck-Razi N, Abadi S, et al: Sonographic detection of pneumothorax by radiology residents as part of extended focused assessment with sonography for trauma. *J Ultrasound Med.* 2009;28(6):749–755 [PMID: 19470815].

Pitetti RD, Walker S: Life-threatening chest injuries in children. *Clin Pediatr Emerg Med.* 2005;6:16-22.

OPEN PNEUMOTHORAX (Sucking Chest Wound)

Open pneumothorax occurs when a penetrating injury creates a direct communication between the pleural space and the outside environment. This results in equal pressures in the atmospheric and intrapleural environments, allowing air to enter directly into the pleural space instead of the lungs. The result is lung collapse with respiratory difficulty and/or insufficiency and ultimately, cardiovascular collapse.

▶ Diagnosis

Open pneumothorax should be identified on the primary survey, with an obvious chest wound, respiratory distress with hypoxia, tachypnea, and decreased breath sounds on the affected side. There may be subcutaneous emphysema palpated close to the wound site, or over the chest wall if more severe. Bedside ultrasound is useful for diagnosis of pneumothorax (see Chapter 2).

▶ Treatment

Administration of the maximal fractional inspired oxygen should be the priority. Definitive treatment consists of preventing more air from entering through the wound site and removing the air already present. An occlusive dressing placed over the wound site will prevent more air from entering the intrapleural space. The dressing should be taped down on three sides to create a one-way valve that allows air to be expelled during expiration and prevents air entry during inspiration. Chest tube placement in the affected side, as described previously, will remove the already present intrapleural air.

Kerr M, Maconochie I: Paediatric chest trauma (part 1)—Initial lethal injuries. *Trauma*. 2008;10:183-194.

HEMOTHORAX

Hemothorax often occurs as a result of blunt chest trauma. The presence of hemothorax may be indicative of great vessel injury, or may be secondary to laceration of lung vessels.

▶ Diagnosis

Respiratory distress as evidenced by tachypnea, dyspnea, and hypoxia may be present. If large enough, there may be decreased breath sounds on the affected side on auscultation. Chest radiography may show pleural fluid accumulation. Ultrasound is another modality useful for diagnosis (see Chapter 2).

▶ Treatment

Chest tube thoracostomy is the treatment of choice for hemothorax (see Chapter 3). Incomplete evacuation of blood within a week of the injury should prompt the provider to consider interval development of an empyema.

Sartorelli KH, Vane DW: The diagnosis and management of children with blunt injury of the chest. *Semin Ped Surg*. 2004;13(2):98 [PMID: 15362279].

CARDIAC TAMPONADE

Cardiac tamponade occurs when blood accumulates in the pericardium, often due to penetrating chest injury, but can also occur in the presence of blunt chest trauma. The pericardium is fibrous and nondistensible, and even a rapid accumulation of a small amount of blood could cause a marked decrease in diastolic filling, and impair cardiac output. This condition will result in cardiovascular collapse if untreated.

▶ Diagnosis

Diagnosis of cardiac tamponade can be difficult because the classic triad of narrowed pulse pressure, jugular venous distension, and muffled heart sounds does not occur often in children. Children have shorter necks compared with adults, such that jugular venous distension may be difficult to identify. Furthermore, the child's thinner chest wall transmits sounds to all areas of the lung fields so muffled heart sounds may not be appreciated. In the pediatric patient with breathing difficulty and signs of shock that fail to respond to adequate ventilation and fluid resuscitation, cardiac tamponade should be considered. A bedside ultrasound may help detect poor contractility as well as pericardial effusion (see Chapter 2). Chest radiography may demonstrate an enlarged cardiac silhouette, suggestive of the diagnosis. An echocardiogram is the diagnostic tool of choice.

▶ Treatment

Needle pericardiocentesis can provide relief without radiographic assistance if emergent bedside echocardiography is unavailable. However, pericardiocentesis may be helpful only if nonclotted blood is obtained using a large-bore plastic-sheathed needle. Ultrasound-guided needle pericardiocentesis has been shown to be safe and reliable. The needle is introduced to the left of the subxiphoid area, directing it upward and toward the left shoulder at a 45-degree angle carefully aspirating until fluid/blood is obtained. The pericardiocentesis cannula can be left in place as needed for repeated aspirations, pending definitive surgical decompression.

Kerr M, Maconochie I: Paediatric chest trauma (part 1)—Initial lethal injuries. *Trauma*. 2008;10:183-194.

FLAIL CHEST

When two or more contiguous ribs are fractured in more than one place, a "free-floating" or "flail" segment results. This section of the chest moves in response to changes in the intrapleural pressure, while the rest of the chest responds to changes in intrathoracic pressure and respiratory muscle activity. The free-floating segment contracts when the chest expands during inspiration, and then bulges outward during expiration when the rest of the chest wall retracts, creating the typical "paradoxical" movement decreasing the efficiency of respiration.

▶ Diagnosis

Flail chest is often difficult to diagnose in pediatric patients. Tachypnea and shallow breathing may be evident in the conscious child, and if the condition has been present for a prolonged period, respiratory fatigue with resultant hypoxia can be seen. Palpation of the chest wall should reveal the flail segment. Chest wall crepitus may also be present. Lateral and posterior chest wall flail segments are potentially more serious and greater impairment of diaphragmatic movement can occur, which can further impede respiration. Chest radiograph often demonstrates multiple displaced rib fractures with underlying pulmonary contusion and subcutaneous emphysema near the flail segment (see Figure 25–2).

▶ Treatment

Administration of maximal fractional inspired oxygen is a priority. Often, elective intubation is undertaken to aid with both initial pain control and aggressive pulmonary toilet. Direct pressure over the flail segment to prevent the paradoxical movement should be done immediately. This can be achieved by taping the flail segment. Aggressive pain control using morphine or fentanyl, and sometimes, intercostal nerve blocks may be utilized. More invasive pulmonary toilet such as suctioning and sometimes bronchoscopy may be necessary.

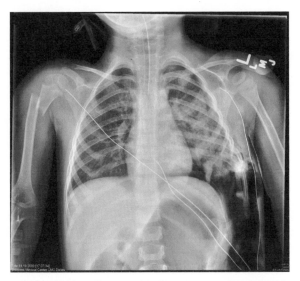

▲ **Figure 25–2.** Left-sided flail chest with underlying pulmonary contusion and associated subcutaneous emphysema. Also noted is a proximal right humerus fracture.

The presence of flail chest should alert the physician to look for other potential injuries, as their presence denotes a significant amount of force applied to the chest wall.

Kerr M, Maconochie I: Paediatric chest trauma (part 1)—Initial lethal injuries. *Trauma*. 2008;10:183-194.

POTENTIALLY LIFE-THREATENING INJURIES

Potentially life-threatening injuries frequently identified on the secondary survey are not immediately life-threatening but can impact morbidity significantly, and may result in increased mortality if not promptly identified and managed appropriately.

PULMONARY CONTUSION

Pulmonary contusion is the most common injury in chest trauma in children. It usually occurs from blunt chest trauma, and has a high association with other intrathoracic and extrathoracic injuries. Injury to the lung parenchyma results in hemorrhage and edema from the lung capillaries, leading to alveolar collapse and lung consolidation. Ultimately, a ventilation perfusion mismatch occurs in addition to a decrease in lung compliance.

▶ Diagnosis

As many as 50% of children may have no symptoms making the diagnosis difficult during the initial evaluation. The

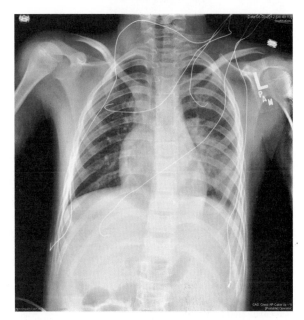

▲ **Figure 25–3.** Pulmonary contusion in the left lower lobe.

degree of symptoms is often directly proportional to the areas involved. Patients may have tachypnea, hypoxia, hypoxemia, tachycardia, decreased breath sounds or adventitial breath sounds (crackles or wheezing), over affected areas. Chest wall bruising may be present. Chest pain may also be present in the conscious, verbal child. Chest radiography may demonstrate areas of consolidation that can initially be in a patchy distribution, or involve a whole lung (Figure 25–3). In children, these patchy areas of consolidation do not conform to anatomical boundaries of segments or lobes. However, chest radiography findings may lag behind clinical findings or underestimate the degree of injury; therefore, serial x rays are recommended if the condition is suspected. Chest computed tomography is more sensitive than chest radiography, but is not routinely recommended. However, it may be helpful if there is a concern for intrathoracic injuries.

▶ Treatment

Administration of 100% oxygen is indicated with treatment as mainly supportive. If respiratory distress is severe, elective intubation may be undertaken, with positive end-expiratory volume. Aggressive analgesia with morphine or fentanyl should be done. Chest physiotherapy including suctioning and postural drainage should be undertaken. Careful fluid management to maintain euvolemia is critical, as hypervolemia can worsen the condition.

Pneumonia is the most common complication and should be managed as clinically indicated.

Hamrick M, Duhn R, Boswell W Ochsner M: Pulmonary contusion in the pediatric population. *Am Surg*. 2010;76 (7):721-724 [PMID: 20698378].

Kerr M, Maconochie I: Paediatric chest trauma (part 2)—Hidden injuries. *Trauma*. 2008;10:195-210.

Moore MA, Wallace EC, Westra SJ: Chest trauma in children: Current imaging guidelines and techniques. *Radiol Clin N Am*. 2011;49:949-968 [PMID: 21889016].

MYOCARDIAL CONTUSION

Myocardial contusion is the most common cardiac injury in pediatric chest trauma, but it occurs less often compared with adults. Myocardial contusion is often due to blunt chest trauma. Many cardiac contusions in children either are underreported because of absence of symptoms at presentation, or are misdiagnosed. In addition, many children with significant injury die before arriving at a hospital. There are distinct areas of hemorrhage within the cardiac muscle and may involve a layer of the muscle. The condition can lead to conduction defects, a decrease in cardiac output, and eventual cardiogenic shock.

▶ Diagnosis

Confirmation of myocardial contusion can be difficult, particularly in the preverbal child. Children may be asymptomatic at presentation. Chest pain, tachycardia, and hypotension, particularly in children not responsive to adequate fluid resuscitation, may be clues to aid in the diagnosis. There is currently no consensus on the ancillary study of choice for determining a definitive diagnosis. However, there are several agreed-upon modalities that can aid in the diagnosis.

Electrocardiography

Electrocardiography is the best screening tool and should be obtained in a child presenting with chest trauma. However, a normal electrocardiography does not rule out the diagnosis. Electrocardiography findings can be varied and nonspecific: T-wave inversions, ST-segment changes, premature ventricular beats, supraventricular and ventricular arrhythmias, and varying degrees of heart block have all been described. However, some reports indicate that if a child with blunt chest trauma is hemodynamically stable at the time of presentation and has a normal sinus rhythm, it is unlikely that the child will develop cardiac pump failure.

Biochemical Markers

Serum levels of cardiac enzymes: creatinine phosphokinase (CPK) and creatinine phosphokinase isoenzyme (CPK-MB) are not cardiac specific and can often be elevated in the presence of trauma due to their presence in skeletal muscle, bowel, and liver. Troponin T and troponin I are more cardiac specific, but are less sensitive.

Echocardiography

Echocardiography should not be used as a screening tool for children with suspected myocardial contusion. This modality is recommended in the presence of persistent hypotension despite adequate fluid resuscitation and abnormal electrocardiographic findings. Echocardiography is usually obtained to exclude other potential cardiac injuries such as myocardial rupture, pericardial effusion, or cardiac pump failure.

Radionuclide Imaging

The labeled radionuclide accumulates in the damaged myocardium allowing rapid, noninvasive assessment of cardiac muscle injury, thus making it the theoretical diagnostic study of choice. It provides a rapid, noninvasive assessment of cardiac muscle damage. However, it may not be readily available, and may be falsely negative in the setting of minor myocardial contusions.

▶ Treatment

Treatment of myocardial contusions is primarily supportive with management of hypotension or cardiac arrhythmias should they occur. Hypotension not responsive to intravenous fluid therapy may require inotropes. However, the clinician should remember that inotropes may increase myocardial oxygen consumption, and hence worsen the already present cardiac contusion. Antiarrhythmics may be necessary for the treatment of persistent arrhythmias.

Brock JS, Benitez R: Blunt Cardiac trauma. *Cardiol Clin*. 2012 30(4):545-555 [PMID: 23102031].

Kerr M, Maconochie I: Paediatric chest trauma (part 2)—Hidden injuries. *Trauma*. 2008;10:195-210.

DIAPHRAGMATIC HERNIA

Diaphragmatic hernia is a very rare occurrence in children, and occurs most commonly on the left side, as the right side is protected by the superior edge of the liver although evidence suggests this observed laterality difference may be an overestimation. It may result from blunt or penetrating chest trauma. A penetrating chest trauma below the nipple line warrants extensive radiological studies to exclude the condition.

▶ Diagnosis

Children may be asymptomatic, particularly if the rupture is small. Herniation of abdominal contents into the chest cavity, causing respiratory compromise, leading to hypoxia and tachypnea can occur if the defect is large enough. The typical "scaphoid abdomen" may not be apparent initially, unless

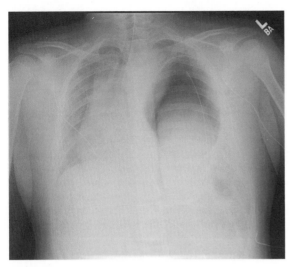

▲ **Figure 25–4.** Left diaphragmatic rupture with displacement of mediastinal stuctures to the right. The nasogastric tube demonstrates that the gastric bubble is intrathoracic.

a substantially large herniation is present. Absent or decreased breath sounds on the affected side may occur. The presence of bowel sounds on the affected side may also be heard. Chest, abdominal, or shoulder pain (from irritation of the phrenic nerve) may be present. Symptoms of bowel obstruction such as vomiting may be observed. If visceral herniation does not occur, diagnosis can be delayed or difficult to make.

Chest radiography is the initial diagnostic study of choice, but lacks high sensitivity. However, findings may be missed in the presence of associated injuries such as lung contusions or right diaphragmatic injuries due to the liver preventing herniation of abdominal contents. Findings of an elevated hemidiaphragm, irregularity of the diaphragmatic border, presence of intrathoracic abdominal contents, or presence of a nasogastric tube in the intrathoracic cavity may indicate the diagnosis (Figure 25–4).

Chest computed tomography is not very sensitive for this diagnosis, even with very small slice cross sections.

Other imaging modalities have been suggested to aid the diagnosis, including magnetic resonance imaging (MRI), fluoroscopy, and diagnostic thoracoscopy. Diagnostic thoracoscopy should be undertaken when a high index of suspicion is present. However, these diagnostic strategies are often not available or convenient in the acute setting.

▶ **Treatment**

Surgical repair is mandatory in patients with diaphragmatic rupture, as the injury will not heal spontaneously, regardless of the size of the rupture.

Kerr M, Maconochie I: Paediatric chest trauma (part 2)—Hidden injuries. *Trauma.* 2008;10:195–210.

ESOPHAGEAL DISRUPTION

Blunt or penetrating trauma can cause esophageal disruption; however, it is rare in children. The distal esophagus, with its lack of surrounding mediastinal structural support is the most affected region with blunt trauma. Perforation leads to spilling of contents directly into the mediastinum and or pleural space. This injury is usually associated with other intrathoracic injuries and has a relatively high mortality rate.

▶ **Diagnosis**

Esophageal disruption can be difficult to diagnose. Symptoms are typically nonspecific and can include chest pain, abdominal pain, dyspnea, dysphagia, and vomiting. If rupture occurs more proximally, neck pain can occur. The presence of chest wall crepitus or subcutaneous emphysema can aid in the diagnosis. Chest radiography is the initial diagnostic study of choice and may demonstrate subcutaneous emphysema, pneumothorax, pneumomediastinum, and/or pleural effusion. A widened mediastinum may also be observed.

Water-soluble esophagogram and rigid esophagoscopy are confirmatory. Rigid esophagoscopy should be performed if the injury is suspected despite a negative esophagogram.

▶ **Treatment**

Treatment is determined by the size and location of the rupture. Several authors advocate primary surgical repair of the rupture. Conservative management with intravenous antibiotics, nutritional support, and drainage is advocated for ruptures that are not associated with mediastinitis.

Kerr M, Maconochie I: Paediatric chest trauma (part 2)—Hidden injuries. *Trauma.* 2008;10:195–210.

AORTIC DISRUPTION

Aortic disruption occurs rarely in children; however, it is associated with a high mortality rate. A considerable amount of energy is required to cause an aortic disruption, usually due to rapid acceleration-deceleration and shearing forces most commonly caused by motor vehicle collisions, motor vehicle pedestrian collisions, and falls. Injuries commonly seen in patients with aortic injury include pulmonary contusions, pelvic or other long bone fractures, abdominal injuries, and central nervous system (CNS) injuries. The aorta is very mobile in children and rupture tends to occur in areas of decreased mobility, such as at the level of the ligamentum arteriosum and the aortic isthmus distal to the left subclavian artery. The injury ranges from a small intimal tear to a full transection. Mortality is near 100% with full transections.

▶ Diagnosis

Partial aortic disruption presents as hypotension, dyspnea, retrosternal chest pain, and decreased pulses particularly in the lower extremities and left upper extremity. Hoarseness, back pain, and scapular pain may also be present. The following diagnostic modalities may be used to evaluate aortic disruption.

Chest Radiography

Findings on plain radiography may be nonspecific; however, it is the diagnostic screening modality of choice. The presence of a widened mediastinum is the most consistent finding but can be obscured by the presence of the thymus in young children. Additional radiographic signs such as an indistinct aortic knob or right tracheal deviation may be present.

Chest Computed Tomography

This modality is the diagnostic study of choice in the hemodynamically stable patient. It has good specificity but not sensitivity. Abnormal findings warrant an aortography.

Transesophageal Echography

This diagnostic modality is recommended in the unstable patient because it is quick, noninvasive, and can be performed at the bedside. However, it may not be readily available.

Aortography

This radiologic modality is used less currently because it is expensive, time-consuming to perform, and not readily or widely available. It is often used when computed tomography is inconclusive.

▶ Treatment

Careful management of blood pressures and prompt surgical repair of aortic disruption are the mainstays of treatment.

Kerr M, Maconochie I: Paediatric chest trauma (part 2)—Hidden injuries. *Trauma*. 2008;10:195–210.

TRACHEOBRONCHIAL INJURY

Tracheobronchial injury is often due to blunt chest trauma. It occurs very infrequently in children. However, it may also occur with penetrating chest trauma. The mortality rate is high. The pliability of the chest wall in children allows the dissipation of great forces into the mediastinum, without disruption of the chest wall. Thus, the absence of rib fractures should not discount the possibility of a tracheobronchial injury. Most injuries occur close to the carina, around the distal trachea or proximal right main-stem bronchus.

▶ Diagnosis

Respiratory distress as evidenced by tachypnea, dyspnea, and hypoxia may be present. Chest pain, hemoptysis, and dysphagia may also be present. Chest radiography may show nonspecific findings such as pneumothorax, pneumomediastinum, and/or rib fractures. Subcutaneous emphysema may also be present. With more proximal injuries, there may be tension pneumothorax. The diagnosis should be considered when there is a persistent air leak after tube thoracostomy. Bronchoscopy can help identify the location of the injury.

▶ Treatment

Administrations of 100% oxygen and tube thoracostomy are indicated early in the management of children with tracheobronchial injury. Early elective intubation is often advocated, preferably with use of a bronchoscope, to prevent the conversion of partial injuries to complete transections. Early surgical debridement and primary anastomosis is the treatment of choice.

Kerr M, Maconochie I: Paediatric chest trauma (part 2)—Hidden injuries. *Trauma*. 2008;10:195–210.

OTHER INJURIES

RIB FRACTURES

Rib fractures rarely occur in the child with chest trauma and, when present, may herald other injuries. Rib fractures are often caused by blunt chest trauma. Non-accidental trauma should be considered a cause in children younger than 1 year, as it accounts for most incidences in this age group. Causes such as bone fragility, birth trauma, and rickets, should be excluded. Most rib fractures occurring as a result of non-accidental trauma are often located posteriorly, as with birth trauma. Rib fractures have been reported to occur with cardiopulmonary resuscitations, but these are mostly located anteriorly, and rarely occur.

▶ Diagnosis

Chest radiography is the screening modality of choice for rib fractures (Figure 24–5). The presence of a fracture of the first rib is highly indicative of non-accidental trauma, and is associated with the presence of other intrathoracic injuries. Multiple rib fractures are a marker of severe injury; associated injuries have a high mortality rate. Accordingly the

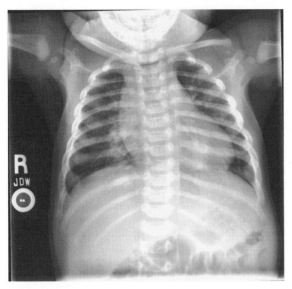

▲ **Figure 25–5.** Chest radiograph demonstrating healing fractures of the posterior eighth and ninth ribs. These fractures are highly suspicious for non-accidental trauma.

physician should strongly consider obtaining a computed tomographic scan of the head as well as other adjunctive studies looking for evidence of non-accidental trauma in a young child with multiple rib fractures.

▶ Treatment

Treatment is primarily supportive. Aggressive pain control, deep-breathing measures are usually sufficient to prevent complications such as atelectasis.

Kerr M, Maconochie I: Paediatric chest trauma (part 2)—Hidden injuries. *Trauma.* 2008;10:195-210.
Moore MA, Wallace EC, Westra SJ: The imaging of pediatric thoracic trauma. *Pediatr Radiol.* 2009;39:485-496 [PMID: 19151969].

STERNAL FRACTURES

Sternal fractures rarely occur in children, due to the pliability of the chest wall. These fractures usually occur with blunt chest trauma and are often a result of considerable force, which alert the physician to the possibility of additional intrathoracic injuries.

▶ Diagnosis

The presence of chest pain, worse with palpation of the sternum, should raise the suspicion of a sternal fracture. Chest radiography may demonstrate the fracture, although this may be subtle and easily missed. If significantly displaced,

accompanying pneumothorax, lung contusions may also be present.

▶ Treatment

Aggressive pain control with morphine and fentanyl, and deep-breathing exercises to prevent atelectasis are treatment priorities.

Garel T, Ince A, et al: The sternal fracture: Radiographic analysis of 200 fractures with special reference to concomitant injuries. *J Trauma Inj Infect Crit Care.* 2003;57(4):837844 [PMID: 15514539].
Mayberry JC, Ham LB et al: Surveyed opinion of American Trauma, orthopedic, and thoracic surgeons on rib and sternal fracture repair. *J Trauma Inj, Infect Crit Care.* 2008;66(3): 875–879 [PMID: 19276767].

TRAUMATIC ASPHYXIA

Direct, severe blow to the chest with a closed glottis can result in traumatic asphyxia. This injury can occur when a motor vehicle runs over a child or a heavy object falls over the chest or abdomen of a child. The increase in pressure dilates the capillary and venous systems. The areas drained by the superior vena cava are particularly affected, hence the marked difference between the head and neck and the rest of the body of the child upon physical examination.

▶ Diagnosis

The child may have significant petechial hemorrhages in the regions of the head and neck, and can also involve the sclera and mucous membranes. Bruising, cyanosis, and edema in the body region above the area of impact may occur, whereas the body region below the area of impact may be normal. Additional associated intrathoracic injuries resulting from the direct impact forces should also be considered.

▶ Treatment

The cutaneous manifestations will resolve with time. Associated injuries including, flail chest, pneumothorax, pulmonary contusion and aortic disrption, should be managed appropriately.

The following conditions have an unusually high mortality rate and thus rarely present to the emergency department.

Pitetti RD, Walker S: Life-threatening chest injuries in children. *Clin Pediatr Emerg Med.* 2005;6:16-22.

COMMOTIO CORDIS

Commotio cordis describes an event when the anterior chest wall is struck by a force that results in ventricular dysrrythmia, without causing structural myocardial damage, potentially leading to sudden cardiac death. Patients are usually previously healthy without underlying cardiac disease. The reported mortality rate of this injury is approximately 85%.

Diagnosis

A complete and accurate history helps determine the diagnosis. Patients may have chest pain, dysrhythmia, or unexplained hypotension. Elevation of troponin I may be very useful in confirming the diagnosis. Electrocardiography may show nonspecific ST-segment elevation, sinus tachycardia, and arrhythmias. There may be associated sternal fracture present on chest radiography.

Treatment

Children with hemodynamic instability should have prompt echocardiography and may require inotropic support. Immediate administration of defibrillation can be lifesaving in children with ventricular fibrillation.

Since the mortality rate is very high, prevention is the mainstay of preventing this injury, such as appropriate protective gear during associated sporting activities like baseball.

Kamdar G, Santucci K, et al: Management of pediatric cardiac trauma in the ED. *Clin Pediatr Emerg Med.* 2011;12(4):323-332.
Pitetti RD, Walker S: Life-threatening chest injuries in children. *Clin Pediatr Emerg Med.* 2005;6:16-22.

PENETRATING TRAUMA WITH EMERGENCY DEPARTMENT THORACOTOMY

The injury is uncommon in children, particularly in children younger than 13 years. These are often the result of high-velocity ballistic projectile wounds or wounds sustained by a sharp object such as a knife. The chest wall in children is more pliable relative to that of adults and offers less protection of the intrathoracic contents. Hence, lacerations of the lung parenchyma, as well as the heart can occur. Lacerations involving the heart are often fatal, resulting from cardiac tamponade and circulatory collapse.

If the child survives to the emergency department, emergency thoracotomy may be lifesaving. Indications for emergency thoracotomy include

1. Improvement in temporary shunting of blood preferentially to the brain by way of open cardiac massage and access to cross-clamping the thoracic aorta

2. Control of subdiaphragmatic hemorrhage caused by intra-abdominal trauma by cross-clamping the thoracic aorta

3. Control of persistent thoracic intravascular hemorrhage as evidenced by persistent bleeding via chest thoracostomy

4. Control of cardiac hemorrhage or alleviation of massive pericardial tamponade that cannot be drained by pericardiocentesis

This arguably heroic, lifesaving procedure is best used in patients with penetrating thoracic injuries who have a witnessed cardiopulmonary arrest in the emergency department, with loss of vital signs during short transport time to the emergency department, or who have persistent severe hypotension or shock with suspected intrathoracic hemorrhage or massive pericardial tamponade.

Mejia JC, Stewart RM, Cohn SM: Emergency department thoracotomy. *Semin Thorac Cardiovas Surg.* 2008;20:13-18 [PMID: 18420121].

Abdominal Trauma

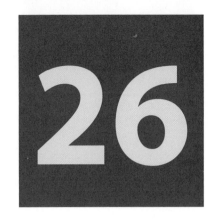

Mercedes Uribe, MD
Halim Hennes, MD, MS

▼ OVERVIEW

Abdominal trauma is the most common unrecognized fatal injury and the third leading cause of pediatric trauma death after injuries to head and thorax. The mortality rate is estimated to be as high as 8.5% and accounts for 8-12% of all deaths of children admitted with abdominal trauma.

Children have anatomic, physiologic, and psychological characteristics in contrast to adults that predispose them to a variety of injuries. Recognition of these characteristics plays a major role in the evaluation and management of pediatric trauma patient. The most pertinent characteristics related to abdominal trauma are outlined in (Table 26–1).

TYPES OF INJURY

BLUNT ABDOMINAL INJURY

More than 80-90% of traumatic abdominal injuries in children result from blunt mechanism. The most common causes of injury are traffic accidents (49%), falls (22%), direct impact trauma (20%), and being run over by a vehicle (9%). Other mechanisms include all-terrain vehicle (ATV) accidents, handlebar injuries from bicycles, and sport or non-accidental trauma. Incidences of solid organ injuries associated with blunt trauma are spleen (46.7%), liver (33.3%), renal (17.5%), and pancreas (2.5%).

Children with non-accidental trauma have the highest risk for morbidity and mortality.

PENETRATING INJURIES

Penetrating abdominal trauma accounts for 4-15% of all pediatric abdominal trauma. In the United States, firearm-related injury and gunshot wounds (GSWs) are the most common causes of penetrating injuries in the pediatric age group and represent the leading cause of death in black males aged 15-24 years. Other penetrating injuries include stab wounds, impalements, dog bites, and machinery-related accidents. Penetrating trauma generally involves injuries to the hollow viscera, primarily the small intestine. The liver is the most common solid organ injured (possibly due to its large size), followed by the kidneys and spleen. While GSWs to the abdomen generally require surgical intervention, a subset of stable children with stab wounds can be managed conservatively.

Tataria M, Nance ML, Holmes JH, et al: Pediatric blunt abdominal injury: Age is irrelevant and delayed operation is not detrimental. *J Trauma*. 2007;63(3):608-614 [PMID: 18073608].

MANAGEMENT OF LIFE-THREATENING INJURIES

Trauma care for all pediatric injuries should follow the Advanced Trauma Life Support (ATLS) guidelines. Airway, breathing, and circulation (ABC) are the first priority. Early recognition and timely initiation of resuscitation, appropriate diagnostic tests, and definitive care can reduce morbidity and mortality in these patients. Radiologic diagnostic tests that require the patient to leave the trauma room should be reserved for hemodynamically stable patients only and in conjunction with the trauma surgeon.

ASSESSMENT

The abdomen is typically evaluated during the secondary survey and begins with decompression of the stomach and bladder and physical examination of the torso. The physical examination should include inspection, auscultation, and palpation. During inspection, abrasions and contusions of the lower thoracic and abdominal wall or distention of the

Table 26–1. Reasons for pediatric susceptibility in trauma.

- The abdomen is wide and short especially in young children.
- The thinner abdominal wall musculature, larger solid organs, and protuberant abdomen increase risk of direct injury.
- The pliable and underdeveloped ribs and pelvis increase the risk of injury to liver, spleen, and urogenital system in the absence of skeletal fracture.
- The internal organs have less insulation from fat, and are suspended by more elastic structures. This reduces the amount of energy absorption and contributes to damage to organs.
- The first part of the duodenum is not well protected and children can have intramural hematoma even with mild trauma.
- High jejunal tears and injuries near the ileocecal valve are also common in children.
- Abdominal distention is more common following trauma due to air swallowing from pain and crying, making examination more difficult.
- Children can maintain blood pressure with up to 25-40% blood volume loss before hypotension results.
- Children have small anteroposterior abdominal cavity diameter and when poorly restrained, the fulcrum of a flexion injury would be at the body of the spine, which exposes it to a flexion-distraction injury (Chance fracture).
- A child's smaller body size leads to traumatic forces that are often distributed over a smaller body mass, increasing the number of systems injured during trauma.
- The larger relative surface area promotes hypothermia complicating shock.

Table 26–2. Indications for laparotomy in abdominal trauma.

- Hemodynamic instability in patients sustaining blunt or penetrating trauma, sign of peritoneal irritation
- Pancreatic transection or avulsion and pancreatic pseudocyst
- Renovascular injury
- Suspected bowel injury with pneumoperitoneum or evidence of fecal or bowel contamination on DPL
- Evisceration of abdominal content
- Rectal or vaginal lacerations
- Intraperitoneal bladder rupture
- Abdominal compartment syndrome
- Traumatic diaphragmatic hernia
- Gunshot wound (GSW) to abdomen

abdomen are markers for solid-organ or intestinal injuries. Percussion is helpful in determining the presence of intraperitoneal fluid or free air with dullness to percussion or tympanic resonance respectively. In a neurologically healthy child, abdominal palpation can reveal abdominal pain, tenderness or guarding as signs of abdominal injury. Some injuries may develop symptoms very slowly (gastrointestinal perforation, pancreatic contusions, duodenal hematoma or hematobilia); therefore repeated physical examinations are necessary.

Children with painful or distracting injuries, an altered sensorium, or those who are uncooperative because of their age or underlying neurologic impairment, may not manifest signs or symptoms of abdominal injury. Areas that are often overlooked in children with possible abdominal injury include the genitourinary region, back or flank, and rectum.

TREATMENT

Fluid resuscitation

The goal of fluid resuscitation in the child is to rapidly correct intravascular volume deficit. Use the ATLS guidelines for trauma resuscitation (see Chapter 22).

Indications for Emergent Laparotomy

Nonoperative management of solid organ injury in hemodynamically stable children with blunt abdominal trauma is well-supported in the literature. The success rate of nonoperative management is near 90% in these patients.

The decision to operate in pediatric patients is based not only on the anatomy or radiographic grade of the injury, but on the physiologic response to the injury and response to resuscitation. Indications for laparotomy in pediatric abdominal trauma are listed in Table 26–2.

The trauma surgeon should be involved in the care of these children upon arrival to the trauma room to prevent delays in diagnosis and definitive care.

Avarello JT, Cantor RM: Pediatric major trauma: An approach to evaluation and management. *Emerg Med Clin North Am.* 2007;25(3):803-846 [PMID: 17826219].

Tataria M, Nance ML, Holmes JH 4th, et al: Pediatric blunt abdominal injury: Age is irrelevant and delayed operation is not detrimental. *J Trauma.* 2007;63(3):608-614 [PMID: 18073608].

DIAGNOSTIC TESTING

Laboratory Evaluation

Laboratory evaluation is dependent upon the severity of trauma and physical examination of the child. A type and cross is needed for transfusion in the unstable patient. Blood type O negative or type specific packed red blood cells can be used until cross-matched blood is available. Essential laboratory tests in abdominal trauma include complete blood count (CBC), liver function tests (LFTs) and urinalysis (UA). Additional tests include amylase, lipase, coagulation studies, and general chemistries as part of trauma patients' workup in many institutions and can be individualized.

Hemoglobin and Hematocrit

The greatest value for a baseline hemoglobin and hematocrit is the ability to follow serial values that reflect ongoing blood loss. Initial values may be normal even with significant bleeding, until equilibration occurs. The goal is to maintain the hematocrit level at 30% and blood transfusion when hemoglobin level drops to 7-8 g/dL.

Liver Function Tests

Hepatic transaminases are elevated in liver injury. Serum aspartate aminotransferase (AST) greater than 400 IU/L or serum alanine aminotransferase (ALT) greater than 250 IU/L are good predictors for unsuspected hepatic injury. Abdominal computed tomography (CT) scan is recommended to identify and grade suspected liver injuries.

Urinalysis

The presence of microscopic or gross hematuria can indicate a genitourinary system injury, but can also represent a nonrenal trauma in children. Hematuria is not specific for renal or ureteral injuries, and may be absent in these injuries. Renal imaging is indicated if greater than 50 RBC/hpf on urinalysis exists.

Amylase & Lipase

Elevated serum amylase and lipase levels are not sensitive markers for pancreatic trauma. They may be elevated in patients with renal failure, and amylase may be elevated with salivary gland injury or inflammation. The sensitivity of these enzymes may increase if serial values are obtained. To date, there are no reliable tests for identifying pancreatic trauma including CT. Some experts continue to recommend measuring amylase and lipase in children with blunt abdominal trauma as the best available mean for identifying suspected pancreatic injury.

Coagulation Studies

Coagulation studies, including platelet count, prothrombin time, and partial thromboplastin time, are seldom useful in acute trauma. However, they should be monitored in children who receive multiple units of blood at risk for developing transfusion-related coagulopathies

Electrolytes

Electrolyte abnormalities are uncommon in acute trauma. Metabolic acidosis, increased lactate, and base deficit (BD) are useful markers for the presence of abdominal injury which may require surgery. Other electrolyte abnormalities that occur primarily following massive transfusions include hyperkalemia, metabolic alkalosis, hyperphosphatemia, and hypocalcemia.

Other Diagnostic Modalities

Laboratory testing and clinical examination lack sufficient sensitivity and specificity to diagnose or exclude intra-abdominal injury in children. Therefore, imaging plays an essential role in evaluating a child with suspected abdominal trauma. These diagnostic modalities are abdominal radiographs, abdominal ultrasound (US), CT, diagnostic peritoneal lavage (DPL), and diagnostic laparoscopy (DL).

Plain Radiography

The American College of Surgeons Committee on Trauma recommends routine series of radiographs in trauma patients including cervical spine, chest, and pelvis. Plain abdominal radiographs are primarily useful in penetrating trauma to detect pneumoperitoneum and foreign bodies. Additional studies, including upper gastrointestinal (UGI) series and endoscopic retrograde cholangiopancreatography (ERCP), are occasionally required to diagnose select injuries like duodenal hematoma and pancreatic duct trauma. However, these are not indicated in the emergency department setting.

Ultrasonography

Ultrasound (US) has been promoted as an effective initial screening tool in the emergency department for evaluating children with suspected blunt abdominal trauma (see Chapter 2 for complete discussion of ultrasound). The FAST(focused assessment with sonography in trauma) technique takes only 2-3 minutes to perform and involves limited examination of four specified abdominal locations: right upper quadrant including Morison pouch (the potential space between Gerota fascia of the kidney and Glisson capsule covering the liver [Figure 26–1A]), and the right pleural space, the left upper quadrant (splenorenal recess) and left pleural space, the subxiphoid area for pericardial fluid and the pelvis and the pouch of Douglas (rectovesical pouch). Other authors have included views, such as the right and left paracolic gutters (Figure 26–1B) and the hemithoraces for blood or pneumothorax. FAST can be performed during the primary survey of trauma resuscitation and could provide timely information regarding the presence of intraperitoneal fluid (hypoechoic area), which suggests intra-abdominal injury. The rapid and timely assessment can aid the physician in identifying children requiring immediate surgical intervention. Studies have shown FAST sensitivity ranging from 46 to 100% and specificity ranging from 84 to 98% when attempting to detect all children with intra-abdominal injuries (regardless of the presence of hemoperitoneum). However, a negative US examination in the unstable child has limited utility as the sole diagnostic test.

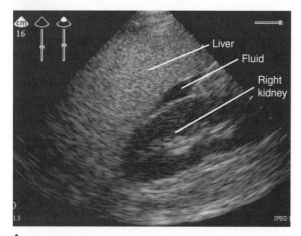

A

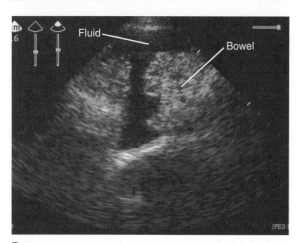

B

▲ **Figure 26–1.** (**A**) Free fluid in hepatorenal interface. (**B**) Demonstration of paracolic gutters.

Diagnostic Peritoneal Lavage

Diagnostic peritoneal lavage (DPL) is an invasive, rapid, and highly accurate test historically used for evaluating intraperitoneal hemorrhage or a ruptured hollow viscus. The indication for DPL in abdominal trauma is to determine the need for emergent laparotomy in hemodynamically unstable or comatose patients. This procedure can detect abnormalities in more than 98% of patients with intra-abdominal injury. DPL is rarely used in pediatric patients currently because of the increasing use of FAST and helical CT. Traditionally, DPL is performed in two steps after decompression of the bladder (Foley catheter) and stomach (NG or OG tube). First, the clinician attempts to aspirate free intraperitoneal fluid. If 10 mL or more of blood is aspirated, the procedure

Table 26–3. Criteria for positive diagnosis of peritoneal lavage.

- 10 mL gross blood on initial aspiration
- > 500 white blood cells/m
- > 100,000 red blood cells/mL
or
- Presence of enteric/vegetable matter

stops because intraperitoneal injury is likely. Second, if little or no blood is detected, the clinician performs a peritoneal cavity lavage with either normal saline or Ringer lactate solution and the effluent is sent for laboratory for Gram stain, red blood cell count, and white blood cell count. The fluid is also examined for enteric pathogen, bilious, or vegetable matter content. The only absolute contraindication to DPL is previous abdominal surgery. Major contraindications include preexisting recent abdominal surgery, coagulopathy, advanced cirrhosis, and morbid obesity. The results of a positive DPL are listed in Table 26–3. However, DPL does not identify retroperitoneal injuries. Complications of DPL include bladder, bowel, or vascular injury or perforation.

Computed Tomography

Abdominal computed tomography (CT) is the radiologic procedure of choice for evaluating hemodynamically stable patients with suspected blunt abdominal trauma. It is considered the gold standard in assessing the extent and severity of intra-abdominal injuries in children and has reduced the incidence of nontherapeutic exploratory laparotomy. Although CT is a noninvasive diagnostic modality, the physician should weigh the risks and benefits for obtaining abdominal CT given concerns regarding risk of potential malignancy from its radiation exposure. For solid organ injuries (liver, spleen, kidneys, and adrenal glands), CT is useful in grading injury severity. CT has the limitation of poor sensitivity for diagnosing pancreatic, bowel, diaphragmatic, bladder, and mesenteric injuries. Double-contrast abdominal CT with intravenous and oral contrast improves the sensitivity for identifying pancreatic, duodenal, and proximal bowel injuries. The indications for abdominal and pelvic CT are listed in Table 26–4.

Laparoscopy

Laparoscopy serves as a rapid diagnostic and treatment tool in abdominal trauma, and it reduces the incidence morbidity and negative laparotomy. It is a safe alternative for evaluating and managing selective injuries in blunt and penetrating abdominal trauma in hemodynamically stable patients. In

Table 26–4. Indications for abdominal computed tomography.

- Suspected blunt abdominal trauma based on injury pattern
- Abdominal pain or tenderness in the hemodynamically stable trauma child
- Significant initial fluid resuscitation requirement without obvious blood loss
- Multisystem trauma such as severe pelvic, thoracic, or cranial injury
- Inability to perform adequate abdominal examination secondary to altered mental status, suspected head injury, spinal cord injury, or alcohol or drug intoxication
- Hemoglobin < 10 g/dL without obvious blood loss
- Gross hematuria or > 50 RBC/hpf
- Penetrating wounds to the back or flank
- Need for emergent surgical intervention that will limit the physician ability to perform serial abdominal examination

blunt trauma, laparoscopy is indicated for hollow viscus injury, exploring the origin of free peritoneal fluid without evidence of solid organ injury and equivocal physical examination. In penetrating trauma, laparoscopy is indicated in hemodynamically stable patients with anterior abdominal stab wounds or tangential GSWs.

Brenner DJ, Hall EJ: Computed tomography—an increasing source of radiation exposure. *N Engl J Med*. 2007;357: 2277-2284 [PMID: 18046031].

Capraro AJ, Mooney D, Waltzman ML: The use of routine laboratory studies as screening tools in pediatric abdominal trauma. *Pediatr Emerg Care*. 2006;22:480-484 [PMID: 16871106].

Donnelly L: Imaging issues in CT of blunt trauma to the chest and abdomen. *Pediatr Radiol*. 2009;39(Suppl 3):S406-S413 [PMID: 19440760].

Fox C, Boysen M, Ghrahbaghian L: Test characteristics of focused assessment of sonography for trauma for clinically significant abdominal free fluid in pediatric blunt abdominal trauma. *Acad Emerge Med*. 2011;18:477-482 [PMID: 21569167].

Gaines BA, Rutkoski JD: The role of laparoscopy in pediatric trauma. *Semin Pediatr Surg*. 2010;19:300-303 [PMID: 20889087].

Holmes J, Gladman A, Chang C: Performance of abdominal ultrasonography in pediatric blunt trauma patients: A meta-analysis. *J Pediatr Surg*. 2007;42:1588-1594 [PMID: 17848254].

Holmes JF, Mao A, Awasthi S, McGahan JP, Wisner DH, Kuppermann N: Validation of a prediction rule for the identification of children with intra-abdominal injuries after blunt torso trauma. *Ann Emerg Med*. 2009;54:528-533 [PMID: 19250706].

Hom J: The risk of intra-abdominal injuries in pediatric patients with stable blunt abdominal trauma and negative abdominal computed tomography. *Acad Emerg Med*. 2010;17:469-475 [PMID: 20536798].

Moore MA, Wallace C, Westra SJ: The imaging of pediatric thoracic trauma. *Pediatr Radiol*. 2009;39:485-496 [PMID: 19151969].

Sivit CJ: Imaging children with abdominal trauma. *AJR Am J Roentgenol*. 2009;192:1179-1189.

Whitehouse J, Weigelt J: Diagnostic peritoneal lavage: A review of indications, technique, and interpretation. *Scand J Trauma Resusc Emerg Med*. 2009;17:13 [PMID: 19267941].

Winslow JE, Hinshaw JW, Hughes MJ: Quantitative assessment of diagnostic radiation doses in adult blunt trauma patients. *Ann Emerg Med*. 2008;52:93-97 [PMID: 18328598].

EMERGENCY MANAGEMENT OF SPECIFIC INJURIES

SPLENIC INJURIES

 ESSENTIAL OF DIAGNOSIS

▶ Spleen is the most common solid organ injury in blunt abdominal traum.

▶ Left shoulder pain (Kehr sign) and left upper quadrant pain are hallmarks of splenic injury

▶ It may cause significant hemodynamic instability.

▶ FAST examination can reliably identify injury in unstable patients.

▶ CT scan is the gold standard for splenic injury in hemodynamically stable patients.

▶ Splenomegaly from any cause increase the risk of injury even with minor trauma.

▶ Non-operative management is the standard of care for all grades of splenic injury.

Findings that suggest splenic trauma on physical examination include left upper quadrant abrasions, tenderness, evidence of left lower rib fracture, grunting, and abdominal distention.

Abdominal CT scan has an important role in guiding management and in determining subsequent conservative management, including level of care, duration of monitoring, and length of activity restriction or need for surgical intervention.

Plain radiographic findings are often unreliable and nonspecific in detecting splenic injury; however, subtle findings may provide early and helpful diagnostic clues. Left lower rib fractures, left diaphragmatic elevation, left lower lobe atelectasis, left pleural effusion, medial displacement of the gastric bubble, and inferior displacement of the splenic colon flexure are subtle findings.

On FAST examination, the presence of free fluid or parenchymal injury may aid the physician in determining the need for immediate laparotomy. When splenic injury is unlikely, a normal FAST may preclude the need for CT and replace it with appropriate clinical observation and serial physical examinations.

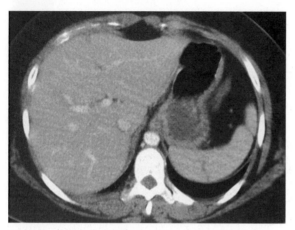

▲ **Figure 26–2.** CT image demonstrates a curvilinear low attenuation laceration involving less than 3 cm of parenchymal depth in the posterior spleen, consistent with grade II injury.

Splenic injuries are graded on abdominal CT (Figure 26–2) using a standardized organ injury scale grades I to V from the American Association for the Surgery of Trauma (AAST) to correlate CT findings with potential morbidity and mortality (Table 26–5).

Table 26–5. Grading of splenic injuries.

Grade	Injury type	Description of injury
I	Hematoma	Subcapsular, < 10% surface area
	Laceration	Capsular tear, < 1 cm parenchymal depth
II	Hematoma	Subcapsular, 10-50% surface area; intraparenchymal, < 5 cm in diameter
	Laceration	Capsular tear, 1-3 cm parenchymal depth that does not involve a trabecular vessel
III	Hematoma	Subcapsular, > 50% surface area or expanding; rupture subcapsular or parenchymal hematoma; intraparenchymal hematoma ≥ 5 cm or expanding
	Laceration	> 3 cm parenchymal depth or involving trabecular vessels
IV	Laceration	Laceration involving segmental or hilar vessels producing major devascularization (> 25% of spleen)
V	Hematoma	Complete shattered spleen
	Laceration	Hilar vascular injury devascularizes spleen

Most splenic injuries require nonoperative management. Nonoperative management decisions are based on the physiological response to the injury and the presence of associated injuries rather than the radiologic features of the injury. Nonoperative management is considered the standard of care in hemodynamically stable patients with all grades of splenic lacerations and the success rate of the approach is 90%. All patients require admission to a pediatric trauma service.

Conservative management includes hospital admission for bed rest, serial abdominal examination, intravenous hydration, antibiotic therapy, and monitoring of hemoglobin and vital signs. Admission to the intensive care unit (ICU) is not mandatory. Complete healing of all grades is seen 3 months after injury.

Children with hemodynamic instability after primary survey, secondary survey, and aggressive resuscitation usually require exploratory laparotomy. Splenectomy is more likely in children with shattered splenic injury or who have a grade IV and/or V injury. Splenorrhaphy and partial splenectomy are two techniques used to control bleeding while preserving spleen parenchyma. Laparoscopic splenectomy has been shown to be safe in children. Vaccination against encapsulated bacteria is recommended after splenectomy or nonoperative management of a severely damaged spleen.

Delayed complications occur at least 48 hours after injury and include pseudocyst, abscesses, pseudoaneurysms, and a delayed rupture.

LIVER INJURIES

 ESSENTIALS OF DIAGNOSIS

▶ Liver injury is the second most common solid organ injury in blunt trauma.

▶ Liver injury is the most common solid organ injury in penetrating trauma.

▶ Liver injury is the most common cause of lethal hemorrhage.

▶ Right shoulder pain and right upper quadrant pain are hallmarks of liver injury.

▶ Check hemoglobin and liver function test to assess ongoing liver bleeding.

▶ Use FAST for unstable patients.

▶ CT scan is the gold standard for liver injury in hemodynamically stable patients.

▶ Compared with splenic injuries, children with liver injuries require more transfusions and surgical interventions.

Hepatic injuries are generally more severe than splenic injuries and are more likely to cause delayed bleeding. The most common mechanisms of injury are traffic accidents, followed by falls and direct impact trauma. The dual blood supply to the inferior vena cava predisposes it to severe hemorrhage after blunt trauma.

Findings that suggest liver trauma on physical examination include right upper quadrant pain or abrasions, right shoulder tenderness, right lower chest tenderness, and abdominal distention.

The most useful laboratory tests in liver trauma are the hemoglobin, hematocrit, and the liver function tests. Repeated serial hematocrit values will identify potential ongoing bleeding. The management goal is to keep a hematocrit of 30% and consider blood transfuse if the hemoglobin drops to 7-8 g/dL. Hepatic transaminases are elevated in liver injury. Serum AST greater than 400 IU/L or serum ALT greater than 250 IU/L are predictors of hepatic injury.

Diagnostic imaging plays an important role in guiding and determining subsequent conservative management, including level of care, duration of monitoring, and length of activity restriction or surgical intervention.

Plain radiographic findings are usually normal. However, subtle radiologic findings include right lower rib fracture, elevation of right hemidiaphragm, and right pleural effusion.

The FAST examination may reveal free fluid or parenchymal damage. These findings should prompt consideration for urgent surgical intervention.

Abdominal CT remains the gold standard in the assessment of blunt trauma in the hemodynamically stable patient. It accurately determines the degree of liver injury, other associated injuries, and the amount of free fluid in the abdomen (Figure 26–3). Liver injuries are classified as subcapsular or intrahepatic hematoma, contusion, vascular injury, or biliary disruption. CT findings are graded I through VI using a standardized organ injury scale (Table 26–6). Classification is from the AAST; however the classification has not correlated with outcomes. Nonoperative management of blunt liver trauma in stable patients is well established, with a success rate of 85-90% in most pediatric trauma centers. Conservative management includes hospital admission to the trauma service for bed rest, serial abdominal examination, intravenous hydration, antibiotic therapy, and monitoring of hemoglobin and vital signs. Unique complications of nonoperative management include bile leaks, delayed bleeding, abscess formation, and development of hemobilia. Complications can be treated with nonoperative intervention such as ERCP or percutaneous drainage.

Indications for exploratory laparotomy include higher grade of injury (grades IV-VI), lower Pediatric Trauma Score owing to multisystem injury, transfusion required within 2 hours of presentation, associated retrohepatic vena cava or major hepatic vein trauma, unresponsive hypotensive patient. Complications from surgery may include

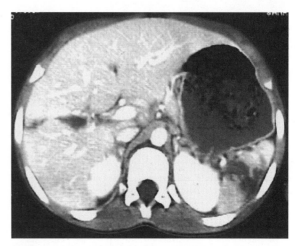

▲ **Figure 26–3.** Abdominal contrast CT scan of a 7-year-old boy with a liver rupture grade II and an associated splenic rupture.

Table 26–6. Grading of hepatic injuries.

Grade	Injury type	Description of injury
I	Hematoma	Subcapsular, < 10% surface area
	Laceration	Capsular tear, < 1 cm parenchymal depth
II	Hematoma	Subcapsular, 10-50% surface area; intraparenchymal, < 10 cm in diameter
	Laceration	Capsular tear, 1-3 cm parenchymal depth, < 10 cm in length
III	Hematoma	Subcapsular, > 50% surface area of ruptured subcapsular or parenchymal hematoma; intraparenchymal hematoma > 10 cm or expanding
	Laceration	> 3 cm parenchymal depth
IV	Laceration	Parenchymal disruption involving 25-75% hepatic lobe or 1-3 Couinaud segments
V	Laceration	Parenchymal disruption involving > 75% of hepatic lobe or > 3 Couinaud segments within a single lobe
	Vascular	Juxtahepatic venous injuries (retrohepatic vena), cava/central major hepatic veins
VI	Vascular	Hepatic avulsion

abscess formation, pancreatic fistula, hematemesis from hemobilia, biliary obstruction, bilioma, stress gastric ulceration, sympathetic pleural effusion, abdominal compartment syndrome, delayed bleeding, wound infection, and bowel obstruction from adhesions. Hepatic arterial embolization via interventional radiology has been used in selected patients. It is recommended that children with these conditions be transferred to pediatric trauma centers where the appropriate resources are available.

Kiankhooy A, Sartorelli K, Vane D, Bhave A: Angiographic embolization is safe and effective therapy for blunt abdominal solid organ injury in children. *J Trauma*. 2010;68(3):526-531 [PMID: 20220415].

Landau A, van As AB, Numanoglu AJ, Millar AJ, Rode H: Liver injuries in children: The role of selective non-operative management. *Injury*. 2006;37(1):66-71 [PMID: 16246338].

Lynn K, Werder G, Callaghan R, et al: Pediatric blunt splenic trauma: A comprehensive review. *Pediatr Radiol*. 2009;39:904-916 [PMID: 19639310].

Thompson SR, Holland AJ: Evolution of nonoperative management for blunt splenic trauma in children. *J Paediatr Child Health*. 2006;42(5):231-234 [PMID: 16712549].

Tinkoff G, Esposito T, Reed J, et al: American Association for the Surgery of Trauma Organ Injury Scale I: Spleen, liver, and kidney, validation based on the National Trauma Data Bank. *J Am Coll Surg*. 2008;207:646-655 [PMID: 18954775].

RENAL INJURIES

 ESSENTIAL OF DIAGNOSIS

▶ Renal trauma is the most common urologic trauma.

▶ Delay in diagnosis can increase morbidity.

▶ Clinical presentation is not specific and can be caused by injury to other organs.

▶ CT scan is the imaging of choice in renal injury.

▶ Nonoperative management can be successful in up to 95% of renal injuries.

After the spleen and liver, the kidney is the most common solid organ to be injured following blunt trauma. Most are minor injuries and are associated with direct flank trauma or rapid deceleration forces that crush the kidneys against the ribs or vertebral column. Motor vehicle collisions (MVCs) are the most common mechanism of injury, followed by pedestrians struck by motor vehicle and falls. Associated abdominal and nonabdominal injuries occur in 80% of children with renal injuries and include liver, spleen, head, and chest trauma. Kidneys with preexisting abnormalities are more easily injured than normal kidneys. Delay in diagnosis of renal injury is associated with increase morbidity, such as hypertension or renal insufficiency.

Clinical manifestations in renal injury are nonspecific. Findings that suggest renal injury on physical examination include dull flank tenderness, flank hematoma, abdominal tenderness, and hematuria. Symptoms of injury to other structures commonly mask or supersede that of renal injury, both early and late in the hospital course. Therefore, a high degree of clinical awareness is necessary to ensure that renal injuries are not overlooked or missed.

The diagnosis of renal injuries is difficult due to its retroperitoneal location and is based on clinical examination, mechanism of injury, radiographic, and laboratory analysis.

Microscopic or gross hematuria can indicate trauma to any location within the genitourinary system, but can also represent a nonrenal trauma in children. Hematuria is not specific for renal or ureteral injuries, and may be absent in these injuries. Renal imaging is indicated only in children with abdominal trauma, with another indication for abdominal CT, or with 50 RBC/hpf on urinalysis. Hematuria doesn't consistently correlate with the severity of the renal injury. High-grade injuries can present with no hematuria. Significant renal injuries are more likely in patients with multiple intra-abdominal injuries and hematuria.

Diagnostic imaging modalities are the key to accurate classification of these injuries and planning appropriate management. Plain radiography is usually normal. However, subtle findings may include obliteration of the renal and psoas shadows, scoliosis with concavity toward the injured side, fractures of lower posterior ribs, or adjacent transverse spinous process or pelvic fractures. Ultrasonography does not detect parenchyma injuries, is not useful in grading injury, and doesn't provide functional assessment. Abdominal CT remains the gold standard in the assessment of blunt trauma in the hemodynamically stable patient. It can accurately delineate extent of renal parenchymal injury, detects extravasation, identifies active bleeding, assesses nonviable tissues, and detects other associated retroperitoneal and abdominal injuries. CT is graded by a standardized organ injury scale I through V, from the AAST, to standardize the severity, diagnosis, and successful management of renal injuries (Figure 26–4).

Management decisions are based on the subjective clinical status of the patient, the presence or absence of associated abdominal injuries, and guided by objective evidence of the severity of injury.

Nonoperative management has become the standard of care in most solid organ injuries, including renal trauma grades I through III. It is successful in up to 95% of renal injuries. In high-grade renal injuries (IV and V), conservative management remains controversial. Conservative

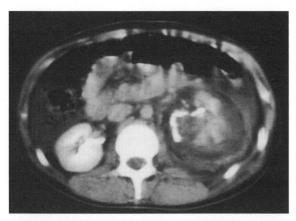

▲ **Figure 26–4.** A CT scan showing disruption of the left kidney accompanied by extravasation of contrast agent and massive left retroperitoneal hemorrhage.

management generally includes hospital admission to the trauma service for bed rest, intravenous hydration, and monitoring of hemoglobin, hematuria, and vital signs. After gross hematuria resolves, limited activity is allowed for 2-4 weeks until microscopic hematuria ceases.

When a child exhibits persistent symptomatic urinary extravasation (urinoma), minimally invasive percutaneous nephrostomy and/or stenting techniques may be considered before open operative intervention. These techniques have an overall renal salvage rate of 98.9%. Angiographic embolization is an alternative to surgery in stable patients with persistent gross hematuria secondary to hemorrhage from the injured kidney. Early surgical exploration should be reserved only for children with extensive renal injury associated with hemodynamic instability and hemorrhage.

Despite the markedly improved renal salvage rates associated with nonoperative management, significant complications are described and include delayed hemorrhage, delayed massive hematuria, nephrectomy, renal scaring with loss of function, renal cyst development, postinjury hypertension, infection, and persistent urinoma.

Bartley JM, Santucci RA: Computed tomography findings in patients with pediatric blunt renal trauma in whom expectant (nonoperative) management failed. *Urology*. 2012;80(6):1338-1344 [PMID: 23206778].

Buckley JC, McAninch JW: Revision of current American Association for the Surgery of Trauma Renal Injury grading system. *J Trauma*. 2011;70(1):35-37 [PMID: 21531196].

Henderson CG, Sedberry-Ross S, Pickard R, et al: Management of high grade renal trauma: 20-year experience at a pediatric level I trauma center. *Urology*. 2007;178(1):246-250 [PMID: 17499798].

VISCERAL INJURY

 ESSENTIAL OF DIAGNOSIS

▸ Intestinal injuries are rare.

▸ Delay or unrecognized diagnosis can increase mortality.

▸ Seat belt use related to accidents have up to 50% risk of intestinal injury.

▸ Jejunum is the most common segment injured.

▸ Clinical manifestation of peritonitis is present in less than 50% of patients.

▸ Imaging studies are not specific for intestinal injuries, including CT.

▸ DPL should be considered in the critically brain-injured child with suspicious CT findings and in whom reliable physical examination is difficult.

▸ If suspicion for visceral injuries exists, patient should be observed on the surgical trauma service.

▸ Confirmed visceral injury requires operative intervention.

Intestinal injury following blunt and penetrating abdominal trauma is rare in children, occurring in 1-15% of patients. The most common mechanism of injury is motor vehicle accident. This form of trauma has increased in incidence since the mandate of safety belt use. Restrained occupants of MVCs with sufficient force to produce a visible abdominal wall contusion and vertebral column fracture have as high as 50% risk of intestinal injury. Other mechanisms include direct trauma, handlebar injuries, or penetrating trauma. The most common site of intestinal injury in both penetrating and blunt trauma is the small intestine, followed by colon and stomach. The jejunum is the most common segment of the small bowel injured, followed by the duodenum, ileum, and cecum. Colonic injury far more often follows penetrating injury of the abdomen with the left colon the most affected. Anorectal injury is the least common intestinal injury in children. The diagnosis of blunt intestinal injury is often difficult, is often delayed, and can result in mortality in up to 15% of patients. The relatively high mortality may be due to the frequency of associated multisystem injury, specifically brain injury. Injuries to the intestines include perforation, intestinal hematomas, and mesenteric tears with bleeding. The "lap belt complex" has been described in children who have a seat belt applied inappropriately. This complex typically occurs in children 4-9 years, who wear seat belts improperly positioned over the immature iliac crests with migration onto the abdomen during rapid deceleration of the car (Figure 26–5). Injuries include small bowel contusions/lacerations and lumbar flexion distraction injuries.

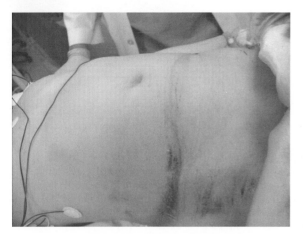

▲ **Figure 26–5.** Abdominal wall contusion or "seat belt sign" in a child involved in a motor vehicle collision.

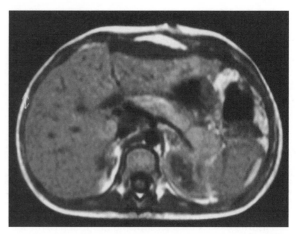

▲ **Figure 26–6.** Abdominal MRI of a 10-year-old girl with a transection of the tail of the pancreas.

The clinical manifestation of intestinal injury is often difficult and may be delayed. In general any contusion or ecchymosis to the abdominal wall on physical examination may imply a significant risk of visceral, solid organ, or spinal column injury. The leakage of intestinal contents results in peritoneal irritation that may or may not be evident on initial physical examination. Despite careful initial physical examination, in children with blunt intestinal perforation, peritonitis is noted in less than 50% of patients. Other signs and symptoms that suggest intestinal injury include abdominal tenderness, fever, and tachycardia. A high clinical awareness is necessary to ensure that intestinal injuries are not overlooked or missed (Figure 26–6). Hematomas of the duodenum and other intestinal sites can cause symptoms of obstruction with pain, vomiting, and abdominal distention.

The diagnosis and potential delay remains problematic in visceral injuries. A high index of suspicion and serial abdominal examinations, coupled with subsequent comparative laboratory and radiographic evaluations, are critical to identifying children with intestinal injury. Laboratory studies may initially be normal. Leukocytosis had been reported to be present in intestinal injuries of greater than 6 hours of presentation.

Plain radiography is usually normal. Less than a third of patients with intestinal perforation exhibit pneumoperitoneum. Additional diagnostic studies will be required in the majority of children with suspected intestinal injury, particularly in those with central nervous system or distracting injuries.

GI contrast studies and ultrasound may be diagnostic in cases of hematoma to duodenum or other parts of intestine. CT remains the gold standard in the assessment of abdominal blunt trauma in the hemodynamically stable patient. Its accuracy decreases in the detection of intestinal injuries.

Pneumoperitoneum or extravasation of contrast by CT is diagnostic of intestinal injury, but these findings are present in less than 50% of patients. In an effort to improve the diagnostic accuracy of CT, additional CT findings of intestinal injury have been described such as unexplained free fluid, bowel wall thickening and enhancement, dilated bowel loops, and mesenteric fat stranding.

Because of the limitations of the physical examination, laboratory studies, and noninvasive diagnostic studies, DPL has been advocated to facilitate early diagnosis of intestinal injury. DPL is rarely employed in children today and suffers its own limitations as described. Despite the limitations and disadvantages, DPL may be considered in the critically brain-injured child with suspicious CT findings and in whom reliable physical examination is difficult, but laparotomy poses substantial risk. Again, the trauma surgeon should be involved early in the management of these patients.

Management decisions are based on the subjective clinical status of the patient, the presence or absence of associated abdominal injuries, and guided by evidence of the severity of injury. It is best that these children be transferred to a pediatric trauma center for evaluation and definitive management by trauma surgeons.

Chidester S, Rana A, Lowell W, et al: Is the 'seat belt sign' associated with serious abdominal injuries in pediatric trauma? *J Trauma.* 2009;67(Suppl 1):S34-S36 [PMID: 19590352].

Paris C, Brindamour M, Quimet A, St-Vil D: Predictive indicators for bowel injury in pediatric patients who present with a positive seat belt sign after motor vehicle collision. *J Pediatr Surg.* 2010;45(5):921-924 [PMID: 20438927].

Sracey S, Forman J, Woods W, Arbogast K, Kent R: Pediatric abdominal injury patterns generated by lap belt loading. *J Trauma.* 2009;67(6):1278-1283 [PMID: 20009678].

Genitourinary Trauma

Eric William Stern, MD
Ryun Summers, DO
Dhriti Mukhopadhyay, MD

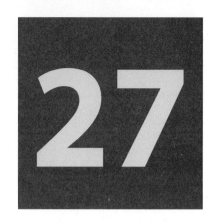

27

GENERAL CONSIDERATIONS

Approximately 10% of multiple trauma patients are diagnosed with genitourinary injury, most commonly in the setting of other multiple blunt force injuries. Significant injury to the genitourinary system is an uncommon cause of serious morbidity or mortality. A number of genitourinary injuries are not immediately apparent and are rarely responsible for significant hemodynamic compromise. Initial evaluation of the trauma patient should focus on stabilization and resuscitation, prioritizing hemodynamic instability. See Chapter 22 for the approach to the multiple trauma patients.

Penetrating injuries to the abdomen and trunk, as well as blunt injuries to the torso should heighten the clinician's suspicion for the possibility of occult genitourinary trauma. Blood at the urethral meatus or vaginal introitus are likely indicators of injury. Gross hematuria noted with the first spontaneous void or with Foley catheter placement should prompt further evaluation.

Greater than 90% of genitourinary injuries are safely managed nonoperatively with a low rate of long-term serious sequelae. A decrease in nephrectomies and laparotomies has coincided with improvements in modern imaging techniques and injury assessment. The role of careful observation, urinary drainage, and selected interventional radiologic procedures has largely supplanted operative management.

Antonis MS, Phillips CA, Bialvas M: Genitourinary imaging in the emergency department. *Emerg Med Clin North Am.* 2011;29(3):553-567 [PMID 21782074].

Ramchandani P, Buckler PM: Imaging of genitourinary trauma. *AJR Am J Roentgenol.* 2009;192(6):1514-1523 [PMID: 19457813].

Shenfeld OZ, Gnessin E: Management of urogenital trauma: State of the art. *Curr Opin Urol.* 2011;21(6):449-454 [PMID: 21897259].

Shewakramani S, Reed KC: Genitourinary trauma. *Emerg Med Clin North Am.* 2011;29(3):501-518 [PMID: 21782071].

BLUNT RENAL TRAUMA

Clinical Findings

Most pediatric renal injuries are a result of blunt force trauma. These injuries are most commonly noted in the multiply injured patient and are less life-threatening than other system injuries. Renal injury should be considered in a patient with significant trauma to the torso. Contusions, abrasions, and lacerations to the flank or abdominal wall should be noted. A "seat belt sign" or contusion over the lower abdomen is concerning. Children with genitourinary trauma have three to five times the rate of congenital renal malformations compared with similar adult cohorts.

Pelvic fractures have a high degree of correlation with both upper and lower genitourinary trauma, including renal injury. Evaluate the stability of the pelvis and observe for blood at the urethral meatus or vaginal introitus. Gross hematuria is major warning for renal, renovascular, and lower genitourinary system trauma. The clinician should observe the first urine (or Foley catheter) output from the patient, as initial obvious hematuria may fade with the dilutional effects of aggressive crystalloid infusion.

Treatment

Resuscitation of the patient in shock with suspected renal injury should follow standard life support algorithms with attention to airway, breathing, and circulation (ABC) and judicious use of crystalloid and packed red blood cells (PRBC) infusion. Diagnostic studies will help stratify severity of injury.

▶ Laboratory Studies

Suspicion of renal injury warrants a urine analysis and measurement of current renal function. Gross hematuria on examination marks a high likelihood of injury. Work-up and management of children with microscopic hematuria (> 50 red blood cells [RBCs] per high-power field [HPF]) remains somewhat controversial. Most hemodynamically stable patients with microscopic hematuria are suitable candidates for expectant management. In hemodynamically unstable children with greater than 50 RBCs per HPF and no other obvious source of hemorrhage, radiologic imaging, and even retroperitoneal exploration may be appropriate.

▶ Radiologic Studies

Studies have demonstrated that it is safe to perform expectant management without imaging in children with microscopic hematuria who are hemodynamically stable and additional imaging is not required to rule out suspected concomitant injuries. In patients with gross hematuria, microscopic hematuria with shock, or microscopic hematuria with a concerning injury mechanism (high-velocity deceleration injuries), diagnostic imaging is recommended.

Computerized tomography (CT) has supplanted the intravenous pyelogram (IVP) as the imaging modality of choice. CT imaging allows screening for concomitant injuries, and contrast enhancement allows for visualization of renal and renovascular perfusion as well as evaluation of the ureters and bladder. Precontrast, immediate postcontrast, and delayed (8-15 min) postcontrast CT images should be obtained when renal trauma is considered. Ultrasound may be helpful in follow-up imaging after initial CT to continue to monitor the evolution of renal injuries while reducing radiation exposure.

Renal injuries are categorized by the nature and severity of injury. Table 27–1 describes the grading of renal trauma

by severity. Up to 70% of children with the American Association for the Surgery of Trauma (AAST) grade II or higher renal injury may have no hematuria. Figure 27–1 illustrates the grades of renal trauma.

Disposition

AAST grade I-III injuries (small renal contusions and lacerations) can be managed expectantly with bed rest, pain control, and close observation in the hospital setting. AAST grade IV and V injuries often require more aggressive management including repeated PRBC infusion for nonlifethreatening bleeding, endovascular intervention, and, in the patient with refractory shock, retroperitoneal exploration with potential nephrectomy. Surgical management may be required for high-grade renovascular injuries. Renal vein disruption may produce a greater degree of shock compared with renal artery disruption, as the renal vein has comparatively limited ability to constrict.

Children who are hemodynamically stable with AAST grade I-III renal injuries may be managed by surgeons and urologists who are familiar and comfortable with pediatric care. Patients with high-grade renal injuries or significant renovascular disruption should be stabilized and possibly transferred to an appropriate tertiary level trauma center for further care. Antibiotics are generally recommended to cover common urinary pathogens.

Unrecognized renal injury may range from no sequelae to delayed complications. Renovascular hypertension usually manifests approximately 1 month after initial injury. A severely nonperfused kidney may result in renal artery constriction, increased renin release, and associated severe renovascular hypertension (Goldblatt kidney).

Table 27–1. The American Association for the Surgery of Trauma renal injury grading system.

AAST grade	Injury pattern
I	Contusion/subcapsular hematoma
II	< 1 cm laceration
III	> 1 cm laceration +/− devascularized fragments, without collecting system rupture or urinary extravasation
IV	Laceration with urinary extravasation, major renovascular injury with controlled hemorrhage
V	Shattered kidney, hilar avulsion, major renovascular injury with uncontrolled hemorrhage

The American Association for the Surgery of Trauma: Injury scoring scale, a resource for trauma care professionals. Chicago, IL; 2013. Also available at http://www.aast.org/library/traumatools/injuryscoringscales.aspx#kidney. Accessed August 17, 2013.

Umbrelt EC, Routh JC, Husmann DA: Nonoperative management of nonvascular grade IV blunt renal trauma in children: Meta-analysis and systematic review. *Urology.* 2009;74(3):579-582 [PMID: 19589574].

URETERAL TRAUMA

Clinical Findings

Ureteral injuries are relatively rare and often are occult, accounting for less than 1% of urologic injuries in children. Ureteral injuries are often a result of a deceleration injury with associated shearing forces. Blunt ureteral disruption is associated with a greater than 30% mortality rate, which

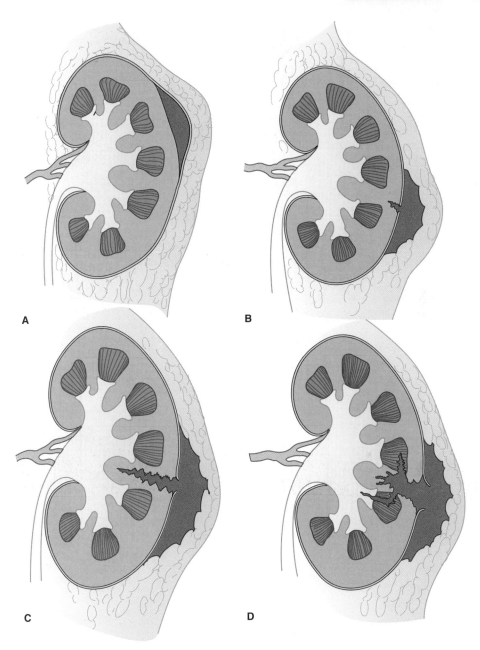

▲ **Figure 27–1.** Classification of renal injuries. Grades I and II are minor. Grades III, IV, and V are major. (**A**) Grade I: Microscopic or gross hematuria; normal findings on radiographic studies; contusion or contained subcapsular hematoma without parenchymal laceration. (**B**) Grade II: Nonexpanding, confined perirenal hematoma or cortical laceration less than 1 cm deep without urinary extravasation. (**C**) Grade III: Parenchymal laceration extending more than 1 cm into the cortex without urinary extravasation. (**D**) Grade IV: Parenchymal laceration extending through the corticomedullary junction and into the collecting system. A laceration at a segmental vessel may also be present. (**E**) Grade IV: Thrombosis of a segmental renal artery without a parenchymal laceration. Note the corresponding parenchymal ischemia. (**F**) Grade V: Thrombosis of the main renal artery. The inset shows the intimal tear and distal thrombosis. (**G**) Grade V: Multiple major lacerations, resulting in a "shattered" kidney. (**H**) Grade V: Avulsion of the main renal artery and/or vein. (Reproduced, with permission, from Tanagho EA, McAninch JW: *Smith's General Urology*, 17th ed. New York: McGraw-Hill, 2007. Copyright © McGraw-Hill Education LLC.)

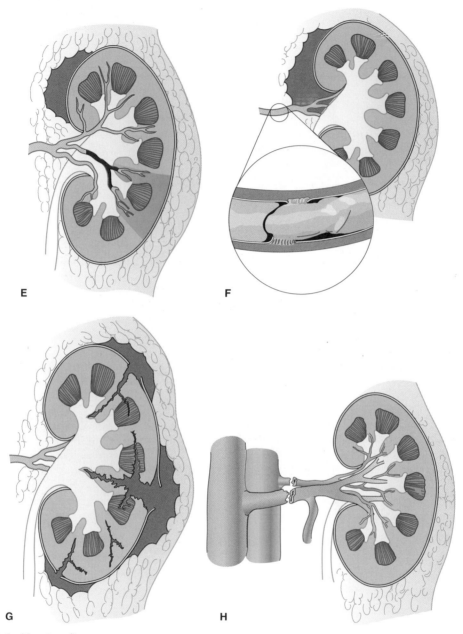

E

F

G

H

▲ **Figure 27–1.** (*Continued*)

is usually attributed to the multisystem injuries from which patients with ureteral disruption often suffer. Up to 70% of cases of ureteral injury may present with no hematuria. Urine output from the unaffected side may be normal in volume and analysis, if complete disruption of the contralateral ureter has occurred. Ureteropelvic disruption may occur after severe blunt force trauma. A high index of suspicion is necessary to diagnose these injuries. Children are at greater risk for ureteropelvic disruption than adults because of their flexible vertebral columns and limited ribcage protection over their low-lying kidneys. Children presenting with major trauma to the torso should be considered at risk for ureteral injury.

Treatment

Obtain a urine analysis and measurement of renal function. Delayed postcontrast images on CT scan may reveal unilateral ureteral filling and possible medial contrast extravasation at the site of the ureteral disruption. If CT scan findings are suspicious for ureteral disruption, a retrograde pyelogram should be performed to determine the patency of the ureteropelvic junction.

Children with multiple trauma may undergo emergent laparotomy, and the injuries not noted initially during exploration. A concerning finding 3-5 days after laparotomy is urine leakage from incisional sites, likely a result of ureteral necrosis or urinoma formation.

Disposition

Confirmed ureteral injury warrants hospital admission and possibly operative repair. Transfer to an appropriate trauma center with an available pediatric urologist is recommended, if the initial evaluation occurs in the absence of these resources. If the ureteropelvic junction is intact, ureteral stenting with or without placement of a nephrostomy tube may be indicated. If the ureteral injury is discovered within 5 days of injury, primary surgical repair may be possible. In unstable patients, the damaged end of the ureter may be clipped and a nephrostomy tube placed, with plans for a delayed surgical repair.

Asali MG, Romanowsky I, Kaneti J: [External ureteral injuries]. *Harefuah.* 2007;146(9):686-689,734 [PMID: 17969305].

Elliot SP, McAninch JW: Ureteral injuries: External and iatrogenic. *Urol Clin North Am.* 2006;33(1):55-66 [PMID: 16488280].

Helmy TE, Sarhan OM, Harraz AM, Dawaba M: Complexity of non-iatrogenic ureteral injuries in children: Single-center experience. *Int Urol Nephrol.* 2011;43(1):1-5 [PMID: 20526809].

Pereira BM, Ogilvie MP, Gomez-Rodgriguez JC, et al: A review of ureteral injuries after external trauma. *Scand J Trauma Resusc Emerg Med.* 2010;18:6 [PMID: 20128905].

TESTICULAR TRAUMA

Clinical Findings

Children may present after blunt or penetrating injury to the testicles and scrotum. A significant blunt force is often required to produce severe testicular injury, given the testicle's freely mobile anatomic nature. At initial examination, a thorough history should be obtained including careful documentation of the degree of pain, the presence

of obvious swelling or bruising to the scrotum or perineum, and an exhaustive search for concomitant injuries. Patients may complain primarily of abdominal pain and/or nausea and vomiting. Note the presence or absence of the cremasteric reflex, position and nature of the prostate, and lie of the testes.

Treatment

Adequate analgesia should be provided. Penetrating injuries warrant immediate consultation with a urologist without delay for diagnostic imaging or other studies. Diagnosis and management of significant blunt testicular trauma remains controversial. Some authors recommend surgical exploration and recommend against reliance on scrotal ultrasound because of its low sensitivity for testicular rupture. The classic findings of testicular rupture including tunica albuginea rupture with seminiferous tubule extrusion can be visualized on ultrasound but sensitivity will vary by operator. It can be quite difficult clinically and ultrasonographically to distinguish between simple hematoma, hematocele, and true testicular rupture. Ultrasound is a safe modality to evaluate testicular injury, but its use should not delay specialist consultation.

Disposition

Patients with penetrating and blunt trauma to the testicle(s) warrant consultation with a urologist to ensure a safe disposition. Penetrating injuries require immediate consultation and likely surgical exploration. Blunt injuries were historically managed conservatively; however, recent studies have shown increased rates of atrophy, infection, and delayed orchiectomy with conservative management. A great number of urologists now explore blunt testicular injures surgically. In the absence of true testicular rupture, the urologist may elect to drain large hematoceles to improve pain and allow a more rapid return to functional status. The primary consideration for the emergency department physician is to provide adequate analgesia and to obtain emergent consultation with a neurologist. Depending on the setting of initial evaluation and the expertise of available urologists, transfer to a trauma center may be necessary.

Chandra RV, Dowling RJ, Ulubasoglu M, Haxhimolla H, Costello AJ: Rational approach to diagnosis and management of blunt scrotal trauma. *Urology.* 2007;70(2):230-234 [PMID: 17826476].

Guichard G, El Ammari J, Cellarier D, et al: Accuracy of ultrasonography in diagnosis of testicular rupture after blunt scrotal trauma. *Urology.* 2008;71(1):52-56 [PMID: 18242364].

Pogorelić Z, Jurić I, Furlan D, et al: Management of testicular rupture after blunt trauma in children. *Pediatr Surg Int.* 2011;27(8):885-889 [PMID: 21387107].

URETHRAL INJURY

Clinical Findings

Children are at increased risk for urethral disruption in comparison with adults. Blood at the urethral meatus, inability to void, blood at the vaginal introitus, a boggy or high-riding prostate, and the presence of pelvic fractures should warn the clinician of possible urethral injury. A retrograde urethrogram (RUG) should precede placement of Foley catheter in the presence of these clinical findings. Pelvic fractures in children are more likely to be unstable than in adults, tending to displace the urethra posteriorly. Complete posterior urethral disruption is more common in boys than in adult men. Prepubertal girls are four times more likely to have urethral injuries with pelvic fractures than women.

Treatment

Boys should be assessed with an RUG if there is suspicion of urethral injury. A 10-15 mL of contrast can be instilled by either Toomey syringe or appropriately sized Foley catheter with slightly expanded balloon placed at the urethral opening, with concomitant KUB taken during the instillation of contrast. If there is evidence of contrast extravasation, do not place an indwelling Foley catheter and consult a urologist emergently. See Figure 27–2 for an example of a positive RUG. In young girls procedural sedation may be necessary to allow vaginoscopy and cystoscopy, as the prepubescent

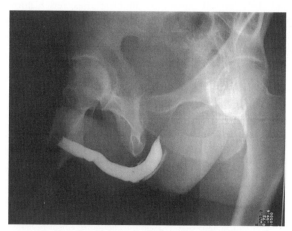

▲ **Figure 27–2.** Straddle injury to the male perineum, blood at the urethral meatus noted on examination. Example of a positive RUG with extravasation of contrast in the bulbous urethra indicating urethral injury. (Reproduced, with permission, from Stone CK, Humphries RL: *Current Diagnosis and Treatment Emergency Medicine*, 7th ed. New York: McGraw-Hill 2011. Copyright © McGraw-Hill Education LLC.)

female urethra is too short to permit retrograde urethroscopy. Patients with suspected urethral injury should receive a rectal examination to assess for blood, the position of the prostate in boys, and the integrity of the rectal mucosa. At least two-thirds of girls with urethral injury have a concomitant vaginal injury, which should be assessed during an emergent cystoscopy. At least one-third of urethral injuries in children are associated with concomitant rectal injuries.

Disposition

A multidisciplinary approach to patients with urethral injuries is essential, often involving the emergency department, surgery, urology, gynecology, and the operating room. All involved consultants should have experience and comfort in treating pediatric patients. Given the frequent association of urethral injuries with multiple system trauma, clinicians in community centers may pursue emergent transport to a trauma center after initial stabilization. For severe urethral disruption, the emergent placement of suprapubic cannula (or in infants, an emergent vesicostomy) may be prudent prior to transfer. Decisions about the emergent needs of patients with urinary diversion should be made in consultation with an appropriate receiving specialist. Antibiotics should be administered for common urinary pathogens, and immediate stabilization of concomitant injuries should not be delayed.

Brandes S: Initial management of anterior and posterior urethral injuries. *Urol Clin North Am.* 2006;33(1):87-95 [PMID: 16488283].

Pichler R, Fritsch H, Skradski V, et al: Diagnosis and management of pediatric urethral injuries. *Urol Int.* 2012;89:136-142 [PMID: 22433843].

Rosenstein DI, Alsikafi NF: Diagnosis and classification of urethral injuries. *Urol Clin North Am.* 2006;33(1):73-85 [PMID: 16488282].

BLADDER INJURY

Clinical Findings

Bladder injuries in children are relatively rare and are usually associated with concomitant abdomino-pelvic trauma. Direct blunt force to the full bladder results in rupture (Figure 27–3). Gross hematuria, the inability to void, and the presence of pelvic fractures should increase the clinician's index of suspicion for bladder injury. Urethral injury may be associated and should be evaluated as described in the Urethral Injury section of this chapter.

Treatment

Before evaluating for bladder injury and placement of Foley catheter, urethral injury should be excluded, including performance of an RUG if indicated. Approximate Foley

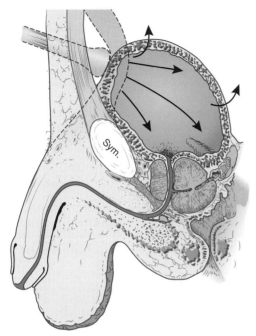

▲ **Figure 27–3.** Bladder injury mechanism: a direct strike to a full bladder increases pressure and results in intraperitoneal rupture. (Reproduced, with permission, from Tanagho EA, McAninch JW: *Smith's General Urology,* 17th ed. New York: McGraw-Hill, 2007. Copyright © McGraw-Hill Education LLC.)

catheter tube sizes are detailed in Table 27–2. After safely placing a Foley catheter and assessing for gross hematuria, a cystogram may be obtained. Use a contrast media such as gastrografin to instill at least one-half of estimated bladder

Table 27–2. Approximate Foley catheter size by age.

Age	Catheter size (French gauge)
Newborn	5 Fr
3 mo	8 Fr
1 y	8-10 Fr
3-6 y	10 Fr
8 y	10-12 Fr
10 y	12 Fr
12 y	12-14 Fr
Young teen	16 Fr
Adult	16-18 Fr

capacity under gravity. Estimated bladder capacity is calculated as follows.

$$\text{Bladder capacity in mL} = (\text{age} + 2) \times 30$$

Images of the cystogram may be obtained on a simple KUB, or a CT cystogram may be obtained. Evidence of clot "filling defects" and intraperitoneal or retroperitoneal extravasation should be assessed. Careful attention should be paid to identify bladder neck injuries, which are twice as likely in children compared with adults.

Disposition

Bladder injury indicates the need for admission or transfer to a trauma center. Absolute indications for surgical repair include urinary retention and the presence of significant pelvic fracture. Bladder neck injuries that are not surgically repaired may result in persistent urinary extravasation and incontinence. Absence of bladder neck injury can be managed with urine drainage and allowance of the bladder to heal expectantly.

Operative repair may be primary or consist of suprapubic drainage with delayed repair. Indications for surgery include significant nonclearing clot retention and perineal hematoma. Retroperitoneal bladder ruptures are managed conservatively with urinary drainage by Foley catheter or suprapubic drainage. Intraperitoneal ruptures are managed with primary surgical repair followed by urinary drainage. Antibiotics covering common urinary pathogens should be administered.

Delbert CM, Glassberg KI, Spencer BA: Repair of pediatric bladder rupture improves survival: Results from the national trauma data bank. *J Pediatr Surg.* 2012;47(9):1677-1681 [PMID: 22974605].

STRADDLE INJURIES

Clinical Findings

Straddle injuries are common in young boys and girls. These injuries generally occur when a child's anus, perineum, or vagina forcefully impacts a hard surface or when the structure is subject to shearing forces. Straddle injuries often cause considerable anxiety to both children and parents; however, most injuries heal without medical or surgical intervention. Straddle injuries most often occur in children younger than 10 years. Assault is the most common cause of injuries in children aged 0-4 years; falls and bicycle accidents cause most injuries in children aged 5-9 years; and motor vehicle accidents cause most injuries in children aged 15 years and older. Detailed history should include assessment for non-accidental trauma. The clinician must be especially concerned about the possibility of abuse in non-ambulatory children (see Chapter 5).

Careful examination of the patient is mandatory. It may be necessary to provide procedural sedation to allow adequate examination, both to relieve pain and patient anxiety. The anus, perineum, vulva, labia, posterior fourchette, hymen, vagina, and urethra must all be visualized. Many facilities employ forensic nursing teams to perform and document the examination in cases of suspected abuse.

Treatment

Abrasions and contusions to the vulva, labia, hymen, and perineum are common in straddle injuries. Unless injuries are large enough to impair urination, are expanding, or have caused hemodynamic instability or decreasing hemoglobin concentration, they generally require local wound care and minimal medical management. Small lacerations to the posterior fourchette, hymen, perineum, and vagina often require supportive therapy only. Lacerations with continued bleeding, large vaginal lacerations, hematoma formation about the urethra, urethral tears, and lacerations or tears through the rectum may require operative management.

Most straddle injuries heal well with no specific intervention; however, 8-15% will require operative management. If the patient does not meet requirements for operative management, symptomatic treatment with analgesia and sitz baths may be helpful, as well as reassurance to the patient's caregivers. Complex injuries may require antibiotic prophylaxis.

When in question about whether laceration repair or operative treatment may be required, consultation with a pediatric surgeon or pediatric gynecologist is recommended. It is advised to involve these specialists early, so that if sedation is needed for examination, the specialist may be able to complete both the examination and potential repair during a single sedation. In the patient with severe vaginal hemorrhage that is causing hemodynamic compromise, packing the vagina with Kerlix or a similar material may provide direct intravaginal pressure and may help to minimize the bleeding. As in all patients with severe hemorrhage, IV access as well as transfusion if necessary should not be delayed.

Disposition

Patients with suspected non-accidental trauma should be evaluated and dispositioned as described in Chapter 5. Continued bleeding and need for operative repair warrant admission. No antibiotic prophylaxis is required for most patients with straddle injuries.

Iqbal CW, Jrebi NY, Zielinski MD, et al: Patterns of accidental genital trauma in young girls and indications for operative management. *J Pediatr Surg.* 2010;45(5):930-933 [PMID: 20438929].

McCann J, Miyamoto S, Boyle C, et al: Healing of hymenal injuries in prepubertal and adolescent girls: A descriptive study. *Pediatrics.* 2007;119(5):e1094-1106 [PMID: 17420260].

Spitzer RF, Kives S, Caccia N, et al: Retrospective review of unintentional female genital trauma at a pediatric referral center. *Pediatr Emerg Care.* 2008;24(12):831-835 [PMID: 19050662].

Spinal Trauma

Mohamed Badawy, MD

MANAGEMENT OF PATIENTS WITH SUSPECTED SPINAL INJURY

Children who present to the emergency department with considerable trauma such as motor vehicle crash, motor vehicle-pedestrian accident, fall from high elevations, sports injuries, and/or neurologic complaints should alert the provider about the potential for spinal cord injury. Management of children with spinal injuries usually starts in the pre-hospital setting and begins with rapid cardiorespiratory resuscitation. Immobilization of the cervical spine must be provided immediately and maintained until evaluation and assessment is performed.

IMMOBILIZATION

Children with suspected spinal injuries should be immobilized on a spine board. The neck should be protected against unwanted movements with a rigid cervical collar and sandbags on the sides with tape across the forehead. Because of the relatively large size of the head compared with the torso in children, immobilization on a spine board may produce an undesirable flexion of the cervical spine. This can be avoided by elevating the torso on additional supports such as a thin mattress or blanket or using a spine board with a recess that allows the head to be lowered relative to the rest of the body. Spine boards are mainly used for extrication and transport to the emergency department, and should be removed once the primary survey is completed. Once in the emergency department, the rigid collar should be changed to a semi-rigid collar (Miami J, Aspen). Some pediatric patients with potential spinal column or cord injuries may present to the emergency department wearing a helmet (football or motorcycle). Using a two-person technique, the helmet should be removed extremely carefully with no movement of the cervical spine.

TECHNIQUE FOR MOVING THE PATIENT

In-line spinal stabilization and axial alignment should be maintained at all times. In order to remove the spine board, three assistants are usually needed. The first assistant holds the head and maintains C-spine stabilization and controls the turn. The second and third assistants stand on one side of the patient to maintain thoracic and lumbar spine alignments. The patient is log-rolled on a count of three. The physician then inspects and palpates the back of the head and the entire length of the spine and removes the board. If the patient will be transferred quickly to computed tomography (CT), a slider board can be introduced at the time the long board is removed, which will minimize patient motion. It is important to remember that immobilization on a backboard or slider board can result in pressure sores and unnecessary discomfort. In addition, rapid removal of the pediatric patient from the spine board is important because the board itself causes pain. Examination of the child who has lain on the spinal board for a prolonged period, will lead to unnecessary radiographic imaging of areas not injured, but are painful just by being immobilized on the hard spine board.

AIRWAY MANAGEMENT

When approaching the trauma patient, assume that an injury to the cervical spine is present. Cervical spine immobilization should be maintained at all times, including attempts to establish an airway The evaluation of the airway starts with a question to the patient to evaluate for response (airway patency), followed by direct visualization of the face and oropharynx. Breathing and adequate ventilation status is evaluated by visual examination of the trachea, thorax, chest expansion, and auscultation of all lung fields. Palpation of the chest can identify rib fractures, and subcutaneous air in the neck and the chest. Children with associated head injury and a Glasgow coma scale (GCS) score less than

9 may require emergent airway intervention. Injuries to the spinal cord above C3 require immediate airway management because of respiratory paralysis. Lower cervical injuries may result in phrenic nerve paralysis or increasing respiratory distress from ascending edema. In addition, injuries to the cervical spine may cause local edema, hematoma, and obstruction of the airway, which may necessitate prompt airway intervention.

Rapid sequence intubation (RSI) using standard drugs for induction paralysis is the preferred method. Manual in-line stabilization reduces cervical spine movement and minimizes potential injury to the spinal cord. This is usually achieved by an assistant who firmly holds both sides of the patient's head with the neck in the midline on a firm surface throughout the procedure. The front of the cervical collar can be removed to increase mouth opening and visualization by direct or indirect laryngoscopy, and should be replaced immediately after intubation is achieved.

Orotracheal intubation is preferred in trauma patients requiring intubation. Airway adjuncts such as a Bougie or stylet, video laryngoscope, or fiber optic bronchoscope may facilitate intubation and minimize airway manipulation. Alternative methods to orotracheal intubation include nasotracheal intubation, cricothyrotomy, laryngeal mask airway, and transtracheal jet insufflation. At minimum, 100% oxygen should be administered by means of a non-rebreather mask to maximize oxygen delivery. Continuous monitoring of respiratory status should continue with the help of pulse oximetry and capnography.

MAINTAINING ADEQUATE CIRCULATION

After airway management, the next step in trauma resuscitation is to maintain adequate hemodynamic support. Hypotension should not be attributed to neurogenic shock but rather to hypovolemic shock until proven otherwise. Regardless of the etiology of the hypotension, aggressive fluid resuscitation is necessary to prevent secondary injury that may result from reduced spinal cord perfusion.

Spinal cord injury resulting in neurogenic shock is defined as inadequate tissue perfusion caused by serious paralysis of vasomotor input below the level of the spinal cord injury. It is characterized by bradycardia and hypotension in contrast to hypovolemic shock that is characterized by tachycardia. This condition does not usually occur with spinal cord injury below the level of T6. It is more common in injuries above T6, secondary to the disruption of the sympathetic outflow from T1-L2 and to unopposed vagal tone. If left untreated, the systemic effects of neurogenic shock, such as ischemia of the spinal cord and other organs may exacerbate neuronal tissue damage. The goal is to maintain adequate tissue perfusion. If hypotension has not responded after fluid resuscitation and transfusion, pressor agents should be administered to maintain the mean arterial pressure in the desired range.

Table 28–1. Spinal cord injuries suspected by examination.

1. Head tilt is associated with a rotary subluxation of C1 on C2 or a high cervical injury.

2. Prayer position (arms folded across the chest) is a fracture in the C4-C6 area.

3. Paresis or paralysis of the arms/legs always suggests spinal injury.

4. Pins and needles sensation or numbness or burning (paresthesia) may indicate spinal injury.

5. Horner syndrome (ptosis and a miotic pupil) is associated with a cervical cord injury.

6. Priapism indicates that the sympathetic nervous system is involved. Priapism is present only in approximately 3-5% of spine-injured patients.

7. Absent Osinski reflex (absence of the bulbocavernosus reflex). Accompanied by flaccid paralysis, may indicate a poor prognosis. The test involves observing for anal sphincter contraction in response to squeezing the glans penis or tugging on an indwelling Foley catheter. This reflex is spinal mediated by and involves S2-S4. Typically this is one of the first reflexes to return after spinal shock.

Agents such as dobutamine, dopamine, or norepinephrine, with both α- and β-agonist properties, are preferred over pure α-agonists such as phenylephrine that can lead to reflex bradycardia. Norepinephrine should be considered first line.

EXAMINATION

Spinal cord injury is suspected in any multiple trauma; for example, significant trauma to the head, neck, or back; high-speed motor vehicle collisions, and falls from heights. Alert cooperative children may have complaint of localized pain to the involved vertebra. Otherwise, observation of the patient's position may indicate a spine injury (Table 28–1).

ROLE OF STEROIDS

Controversy exists currently concerning effectiveness of steroids in the management of acute spinal cord injury. Several studies titled National Acute Spinal Cord Injury Study (NASCIS) have investigated the effectiveness of pharmacologic intervention in spine injury. Based on these studies, recommendations were made to administer high-dose steroids for 24 hours if started within 3 hours of spinal cord injury. If steroids were begun between 3-8 hours post spinal trauma, they were continued for 48 hours. The cut off times of 8 hours and 3 hours were arbitrary. The beneficial effect of methylprednisolone compared with placebo was linked to a posthoc subgroup analysis. The gain in motor scores was at best marginal without any improvement in disability. Several authors theorize that the potential adverse effects of steroids were underemphasized in these studies. Currently, the American Association of Neurological Surgery, Canadian Association of Emergency Physicians, and American College of Surgery have revised their recommendation from routine use to a treatment option, stating "evidence suggesting harmful side effects is more consistent than any suggestion of clinical benefit from methylprednisolone use in the management of spinal cord injury." Furthermore, no children were involved in the NASCIS studies. Therefore routine use of steroids in spinal cord injury is not supported. Consultation with neurosurgical or orthopedic specialists is recommended. If chosen as a treatment, administer methylprednisolone as a 30 mg/kg bolus over 15 minutes, followed by a maintenance infusion of 5.4 mg/kg/hour, for 24 hours if started within 3 hours, or 48 hours if started 3-8 hours after the injury. Steroids have no role in penetration of spinal injuries.

ANATOMY/PHYSIOLOGY

Patterns of spinal injury in children can be explained by their changing anatomy. In children younger than 8 years, cervical fractures occur from the occiput to C2 (Table 28–2).

American College of Surgeons Committee on Trauma: *Advanced Trauma Life Support for Doctors Student Course Manual*, 8th ed. Chicago, Illinois;2008.

Avarello JT, Cantor RM: Pediatric major trauma: An approach to evaluation and management. *Emerg Med Clin North Am.* 2007;25:803-836 [PMID: 17826219].

Table 28–2. Anatomical explanations for pediatric cervical spinal injuries.

Larger and heavier head in relation to body height and weight
Fulcrum at C2-3 in children vs C5-6 in adolescents and adults
Weak neck muscles
More elasticity and laxity of the spinal column ligaments and joint capsules
Intervertebral disc and annulus can stretch longitudinally ($\geq$ 2 in) without rupture
Horizontal orientation of facet joints
Physiologic anterior wedging of vertebral bodies in infants and young children
Incomplete ossification of the odontoid process
Uncinate process of the adult vertebrae (restrict lateral and rotational motion) is absent in children < 10 yr

Boswell K, Menaker J: An update on spinal cord injury: Epidemiology, diagnosis, and treatment for the emergency physician. *Trauma Reports.* 2013;14(1):1-11.

Kenefake ME, Swarm M, Wlathall J: Nuances in pediatric trauma. *Emerg Med Clin North Am.* 2013;31:627-652 [PMID: 23915597].

Leonard JC: Cervical spine injury. *Pediatr Clin North Am.* 2013;60:1123-1137 [PMID: 24093899].

Vogel LC, Hickey KJ, Klaas SJ, Anderson CJ: Unique issues in pediatric spinal cord injury. *Orthop Nurs.* 2004;23(5):300-308 [PMID: 15554466].

ASSESSMENT & CLASSIFICATION OF SPINAL CORD INJURY

Evaluation of children with spinal cord injury includes assessment of mental status, cranial nerves, motor and sensory functions. The American Spinal Injury Association (ASIA) published the International Standards for Neurological and Functional Classification of Spinal Cord Injury (ISNCSCI) to assess sensory and motor deficits following spinal cord injury (Figure 28–1). Classification is based on neurological responses: touch and pinprick sensations tested in each dermatome, and strength of the muscles of 10 key motions on both sides of the body, including elbow flexors (C5), wrist extensors (C6), elbow extensors (C7), finger flexors (C8), finger abductors (little finger) (T1), hip flexors (L2), knee extensors (L3), ankle dorsiflexors (L4), long toe extensors (L5), and ankle plantar (S1). Traumatic spinal cord injury is classified in five categories (A-E) on the ASIA Impairment Scale (AIS).

A = Complete. No sensory or motor function is preserved in the sacral segments S4-5.

B = Sensory incomplete. Sensory but not motor function is preserved below the neurological level and includes the sacral segments S4-5 (light touch or pin prick at S4-5 or deep anal pressure) *and* no motor function is preserved more than three levels below the motor level on either side of the body.

C = Motor incomplete. Motor function is preserved below the neurological level, and more than one-half of key muscle functions below the neurological level of injury (NLI) have a muscle grade less than 3 (grades 0-2).

D = Motor incomplete. Motor function is preserved below the neurological level and at least one-half (one-half or more) of key muscle functions below the NLI have a muscle grade at or greater than 3.

E = Normal. If sensation and motor function as tested with ISNCSCI are graded as normal in all segments, and the patient had prior deficits, the AIS grade is E. An individual without an initial SCI does not receive an AIS grade.

Patient Name _____   Date/Time of Exam _____

Examiner Name _____

AMERICAN SPINAL INJURY ASSOCIATION

INTERNATIONAL STANDARDS FOR NEUROLOGICAL
CLASSIFICATION OF SPINAL CORD INJURY

ISCOS

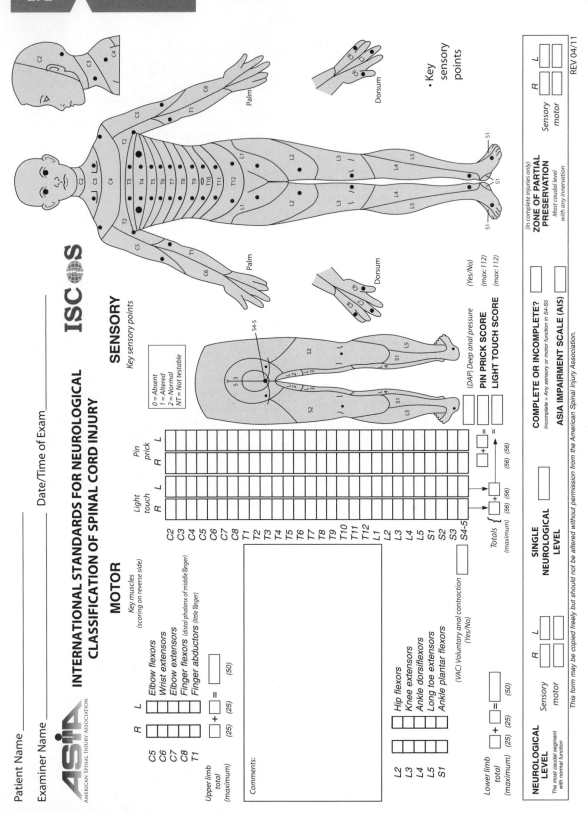

MOTOR

Key muscles
(scoring on reverse side)

	R	L
C5		Elbow flexors
C6		Wrist extensors
C7		Elbow extensors
C8		Finger flexors *(distal phalanx of middle finger)*
T1		Finger abductors *(little finger)*

Upper limb total
(maximum)   __ + __ = __
             (25) (25) (50)

Comments:

	R	L	Hip flexors
L2			Hip flexors
L3			Knee extensors
L4			Ankle dorsiflexors
L5			Long toe extensors
S1			Ankle plantar flexors

(VAC) Voluntary anal contraction __
(Yes/No)

Lower limb total
(maximum)   __ + __ = __
             (25) (25) (50)

SENSORY

Key sensory points

0 = Absent
1 = Altered
2 = Normal
NT = Not testable

• Key sensory points

Light touch | **Pin prick**
R L | R L

C2, C3, C4, C5, C6, C7, C8, T1, T2, T3, T4, T5, T6, T7, T8, T9, T10, T11, T12, L1, L2, L3, L4, L5, S1, S2, S3, S4-5

Totals { __ + __ } = __   __ + __ = __
        (56)(56) (max:112) (56)(56)

(maximum)

(DAP) Deep anal pressure (Yes/No)

PIN PRICK SCORE (max: 112) __

LIGHT TOUCH SCORE (max: 112) __

NEUROLOGICAL LEVEL

The most caudal segment with normal function

	R	L
Sensory		
motor		

SINGLE NEUROLOGICAL LEVEL

__

COMPLETE OR INCOMPLETE?

Incomplete = Any sensory or motor function in S4-S5

__

ZONE OF PARTIAL PRESERVATION

(In complete injuries only)

Most caudal level with any innervation

	R	L
Sensory		
motor		

ASIA IMPAIRMENT SCALE (AIS)

__

REV 04/11

This form may be copied freely but should not be altered without permission from the American Spinal Injury Association.

Muscle Function Grading

0 = Total paralysis

1 = Palpable or visible contraction

2 = Active movement, full range of motion (ROM) with gravity eliminated

3 = Active movement, full ROM against gravity

4 = Active movement, full ROM against gravity and moderate resistance in a muscle specific position.

5 = (Normal) active movement, full ROM against gravity and full resistance in a muscle specific position expected from an otherwise unimpaired person.

5* = (Normal) active movement, full ROM against gravity and sufficient resistance to be considered normal if identified inhibiting factors (i.e. pain, disuse) were not present.

NT = Not testable (i.e. due to immobilization, severe pain such that the patient cannot be graded, amputation of limb, or contracture of > 50% of the range of motion).

ASIA Impairment (AIS) Scale

☐ **A = Complete.** No sensory or motor function is preserved in the sacral segments S4-S5.

☐ **B = Sensory incomplete.** Sensory but not motor function is preserved below the neurological level and includes the sacral segments S4-S5 (light touch, pin prick at S4-S5; or deep and pressure (DAP)), AND no motor function is preserved more than three levels below the motor level on either side of the body.

☐ **C = Motor incomplete.** Motor function is preserved below the neurological level**, and more than half of key muscle functions below the single neurological level of injury (NLI) have a muscle grade less than 3 (Grades 0-2).

☐ **D = Motor incomplete.** Motor function is preserved below the neurological level**, and at least half (half or more) of key muscle functions below the NLI have a muscle grade ≥ 3.

☐ **E = Normal.** If sensation and motor function as tested with the ISNCSCI are graded as normal in all segments, and the patient had prior deficits, then the AIS grade is E. Someone without an initial SCI does not receive an AIS grade.

**For an individual to receive a grade of C or D, i.e. motor incomplete status, they must have either (1) voluntary anal sphincter contraction or (2) sacral sensory sparing with sparing of motor function more than three levels below the motor level for that side of the body. The Standards at this time allows even non-key muscle function more than 3 levels below the motor level to be used in determining motor incomplete status (AIS B versus C).

NOTE: When assessing the extent of motor sparing below the level for distinguishing between AIS B and C, the **motor level** on each side is used; whereas to differentiate between AIS C and D (based on proportion of key muscle functions with strength grade 3 or greater) the **single neurological level** is used.

Steps in Classification

The following order is recommended in determining the classification of individuals with SCI:

1. Determine sensory levels for right and left sides.

2. Determine motor levels for right and left sides.
   Note: *In regions where there is no myotome to test, the motor level is presumed to be the same as the sensory level, if testable motor function above that level is also normal.*

3. Determine the single neurological level.
   This is the lowest segment where motor and sensory function is normal on both sides, and is the most cephalad of the sensory and motor levels determined in steps 1 and 2.

4. Determine whether the injury is complete or incomplete.
   (i.e. absence or presence of sacral sparing)
   If voluntary anal contraction = No AND all S4-5 sensory scores = 0 AND deep anal pressure = No, then injury is COMPLETE. Otherwise injury is incomplete.

5. Determine ASIA Impairment Scale (AIS) Grade:

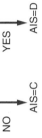

Is injury Complete? If **YES**, AIS=A and can record ZPP (lowest dermatome or myotome on each side with some preservation)

NO

Is injury motor Incomplete? If **NO**, AIS=B
(Yes=voluntary anal contraction OR motor function more than three levels below the motor level on a given side, if the patient has sensory incomplete classification)

YES

Are at least half of the key muscles below the single neurological level graded 3 or better?

NO → AIS=C   YES → AIS=D

If sensation and motor function is normal in all segments, AIS = E
Note: *AIS E is used in follow-up testing when an individual with a documented SCI has recovered normal function. If at initial testing no deficits are found, the individual is neurologically intact; the ASIA Impairment Scale does not apply.*

▲ **Figure 28–1.** International standards for neurological and functional classification of spinal cord injury. (From American Spinal Injury Association. International Standards for Neurological Classification of Spinal Cord Injury. Atlanta, 2011.)

Kirshblum SC, Burns SP, Biering-Sorensen F, et al: International standards for neurological classification of spinal cord injury (revised 2011). *J Spinal Cord Med*. 2011;34:535-546 [PMID: 22330108].

GENERAL CONCEPTS: IMAGING IN SPINAL TRAUMA

If a pediatric patient has a spinal column injury at one level, there is approximately 11-34% chance that additional injuries exist in other areas of the spinal column and a 6-7% chance of injury in a noncontiguous area. For this reason, plain radiographs of the entire spine are necessary when a spinal injury is noted. In general, CT should not be used as a screening tool for spinal trauma in pediatric patients. The dose of radiation delivered to the thyroid gland is a major concern. If fractures are identified on plain radiography, CT can be used to identify the extent of bony injuries. If spinal cord injury is suspected, MRI is the test of choice.

CERVICAL SPINE IMAGING

Plain Radiographs

Three-view spine series (cross table lateral, anteroposterior (AP), and open mouth odontoid) have been traditionally used to screen for cervical spine injuries. Approximately 80% of cervical spine injuries can be identified on lateral views. Obtaining AP and odontoid views, when possible, increase the sensitivity of plain radiographs to detect cervical spine injuries (92-99%).

Lateral views are not considered adequate unless the seven cervical vertebrae and the superior aspect of T1 are visualized. If the C7-T1 portion is not seen, techniques such as pulled arms, or swimmer's view can be attempted to obtain adequate lateral images. The physician should follow the acronym ABCS to interpret cervical spine images: **A**, alignment of the vertebral bodies and the posterior cervical line; **B**, bones should be assessed for height, contour, and fracture; **C**, cartilage or disc spaces for anterior or posterior widening and any loss of height; **S**, soft tissue should be assessed such as predental space and prevertebral soft tissue space at C3. The predental space, which is the space between the posterior surface of the anterior arch of C1 and the anterior surface of the odontoid process (C2), should be less than 4 mm in children younger than 8 years and less than or as great as 3 mm in older children and adults. Measurement of the prevertebral soft tissue can be inaccurate and is particularly difficult in crying children. The prevertebral space should be no more than one-third of the anteroposterior diameter of the vertebral body at C3 in children younger than 8 years or 7 mm in older children and adults.

The AP view should be assessed for alignment of the spinous processes' tips and symmetry of the vertebral bodies. The open mouth odontoid view should be assessed for fractures and misalignment of the lateral mass of C1 and C2.

The usefulness of open mouth odontoid views, in the evaluation of young children with suspected cervical spine injury, has been questioned by several authors. Open mouth images require cooperation and can be difficult to obtain in young children. A multi-institutional retrospective review of cervical spine injuries in children younger than 16 years revealed 51 children with C-spine injuries. Lateral radiographs of 13/15 children younger than 9 years revealed the injury. The odontoid view did not add more information in these 15 patients. In only 1 of 36 patients 9 years or older was the odontoid view diagnostic and revealed grade III odonoid fracture. The authors concluded that odontoid views are not necessary to clear cervical spine injuries in children younger than 9 years.

Flexion-extension (FE) films have been advocated previously to assess ligamentous injuries. However, their utility has been questioned recently. Ligamentous injuries are very rare without bony fractures. In the National Emergency X-Radiography Use Study (NEXUS), FE films added little value to the acute evaluation of patients with blunt trauma. There were 818 spine injuries in 34,069 patients. Two of 818 patients had stable bony injuries that were detected only with flexion-extension images. Four of 818 patients had subluxation detected on flexion extension views; however, all had other injuries clearly shown on the routine three views (lateral, AP, and odontoid views).

Cervical Spine Clearance

Decision rules have been developed to guide the use of cervical spine radiography in patients with trauma. The most widely used is NEXUS, designed to identify patients who do not need radiographic imaging to exclude a clinically significant cervical spine injury. The study uses five low-risk criteria, which are the *absence of*

1. Cervical tenderness,

2. Evidence of intoxication,

3. Altered level of alertness,

4. Focal neurological deficit, and

5. Painful distracting injury.

At the discretion of the treating physician, x-rays were obtained. When x-rays were obtained, three views were ordered: lateral, AP, and odontoid. Of 3065 children evaluated, 603 fulfilled low-risk criteria, and none had a radiographic abnormality by x-ray. Thirty injuries (0.80%) were identified in children who did not fulfill low-risk criteria. The authors concluded that using NEXUS criteria for the evaluation of cervical spine injury in children would reduce imaging by 20% and would not result in missed injuries.

Frohna W: Emergency department evaluation and treatment of the neck and cervical spine injuries. *Emerg Med Clin North Am.* 1999;17:739-791 [PMID: 10584102].

Hoffman JR, Mower WR, Wolfson AB, et al: Validity of a set of clinical criteria to rule out injury to the cervical spine in patients with blunt trauma. National Emergency X-Radiography Utilization Study Group. *N Engl J Med.* 2000;343:94-99 [PMID: 10891516].

Pollack CV Jr, Hendey GW, Martin DR, Hoffman JR, Mower WR; NEXUS Group: Use of flexion-extension radiographs of the cervical spine in blunt trauma. *Ann Emerg Med.* 2001;38:8-11 [PMID: 11423804].

Viccellio P, Simon H, Pressman BD, et al: NEXUS Group. A prospective multicenter study of cervical spine injury in children. *Pediatrics.* 2001;108:E20 [PMID: 10584102].

ADJUNCT IMAGING STUDIES

COMPUTED TOMOGRAPHY

Computed tomography (CT) is not routinely used in the initial evaluation of spine injuries in children. The CT scan delivers a significant amount of radiation compared with plain films. Children, specifically those younger than 5 years, are particularly sensitive to radiation exposure and have longer time during which malignancies can develop. Although CT has a very high sensitivity, as high as 98%, to detect bony injuries, it is not ideal to detect ligamentous injuries that are more common in children than in adults. CT should be obtained in the following situations: inadequate plain films, suspicious findings on plain films such as fracture and/ or dislocation, and high index of suspicion despite normal plain films. CT is particularly useful to examine areas of the cervical spine that are commonly missed and frequently injured in children, such as the occipitoatlantal and cervicothoracic junctions. Limited CT can be used in conjunction with plain radiographs to reduce radiation exposure. CT may detect injuries not readily apparent on plain radiographs. Thin-cut sections (2-3 mm) with sagittal and coronal three-dimensional reconstruction are recommended and should be tailored to the plain radiographic findings.

Because children are more likely than adults to suffer ligamentous injury, CT scanning in children younger than 8 years may have limited benefit. Magnetic resonance imaging (MRI) best assesses spinal cord, disc, and ligamentous disruption. MRI can also detect soft tissue injury and hematoma not visualized by other imaging modalities.

MAGNETIC RESONANCE IMAGING

Magnetic resonance imaging (MRI) is the imaging of choice in evaluation of the patient with neurological symptoms and signs whose plain films are normal. MRI is superior to CT in identification of ligamentous injuries, intervertebral disc herniation, cord edema and/or hemorrhage. Discrimination of cord hemorrhage from cord edema has an important prognostic factor as cord edema resolves, whereas cord hemorrhage is associated with poor outcome. MRI is especially helpful in evaluating C-spine injuries in uncooperative, comatose or unconscious patients to rule out C-spine injuries thereby allowing for the safe removal of cervical collar. Children require sedation for MRI studies; therefore, coordination of care with anesthesiologists and pediatric critical care specialists is important to obtain imaging results in a timely fashion.

Condition of the spinal cord on MRI is predictive of neurologic outcome. Spinal cord transection and major hemorrhage are associated with poor outcome and significant neurologic sequelae. Minor hemorrhage or edema is associated with moderate to good recovery. The absence of an abnormal signal is associated with full recovery.

Reynolds R: Pediatric spinal injury. *Curr Opin Pediatr.* 2000;12:67-71 [PMID: 10676777].

Slotkin J, Lu Y, Wood KB: Thoracolumbar spinal trauma in children. *Neurosurg Clin N Am.* 2007;18(4):621-630 [PMID: 17991587].

Sundgren PC, Philipp M, Maly PV: Spinal trauma. *Neuroimaging Clin N Am.* 2007;17:73-85 [PMID: 17493540].

SYNDROMES OF SPINAL CORD INJURY

It is important for the physician to classify the pattern of neurologic deficit into one of the cord syndromes. In most clinical situations, the physician may use a best fit model to describe the spinal cord injury syndrome.

Clinical presentation of complete spinal cord injuries depends on the level of the injury. A high cervical injury results in cessation of breathing, quadriplegia with upper and lower extremity areflexia, loss of sphincter tone, and anesthesia caused by neurogenic shock. If the injury affects the lower cervical region, the patient's respiratory function is preserved. High thoracic injuries result in paraplegia with preservation of the functions of upper extremities and breathing. Lesions above the T6 spinal cord level can result in autonomic dysreflexia. Lower thoracic and lumbosacral injuries present with bladder and bowel dysfunction.

Incomplete cord syndromes have variable neurologic findings with partial loss of motor and/or sensory functions below the level of the traumatic injury, including anterior cord syndrome, central cord syndrome, and Brown-Sequard syndrome.

Anterior cord syndrome (Figure 28–2) results from compression or disruption of the anterior spinal artery, direct compression of the anterior cord, or compression by fragments from burst fractures. The syndrome is characterized by complete motor paralysis below the level of the injury, and/or loss of pain and temperature sensation with preservation of proprioception.

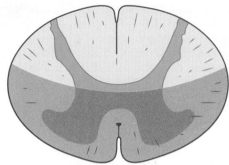

▲ **Figure 28–2.** Anterior cord syndrome.

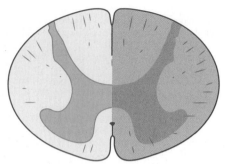

▲ **Figure 28–4.** Brown-Sequard syndrome.

Central cord syndrome (Figure 28–3), induced by damage to the corticospinal tract, is characterized by greater motor weakness in the upper rather than in the lower extremities, with sacral sensory sparing. In the affected extremities, motor weakness is more profound in the distal than in the proximal group of muscles. Sensory loss can be variable. Patients are more likely to lose pain and/or temperature sensation than proprioception.

Brown-Sequard syndrome (Figure 28–4) is characterized by ipsilateral paralysis and loss of proprioception, with contralateral loss of pain and temperature sensation. Symptoms and signs result from hemisection of the spinal cord, most often from penetrating trauma or compression from a lateral fracture.

CERVICAL SPINE INJURIES

ATLANTO-OCCIPITAL DISLOCATION

Atlanto-occipital dislocation (AOD) is a frequently fatal injury that occurs in high-energy trauma. Children are particularly susceptible to this injury because of their large head-to-body size ratio and the immature osseous and musculoligamentous components of their growing cervical spine. Children aged

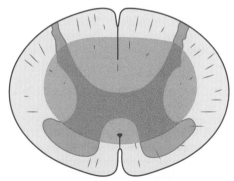

▲ **Figure 28–3.** Central cord syndrome.

5-9 years are more likely to be diagnosed with this injury. Two common mechanisms that cause pediatric AOD are unrestrained occupant in a motor vehicle collision with ejection, and pedestrian struck by a motor vehicle. Injuries to the upper cervical spinal cord are common when AOD occurs and patients who survive the injury are often left with permanent neurologic deficits. Because of the high-energy mechanism, other injuries are common in patients with AOD, including traumatic brain injury, thoracoabdominal, and skeletal injuries. AOD can occur in one of three ways: type 1 occurs with anterior displacement of the occiput over the atlas (C1), type II is longitudinal distraction, and type III is posterior displacement of the occiput over C1. For patients who survive, hydrocephalus is a complication that occurs commonly. The lateral C-spine is the most useful view to diagnose AOD (Figure 28–5).

Astur N, Klimo P, Sawyer J, et al: Traumatic atlanto-occipital dislocation in children. *J Bone and Joint Surg.* 2013;9(24):e194(1-8) [PMID: 24352780].

C1 Injury

This cervical spine injury, also known as Jefferson fracture, is very uncommon in children. It results from axial loading causing fractures in the ring of the first cervical spine in two to four places and is frequently associated with head injury and/or fracture of C2. This fracture can be detected in an odontoid view of the cervical spine which manifests as displacement of the lateral mass of C1 over the lateral mass of C2. A CT scan is more sensitive imaging than plain radiographs for the diagnosis of these fractures.

C2 Injury

▶ Atlanto-Axial Rotatory Displacement

Atlanto-axial rotatory displacement is one of the most common causes of childhood torticollis; however, diagnosis is commonly delayed or missed. Onset may be spontaneous or

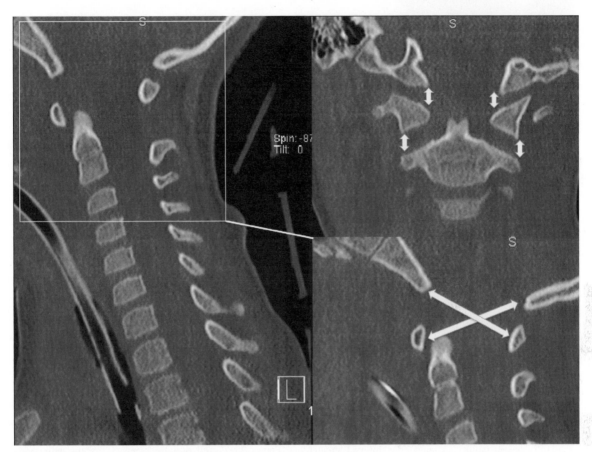

▲ **Figure 28–5.** Atlanto-occipital dislocation in 5½-year-old female pedestrian struck by a car. Severe craniocervical junction injury; abnormal widening of the craniocervical junction (diagonal arrows and upper vertical arrows) as well as the space between C1 and C2 (lower vertical arrows).

may follow an upper respiratory tract infection or may rarely be caused by minor or major trauma. The torticollis position is typically similar to that of a robin listening to a worm with its head cocked and flexed. The child's head is tilted to one side and rotated to the opposite side with slight flexion. The child resists attempts to move the head with associated muscle spasm. Neurologic examination is usually normal.

Rotatory displacement of C1 over C2 is often difficult to identify radiographically, due to difficulty in positioning the child because of pain and rotational deformity. Diagnosis is best conducted with dynamic CT scans. The CT is done with neck turned as far right as possible and then compared with CT scan of the neck turned as far left as possible. If the relationship between C1 and C2 vertebrae is unchanged, rotatory displacement has occurred.

Treatment of atlanto-axial rotatory displacement must be tailored to the degree of the severity of the individual patient. Many patients benefit from conservative therapy

such as the administration of nonsteroidal anti-inflammatory drugs or muscle relaxants and use of a soft collar or hard cervical collar. Some patients may need Halter traction, cervico-thoracic orthotics, or halo traction. Studies have shown that the duration of symptoms before treatment is an important factor in determining the response to more conservative treatment.

▶ Odontoid Fracture & Associated Ligamentous Injury

Odontoid fracture is the most common fracture of C2 (axis) that may result from blunt trauma to the head leading to cervical hyperextension or hyperflexion. The fracture must not be confused with the normal anatomic variations in the odontoid due to synchondrosis between the body of the axis and the odontoid, seen in children as old as 7 years. The displacement may be anterior (hyperflexion) or posterior

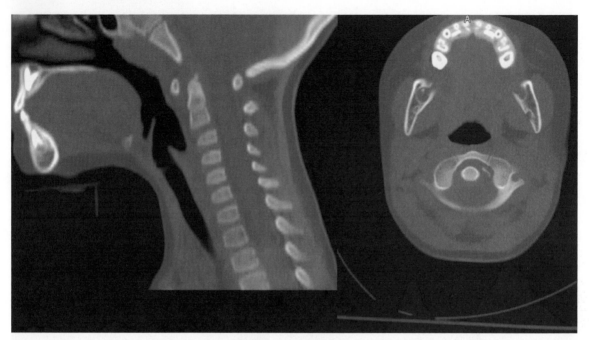

▲ **Figure 28–6.** C2 transverse ligament fracture in a 3-year-old female unrestrained front seat passenger who struck the windshield sustaining an avulsion fracture of the left tubercle of the lateral mass of C1 at the attachment site of the transverse ligament. There is also widening of the anterior atlantoaxial distance.

(hyperextension). Posterior displacement of the odontoid (dens) is associated with transverse atlantal ligament failure and atlantoaxial instability. Atlanto-dens interval greater than 5 mm suggests transverse atlantal ligament injury (Figure 28–6). There are three types of odontoid fracture: Type I is avulsion fracture of the tip of the dens; type II fracture is the most common of the three and is localized to the waist of the dens. Because of interruption of blood supply, the fracture is associated with a high nonunion rate; type III fracture extends into the body of C2. Most patients are managed conservatively with halo immobilization.

The odontoid is separated from the body of C2 by a cartilaginous line that represents growth plate. The epiphyseal line is present in most children at 3 years of age, 50% of children at 4 years of age, and closed by 6 years of age. The presence of the basilar odontoid growth plate may result in a false impression of fracture of the base of the odontoid process. However, most fractures occur at the base of the odontoid, whereas the epiphyseal line lies lower within the body of the axis.

▶ **Hangman Fracture**

Hangman fracture occurs as a hyperextension injury in association with sudden axial loading, as is achieved in judicial hanging. The injury can occur through the synchondroses

between the odontoid and the arch of C2. The fracture can be detected by plain films of the cervical spine lateral view (Figure 28–7) and odontoid view. CT scans with sagittal reconstructions or MRI is very helpful for diagnosis.

▶ **Pseudosubluxation of C2 on C3**

Physiological motion of the cervical vertebrae in children is greater than that in adults, and normal pediatric cervical spine may appear to have a subluxation. When a subluxation is not present, the movement is referred to as pseudosubluxation and does not need treatment. Pseudosubluxation of C2 on C3 may occur in up to 40 % of children younger than 8 years and may persist up to 16 years of age. Pseudosubluxation of C3 on C4 may also occur but is far less common than C2 on C3. Causes of pseudosubluxation seen only in children are ligamentous laxity, relative horizontal configuration of the facet joints, and the anterior wedged configuration of the growing vertebral bodies. The differentiation of pseudosubluxation from true injury can be aided by the use of Swischuk line (Figure 28–8), which is drawn along the posterior arch (the spinolaminar line) from the first cervical vertebra to the third. The line should pass within 1.5 mm of the posterior arch of the second cervical vertebra. When a fracture is present, the line is disrupted. As children grow, most achieve the adult configuration, and the pseudosubluxation disappears.

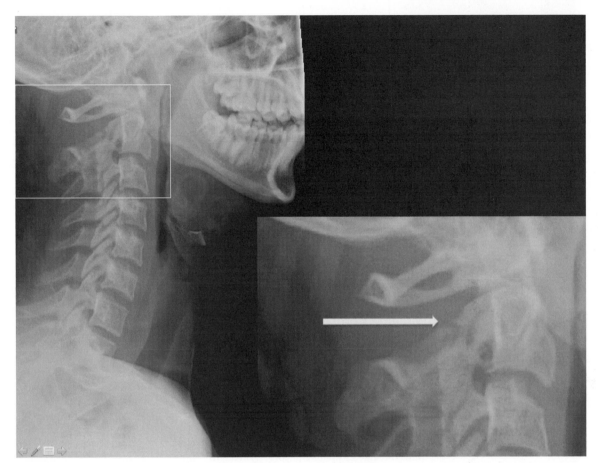

▲ **Figure 28–7.** Hangman fracture in a 13-year-old female involved in a motor vehicle collision who was neurologically intact with complaint of severe neck pain. Note the lucency at the lamina of C2 (white arrow) demonstrating bilateral laminar fractures; additional findings include widening of the interspinous distance at C1-C2 and mild anterolisthesis of C2 on C3.

C3-C7 Fractures

Lower cervical injuries in children are less common than in adults (Figure 28–9). They are usually ligamentous injuries and are thus difficult to recognize without MRI.

THORACIC FRACTURES

COMPRESSION FRACTURES

Because of the immature musculature, wedge shape of the thoracic spine, and the normal kyphosis, compression fractures are the most common injury pattern seen in children with thoracic spine injuries. Axial loading and hyperflexion mechanisms, such as football injuries, falls, and diving rather than hyperextension mechanisms or dislocation injuries,

more often result in compression of the vertebral body. Compression fractures are usually simple and require no specific treatment other than pain control.

SHEAR FRACTURES

Shear fractures are usually associated with more violent mechanisms than those observed with compression fractures. They cause fractures through the cartilaginous end plates, which when coupled with distraction injuries, may result in spinal cord injuries because of stretching.

BURST FRACTURES

Burst fractures in children usually occur at the thoracolumbar junction and can include the annular epiphysis and the intervertebral disc. In young children, burst fractures can

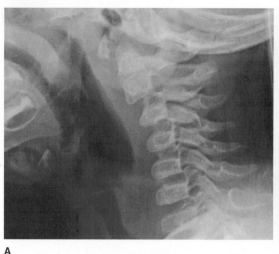 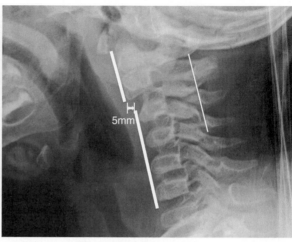

A   B

▲ **Figure 28–8, A and B.** Pseudosubluxation of the pediatric spine demonstrated in this lateral C-spine of a 15 month-old female toddler was restrained in a rear-facing child seat when her vehicle was involved in a collision. She had no loss of consciousness but sustained a laceration to her forehead. Radiograph showed 5 mm of anterolisthesis of C2 on C3 (thick lines). The spinolaminar line (thin line) demonstrates good alignment of the posterior elements of C1, 2, and 3.

also damage the germinative layer which may result in premature epiphyseal fusion. Burst fractures are identified by a combination of a wedge compression of the anterior column with propulsion of fractured bony fragments into the spinal canal (Figure 28–10). On plain films, burst fractures may be misdiagnosed as stable compression fractures. Therefore, in patients with significant blunt trauma to the spine and/or high clinical suspicion CT scans are often ordered to evaluate abnormalities in the thoraco-lumbar spine. Reformatted images from standard CT studies of the chest and abdomen are sufficient to assess for spine injuries and have been shown to have a superior sensitivity in detecting spine injuries compared with plain films.

LUMBAR SPINE INJURIES

SEAT BELT INJURY

Chance fracture is a form of flexion distraction injury and is one of the most commonly reported lumbar spine injuries in children. It may result from the inappropriately applied lap seat belt across the abdominal wall and can be associated with severe abdominal trauma such as contusions and/or lacerations of the pancreas, duodenum, and mesentery. A classic presentation of this injury would be that of a child, who was injured in a motor vehicle collision and who was inappropriately restrained with a lap belt across the abdomen. Such a patient may have ecchymosis across the abdominal wall ("seat belt" sign) and tenderness along

the lumbar spine raising the suspicion for lumbar spine injury and intra-abdominal injuries. Intra-abdominal injuries are relatively common (noted in 1/3 of Chance fracture patients in some series). Such injuries result from the sudden forward propulsion of the upper portion of the body while the lower abdomen is harnessed by the lap belt. The spinal column elasticity in children is greater than that of the spinal cord. Distraction of the posterior and middle spinal columns may occur over the lap belt during rapid deceleration. The anterior spinal column may or may not be injured depending on the distance of displacement from the anterior surface of the vertebral body.

Plain films are often used to evaluate lumbar spine injuries. On lateral films, a fracture can be seen through the spinous process, lamina, pedicles and portion of the vertebral body. Lamina fractures can be also demonstrated on AP views. In addition, CT scans of the abdomen and pelvis with reconstruction images of the spine are frequently ordered because of the high association between Chance fractures and internal abdominal injuries (Figure 28–11).

SLIPPED VERTEBRAL APOPHYSIS

Slipped vertebral apophysis injuries most commonly occur in adolescent boys and are often associated with disc protrusions. These most commonly occur at L4 but may also occur at L3 or L5 and may result from a single traumatic event or cumulative injuries in sports such as weightlifting, gymnastics, or wrestling.

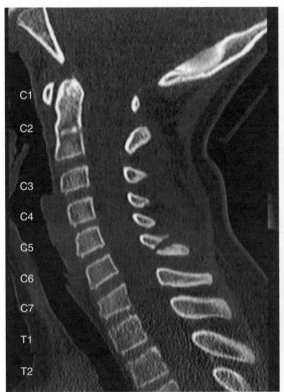 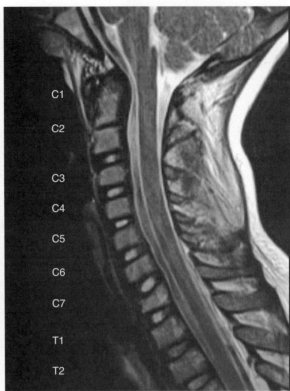

A   B

▲ **Figure 28–9.** (**A**) CT reconstruction lateral cervical spine demonstrating compression fracture and spinous process fracture from motor vehicle collision flexion injury in a 9½-year-old boy. There is a displaced and distracted fracture involving the C6 spinous process (although not visualized, this fracture extends into the lamina on left side). Also not visualized in these images, the C6-C7 facet joints show mild widening, especially on right side with uncovering of the superior facet of the C7. There is associated widening of the C6-C7 disc space with anterior compression deformity of C7 vertebral body. Findings are compatible with a hyperflexion injury of the cervical spine. (**B**) MRI demonstrating compression fracture and spinous process fracture. A 20-30% compression deformity superior aspect of the vertebral body at C7. No traumatic injury at the C6-C7 disc.

SPINAL CORD INJURY WITHOUT RADIOGRAPHIC ABNORMALITY

Spinal cord injury is most often associated with radiographic findings such as fractures, ligamentous injuries, or subluxations. However, a spinal cord injury can occur without radiographic abnormalities. Spinal cord injury without radiographic abnormality (SCIWORA) was first described by Pang and Willberger in 1982. With SCIWORA, symptoms may not be present initially but may be delayed up to 48 hours after the initial injury. Associated symptoms in SCIWORA patients include weakness, numbness, paresthesias, or an electric "shock-like" sensation in the extremities.

MRI is indicated to differentiate cord edema from hemorrhage as well as to assess ligamentous injury.

SCIWORA originally referred to spinal cord injury without radiographic or CT scanning evidence of fracture or dislocation. However, with advent of MRI and its widespread application and availability, the term has become ambiguous, because most patients have radiographic abnormality of the soft tissues (ligaments and spinal cord) detectable on MRI. The proper term should be spinal cord injury without *bony* radiographic abnormality. Although SCIWORA was initially described in children, it is now found to occur in adults. Based on the database of NEXUS, of the 34,069 patients enrolled, there were 818 (2.4%) with cervical spine

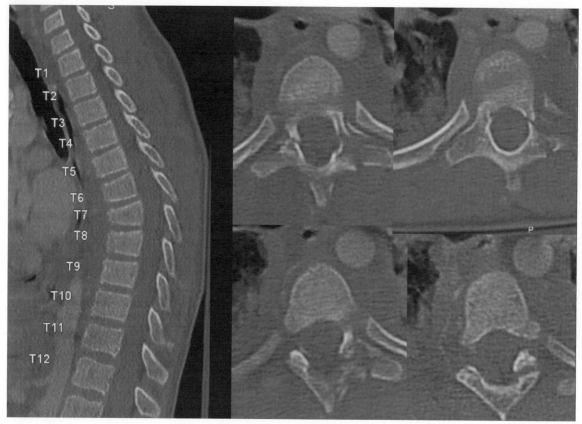

▲ **Figure 28–10.** Burst fracture in a 10-year-old unrestrained female in a motor vehicle collision who was ejected from the vehicle; burst type fracture of T7 with extension into the bilateral pedicles, transverse processes, and spinous process. Patient did not have a spinal cord injury and was treated with bracing.

injury, including 27 (0.08%) adult patients with SCIWORA. The most common abnormalities seen on MRI among SCIWORA patients were central disc herniation, spinal stenosis, and cord edema or contusion. As the pediatric spinal column takes on more and more adult morphology, SCIWORA of the upper cervical cord is very rare in children older than 9 years.

TRANSIENT QUADRIPARESIS & STINGERS

Patients with transient quadriparesis (TQ) will have complaint of neurological symptoms in two to four limbs. Symptoms include weakness, paralysis, and sensory complaints including, burning, tingling, diminished or absent sensation. Symptoms of TQ usually last less than 15 minutes but may persist up to 2 days. Patient with TQ will require CT imaging of the cervical spine to identify cervical fractures or

dislocations, and MRI to evaluate for ongoing spinal cord and nerve root compression.

Stingers are known as burners and are common peripheral nerve injuries occurring at any point from the cervical nerve root to the brachial plexus. Because these injuries often resolve quickly, they are likely underreported. Stingers involve only one limb and if bilateral symptoms (no matter how transient) occur, a spinal cord injury should be strongly suspected. Nerve roots are C5 and C6, which are most commonly involved in stinger injuries. A stinger patient presents with pain and/or paresthesia in a limb and may also have weakness. If symptoms completely resolve quickly (within minutes), no imaging is required. If symptoms persist, imaging that includes plain radiography or CT and MRI are warranted to identify foraminal stenosis, disc herniation, or disc osteophyte complexes.

For patients whose symptoms have completely resolved and have had an appropriate evaluation in the emergency

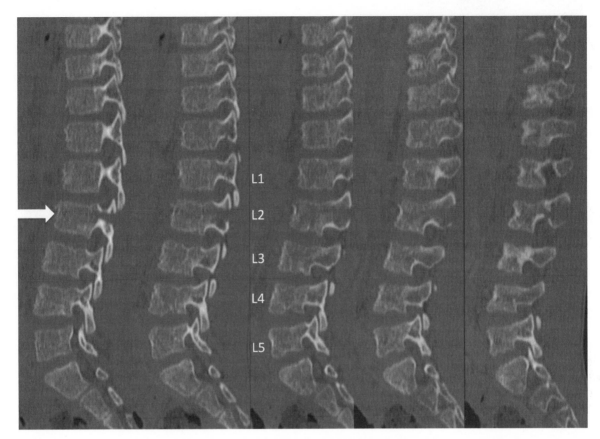

▲ Figure 28–11. Chance fracture through the L2 vertebral body and posterior elements. There is mild focal kyphosis at this level. It appears to be extra dural hemorrhage posterior to the thecal sac on the left which causes mild narrowing at the L1-L2 disc space level; patient did not have a spinal cord injury and was treated with bracing. Patient also had a small bowel perforation requiring exploratory laparotomy and repair of enterotomy; the arrow demonstrates the area of the fulcrum around which the flexion injury occurred.

department, follow-up with a spinal surgeon should occur as outpatient.

Concannon LG, Harrast MA, Herring SA: Radiating upper limb pain in the contact sports athlete: An update on transient quadriparesis and stingers. *Curr Sports Med Rep.* 2012;1:28 [PMID: 22236823].

Daniels AH, Sobel AD, Eberson CP: Pediatric thoracolumbar spinal trauma. *J Am Acad Orthop Surg.* 2013;21:707-716 [PMID: 24292927].

Pang D: Spinal cord injury without radiographic abnormality in children, 2 decades later. *Neurosurgery.* 2004;55:1325-1342 [PMID: 15574214].

Tyroch AH, McGuire EL, McLean SF, et al: The association between chance fractures and intra-abdominal injuries: A multicenter review. *Am Surg.* 2005;71:434-438 [PMID: 15986977].

MANAGEMENT OF DELAYED COMPLICATIONS OF SPINAL CORD INJURY

NEUROGENIC BLADDER

Manifestations of neurogenic bladder include loss of sensation of fullness and inability to voluntarily initiate urination and to completely empty the bladder. These need to be related to the child's developmental level, lifestyle, and family needs. In the early acute phase of spinal cord injury an indwelling urinary catheter will be used. This helps prevent urinary retention and to monitor output. Long-term management includes intermittent catheterization in order to provide regular, predictable, and complete emptying of the bladder. The aim of bladder care is to prevent infections, renal complications, and provide continence.

GASTROINTESTINAL STRESS ULCERATION

Patients with spinal cord injuries, especially those that involve the cervical cord, are at high risk for stress ulceration. Prophylaxis with proton pump inhibitors upon admission is recommended for up to 4 weeks.

PARALYTIC ILEUS

The bowel may be affected by damage to the nerves that control its function (neurogenic bowel), as well as the impact of medical care such as the use of opioids. Patients should be monitored for bowel sounds and bowel emptying and should not be given food or liquids until motility is restored. If patients are nauseated acutely after a spinal cord injury, strongly consider nasogastric (NG) or orogastric (OG) tube decompression of the stomach to reduce the volume of emesis associated with gastric distention and intestinal ileus.

RESPIRATORY COMPLICATIONS

Respiratory complications depend on the injury level: paralysis of the diaphragm (C1-C4), paralysis of intercostal muscles (C5-C6), and paralysis of abdominal muscles (T6-T12). Weakness of the diaphragm and intercostal muscles may lead to impaired clearance of secretions, ineffective cough, and hypoventilation. Frequent suctioning is often necessary to clear secretions, coupled with chest physiotherapy aiming at preventing atelectasis and pneumonia.

SKIN CARE

Children with spinal cord injuries are at higher risk for damage to skin integrity. Spinal cord injury causes loss of pain, pressure, and temperature sensation. This may result in a lack of sensory warning mechanisms, inability to move, and circulatory changes that will impact skin integrity. Pressure sores are most common on the buttocks and may develop within hours in immobilized patients. Backboards and slider boards should be discontinued as soon as possible. After spinal stabilization, patients should be turned side to side (log-rolled) every few hours to avoid pressure sores. Patients with cervical spine injury may lack vasomotor control and cannot sweat below the lesion. Their temperature may vary with the environment and it should be monitored closely.

Extremity Trauma

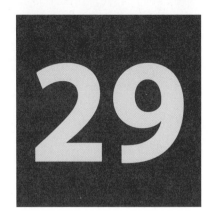

Jessica Kanis, MD
Timothy E. Brenkert, MD

▼ SALTER-HARRIS CLASSIFICATION OF PEDIATRIC FRACTURES

Salter-Harris classification describes injuries of the physis, or growth plate, in children (Figure 29–1). There are five types with severity of injury to the growth plate increasing with each type. All suspected Salter-Harris fracture require follow up with a orthopedic physician. They are described as follows.

Type I—Fracture line extends through the physis, separating epiphysis from metaphysis. There may be no radiographic evidence of the injury if no displacement is present. Therefore, diagnosis is based on clinical suspicion and point tenderness over the growth plate. If suspected, patients should be appropriately splinted with follow up with and orthopedic physician.

Type II—Most common of physeal fractures, these injuries begin in the physis and extend into the metaphysis. Low risk of growth disturbances in group I and II injuries.

Type III—Fracture extends from physis through epiphysis and into intra-articular space. It frequently requires operative fixation, therefore consultation with orthopedist should be sought.

Type IV—More commonly due to compressive forces with fracture extension from articular surface, through epiphysis and physis and involving metaphysis. Operative fixation is required with risk of partial or complete growth arrest despite appropriate treatment.

Type V—Crush injury to the physis most often seen in knee and ankle. These injuries have the highest risk of subsequent growth arrest and may be missed on initial radiographs due to lack of visible fracture. Diagnosis is often made in retrospect after growth arrest is noted. If suspected, extremity should be immobilized and follow-up with orthopedist should be arranged.

TRAUMATIC AMPUTATIONS

 ESSENTIALS OF DIAGNOSIS

▶ Sharp, clean amputations are best candidates for reimplantation.

▶ Amputated parts should be cleaned gently, kept moist with saline, and placed on ice.

▶ Cooling of amputated part helps to increase viability.

▶ General Considerations

All traumatic amputations should be considered for reimplantation surgery. Sharp, complete amputations with minimal crush injury are the best candidates for successful reimplantation. Amputated parts should always accompany the patient. The part should be rinsed gently to clean a dirty wound, covered with saline-moistened gauze, placed in a bag, and then kept on ice (do not place amputated part directly on ice). Cooling of the amputated part improves viability from 6-8 hours to 12-24 hours. Significant blood loss can occur with amputations and close monitoring of vital signs is imperative.

▶ Clinical Findings

Symptoms and Signs

When a patient presents with an amputated digit or limb, evaluation should include crush injury to both sides of the amputation. Monitor vital signs closely for signs of hemorrhagic shock.

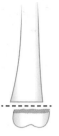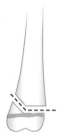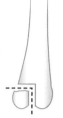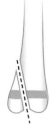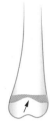

I. Through growth plate

II. Through metaphysis and growth plate

III. Through growth plate and epiphysis into joint

IV. Through metaphysis, growth plate, and epiphysis into joint

V. Crush of growth plate, may not be seen on x-ray

▲ **Figure 29–1.** Salter-Harris classification. (Reproduced, with permission, from Stone CK, Humphries RL: *Current Diagnosis & Treatment Emergency Medicine*, 7th ed. New York: McGraw-Hill, 2011. Copyright © McGraw-Hill Education LLC.)

X-ray Findings

Amputation is a clinical diagnosis. X-rays can be used to detect underlying fractures. X-rays should be taken of both the amputated digit or limb and extremity.

▶ Treatment

Evaluate and manage abnormal alignment, bones-periarticular osteoporosis, cartilage-joint space loss, deformities, marginal erosions, soft tissue swelling (ABCDEs). Strongly consider antibiotics and tetanus prophylaxis for all amputations. Antibiotic choices should follow the options for open fracture coverage recommendations. The amputated part should be kept clean, wrapped in a sterile dressing, moistened with sterile saline, placed in a plastic bag, and put on ice.

▶ Disposition

Prompt consultation with surgeon (orthopedic, plastic, or trauma) for limb amputations is often necessary. Patients will often need surgical management followed by inpatient monitoring with frequent neurologic and vascular examinations. Patients with small digit amputations frequently may be managed in the emergency department and discharged with close follow-up.

OPEN FRACTURES

 ESSENTIALS OF DIAGNOSIS

▶ Fracture with associated break in the skin.

▶ If wound exists in proximity to a fracture, strongly consider open fracture.

▶ Early antibiotics and tetanus prophylaxis.

▶ Surgical washout and debridement.

▶ General Considerations

Open fractures can be classified by the extent of skin injury, soft tissue damage, fracture severity, and degree of contamination. Type I fractures involve skin opening of less than or equal to 1 cm, clean wound, minimal muscle contusion, and simple transverse or oblique fractures. Type II fractures involve skin opening of greater than 1 cm, extensive soft tissue damage, flaps or avulsion with a moderate crushing component, and simple transverse or oblique fractures with minimal comminution. Type III fractures have extensive soft tissue damage including muscle, skin, and neurovascular structures, or fractures open for greater than 8 hours.

▶ Clinical Findings

Symptoms and Signs

Patient presents with pain, swelling, and deformity to the extremity with overlying break in the skin. Open fractures may present as large open wounds with underlying fracture.

X-ray Findings

X-rays of the affected limb should be performed to characterize the fracture.

▶ Treatment

Management of open fractures in the emergency department should include early administration of antibiotics. Systemic antibiotic coverage is directed at gram-positive organisms (typically first- or second-generation cephalosporins). Additional gram-negative coverage should be added for type III fractures. High-dose penicillin should be added for potential fecal or clostridial contamination. Tetanus prophylaxis is advised. Surgical debridement and skeletal stabilization may be indicated if surgical management may be delayed.

Disposition

Patients with large or contaminated wounds should be admitted to the hospital for continued antibiotic therapy and possible surgical debridement. Discharge can be considered in patients with smaller wounds and stable fractures following consultation with the surgical team.

Hoff W, Bonandier J, Cachecho R, Dorlac W: East Practice Management Guidelines Work Group: Update to practice management guidelines for prophylactic antibiotics use in open fractures. *J Trauma, Inj, Infect Crit Care.* 2011;70(3):751-754 [PMID: 21610369].

ACUTE COMPARTMENT SYNDROME

ESSENTIALS OF DIAGNOSIS

▶ Most frequently occur in the leg.

▶ Often associated with fractures, crush injuries, or constrictive splints.

▶ Severe, poorly localized pain out of proportion to the injury.

▶ Paresis, paresthesias, and diminished pulses are late findings.

General Considerations

Compartment syndrome can lead to devastating long-term conditions without prompt recognition and treatment. Ischemic contractures can result due to muscle and nerve ischemia when not treated. The leg is the most common location to develop compartment syndrome, specifically the anterior compartment.

Clinical Findings

Symptoms and Signs

Patients will have severe pain out of proportion to the injury that worsens despite rest. Pain is poorly localized and worsens with passive stretch. Palpation will reveal a painful, tense compartment with associated weakness and sensory loss over the distribution of affected nerves. Paresis, paresthesia, pallor, and diminished pulses are late findings. Patients with altered mental status or coma should be examined carefully for extremity injuries with associated swelling as compartment syndrome can be easily missed in these patients. Confirmatory diagnosis is based on measurement of the compartment pressure. Normal pressures are less than 10 mm Hg.

X-ray Findings

Films of the affected limb can identify an underlying fracture.

Treatment

Pressures greater than 20 mm Hg should prompt admission and surgical consultation. A compartment pressure of 30-40 mm Hg will likely require emergent fasciotomy in the operating room.

Disposition

Patients with true compartment syndrome require immediate consultation with an orthopedist and admission.

▼ MANAGEMENT OF SPECIFIC ORTHOPEDIC INJURIES

SHOULDER GIRDLE INJURIES

CLAVICLE FRACTURES

ESSENTIALS OF DIAGNOSIS

▶ Pain and deformity over clavicle.

▶ X-ray confirmation of fracture.

General Considerations

Clavicle injuries are very common in children. Most occur as result of fall onto shoulder. Clavicle injuries are often seen in newborns as a result of shoulder compression during birth. The middle third of the clavicle is most frequently fractured with the medial third least commonly injured.

Clinical Findings

Symptoms and Signs

Pain, swelling, and possibly deformity are present over the clavicle. Pain is worsened with attempts at movement of the ipsilateral arm.

X-ray Findings

Anteroposterior (AP) view is often sufficient to detect most middle third fractures. An apical lordotic view, with tube directed 45 degrees cephalad, may be needed to visualize fractures of the medial third.

Treatment

Conservative treatment is best as rapid healing and remodeling with full return to function is typical. Sling, or sling and swathe, is recommended and more comfortable than the figure-eight harness. Consultation with an orthopedist is needed for open fractures or concern for neurovascular compromise.

Disposition

Surgical correction is indicated for open fractures, presence of significant neurovascular compromise, or threatened skin from fracture displacement. However, most patients may be discharged with follow-up to an orthopedist.

ACROMIOCLAVICULAR JOINT SEPARATION

ESSENTIALS OF DIAGNOSIS

▶ Pain with palpation over joint.

▶ Deformity to superior shoulder.

▶ Pain with adduction of ipsilateral arm across chest.

▶ X-ray helpful in type 2-6 injuries.

General Considerations

Many injuries are the result of a direct fall on the point of the shoulder. Injuries are classified in the following manner (Figure 29–2).

Type 1—Sprain of the acromioclavicular (AC) ligament with normal radiographs.

Type 2—Rupture of the AC ligament with an intact coracoclavicular (CC) ligament.

Type 3—Rupture of AC and CC ligaments resulting in upward displacement of clavicle.

Types 4-6—Rupture of AC and CC ligaments with additional muscular facial disruption and displacement of the clavicle posteriorly (type 4), superiorly (type 5), or inferiorly (type 6).

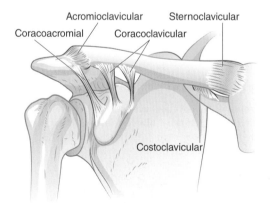

▲ **Figure 29–2.** Ligamentous attachments of the clavicle to the sternum medially and the acromion laterally. (Reproduced, with permission, from Simon RR, Sherman SC: *Emergency Orthopedics*, 6th ed. New York: McGraw-Hill, 2011. Copyright © McGraw-Hill Education LLC.)

Clinical Findings

Symptoms and Signs

Examine the patient in the upright, sitting position. Swelling and tenderness may be present at the location of the AC joint. Look for deformity as well (≥ type 3 injuries) representing elevation of the distal clavicle as the weight of the arm pulls the shoulder inferiorly with rupture of the CC ligament.

X-ray Findings

X-rays obtained should include AP and axial views. Additionally, obtaining a view by tilting the beam 10-15 degrees in the cephalic direction can allow for detection of subtle injuries. Bilateral views may be obtained to compare with uninjured joint. Type 1 injuries will show normal radiographs. However, type 2 x-rays may demonstrate elevation of distal clavicle due to AC ligament rupture, films obtained in type 3 injuries will display clavicular elevation due to tearing of the AC and CC ligaments.

Treatment

Conservative treatment is instituted for type 1 and 2 injuries with application of sling and ice. Brief immobilization (3-7 days) is recommended for type 2 injuries; however, return to activity should begin as soon as tolerated by patients with type 1 injuries. These days most patients with type 3 injuries also do well with conservative management, whereas traditionally they were managed surgically. Surgical management is required for type 4-6 injuries.

Disposition

Most patients can be discharged home from the emergency department with follow-up to an orthopedist.

Mazzoca AD, Arciero RA, Bicos J: Evaluation and treatment of acromioclavicular joint injuries. *Am J Sports Med.* 2007;35:316 [PMID: 17251175].

SHOULDER DISLOCATION

ESSENTIALS OF DIAGNOSIS

▶ Pain, swelling, and deformity to shoulder.

▶ Majority are anterior dislocations.

▶ Rare in children younger than 12 years.

▶ Include scapular Y view to standard shoulder films for detection.

▶ General Considerations

Dislocations of the shoulder are rare in young children; injuries that cause dislocation in adults result in fractures in the skeletally immature. Most (> 95%) are dislocated anteriorly as in adults and are the result of trauma to an abducted, externally rotated arm.

▶ Clinical Findings

Symptoms and Signs

Patients with anterior shoulder dislocations present with the arm held in adduction and pain with attempted movement of the shoulder. The shoulder exhibits loss of its normal rounded contour and a prominent acromion is present. The humeral head may be palpated in the anterior shoulder or fullness appreciated in this area. A thorough nerve examination of the upper extremity should be performed with specific attention to the axillary nerve. Motor and sensory functions of the nerve can be tested on the lateral shoulder and should be compared with the opposite shoulder. Distal pulses should be tested and documented.

X-ray Findings

In addition to standard shoulder views, a scapular Y view (Figure 29–3) should be included to assess the direction of dislocation. Films should be obtained prior to reduction attempts to assess for presence of associated fractures and direction of dislocation as well as follow-up of reduction to demonstrate success and evaluate for fractures caused by the procedure. Axillary view of the shoulder should be obtained if the diagnosis remains in question after initial films. A defect in the posterior lateral portion of the humeral head,

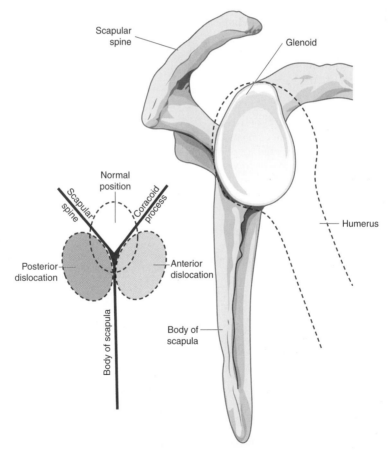

▲ **Figure 29–3.** Sketch of view on the scapular Y view x-ray. The position of the humeral head in relationship to the Y created by the scapula can tell direction of dislocation versus normal position. (Reproduced, with permission, from Stone CK, Humphries RL: *Current Diagnosis & Treatment Emergency Medicine,* 7th ed. New York: McGraw-Hill, 2011. Copyright © McGraw-Hill Education LLC.)

or Hill-Sachs deformity, is created by the glenoid rim during dislocation and is present in up to 50% of anterior dislocations. A fracture of the anterior glenoid rim during dislocation, or Bankart fracture, is less common.

▶ Treatment

A number of methods of shoulder reduction have been described and the emergency physician should be familiar with more than one. Sedation may be required in the reduction attempt as overcoming muscle spasm is imperative to successful reduction.

External Rotation Technique

The patient may be in a supine or upright position with the affected arm flexed 90 degrees at the elbow. The proceduralist slowly externally rotates the arm while supporting the elbow and maintaining adduction. The process should be slow and gradual and may take 5-10 minutes. The examiner should stop at the presence of any pain and wait for the muscles to relax. This technique does require significant force and can be accomplished without the aid of an assistant (Figure 29–4).

Scapular Manipulation Technique

The method may be utilized on its own or in combination with other techniques. The examiner pushes the tip of the scapula medially while rotating the acromion inferiorly in attempts to rotate the glenoid fossa.

Stimson Technique

The patient is in the prone position with the affected arm extending over the side of the bed. Ten to 15 pounds are suspended from the patient's wrist for 20-30 minutes until reduction is achieved.

Traction and Countertraction

As linear traction is applied to the patient's affected arm, an assistant applies countertraction with a sheet wrapped under the axilla. This method requires the application of physical force as well as the presence of an assistant (Figure 29–5).

FARES Method

With the patient in the supine position, the examiner grasps the affected limb at the wrist with the elbow extended and forearm in neutral rotation. Longitudinal traction is applied while making small vertical oscillating movements with the patient's arm of approximately 5 cm up and down. The arm

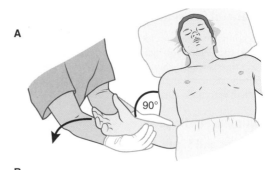

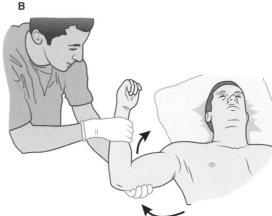

▲ **Figure 29–4.** External rotation method for reduction of anterior shoulder dislocation. The patient may be supine or sitting up during this procedure. (Reproduced, with permission, from Reichman EF, Simon RR: *Emergency Medicine Procedures*. New York: McGraw-Hill, 2004. Copyright © McGraw-Hill Education LLC.)

is slowly abducted while continuing the movements with external rotation added once greater than 90 degrees.

▶ Disposition

Following successful reduction, place the patient in a shoulder immobilizer/sling, and discharge home with adequate analgesia and close follow-up with an orthopedist. Consultation with an orthopedist in the emergency department is indicated for patients with neurological or vascular complications, or patients with failed reduction attempts.

Maity A, Roy DS, Mondal BC: A prospective randomized clinical trial comparing FARES method with the Eachempati external rotation method for reduction of acute anterior dislocation of shoulder. *Injury*. 2012;43:1066 [PMID: 22333561].

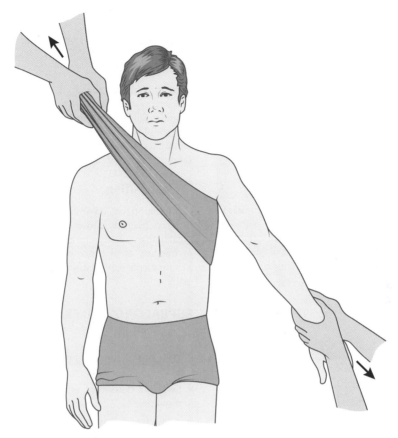

▲ **Figure 29–5.** Traction and countertraction method for reduction of anterior shoulder dislocation. (Reproduced, with permission, from Stone CK, Humphries RL: *Current Diagnosis & Treatment Emergency Medicine,* 7th ed. New York: McGraw-Hill, 2011. Copyright © McGraw-Hill Education LLC.)

UPPER EXTREMITY INJURIES

PROXIMAL HUMERUS FRACTURES

 ESSENTIALS OF DIAGNOSIS

▶ Pain to upper arm with limited range of motion of shoulder.

▶ Potential site for pathologic fractures.

▶ Consider abuse if mechanism inconsistent with injury.

▶ X-rays are confirmatory.

▶ General Considerations

Fractures of the proximal humerus typically occur following a fall on outstretched hand or direct blow to the area. Bone cysts and other benign lesions are common in the humerus increasing the risk of pathologic fractures. Forcible twisting or pulling of the extremity may result in metaphyseal corner fractures at the proximal humeral physis, or bucket handle fractures, and their presence should raise suspicion of non-accidental trauma.

▶ Clinical Findings

Symptoms and Signs

Pain and swelling at site of injury with limited movement of shoulder. Assess axillary nerve function with sensation over deltoid and shoulder abduction.

X-ray Findings

Routine AP and axillary views are sufficient for diagnosis.

Treatment

Management of proximal humerus fractures is often conservative due to the high activity of the proximal humeral growth plate and its excellent remodeling potential. Sling, ice, and pain management is common in older children with open physes. Younger children and infants may require swathe for further stabilization (see Table 29-1). Adolescents with closed physes are managed similar to adults, with surgical repair dependent upon the location of the fracture and degree of displacement and/or angulation.

Disposition

Prompt consultation with an orthopedist should be made in the presence of open fracture (rare), concern for neurovascular compromise, intra-articular Salter-Harris IV fracture, associated shoulder dislocation, or significant displacement or angulation in an older child. Younger children may be discharged home with follow-up to an orthopedist.

HUMERAL SHAFT FRACTURES

ESSENTIALS OF DIAGNOSIS

▸ Swelling and pain to midarm.

▸ Potential site for pathological fractures.

▸ Consider abuse if mechanism inconsistent or in otherwise healthy child younger than 3 years with normal bone by x-ray.

▸ X-rays are confirmatory.

▸ Conservative management.

General Considerations

Humeral shaft fractures are uncommon in children, representing less than 10% of fractures in children less than 12 years. When present, humeral shaft fractures are typically secondary to fall on an outstretched hand or to a direct blow to the arm. Pathologic fractures may occur in presence of bone cysts, which are common in the humerus. This injury may be seen in patients with non-accidental trauma due to traction with humeral rotation or twisting resulting in oblique fractures.

Clinical Findings

Symptoms and Signs

Pain at site of injury. Assess radial nerve function with sensation over dorsum of hand between first and second metacarpals and wrist extension or forearm supination.

X-ray Findings

Routine humeral films (AP and lateral views) are sufficient.

Treatment

Most patients are managed conservatively with pain control and immobilization by means of sling and swathe or shoulder immobilization. Sugar tong splints to the upper arm should accompany a sling in patients with complete or moderately displaced fractures (Table 29-1). Need for surgical repair is rare due to high potential for remodeling.

Disposition

Consultation with an orthopedist should be made in presence of open fracture, concern for neurovascular compromise, greater than 15 degrees angulation, complete displacement of fracture, or evidence of compartment syndrome (rare). Most patients may be discharged home with follow-up to an orthopedist.

SUPRACONDYLAR FRACTURES

ESSENTIALS OF DIAGNOSIS

▸ Swelling, deformity, and pain to elbow with decreased movement.

▸ X-rays findings may be subtle; look for posterior fat pad on lateral film.

▸ Potential for neurovascular compromise.

General Considerations

Supracondylar fractures are the most frequent pediatric elbow fractures and typically occur as a result of a fall on outstretched hand (FOOSH) with hyperextension of the elbow, most commonly in children aged 5-10 years.

Clinical Findings

Symptoms and Signs

Pain and swelling at the elbow is typical. Rapid neurovascular assessment is essential due to risk of complications. Motor function of the main nerves of the upper extremity can be assessed with three motions: the "thumbs up sign" (radial nerve), finger spreading against resistance or holding paper between middle and ring fingers (ulnar nerve), and the "OK sign" (median nerve). The anterior interosseous branch of the median nerve is the most common nerve injury with FOOSH injuries resulting in a weak "OK sign" that appears more like a pincer due to limited use of the flexor digitorum profundus of the index finger and flexor pollicis longus. Sensation can be determined

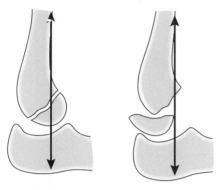

▲ **Figure 29–6.** The anterior humeral line drawn on the lateral radiograph along the anterior surface of the humerus. This should extend through the middle of the capitellum, but may transect the anterior third of the capitellum or pass completely anterior to it in the case of a supracondylar fracture. (Reproduced, with permission, from Simon RR, Sherman SC: *Emergency Orthopedics*, 6th ed. New York: McGraw-Hill, 2011. Copyright © McGraw-Hill Education LLC.)

by two-point discrimination over the palmar surface of thumb and first two fingers (median nerve), the dorsal surface of web space between thumb and index finger (radial nerve), and the pinky finger and ulnar aspect of ring finger (ulnar nerve).

X-ray Findings

AP and lateral views of the elbow are essential, and appropriate analgesia should be administered prior to x-rays to ensure ideal images. Films should be evaluated for the presence of a posterior fat pad, suggesting fluid in the elbow joint and an occult fracture if films otherwise unremarkable. The location of the anterior humeral line, drawn down cortical surface of anterior humerus on the lateral x-ray (Figure 29–6), should be determined. It should bisect the middle third of the capitellum and its movement from this point suggests the presence of fracture with displacement.

▶ Treatment

Supracondylar injuries frequently require consultation with an orthopedist, particularly if there is evidence of displacement or periosteal involvement. Attempts at reduction should be withheld until consultation is made at risk of creating or worsening neurovascular compromise.

▶ Disposition

Consultation with an orthopedist is required for all supracondylar fractures. Fractures with significant displacement require admission for operative repair. Patients may be discharged with proper splinting if there is no evidence of displacement or presence of complications. Patients who are discharged home should have follow-up with an orthopedist.

Allen SR, Hang JR, Hau RC: Review article: Paediatric supracondylar humeral fractures: Emergency assessment and management. *Emerg Med Australas.* 2010;22:418 [PMID: 20874821].

LATERAL CONDYLE FRACTURES

ESSENTIALS OF DIAGNOSIS

▶ Pain and swelling to lateral elbow.

▶ Obtain oblique x-rays for fracture delineation.

▶ General Considerations

Lateral condyle fractures occur after fall on outstretched hand with varus stress at the elbow or onto a flat hand with flexed elbow. They are transphyseal and intra-articular and are classified as Salter-Harris type IV fractures.

▶ Clinical Findingss

Symptoms and Signs

Pain and swelling over the lateral elbow is present with decreased range of motion. Neurovascular injury is uncommon in these injuries.

X-ray Findings

Oblique views are needed in addition to AP and lateral films to detect nondisplaced fractures (Figure 29–7).

▶ Treatment

Open reduction is often needed for displaced fractures; nondisplaced fractures may be splinted with long-arm posterior splint and forearm in pronation (Table 29-1).

▶ Disposition

Consultation with an orthopedist should be made for all injuries with disposition per orthopedic recommendations. Patients may be discharged home with splint and follow-up to an orthopedist.

MEDIAL EPICONDYLAR FRACTURES

ESSENTIALS OF DIAGNOSIS

▶ Often associated with elbow dislocation.

▶ Pain and swelling over medial elbow.

▶ Evaluate ulnar nerve function.

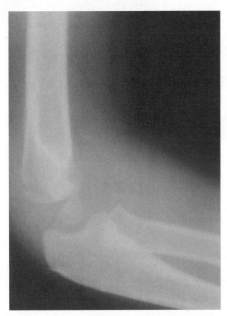

▲ **Figure 29–7.** Lateral condyle fracture of the humerus. (Reproduced, with permission, from Skinner HB: *Current Diagnosis & Treatment in Orthopedics,* 4th ed. New York: McGraw-Hill, 2006. Copyright © McGraw-Hill Education LLC.)

▶ General Considerations

Medial epicondylar fractures are typically seen following a direct fall onto the elbow or fall on outstretched hand with valgus stressing of the elbow. Avulsion fractures at this location may also be seen as a result of repeated valgus strain to the elbow. In conjunction with other local injuries, this is known as "little league elbow" which is often seen in adolescent throwers.

▶ Clinical Findings

Symptoms and Signs

Patient will exhibit swelling and tenderness to palpation over medial elbow. Pain is worsened with pronation or flexion of the wrist. An isolated fracture is less common, with the injury more often associated with posterior elbow dislocation. Assessment of ulnar nerve function is imperative as associated injury may be seen. Motor function of the nerve can be tested by having the patient spread fingers against resistance or hold a piece of paper between the middle and ring fingers. The sensory distribution of the ulnar nerve is the pinky finger and ulnar aspect of the ring finger.

X-ray Findings

In addition to AP and lateral views of the elbow, oblique views and comparison views may be required to detect subtle changes. If injury occurs prior to onset of ossification of the medial epicondyle (typically 4-6 years), MRI may be needed (Figure 29–8).

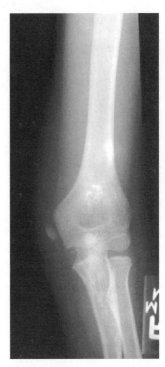

▲ **Figure 29–8.** Medial condyle fracture of the humerus. (Reproduced, with permission, from Simon RR, Sherman SC: *Emergency Orthopedics,* 6th ed. New York: McGraw-Hill, 2011. Copyright © McGraw-Hill Education LLC.)

▶ Treatment

Open reduction is often needed in children with displaced fractures; nondisplaced fractures may be splinted with long-arm posterior splint (Table 29-1).

▶ Disposition

Consultation with orthopedist should be made for all injuries with disposition per orthopedic recommendations. Patients may be discharged home with splint and follow-up to an orthopedist.

FRACTURE SEPARATION OF THE DISTAL HUMERAL PHYSIS

ESSENTIALS OF DIAGNOSIS

▶ Elbow swelling without deformity in most patients.

▶ Comparison films may be needed to demonstrate displacement.

▶ Consider non-accidental injury in patients younger than 3 years.

General Considerations

This fracture is uncommon injury, with most in children younger than 7 years. It often results from a fall onto an outstretched hand with hyperextension of the elbow in children 5-7 years. In infants, it typically results from non-accidental trauma with forceful twisting of the arm. Neurovascular complication is rare.

Clinical Findings

Symptoms and Signs

Patients often exhibit elbow swelling without deformity. If there is large displacement of the fracture, physical examination may mimic a posteriorly displaced elbow dislocation.

X-ray Findings

AP and lateral views of the elbow are needed to evaluate for posteromedial displacement of the radius and ulna in relation to the distal ulna. Diagnosis in children may be difficult, especially those in whom capitellar ossification has not yet begun (< 1 year). Comparison films may be needed to detect subtle displacement.

Treatment

Closed reduction and pinning are often required; therefore, consultation with orthopedist is required in all patients.

Disposition

Disposition is per orthopedist recommendation because of the frequent need for operative repair.

ELBOW DISLOCATIONS

ESSENTIALS OF DIAGNOSIS

▶ Pain and deformity to elbow with limited movement.

▶ Majority demonstrate posterior displacement of ulna in relation to humerus.

▶ High risk of associated fractures.

General Considerations

Elbow dislocation is the most common dislocation in children younger than 10 years. Posterior elbow dislocation, where the olecranon is displaced posteriorly in relation to the humerus, represents 90% of patients. This dislocation typically occurs after a fall or twisting injury to the elbow.

Clinical Findings

Symptoms and Signs

Elbow is usually held in 45 degrees of flexion with deformity noted to elbow. Distal nerves and peripheral pulses should

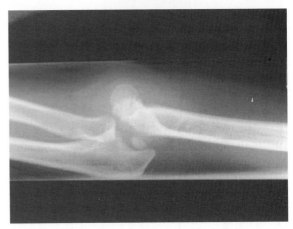

▲ **Figure 29–9.** Posterior elbow dislocation with avulsion of the medial epicondyle. (Reproduced, with permission, from Strange GR, Ahrens WR, Schafermeyer RW, Wiebe R: Pediatric Emergency Medicine, 3rd ed. New York: McGraw-Hill, 2009. Copyright © McGraw-Hill Education LLC.)

be examined due to risk of associated neurovascular injury. Particular attention should be paid to the ulnar nerve as this represents the most frequently injured nerve in posterior dislocations. Brachial artery injury is associated with anterior dislocations.

X-ray Findings

In posterior elbow dislocation, the capitellum is displaced anteriorly out of the olecranon fossa and is best seen on the lateral elbow radiograph. Associated fractures can occasionally occur simultaneously as demonstrated in Figure 29–9.

Treatment

Emergent reduction should commence in the presence of neurovascular compromise. Reduction can be attempted with the assistance of procedural sedation and is best achieved by axial traction on the forearm while stabilizing the humerus. Following reduction, a long-arm posterior splint with the elbow at 90 degrees of flexion should be applied (Table 29-1).

Disposition

Consultation with orthopedist should be sought in the presence of open fracture, significant associated fractures, or neurovascular compromise. Patients may be discharged home with splint and sling and follow-up to an orthopedist assuming uncomplicated reduction.

Parsons BO, Ramsey ML: Acute elbow dislocations in athletes. *Clin Sports Med.* 2010;29:599 [PMID: 20883899].

CHAPTER 29

APOPHYSITIS OF MEDIAL EPICONDYLE

ESSENTIALS OF DIAGNOSIS

▶ Pain over medial epicondyle that is worsened with resistance to wrist flexion.

▶ X-ray demonstrates open ossification center without evidence of separation.

▶ General Considerations

Overuse injury with complaints of medial elbow that pain that initially begins after throwing. Symptoms can worsen to point of persistent pain.

▶ Clinical Findings

Symptoms and Signs

Pain with palpation over the medial epicondyle. Pain to the area is worsened with resistance of ipsilateral wrist flexion.

X-ray Findings

AP and lateral elbow films will demonstrate an open ossification center at the medial epicondyle with no separation.

▶ Treatment

Conservative treatment is curative. Child should refrain from throwing for 4-6 weeks with attempts to correct throwing mechanics once able to return to activity. Symptomatic care with ice and NSAIDs as needed.

▶ Disposition

Patients may be managed on an outpatient basis and may benefit from follow-up to a sports medicine physician.

FOREARM INJURIES

RADIAL HEAD SUBLUXATION

ESSENTIALS OF DIAGNOSIS

▶ Peak incidence during toddler years (ages 1-4 years).

▶ Mechanism is often axial traction on extended and pronated arm.

▶ X-rays not needed prior to reduction attempt in classic cases.

▶ Reduce with either hyperpronation or supination and flexion of the elbow.

▶ General Considerations

The injury known as "nursemaid's elbow" or "pulled elbow" is the most common elbow injury in children. Peak incidence in children is 1-4 years but has been reported in infants younger than 6 months and in children as old as 8 years. Incidence decreases after 5 years of age when the annular ligament has strengthened significantly. Axial traction on a pronated, extended arm causes displacement of the annular ligament to the radiohumeral joint where it becomes trapped. A "pull" injury is most common, but injury may also be seen after fall or direct trauma to the elbow. In infants, a history of rolling over with arm being trapped underneath may be given. Recurrence is common.

▶ Clinical Findings

Symptoms and Signs

The main complaint is disuse of the affected arm. Patients classically hold the arm pronated and extended or slightly flexed at the elbow and are rarely distressed unless examination of the elbow is attempted. The presence of significant tenderness, swelling, or ecchymosis suggests an alternative diagnosis and imaging should be pursued in these patients. Full examination of the remainder of the upper extremity should be completed to assess for tenderness over the clavicle, ulna, or distal humerus especially if the history is not consistent with radial head subluxation.

X-ray Findings

Films are not needed when history and examination are classic as this is a clinical diagnosis. If repeated attempts at reduction are unsuccessful or history or examination is not consistent, AP and lateral films of the elbow should be obtained as well as x-rays of other parts of the upper extremity that exhibit concern for injury on examination.

▶ Treatment

Two methods at reduction are hyperpronation (Figure 29–10) and supination/flexion (Figure 29–11). Although both techniques are effective, hyperpronation has shown to be more successful on first attempt. Each technique requires stabilization of the patient's elbow by the examiner with one hand, placing pressure over the radial head with a thumb or finger. In hyperpronation, the examiner then hyperpronates the forearm; a click may be felt at the site of the radial head. In supination/flexion, the examiner uses his or her other hand to provide gentle traction to the patient's forearm. This is followed by full supination and then flexion at the elbow in a single smooth motion. A click may be heard or felt at the location of the radial head. Use of the extremity should be seen within 10-15 minutes.

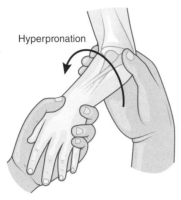

▲ Figure 29–10. Hyperpronation method for reduction of radial head subluxation. (Reproduced, with permission, from Simon RR, Sherman SC: *Emergency Orthopedics*, 6th ed. New York: McGraw-Hill, 2011. Copyright © McGraw-Hill Education LLC.)

▶ Disposition

Patients may be discharged home with no follow-up needed for those whose fractures are successfully reduced. If reduction is unsuccessful and no other injuries are found on imaging, placement in a sling with close follow-up with the primary physician

is indicated. In patients with failed reduction, spontaneous reduction typically occurs. Outpatient referral to an orthopedist is indicated for patients with recurrent subluxation.

MONTEGGIA FRACTURES

 ESSENTIALS OF DIAGNOSIS

▶ Presence of proximal ulnar fracture and pain over radial head.

▶ Ensure sufficient visualization of elbow on films with presence of true lateral.

▶ Consultation with orthopedist for all patients.

▶ General Considerations

Monteggia fracture is a proximal ulnar fracture with radial head dislocation. This injury may result after a direct blow to the ulna or after a fall. The associated radial head dislocation can be missed if suspicion is not high. True lateral films that include the elbow should always be obtained in children with forearm fractures.

▶ Clinical Findings

Symptoms and Signs

Pain with palpation over ulna as well as lateral elbow pain over the radial head is demonstrated. Patients have increased pain with supination and pronation in contrast to those with isolated ulnar fractures.

X-ray Findings

AP and lateral films of the forearm that include a true lateral of the elbow are needed. If pain with palpation of the elbow is present, elbow films should be obtained as well. A line drawn through the axis of the radius should pass through the center of the capitellum on all projections, if this is not seen, dislocation of the radial head should be suspected (Figure 29–12).

▶ Treatment

Consultation with the orthopedist is required for all patients with reduction of the dislocation and/or fracture as needed.

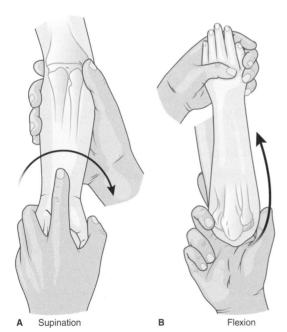

A Supination   **B** Flexion

▲ Figure 29–11. Supination and flexion method for reduction of radial head subluxation. (Reproduced, with permission, from Simon RR, Sherman SC: *Emergency Orthopedics*, 6th ed. New York: McGraw-Hill, 2011. Copyright © McGraw-Hill Education LLC.)

Krul M, van der Wouden JC, van Suijlekom-Smit LWA, et al: Manipulative interventions for reducing pulled elbow in young children. *Cochrane Database Syst Rev.* 2012;1:CD007759 [PMID: 22258973].

▶ Disposition

Patients with successful closed reduction may be discharged home with a posterior long-arm splint with follow-up to an orthopedist (Table 29–1).

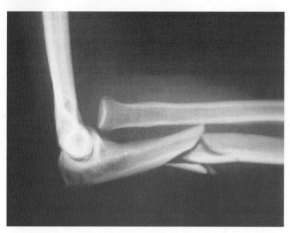

▲ **Figure 29–12.** Monteggia fracture. Proximal ulnar fracture with associated radial head dislocation. Note that a line drawn through the radius does not transect the center of the capitellum. (Reproduced, with permission, from Simon RR, Sherman SC: *Emergency Orthopedics,* 6th ed. New York: McGraw-Hill, 2011. Copyright © McGraw-Hill Education LLC.)

GALEAZZI FRACTURE

 ESSENTIALS OF DIAGNOSIS

▶ Presence of radial fracture with distal radioulnar joint tenderness or prominence of distal ulna.

▶ X-rays are confirmatory.

▶ Consultation with orthopedist for all patients.

▶ **General Considerations**

Relatively rare in children, the Galeazzi fracture is the presence of a radial fracture with distal radioulnar joint disruption. It typically results from a fall onto an outstretched hand.

▶ **Clinical Findings**

Symptoms and Signs

Patients present with pain at fracture site as well as prominence of the distal ulna or suspected instability of distal radioulnar joint.

X-ray Findings

AP and lateral films of the forearm are confirmatory (Figure 29–13).

▶ **Treatment**

Consultation with an orthopedist for closed reduction is required in the emergency department for patients with displaced injuries. Patient with nondisplaced injuries or postreduction may be placed in a sugar tong splint (see Table 29-1).

▶ **Disposition**

Patients with nondisplaced injuries or successful reduction may be discharged home with splint and sling for close follow-up to an orthopedist.

DISTAL RADIUS AND ULNA FRACTURES

 ESSENTIALS OF DIAGNOSIS

▶ Most common fractures of children and adolescents.

▶ Pain and swelling present at fracture site.

▶ Neurovascular complications rare.

▶ **General Considerations**

Distal radius and ulnar fractures are the most common fractures in children and adolescents.

▶ **Clinical Findings**

Symptoms and Signs

Pain and swelling at the site of the fracture are typically seen with decreased mobility at the wrist. Vascular integrity should be evaluated by the strength of the radial pulse as well as perfusion distally to the hand.

X-ray Findings

Standard forearm views are sufficient for diagnosis. The entirety of the forearm should be visualized radiographically as wrist pain may be seen in some proximal forearm injuries.

▶ **Treatment**

Patients with nondisplaced fractures and those with minimal angulation should be stabilized with a sugar tong splint (see Table 29-1). Closed reduction in the emergency department is indicated for displaced fractures or those with at least 10 degrees of angulation of the distal fracture fragment.

▶ **Disposition**

Consultation with orthopedist is indicated in the presence of an open fracture, in patients displaying vascular compromise or in those with displacement or angulation. Patients

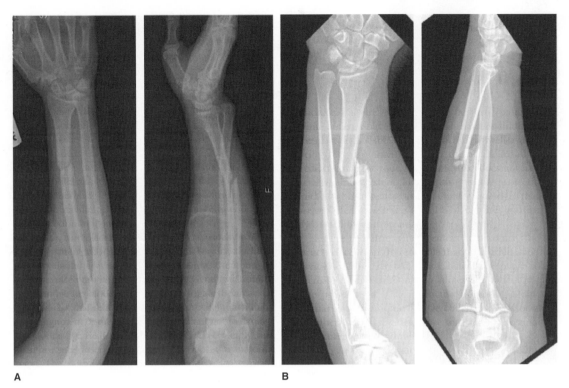

A   **B**

▲ **Figure 29–13.** Galeazzi fracture. Radial fracture with associated distal radioulnar joint disruption. Note the widening of the distal radial ulnar joint space on AP view and dislocation of the distal radius relative to the ulna on the lateral film. (Reproduced, with permission, from Simon RR, Sherman SC: *Emergency Orthopedics*, 6th ed. New York: McGraw-Hill, 2011. Copyright © McGraw-Hill Education LLC.)

with nondisplaced fractures may be splinted and discharged home with outpatient follow-up to an orthopedist.

TORUS (BUCKLE) FRACTURE

 ESSENTIALS OF DIAGNOSIS

▶ Fracture of the distal metaphysis seen after fall on outstretched hand.

▶ X-rays are confirmatory.

▶ Treat with well-padded volar or sugar tong splint and follow-up with an orthopedist.

▶ General Considerations

Torus (buckle) fractures are seen in the area of the distal metaphysis and are so named because of the buckling of the cortex that occurs due to failure of compression after a fall on an outstretched hand. Radiographic evidence of their presence may be subtle and all angles should be evaluated for this irregularity.

▶ Clinical Findings

Symptoms and Signs

Pain over the fracture site is present with a variable degree of swelling and immobility.

X-ray Findings

Standard films of the wrist demonstrate disruption of the smooth contour of the distal metaphyseal cortex (Figure 29–14).

▶ Treatment

A well-padded volar or sugar tong splint is indicated (see Table 29-1).

▶ Disposition

Patients may be discharged home with follow-up in 1 week to an orthopedist.

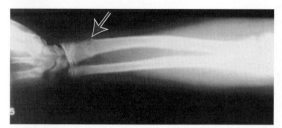

▲ **Figure 29–14.** Torus (buckle) fracture. (Reproduced, with permission, from Strange GR, Ahrens WR, Lalyveld S, Schafermeyer RW: *Pediatric Emergency Medicine*, 2nd ed. New York: McGraw-Hill, 2002. Copyright © McGraw-Hill Education LLC.)

CARPAL FRACTURES

SCAPHOID FRACTURES

ESSENTIALS OF DIAGNOSIS

► Seen after fall on hand with hyperextension of wrist.

► Patients with pain over snuffbox or pain with supination against resistance.

► Rates of nonunion lower in children compared with adults.

► Thumb spica immobilization if suspected clinically.

▶ General Considerations

Carpal fractures are rare in children; most common are scaphoid fractures in adolescents. Fractures to the scaphoid in adolescents traditionally are seen commonly in the distal third of the bone, as opposed to middle third in adults. Recent literature suggests a trend toward adult injury patterns, possibly due to a change in size and activities of adolescents. The injury is seen after a fall on the hand with hyperextension of the wrist.

▶ Clinical Findings

Symptoms and Signs

The presence of tenderness over the snuffbox or pain with resisted supination suggests the possibility of a scaphoid fracture.

X-ray Findings

In addition to a standard wrist series, an AP of the scaphoid with 30 degrees of ulnar deviation of the wrist may assist in visualization of a fracture; however, detection may still be difficult (Figure 29–15).

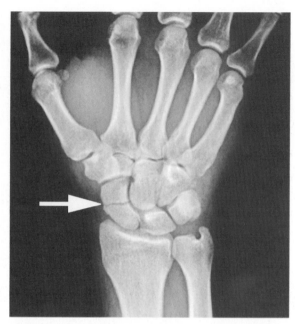

▲ **Figure 29–15.** Scaphoid fracture. (Reproduced, with permission, from Simon RR, Sherman SC: *Emergency Orthopedics*, 6th ed. New York: McGraw-Hill, 2011. Copyright © McGraw-Hill Education LLC.)

▶ Treatment

Immobilization should be achieved with the application of a thumb spica in all patients with suspected scaphoid fracture due to the risk of malunion (see Table 29-1).

▶ Disposition

Patients may be discharged home with follow-up in 10-14 days to an orthopedist if suspected or nondisplaced fracture exists, or sooner if there is fracture displacement.

Gholson JJ, Bae DS, Zurakowski D, Waters PM: Scaphoid fractures in children and adolescents: Contemporary injury patterns and factors influencing time to union. *J Bone Joint Surg Am.* 2011;93:1210 [PMID: 21776574].

PHALANX DISLOCATIONS

ESSENTIALS OF DIAGNOSIS

► Pain, swelling, and deformity of affected finger.

► Often seen when an extended finger is struck by a ball.

► X-rays of finger are confirmatory.

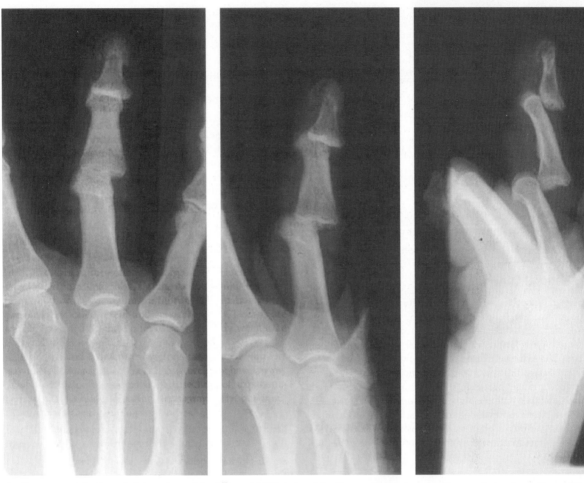

▲ **Figure 29–16.** Dorsal dislocation of the PIP and DIP joints of the finger. (Reproduced, with permission, from Simon RR, Sherman SC: *Emergency Orthopedics*, 6th ed. New York: McGraw-Hill, 2011. Copyright © McGraw-Hill Education LLC.)

▶ General Considerations

Phalanx dislocations often are the result of joint hyperextension, seen when an outstretched finger is struck by an object. Dorsal displacement of the distal segment is the most common scenario. (See Chapter 30.)

▶ Clinical Findings

Symptoms and Signs

Patients present with pain, swelling, deformity, and decreased range of motion to the affected finger. There is point tenderness over the area as well. Neurovascular integrity of the finger distally should be assessed by capillary refill time and two-point discrimination.

▶ X-ray Findings

AP and lateral views of the injured hand or finger are sufficient to evaluate for dislocation. Films should be studied for the presence of associated fractures (Figure 29–16).

▶ Treatment

Most dislocations are easily reduced with longitudinal traction applied to the distal segment. Local anesthesia or digital blocks should be considered for patient comfort prior to reduction attempts. Successful reductions should be placed in aluminum finger splints as ligamentous injury accompanies these injuries (see Table 29-1).

Disposition

Patients may be discharged home with close follow-up with a hand surgeon.

HIP INJURIES

PELVIS FRACTURES

ESSENTIALS OF DIAGNOSIS

▶ The pediatric pelvis is pliable which allows for significant displacement without fracture.

▶ May have large amount of bleeding.

▶ Consider if hematuria or scrotal hematoma.

▶ Anteroposterior films are usually confirmatory.

General Considerations

The pediatric pelvis is elastic allowing for more displacement without fracture. Pelvic fractures can be severe injuries with associated morbidity and mortality. Mechanism of injury is often a high-velocity trauma with other significant injuries. Disruption to the pelvic ring can tear pelvic veins and arteries leading to significant bleeding and hemodynamic instability. Isolated or single breaks in the pelvic ring are considered stable fractures; multiple points of disruption render the pelvis unstable. Compression injuries cause acetabular fractures or cartilage injuries often associated with hip dislocations. Avulsion fractures can occur due to muscle traction stress in adolescents. These are usually due to strong contraction of the sartorius and hamstring muscles damaging the anterior superior and inferior iliac spines or ischial tuberosity.

Clinical Findings

Symptoms and Signs

Pelvic fractures can be indicated by pain or instability on palpation. There also may be perianal edema, pelvic edema, ecchymoses, deformities, or hematomas over the inguinal ligament or scrotum. Careful examination of trauma patients for rectal or urethral bleeding is seen in pelvic fracture. Compression to determine pelvic stability should be accomplished with gentle anteroposterior and lateral pressure (Figure 29–17).

X-ray Findings

Anteroposterior view of the pelvis is often diagnostic. A CT scan should be obtained to classify the extent of injury and to plan for treatment.

Treatment

Unstable fractures are frequently associated with massive bleeding into the pelvis. The patient's vital signs and hemodynamics should be monitored closely to ensure adequate resuscitation. Pelvic binders may be initiated in the prehospital setting and should be continued in the emergency department. A sheet wrapped tightly around the pelvis may be used to stabilize the fracture and tamponade the bleeding. The orthopedist can place an external fixator device. In

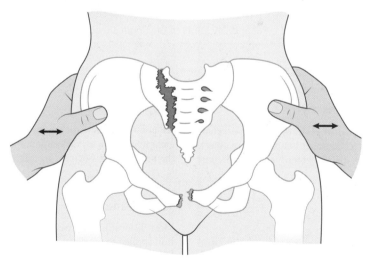

▲ **Figure 29–17.** Compression distraction test for stability of the pelvic ring. (Reproduced, with permission, from Stone CK, Humphries RL: *Current Diagnosis & Treatment Emergency Medicine,* 7th ed. New York: McGraw-Hill, 2011. Copyright © McGraw-Hill Education LLC.)

cases of severe bleeding and fracture, the patient may need emergent arteriography and embolization in radiology or open reduction with internal fixation (ORIF).

Disposition

Consultation with an orthopedist is indicated for all patients. Many patients will require hospitalization. Simple nondisplaced fractures and avulsion fractures may be managed conservatively as outpatient. Unstable fractures may require urgent or emergent intervention. Consultation with urologist or gynecologist may be necessary for some patients.

HIP FRACTURES

ESSENTIALS OF DIAGNOSIS

► Rare in children unless high-energy mechanism.

► Leg shortening and external rotation.

► X-ray confirms the diagnosis.

► True surgical emergencies.

General Considerations

Hip fractures are much less common in children than in adults and are associated with a high-impact mechanism. Hip fractures in a child younger than 2 years without history of a significant trauma should cause concern for inflicted injury. Hip fractures account for less than 1% of pediatric fractures; however, the fractures are associated with a high risk of late complications including osteonecrosis, coxa vara, nonunion, and premature physeal closure. Aggressive management is needed to prevent complications. Hip fractures are divided into four types as shown in Figure 29–18.

Type I—Transepiphyseal, extends through the proximal femoral physis.

Type II—Transcervical, most common type (40-50%), extends through the mid portion of the femoral neck.

Type III—Cervicotrochanteric (25-35%) occurs through the base of the femoral neck.

Type IV—Intertrochanteric (6-15%) occurs between the greater and lesser trochanters; best outcome.

Clinical Findings

Symptoms and Signs

Physical examination may reveal hip tenderness to palpation with limited range of motion. If the fracture is displaced, the leg will often be shortened and externally rotated. Nondisplaced fractures may present with subtle limp, knee pain, or pain with extreme range of motion.

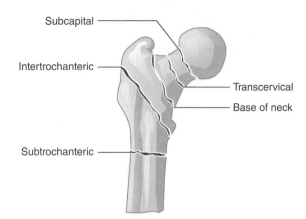

▲ **Figure 29–18.** Femoral neck fractures. (Reproduced with permission from Simon RR, Sherman SC. *Emergency Orthopedics*, 6th ed. Copyright © 2011 McGraw-Hill Education LLC.)

X-ray Findings

X-rays of the affected hip, AP and lateral views are diagnostic for fracture. Subtle fractures may not be visualized on plain films; CT, MRI, or bone scan may be warranted.

Treatment

Obtain urgent consultation with an orthopedist. Most hip fractures will require closed reduction and internal fixation. Nondisplaced type III and IV fractures may be placed in abduction spica cast.

Disposition

Pending consultation with orthopedist, admission for intraoperative repair or cast education is indicated.

Boardman MJ, Herman MJ, Buck B, Pizzutillo PD: Hip fractures in children. *J Am Acad Orthop Surg.* 2009;17:162 [PMID: 19264709].

HIP DISCLOCATION

ESSENTIALS OF DIAGNOSIS

► Pain and deformity at the hip.

► Posterior dislocations are most common.

► Pelvic or hip x-rays confirm the diagnosis.

► Early reduction to prevent complications.

General Considerations

Hip dislocations in children occur more frequently than hip fractures, although both are rare. A low-energy mechanism may cause a hip dislocation in children due to cartilage pliability and ligamentous laxity. Hip dislocations are typically caused by high-energy mechanisms and may occur in an anterior or posterior direction. As in adults, posterior dislocations are more common accounting for 80-90% of injuries occurring after impact to the knee while the hip and knee are flexed. Anterior dislocations are less common and the result of forced abduction resulting in impingement of the femoral neck or trochanter against the acetabulum. Central dislocation refers to dislocation of the femoral head caused by a fracture of the acetabulum. Posterior hip dislocations are classified as grades I-IV as shown in Figure 29–19.

Grade I—Simple dislocation without fracture.

Grade II—Dislocation associated with a large acetabular rim fracture stabilized after reduction.

Grade III—Dislocation associated with an unstable or comminuted fracture.

Grade IV—Dislocation associated with a femoral head/ neck fracture.

▶ Clinical Findings

Symptoms and Signs

Posterior dislocations present with limb shortening, hip adduction, and internal rotation of the extremity with hip and knee held in flexion. Anterior dislocations usually present with the affected limb abducted, externally rotated, and hip and knee flexion. Physical examination should include

evaluation of sensory and motor functions. Vascular injury is rare with posterior dislocation.

X-ray Findings

AP and lateral hip films will confirm the diagnosis. Evaluation is warranted for associated fractures.

▶ Treatment

Timely reduction of the dislocation is imperative to reduce the risk of further damage to the hip, including avascular necrosis, sciatic nerve injury, and traumatic arthritis. The Allis technique is a common method of closed reduction (Figure 29–20). After the patient is sedated and placed in supine position, an assistant immobilizes the pelvis by holding down the iliac crests. The physician applies traction in line with the deformity with flexion of the hip to 90 degrees. While maintaining traction, the external rotation, abduction, and extension of the hip are performed. Stimson technique is an alternative method in which the patient is placed prone with the hip flexed over the edge of the stretcher. As an assistant stabilizes the pelvis, the physician applies downward pressure with gentle rotation. The assistant aids in the

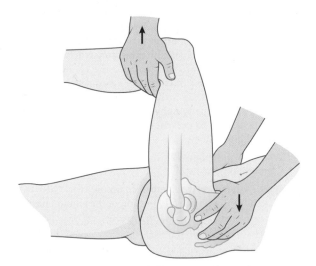

▲ **Figure 29–20.** The Allis technique for reduction of posterior hip dislocation. Both hip and knee are flexed 90 degrees. An assistant stabilizes the pelvis while the operator pulls the femur anteriorly, rotating it slightly internally and externally to aid reduction, which is achieved mainly by firm steady traction. (Reproduced, with permission, from Stone CK, Humphries RL: *Current Diagnosis & Treatment Emergency Medicine,* 7th ed. New York: McGraw-Hill, 2011. Copyright © McGraw-Hill Education LLC.)

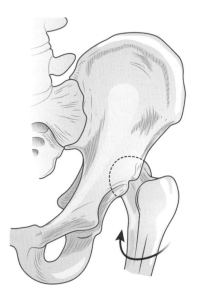

▲ **Figure 29–19.** Posterior hip dislocation. (Reproduced, with permission, from Simon RR, Sherman SC: *Emergency Orthopedics,* 6th ed. New York: McGraw-Hill, 2011. Copyright © McGraw-Hill Education LLC.)

reduction by directly manipulating the femoral head into a reduced position. Following reduction, the leg is placed in traction until postreduction films are obtained. Evaluate distal pulses, sensation, and motor function postprocedure.

Disposition

Consultation with an orthopedist is recommended for patients with hip dislocations.

SLIPPED CAPITAL FEMORAL EPIPHYSIS

 ESSENTIALS OF DIAGNOSIS

▸ Often in overweight children, aged 10-16 years.

▸ Affected limb held in external rotation.

▸ X-rays for diagnosis confirmation.

▸ Immediate consultation with orthopedist for reduction and fixation.

General Considerations

Slipped capital femoral epiphysus (SCFE) occurs in children aged 10-16 years with a male predominance. Children with endocrine disorders are at increased risk. Patients are typically overweight and approximately 25% have both hips affected. SCFE can occur insidiously or from minor trauma. There are three clinical stages: preslipping state, chronic slipping, and fixed deformity. School-aged children with knee pain and no effusion should be evaluated for SCFE. (See Chapter 43 Orthopedic Emergencies.)

Clinical Findings

Symptoms and Signs

In the preslipping stage, symptoms are usually vague and the patient may have no objective findings on examination. The patient may complain of slight groin discomfort, worse with activity and subsides with rest, and may have stiffness or slight limp. With chronic slipping or fixed deformity, the patient has tenderness around the hip. On examination, the hip is externally rotated with adduction. There is often pain and limited range of motion with internal rotation, abduction, and flexion. With bilateral involvement, the patient may have a waddling gait.

X-ray Findings

X-rays of bilateral hips confirm the diagnosis. Obtain AP and lateral views in a lateral position. Kline line, a line drawn through the superior border of the proximal femoral metaphysis, should intersect the proximal femoral epiphysis. If it does not, SCFE should be suspected (Figure 29–21).

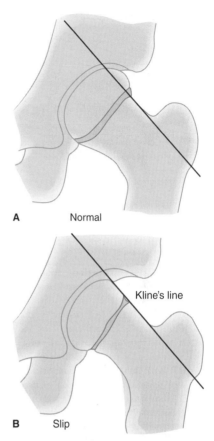

A Normal

B Slip

▲ **Figure 29–21.** Kline line on hip films to evaluate for SCFE. A normal Kline's line should intersect the epiphysis of the femoral head. (Reproduced, with permission, from Simon RR, Sherman SC: *Emergency Orthopedics,* 6th ed. New York: McGraw-Hill, 2011. Copyright © McGraw-Hill Education LLC.)

Treatment

Management involves immediate consultation with an orthopedist for operative reduction and fixation. Unstable or acute slips are more urgent to avoid avascular necrosis, chondrolysis, and to prevent further slip.

Disposition

Orthopedic consultation is required. Admission for operative repair is often indicated.

Kienstra AJ, Macias CG: Slipped capital femoral epiphysis (SCFE). *In: UpToDate, Philips W, Singer JI (ed): UpToDate:* Waltham, MA, 2012.

Murray AW, Wilson NI: Changing incidence of slipped capital femoral epiphysis: A relationship with obesity? *J Bone Joint Surg Br.* 2008;90:92-94 [PMID: 18160507].

Riad J, Bajelidze G, Gabos PG: Bilateral slipped capital femoral epiphysis: Predictive factors for contralateral slip. *J Pediatr Orthop.* 2007;27:411 [PMID: 17513962].

FEMORAL FRACTURES

FEMORAL SHAFT FRACTURES

ESSENTIALS OF DIAGNOSIS

▶ Swollen, deformed, tender thigh.

▶ Potential for large volume blood loss.

▶ X-ray is diagnostic.

▶ Consider abuse in nonambulatory children without adequate mechanism of injury.

▶ General Considerations

Femoral shaft fractures are common childhood fractures. The femur has an excellent blood supply and thus has good healing potential as well as potential for large volume of blood loss. Femoral shaft fractures occur in a bimodal distribution, peaking in toddlers due to falls and in adolescents due to motor vehicle accidents. Femur fractures in children who are nonambulatory without a significant mechanism raise suspicion for abuse.

▶ Clinical Findings

Symptoms and Signs

Physical examination often reveals a swollen, deformed, tender thigh. With significant bleeding, the patient may have tachycardia and hypotension.

X-ray Findings

AP and lateral films confirm the diagnosis and characterize the type of fracture.

▶ Treatment

Establish IV access and consider fluid resuscitation for unstable vital signs. Treatment options depend on the child's age and consultation with an orthopedist. Infants younger than 6 months may be treated with a padded splint or Pavlik harness, whereas older infants, toddlers, and children younger than 5 years are often placed in a hip spica cast. Closed reduction is indicated for angulation greater than 10 degrees. Surgical fixation is often used for older children: intramedullary flexible rod for children aged 5-11 years and intramedullary fixation with a rigid locked rod for children older than 11 years.

▶ Disposition

Consultation with an orthopedist. Admission for surgical management or cast care/teaching is often indicated.

▶ TRACTION

Traction can be used in fractures and dislocations that are displaced by muscle tension when they cannot be controlled with simple splints. Traction is most commonly employed to immobilize injuries of the pelvis, hip dislocations, acetabular fractures, and proximal femur or femoral shaft fractures. Buck traction boots apply traction through the skin and are often used in pediatric injuries that require less force. The Hare traction splint applies force through an ankle stirrup and can be used to immobilize a femoral shaft fracture (Figure 29–22). Hare traction splint can be applied in the field for transport but should be used briefly as it can lead to skin breakdown. Skeletal traction involves a pin placed through the bone distal to the fracture and is used in injuries that require more force to prevent skin damage. Skeletal traction can withhold up to 10% of body weight in applied force and can be used for a longer duration.

Hui C, Joughin E, Goldstein S, et al: Femoral fractures in children younger than three years: The role of nonaccidental injury. *J Pediatr Orthop.* 2008;28:297 [PMID: 18362793].

Kanlic E, Cruz M: Current concepts in pediatric femur fracture treatment. *Orthopedics.* 2007;30(12):1015-1019 [PMID: 18198772].

Loder RT, O'Donnell PW, Feinberg JR: Epidemiology and mechanisms of femur fractures in children. *J Pediatr Orthop.* 2006; 26:561 [PMID: 16923091].

KNEE INJURIES

KNEE DISLOCATION

ESSENTIALS OF DIAGNOSIS

▶ Dislocation of the tibiofemoral joint is a surgical emergency

▶ High or low energy mechanism

▶ Visible deformity to the knee

▶ At risk for vascular and nerve injury

▶ General Considerations

Tibiofemoral dislocations are infrequent but are potentially limb-threatening injuries. They can be due to high- or low-energy mechanisms that also involve injury to multiple ligaments of the knee. The popliteal artery runs across the popliteal space making it highly susceptible to injury during

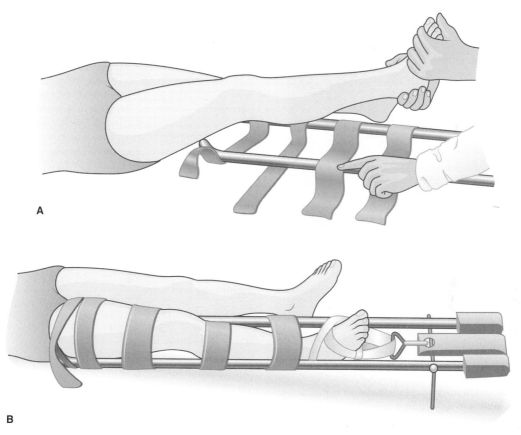

▲ Figure 29-22. Hare traction splint. **(A)** Hare traction is applied as shown by applying traction to the lower limb and elevating it with the knee held in extension. **(B)** The splint is then inserted under the limb and the foot secured in the traction apparatus. (Reproduced, with permission, from Simon RR, Sherman SC: *Emergency Orthopedics,* 6th ed. New York: McGraw-Hill, 2011. Copyright © McGraw-Hill Education LLC.)

knee dislocation. Approximately 40% of patients with knee dislocations have associated vascular injury. The peroneal nerve winds around the fibular neck and is injured in up to 23% patients with knee dislocations.

▶ Clinical Manifestations

Signs and Symptoms

Tibiofemoral dislocations may be clinically obvious with history of acute trauma and grossly abnormal position of the knee. Injury is often associated with significant hemarthrosis and ecchymosis, pain, and swelling. Initial physical examination may be limited due to pain but assessment of direction of the dislocation can be made. Careful assessment of distal pulses, sensation, and motor function should be performed frequently to assess for popliteal artery and peroneal nerve damage.

▶ Diagnosis

AP and lateral films of the knee can characterize degree and directions of dislocation and assess for fractures. CT or MRI may be performed to delineate the extent of injury (Figure 29–23).

▶ Treatment

Closed reduction should be performed immediately if there is evidence of vascular compromise. Imaging may be done pre-reduction if distal pulses are strong. Posterolateral dislocations cannot be reduced by closed reduction due to two factors: buttonholing of the medial femoral condyle through the medial capsule and medial collateral ligament invagination into the joint. Following closed reduction, look closely for signs of vascular injury, such as diminished or absent pulses, pale or dusky skin, paresthesias, or paralysis. The knee is then immobilized at 15-20 degrees of flexion.

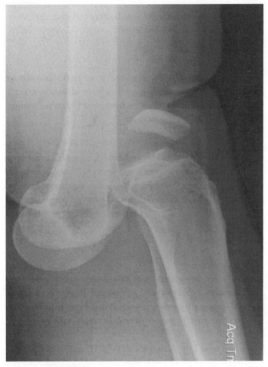

▲ **Figure 29–23.** Anterior dislocation of the knee.
(Reproduced, with permission, from Simon RR, Sherman SC: *Emergency Orthopedics*, 6th ed. New York: McGraw-Hill, 2011. Copyright © McGraw-Hill Education LLC.)

▶ Disposition

Obtain prompt consultation with orthopedist for closed reduction. After reduction, the patient is admitted to the hospital for close monitoring of the limb's vascular function with serial reassessment. After hospital discharge, the patient will follow-up with orthopedist to assess and repair ligamentous injury.

DISTAL FEMUR FRACTURES

 ESSENTIALS OF DIAGNOSIS

▶ Often high-energy mechanism with associated injuries.

▶ Pain, swelling near the distal femur and inability to bear weight.

▶ Monitor closely for neurovascular compromise and compartment syndrome.

▶ Consider abuse in nonambulatory children without adequate mechanism of injury.

▶ General Considerations

Distal femur fractures are relatively uncommon fractures accounting for 12-18% of femur fractures in children. Femur fractures are typically due to a high-energy mechanism involving direct force and often have additional injuries including fractures of the hip and proximal femur, ligamentous injury, vascular injury, peroneal nerve injury, and damage to the quadriceps. Due to the risk of vascular compromise, it is necessary to monitor closely for compartment syndrome on initial presentation with frequent repeat assessments. Transverse fractures through the metaphysis are the most common site of injury followed by Salter-Harris II fractures of the epiphysis. Condylar fractures are partially intra-articular and often disrupt the articular surface with long-term complications, including arthritis.

▶ Clinical Findings

Symptoms and Signs

Patients exhibit pain and swelling near the distal femur and are unable to bear weight. Physical examination may reveal shortening, rotation, and angulation with tenderness upon palpation along the joint line. Leg is often held in flexion due to hamstring muscle spasm. Swelling in the popliteal fossa, diminished distal pulses, delayed capillary refill, and a cold pale foot may be seen with injury to the popliteal vessels. Foot drop and sensory deficits to the foot may indicate injury to the peroneal or posterior tibial nerves.

X-ray Findings

AP and lateral films that include the entire femur and hip are diagnostic. Angiography or computed tomography may be indicated with neurovascular compromise.

▶ Treatment

Treatment options depend on the child's age and consultation with an orthopedist. Infants younger than 6 months may be treated with a padded splint; older infants, toddlers, and children younger than 6 years are often placed in a high long leg cast. Closed reduction is indicated for angulation greater than 10 degrees. Pins, screws, intramedullary flexible rods, plates, and external fixators may be used in children older than 6 years.

▶ Disposition

Consult orthopedist regarding treatment options. Children with stable fractures that are splinted may be followed up as outpatient.

PATELLA FRACTURES

ESSENTIALS OF DIAGNOSIS

▶ Caused by direct blunt trauma or indirect pulling force.

▶ Swollen, tender knee.

▶ May disrupt extensor mechanism.

▶ X-rays are diagnostic.

General Considerations

Patella fractures are uncommon in children. Most fractures are due to a direct blow to the patella, such as falling on a flexed knee or striking the dashboard during a motor vehicle collision. Indirect force from a sudden, forceful pull of the quadriceps muscle is a potential mechanism, typically resulting in a transverse fracture or upper/lower pole avulsion. Patella fractures may be associated with disruption of the extensor mechanism of the knee.

Clinical Findings

Symptoms and Signs

Examination reveals tenderness over the patella with an acutely swollen knee. Joint effusion may also be present. Inability to extend the knee indicates disruption to the extensor mechanism.

X-ray Findings

X-rays of the knee, including AP, lateral, and sunrise views, are often adequate to define the fracture, as shown in Figure 29–24. Magnetic resonance imaging may be useful if associated soft tissue injury or occult fracture is suspected.

Treatment

Obtain consultation with an orthopedist. Simple or non-displaced fractures with intact extensor mechanism may be splinted in extension and non–weight-bearing.

Disposition

Simple fractures require outpatient management with and orthopedic physician. Displaced, comminuted fractures or disrupted extensor mechanism are repaired operatively.

PATELLA DISLOCATION

ESSENTIALS OF DIAGNOSIS

▶ History of twisting mechanism with a pop.

▶ Obvious deformity of the knee held in flexion.

▶ Lateral dislocation is most common.

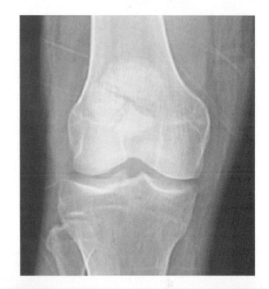

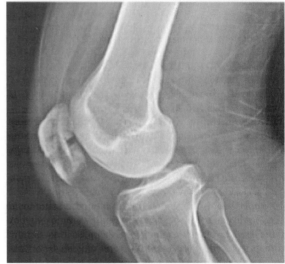

▲ **Figure 29–24.** X-ray patella fracture. (Reproduced, with permission, from Simon RR, Sherman SC: *Emergency Orthopedics,* 6th ed. New York: McGraw-Hill, 2011. Copyright © McGraw-Hill Education LLC.)

General Considerations

Patella dislocation is typically due to a twisting mechanism, though less commonly results from direct trauma. Lateral dislocation is most common and approximately 40% of children have associated fractures. Children younger than 15 years have a high rate of recurrent dislocation ($\geq$ 60%). Patients often describe severe acute pain and hearing a pop or tear.

▶ Clinical Findings

Symptoms and Signs

Physical examination reveals a grossly deformed knee held in 20-30 degrees of flexion with palpable patella laterally. The dislocation is usually obvious unless the patella has spontaneously reduced with knee extension.

X-ray Findings

AP, lateral, and patellar sunrise radiographs should be obtained after the reduction to assess for fracture or avulsion.

▶ Treatment

To reduce a lateral patella dislocation manually, flex the hip slightly to relax the quadriceps. The knee is then slowly extended while applying pressure to the lateral aspect of the patella. A successfully reduced patella should then be in line with the tibiofemoral tract with normal function.

▶ Disposition

Following successful reduction and postreduction films, the patient is placed in a knee immobilizer held in extension and kept non–weight-bearing with outpatient follow-up to an orthopedist.

KNEE INJURIES: SOFT TISSUE INJURIES

GENERAL CONSIDERATIONS

The knee is a large, complex joint that is capable of a wide range of movements including flexion, extension, internal and external rotation, abduction, and adduction. It is composed of three articulations: the medial and lateral condylar joints and the patellofemoral joint. Multiple stabilizing structures are necessary to allow for movement without compromising the strength of the joint, including articular capsule and its tendinous attachments, the collateral ligaments, and the intra-articular cruciate ligaments (Figure 29–25). Disruption to these ligaments can be classified according to severity.

  Grade 1—Small incomplete tear: focal tenderness, minimal swelling, no stress test instability with firm end point.

  Grade 2—Moderate incomplete tear: local tenderness, moderate swelling, 1+ instability with firm end point, moderate disabling.

  Grade 3—Complete rupture: local tenderness with significant pain, minimal to marked swelling, 2-3+ stress instability with mushy end point, severe disability.

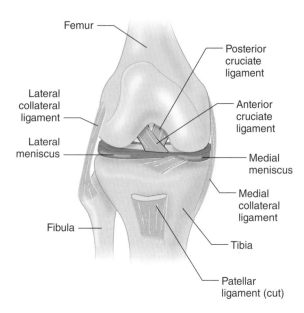

▲ **Figure 29–25.** The ligamentous and meniscal structures of the knee. (Reproduced, with permission, from Spence, *Basic Human Anatomy*, 3rd, ©1991. Printed and Electronically reproduced by permission of Pearson Education, Inc., Upper Saddle River, New Jersey.)

EXTENSOR MECHANISM DISRUPTION: QUADRICEPS/PATELLAR TENDON RUPTURE

 ESSENTIALS OF DIAGNOSIS

▶ Knee buckles or "gives out" and severe pain.

▶ Consider in young athletes who perform repetitive movements.

▶ Patella displacement with associated swelling and pain.

▶ Plain films often indicative of the injury.

▶ General Considerations

Extensor mechanism of the knee can become disrupted by injury to the following: quadriceps tendon, patella, patellar tendon, and tibial tubercle. Acute tendon rupture injury may be direct or indirect. Indirect is most common resulting from forced flexion when the quadriceps is contracted, such as falling down a staircase. Patients often report sudden buckling of the knee followed by severe pain. Rapid repetitive acceleration, deceleration, jumping, and landing result in small tears of the extensor tendons. Proximal patellar tendonitis progressing to tendon rupture or "jumper's knee" typically occurs in young athletes. Jumper knee is divided into four stages, from stage I (pain after activity) to stage IV (tendon rupture).

 Clinical Findings

Symptoms and Signs

The patella may be inferiorly displaced with proximal ecchymosis and swelling indicating quadriceps rupture. Superior displacement of the patella with inferior swelling and tenderness indicates a patellar tendon rupture. The patient often will have inability to actively extend or hold passive extension of the knee against gravity. Rarely the patient will have very weak intact extension.

X-ray Findings

AP and lateral knee films often suggest the injury. MRI is used to further characterize the injury.

Treatment

Knee is maintained in extension with a knee immobilizer and patient is kept non–weight-bearing.

Disposition

Definitive treatment for a partial rupture requires early referral to an orthopedist for casting. A complete tendon tear is treated surgically within 1-2 weeks of injury.

MENISCUS TEARS

ESSENTIALS OF DIAGNOSIS

▶ Associated with twisting injuries.
▶ History of locking or giving way.
▶ Joint line tenderness, effusion, inability to squat.
▶ MRI or arthroscopy is diagnostic.

General Considerations

The two menisci in the knee are crescent-shaped pads of cartilage between the femoral condyles and tibial plateaus that dissipate loading forces placed on the knee, stabilize the knee during rotation, and lubricate the joint. Meniscal injuries of the knee are common. Acute meniscal tears in children and adolescents occur most often from twisting injures or rotational force that occurs when the foot is planted. The medial meniscus is most commonly affected. Patients with untreated tears may present with complaint of the affected knee popping, locking, giving out, or catching.

 Clinical Findings

Symptoms and Signs

Examination findings depend on the location and extent of the tear. Physical examination may show joint line tenderness, joint effusion, and inability to squat or kneel. Knee motion may be abnormal with a loss of smooth passive motion or inability to fully extend the knee. Palpable catching at the joint line during extension may be detected by the McMurray maneuver. To perform the McMurray test, the patient is supine with the hip and knee flexed while the examiner extends in internal rotation (lateral meniscus) or external rotation (medial meniscus). A painful click, popping, or thud felt in early extension is abnormal. Apley test is performed on a prone patient with the knee flexed. The examiner extends the knee while in external rotation while providing distraction then compression. Pain worse with compression may indicate a meniscal tear.

X-ray Findings

Plain films of the knee, AP, lateral, and sunrise views, are often negative. MRI may be obtained if symptoms persist and is useful in characterizing tears and detecting small tears.

Treatment

Immobilize the knee, non–weight-bearing with repeat examination in 24 hours to assess for ligamentous injury. Limit immobilization to 2-4 days to begin quadriceps strengthening.

Disposition

Patients with meniscal tears may be discharged home with knee immobilization and follow-up to orthopedist. MRI or arthroscopy may be indicated for significant effusion, joint instability, or chronic symptoms.

CRUCIATE LIGAMENTS

ESSENTIALS OF DIAGNOSIS

▶ Often low-energy, non contact sports injuries.
▶ Pop followed by rapid development of large joint effusion.
▶ ACL tears much more common than PCL tears.
▶ X-rays with a Segond fracture indicate likely ACL tear.

General Considerations

Anterior cruciate ligament (ACL) tears are common. They often occur in noncontact sports with a female predominance. The typical noncontact mechanism is a running or jumping athlete who suddenly decelerates or pivots causing rotation or valgus stress of the knee. Injuries that occur during contact involve a direct blow causing hyperextension or valgus stress to the knee. History of a pop or snap at the time of injury with rapid development of knee effusion is an ACL injury until proven otherwise. Posterior cruciate ligament (PCL) injury is less common than ACL injury and occurs from a fall forward onto the knee when the foot is plantar flexed or from a direct blow to the anterior proximal tibia, often during a contact sport or motor vehicle crash.

▶ Clinical Findings

Symptoms and Signs

Knee examination will likely show pain, effusion, and often hemarthrosis. Three tests commonly used to assess for ACL tear include the anterior drawer, the Lachman, and the pivot shift. Each test must be performed in comparison with the uninjured knee. Anterior drawer test detects movement of the tibia anteriorly relative to the femur while the knee is flexed at 90 degrees and the patient is supine. Lachman test signifies injury when an increase in laxity is noted when attempting to pull the tibia forward relative to the femur while the knee is slightly flexed. Pivot shift test is used to detect anterolateral rotatory instability. A positive posterior drawer test (increased knee laxity when the tibia is pushed posteriorly) suggests a PCL injury.

X-ray Findings

Plain films are obtained to rule out associated fractures. Segond fracture is a small avulsion fracture of the lateral tibial condyle that suggests an ACL tear as shown in Figure 29–26. MRI can delineate soft-tissue injuries although it is often unnecessary in the emergency department.

▶ Treatment

Isolated ACL injuries can be treated with partial weight-bearing with crutches. Immobilization is used in patients with ligamentous injury and joint instability.

▶ Disposition

Patients may be discharged home, partial weight-bearing, with follow-up to orthopedist. Surgical repair may be considered depending on the patient's age, activity level, and associated injuries.

Spindler KP, Wright RW: Clinical practice. Anterior cruciate ligament tear. *N Engl J Med.* 2008;359:2135 [PMID: 19005197].

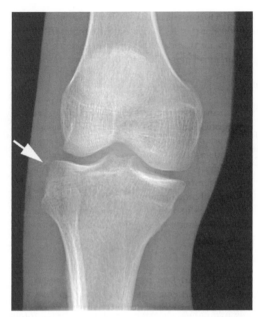

▲ **Figure 29–26.** X-ray of Segond fracture. (Reproduced, with permission, from Simon RR, Sherman SC: *Emergency Orthopedics,* 6th ed. New York: McGraw-Hill, 2011. Copyright © McGraw-Hill Education LLC.)

COLLATERAL LIGAMENTS

 ESSENTIALS OF DIAGNOSIS

▶ Medial collateral ligament is most often affected.

▶ Often sports-related injuries involving direct force to lateral knee.

▶ Initial examination may be limited by pain and swelling.

▶ X-rays often normal.

▶ General Considerations

Medial collateral ligament (MCL) is most commonly injured ligament in the knee and is often associated with ACL injury. Injuries to MCL are frequently sports injuries that involve a direct blow to the lateral knee. Lateral collateral ligament (LCL) injuries are less common and occur in high-energy trauma such as motor vehicle collisions. Initial examination may be limited due to pain, swelling, and muscle spasm.

▶ Clinical Findings

Symptoms and Signs

Patient will have pain along the area of the injured ligament. Joint effusion may be present. Joint opening palpable on valgus stress test indicates an injury to MCL, whereas joint opening on varus stress test suggests injury to LCL.

X-ray Findings

Plain films are obtained to rule out associated fractures. MRI can delineate soft-tissue injuries although is often unnecessary in the emergency department.

▶ Treatment

For mild sprains, ice, elevation, and compression with early ambulation are recommended.

▶ Disposition

Patients may be immobilized and discharged home with close follow-up to orthopedist. Unstable knees will often need MRI and surgical repair.

> Louw QA, Manilall J, Grimmer KA: Epidemiology of knee injuries among adolescents: A systematic review. *Br J Sports Med.* 2008;42:2 [PMID: 17550921].

TIBIA/FIBULA INJURIES

TIBIAL TUBEROSITY FRACTURES AND OSGOOD-SCHLATTER

ESSENTIALS OF DIAGNOSIS

▶ Pain when squatting, kneeling, or climbing stairs.

▶ Painful, swollen knee, with tenderness over the tibial tubercle.

▶ General Considerations

Osgood-Schlatter disease, or tibial tubercle apophysitis, is due to a disturbance in the development of the tibial tuberosity due to chronic repetitive trauma to the proximal tibial growth plate. The disease is most commonly found in pubertal adolescents, 8 to 13-year-old-girls and 10 to 15-year-old-boys, who participate in sports that involve repetitive jumping. There is a male predominance and is usually unilateral. Pain is worse with quadriceps use against resistance such as climbing stairs, squatting, or kneeling.

▶ Clinical Findings

Symptoms and Signs

On physical examination, the knee is painful, swollen, and tender over the tibial tubercle. Joint effusion is absent.

X-ray Findings

X-rays of the knee are typically diagnostic. MRI and ultrasound of the knee may be used if diagnosis is uncertain or patient does not respond to typical therapy.

▶ Treatment

Treatment includes reduced activity for 2-4 months, ice after exercise, and a short course of nonsteroidal anti-inflammatory medications. Consultation with orthopedist is necessary for tibial tuberosity fractures as they may require open reduction.

▶ Disposition

Patients are discharged home with primary care physician follow-up. Referral to orthopedist for patients with tibial tuberosity fractures, and for those with persistent pain not improved with rest.

TIBIAL PLATEAU FRACTURES

ESSENTIALS OF DIAGNOSIS

▶ Painful, swollen knee with point tenderness and effusion.

▶ May have associated nerve or popliteal artery injury.

▶ High risk for compartment syndrome.

▶ CT/MRI may be needed to fully delineate the injury.

▶ General Considerations

Tibial plateau fractures involve the articular surface and are frequently associated with other severe injuries, including ligamentous, meniscal, vascular injuries, and compartment syndrome. The mechanism of injury is often a direct force to the proximal tibia such as a fall from height, an automobile-pedestrian accident, or an axial load with varus or valgus force.

▶ Clinical Findings

Symptoms and Signs

On physical examination, the knee is painful, swollen and often held in flexion. There is often a large effusion and hemarthrosis.

X-ray Findings

AP, lateral, and oblique views of the knee on x-ray are often adequate for characterizing these fractures (Figure 29–27). Widened spaces or small avulsion fragments may indicate a ligamentous injury, and a CT scan or MRI may be necessary

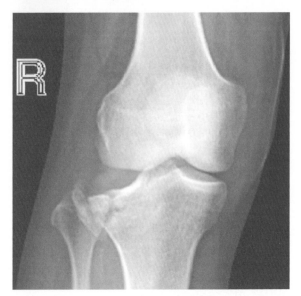

▲ **Figure 29–27.** Tibial plateau fracture. (Reproduced, with permission, from Simon RR, Sherman SC: *Emergency Orthopedics*, 6th ed. New York: McGraw-Hill, 2011. Copyright © McGraw-Hill Education LLC.)

to fully determine the extent of the injury. Arteriogram may be obtained if vascular injury is suspected.

▶ **Treatment**

Treatment includes knee immobilization, non–weight-bearing and early consultation with orthopedist. Close monitoring is needed for signs of compartment syndrome.

▶ **Disposition**

Nondisplaced, stable fractures without depression may be treated nonoperatively, discharged home with protected immobilization and orthopedist follow-up. Articular fracture that results in instability of the knee joint requires operative fixation.

TIBIAL SPINE FRACTURES

 ESSENTIALS OF DIAGNOSIS

▶ Occur in adolescents.

▶ Painful, swollen knee with effusion.

▶ Typically avulsion fracture from the cruciate ligament.

▶ **General Considerations**

Tibial spine fractures typically occur in children, aged 8-14 years, and are analogous to ACL injury in skeletally mature adults. Tibial spine fractures are often the result of indirect trauma when anterior or posterior force is directed against the flexed proximal tibia. This causes cruciate ligament tension and avulsion of the spine. Collateral and cruciate ligamentous injuries are commonly associated.

▶ **Clinical Findings**

Symptoms and Signs

On physical examination the knee is painful and swollen with effusion. Inability to fully extend the knee indicates a displaced or complete fracture.

X-ray Findings

AP, lateral, and sunrise x-rays of the knee are often adequate for characterizing these fractures as shown in Figure 29–28. Widened spaces or small avulsion fragments may indicate a ligamentous injury, and a CT scan or MRI may be necessary to determine the extent of the injury.

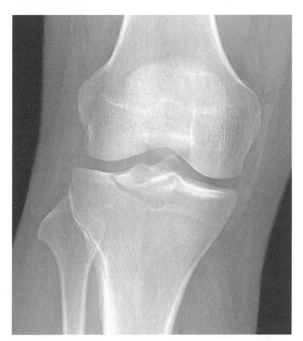

▲ **Figure 29–28.** Tibial spine fracture. (Reproduced, with permission, from Simon RR, Sherman SC: *Emergency Orthopedics*, 6th ed. New York: McGraw-Hill, 2011. Copyright © McGraw-Hill Education LLC.)

Treatment

Nondisplaced fractures with no ligamentous injury can be treated with immobilization.

Disposition

Incomplete avulsions with displacement without ligamentous injury undergo closed reduction with subsequent cast immobilization. Operative repair is indicated for complete fractures.

TIBIAL/FIBULA SHAFT FRACTURES

 ESSENTIALS OF DIAGNOSIS

- ▶ May be due to direct or indirect trauma.
- ▶ Third most common fracture in children.
- ▶ X-rays are diagnostic.
- ▶ High risk for open fractures and compartment syndrome.

General Considerations

Tibial shaft fractures are the third most common long bone fracture in children with associated fibula fracture in 30% of patients. Multiple mechanisms result in fractures of the tibia shaft. Older children are more likely to have transverse or comminuted fractures due to high-energy direct trauma, whereas younger children are more likely to have spiral or oblique fractures from a low-energy fall or twisting mechanism. The anterior tibia is close to the skin surface making open fractures more common. Compartment syndrome is relatively frequent after tibial fracture accounting for approximately 35% of patients with compartment syndrome. Toddler fractures are specific nondisplaced spiral fractures of the distal tibia that occur in children aged 9 months-3 years that result from relatively minor trauma and falls. Tibia shaft fractures in a nonambulatory child without a mechanism should raise suspicion for non-accidental trauma. Isolated fibula fractures are typically due to a direct injury to the lateral distal leg.

Clinical Findings

Symptoms and Signs

Physical examination reveals pain, swelling, and deformity to the lower leg. Assess for open fractures and neurovascular compromise due to compartment syndrome. Toddler fractures and isolated fibula fractures may present with limp or refusal to bear weight.

X-ray Findings

AP and lateral films, including the knee and ankle, are often adequate to define the fracture.

Patients with open fractures, evidence of compartment syndrome, or fractures with greater than 10 degrees of anterior angulation, greater than 5 degrees varus/valgus angulation, or greater than 1 cm shortening should have prompt consultation with orthopedist.

Treatment

Simple, nondisplaced fractures can be placed in a long posterior splint (Table 29–1). Open fractures require prompt antibiotics with broad coverage and tetanus.

Disposition

Those with simple non-displaced fractures should be kept non weight-bearing with outpatient follow-up with and orthopedist.

Podeszwa DA, Mubarak SJ: Physeal fractures of the distal tibia and fibula (Salter-Harris Type I, II, III, and IV fractures). *J Pediatr Orthop.* 2012;32:S62 [PMID: 22588106].

ANKLE INJURIES

ANKLE DISLOCATION

 ESSENTIALS OF DIAGNOSIS

- ▶ Often has an associated fracture.
- ▶ Assess neurovascular status closely.
- ▶ May need urgent reduction prior to imaging.

General Considerations

Ankle dislocation represents displacement of the talus and foot from the tibia. Dislocations are described by the relationship of the talus to the tibia with posterior dislocations being the most common. Associated fractures are often present. Dislocations can occur from axial loading to the foot in plantar flexion and are seen in sporting injuries and in high-energy trauma such as motor vehicle collisions.

Clinical Manifestations

Signs and Symptoms

Patient will have gross deformity of the ankle with significant swelling and pain. Assess quickly distal pulses, perfusion, and sensation. Skin tenting may be noted over the malleoli.

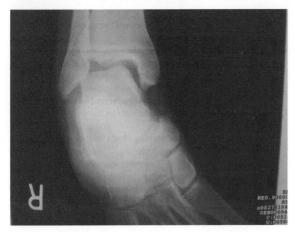

▲ **Figure 29–29.** Ankle dislocation.

Diagnosis

X-rays of the ankle are diagnostic (Figure 29–29). Do not delay reduction for imaging in the setting of neurovascular compromise or skin tenting. Subsequent CT is often performed to characterize the extent of injury.

Treatment

Following closed reduction and reassessment of the neurovascular status, splint the ankle and obtain radiographs. Consultation with orthopedist should be obtained in patients with ankle dislocation.

Disposition

Patients should be admitted to the hospital for close monitoring of neurovascular status overnight, and follow-up with orthopedist after discharged home.

MALLEOLAR FRACTURES

 ESSENTIALS OF DIAGNOSIS

▶ Swelling, ecchymosis, and point tenderness.

▶ Range from simple fractures to complete joint disruption.

▶ X-rays are diagnostic.

General Considerations

The ankle bears more weight per size than any joint in the body. Ankle bones include the distal tibia, distal fibula, and talus. The mortise is formed by the medial and lateral malleoli and the articular surface of the distal tibia. Inversion injuries typically affect the lateral malleolus, whereas forces applied during eversion stress the medial malleolus. However, significant force can cause disruption to both. Malleolar fractures range from simple avulsion fractures to unstable fractures through multiple planes that lead to disruption of the ankle mortise. When fractures are present through the lateral and medial malleoli, they are referred to as bimalleolar fractures. The presence of a third fracture through the posterior malleolus is classified as a trimalleolar fracture.

Clinical Findings

Symptoms and Signs

Physical examination reveals inability to bear weight with ankle swelling, ecchymoses, and tenderness. Isolated fracture will have predominance of swelling and tenderness over the affected side. Careful examination of the foot and knee should be performed to assess for associated fractures.

X-ray Findings

X-rays of the ankle including AP, lateral, and mortise views are usually diagnostic.

Treatment

Simple fractures of the fibula and some nondisplaced fractures of the distal tibia may be placed in a short posterior leg splint with ankle stirrup and non–weight-bearing with orthopedic follow-up. Consultation with orthopedist should be obtained for Salter-Harris fractures that may affect subsequent growth. Unstable fractures that are displaced should undergo prompt closed reduction and splinting (see Table 29-1).

Disposition

Definitive management of an unstable ankle fracture is surgical fixation. If unstable fractures cannot be reduced in the emergency department, urgent surgical reduction is required to prevent long-term complications.

TRIPLANE FRACTURES

 ESSENTIALS OF DIAGNOSIS

▶ Occurs in adolescents prior to growth plate fusion.

▶ Eversion injury.

▶ X-rays often adequate.

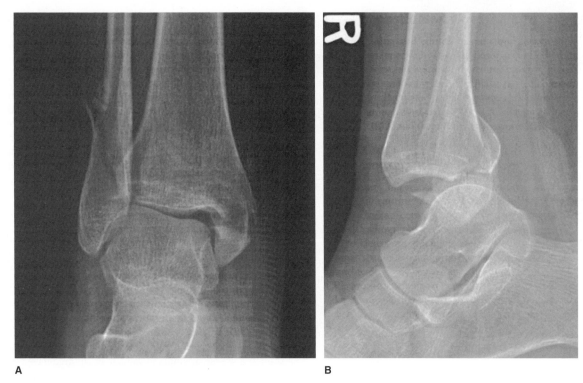

A   B

▲ **Figure 29–30.** Triplane fracture of the ankle. (Reproduced, with permission, from Simon RR, Sherman SC: *Emergency Orthopedics*, 6th ed. New York: McGraw-Hill, 2011. Copyright © McGraw-Hill Education LLC.)

► General Considerations

Triplane fractures of the distal tibia typically occur in adolescents (12–15 years) prior to fusion of the distal tibia growth plate. Triplane fractures extend through a number of planes: transverse (through the growth plate), sagittal (epiphysis), and coronal (distal tibial metaphysis). This results in three distinct fragments, disrupting the tibial plafond and often extending into the joint. Combination of Salter-Harris type II fracture plus Tillaux fracture results in a type IV fracture. This distinct fracture occurs due to the unequal fusion of the growth plate. When eversion of the foot on the tibia is applied, it places stress on the open distal lateral tibial growth plate initiating the fracture. The other fracture lines are propagated through the coronal and sagittal planes as the foot is plantar flexed with variable axial load. Fibula fractures are often associated with triplane fractures.

► Clinical Findings

Symptoms and Signs

Physical examination reveals swelling, ecchymosis, tenderness, and inability to bear weight. Deformity may be present. Inspect carefully for sites of open fracture. Tenderness over associated fibula fractures may be present.

X-ray Findings

X-rays of the ankle including AP, lateral, and mortise views are usually diagnostic. CT may be obtained to further characterize complex fractures (Figure 29–30).

► Treatment

Nondisplaced fractures (< 2 mm displacement) that are extra-articular may be placed in posterior leg splint with ankle stirrup, non–weight-bearing with follow-up to orthopedist. Closed reduction may be attempted for displacement of greater than 3 mm.

► Disposition

Triplane fractures with greater than 2-mm displacement after attempted closed reduction are treated with open reduction and internal fixation by the orthopedic physician.

ANKLE SPRAINS

ESSENTIALS OF DIAGNOSIS

▶ Most common ankle injury.

▶ Frequently inversion injuries with lateral ligamentous sprain.

▶ Pain and swelling.

▶ Ottawa ankle rules to determine if imaging is necessary.

General Considerations

Ankle sprain are the most common ankle injury that presents to the emergency department, accounting for 75% of ankle injuries. Sprains are due to forced inversion or eversion of the ankle typically while the ankle is plantar-flexed. Inversion injuries resulting in lateral ligamentous injury account for 85% of ankle sprains. Eversion injuries are much less likely to result in sprains; avulsion of the medial malleolus occurs more frequently. Ankle sprains can be categorized by level of injury and instability. Stress testing is often limited due to pain and swelling.

Clinical Findings

Symptoms and Signs

First-degree injuries: Ligament injury without tear. Patient is able to ambulate with minimal pain; little to no swelling with mild tenderness over the affected ligament. No abnormal motion or pain with stress testing

Second-degree injuries: Incomplete tear of a ligament. Patient is able to bear weight with pain; moderate swelling, ecchymosis, and tenderness. Pain with normal range of motion and mild instability. Moderate pain with stress testing.

Third-degree injuries: Complete tear of a ligament. Patient is unable to bear weight; large amount of swelling within 1-2 hours. Positive stress test.

Stress testing of the ankle can determine the extent of injury and identify ligament involved. Tests are performed with patient seated with knee flexed to 90 degrees and ankle in neutral position. Anterior drawer test examines the anterior talofibular ligament. The heel is gently pulled forward while pushing the lower leg posteriorly assessing for visual deformity or palpable clunk. Talar tilt test assesses the anterior talofibular and calcaneofibular ligaments. The heel is inverted while examining for displacement of the talar head or laxity. External rotation test evaluates the distal talar syndesmotic ligaments. The foot is rotated, observing for laxity and pain laterally.

X-ray Findings

X-rays, including AP, lateral, and mortise views of the ankle, should be taken to assess for associated fractures. Films may be avoided by applying the Ottawa Ankle Rules, typically in cases of first-degree sprains. CT or MRI may be indicated if later complications develop.

▶ Treatment

First-degree sprains can be treated with ice, elevation, and compression (using air casts or Ace bandages) with early mobilization, weight-bearing as tolerated. Second-degree sprains are treated similarly; however, they are kept non–weight-bearing for 48-72 hours with progression to ambulation as tolerated. Patients with complete ligamentous tear should be splinted and kept non–weight-bearing with follow-up in 5 days with orthopedist when swelling has lessened.

▶ Disposition

Patients with ankle sprains can be discharged home with follow-up to orthopedist if indicated.

▶ Ottawa Ankle Rules

The Ottawa Ankle Rules were developed to prevent unnecessary imaging in ankle injuries by predicting likelihood of fracture. They have been shown to identify 100% of significant malleolar fractures and have been validated in multiple studies; however, attempts to validate in children have been inconclusive.

Ankle x-ray series is required only if there is pain in the ankle plus one of the following.

1. Lateral malleolus (posterior aspect) tenderness

2. Medial malleolus (posterior aspect) tenderness

3. Inability to bear weight immediately and in the emergency department for four steps

Boutis K, Willan AR, Babyn P, et al: A randomized, controlled trial of a removable brace versus casting in children with lowrisk ankle fractures. *Pediatrics.* 2007;119:e1256 [PMID: 17545357].

Dowling S, Spooner CH, Liang Y, et al: Accuracy of Ottawa Ankle Rules to exclude fractures of the ankle and midfoot in children: A meta-analysis. *Acad Emerg Med.* 2009;16:277 [PMID: 19187397].

FOOT INJURIES

ACHILLES TENDON RUPTURE

ESSENTIALS OF DIAGNOSIS

▶ Due to sudden force on the Achilles tendon.

▶ Weakness of plantar flexion and palpable defect.

▶ Positive calf-squeeze and knee flexion tests.

▶ Clinical diagnosis.

General Considerations

Achilles tendon rupture is typically due to a mechanism of injury that includes an extra stretch applied to a taut tendon, forceful dorsiflexion with the ankle in a relaxed state, or direct trauma to a taut tendon. Patients often participate in a strenuous sport that involves pivoting or sudden acceleration. Patients are typically asymptomatic prior to rupture and report a sudden onset of pain and sensation that they sustained a direct blow to the back of the leg. They may report hearing a snap or pop. Tendon rupture is commonly misdiagnosed as ankle sprain due to incomplete examination or vague pain symptoms; pain in ankle sprains often begins with landing, whereas pain in Achilles tendon rupture begins with pushing off. Oral steroids and fluoroquinolones predispose patients to injury.

Clinical Findings

Symptoms and Signs

Physical examination may reveal bruising and swelling in the area of the Achilles tendon. There may be weakness of plantar flexion with a palpable defect.

Calf-squeeze or Thompson test is helpful in detecting complete tendon rupture as some patients may not have weakness of plantar flexion or inability to bear weight. The patient lies prone with feet off the table or kneels on a chair; the calves are squeezed bilaterally and the foot is observed for plantar flexion. A complete rupture is indicated by little or no foot movement.

Knee flexion test is performed by asking the patient to flex the knees to 90 degrees while lying prone. In cases of Achilles tendon rupture, the foot will be dorsiflexed or neutral.

X-ray Findings

X-rays are not helpful in diagnosing Achilles tendon rupture but may show associated stress fractures. Ultrasound and MRI may be utilized if needed to further detail the rupture.

Treatment

Ice, analgesics, immobilization with the ankle plantar flexed to a position of comfort and non–weight-bearing (see Table 29-1).

Disposition

Patients may be discharged home with immobilization and non–weight-bearing with urgent follow-up within 48 hours to an orthopedist. Surgical treatment is preferred over casting in younger or athletic patients.

CALCANEAL/TALAR FRACTURES

ESSENTIALS OF DIAGNOSIS

- ▶ Rare fractures in children.
- ▶ Risk for disrupted vascular supply and AVN.
- ▶ Pain, swelling, and inability to bear weight.
- ▶ May need CT or MRI to identify subtle fractures.

General Considerations

Fractures of the hindfoot in children are uncommon due to skeletal immaturity and the large amount of cartilage present. However, fractures of the hindfoot have the greatest potential for causing permanent deformity and disability. Talar neck fractures are the most common. Fractures of the calcaneus, as well as the cuboid, navicular, and cuneiform are rare and often associated with high-energy mechanisms involving motorized recreational vehicles. Talar neck fractures are often associated with forced dorsiflexion. These fractures may disrupt the vascular supply to the talus placing it at risk for avascular necrosis as well as compartment syndrome. Calcaneus fractures can occur after trivial falls in toddlers and young children and after falls from height or high-energy mechanisms in adolescents. Approximately 50% of calcaneal fractures in children have associated tibia fractures (Figure 29–31).

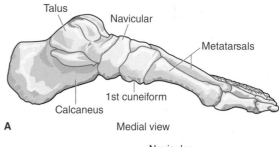

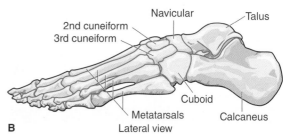

▲ **Figure 29–31.** Diagram of bones of the ankle/foot. (Reproduced, with permission, from Simon RR, Sherman SC: *Emergency Orthopedics*, 6th ed. New York: McGraw-Hill, 2011. Copyright © McGraw-Hill Education LLC.)

Clinical Findings

Symptoms and Signs

Physical examination will reveal pain, swelling, deformity, and inability to bear weight. Careful examination of the entire extremity should be performed to assess for associated injuries. Examination of talus fractures shows pain and swelling distal to the anterior ankle joint, whereas calcaneus fractures localize to the sole of the foot.

X-ray Findings

X-rays of the foot including AP, lateral, and oblique views will identify most fractures. Additional views may be performed if fracture is suggested on initial x-rays. CT scan may be used to further characterize talar fractures, intra-articular calcaneus fractures, and tarsometatarsal fractures/dislocations (Figure 29–32).

Treatment

Urgent consultation with orthopedist should be obtained for open fractures or if there is evidence of vascular compromise or compartment syndrome in addition to talar fractures, intra-articular calcaneus fractures, and tarsometatarsal fractures/dislocations. Extra-articular calcaneus fractures may be immobilized and non–weight-bearing with follow-up to orthopedist (see Table 29-1).

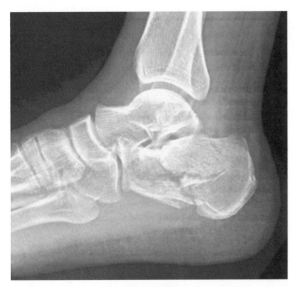

▲ **Figure 29-32.** Calcaneus fracture. (Reproduced, with permission, from Simon RR, Sherman SC: *Emergency Orthopedics*, 6th ed. New York: McGraw-Hill, 2011. Copyright © McGraw-Hill Education LLC.)

Disposition

Consultation with an orthopedist is necessary to determine surgical versus conservative management.

Schneidmueller D, Dietz HG, Kraus R, Marzi I: [Calcaneal fractures in childhood: A retrospective survey and literature review]. *Unfallchirurg.* 2007;110:939 [PMID: 17492498].

METATARSAL FRACTURES

 ESSENTIALS OF DIAGNOSIS

▶ Often crush injuries.

▶ Point tenderness over site of fracture.

▶ X-rays are diagnostic.

General Considerations

Metatarsal fractures account for most pediatric foot fractures. The first metatarsal is most frequently fractured in children younger than 5 years, whereas the base of the fifth metatarsal (Jones fracture) is most common in older children and adolescents. Injuries to the open growth plate are at risk for growth arrest and permanent deformity though rare. Metatarsal injuries can occur from multiple mechanisms: axial loading, abduction injuries, which often involve the fifth digit, or crush injuries. Metatarsal stress fractures may also occur, most commonly in endurance athletes with repetitive intense training.

Clinical Findings

Symptoms and Signs

Children often present due to pain and difficulty ambulating with point tenderness over the fracture site. Diffuse ecchymosis and swelling may be present that limit the examination.

X-ray Findings

X-rays of the foot including AP, lateral, and oblique views are often diagnostic. Stress fractures may require follow-up imaging to be detected.

Treatment

Consultation with the orthopedist should be obtained in the emergency department for open fractures, displaced Salter-Harris I or II fractures, Salter-Harris III, IV, or V fractures, completely displaced metatarsal fractures, and children with greater than 20 degrees of angulation, or acute fractures of the proximal diaphysis.

Disposition

Nondisplaced or minimally displaced metatarsal fractures may be placed in a posterior leg splint, non–weight-bearing, and discharged home with follow-up in 1 week to orthopedist (see Table 29-1). Fractures that are significantly displaced or have greater than 20 degrees of angulation should undergo closed reduction, then are splinted, and patients discharged home with follow-up to orthopedist.

Herrera-Soto JA, Scherb M, Duffy MF, Albright JC: Fractures of the fifth metatarsal in children and adolescents. *J Pediatr Orthop.* 2007;27:427 [PMID: 17513965].

Singer G, Cichocki M, Schalamon J, et al: A study of metatarsal fractures in children. *J Bone Joint Surg Am.* 2008;90:772 [PMID: 18381315].

PHALANGEAL FRACTURES

ESSENTIALS OF DIAGNOSIS

▶ Mechanism of axial loading or "stubbing the toe."

▶ Subungual hematoma often indicates underlying fracture of distal phalanx.

▶ X-rays are often diagnostic.

General Considerations

Toe fractures commonly occur in children involving the first phalanx or the great toe. Fractures of the distal phalanx may be complicated by nail bed injuries. Salter-Harris type III or IV of the proximal phalanx are often intra-articular and at risk for long-term complications.

Clinical Findings

Symptoms and Signs

Physical examination will reveal swelling and point tenderness at the fracture site. Deformity may be present in displaced fractures. Subungual hematomas are frequently present with fractures of the distal phalanx.

X-ray Findings

X-rays of the foot including AP, lateral, and oblique views are often diagnostic. Salter-Harris type I fractures may require follow-up imaging to be detected.

Treatment

Nondisplaced fractures can be buddy taped to an adjacent toe. Patients can then ambulate wearing a hard-soled shoe. Salter-Harris type III or IV of the proximal phalanx that

involves more than one-third of the joint surface or displace more than 2-3 mm should be seen by an orthopedist for closed or open reduction with pinning. Subungual hematomas should be drained within 24 hours if painful. Removal of the nail for nail bed laceration repair is controversial and should be reserved for patients with obvious misalignment of the nail bed.

Disposition

Simple fractures do not need follow-up with orthopedist. Patients with subungual hematomas and underlying distal phalanx fracture have open fractures and are discharged home on antibiotics for 5-7 days.

SEVER DISEASE/CALCANEAL APOPHYSITIS

ESSENTIALS OF DIAGNOSIS

▶ Common cause of heel pain in children aged 8-12 years.

▶ Heel pain is chronic with insidious onset and relates to physical activity.

▶ May need CT or MRI to define subtle fractures.

General Considerations

Calcaneal apophysitis, known as Sever disease, is one of the most common causes of heel pain in young athletes. Sever disease is male predominant and typically presents in children aged 8-12 years. Bilateral disease is present in approximately one-half of patients. Pain is due to inflammation that can be due to multiple factors: increased metabolism in the growth plate during growth spurts, use of footwear that lacks heel cushioning or with heel cleats, and overuse in sports that involve repetitive jumping and running.

Clinical Findings

Symptoms and Signs

Patients typically have complaint of the onset of chronic heel pain that correlates with physical activity. Physical examination reveals decreased gastrocnemius-soleus flexibility with a flat foot or rigid foot alignment. Heel pain may be reproducible on palpation over the apophysis. Pain on the calcaneal compression test may also be used to make the diagnosis. The examiner holds the affected heel with fingers surrounding the upper heel and then squeezes the heel.

X-ray Findings

X-rays are not necessary for diagnosis but may be used to exclude other injuries if suspected or the patient fails to respond to therapy.

▶ Treatment

All management is outpatient. Treatment of Sever disease is primarily rest with reduction of amount and intensity of activity. Initial treatment may include daily ice and NSAIDs. Gentle calf stretching or the use of a heel cup or lift with proper footwear will also help decrease the stress on the apophysis.

▶ Disposition

For patients who fail to improve within 4-8 weeks despite adequate rest, short-term casting may help. Physical therapy and slow progressive return to activity may also be necessary for recovery.

Rachel JN, Williams JB, Sawyer JR, et al: Is radiographic evaluation necessary in children with a clinical diagnosis of calcaneal apophysitis (sever disease)? *J Pediatr Orthop.* 2011;31:548 [PMID: 21654464].

Splinting

Splints are frequently used to immobilize an injury initially in the emergency department. Splints are not circumferential and allow swelling of the extremity without causing a significant increase in tissue pressure. Once swelling has decreased, casting is performed to provide more stability to keep the fractured bone in a fixed position.

Green NE, Swiontkowski MF: *Skeletal Trauma in Children*, 4th ed. Philadelphia: Saunders, 2009.
Herring JA: Tachdjian's *Pediatric Orthopadeics*, 4th ed. Philadelphia: Saunders, 2007.

Table 29–1. Splinting chart.

Type of splint	Indications
Ulnar gutter	4th and 5th proximal/middle phalangeal shaft fractures Select metacarpal fractures
Thumb spica	Injuries to the scaphoid/trapezium Stable thumb fractures Nondisplaced, nonangulated first metacarpal fractures
Volar	Carpal bone fractures (excluding scaphoid/trapezium) Buckle fracture of distal radius
Sugar tong	Distal radial and ulnar fractures
Posterior long arm	Distal humeral and proximal/midshaft forearm fractures Elbow fractures
Short leg	Isolated, nondisplaced malleolar fractures Acute foot fractures
Stirrup	Ankle sprains Isolated, nondisplaced malleolar fractures
Posterior long leg	Proximal/midshaft tibia fractures

Simon RR, Sherman SC: *Emergency Orthopedics*, 6th ed. New York: McGraw-Hill Medical, 2011.
Stone CK, Humphries RL: *Current Diagnosis and Treatment Emergency Medicine*, 7th ed. New York: McGraw-Hill, 2011.

Hand Trauma

Brian Adkins, MD
Adam Scrogham, MD
Terren Trott, MD

30

Hand trauma is one of the more common reasons for emergency department evaluations of individuals and specifically of children. Studies suggest that hand and upper extremity injuries comprise over 31% of all traumatic injuries in children younger than 12 years. There is bimodal distribution of injuries with the highest incidence between 1 and 2 years of age, and the second highest incidence at 12 years. In addition to the potential functional loss associated with hand injuries, a review of the psychiatry of injuries indicates that a child's "self esteem and skill are associated with hand sensation, appearance, and functions." Because of the potential mechanical and developmental consequences, appropriate initial evaluation and management of hand injuries is crucial.

PATIENT POSITION

The hand is a complex body part to examine because of the number of mechanical and neurovascular components in a small area. Examination of the hand is detailed to isolate the integrity of individual structures. Positioning of the patient's body and hand must be optimized to allow for a thorough examination. Ideally the patient should be supine on a stretcher with the hand outstretched as comfortably as possible on a clean, illuminated area such as a bedside table. Examination of a pediatric patient can be challenging; therefore placement of the child in parent's lap with the hand extended on a table may be the best positioning available.

STABILIZATION

Hemostasis

Although injuries to the hand are often accompanied by significant morbidity, they are fortunately not a source of great

mortality in isolation. However, bleeding can be brisk from the well-vascularized hand and particularly in the setting of laceration of the distal forearm involving the radial and ulnar arteries. Hemostasis is typically the most emergent intervention necessary for the hand. Elevation and direct pressure are primary strategies and are usually successful. If necessary, an arterial tourniquet such as a manual blood pressure cuff inflated on the forearm above the systolic blood pressure can be helpful. Clamps should be avoided if possible because it can be extremely difficult to distinguish nerves from blood vessels in a bloody wound. Intravenous (IV) access should be established for patients with heavy bleeding, need for IV antibiotics, sedation, or potentially surgery.

Analgesia

Analgesia can be attained by several methods and can improve patient comfort and cooperation to optimize ease of examination and treatment. Splinting, oral analgesia, and nerve blocks are discussed in detail later.

Tissue Preservation

Amputated tissues must be preserved immediately. Strategies for effective storage are discussed below.

HISTORY

Details gathered from a full description of the incident can be integral. As with any childhood illness, engaging the family and witnesses can be very helpful in obtaining the necessary elements of the incident.

Immediate History

- Timing of injury: of particular interest in wound repair and amputations.
- Nature of injury: blunt, sharp, crush, blast, etc.

- Possible coexisting injuries: fall, head injury, or impact to other locations of the body.

- Positioning of the digits and wrist at impact.

- Locations of pain, paresthesia, discoloration, motor weakness, difficulty performing certain tasks, foreign body sensation in the wound.

- Wounds: What tool, device, or structure created the laceration, avulsion, or abrasion? Was the environment clean or contaminated? Was there a fight, bite, a dirty blade, or pond water?

- Estimated blood loss since the injury.

Pertinent Past History

- History of congenital structural abnormalities of the hand or prior trauma creating functional loss.

- Bleeding disorders or therapeutic anticoagulation.

- Allergies.

- Illness or therapies that may impact wound healing or compliance: chronic steroid use, immunocompromise, diabetes, smoking in adolescents.

- General medical history.

- Dominant handedness, involvement in school and athletic activities that may influence compliance and use of the affected limb.

- Tetanus and rabies immunization status.

HAND EXAMINATION

Hand examination should begin as the history is taken. Sterile equipment should be readily available as hemostasis and minor exploration may be necessary even in the early stages. Rings and jewelry should be removed prior to examination and radiography. Although it is tempting to provide local anesthesia immediately for patient comfort and to expedite evaluation, the physician should first perform a sensory examination including two-point discrimination if the child is old enough to cooperate and understand instructions.

Anesthesia

Performing an adequate local exploration and evaluation of the underlying structures can be extremely difficult in a child, particularly without anesthesia. The short-term agent of choice for the hand and digits has been lidocaine without epinephrine. It has been assumed that anesthetics with epinephrine could create digital ischemia due to the vasoconstrictive properties of epinephrine. Recent literature does not support these historical concerns. However, for purposes of basic practice, most clinicians continue to avoid epinephrine-containing anesthetics in distal extremities and appendages.

Digital Blocks

For injuries distal to the proximal interphalangeal joint (PIP), digital blocks are typically preferred. Injections of small volumes (0.5-1 mL) of 1% lidocaine without epinephrine or 0.5% bupivacaine are placed around the digital nerve using a 25-gauge or smaller needle. Aspiration should be performed prior to injection to ensure that the needle is not in the digital artery. Care should be taken not to infiltrate a high volume that creates a circumferential tamponade of the soft tissues (Figure 30–1).

Transthecal Digital Block

Transthecal digital blocks are often used for injuries to the distal phalanx, volar tip, and nail bed. Block is performed by a palmar percutaneous injection of local anesthetic into the flexor tendon sheath. The metacarpophalangeal (MCP) flexion crease is identified in the extended digit and the needle is inserted at 90 degrees until striking bone. The needle is then angled 45 degrees distally and approximately 2-3 cc of a 50:50 mix of lidocaine without epinephrine and bupivacaine, is injected into flexor tendon sheath while the opposite hand's index finger palpates the infusion. The finger will then assume a flexed position (Figure 30–2). This block should not be performed if infection or tenosynovitis is present.

Wrist Blocks

The ulnar nerve is located in a superficial position to the ulnar artery in most patients. Ulnar block can provide excellent anesthesia to the ulnar side of the hand including the fifth digit and the ulnar half of the fourth digit (Figure 30–3). The radial nerve can be blocked at the wrist as shown in Figure 30–4. The radial nerve is located in a more dorsal position along the radial aspect of the wrist. A radial nerve block will anesthetize the dorsum of the hand proximal to the second and third digits as well as the entire dorsal surface of the thumb. The median nerve can be blocked at the volar surface of the wrist (see Figure 30–3) and will provide anesthesia to the palmar surface of the hand from the ulnar half of the thenar eminence to the radial half of the fourth digit. It covers the extensor and flexor surfaces of the distal portions of the first, second, and third digits and radial half of the fourth digit. Although clinicians have been taught to perform the three wrist blocks using well-established anatomic landmark techniques, emergency medicine physicians are utilizing ultrasound to rapidly and precisely locate the nerve and, under direct ultrasound visualization of the needle, deposit local anesthetic around the nerve. Utilizing ultrasound to facilitate these blocks will likely lead to faster setup of the block, less failure of the block after the initial injection, and less discomfort for patients. Young children usually require sedation to accomplish a successful wrist block.

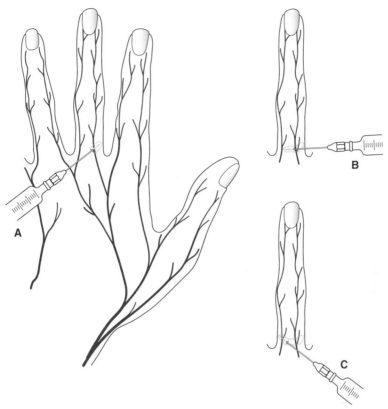

▲ **Figure 30–1.** Digital block. A small gauge needle (25 gauge or smaller) is used to infiltrate 0.5-1 mL of local anesthetic around the digital nerve. Avoid a large volume injection which can tense the tissues and decrease perfusion. (Reproduced, with permission, from Stone CK, Humphries RL: Current *Diagnosis & Treatment Emergency Medicine*, 7th ed. New York: McGraw-Hill, 2011. Copyright © McGraw-Hill Education LLC.)

Cautions Regarding Local Anesthesia Use

- Although performing local anesthesia on the hand is unlikely to require a large volume of lidocaine, the physician must avoid toxicity associated with high doses of subcutaneous infiltration with larger wounds. The maximum dosage of lidocaine administration is 5 cc/kg without epinephrine and 7 cc/kg with epinephrine.

- Avoid creating soft tissue tension and vessel tamponade of the digits when infiltrating lidocaine for a digital block.

- Anesthetic solutions should be avoided over inflamed tissue sites except when used directly over an abscess that is to be incised and drained. The vascularity of infected and inflamed skin can lead to increased systemic absorption, and the acidity of the tissue may prevent appropriate anesthetic activity.

Tourniquets

If there is excessive bleeding from the limb, a tourniquet can be applied temporarily to permit appropriate examination and intervention. A blood pressure cuff should be placed on the arm and inflated until bleeding is reduced or stopped. The cuff will be painful after a brief time and should be avoided for long periods. When a tourniquet is used, the clinician should document the time the cuff was inflated and the pressure utilized to achieve cessation of bleeding from the limb.

PERFORMING THE EXAMINATION

A four-step examination of the hand can assess the anatomical structures without missing vital information. Age and maturity level of the pediatric patient may present a challenge for evaluation of the structural integrity and neurovascular status of the hand. Sedation may assist with wound repair and

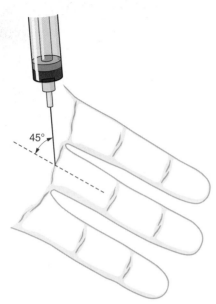

▲ **Figure 30–2.** Transthecal digital nerve block. The needle is inserted at a 90-degree angle to the level of the bone at the proximal digital crease. The needle is then withdrawn 2-3 mm and angled 45 degrees to the long axis of the digit. Local anesthetic is injected along the flexor tendon sheath. (Reproduced, with permission, from Stone CK, Humphries RL: Current *Diagnosis & Treatment Emergency Medicine*, 7th ed. New York: McGraw-Hill, 2011. Copyright © McGraw-Hill Education LLC.)

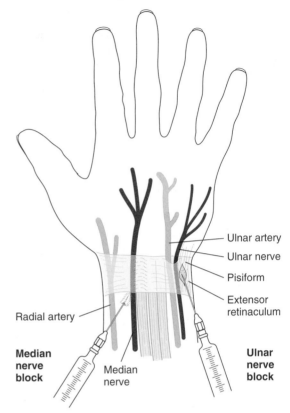

▲ **Figure 30–3.** Median and ulnar nerve blocks performed on the dorsum of the hand. (Reproduced, with permission, from Stone CK, Humphries RL: Current *Diagnosis & Treatment Emergency Medicine*, 7th ed. New York: McGraw-Hill, 2011. Copyright © McGraw-Hill Education LLC.)

inspection, but it is necessary for the patient to follow directions for a complete assessment. A calm patient approach, a peaceful environment, adequate analgesia, and parental cooperation are needed to optimize examination outcome.

1. Observe the posture of the hand at rest in supine position for apparent deformity.

2. Test the active function of the skeletal structures and musculotendinous junctions.

3. Evaluate for loss of sensation with two-point discrimination (if possible).

4. Examine the wound in a sterile and bloodless environment. A 2.5 power magnifying loupe can be helpful if available. Examination will often occur during the process of debridement and cleaning. Inspect for foreign body and structural damage. Investigate integrity of the soft tissue fragments for viability and circulation. In wounds with active hemorrhage, a tourniquet applied as described can improve visibility. Removal of thrombus and debris are also important prior to wound closure.

EXAMINATION & ASSESSMENT OF FUNCTION

The hand is a remarkable instrument due to its fine movement, precision, sensation, and adaptability. It is a complex structure that must be understood for appropriate care.

TERMINOLOGY

The emergency department physician's ability to communicate with the hand surgeon is paramount. A basic knowledge of anatomic nomenclature is most helpful in discussion of injuries with a hand surgeon regarding acute treatment or follow-up of patients. The injured hand must be specified and identified as the dominant or nondominant hand. The gripping side of the hand is referred to as the palmar surface and the "back" of the hand and fingers with the nail is referred to as the dorsal surface. Lateral location is usually

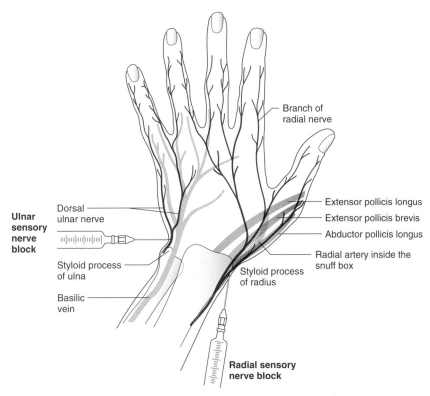

▲ **Figure 30–4.** Ulnar and radial sensory nerve block. (Reproduced, with permission, from Stone CK, Humphries RL: *Current Diagnosis & Treatment Emergency Medicine*, 7th ed. New York: McGraw-Hill, 2011. Copyright © McGraw-Hill Education LLC.)

described as ulnar or radial in relation to the side closest to the ulna or radius. The fingers (digits) were formerly numbered one through five, but are now more commonly named the thumb, index, long or middle, ring, and little finger.

ANATOMY

Age-Specific Anatomy

▶ Integument

The palmar surface is covered by thick skin, cushioned by fat, and is highly vascularized by arterial supply and innervated. The dorsum is protected by a thin skin layer which has less sensation and sweating capabilities. Most of the venous and lymphatic drainage of the hand is dorsal.

▶ Extrinisic Flexors

Wrist Flexors

Flexor carpi ulnaris (FCU), which is innervated by ulnar nerve; palmaris longus, median nerve; and flexor carpi radialis (FCR), median nerve, serve to flex the wrist.

The FCR is palpable on the radial aspect of the wrist and can be tested by flexion of the wrist. During flexion, the FCU can be palpated on the ulnar portion of the volar wrist. The palmaris longus can be palpated when the thumb and small finger are opposed during wrist flexion.

Digital Flexors

Each of the nine interphalangeal joints has a primary flexor. A flexor digitorum profundus (FDP) moves each distal interphalangeal joint (DIP). The median nerve innervates the index and long finger, and the ulnar nerve innervates the ring and small finger FDP activity. The PIPs are flexed by the flexor digitorum superficialis (FDS), which is innervated by the median nerve. The thumb interphalangeal joint is flexed by the flexor pollicis longus (FPL) and is innervated by the median nerve (Figure 30–5). Flexor tendon injuries are best identified with opposition testing.

Profundus Flexors

The FDP flexors are assessed by immobilizing the PIP joint and asking the patient to flex the distal tip.

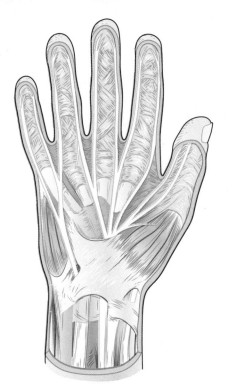

▲ **Figure 30–5.** The palmar aspect of the left hand is shown, revealing the flexor tendon sheaths and the branches of the ulnar and median nerves. (Reproduced, with permission, from Way LW: *Current Surgical Diagnosis & Treatment,* 9th ed. Norwalk, CT: Appleton & Lange, 1991. Copyright © McGraw-Hill Education LLC.)

Superficialis Flexors

The FDS flexors of an individual digit are evaluated by immobilizing the other three fingers and asking the patient to flex the isolated digit.

Flexor Pollicis Longus

The FPL is assessed by flexion of the distal phalanx of the thumb.

Extrinsic Extensors

There are 12 extrinsic extensors and all are innervated by the radial nerve

Central Wrist Extensors

The extensor carpi radialis brevis attaches to the base of the second metacarpal, and the extensor carpi radialis longus inserts into the third metacarpal base.

Extensor and Ulnar Deviator

The extensor carpi ulnaris attaches the fifth metacarpal base.

Abductor Pollicis Longus

The APL stabilizes the base of the thumb and radially deviates the wrist. This can be tested by radially abducting the thumb.

Four Finger Extensors

On each finger, an extensor digitorum communis forms the central slip of the extensor hood.

Two Thumb Extensors

The extensor pollicis brevis mainly works at the MP joint. The extensor pollicis longus mostly extends at the IP joint along with assistance with the intrinsics. The EPL can extend with force unlike the intrinsics.

Testing of the Extensors

Testing the extensors is relatively straightforward. The patient is asked to extend the fingers at the MP joints and then at the IP joints. Interphalangeal joint extension is performed by the extensor in concert with the intrinsic tendons of the extensor hood (Figure 30–6).

Intrinsic Muscles

Fifteen of the 20 intrinsic muscles are innervated by the ulnar nerve and five by the median nerve. They combine with the extensor tendon to form the extensor hood mechanism, a proximal triangular sheet of three connected tendons. The lateral bands are the small lateral extensor tendon (LETs) from the intrinsic muscles. The central slip (central large tendon) from the extrinsic extensors is called the middle extensor tendon (MET) and inserts on the middle phalanx of each finger. The METs and the LETs combine to form the terminal extensor tendon (TET), a very thin tendon that inserts on the distal phalanx. The thumb only has two phalanges and the extensor pollicis brevis acts as the MET, whereas the extensor pollicis longus acts as the TET. The intrinsics allow for one to cup the palm, by flexing the MP joints, extending the IP joints, and abducting and adducting the digits.

▶ **Testing the Intrinsics**

The hypothenar and the intrinsics allow the little finger and thumb to pronate and cup the palm. The intrinsics can be assessed by touching the little finger pad to the thumb pad. The other intrinsics can be evaluated by having the patient extend the IP joints and flex at the MP joints, while abducting the second through fifth digits.

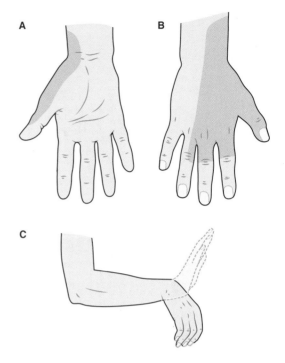

▲ **Figure 30–7.** (**A**) Palmar and (**B**) dorsal sensory areas of the radial nerve. (**C**) Testing for radial nerve paresis by wrist extension. (Reproduced, with permission, from Stone CK, Humphries RL: *Current Diagnosis & Treatment Emergency Medicine*, 7th ed. New York: McGraw-Hill, 2011. Copyright © McGraw-Hill Education LLC.)

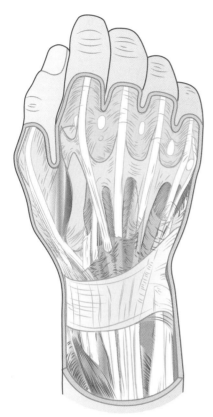

▲ **Figure 30–6.** A view of the dorsal hand, revealing the extensor tendons. (Reproduced, with permission, from Way LW: *Current Surgical Diagnosis & Treatment*, 9th ed. Norwalk, CT: Appleton & Lange, 1991. Copyright © McGraw-Hill Education LLC.)

▶ Examination of Nerve Injuries to the Hand

Radial Nerve: All extensors are innervated by the radial nerve.

Motor examination: The patient is asked to extend the wrist and the digits.

Sensory examination: The dorsal and radial aspects of the hand can be assessed with touch as illustrated in Figure 30-7A and B.

Median Nerve: Nine of the twelve extrinsic flexors, the index and long finger lumbricals, and the three muscles of the thenar eminence are innervated by the median nerve.

Motor examination: High median nerve assessment for injuries proximal to the wrist: The patient is asked to flex the DIP joint of the index finger and the IP joint of the thumb. While holding the fourth and fifth digits in flexion to the palm, ask the patient to flex the second and third fingers.

Low median nerve assessment for injuries distal to the wrist: The patient is asked to press the thumb pad against the index finger pad. You want to feel for a firm contracted adductor pollicis brevis alongside the thumb and metacarpal.

Sensory examination: (Figure 30-8A and B). The clinician may opt for sensory assessment at the index finger tip.

Ulnar Nerve: Fifteen of the 20 intrinsic muscles, and only three extrinsic muscles are innervated by the ulnar nerve.

Motor examination: The intrinsics can be assessed by instructing the patient to abduct and adduct the digits or simply move the pointed index finger in a radial direction.

Sensory examination: Figure 30-9A and B shows distribution. A simple sensory assessment of the small finger is often appropriate for physicians.

▶ Radiographic Evaluation of the Hand

Most significant injuries of the hand should be imaged with an x-ray for assessment of fracture, dislocation, foreign

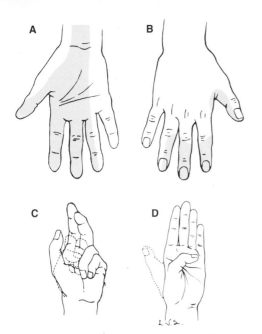

▲ **Figure 30–8.** (**A, B**) Sensory distribution of the median nerve. (**C**) Median nerve motor innervation of the profundi of the index and long fingers. (**D**) Median nerve inner-vated flexor pollicis longus. (Reproduced, with permission, from Stone CK, Humphries RL: *Current Diagnosis & Treatment Emergency Medicine*, 7th ed. New York: McGraw-Hill, 2011. Copyright © McGraw-Hill Education LLC.)

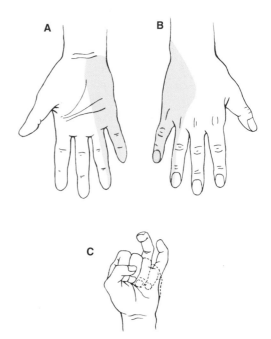

▲ **Figure 30–9.** (**A, B**) Sensory distribution of the ulnar nerve. (**C**) Ulnar nerve innervates the terminal phalangeal flexion of the fourth and fifth digits. (Reproduced, with permission, from Stone CK, Humphries RL: *Current Diagnosis & Treatment Emergency Medicine*, 7th ed. New York: McGraw-Hill, 2011. Copyright © McGraw-Hill Education LLC.)

bodies, and gas. Imaging such as CT or MRI is commonly used in the specialty or outpatient setting but is not a rou-tine examination by an emergency department physician unless in consultation with a hand surgeon. Ultrasound is used more commonly, particularly for assessment of foreign bodies (Figure 30–10).

SPLINTS, SLINGS, & DRESSINGS

Dressings

There is variability among physicians in selection of wound dressings for hand injuries. Petrolatum-impregnated gauze lined by a wet surgical gauze can serve as an effective pri-mary bandage and should be applied noncircumferentially. The core dressing can be wrapped with soft elastic gauze such as Kerlix.

Splint

Significant hand and even single-digit injuries should include a splint that immobilizes the wrist. This is particularly true in the pediatric patient where wound care compliance can

be difficult in an active child. Distal digital injuries can be treated with less occlusive splinting that only immobilizes the IP joint. Molded or prefabricated aluminum and foam splints can be effective in phalangeal and IP joint injuries. Gauze circumferentially wrapped around an appropriate length fragment of a tongue depressor can be used as an alternative. A common and useful wrist and hand immobili-zation technique is a palmar splint with the hand in the "posi-tion of function." The "position of function" describes slight wrist extension and MP flexion with the PIP and DIP joints in partial extension and the thumb open, similar to holding a drink can (Figure 30–11). Approximately 10 layers of plaster can be cut to fit the digit and extend about halfway up the volar forearm. It is padded with soft dressing and molded to fit with an overlying elastic dressing.

Sling

A sling can be very helpful for a splinted hand injury for therapeutic and comfort purposes. Elevation of the injured limb at or above heart level can decrease edema by promot-ing venous and lymphatic drainage. Also, the sling assists with the potentially cumbersome weight of a splint placed on a child's distal extremity.

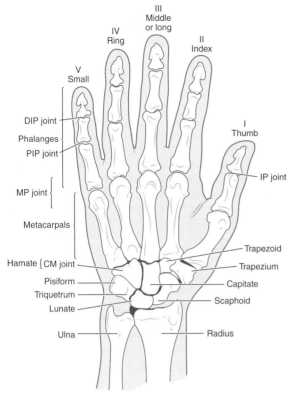

▲ **Figure 30–10.** Skeletal anatomy and terminology of the bones and joints of the hand. (Reproduced, with permission, from Stone CK, Humphries RL: *Current Diagnosis & Treatment Emergency Medicine*, 7th ed. New York: McGraw-Hill, 2011. Copyright © McGraw-Hill Education LLC.)

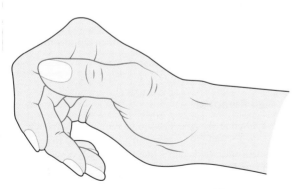

▲ **Figure 30–11.** The hand in "position of function." (Reproduced, with permission, from Stone CK, Humphries RL: *Current Diagnosis & Treatment Emergency Medicine*, 7th ed. New York: McGraw-Hill, 2011. Copyright © McGraw-Hill Education LLC.)

MANAGEMENT OF HAND INJURIES

Lacerations

Small lacerations are a very common presentation to the emergency department. It is vital to evaluate fully the neurological, tendonous, and vascular functions of the hand. Tendons are the most common underlying injury in lacerations less than 3 cm. Once other injuries have been excluded, superficial lacerations that are not perpendicular to skin tension lines and not extending into deep structures can often be managed with a dressing, adhesives, or surgical tape. In one study, wounds of 2 cm or less on the hand can be managed without sutures with equal cosmetic and functional result.

Topical adhesives were found to be effective for pediatric extremity lacerations when combined with immobilization in one small study. Wounds requiring sutures should be followed up for suture removal in 7-10 days. Typically, size 4-0 or 5-0 nonabsorbable monofilament suture is used on the hand in pediatric patients when sutures are required.

Splinting and elevation can assist in pain relief of small lacerations and can promote wound care compliance in a child.

Extensive lacerations should prompt heavy irrigation and exploration. Sutures should be placed without great tension. Delayed presentations and high-tension wounds should be considered for delayed closure.

Prophylactic antibiotics that cover typical skin pathogens should be considered in contaminated and macerated wounds, although there is no proof of benefit.

Valencia J, Leyva F, Gomez-Bajo GJ: Pediatric hand trauma. *Clin Orthop.* 2005;432:77-86 [PMID: 15738807].
Zehtabchi S: Evidence-based emergency medicine/critically appraised topic. The role of antibiotic prophylaxis for prevention of infection in patients with simple hand lacerations. *Ann Emerg Med.* 2007;49(5):682-689, 689.e1 [PMID:17452265].

FINGERTIP INJURIES

FINGERTIP AMPUTATIONS

▶ **Clinical Findings**

Fingertip amputations are the most common type of upper extremity amputations, which result from injuries that occur frequently in children as a result of fingers getting caught in closing doors. There are four zones that classify fingertip injuries based on the location of the injury.

Zone 1 lesions consist of the area distal to the distal phalanx tubercle and do not affect the nail bed or bone.

Zone 2 lesions involve the nail bed and usually also involve phalangeal bone disruption or exposure.

Zone 3 lesions involve the nail matrix in a way that nail growth will be disrupted by the deformation.

Zone 4 amputations occur at the distal phalanx near the DIP joint. These injuries can limit the active motion of the distal remnant despite possible intact distal attachments of the flexor and extensor tendons at the site.

A thorough history is helpful in the treatment of fingertip injuries. Important questions include age, location of the wound, mechanism and timing of the injury, hand dominance in toddlers and older children, and level of patient involvement in sports and other activities. The treatment planning for each digit can be different as well. The hand surgeon's primary focus is maintaining the length of the thumb and working to optimize the pincer grasp. The index finger is the second most important and other digits are of lesser concern to function.

▶ Treatment & Disposition

Zone 1 injuries with minimal pad loss may be treated conservatively, allowing healing by secondary intention. This is simple, effective, and the treatment of choice for the pediatric patient particularly if there is no bone exposure. Treatment in the emergency department includes wound cleansing, coverage with a sterile nonadherent dressing, and placement of a protective splint or bulky dressing. Injuries that include exposure of the distal phalanx should be treated as a contaminated open fracture with an IV dose of a cephalosporin with an outpatient oral course and tetanus prophalxis if indicated. Close follow-up for wound check is indicated within 1-3 days.

Zone 2-4 injuries require more aggressive treatment. Injuries include significant pad, soft tissue, or bone loss, and require surgical expertise for proper repair. Transfer to a hand surgeon should be pursued promptly. The surgeon may employ a number of techniques including closure, grafts, and replantation.

SUBUNGUAL HEMATOMA

Clinical Findings

Hematoma from a blunt injury or crush injury (such as a hammer blow or slam in a door) may rupture blood vessels beneath the nail causing a dark red to black discoloration of the nail bed. Crush injuries are common in the toddler age group due to fingers caught in closing doors. Appropriate analgesia should be considered and imaging is required to rule out an underlying fracture.

Treatment

Large subungual hematomas may cause severe pain and should be evacuated. Nail trephination (boring a hole in the nail) is usually effective. A high temperature microcautery device (after cleaning the nail with a non-alcohol based prep to avoid accidental fire) or a sharp 18-guage needle can be effective in boring a small hole in the nail to release the blood and pressure. The nail can be removed as well in certain circumstances but this is obviously much more invasive. Avoid use of heated paper clips as they may lead to the introduction of carbon particles, known as lampblack. Anesthesia is usually not required, as the procedure can be done quickly. Pain relief should be immediate following decompression. Large hematomas are often coincident with nail bed lacerations and many surgeons recommend removal of the nail and repair of nail bed injuries. This promotes proper healing and avoids a curved nail and abnormal nail growth in the future. The nail should be cleaned and sutured into place to keep the nail fold open and provide a tract for new nail growth. Traditionally, nail bed lacerations had been sutured for closure, but research has shifted the culture to utilization of topical adhesives. A prospective randomized trial found that 2-octylcyanoacrylate is faster than sutures while providing equivalent functional and cosmetic outcomes.

A fracture of the distal phalanx on imaging is technically an open fracture but usually heals without complication, and the incident of osteomyelitis with subungual tuft fractures is low. Despite this, a broad-spectrum antibiotic and close follow-up is recommended.

Disposition

Patients with subungual hematomas may be discharged safely from the emergency department following treatment. Depending on the child's age, the patient, as well as the family, should be informed of the risk for nail loss or deformity. Close follow-up is highly recommended.

NAIL AVULSION

Clinical Findings

Avulsion of the nail results from dorsal elevation of the tip of the nail or from a downward force sufficient to tear the nail away from the bed.

Treatment

▶ Nail Removal

Nails avulsed at the base need to be removed completely. A digital block should be implemented for analgesia in removal of avulsed nail. Removal of the avulsed nail via advancing a clamp underneath the nail and spreading toward the still attached site is usually effective. The nail bed needs to be covered either with the nail itself or with a piece of sterile petrolatum gauze. A portion of either should be tucked into the nail sulcus to keep an open tract at that site. If the nail bed is lacerated, it may be closed with 5-0 or 6-0 absorbable suture or with tissue adhesive after careful cleansing of the site.

▶ Reattachment of a Torn Finger Flap

If the distal portion of the finger has been torn away with the nail and left attached by a volar pedicle, the flap needs to be anatomically reduced and sutured in place with 6-0 absorbable suture. Prophylactic antibiotics should be administered.

▶ Fractures

Open fractures of the distal phalanx require reduction and soft tissue suturing for proper healing and realignment. Displaced fractures may require realignment via internal fixation with a Kirschner wire by a hand surgeon.

Disposition

The patient should be recommended for close follow-up in 2-3 days for a wound check and dressing change when not referred to a hand surgeon. Complicated problems requiring surgical expertise should be referred and appointments made without delay. Broad-spectrum antibiotics are recommended as well as tetanus prophylaxis if indicated.

DISTAL EXTENSOR TENDON INJURIES

LACERATION OF EXTENSOR TENDONS

Clinical Findings

Dorsal hand and finger wounds commonly result in a completely or partially lacerated extensor tendon(s). It is imperative to examine the injury with adequate exposure and direct examination through a full range of motion. A 90% lacerated tendon can retain function; therefore, appropriate visualization is warranted. Partial tendon lacerations usually show diminished strength against resisted extension and the patient will note pain with resistance. The eight zones of extensor tendon injuries help assess and guide treatment (Figure 30–12).

Treatment

Partial tendon laceration less than 50% may require no repair and be treated effectively with a simple protective splint. Minor repairs may be treated in the emergency department following irrigation, inspection, and debridement, or handled later by a consultant if desired.

If the tendon ends are easily retrievable, the tendon should be repaired by figure-of-eight suturing techniques or crisscross suture technique with 4-0 or 5-0 suture (infants requiring 6-0 nylon). Tendon repair is ideally performed by a hand surgeon experienced in this type of repair (Figure 30–13). Proper splinting following tendon repair should be observed. Forearm splint should be applied to position the hand in neutral position. One or more neighboring fingers should be immobilized with the injured digit.

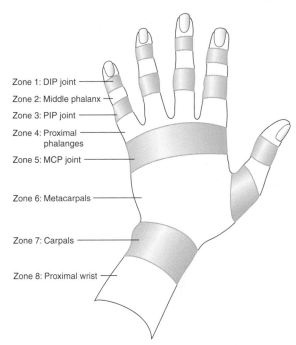

▲ **Figure 30–12.** Extensor tendon injury zones. (Reproduced, with permission, from Stone CK, Humphries RL: *Current Diagnosis & Treatment Emergency Medicine*, 7th ed. New York: McGraw-Hill, 2011. Copyright © McGraw-Hill Education LLC.)

Zone 1: DIP joint
Zone 2: Middle phalanx
Zone 3: PIP joint
Zone 4: Proximal phalanges
Zone 5: MCP joint
Zone 6: Metacarpals
Zone 7: Carpals
Zone 8: Proximal wrist

Disposition

If the tendon ends are not easily visible or retrieved, a hand surgeon should be consulted for prompt follow-up within 1-2 days, and antibiotic treatment initiated in the interim.

MALLET FINGER

 ESSENTIALS OF DIAGNOSIS

▶ Bruising at DIP joint.

▶ X-ray may be normal or show avulsed chip at DIP joint.

▶ Carefully test extension at DIP joint.

▶ Swan neck deformity may occur if untreated.

Clinical Findings

Mallet finger occurs following avulsion or laceration of the extensor tendon at its insertion on the dorsum of the distal phalanx. Injury results if the finger is forcibly flexed usually from a sudden blow to the tip of the finger while extended. There may be bruising at the DIP joint but edema and

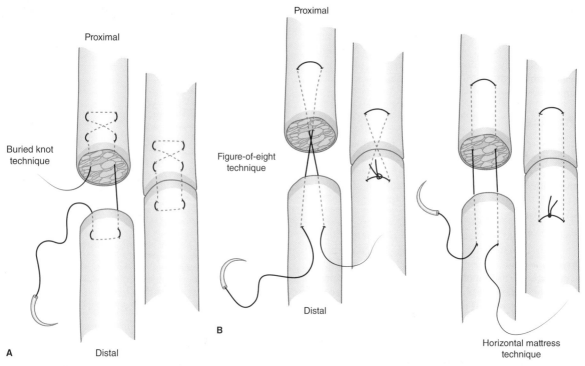

▲ **Figure 30–13.** Methods of tendon repair for (**A**) large tendons and (**B**) thin tendons. (Reproduced, with permission, from Stone CK, Humphries RL: *Current Diagnosis & Treatment Emergency Medicine*, 7th ed. New York: McGraw-Hill, 2011. Copyright © McGraw-Hill Education LLC.)

tenderness at the site may be less than expected. Imaging may be normal or possibly show an avulsed chip fragment at the DIP joint. If articular fracture involves 40% or more of the joint surface, referral to a hand surgeon for open reduction is required. Extensor lag may not be present on initial presentation; therefore, careful testing of extension at the DIP joint is vital for diagnosis. If left untreated, swan neck deformity will develop noted by flexion deformity at the DIP with hyperextension at the PIP (Figure 30–14).

Treatment

▶ Open Mallet Injuries

Open mallet injuries require reduction by a hand surgeon. Antibiotic coverage and prompt consultation are the focus of care in the emergency department.

▶ Closed Mallet Injuries

Closed mallet injuries can be treated nonoperatively but require a prolonged course of treatment. Treatment includes splint fixation of the DIP joint extension for 8 weeks followed by 1 month of night splinting. The digit should be

held up in extension during splint changes to avoid any bending as this sets the healing process back to time zero.

Disposition

Mallet injuries are an important diagnosis to make and treat properly to avoid chronic problems and long-term deformity. Close follow-up with a hand surgeon is highly recommended.

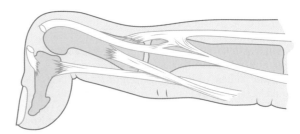

▲ **Figure 30–14.** Mallet finger with swan neck deformity. (Reproduced, with permission, from Way LW: *Current Surgical Diagnosis & Treatment*, 9th ed. Norwalk, CT: Appleton & Lange, 1991. Copyright © McGraw-Hill Education LLC.)

BOUTONNIÈRE DEFORMITY

ESSENTIALS OF DIAGNOSIS

▶ Swollen and painful PIP joint secondary to trauma.

▶ Normal imaging studies are common.

▶ Deformity is rarely present directly after the inciting event.

Clinical Findings

Middle extensor tendon rupture or avulsion leads to boutonnière deformity but early diagnosis can be difficult as early presentation rarely shows obvious deformity. High index of suspicion needs to be observed in patients with a swollen and painful PIP joint following hand trauma. Rarely, volar dislocations of the PIP joint can cause tendon MET rupture but unless dislocation is present, radiographs are typically unremarkable.

Findings of boutonnière deformity include a flexed PIP joint and hyperextended distal joint. Deformity results from a gradual stretching of the injured extensor hood and thus is rarely present on initial evaluation in the emergency department. As the bone protrudes through the injured extensor hood, it pushes aside the MET and the lateral extensor tendons act as flexors of the PIP and hyperextensors of the DIP as they slip volarly (Figure 30–15).

Treatment

▶ Open Injuries

Injuries with open exposure should be repaired by a hand surgeon if possible with figure-of-eight nylon sutures. The joint is then placed in full extension in a palmar digital splint.

▶ Closed Injuries

Closed injuries require a high index of suspicion and usually respond well to a 4-week course of splinting in extension.

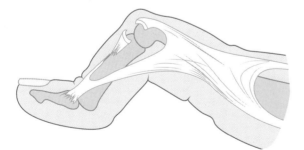

▲ **Figure 30–15.** Boutonnière deformity. (Reproduced, with permission, from Way LW: *Current Surgical Diagnosis & Treatment*, 9th ed. Norwalk, CT: Appleton & Lange, 1991. Copyright © McGraw-Hill Education LLC.)

Long-term deformity is rare when the injury is treated promptly and correctly. If missed for a length of time, long-term repair may be difficult due to tendon contracture.

Disposition

Open injuries require emergent consultation with a hand surgeon following careful irrigation and clean dressings. Closed injuries require prompt follow-up in clinic with a hand surgeon. Proper splinting is performed with the PIP joint held in extension and DIP and MP joints mobile.

BONE & JOINT INJURIES

Bone injuries are discussed in more detail in Chapter 29; however, some important principles apply to pediatric hand trauma.

Clinical Findings

When you have concern for a bone or joint injury on radiograph without an obvious answer, try alternative views or comparison to the opposite extremity. This is particularly helpful in the pediatric patient due to ossifying centers and growth plate changes. Also, follow-up for repeat x-rays at a 7- to 10-day interval can be helpful.

Treatment

▶ Splinting

The wrist joint governs mobility and should be properly immobilized in carpal and metacarpal fractures. As such it should be splinted initially and carefully in mild extension with functional finger flexion and opposition of the thumb. When splinting one finger, an adjacent finger should be immobilized with it for proper healing. Be careful to ensure that after a splint has been applied the digits are visible and have intact sensation and capillary refill prior to discharge (this may be complicated by a nerve block). As always, place adequate padding for any splint, particularly in the pediatric patient.

▶ Stable Injuries

Stable fractures can be treated safely and effectively by the emergency department physician by means of reduction and splinting techniques. Adequate analgesia should be provided and proper technique, not force, should be used for reduction.

Articular injuries are common in children as well, with and without fracture. The most common injuries are stable ligamentous injuries that present without radiographic abnormality. They usually present with pain, tenderness, and occasionally a joint effusion. Sprains can usually be treated supportively with brief immobilization followed by early mobilization. Dislocations, although common in children, are less frequent than in adults. The pediatric ligaments are stronger than physis plates and usually lead to volate plate avulsion fractures. Complete dislocations and resulting ligamentous injuries can usually be treated by closed reduction, splinting, and follow-up. Following local anesthesia, reduction of finger dislocations can usually be accomplished by proximal stabilization in combination with gentle distal traction.

▶ Open or Unstable Injuries

These injuries require special attention and close consultation with a hand surgeon. Temporizing measures including cleansing, dressing, temporary splinting, antibiotics, and tetanus immunization (if necessary) are the mainstay of treatment in the emergency department. Emergency referral to a hand surgeon is required and should be adequately stressed to the patient and family. Any structure with neurologic or vascular compromise requires prompt surgical intervention.

Disposition

Patients with closed or stable injuries can be discharged safely with follow-up in 1-3 days with a hand surgeon for reassessment. Patients with open or unstable injuries require emergent referral to a hand surgeon. Difficult or inadequate reductions require similar emergent referral.

INFECTIONS

Hand infections are common in the emergency department and many infections arise from neglect following trauma. They are worsened by tissue edema and venous congestion. Prompt early care of the injury may prevent infections and is more effective than secondary measures such as antibiotics. Severe hand infections may require admission for close observation or rapid referral. However, many minor hand infections may treated by an emergency department physician.

PARONYCHIA & EPONYCHIA

ESSENTIALS OF DIAGNOSIS

- ▶ Collection of pus or swelling at the nail fold.
- ▶ Consider antibiotics if there is associated lymphangitis or cellulitis.
- ▶ X-rays may be utilized if there is concern for osteomyelitis or foreign body.

Clinical Findings

Following minor trauma, it is possible for inflammation to lead to infection inside the nail fold. The usual pathogen is *Staphylococcus aureus* and culture is rarely required. *Candida albicans* is most commonly the cause of chronic paronychia found in individuals with exposure to moisture or cleaning solutions (older children as dishwasher in a restaurant). An x-ray may be ordered if there is clinical concern for a foreign body or underlying osteomyelitis.

Treatment

Simple incision, drainage, and nail fold elevation is the mainstay of treatment. Use of a No. 11 scalpel is generally effective (Figure 30–16). Digital block should be considered for treatment, particularly in the younger pediatric patient who is less likely to allow mild probing of a digit. Elamax can be used prior to placement of the block to reduce pain during injection.

Antibiotics are not indicated unless there is surrounding cellulitis. Chronic paronychia may require further care including nail removal, antibiotics, and topical antifungals.

Disposition

Close follow-up is preferred within 24-48 hours and hand elevation is desired. Osteomyelitis of the distal phalanx may

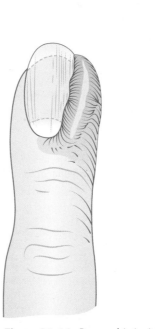

▲ **Figure 30–16.** Paronychia incision and drainage. (Reproduced, with permission, from Way LW: *Current Surgical Diagnosis & Treatment*, 9th ed. Norwalk, CT: Appleton & Lange, 1991. Copyright © McGraw-Hill Education LLC.)

develop as a complication, and chronic paronychia requires referral to a hand surgeon for possible marsupialization of the eponychial fold.

HERPETIC WHITLOW

ESSENTIALS OF DIAGNOSIS

▶ Collection of grouped vesicles on the fingertip.

▶ Use of oral acyclovir in the immune-compromised patient is indicated.

Herpetic whitlow is a self-limited herpes simplex infection of the distal finger. It is the most common viral infection of the hand. This infection is commonly overlooked if not considered when diagnosing a rash on the hand. It presents as a group of clear vesicles with an erythematous base. Incision and drainage is contraindicated and regular treatment is supportive. Immunocompromised patients require oral acyclovir if tolerated based on age and ability to swallow medications.

FELON

ESSENTIALS OF DIAGNOSIS

▶ Fat pad of the distal phalanx is painful and swollen.

▶ Most felons may be drained with a simple incision.

▶ *Staphylococcus aureus* is the most common pathogen.

Clinical Findings

Patients usually present with a swollen and painful distal phalanx fat pad. Infection is most commonly caused by *S. aureus*. This is a clinical diagnosis and imaging is not necessary.

Treatment & Disposition

Treatment of felons is via incision and drainage of the infection, which relieves pressure and improves pain control. The pediatric patient may require more aggressive pain control with a digital block than the adult patient requires. Central longitudinal incision is the classic method of incising felons, but these infections can be drained where they point. If a lateral incision is used, care should be taken to avoid the neurovascular bundle. Irrigate and loosely pack the wound, and immobilization of the finger is recommended (Figure 30–17). Complications include damage to nerves and blood vessels, as well as painful neuromas or anesthetic

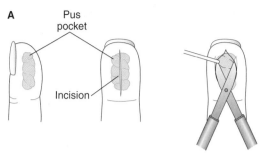

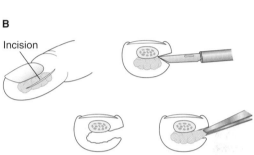

▲ **Figure 30–17.** Felon incision and drainage. (**A**) The recommended central longitudinal incision. (**B**) The classic lateral incision which bears a higher risk of complication. (Reproduced, with permission, from Stone CK, Humphries RL: *Current Diagnosis & Treatment Emergency Medicine*, 7th ed. New York: McGraw-Hill, 2011. Copyright © McGraw-Hill Education LLC.)

fingertips. Empiric treatment with antistaphylococcal antibiotics and close follow-up for wound checking is appropriate.

DEEP FASCIAL SPACE INFECTIONS

ESSENTIALS OF DIAGNOSIS

▶ Antibiotics should be initiated in the emergency department.

▶ Deep space abscesses require referral to a hand surgeon.

There are four potential deep fascial space infections of the hand. They include the thenar space, midpalmar space, dorsal subaponeurotic space, and subfascial web space. These infections are frequently caused by *S. aureus*, streptococci, and coliforms. Antibiotic therapy should be initiated in the emergency department and referral to a hand surgeon for exploration and drainage is the mainstay of care.

CELLULITIS

▶ Cellulitis usually takes 2-3 days from the inciting incident to become apparent clinically.

▶ *Capnocytophaga*, associated with animal bites, can cause overwhelming sepsis in the immunocompromised.

Closed fist bite wounds following altercation should be treated with care as they can rapidly progress into serious infections. This injury may be complicated by an infected open metacarpal phalangeal joint.

Treatment

▶ Uncomplicated Cellulitis & Antibiotic Prophylaxis

Typical antibiotic coverage for simple wounds or cellulitis includes first-generation cephalosporins (cephalexin or trimethoprim-sulfamethoxazole) for penicillin-allergic patients. Wounds with increased infectious risk such as bites or soiled wounds should prompt leaning toward antibiotic coverage. Diabetics and potential drug users in the older pediatric patient should warrant extra consideration.

▶ Animal Bites

Animal bites may cause severe infections if not treated promptly and properly. Dogs and cats carry *Pasteurella multocida*, which often causes a rapidly progressive cellulitis, and can be identified within 24 hours of injury. Other pathogens may not cause clinical findings for 2-3 days. Augmentin (Amoxicillin-clavulanate) is the suggested antibiotic coverage in children with rapidly evolving infections suggestive of *Pasteurella*. Alternative treatments for delayed infections include clindamycin plus trimethoprim-sulfamethoxazole and close follow-up for wound checks. Cleaning the wounds out thoroughly to remove contamination and check for foreign bodies is advised. Do not close animal bite wounds as it may cause worsening infection rather than appropriate healing.

▶ Human Bites

These injuries are more common in older pediatric patients and are typically the result of the "fight-bite" injury. However, other incidences occur for human bites in children. Close examination of the wound to evaluate for tendon involvement and depth of injury is paramount. Thorough irrigation and checking for foreign bodies such as a tooth or

tooth fragment are recommended. These wounds should be left open and not sutured.

Infections from human bites may be treated as outpatient but must be given a low threshold for admission. Children should be observed with a high level of suspicion for abuse or if parents seem unreliable for close follow-up care. Antibiotic coverage with amoxicillin-clavulanate or second-generation cephalosporins provides good prophylaxis. Severe infections require admission and IV antibiotics. Penicillin-allergic patients may be treated with clindamycin plus trimethoprim-sulfamethoxazole. Typically microbes include mixed anaerobes, *S. aureus*, streptococci, and *Eikenella*. Admission or follow-up daily is recommended.

Disposition

Obvious infections require admission and referral to a hand surgeon. Injuries to the tendon or tendon sheaths, those with systemic symptoms, or presence of extensive cellulitis fall into this category. Other considerations for admission are those with stories concerning for possible abuse (and need for social services consult) or unreliable follow-up. Children managed as outpatients need daily follow-up for wound checks.

SUPPURATIVE TENOSYNOVITIS

Clinical Findings

Infection may be caused by a nearby open wound to the affected tendon site. Localized swelling, erythema, and pain to palpation along the tendon sheath are indicators. Specifically, pain with passive stretch will cause severe pain in these patients.

Treatment & Disposition

Concern for suppurative tenosynovitis such as a flexor tenosynovitis requires prompt antibiotic treatment and hospitalization for surgical drainage. Intravenous cephalosporins are effective first-line treatment in the emergency department. Immobilization in a supportive splint and use of a sling are suggested until surgical intervention can be achieved. Care should not be delayed.

DISSEMINATED GONOCOCCAL INFECTION

Pustular skin lesions in the older pediatric patient with associated tenosynovitis may represent gonococcal infection. There is typically not an associated nearby wound to the affected site as this is caused by hematogenous spread. Immediate hospitalization and IV antibiotic therapy is indicated. Gonococcal infections diagnosis and treatment are discussed in Chapter 39.

MINOR CONSTRICTIVE PROBLEMS

Constrictive problems are uncommon in the pediatric patient but may occur in the adolescent pediatric subset. These types of injury are typically the result of overuse and symptoms may occur due to increasing use of computers and gaming consoles both for school and for play. A brief discussion of the most common topics follows.

CARPAL TUNNEL SYNDROME (COMPRESSION OF MEDIAN NERVE)

Patients will note symptoms in the median nerve distribution sparing the fifth finger and commonly note numbness, tingling, or aching. Use of the Phalen maneuver may elicit symptoms by placing the wrist in full flexion for 30 seconds. The Tinel sign, described as a sensation of an electric shock when the physician taps the wrist over the median nerve, may be present. Initial treatment involves NSAIDs and possibly wrist splinting as well as activity modification or cessation. Steroid injections may be considered later in the course of therapy. Similar to other constrictive pathologies, carpal tunnel syndrome is usually seen in adults. When seen in children, it is often the result of overuse during sports.

STENOSING FLEXOR TENOSYNOVITIS (TRIGGER FINGER)

Repetitive strain is the common cause of this condition that is characterized by tenderness at the MP joint, referred pain to the PIP joint, and a snapping during active range of motion of the thumb or finger. NSAIDs and splinting the finger in extension should be considered as primary treatment. Although this condition is worth mentioning, it is very rare in children and usually involves the thumb when present.

DE QUERVAIN TENOSYNOVITIS

De Quervain tenosynovitis is a painful inflammation of tendons in the thumb that extend to the wrist (tenosynovitis). Finkelstein test may elicit the inflammation by putting the wrist into marked ulnar deviation with a clenched fist over the thumb. Pain should be noticed on the radial side of the wrist caused by stretching of the tendons. Treatment includes NSAIDs, rest, and possibly splinting with a thumb spica splint. This condition is very uncommon in children, but may occur in adolescents.

Minor constrictive problems may be treated in a conservative manner in the emergency department, including splinting in a thumb spica splint (see Chapter 29) to rest the tendon and referred to a hand surgeon for follow-up and long-term care regarding the steroid injections and in some cases tendon releases.

THERMAL INJURIES

FIRST-DEGREE BURNS

First-degree burns are classified as redness of the skin without blister formation. These may be treated with simple cleansing with cold water and appropriate analgesia. Avoid constricting with tight wraps or tight-fitting clothing. First-degree burns typically heal well without complication and a follow-up visit is recommended after 1-2 days with a primary care physician.

SECOND-DEGREE BURNS

Second-degree burns are signified by blistering of the skin that retains sensation and is therefore painful. Second-degree burns are known as partial-thickness burns and are variable in depth and severity. In many patients, the injuries may be treated and dispositioned to home, but those with extensive burns or severe swelling should be referred emergently for evaluation by a hand surgeon as well as possible hospitalization. Treatment in the emergency department consists of aspiration or unroofing of larger blisters and silver sulfadiazine should be applied topically to the affected site. Bacitracin may be substituted in those with sulfa allergy. Tetanus immunization should be updated. Bulky dressing and splinting in functional position are recommended to avoid contracture issues.

THIRD-DEGREE BURNS

Third-degree burns known as full-thickness burns require aggressive treatment with topical silver sulfadiazine or bacitracin, loose dressings, splinting, and elevation. Tetanus immunization status must be up to date. Circumferential burns or those overlying a joint should be transferred to a burn center. These injuries are classically painless but may be associated with painful surrounding first- or second-degree burns.

ELECTRICAL BURNS

Electrical burns come in two varieties: conduction and crossed circuit. High-voltage conduction burns typically have points of entry and exit and injure the deep tissues disproportionately to the skin appearance. Crossed circuit electricity produces arc heat and may cause blackening of the skin surface due to carbon deposition. These injuries are typically less extensive than they are frightening to the patient and family. Arc heat burns are treated in the same manner as other thermal injuries.

Conduction burns may cause ischemia and paralysis. They should be treated by a hand surgeon as they will possibly require fasciotomy, debridement, grafting, and sometimes amputation.

As with all burns, consideration of systemic effects of potassium release and rhabdomyolysis are possible. Particular concern should be given to the possible myocardial injury associated with conduction injury.

FROSTBITE

Frostbite is a disorder of vasoconstriction and microvascular thrombotic events. Extent of injury depends on the temperature, windchill, moisture exposure, and duration of exposure. Injuries may be superficial or deep. Appropriate protective gear should be worn to avoid exposure preemptively when possible.

Superficial frostbite may be treated readily in the emergency department but should be treated rapidly and with care to avoid further injury. Frostbite is limited to the skin layer and the typical progression is pain replaced by numbness of the digits over time. Reversal by warming is required urgently and improvement is identified by a tingling sensation in the affected areas.

Deep frostbite requires emergent care by a hand surgeon. Frostbite is signaled by pain and swelling of the entire hand with associated blister formation and later complete dysesthesia. Rewarming both the hands and the core are recommended, immersion in water for a short duration may be helpful. Water temperature should be kept 37°C-40°C (98.6°F-104°F) and soaking less than 20 minutes is recommended. Blisters require debridement and sterile dressings. Sympathic blockade should be considered. Following rewarming and consideration of the patient's associated injuries, appropriate disposition to a hand surgeon is required.

FIREWORKS INJURIES

Pediatric thermal injuries to the hand due to seasonality and fireworks cause significant burden on medical resources. The age at which injuries occur may cause long-term morbidity compared with similar injuries in adults. When these injuries occur, prompt treatment and disposition to a level 1 trauma center with appropriate hand surgeon is often necessary.

Strauss EJ, Weil WM, Jordan C, Paksima N: A prospective, randomized, controlled trial of 2-octylcyanoacrylate versus suture repair for nail bed injuries. *J Hand Surg Am.* 2008 Feb;33(2):250-253.

▼ FOREIGN BODIES

Foreign body injuries are not uncommon in pediatric patients and should be treated delicately and with care to avoid infections or long-term disability of the hand. X-ray imaging may help identify location and type of foreign body in addition to a good history and examination. Ultrasound may be helpful for identifying nonradiopaque foreign bodies as CT and MR imaging studies take longer to perform.

Foreign bodies such as splinters, fishhooks, or arrowhead tips may have ends or barbs that prevent or discourage retrograde withdrawal. In these patients, attempting to push the foreign body along the current track and removal by counter-incision may be possible. Small foreign bodies may be left alone and followed up with hand surgeon. In some patients, attempt at acute retrieval may be more difficult than therapeutic.

When attempting removal, appropriate use of tourniquet (remember to take it off the patient), regional anesthesia, magnification if possible, and sterile technique are recommended. Nerve blocks are particularly helpful for foreign bodies in an isolated digit. Sterile dressings, elevation, and immobilization are recommended following removal or attempted removal. Prophylactic antibiotics and tetanus immunization should be followed by nonemergent referral to a hand surgeon unless the injury threatens the neurovascular status of the extremity.

COMPLEX HAND INJURIES

CLASSIFICATION

Amputations, flexor and proximal extensor tendon lacerations, nerve disruptions, high-pressure injections, compartment syndrome, and mangling and blast injuries require rapid evaluation and referral to specialty care.

PRIMARY ASSESSMENT & STABILIZATION

The initial evaluation should include rapid examination, diagnosis, supportive therapy, and referral to a hand surgeon if appropriate. Following are measures that should be considered in these patients.

Avoid Unnecessary Manipulation

A significant injury requiring transfer to specialty care should be handled gently, avoiding extensive probing or manipulation. Removal of easily accessible debris and gross contamination is appropriate but excessive tissue probing is not recommended. Easily removable sterile dressings and temporary splinting should be utilized for transport.

Surgical Preparation

Patients planning to undergo urgent surgery should be made NPO and IV fluids started. Preoperative labs should be collected, and the patient and family should be informed of the possibility of surgery. In cases of transfer by privately owned vehicle to definitive care, NPO status should be emphasized to the family.

Antibiotic Administration

Parenteral antibiotics should be administered as early as possible in significant open wounds to reduce infectious complications. Cefazolin can be given intravenously or intramuscularly and provides adequate coverage for most wounds. Clindamycin can be used for patients with a severe penicillin allergy.

AMPUTATIONS

Background & Considerations

Pediatric amputations are fairly common injuries requiring assessment for reimplantation. Because the younger patient has the possibility for lower morbidity and mortality compared with adult counterparts, aggressive action and evaluation is recommended. The diagnosis is obvious on inspection of the hand and may be generally classified into partial or complete and are caused by crush, avulsion, or laceration.

Definitive conversations about the risks and benefits of replantation should be addressed by the hand surgeon.

Treatment

▶ Replantation Possible

Because children tend to heal and adapt to trauma quickly, broader selection criteria should be used for quick referral to a hand surgeon. Determinants of outcome are primarily based on type of injury and body mass, and not necessarily age.

The amputated member can be safely kept at 4°C (39.2°F), wrapped in sterile saline-moistened gauze and sealed in a plastic bag or container, which is then placed in a cooler or bag of ice. It should be noted that freezing the amputated part is not recommended as it destroys tissue viability.

After stabilization of the patient and amputated fragment, a pediatric hand surgeon should be contacted for definitive care.

▶ Replantation Impossible

If the amputated digit is not salvageable or recoverable, the stump should be closed appropriately. Only simple fingertip pad amputations should be closed in the emergency department, as all other injuries should likely be discussed with a hand surgeon.

FLEXOR & PROXIMAL EXTENSOR INJURIES

General Considerations

Common etiologies in pediatric tendon ruptures include fights, extended use (such as gymnastics), trauma, suicide attempts and self-mutilation, and farmyard injuries. Rarely do tendons tear intratendinously, but more frequently at the musculotendinous junction or in the belly of the muscle. This leads to tendons that have retracted out of reach of investigation.

Most flexor tendon injuries, and extensor injuries where the proximal tendon has retracted, are considered complex hand injuries.

Clinical Findings

Incomplete tendon injuries are not always easy to identify and the physician must keep a level of suspicion. Partial injuries and occasionally complete injuries do not reveal functional debility immediately and sometimes present at a later date. To discriminate between partial-thickness and full-thickness tears, ultrasound is an ideal imaging modality. Ultrasound can identify the anatomy of tendon avulsion when no bony abnormalities are present.

Open tendon lacerations can frequently be identified by abnormal posturing and function of the digits. Direct visual examination of the tendon is always the best assessment if the open soft tissue defect is in a location that could create a tendon laceration. Observation of the tendon through full range of motion should be performed on every examination.

A common closed tendon injury seen in pediatric patients is a rupture of the flexor digitorum profundus (jersey finger) that results from hyperextension of the flexed ring finger that occurs when grabbing an opponent's jersey. This clinically manifests as an inability to flex the finger at the DIP joint. Partial tears can be managed conservatively with appropriate follow-up with a hand surgeon. Complete injuries require more prompt referral for definitive repair.

Treatment

Flexor and proximal extensor injuries warrant consultation with a hand surgeon. Immediate supportive therapy includes appropriate irrigation, dressing, and splinting of the hand and wrist. If definitive management is postponed, closure of the wound and administration of antibiotics is recommended (cefazolin, 25-100 mg/kg/day IV, followed by cephalexin 25 mg/kg/day orally, divided into four doses). Flexor tendons can be repaired up to days after the injury without functional compromise. Deep lacerations with concern of partial or poorly visualized tendon lacerations should be immobilized and referred to a hand surgeon for follow-up.

NERVE INJURIES

Clinical Findings

In pediatric patients, nerve injuries are frequently the product of fractures, dislocations, or crush injuries. (Figure 30–18). Because of their complex nature, a thorough physical examination is crucial. With careful motor and sensory examination (Figure 30–19), few significant nerve injuries will be missed. However, the limitations of a child's cooperation and ability to follow directions make follow-up imperative.

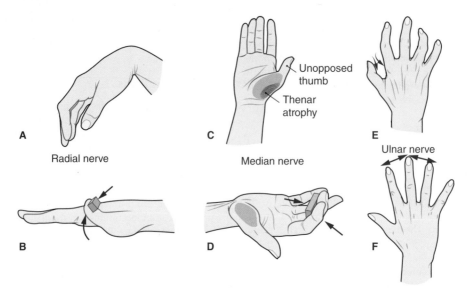

▲ **Figure 30–18.** Disabilities associated with peripheral nerve injuries. (**A**) Wrist drop from radial nerve injury. (**B**) Inability to forcefully extend the thumb due to radial nerve injury. (**C**) "Ape hand" from median nerve injury. (**D**) Loss of forceful index finger from median nerve injury. (**E**) Ring and small fingers "clawing" and thenar atrophy from an ulnar nerve injury. (**F**) Ulnar nerve injury resulting in loss of finger adduction and abduction. (Reproduced, with permission, from Stone CK, Humphries RL: *Current Diagnosis & Treatment Emergency Medicine*, 7th ed. New York: McGraw-Hill, 2011. Copyright © McGraw-Hill Education LLC.)

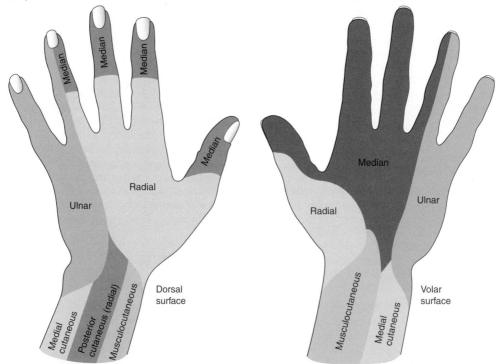

▲ **Figure 30–19.** Sensory innervation of the hand. (Reproduced, with permission, from Stone CK, Humphries RL: *Current Diagnosis & Treatment Emergency Medicine*, 7th ed. New York: McGraw-Hill, 2011. Copyright © McGraw-Hill Education LLC.)

Treatment

The injury should be appropriately dressed and splinted. Imaging should be performed as necessary. Patient and family should be educated about the possibility of injuries to anesthetized skin that may go unrecognized due to lack of sensation.

Disposition

Nerve injuries should prompt immediate consultation with a hand surgeon to identify the time course of evaluation and possible required interventions. Typically, closed nerve injuries are associated with soft tissue damage and neurapraxia. These are sometimes managed conservatively until swelling and inflammatory response can resolve. However, open wounds with nerve injuries are more likely to represent a severed nerve and may require emergent repair.

HIGH-PRESSURE INJECTION INJURIES

 ESSENTIALS OF DIAGNOSIS

▶ Recognize the puncture at the site of entry.
▶ Radiographic imaging with x-ray.
▶ Inquire about timing and the quantity, quality, and suspected velocity of the intruding substance.

Clinical Findings

Severity of high-pressure injection injuries is often underestimated because of a lack of overt clinical findings. At initial presentation, only a pin point entry portal may be appreciated; however, massive damage may have occurred subcutaneously and along fascial planes. An x-ray should be obtained; if the material is radiopaque, the extent of distribution can be determined. With many substances, massive tissue necrosis may be seen within 4-12 hours of injury. The injected material (paint thinner, gasoline, steam) plays a role in determining outcome, and a thorough history should be obtained including velocity and amount of injected solution.

Treatment & Disposition

Immediate referral to a hand surgeon is required. Often, high-pressure injuries carry a dismal outcome with amputation rates as high as 30%. Analgesics may be necessary for pain control and the extremity should be slung for comfort.

1. Obtain x-rays.
2. Give nothing by mouth and provide appropriate tetanus prophylaxis and systemic antibiotics. Frequently decompressive treatment must be made ready.

3. Avoid digital blocks to prevent increased elevated tissue pressure and compressive ischemia.

CLOSED COMPARTMENT SYNDROMES

 ESSENTIALS OF DIAGNOSIS

▶ Progressive swelling, pain, and palpably tense soft tissues.
▶ Disproportional pain response to passive flexion and extension.
▶ Symptoms of hypoesthesia and sensory disturbances of the digits are common but may be difficult to elicit in history from small children.

General Considerations

Compartment syndrome is a limb-threatening event defined as the compression of nerves and blood vessels in a confined space. Compression leads to local tissue ischemia, fat necrosis, and accumulation of toxic end-products. Frequently involving the upper extremities, any single space of the digit, hand, forearm, or arm may be involved. Etiology of compartment syndrome can arise from an external compression (prolonged pressure, constrictive casting), or internal expansion within the inelastic connective tissue (crush injuries, fractures, intracompartmental hemorrhage). Without quick assessment and treatment, compartment syndrome results in dysfunction and potentially systemic consequence including rhabdomyolysis.

Clinical Findings

In contrast to adult patients, where pain with passive stretch, pressure, paresthesias, paralysis, and pulselessness (5 Ps) of compartment syndrome hold true, in pediatric patients increasing anxiety, agitation, and analgesia (3 As) can lead to a detection of compartment syndrome. Pediatric patients have difficulty describing classical symptoms such as paresthesia, so a high clinical suspicion and objective findings are necessary to make a diagnosis. Identification of increasing doses of analgesia over the emergency department course, for example, may identify a case of compartment syndrome in ample time for treatment.

Treatment

Definitive management of compartment syndrome is surgical and supportive measures such as analgesia, elevation, and sling application are recommended. The affected hand should be reassessed frequently for signs of circulatory compromise. Increasing pain and physical examination signs concerning for extremity hypoperfusion including decreased capillary refill, pallor, loss of Doppler pulses, and increased pain should prompt immediate action. If surgical care cannot be accessed, an escharotomy along the hand's dorsal interosseus muscle compartments can temporize the situation and alleviate pressure. Incisions should be made down to the fatty tissue along the length of the eschar. Mid-lateral incisions of the forearm can be utilized for extension of eschar to the forearm. Emergency department bedside fasciotomy is recommended only in unique situations where there is no accessible surgical consultation and prolonged ischemia would result from inaction.

Disposition

Immediate consultation with hand surgeon for surgical decompression is recommended.

MANGLING INJURIES

General

Mangling injuries (blasts, gunshots, bites, machinery-related) present a complicated picture in the pediatric patient from a physical and psychosocial perspective. Children will often hide the mangled limb, shy from physical activity, and generally become more reserved. A strong alliance among physician, parents, and hand surgeon has been shown to decrease the effects from such a traumatic injury.

Clinical Findings

Typically obvious on inspection, mutilation injuries share common features of disfigurement, contamination, and damage to multiple types of tissues.

Treatment

Effort should be made to prompt supportive care until definitive surgical management is available. This involves loose, bulky sterile dressing and splinting, as well as immediate intravenous antibiotics (cefazolin 25-100 mg/kg/day).

Goodson A, Morgan M, Rajeswaran G, Lee J, Katsarma E: Current management of jersey finger in rugby players: Case series and literature review. *Hand Surg.* 2010;15(2)103-107 [PMID:20672398].

Mohan R, Panthaki Z, Armstrong MB: Replantation in the pediatric hand. *J Craniofac Surg.* 2009;20:996-998 [PMID: 19553830].

Tuttle H, Olvey S, Stern P. Tendon avulsion injuries of the distal phalanx, *Clin Orthop Rel Res.* 2006;447:157-168 [PMID: 16601414].

Wu TS, Roque PJ, Green J, et al: Bedside ultrasound evaluation of tendon injuries. *Am J Emerg Med.* 2012;30(8):1617-1621 [PMID: 22244220].

Soft Tissue Injuries & Wound Care

Shawn Horrall, MD, DTM&H

Jonathan Wheatley, MD

IMMEDIATE MANAGEMENT OF LIFE-THREATENING PROBLEMS

Hemorrhaging wounds can easily divert attention from more important considerations in the trauma patient. It is unlikely that a bleeding wound will alter the immediate outcome of a trauma patient; however, unverified and compromised airway, breathing, and systemic circulation (ABCs of trauma) most certainly will. Although major wounds require prompt attention of the resuscitation team in evaluation of the patient, the ABCs must be addressed first. Only after the primary survey has been conducted should proper hemostasis be applied and wounds managed appropriately. Primary methods for hemostasis by the emergency physician include direct pressure, tourniquets, epinephrine-containing anesthetics, and suture ligation.

DIRECT PRESSURE

A simple approach is often best. Direct pressure on a bleeding wound is easy, effective, and cost-efficient. Although large-vessel bleeding requires more advanced methods of hemostasis, bleeding from small vessels can often be contained with a pressure dressing made of a bulky dressing held by hand or with an elastic or self-adherent bandage. Direct pressure in the wound compartment often helps contain bleeding after a wound has been firmly closed with suture material.

TOURNIQUETS

Application of tourniquets to extremity sites can be fraught with complications, but proper use can provide adequate hemorrhage control in patients where direct pressure is ineffective. Commercial products are available; however, a simple well-placed blood pressure cuff can provide similar results. Gauze should be placed underneath the cuff to protect intact skin, and the cuff should be inflated initially to 20 mm Hg above patient's blood pressure. Higher pressure

may be required. It is advised that a tourniquet be in place for no longer than 60 minutes total, and no longer than 20-30 minutes before releasing for 5 minutes for temporary restoration of blood flow to prevent distal tissue ischemia.

Finger tourniquets require a different approach in a difficult-to-control situation. Three primary methods are typically employed: (1) a commercially available finger tourniquet (Tourni-cot, T-Ring Digital Tourniquet); (2) a Penrose drain is placed under the base of the finger can be effective; and (3) a sterile glove is placed over the injured hand. After cutting the tip of the glove of the affected finger, the finger of the glove is rolled toward the base of the finger providing a hemostatic and sterile field.

EPINEPHRINE-CONTAINING ANESTHETICS

Lidocaine mixed with a standard concentration of epinephrine to provide hemostasis is effective for many bleeding wounds. Historically, physicians avoided this practice for concern of ischemia in the digits, ears, nose, and genitals, although no evidence of harm may have been found. Studies demonstrate the absence of complications, improved hemostasis, increased duration of anesthesia, and decreased anesthesia requirements. In addition, surgical subspecialists conclude that benefits of epinephrine-containing anesthetics outweigh perceived harm and advocate their use to obtain a hemostatic field in otherwise difficult-to-control areas. Despite more modern approaches, many physicians continue to avoid the use of epinephrine-containing anesthetics in the body areas noted above.

SUTURE LIGATION

A vessel 2 mm or larger may require ligation with sutures. Ligation should be performed with caution, but it may be the appropriate method to achieve hemostasis. The bleeding ends of the vessel should be visualized and clamped with the end of a hemostat. Three ties with synthetic absorbable suture are usually sufficient to provide adequate holding power. The ends of the suture should be trimmed closely to reduce the amount of foreign material that will remain in the wound. Occasionally veins are recalcitrant to simple tying and require a modified technique. The operator can pass the suture needle through the vessel wall and then tie it circumferentially around the vessel.

Consultation with a vascular surgeon is required for many arterial injuries, especially those of the proximal extremity. Although not all arterial injuries require operative repair, proximal extremity arterial injuries tend to be at higher risk of distal blood flow disruption.

Waterbrook AL, Germann CA, Southall JC: Is epinephrine harmful when used with anesthetics for digital nerve blocks? *Ann Emerg Med.* 2007;50(4):472-475 [PMID: 17886362].

WOUND ASSESSMENT

HISTORY

Traumatic wounds are among the most common presenting complaints in the emergency department. A thorough history, including the surrounding circumstances of the injury, is necessary in the evaluation of all traumatic wounds to develop a treatment plan. Emergency department physician obtains the history including: time the injury happened, location of the injury, mechanism by which the injury occurred, and evaluation for an apparent pattern.

When

Timing of the injury is very important to determine the proper treatment plan. The interval between injury and treatment will often dictate whether to treat with closure in the emergency department versus delayed closure. There is a higher risk of infection and complications associated with prolonged interval between injury and treatment. The generally accepted time frame for primary closure for lacerations, with the exception of injuries to the face and scalp, is less than 6 hours. Face and scalp injuries may be closed within 24 hours after injury. These rules are not absolute, as locations with good blood supply may be closed later, while those with decreased blood supply should be considered for delayed closure or closure by secondary intention.

Where

Location of the injury may determine the decision to close primarily versus delayed closure. Other considerations are risk of infection by contamination with bodily substances (feces, pus), or environment contaminants where the injury occurred, (soil, rust).

How

Determine the mechanism by which the injury occurred. Simple lacerations have a relatively low risk of complication. High-energy projectile wounds and crush injuries have a greater risk of vascular compromise and associated fractures, which may predispose to compartment syndrome or failure to heal. Animal or human bites have a high risk of infection and may contraindicate primary closure. High-pressure injection injuries will likely require surgical consultation. Maintain a high level of suspicion for foreign bodies as they commonly complicate wounds.

Patterns

Evaluate for patterns of injury that indicate non-accidental trauma. Loop patterns or right angles are suggestive of man-made objects striking the skin in contrast to typical trips and falls. Injuries on the posterior aspects of the forearms are indicative of abuse, as these patterns of injury are infrequent in accidents. For discussion of non-accidental trauma, see Chapter 5.

PHYSICAL EXAMINATION

Type & Extent of Injury

Thorough wound assessment is imperative in management of acute wounds in the emergency department. Extensive wounds may require consultation with a surgeon for effective closure. Highly contaminated wounds will require copious irrigation and possible debridement to reduce risk of infection. It is important to determine viability of the affected body part, whether any tissue is missing, and adequacy of the blood supply.

Optimize the setting surrounding wound examination, including adequate lighting, hemostasis, and a calm patient. Wound hemostasis should be obtained while examining the wound to evaluate for foreign bodies or damaged underlying tissue such as vessels, nerves, or tendons. Extent of the injury should be determined upon initial examination, which occasionally may require revision or widening of the wound margins to assess the underlying tissue. Better visualization of the wound will help minimize further complications by avoidance of missing more extensive injuries. Several basic categories of acute wounds are encountered in the emergency department.

▶ Abrasion

Abrasion is superficial damage to the skin, involving only the epidermis and occasionally the underlying dermis. Abrasions generally do not require interventions other than covering and moisturizing to prevent secondary infection.

Laceration

A torn or jagged wound, usually linear, although it may be of various shapes and sizes. It is often caused by sharp objects; relatively resistant to infection.

Avulsion

Forcible tearing away of a body part from adjacent tissue, often to be devitalized. The viability of an avulsion flap is dependent upon the blood supply to its base and surrounding tissue.

Puncture

High risk of infection due to contamination and foreign bodies.

Stretch Injury

May produce underlying damage to vasculature, nerves, and other soft tissues that may not be seen superficially.

Crush Injury

Often a complicated injury that may result in lacerations, fractures, bleeding, hematoma, or compartment syndrome. Significant tissue necrosis may occur due to loss of blood supply. Progression of swelling compresses local vasculature and nerves that may lead to further tissue loss.

Bites

Mammalian bites are often heavily contaminated with oral bacterial flora and at the highest risk of infection. These wounds may have puncture components making them difficult to clean and that increase risk of infection.

Location of Injury

The location of an injury requires attention to the unique differences between different body areas. Different locations will require knowledge of varying likely mechanisms of injury, as well as complications specific to each site.

Scalp

The scalp is highly vascularized, making for optimal healing conditions and very low infection rate. Wounds are most often hidden by hair, making cosmesis less important than other areas such as the face. It is important to determine if the underlying galea is involved; large galeal lacerations should be repaired with absorbable suture prior to closure of the dermis and epidermis. Hair removal is discussed in the Cleaning and Debridement section later in this chapter.

Face

Facial lacerations often require a high degree of care and knowledge of skin tension lines in order to reduce the incidence of scarring and poor cosmetic results. Facial wounds that are overly complex or interfere with facial symmetry should give the physician a low threshold for consultation with a plastic surgeon.

Neck

Deep neck injuries may involve important underlying structures. These wounds often require consultation with a trauma or general surgeon for operative exploration and closure to minimize complications.

Chest & Abdomen

Wounds to the chest and abdomen should be explored to determine involvement of, or communication with, underlying structures and cavities.

Extremities

Soft tissue injuries to the extremities are common presenting complaints to the emergency department. These injuries often involve a significant amount of morbidity; thus adequate assessment and treatment is necessary to optimize the patient's functional capacity. Extremity injuries require a thorough neurovascular examination, including pulses, capillary refill, light touch, two-point discrimination, and motor strength.

Forsch RT: Essentials of skin laceration repair. *Am Fam Physician.* 2008;78(8):945-951 [PMID: 18953970].

Singer AJ, Dagum AB: Current management of acute cutaneous wounds. *N Engl J Med.* 2008;359(10):1037-1046 [PMID: 18768947].

Spiro DM, Zonfrillo MR, Meckler GD: Wounds. *Pediatr Rev.* 2010;31(8):326-334 [PMID: 20679098].

Waseem M, Lakdawala V, Patel R, et al: Is there a relationship between wound infections and laceration closure times? *Int J Emerg Med.* 2012;5(1):32 [PMID: 22835090].

WOUND MANAGEMENT

ANESTHESIA

Effective anesthesia is important to optimize conditions for wound closure, to prevent patient movement, morbidity, and to aid in hemostasis. Perform a thorough neurological examination of the affected region prior to anesthesia.

There are a number of anesthesia agents to choose from, each with a unique set of attributes. Appropriate use of an agent includes consideration of duration of action, potency, and safety. A common emerging practice is use of topical anesthetics in the pediatric patient to avoid unnecessary injections, with near-equivalent efficacy to locally injected anesthetic agents. Use of regional anesthetics is limited by their cardiovascular and systemic toxicity.

Topical Anesthetics

Topical anesthetics are useful in patients with small, uncomplicated wounds. Use of tetracaine, adrenaline, and cocaine (TAC) has fallen out of favor due to toxicity and abuse potential. Current preferred preparations are listed following.

LET (lidocaine 2%, epinephrine 1:1,000, and tetracaine 2%): Apply to wound, cover with an occlusive dressing, and wait 20 minutes for absorption and anesthesia. Duration of action is 20 minutes.

LMX-4 (4% liposomal lidocaine): 30 minutes to achieve anesthesia, 45 minutes duration.

EMLA (5% preparation of 2.5% lidocaine and 2.5% prilocaine): 1 hour to achieve anesthesia.

Inhalation Anesthetic

Inhalation anesthetic is used to provide general sedation of the patient to aid in procedure. Nitrous oxide is often used as the inhalant of choice, but use is uncommon in the emergency department.

Local Anesthetic

Local anesthetic is injected, usually from within the wound margin, to infiltrate into the bordering tissue (Figure 31–1). A 25- to 30-gauge needle is preferred, with the smallest needle providing the least discomfort. The minimum volume needed to achieve adequate anesthesia

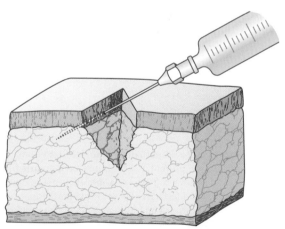

▲ **Figure 31–1. Injection of local anesthetic.**
(Reproduced, with permission, from Dunphy JE, Way LW: *Current Surgical Diagnosis & Treatment*, 5th ed. Los Altos, CA: Lange Medical Publications, 1981. Copyright © McGraw-Hill Education LLC.)

should be used to prevent toxicity and to prevent distortion of the wound borders that may interfere with cosmesis. The pH of the anesthetic preparation causes a local burning sensation, which can be reduced by slow infiltration or by buffering with sodium bicarbonate (add 1 mL sodium bicarbonate to 9 mL lidocaine). Warming the anesthetic prior to administration can reduce pain. Epinephrine preparations will provide a longer duration of action and help constrict local capillaries, providing additional hemostasis. Local anesthesia durations and maximum doses are listed in Table 31–1.

Regional Anesthesia

Regional anesthesia is sensory nerve blockade at a location proximal to the wound. This has the advantage of anesthetizing a larger area with less volume, does not typically

Table 31–1. Local anesthesia duration and maximum dose.

Agent	Duration of Action	Maximum Dosage Guidelines
AMIDES		
Lidocaine	Medium (30-60 min)	Without epinephrine 4.5 mg/kg; ≥ 300 mg
Lidocaine with epinephrine	Long (120-360 min)	With epinephrine: 7 mg/kg
Mepivacaine	Medium (45-90 min) Long (120-360 min with epinephrine)	5 mg/kg; ≥ 400 mg
Bupivacaine	Long (120-240 min)	Without epinephrine: 2.5 mg/kg; 175 mg
Bupivacaine with epinephrine	Long (180-420 min)	With epinephrine: ≥ 225 mg
Prilocaine	Medium (30-90 min)	Body weight < 70 kg: 8 mg/kg; ≥ 500 mg Body weight > 70 kg: 600 mg
Ropivacaine	Long (120-360 min)	2-4 mg/kg; ≥ 200 mg
ESTERS		
Procaine	Short (15-60 min)	7 mg/kg; not to exceed 350-600 mg
Chloroprocaine	Short (15-30 min)	Without epinephrine: 11 mg/kg; ≥ 800 mg With epinephrine: 14 mg/kg; ≥ 1000 mg

distort anatomy, and may have a longer duration of action. Common regional anesthesia sites are digital blocks, extremity nerve blocks, infraorbital, and supraorbital nerve blocks.

Digital Nerve Block

This block requires infiltrating about 0.5 mL of lidocaine or bupivacaine into base of the digit in the area of each of the four nerve sheaths. There are two nerves on the dorsum and two on the palmar aspect of the digits. The duration to adequate anesthesia for lidocaine is approximately 10 minutes. Newer literature supports the use of epinephrine for digital blocks as needed.

Radial Nerve Block

This nerve block will anesthetize the lateral dorsum of the hand in the distribution of the radial nerve. Approximately 2 mL of lidocaine is instilled just proximal to the Lister tubercle, where the radial nerve emerges from beneath the brachioradialis (Figure 31–2).

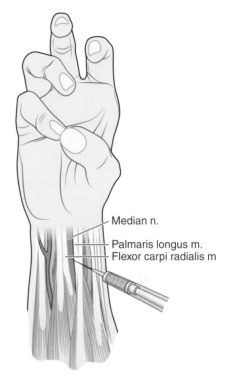

▲ **Figure 31–3.** Median nerve block, in which 2 mL of anesthetic is injected into the carpal tunnel between the tendons of the palmaris longus and flexor carpi radialis. (Reproduced, with permission, from Stone CK, Humphries RL: *Current Diagnosis & Treatment Emergency Medicine*, 7th ed. New York: McGraw-Hill, 2011. Copyright © McGraw-Hill Education LLC.)

Median Nerve Block

This nerve block will anesthetize the lateral palmar aspect of the hand in the distribution of the median nerve. This is achieved by injecting 2 mL of lidocaine into the carpal tunnel between the tendons of the palmaris longus and flexor carpi radialis (Figure 31–3).

Ulnar Nerve Block

This nerve block will anesthetize the medial palmar surface of the hand in the distribution of the ulnar nerve. This is performed by injecting 2 mL of lidocaine just medial to the flexor carpi ulnaris tendon (Figure 31–4).

Infraorbital Nerve Block

This nerve block will anesthetize the infraorbital branch of the maxillary nerve (V^2) as it exits the infraorbital canal. This is located inferior to the eye on an imaginary line between

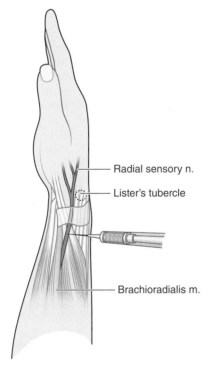

▲ **Figure 31–2.** Radial nerve block, in which 2 mL of anesthetic is injected just proximal to the Lister tubercle on the radial aspect of the forearm. (Reproduced, with permission, from Stone CK, Humphries RL: *Current Diagnosis & Treatment Emergency Medicine*, 7th ed. New York: McGraw-Hill, 2011. Copyright © McGraw-Hill Education LLC.)

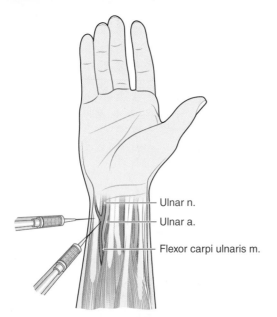

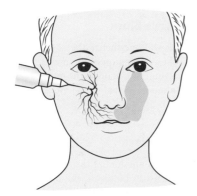

- Ulnar n.
- Ulnar a.
- Flexor carpi ulnaris m.

▲ **Figure 31–4.** Ulnar nerve block, in which 2 mL of anesthetic is just medial to the flexor carpi ulnaris tendon. (Reproduced, with permission, from Stone CK, Humphries RL: *Current Diagnosis & Treatment Emergency Medicine*, 7th ed. New York: McGraw-Hill, 2011. Copyright © McGraw-Hill Education LLC.)

the pupil and the ipsilateral canine. Infiltrate 1-2 mL of lidocaine to achieve anesthesia of this nerve distribution (Figure 31–5).

▲ **Figure 31–5.** Infraorbital nerve block, in which intra-oral or percutaneous injection around the palpable infra-orbital foramina will result in anesthesia within the shaded area. (Adapted, with permission, from Stone CK, Humphries RL: *Current Diagnosis & Treatment Emergency Medicine*, 7th ed. New York: McGraw-Hill, 2011. Copyright © McGraw-Hill Education LLC.)

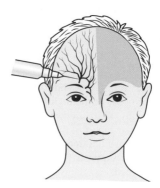

▲ **Figure 31–6.** Supraorbital nerve block, in which anesthetic is injected superior to the orbital ridge at the supraorbital notch. The shaded area will be anesthetized on the ipsilateral side of injection. (Adapted, with permission, from Stone CK, Humphries RL: *Current Diagnosis & Treatment Emergency Medicine*, 7th ed. New York: McGraw-Hill, 2011. Copyright © McGraw-Hill Education LLC.)

► Supraorbital Nerve Block

This nerve block will anesthetize the supraorbital branch of the ophthalmic nerve as it exits the supraorbital foramen. This is performed by palpating the notch of the supraorbital foramen on the superior orbital ridge, then injecting 1-2 mL of lidocaine to achieve anesthesia of this nerve distribution (Figure 31–6).

Procedural Sedation

Procedural sedation has proven safe and effective for pediatric wound care. Sedation creates an environment in which the provider can carefully examine and treat wounds. This limits the risk of further injury to the patient caused by anxiety or pain. (See Chapter 4.)

Of particular note are parental concerns regarding whether their child will suffer during the procedure. Parents may demand sedation without regard to whether the risks of sedation outweigh the perceived benefits of being "asleep" during the procedure. Parents should be advised when it may be more efficacious, timely, and safe to defer procedural sedation and utilize a child life specialist or staff member to divert the patient's attention for a simpler and more straight-forward wound assessment and management.

CLEANING & DEBRIDEMENT

Cleaning of an acute wound is vital to prevent infection and complications. The objective of wound cleaning is to remove as much bacteria, contaminants, and devitalized tissue as possible. There is a spectrum of approaches from wound irrigation, to scrubbing, to complete excision of the initial wound that may be utilized to optimize a clean wound. In the emergency department, copious irrigation is the most common method.

Hair Removal

Wounds in hairy areas pose a unique difficulty as the native hair can become embedded in the wound and act as a foreign body. This can prevent adequate healing and promote infection. A simple solution is to clip the hair short enough to prevent interference with the wound, but not to shave the hair. Shaving exposes the hair follicle and predisposes to more infection. Eyebrows and eyelashes are an exception. It is not recommended to remove these hairs as they have significant cosmetic effect and may cause disruption of anatomic alignment needed to properly approximate wound margins. In a small subset of patients, eyebrows may regrow irregularly after being removed.

Irrigation

Irrigation is the most important intervention to prevent infection and promote wound healing. Wound irrigation is the steady flow of solution across exposed tissue to wash away particulate matter, to hydrate, and enable effective visualization. There is continued debate regarding the need for pressured irrigation versus gentle irrigation to adequately clean wounds. It is generally accepted that pressures of 7-11 lb/in^2 are needed to adequately remove bacteria and particulate matter.

A number of commercial devices are available that provide either constant pressurized flow or pulsatile flow, although no clinical difference has been identified. In the emergency department, a 50 mL syringe and a 19-gauge needle are shown to provide ideal pressure and stream for thorough irrigation. Bulb syringes as well as fluid bottles or bags that have holes poked in them have been shown to be ineffective for adequate wound cleansing.

Recent studies have compared the use of chlorinated tap water versus saline to irrigate wounds. Tap water is shown to an effective alternative to saline to irrigate acute wounds.

Do not mix alcohol, peroxide, or iodine with the irrigation solution as these products are bactericidal, but they also exhibit significant cytotoxicity and can delay wound healing. Diluted hydrogen peroxide is effective for removing dried blood and debris from the surrounding skin. Ionic soaps and detergents are also not recommended for wound cleansing as they are irritating and may increase risk of infection.

Mechanical Scrubbing

High-porosity sponges may be used on the wound surface to gently remove debris. Brushes may further damage the tissue and decrease infection resistance but are effective for removing imbedded foreign bodies that would interfere with normal wound healing.

Debridement

Removal of contaminating foreign matter and devitalized tissue is important to promote wound healing. Devitalized tissue should be excised with a sterile scalpel to expose healthy tissue underneath. Irregularities of the wound margins may be revised to encourage adequate approximation of wound margins and prevent tenting of the wound edges. Debridement of the face and other areas of cosmetic significance should be deferred to a plastic surgeon.

WOUND CLOSURE

After careful examination, anesthesia, and irrigation, a decision about closing the wound must be made. Closing the wound in the acute setting is referred to as primary closure and is the preferred method to reduce scarring, encourage healing, and promote a rapid return to functional state. If electing not to close the wound in the acute setting, closing 48-96 hours later is referred to as delayed primary closure.

Delayed primary closure may be preferred for heavily contaminated wounds, wounds requiring significant debridement, and bite wounds. This is performed by packing the wound with moist saline after initial cleansing, which allows the tissue to develop resistance to infection that it would otherwise not have with primary closure. The moist gauze should be changed three times daily, while inspecting for signs of infection. After the interval period, if no signs of infection are identified, the wound may be closed in the same fashion as primary closure.

Contraindications

Not all wounds should be primarily closed in the emergency department. Heavily contaminated wounds, such as feces or pus, have such a high risk of infection that they are destined to fail and will benefit from delayed closure. Wounds that fall outside of the recommended interval period (> 6 hours) should prompt consideration of delayed closure to minimize infection risk. Any active wound infection evident on the initial examination should not undergo primary closure.

Major tissue defects, such as gaping wounds requiring high suture tension, should be considered for healing by secondary intention. These wounds have a high risk of dehiscence and wound cavity development. They are often best managed by regular dressing changes and allowing granulation tissue to fill the wound. Do not close wounds that result in an empty void under the closure—these spaces predispose to infection and possible abscess formation. Retained foreign bodies are a contraindication to primary closure and need to be addressed first. Crush wounds are high risk for complications such as compartment syndrome, hematoma formation, and dehiscence. Consider allowing these wounds to heal by secondary intention.

Timing

Wounds less than 6 hours old may undergo primary closure unless otherwise contraindicated and have a high likelihood of satisfying results. Primary closure of wounds with intervals greater than 6 hours is at the discretion of the provider. Resistance to infection is directly related to adequacy of blood supply. If the location has sufficient blood supply, closure may be performed at a longer interval, although there is increased risk of infection which should be communicated with the patient and parents. Some patients may have decreased blood flow, such as diabetics; such wounds may be best managed with a shorter interval window for primary closure. Facial and scalp wounds may be considered for primary closure up to 24 hours after initial injury, owing to the region's excellent blood supply.

Methods of Closure

Four methods are available for wound closure: sutures, adhesive wound tape, staples, and tissue wound tape. The modality to choose is determined by the location and characteristics of the wound. There is often no cosmetic difference among the available selections, and outcome depends largely on the patient's individual healing. For simple low-tension linear lacerations, any of the four methods described may be utilized with equivalent cosmetic outcome. For irregular lacerations, areas with movement, or those with high tension, suture is the modality of choice. Staples are frequently used in situations of time restraint or with uncomplicated scalp lacerations. Tissue adhesive is commonly used in the pediatric patient for uncomplicated facial lacerations in regions of low tension.

▶ Suture

Suture selection is generally dependent on the location of the injury and the degree of tension that the sutures will need to maintain. Smaller suture and needle sizes are used for facial wounds to minimize scarring, generally with 5-0 or 6-0 suture. Layered wound closures require a fine absorbable deep suture. Dermal and epidermal closures in locations elsewhere on the body are commonly managed with a 3-0 or 4-0 suture, with 3-0 preferred for areas of higher tensile strength requirement. Scarring related to the suture depends on size of the suture, the wound tension, and the duration that the suture remains in place. All suture materials will cause a local foreign body tissue reaction with variations based upon the type of material.

Decision regarding use of absorbable or nonabsorbable suture is determined on a case-by-case basis. For dermal and epidermal closures, absorbable or nonabsorbable may be used and choice is often determined by the patient's preference, reliability of follow-up, and degree of tensile strength required. For a patient with poor reliability for follow-up, closure with absorbable suture may be preferred to prevent long-term consequences of prolonged suture duration and even retained suture. Common sutures are listed in Table 31-2.

Nonabsorbable Suture

Nonabsorbable sutures are commonly used for superficial closures, for tendon repair, and for regions of high tension. Most nonabsorbable suture will maintain tension for up to 60 days. The following materials are not used in deep sutures due to high tissue reactivity and foreign body response.

Silk. A naturally produced braided material that has been used throughout history for wound closure. Silk is notorious for its high tissue reactivity, the highest of all nonabsorbable suture, as well as its propensity to lose tension with time. The use of silk has largely been replaced by synthetic suture material in developed countries.

Nylon. A monofilament suture material with relatively low tissue reactivity. This suture is progressively degraded by hydrolysis over time, resulting in loss of tensile strength. It is notoriously stiff and does not maintain a knot as well as other suture materials.

Polypropylene. Available as monofilaments that provide long-term tensile strength without a loss of tension, and cause the least tissue reactivity of all sutures. It is commonly used in superficial wound closures.

Polyester. Available as monofilament and braided applications. It is the suture of choice for tendon repair, has minimal tissue reactivity, and does not undergo degradation or weakening with time.

Absorbable Suture

Absorbable suture is often used for deep closure of dermal wounds and fascial layers. It causes a high degree of local tissue reactivity that contributes to its degradation. These suture materials maintain tensile strength for less than 60 days. Many varieties are available for use with the selection decision based on duration of tensile strength. Rapidly absorbing sutures such as fast-acting gut, polydioxanone, or poliglecaprone are effective options for laceration repairs in children who are not candidates for tissue adhesive. This often eliminates a return visit for suture removal.

Gut. Commonly created from bovine serosa, these sutures are degraded by proteolytic enzymes and have inconsistent tensile duration. Available as plain gut or chromic gut, they are selectively used in the emergency department. Plain gut holds tension for approximately 2 weeks with a high degree of tissue reactivity. Chromic gut is treated with chromium salts, offering

Table 31–2. Common suture materials.

Nonabsorbable Suture	Filament	Classification	Duration of Tensile Strength
Silk	Braided	Biological	Many months
Nylon (Ethilon, Dermalon)	Monofilament	Synthetic	Many years
Polypropylene (Prolene, Surgipro)	Monofilament	Synthetic	No degradation
Polyester (Ticron, Mersilene)	Braided and monofilament	Synthetic	No degradation
Polybutester (Novafil)	Monofilament	Synthetic	No degradation
Absorbable suture			
Plain gut	Monofilament	Biological	50% at 5 d
Chromic gut	Monofilament	Biological	50% at 10 d
Poliglecaprone (Monocryl)	Monofilament	Synthetic	60% for 1 wk
Polydioxanone (PDS)	Monofilament	Synthetic	50% at 4 wk
Polyglactin (Vicryl)	Braided	Synthetic	65% at 2 wk
Polyglyconate (Maxon)	Monofilament	Synthetic	70% at 28 d
Polyglytone (Caprosyn)	Monofilament	Synthetic	50% at 10 d

more predictable absorption and loss of tensile strength with a duration of up to 4 weeks.

Synthetic. Available in multiple applications including polyglycolic acid, polyglactin, polydioxanone, poliglecaprone, polyglytone and polyglyconate. They produce minimal tissue reactivity and are often used for deep closures and vascular repairs. Polyglycolic acid and polyglactin retain approximately 50% of tensile strength at 10-14 days. Polydioxanone retains 50% of tensile strength at 4 weeks. Poliglecaprone retains 60% of tensile strength at 1 week. Polyglyconate retains 70% of tensile strength at 1 month.

▶ **Adhesive Wound Tape**

Forgoing the use of suture for wound repair will provide the lowest risk of infection, as there is no foreign body reaction. Wound tapes are highly effective in closure of uncomplicated linear lacerations with low tension. They are also effective for epidermal approximation in wounds that have been closed with deep dermal sutures. Because of very low infection rates, wound tapes are very effective in contaminated wounds as well. The wound must be prepped clean and dry before placement of wound tapes to prevent early failure. Tincture of benzoin is effective in promoting tape adhesion and tension. Wound tapes allow for tension only in the most superficial layers of skin; thus deep dermal sutures may be required to maintain adequate approximation of the wound with the epidermal layer closed with tape.

▶ **Staples**

The ease of use, speed, and good cosmetic outcome makes closing of wounds with staples an acceptable choice. There are a variety of commercially available staple applicators. Staples may be used in relatively simple lacerations without a significant deep component, as they close only the superficial layer of the skin. They are most commonly used in scalp lacerations as both application and removal are uncomplicated by hair. Infection rate and long-term scarring are similar to sutures. Staple removal is slightly more painful than removing suture. It is performed with a commercially available staple remover to evert the penetrating arms of the staple.

▶ **Tissue Adhesives**

Cyanoacrylate tissue adhesive is a commonly used method of closing small uncomplicated wounds in pediatric patients, usually facial lacerations. Cyanoacrylate adhesive polymerizes to maintain approximation of wound edges, providing effective cosmesis and infection prevention while treatment is nearly painless. Adhesives are recommended for lacerations that are less than 5 cm in length, and less than 0.5 cm in width and that are easily approximated with minimal tension.

They are not recommended in areas close to eyes, mucous membranes, or active infection. Adhesive application is performed by approximating wound edges and applying two layers of adhesive over the entire surface of the wound and extending 5-10 mm beyond the wound border. The wound is held in approximation for 45-60 seconds while the adhesive polymerizes and is followed by a second application. To prevent runoff into eyes or hair, cover eyes with gauze and apply petroleum jelly to nearby hair.

Suture Technique

There are a number of suture techniques for wound closures. The goal is to optimize wound margin approximation and reduce the incidence of infection and scar formation. Most often in the emergency department, simple interrupted suture technique is sufficient to obtain optimal repair results. Running sutures may be performed in linear lacerations with low tension, especially during time constraint. Deep or gaping wounds may be closed with vertical and horizontal mattress sutures, respectively. Occasionally, the wound may require multiple layers of suture to close the wound defect, especially in patients with fascia involvement or tissue loss. The specific technique required will vary with patient and provider.

POSTMANAGEMENT WOUND CARE

Dressings

The role of a wound dressing is to protect from contamination and forceful wound disruption, and to optimize the wound-healing environment. An occlusive dressing is a cost-effective means to prevent failure of the wound repair. It can be used to maintain moisture and ointments, and is simple and easy to change. A dressing consists of a simple adhesive bandage or a complex organization of gauze and antibacterial components. Dressing changes should be performed at least daily.

Ointments

Studies have indicated no difference between antibacterial ointment and petrolatum ointment in the prevention of wound infections. Both ointments maintain moisture on the healing tissue, preventing it from drying and delaying healing. Ointments may help prevent and reduce scar formation. Maintaining a moist wound is preferred over the historical recommendation of keeping the wound clean and dry.

Immobilization

Very large wounds and those that overlie joints should be immobilized in a splint. A splint prevents dehiscence and wound disruption caused by the stretching and stress on the wound. Immobilization should be continued for at least 1 week to allow for sufficient wound healing to withstand separation by movement. Avoid prolonged splinting, which will contribute to joint stiffness.

Suture & Staple Removal

Skin lacerations require an average of 7 days to achieve adequate tissue strength to prevent spontaneous dehiscence. General recommendations for suture duration depend on the location of suture due to variations in tissue tension, movement, and cosmetic concerns.

Sutures in the face should be removed after 3-5 days—longer increases the risk of scarring. Sutures or staples in the scalp and arms should be removed after 7-10 days. Sutures of the trunk, legs, hands, and feet should be removed after 10-14 days. Sutures on the palms and soles should be allowed 14-21 days before removal. Each wound should be assessed individually, and dependent on the progress of the wound, suture duration varies. Allow more time for wounds that do not appear to have healed well enough to maintain closure. Table 31–3 lists recommended duration of suture by location.

ADDITIONAL CONSIDERATIONS

Antibiotics

Development of a wound infection is a serious consideration in determining management of an acute wound. From decreasing inflammatory cell actions and tissue oxygenation to increasing inflammation, infection retards healing and worsens outcomes. For outpatient management, topical and enteral antibiotics are the mainstay of treatment.

Irrigation should take priority over antibiotics in the majority of wound management patients where it can be employed. Antibiotics should be employed as an adjunct. An average of 4.5-6.3% of wounds will become infected,

Table 31–3. Duration of suture by location.

Location	Duration of Suture (days)
Face and scalp	3-5
Arms	7-10
Trunk	7-10
Legs	10-14
Hands and feet	10-14
Palms and soles	14-21

but no evidence exists to support the widespread use of prophylactic antibiotics. Patients with comorbidities (AIDS, uncontrolled diabetes), specific type of wounds (crush and compression injuries), grossly contaminated wounds, deep structure involvement, bite wounds, and delayed presentation are candidates to receive antibiotics.

Choice of antibiotic should be tailored to the presumed organism(s). Most wound infections are due to staphylococcal and streptococcal species. Salt-water wounds have increased risk of *Vibrio* species, fresh water wounds have increased risk of *Aeromonas*, and soil-contaminated wounds are at risk of *Clostridium* species. Although community-associated methicillin-resistant *Staphylococcus aureus* (CA-MRSA) is a main cause of cutaneous infection, the overall carriage rates are low and should not impact antibiotic choice for the otherwise healthy patient.

Topical antibiotics have historically been used as basic wound management. However, there is a paucity of data to specifically recommend their use. It has been demonstrated that topical antibiotic administration in the emergency department may decrease the risk of wound infection in comparison with petroleum jelly. The optimum choice of topical antibiotic is unknown. Commonly used and over-the-counter topical ointments include bacitracin or a combination of bacitracin, neomycin, and polymyxin (triple antibiotic ointment). Neomycin is known to cause allergic dermatitis in patients. Ointments are not recommended after a wound has been closed with a tissue adhesive as they can cause early weakening of the polymerized film.

Tetanus Prophylaxis

Tetanus is a potentially life-threatening disease resulting from wound infection by *Clostridium tetani*. In the United States, routine immunization for tetanus is common in children. Tetanus prophylaxis has become standard-of-care in routine wound management and should be considered for a wound with potential skin or mucosal loss of integrity. A three-part immunization series is recommended for adequate background coverage. If a patient has not had an immunization for tetanus in greater than 5 years, it should be updated while in the emergency department. Table 31–4 summarizes tetanus prophylaxis recommendations.

Table 31–4. Summary of tetanus prophylaxis recommendations.

Prior Doses of Tetanus Toxoid	Minor Wounds, Minimal Contamination	Major or Heavily Contaminated Wounds
< 3 or unknown	Tetanus toxoid only	Tetanus toxoid + tetanus immune globulin
≥ 3	No therapy	No therapy

Age of the patient and vaccination status will determine the tetanus toxoid-containing booster. Patients aged 6 weeks to 6 years should be given the diphtheria and tetanus toxoids and acellular pertussis (DTaP) vaccine. For children aged 7-10 years, who are previously vaccinated, the tetanus and diphtheria toxoids (Td) vaccine is preferable. Patients aged 10-18 years, the tetanus toxoid, reduced diphtheria toxoid, and acellular pertussis (Tdap) vaccine are recommended.

Tetanus immunoglobulin (TIG) is considered safe and standard of care for appropriate wounds. High-risk wounds that increase the risk of tetanus include those contaminated with dirt, feces, soil, saliva, and wounds associated with frostbite, crush or avulsion wounds. For infants younger than 6 months, it is appropriate to utilize the mother's immunization status in addition to recommendations in Table 31–4 TIG use. Additionally, TIG should be considered in tetanus-prone wounds for patients with HIV infection regardless of immunization status.

Rabies Prophylaxis

Rabies remains a serious problem in the United States and abroad. It is a nearly universal fatal viral infection caused by an RNA virus transmitted after inoculation into a wound from an infected reservoir. Proximity of inoculation site to the recipient's brain will partially determine time to onset of disease, often weeks to months. Once symptoms of rabies have begun, rabies prophylaxis will no longer be beneficial.

More than 23,000 doses of rabies post-exposure prophylaxis (RPEP) are given annually in the United States. Management of a potential exposure is an essential element in proper wound care.

▶ Assessment of Risk

Type of Animal

Animals considered high-risk include bats, raccoons, skunks, foxes, coyotes, and other carnivores.

Note: Bats are considered high-risk reservoirs and have been linked to many cases in the United States. In situations where it is possible that there was contact with a bat (sleeping areas, children present, mentally disabled patients), even without obvious evidence of a bite, it is recommended that RPEP be administered.

Animals considered low-risk include mice, rats, squirrels, rabbits, gerbils, other small rodents, birds, and reptiles. Domestic cats and dogs are less concerning because of high vaccination penetration in the United States.

Circumstances of Exposure

Unprovoked bite by a domestic animal is considered high-risk for rabies. Normal defensive behavior is conversely low-risk. It can be difficult to discriminate normal defensive behavior from rabid behavior.

Method of Exposure

Violation of skin integrity is considered potential for virus transmission. In addition to teeth breaking through the skin barrier, contamination of previously open wounds with animal saliva is considered higher risk.

Determine if Animal Is (or likely is) Rabid

Rabies vaccination status of the offending animal should be determined quickly. If the domestic animal has up-to-date vaccinations, the risk of rabies transmission is very low. If status cannot be verified, the animal should be observed for 10 days to watch for a change in condition or should be sacrificed to have the brain examined for evidence of rabies. If the animal cannot be found, or is otherwise considered high-risk, RPEP should be administered. Behavior of the offending animal is not a reliable sign of rabies: 80% of rabies cases are "furious" rabies; 20% are "dumb" rabies.

Geography

In the United States, rabies is concentrated in the eastern and southern geographic areas, but is found in all areas. Consult local public health officials to determine risk of exposure.

▶ Management of High-Risk Exposures

Wound Care

Adequate irrigation is essential. Combined with proper RPEP, irrigation is the cornerstone of proper rabies prophylaxis.

Active Immunization

Two forms of vaccine are available in the United States for use in humans for postexposure prophylaxis to confer active immunity. Immunizations are given on days 0, 3, 7, and 14 IM at a site distant from the rabies immune globulin (see RIG, next section). If a patient has received the vaccine prior to exposure, the vaccine should be given on day 0 and 3.

Passive Immunization

Rabies immune globulin (RIG) is given to confer passive immunity to the patient while the patient's immune system generates antibodies through active immunization with the rabies vaccine. RIG is not indicated for those who have been fully immunized pre-exposure.

RIG is given as an injection of 20 IU/kg. As much of the RIG should be infiltrated around the wound edges as is feasible, which may represent an increased challenge in the pediatric patient depending on the volume of the solution. The remaining dose should be given IM at a site distant from the vaccine site.

Follow-up Instructions

Patients and their families should be given clear and concise discharge instructions. There is increasing evidence that patients do not comprehend the instructions they are given and are inappropriately confident in their misunderstandings. Patients should receive written instructions, which are reinforced by oral discussion of the information. Instructions should be given in common vernacular, appropriate for the level of understanding of the patient and family. Salient features include proper home wound care, the date sutures or staples will be removed, as well as what to do if concerning symptoms develop.

Eidelman A, Weiss JM, Baldwin CL, et al: Topical anaesthetics for repair of dermal laceration. *Cochrane Database Syst Rev.* 2011;(6):CD005364 [PMID: 21678347].

Engel KG, Heisler M, Smith DM, et al: Patient comprehension of emergency department care and instructions: Are patients aware of when they do not understand? *Ann Emerg Med.* 2009;53(4):454-461 [PMID: 18619710].

Fernandez RS, Griffiths R, Ussia C: Water for wound cleansing. *Int J Evid Based Health.* 2007;5(3):305-323 [PMID: 21631794].

Garcia-Gubern CF, Colon-Rolon L, Bond MC: Essential concepts of wound management. *Emerg Med Clin N Am.* 2010;28(4): 951-967 [PMID: 20971399].

Luck RP, Flood R, Eyal D, et al: Cosmetic outcomes of absorbable versus nonabsorbable sutures in pediatric facial lacerations. *Pediatr Emerg Care.* 2008;24(3):137-142 [PMID: 18347489].

Moran GJ, Talan DA, Abrahamian FM: Antimicrobial prophylaxis for wounds and procedures in the emergency department. *Infect Dis Clin N Am.* 2008;22(1):117-143 [PMID: 18295686].

Rupprecht CE, Briggs D, Brown CM, et al: Use of a reduced (4-dose) vaccine schedule for postexposure prophylaxis to prevent human rabies: Recommendations of the advisory committee on immunization practices. *MMWR Recomm Rep.* 2010;59(RR-2):1-9 [PMID: 20300058].

Spiro DM, Zonfrillo MR, Meckler GD: Wounds. *Pediatr Rev.* 2010;31(8):326-334 [PMID: 20679098].

Waseem M, Lakdawala V, Patel R, et al: Is there a relationship between wound infections and laceration closure times? *Int J Emerg Med.* 2012;5(1):32 [PMID: 22835090].

EMERGENCY TREATMENT OF SPECIFIC WOUNDS

ORAL LACERATIONS

Most intraoral and perioral lacerations will not require primary closure. Certain situations require special consideration. Some oral injuries will necessitate airway management, and intubation may need to be performed before closure of a hemorrhaging wound. A sedated and immobilized patient may make a difficult encounter more manageable. If the patient's airway is intact, procedural sedation may still be required to allow for a meticulous repair. Adequate anesthesia for wound management may be acceptable with local anesthesia alone, but appropriate regional anesthesia may give superior pain relief with less distortion of local anatomy. Most oral injuries will not require antibiotics for infection prevention as postinjury infection is a rare, even in the relatively flora-rich environment of the mouth. Specific injuries include the following.

Vermillion Border Laceration

This location requires meticulous closure. If the appropriate wound margins are misplaced by 1 mm or more, an unacceptable cosmetic result may occur.

Frenulum Tear

Laceration likely does not require repair. However, this injury (especially in infants) is strongly suggestive of non-accidental trauma.

Tongue Laceration

In most oral mucosa wounds, small, linear tongue lacerations heal rapidly on their own. However, bifid lacerations or hemorrhaging wounds will require repair and can be challenging. A retention suture or a towel clip may be needed to stabilize the tongue. Chromic gut suture will typically provide better outcome.

Through-and-Through Laceration of Cheek

If the laceration is large enough to repair, a multilayered approach is needed. After adequate irrigation, close the mucosal layer first using chromic gut or other rapidly absorbing suture. Irrigate the wound again from the exterior. The deep structures can then be approximated using a polyglycolic acid suture (Vicryl). The epidermis should be closed using an appropriate skin suture for the face.

HIGH-PRESSURE INJECTION INJURIES

Although this injury pattern is less likely in the pediatric patient, a basic understanding of this potentially high-morbidity injury is important. Industrial equipment can produce significant pressures (>10,000 psi) which are considerably more than enough to break clothing, skin, and to instill the delivered agents deep into patient's hand, forearm, or foot. Depending on the agent, pressure, anatomy, and time-to-treatment, amputation may be necessary. If this injury is encountered, immobilize the extremity, administer broad-spectrum antibiotics, obtain radiographs, and consult the appropriate orthopedic, trauma, or plastic surgeon emergently.

AMPUTATIONS

Amputations are more common in the upper extremities (crush or guillotine mechanism), but the lower extremity and other appendages may be affected. Amputations can be classified as complete or partial, depending on the integrity of interconnecting tissue. Replantation (for complete) or revascularization (for partial) will be required, respectively.

After a completed primary survey, attention should be directed toward the amputated appendage. Appropriate prehospital care tips the balance in the right direction for appropriate restoration of the affected tissue. After controlling for hemorrhage, the amputated body part should be wrapped in saline-moistened gauze, sealed in a plastic bag, and then placed in ice water. The wound and the amputated part should not be manipulated and rather only irrigated gently with normal saline. Subjecting the affected tissue to additional trauma, oversaturation with fluids, or freezing by direct contact with ice will reduce the viability of the tissue. Time constraints for replantation have been published: warm ischemia can be tolerated for 6-8 hours and cool ischemia for 12-24 hours.

The decision on replantation and revascularization is best made by the consulting surgeon. Amputated parts should not be discarded until they have been deemed not useful. Occasionally the tissue can be used for grafting.

BLAST INJURIES

Wounds sustained from blasts or high-velocity missiles can be severe, resulting in tremendous injury. Extensive disruption of soft and hard tissues can result in a wound cavity that deceptively hides the extent of the injury. Because the force may be transmitted to sites distant, examination of the entire patient is essential to reduce the likelihood of missed concomitant injuries.

Blast injuries tend to be complicated and have severe pathology; hospital admission is the usual disposition. Initial evaluation should follow a traditional trauma approach: airway, breathing, circulation, hemorrhage control, and complete physical examination. Appropriate surgical consultation will be needed for evaluation and admission; if this is unavailable, transfer to an appropriate referral center should be undertaken expeditiously. These patients will often require staged exploration, debridement, irrigation, and secondary closure technique. Broad-spectrum antibiotics should be given.

BITE WOUNDS

It is estimated that nearly 1% of all emergency department visits in the United States are for mammalian bite wounds. Depending on the etiology and pattern of the bite wound, complications range from immediate (fracture, hemorrhage, death) to long-term (infection, loss of use, disfigurement). An understanding of different bite wounds and proper management is essential. Choices of antibiotics for bite wound infection prophylaxis are listed in Table 31–5.

Table 31–5. Choice of oral antibiotics for treatment or prophylaxis of wound infection based on source of bite.

Bite source	Antibiotic of Choice	Alternative
Human bite	Amoxicillin/clavulanic acid	Macrolides
Dog bite	Amoxicillin/clavulanic acid	Clindamycin + trimethoprim/ sulfamethoxazole
Cat bite	Amoxicillin/clavulanic acid	Clindamycin + trimethoprim/ sulfamethoxazole

Dog Bites

Dog bites are the most common animal bite wounds. Adults are more frequently bitten on the hand, and children more frequently on the face. Avulsions, abrasions, tears, and crush injuries are often encountered secondary to the more blunt teeth of dogs and the high pressures their jaws can generate.

After initial stabilization, irrigation is the mainstay for prevention of infection. Primary closure of wounds has been a controversial issue. Primary closure will likely result in reduction in scar size, but infection may be more likely. A recent study describes the increasingly common physician preference to avoid primary closure. If cosmesis is a concern, primary closure is acceptable if it is not on the patient's hand and patient understands the increased risk of infection. Amoxicillin/clavulanic acid is the preferred antibiotic for coverage of *Pasteurella, Staphylococcus, Streptococcus*, and all species of bacteria that might cause infection. Clearly infected wounds require antibiotics, whereas prophylaxis of acute wounds remains undecided. Current literature supports treating high-risk wounds, especially those of the hand. Rabies and tetanus immunization should follow normal guidelines.

Disposition should include close patient follow-up due to the likelihood of wound infection, especially if closed primarily. Patient should return to the emergency department in 48 hours or follow up with primary care physician. If the cosmetic outcome is unacceptable, referral to a plastic surgeon may be indicated.

Cat Bites

Wounds from cat bites are less commonly encountered than those from dog bites but have higher potential for infection. Cats have a lower biting force and teeth that are sharp and fine, which result in puncture wounds that may deposit oral flora deep into the wound. Wound patterns tend toward upper extremity injury, followed by facial injuries. Wound care should mimic that for dogs, including choice of antibiotic prophylaxis. However, estimated rates of wound infection are 60-80%, and many physicians support antibiotic prophylaxis regardless of site. Infectious etiologies are similar to dog bites, with *Pasteurella* being the most common, followed by *Streptococcus* and *Staphylococcus*. Close follow-up is highly recommended.

Human Bites

Two types of human bite wounds are encountered: occlusive bite wounds and clenched-fist "fight-bite" wounds. In the pediatric patient, occlusive bite wounds can result from aggressive play, sporting events, or non-accidental trauma. Clenched-fist wounds tend to be more common in the older adolescent. Usually they result from a fight where the patient strikes an individual in the mouth, which causes a laceration over the metacarpophalangeal joint by a tooth. These injuries are at great risk of infection as oral flora can be inoculated directly into the nearby joint and tendon structures. Radiographs may reveal fractures or retained foreign bodies.

Irrigation should be the primary means for infection control. One scenario requiring suspicion is that if the tendon was violated with the oral flora when the fist was in the clenched position, the violated area may not be visible when the hand is relaxed.

Oral flora is diverse: *Streptococcal, Staphylococcal*, and *Eikenella* species are the most common, but other species can be encountered. Amoxicillin/clavulanic acid is the preferred antibiotic. These wounds should not be closed primarily. After irrigation, bandage the wound loosely and splint in an anatomical position. Tetanus prophylaxis should be addressed.

In the absence of joint or tendon involvement, retained foreign body, fracture, or signs of infection, and patient has reliable and verified follow-up, the patient/family can be treated solely in the emergency department and discharged. Given the high-risk nature of these wounds, the emergency department physician should have a low threshold to consult a hand surgeon. Human bite wounds commonly require operative debridement and parenteral antibiotics.

PLANTAR PUNCTURE WOUNDS

Plantar puncture wounds are commonly found in children. Patients often report stepping on a rusty nail, although wounds can occur from glass, wood, or other sharp materials. Infection appears to be a common problem, as feet tend to be dirty and the violating material is often contaminated. Infectious complications range from simple cellulitis to more serious abscess, septic arthritis, and osteomyelitis. Retained foreign bodies can occur, which may lead to infection.

Treatment can be slightly more challenging than retained foreign body, although patients and their families should be aware that radiolucent foreign bodies might be missed. Allowing the wounds to heal by secondary intention or with secondary closure techniques may help reduce the risk of infection. There is a paucity of data regarding antibiotic prophylaxis. Usual skin flora tends to be the etiology for cellulitis, and standard skin flora coverage is reasonable. *Pseudomonas* has been found to be the common cause of osteomyelitis, often in puncture wounds that go through a tennis shoe or in those patients with impaired wound healing (particularly in diabetics). If *Pseudomonas* is suspected, fluoroquinolones are a reasonable enteral antibiotic. Fluoroquinolones were previously feared to cause cartilaginous failure in children; however, they have recently been accepted for use in various indications. Use for pseudomonal prevention is not routinely recommended.

Unless a foreign body is found or the patient presents with an already infected foot, most patients can be discharged home after emergency department care. Unless the wound is minimal, it is prudent to have the patient follow-up to the emergency department or primary care physician for a wound check. Referral to an orthopedist or podiatrist for further intervention is warranted for any additional concerns.

Ball V, Younggren BN: Emergency management of difficult wounds: part I. *Emerg Med Clin North Am.* 2007;25(1):101-121 [PMID: 17400075].

Morrison WA, McCombe D: Digital replantation. *Hand Clin.* 2007;23:1-12 [PMID: 17478248].

Wolf SJ, Bebarta VS, Bonnett CJ, et al: Blast injuries. *Lancet.* 2009;374: 405-415 [PMID: 19631372].

Eye Emergencies

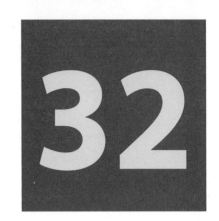

Robert D. Greenberg, MD, FACEP

Cassandra Zhuang, BS

EMERGENCY EVALUATION OF IMPORTANT OCULAR SYMPTOMS

EVALUATION OF THE RED OR PAINFUL EYE

HISTORY & EXAMINATION

Historical factors are important to determine the cause of ocular complaints in the pediatric patient. History, when correlated with characteristic ocular findings on focused physical examination, often makes the diagnosis. History includes a child's activity and behavior, and the usual historical items, including previous episodes, onset of symptoms, contact lens use, concurrent illnesses or complaints, and associated symptoms (Table 32–1) (Figures 32–1, 32–2).

Complete eye examination includes the following components, which need to be tailored to the age and capabilities of each patient

Visual Acuity

Visual acuity testing of the neonate, infant, or toddler is performed by testing the pupillary reaction to light. The ability of the child to track and fixate on a light source 1-3 feet away determines adequate visual acuity. Steady fixation roughly indicates 20/40, unsteady fixation 20/100, and inability to fixate 20/400. Formal visual acuity testing of a child 2-3 years of age is performed by means of a Snellen chart, Allen chart, or rotating "E" chart at 20 feet. An acute change in vision usually indicates disease of the globe or visual pathway. Pain and decreased acuity indicate corneal disease, or iritis.

Inspection

Inspect the eye, including conjunctiva, cornea, sclera, lens, pupil, external eyelids, lashes, lacrimal ducts, orbits, and periorbital areas for sign of trauma, infection, exudate, or irritation.

Pupillary Function

Check pupillary function for shape, symmetry, and reactivity to light and accommodation.

Extraocular Muscle Function

Check the extraocular muscles for sign of entrapment or palsy. This can be challenging in young or frightened children so creative methods of distraction or tracking to an item of interest may be employed to assist the examiner.

Visual Fields

Check for abnormalities in the visual fields, which is generally done by confrontation, but can be challenging in the young child.

Fundoscopy

Direct fundoscopy is used to check the retina, optic disc, and retinal vessels. Confirmation of the red reflex may be all that is possible in a frightened or young child, but an attempt should be undertaken.

Slit-Lamp Examination

Slit-lamp examination should be done before and after fluorescein staining to check for corneal abnormalities and to examine the anterior chamber. Examination of a younger child may be facilitated by having the child sit on the parent's lap during the examination. For examination of an infant, have the parent sit with one hand supporting the infant's buttocks and the other hand placed on the back of the infant's head. A Wood lamp may be used as an alternative to diagnosing corneal defects and may be attempted first if the child cannot cooperate for a slit-lamp examination.

Table 32–1. Causes of unilateral red or painful eye.

History and Clinical Findings	Conjunctivitis	Iritis	Acute Glaucoma	Corneal Infection (bacterial ulcer)	Corneal Erosion
Incidence	Extremely common	Common	Uncommon	Uncommon	Rare
Onset	Insidious	Insidious	Sudden	Slow	Sudden
Vision	Normal to slightly blurred	Slightly blurred	Markedly blurred	Usually blurred	Blurred
Pain	None to moderate	Moderate	Severe	Moderate to severe	Severe
Photophobia	None to mild	Severe	Minimal	Variable	Moderate
Nausea and vomiting	None	None	Occasional	None	None
Discharge	Moderate to copious	None	None	Watery	Watery
Ciliary injection	Absent	Present—perilimbal	Present	Present	Present
Conjunctival injection	Severe diffuse in fornices	Minimal	Minimal, diffuse	Moderate, diffuse	Mild to moderate
Cornea	Clear	Usually clear	Steamy	Locally hazy	Hazy
Stain with fluorescein	Absent	Absent	Absent	Present	Present
Hypopyon	Absent	Occasional	Absent	Occasional	Absent
Pupil size	Normal	Constricted	Mid-dilated, fixed, and Irregular	Normal	Normal or constricted
Intraocular pressure (IOP)	Normal	Normal	Elevated	Normal	Normal
Gram-stained smear	Variable; depending on cause	No organisms	No organisms	Organisms in scrapings from ulcers	No organisms
Pupilary light response	Normal	Poor	None	Normal	Poor to normal

Reproduced, with permission, from Stone CK, Humphries RL: *Current Diagnosis & Treatment Emergency Medicine*, 7th ed. New York: McGraw-Hill, 2011. Copyright © McGraw-Hill Education LLC.

Intraocular Pressure

Intraocular pressure (IOP) can be tested with an electronic or Schiotz tonometer (described later in this chapter) if necessary. Abnormally high pressure may be grossly estimated by palpation (tactile tonometry).

Additional Studies

Further diagnostic studies including blood tests, cultures, plain x-rays, bedside ultrasound, computed tomography (CT) scan, or magnetic resonance imaging (MRI) of the orbits may be needed to determine a diagnosis.

▶ Disposition

Children thought to have acute ocular conditions that may permanently decrease visual acuity should have urgent consultation with an ophthalmologist. Children with other conditions may receive treatment and be discharged with appropriate follow-up.

EVALUATION OF ACUTE UNILATERAL VISUAL LOSS

LOOK FOR TRAUMA

Exclude trauma as a cause of visual loss. Both blunt and penetrating ocular injuries may result in blindness.

HISTORY & EXAMINATION

Obtain a history from the child, parent, or individuals familiar with the child. Crucial questions include rate of onset of visual loss; if it is unilateral or bilateral, painful or painless, with or without redness.

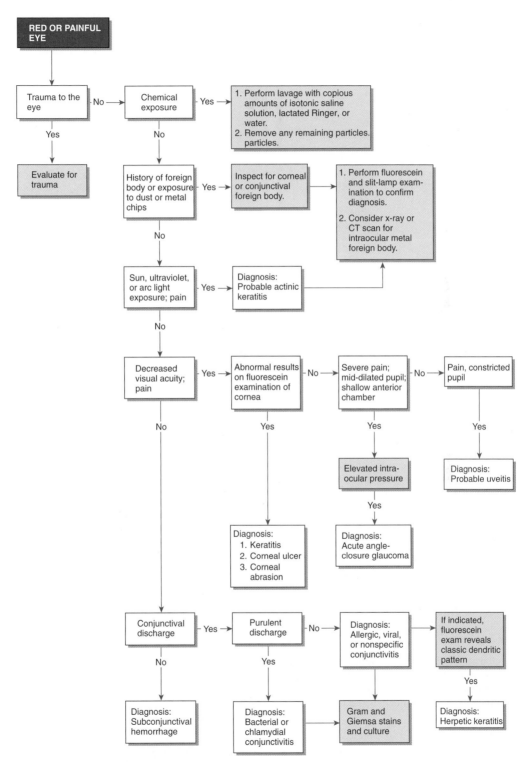

▲ **Figure 32–1.** Red or painful eye. Reproduced, with permission, from Stone CK, Humphries RL: Current Diagnosis & Treatment Emergency Medicine, 7th ed. New York: McGraw-Hill, 2011. Copyright © McGraw-Hill Education LLC.

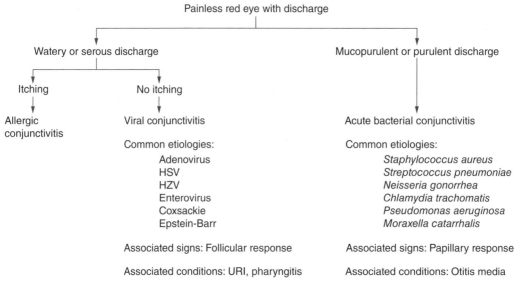

▲ **Figure 32–2.** Differential diagnosis for the painless red eye with discharge.

Inability to Visualize Retina

Cloudy media (cornea, lens, aqueous or vitreous humor) may partially or completely obscure the retina (red reflex blunted or absent), making it difficult to visualize retinal landmarks such as the optic disc.

Abnormal Visual Fields

Grossly abnormal visual fields are usually caused by central nervous system disease and thus generally affect both eyes (though not always to the same degree). The retinas are usually normal on ophthalmoscopic examination.

▶ Hemianopia

Hemianopia (decreased vision or blindness of one-half the visual field of one or both eyes) is usually due to postchiasmal neurologic disorders (tumor, aneurysm, migraine, stroke), in which case other acute neurologic lesions are likely present as well. Rarely, it is functional in origin.

▶ Central Scotoma

A central scotoma (area of partial alteration of the visual field surrounded by a field of normal or relatively preserved vision) indicates isolated macular involvement typical of retrobulbar neuritis and may or may not be associated with pain.

▶ Tubular vision

Tubular vision that is not in conformity with the laws of optics is characteristic of functional visual loss.

Abnormal Retina

Abnormal retina, isolated in the eye with visual loss, is characteristic of rare but serious conditions.

▶ Retinal Hemorrhage

Retinal hemorrhage from other causes (anticoagulation, hemophilia) may produce visual loss.

▶ Retinal Detachment

Retinal detachment produces visual loss preceded by visual flashes. If visual acuity is affected, detachment is large and may be easily visible on direct ophthalmoscopy; however, small detachments may require indirect ophthalmoscopy for visualization. Flashes of light may occur in children with migraine or as a result of posterior vitreous detachment. Ultrasound may be employed to confirm the presence of a retinal detachment.

DIFFERENTIAL DIAGNOSIS

Corneal Edema

Severe corneal edema of diverse causes (abrasion, keratitis, postoperative) may cause visual loss with eye pain.

Hyphema

Hyphema is the presence of blood in the anterior chamber. This is generally traumatic in nature, although spontaneous hyphema may occur especially in children with coagulopathies.

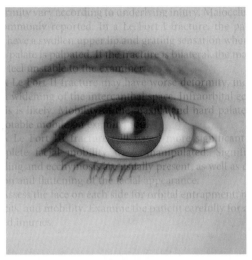

Hyphema

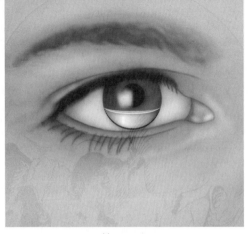

Hypopyon

▲ **Figure 32–3.** Examination appearance of hyphema (blood) or hypopyon (pus) in the anterior chamber.

Vitreous Hemorrhage

Vitreous hemorrhage causes painless visual loss due to accumulation of blood in the posterior chamber. The anterior chamber is clear. The red reflex is often absent.

Endophthalmitis

Endophthalmitis (intraocular infection) is a rare condition usually associated with eye pain and decreased visual acuity. Eye examination will disclose a hypopyon which is pus in the anterior chamber (Figure 32–3) or vitreous. Systemic illnesses associated with endophthalmitis include ankylosing spondylitis, ulcerative colitis, other seronegative arthropathies, sarcoidosis, toxoplasmosis, tuberculosis, syphilis, and herpes zoster.

▶ Disposition

Children with sudden visual loss due to ocular disease should have timely consultation with ophthalmologist.

Canadian Ophthalmological Society: *Assessment of the Red Eye.* Available at http://www.eyesite.ca/7modules/Module2/html/Mod2Sec1.html, Ottawa, ON. Accessed July 12, 2013.

Dargin JM, Lowenstein RA: The painful eye. *Emerg Med Clin North Am.* 2008;26:199-216 [PMID: 18249263].

Seth D, Khan FI: Causes and management of red eye in pediatric ophthalmology. *Curr Allergy Asthma Rep.* 2011;11:212-219 [PMID: 21437648].

Sethurman U, Kamar D: The red eye: Evaluation and management. *Clin Pediatr.* 2009;48:588-600 [PMID: 19357422].

Vortmann M, Schneider JI: Acute monocular visual loss. *Emerg Med Clin North Am.* 2008;26:73-96 [PMID: 18249258].

OCULAR CONDITIONS REQUIRING IMMEDIATE TREATMENT

ORBITAL CELLULITIS

General Considerations

Acute infection of the orbital tissues is generally caused by *Streptococcus pneumoniae,* other streptococci, *Staphylococcus aureus*, and, prior to widespread vaccination, *Haemophilus influenzae*. Obtaining immunization history may be critical in these patients. Less frequently, certain fungi of the Phycomycetes group may cause orbital infections (rhinoorbitocerebral mucormycosis), particularly in immunocompromised children. Most causative organisms enter the orbit by direct extension from the paranasal sinuses (primarily ethmoid) or through the vascular channels draining the periorbital tissues. Rarely, infection spreads to the cavernous sinus or meninges.

Clinical Findings

Patient may have a history of sinusitis or periorbital injury, pain in or around the eye, and possibly reduced visual acuity. Examination may demonstrate swelling and redness of the eyelids and periorbital tissues, chemosis of the conjunctiva, rapidly progressive exophthalmos, and ophthalmoplegia. Disc margins may be blurred, and fever is commonly present. Radiographic evaluation may demonstrate sinusitis with or without soft tissue orbital infiltration, but CT scanning or MRI is essential in establishing the full extent of disease.

Children with invasive infection due to the Phycomycetes group (*Mucor, Rhizopus,* and other genera) may present with rapidly progressive orbital cellulitis, often with cavernous sinus thrombosis. Diabetic and immunocompromised children are at increased risk. Examination often reveals coexisting maxillary and/or ethmoid sinusitis and palatal or nasal mucosal ulceration.

Treatment & Disposition

Obtain cultures of blood and periorbital tissue fluid. Obtain CT scan of the orbit to rule out orbital abscess and intracranial involvement. Child should be admitted and appropriate broad-spectrum intravenous antibiotics started (vancomycin 15-20 mg/kg twice daily plus piperacillin/tazobactam 100 mg/kg four times daily is a reasonable regimen). Obtain immediate consultation with ophthalmologist and/or otolaryngologist (ENT). Child with orbital phycomycosis should receive intravenous antifungal medications and requires surgical intervention for debridement of infected tissue. Consultation with neurosurgeon may be needed for intracranial involvement.

CAVERNOUS SINUS THROMBOSIS

General Considerations

Cavernous sinus thrombosis is often associated with orbital and ocular signs and symptoms. Infection results from hematogenous spread from a distant site or from local extension from the throat, face, paranasal sinuses, or orbits. Cavernous sinus thrombosis begins as a unilateral infection and commonly spreads to involve the other cavernous sinus.

Clinical Findings

Child may have complaint of or exhibit chills, headache, lethargy, nausea, pain, and decreased vision. Fever, vomiting, and systemic signs of infection may be present. Examination by an ophthalmologist discloses unilateral or bilateral exophthalmos, absent pupillary reflexes, and papilledema. Involvement of the third, fourth, and sixth cranial nerves leads to limitation of ocular movement whereas involvement of the ophthalmic branch of the fifth cranial nerve results in a decrease in corneal sensation.

Treatment & Disposition

Obtain blood cultures and start appropriate antibiotics, (nafcillin, plus a third-generation cephalosporin). Consider vancomycin if methicillin-resistant *S. aureus* is suspected or prevalent. Obtain CT scan of the head and orbits. Obtain consultation with ophthalmologist, and neurologist, early. Although controversial, anticoagulation with heparin can be safely considered for children with a deteriorating clinical condition after excluding intracranial hemorrhage.

RETINAL DETACHMENT

General Considerations

Detachment of the retina is actually separation of the neurosensory layer from the retinal pigment epithelium. Subretinal fluid accumulates under the neurosensory layer. Detachment may become bilateral in 25% of patients. Nontraumatic retinal detachment is unusual in children but does occur in those who are highly myopic or who have a family history. Three types of primary retinal detachment are recognized: (1) rhegmatogenous detachment, the most common, from retinal holes or breaks; (2) exudative detachment, usually from inflammation; and (3) traction detachment, which occurs when vitreous bands pull on the retina.

Minimal to moderate trauma to the eye may cause retinal detachment, but in such cases predisposing factors such as changes in the vitreous, retina, and choroid play an important role in pathogenesis. Severe trauma may cause retinal tears and detachment when there are no predisposing factors.

Clinical Findings

Child has complaint of painless decrease in vision and may give a history of flashes of lights or sparks. Loss of vision may be described as a curtain in front of the eye, or as cloudy or smoky. Central vision may not be affected if the macular area is not involved, which frequently causes a delay in seeking treatment. Children in whom the macula is detached present to the emergency department with sudden deterioration of vision. IOP is normal or low. The detached retina appears gray, with white folds and globular bullae (Figure 32–4).

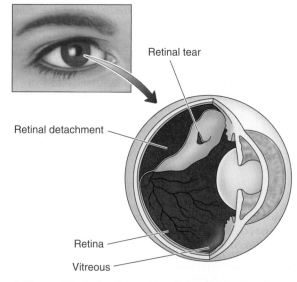

Retinal tear

Retinal detachment

Retina

Vitreous

▲ **Figure 32–4.** Fundoscopic examination findings in retinal detachment.

Round holes or horseshoe-shaped tears may be seen by indirect ophthalmoscopy in the rhegmatogenous detachment. Vitreous bands or other changes may be seen in the traction type of detachment.

Treatment & Disposition

Arrange for urgent or emergent referral to an ophthalmologist. If the macula is attached and central visual acuity is normal, urgent surgery, which is successful in approximately 80% of patients, may be indicated. If the macula is detached or threatened, surgical treatment should be scheduled on an urgent basis, as prolonged detachment of the macula results in permanent loss of central vision.

Bertino JS: Impact of antibiotic resistance in the management of ocular infections: The role of current and future antibiotics. *Clin Ophthalmol.* 2009;3:507-521 [PMID: 19789660].

Magauran B: Conditions requiring emergency ophthalmologic consultation. *Emerg Med Clin North Am.* 2008;26:233-238 [PMID: 18249265].

Prentiss KA, Dorfman DH: Pediatric ophthalmology in the emergency department. *Emerg Med Clin North Am.* 2008;26:181-198 [PMID: 18249262].

NONTRAUMATIC OCULAR EMERGENCIES

ACUTE DACRYOCYSTITIS

General Considerations

Acute infection of the lacrimal sac occurs in children as a complication of nasolacrimal duct obstruction. The most frequently encountered causative organism is *S. pneumoniae.*

Clinical Findings

The child has complaint of pain. There may be a history of tearing and discharge. Examination discloses swelling, redness, and tenderness over the lacrimal sac. Apply pressure over the lacrimal sac to collect pus for Gram-stained smear and culture.

Treatment

Begin systemic antibiotics with an oral cephalosporin or amoxicillin/clavulanate. Topical antibiotic drops may also be used, but not alone. Use warm compresses three to four times daily. Incision and drainage of a pointing abscess should be arranged by consultation with an ophthalmologist.

Disposition

Child can be discharged to home care with a prescription for systemic antibiotics and instructions to the parent how to apply warm local compresses. Consult an ophthalmologist for consideration of surgical correction. The child should be seen again, either by primary care physician or consulting ophthalmologist, within 1-3 days.

ACUTE DACRYOADENITIS

Clinical Findings

Infection and inflammation of the lacrimal gland is characterized by swelling, pain, tenderness, and redness over the upper temporal aspect of the upper eyelid.

Differential Diagnosis

Acute dacryoadenitis must be discriminated from viral infection (mumps), tumors, leukemia, and lymphoma.

Treatment

Purulent bacterial infections should be treated by incision and drainage of localized pus collections, antibiotics, warm compresses, and systemic analgesics. Viral dacryoadenitis (mumps) is treated conservatively.

Disposition

Child should be referred to an ophthalmologist for follow-up care in 2-3 days.

ACUTE HORDEOLUM (STYE)

General Considerations

Acute hordeolum is a common infection of the eyelid glands: the Meibomian glands (internal hordeolum) and the glands of Zeis or Moll (external hordeolum). The most frequent causative organism is *S. aureus.*

Clinical Findings

A stye is characterized by pain and redness with variable swelling over the eyelid. A large hordeolum may rarely be associated with swelling of the preauricular lymph node on the affected side, fever, and leukocytosis.

Treatment

If pus is localized and pointing out to the skin or conjunctiva, a horizontal incision may be made through the skin or a vertical incision through the conjunctiva.

Disposition

Child can be discharged home to continue treatment with warm compresses three times daily and topical antibiotic ointment (erythromycin 0.5% or gentamicin 0.3%) twice daily.

CHALAZION

General Considerations

Chalazion is a blocked Meibomian gland that forms a cyst.

Clinical Findings

In contrast to a stye, a chalazion has usually been present for quite some time and is painless. There are no associated systemic features. Vision is not compromised unless the cyst is very large. The conjunctiva should be clear.

Treatment

Routine, outpatient excision is curative. Injection with corticosteroids may be used for a small chalazion.

Disposition

Child can be sent for routine follow-up for the above treatment with an ophthalmologist.

EYELID INFECTIONS (PERIORBITAL CELLULITIS)

General Considerations

Periorbital cellulitis is an infectious process of the eyelid that may occur from local or hematogenous spread. Common causative organisms are *S. aureus*, streptococci, and *H. influenzae*, although the incidence of invasive *Haemophilus* disease has nearly disappeared with the widespread use of vaccination. Viral causes should be considered if associated with a skin rash (herpes zoster).

Clinical Findings

There is tenderness, erythema, and edema of the eyelid. No proptosis, pain with ocular movement, or restriction of extraocular motility is present. If any of these are present, consider orbital cellulitis.

Treatment

Give amoxicillin-clavulanate or cephalexin for 10 days. Topical eye drops or ointment may be prescribed in addition to oral antibiotics. Antivirals may be considered if herpes zoster is suspected. Incision and drainage may be indicated for patients with more severe infection.

Disposition

Child can be discharged home with daily follow-up. If the child fails antibiotics or has worsening symptoms, administer intravenous antibiotics and obtain consultation with ophthalmologist or otolaryngologist (ENT).

SPONTANEOUS SUBCONJUNCTIVAL HEMORRHAGE

General Considerations

Rupture of small subconjunctival vessel that occurs spontaneously or is preceded by a bout of crying, coughing, sneezing, or vomiting.

Clinical Findings

Bright red to dark maroon blood underneath the conjunctiva. It is painless with no visual loss.

Treatment & Disposition

The best treatment is observation, although many parents are concerned and require extensive reassurance before leaving the emergency department. Consider using artificial tear drops or ointment if needed for protruding chemotic tissue.

CONJUNCTIVITIS

General Considerations

Conjunctivitis is the most frequent cause of red eye. It should be dealt with as an urgent medical problem until it is certain that the process is under control (Table 32–2).

Causes of Acute Conjunctivitis

▶ Infection

Acute conjunctivitis may be caused by bacterial, viral, parasitic, fungal, or chlamydial infection.

▶ Chemical Irritation

Chemical irritations that cause acute conjunctivitis include chlorine gas and tear gas.

▶ Allergy

Allergic causes of acute conjunctivitis include vernal keratoconjunctivitis, hay fever, and other common allergens.

▶ Skin Disorders

Skin disorders such as Stevens-Johnson syndrome, acne rosacea, Lyell disease, Kawasaki disease, and psoriasis may cause acute conjunctivitis.

▶ Systemic Disorders

Sjögren syndrome and vitamin A deficiency may cause acute conjunctivitis.

Table 32–2. Differential diagnosis of conjunctivitis.

Clinical Features	Bacterial	Chlamydial	Viral	Allergic	Irritant
Onset	Acute	Acute or subacute.	Acute or subacute	Recurrent	Acute
Pain	Moderate	Mild to moderate	Mild to moderate	None	None to mild
Discharge	Copious, purulent	Moderate, purulent	Moderate, seropurulent	Moderate, clear	Minimal, clear
Gram-stained smear	PMNs, bacteria	PMNs, monocytes, no bacteria	PMNs, monocytes, no bacteria	Eosinophils present	Negative
Routine culture	Usually *Staphylococcus aureus*, pneumococci	Negative	Negative	Negative	Negative
Special culture	—	*Chlamydia*	Adenoviruses; occasionally enteroviruses; rarely others	Negative	Negative
Preauricular adenopathy	Common	Common	Common	No	Rare

PMNs, polymorphonuclear neutrophils.
Reproduced, with permission, from Stone CK, Humphries RL: *Current Diagnosis & Treatment Emergency Medicine*, 7th ed. New York: McGraw-Hill, 2011. Copyright © McGraw-Hill Education LLC.

Clinical Findings

Child has complaint of a "scratchy" sensation or pain, with conjunctival discharge. One or both eyes may be affected. Adherence of the eyelids upon awakening is common in bacterial conjunctivitis. Examination discloses conjunctival hyperemia, purulent or mucopurulent discharge, and variable degrees of eyelid swelling. In appropriate patients, material may be taken from the conjunctival sac for smear (Gram and Giemsa stains) and culture. Viral cultures may also be indicated.

Treatment

Prescribe erythromycin or gentamicin ophthalmic ointment for suspected bacterial conjunctivitis. It is difficult to get young children to cooperate for application of eye drops, so ointment is generally preferred. For suspected chlamydial infection (Ophthalmia neonatorum or history of urethritis), prescribe topical and systemic macrolides. Consider treatment for gonorrhea or gonococcal conjunctivitis as well.

Disposition

Discharge the child to home care with instructions to return for follow-up in 48-72 hours. Children who do not respond to treatment should be referred to an ophthalmologist.

BACTERIAL CORNEAL ULCER

General Considerations

Corneal infections may be due to bacteria, viruses, chlamydia, or fungi. The conjunctiva may or may not be involved. Bacterial corneal ulcers are serious, because rapid perforation of the cornea and loss of aqueous humor may occur; bacterial endophthalmitis may occur if bacterial ulcers are not treated properly.

Clinical Findings

Child has complaints of pain and photophobia, blurring of vision, and eye irritation. Examination discloses conjunctival hyperemia and chemosis, corneal ulceration, or whitish-yellowish infiltration. Examination is facilitated by fluorescein staining and inspection with ultraviolet light. Hypopyon may be present (see Figure 32–3). Scrapings from the cornea should be taken for culture and staining with Gram and Giemsa stains.

Treatment & Disposition

Management of bacterial corneal infections that cause corneal ulcers must be instituted as early as possible. Urgent consultation with an ophthalmologist should be obtained.

HYPHEMA

General Considerations

Hyphema (blood in the anterior chamber) is usually caused by nonperforating trauma to the eye. In rare instances, hyphema may occur spontaneously as a complication of an ocular or systemic disorder or coagulopathy.

Clinical Findings

Hyphema is characterized by sudden decrease in visual acuity (see Figure 32–3). If the IOP is elevated, there may be pain in the eye with or without headache. The anterior chamber may be completely filled with blood, or a blood level may be seen in a sitting or standing child. The conjunctiva may be hyperemic with perilimbal injection.

Treatment

Elevate the child's head to 30 degrees. Cover the affected eye with a shield. Consultation with an ophthalmologist is needed. Recently, intracameral injection (performed by an ophthalmologist) of 25 mcg of tissue plasminogen activator (t-PA) has been shown to expedite the resorption of blood clots in the anterior chamber. Aminocaproic acid can be used topically to stabilize the clot and decrease the rate of rebleeding.

Disposition

Acute care and evaluation by an ophthalmologist is essential. Operative evacuation of nonabsorbed blood clots may be required. Recurrence of bleeding on days 3-5 following injury is common. Children with hyphema should have daily follow-up as directed to the ophthalmologist.

Bremond-Gignanc D, Mariani-Kurkdijan P, Beresniak A, et al: Efficacy and safety of azithromycin 1.5% eye drops for purulent bacterial conjunctivitis in pediatric patients. *Pediatr Infect Dis J.* 2010;29:222-226 [PMID: 19935122].

Dargin JM, Lowenstein RA: The painful eye. *Emerg Med Clin North Am.* 2008;26:199-216 [PMID: 18249263].

eMedicine. *Ophthalmology.* Omaha, NE; 2010. Also available at http://emedicine.medscape.com/emergency_medicine#ophth. Accessed March 23, 2010.

German CA, Baumann MR, Hamzavi S: Ophthalmic diagnosis in the ED: Optic neuritis. *Am J Emerg Med.* 2007;25:834-837 [PMID: 17870491].

Gold RS: Treatment of bacterial conjunctivitis in children. *Pediatr Ann.* 2011;40:95-105 [PMID: 21323206].

Gupta N. Dhawan A, Beri S, et al: Clinical spectrum of pediatric blepharokera to conjunctivitis. *J AAPOS.* 2010;14:527-529 [PMID: 21093331].

Marco C, Marco J: Pediatric eye infections. *Pediatric Emergency Medicine Reports.* 2011;16:105-115.

Richards A, Guzman-Cottrill JA: Conjunctivitis. *Pediatr Rev.* 2010;31:196-208 [PMID: 20435711].

Rudloe TF, Harper MB, Prabu SP, et al: Acute periorbital infections: Who needs emergent imaging? *Pediatrics.* 2010;125:e719-726 [PMID: 20194288].

Sethurman U, Kamar D: The red eye: Evaluation and management. *Clin Pediatr.* 2009;48:588-600 [PMID: 19357422].

Soon VT: Pediatric subperiosteal orbital abscess secondary to acute sinusitis: A 5-year review. *Am J Otolaryngol.* 2011;32(1):62-68 [PMID: 20031268].

Upile NS, Munir N, Leong SC, et al: Who should manage acute periorbital cellulitis in children? *Int J Pediatr Otorhinolaryngol.* 2012;76:1073-1077 [PMID: 22572409].

OCULAR BURNS & TRAUMA

OCULAR BURNS

General Considerations

In conjunction with the history, diagnosis of burns is based on the presence of swollen eyelids with marked conjunctival hyperemia and chemosis. The limbus may show patchy balanced areas with conjunctival sloughing, especially in the interpalpebral area. There is usually corneal haze and diffuse edema, with wide areas of epithelial cell loss and corneal ulcerations. Corneal ulcerations can be better visualized with blue light following instillation of fluorescein.

ALKALI BURNS

Clinical Findings

Alkali burns (especially particulate alkali such as lime) are very serious, because even after apparent removal of the offending agent, tiny particles may remain lodged within the cul-de-sac and cause progressive damage to the eye.

Treatment

Instill a topical anesthetic *immediately* (proparacaine, 0.5%; or tetracaine, 0.5%), and then irrigate the eye copiously with 2-3 L isotonic saline solution, water, or lactated Ringer solution. An eyelid retractor may be useful.

Double eversion of the eyelids should be performed to look for and remove material lodged in the cul-de-sac. Solid particles of alkali should be removed with forceps or a moist cotton swab. After particles have been removed, irrigate again. *Do not attempt to neutralize the alkali with acid, because the exothermic reaction can cause further injury.*

After irrigation, the pH of the eye should be checked and the range should be 6.8-7.4. If the pH is still high, continue with irrigation. Parenteral narcotic analgesia is often required for pain relief. If the IOP is elevated, begin treatment with acetazolimide. Instill cycloplegic eye drops and antibiotic ointment.

Disposition

Obtain urgent consultation with ophthalmologist.

ACID BURNS

Clinical Findings

Acid burns can cause damage more rapidly but are generally less serious than alkali burns since acid burns do not cause progressive destruction of ocular tissues.

Treatment

Immediately after exposure, irrigate the eyes copiously with sterile isotonic saline solution, lactated Ringer solution, or tap water. Topical anesthetic (proparacaine, 0.5%) may be instilled to minimize pain during irrigation. Do not attempt to neutralize the acid with alkali.

Parenteral or oral narcotic analgesics may be necessary. Patch the eye if corneal defects are present.

Disposition

Obtain consultation with an ophthalmologist.

THERMAL BURNS

Clinical Findings

Injury due to thermal burns of the eyelids, cornea, and conjunctiva may range from minimal to extensive. Superficial corneal burns have a good prognosis, though corneal ulcers may occur as a result of loss of corneal epithelium.

Thermal burns of the skin of the eyelids may be partial-thickness or full-thickness. Conjunctival hyperemia is noted. The cornea may show diffuse necrosis of the exposed corneal epithelium in the interpalpebral area. Corneal haze due to corneal edema is frequently seen in thermal burns of the cornea and may lead to decrease in vision.

Treatment

Treatment of ocular burns is similar to the treatment of burns occurring elsewhere on the body (see Chapter 44). Provide systemic analgesia. Instill proparacaine, 0.5%, or tetracaine, 0.5% drops, to minimize pain during manipulation.

Disposition

Obtain consultation with an ophthalmologist.

MECHANICAL TRAUMA TO THE EYE

General Considerations

Ocular trauma is classified as penetrating or nonpenetrating. Trauma can lead to serious damage and loss of vision. Eye injuries are common in spite of the protection afforded by the bony orbit and the cushioning effect of orbital fat. Prevention as well as recreational and household safety measures should be stressed.

Evaluation

Obtain a history of the injury from the child, parent, or witness. If possible, measure and record visual acuity with and without correction. Inspect the eyelids, conjunctiva, cornea, anterior chamber, pupils, lens, vitreous, and fundus for breaks in tissue and hemorrhage. Search for corneal lesions (abrasion) by instilling fluorescein dye and examining the eye using a light with a light-blue filter (Wood lamp or slit lamp). X-ray, ultrasound, or CT scan may be indicated to rule out radiopaque foreign bodies, look for fractures of orbital bones, and delineate the internal globe structures.

Treatment & Disposition

Consult an ophthalmologist immediately for child with vision-threatening injuries. Avoid causing further damage by manipulation. For discussion of treatment and disposition, see the specific type of injury.

For severe pain, photophobia, or foreign body sensation, instill a topical anesthetic (proparacaine, 0.5%, or tetracaine, 0.5% drops, one or two drops once or twice). Systemic analgesics may be required. Cover the eye with an eye shield.

PENETRATING OR PERFORATING INJURIES

General Considerations

Penetrating or perforating ocular injuries require immediate careful attention and prompt surgical intervention to prevent possible loss of the eye and to attempt vision preservation.

Facial injuries, especially those occurring in motor vehicle collisions, may be associated with penetrating ocular trauma. Injuries may be concealed and not apparent due to eyelid swelling or because the child's other life-threatening injuries have (appropriately) taken precedence. Such injuries, if not promptly attended to, may result in partial or permanent loss of vision. Unfortunately, an unconscious or impaired child may have occult or untreated injuries as a conscious, cooperative child is needed for an appropriate eye examination.

Evaluation

Obtain and record a description of the mechanism of injury. Examine the eye and ocular adnexa, including vision testing if the child's condition permits. Do not apply pressure on the globe. In the appropriate setting, CT scan is indicated to rule out intraocular radiopaque foreign body and to look for fractures of orbital bones.

Clinical Findings

Penetrating injuries are those that cause disruption of the outer coats of the eye (sclera, cornea) without interrupting the anatomic continuity of that layer, thus preventing prolapse or loss of ocular contents. Perforating injuries are those resulting in complete anatomic disruption (laceration) of the sclera or cornea. Wounds may or may not be associated with prolapse of uveal structures. Wounds of the sclera or cornea may be associated with intraocular or intraorbital foreign bodies.

Treatment

Objectives of emergency management of ocular penetrating or perforating injuries are to relieve pain, preserve or restore vision, and achieve a good cosmetic result. Relieve pain with systemic analgesia, as needed. Sedatives may be required. Cover the eye with an eye shield. Patch the uninjured eye to minimize ocular movements. Do not manipulate the globe, instill eye drops, or apply topical antibiotic treatment.

Give tetanus prophylaxis, if needed. Prohibit oral intake until the child is examined by an ophthalmologist, since urgent surgery may be required. Provide hydration with intravenous fluids. Give parenteral antibiotics effective against Gram-negative and Gram-positive organisms. Give antiemetic agents to prevent further injury from IOP increase caused by vomiting.

Disposition

Child should be seen on an emergent basis by an ophthalmologist for management of severe injuries, investigation of intraocular foreign bodies, and immediate surgical repair as required. Prompt repair of uveal prolapse decreases the risk of sympathetic ophthalmia in the uninjured eye. Delay in management of corneal lacerations may increase the risk of surgical and postoperative complications.

BLUNT TRAUMA TO THE EYE, ADNEXA, & ORBIT

Contusions of the eyeball and ocular adnexa result from blunt trauma, most commonly in pediatric patients from sporting and recreational events. The outcome of blunt trauma injury cannot always be determined, and the extent of damage may not be obvious upon superficial examination. Careful eye examination is needed, as well as x-ray examination or CT scan when indicated.

Types of Injury

▶ Eyelids

Examine the eyelids for ecchymosis, swelling, laceration, and abrasions.

▶ Conjunctiva

Examine the conjunctiva for subconjunctival hemorrhages or laceration of the conjunctiva.

▶ Cornea

Examine the cornea for abrasion, edema, laceration, or rupture.

▶ Anterior Chamber

Examine the anterior chamber for hyphema, recession of angle, or secondary glaucoma.

▶ Iris

Examine the iris for iridodialysis (localized separation of the iris), iridoplegia, rupture of iris sphincter, iris prolapse through corneal or scleral lacerations, or iris atrophy.

▶ Ciliary Body

Examine the ciliary body for hyposecretion of aqueous humor or for ciliary body prolapse through scleral lacerations.

▶ Lens

Examine the lens for dislocation or cataract.

▶ Vitreous

Examine the vitreous for hemorrhage or prolapse.

▶ Ciliary Muscle

Examine the ciliary muscle for paralysis or spasm.

Treatment & Disposition

Injury severe enough to cause intraocular hemorrhage (vitreous hemorrhage or hyphema) places the child at risk of delayed secondary hemorrhage from a damaged uveal vessel, which may cause intractable glaucoma and permanent damage to the globe. Consultation with an ophthalmologist is necessary to rule out other eye injuries. Except for rupture of the globe, contusions do not require immediate definitive treatment. Apply an eye shield if the globe has been perforated, and consult an ophthalmologist.

ECCHYMOSIS OF THE EYELIDS (Black Eye)

Clinical Findings

Blood in the periorbital tissues may occur from direct trauma or a blow to adjacent areas. The loose subcutaneous tissue around the eye permits blood to spread extensively. The diagnosis is usually obvious. Always rule out trauma to the eye itself (hyphema, blowout fracture, or retinal detachment).

Treatment

Apply cold compresses to decrease swelling and help stop bleeding. Exclude more serious ocular injury by careful examination.

Disposition

If the eye is uninjured, no follow-up is necessary.

LACERATIONS OF THE EYELIDS

Clinical Findings

Lacerations or other wounds of the eyelids may be associated with serious ocular injuries not apparent at first examination. These include injury to the lacrimal system, levator muscle, or optic nerve. A meticulous search for such injuries is indicated in children with eyelid lacerations.

Treatment & Disposition

Children with lacerations of the eyelids require suturing and an extensive eye evaluation, including visual acuity, slit-lamp examination, IOP measurement, and facial nerve function. Superficial wounds that do not involve the eyelid margins may be repaired with single- or two-layer closures. Lacerations involving the tarsal plate, the upper eyelid levator mechanism, medial canthal area, and all through and through lacerations should be repaired by an ophthalmologist or oculoplastics specialist. If indicated, tetanus toxoid should be administered.

ORBITAL HEMORRHAGE

Clinical Findings

Exophthalmos and subconjunctival hemorrhage in a child with a history of blunt trauma to the face suggest rupture of orbital blood vessels. There may be conjunctival chemosis or ecchymosis of the eyelids.

Treatment & Disposition

Apply cold compresses, and obtain urgent consultation with an ophthalmologist.

CORNEAL ABRASIONS

Clinical Findings

Child may have complaints of pain, photophobia, and blurring of vision. There is usually a history of trivial trauma. Children with severe pain and blepharospasm may require topical anesthetic proparacaine, 0.5%, or tetracaine, 0.5% drops, instilled in the eye to facilitate eye examination. In severe cases, the eye is red and the corneal surface is irregular and loses its normal luster. Staining with fluorescein, sometimes even without blue light enhancement, reveals a defect in the corneal epithelium. Rule out infection or perforation of the globe.

Treatment

Irrigate the eye gently with sterile saline solution if needed to remove debris and loose foreign bodies. In patients with severe infection, instill tropicamide to relax the ciliary muscle and relieve pain. Instill ophthalmic antibiotic ointment. *Caution:* Do not use ointment containing corticosteroids. Consider nonsteroidal anti-inflammatory ophthalmic drops for pain control in the child who can tolerate drops at home. Provide systemic analgesia as needed. Never give the child topical anesthetics, which may lead to irreversible corneal damage.

Disposition

Refer the child for daily outpatient follow-up care. Consultation with an ophthalmologist should be obtained for corneal abrasions that fail to resolve in 48-72 hours.

CORNEAL & CONJUNCTIVAL FOREIGN BODIES

Clinical Findings

There may be a history of being in the presence of high-speed tempered steel tools (drilling), or there may be no history of trauma to the eye and the child may be unaware of a foreign body in the eye. In most patients, however, the child has complaint of a foreign body sensation in the eye or under the eyelid, or irritation only in the eye. Some corneal foreign bodies may be grossly visualized but can be seen with the aid of a loupe and well-focused diffuse light or slit lamp. Conjunctival foreign bodies often become embedded in the conjunctiva under the upper eyelid. The eyelid must be everted to facilitate inspection and removal.

Fluorescein should be instilled to visualize minute foreign bodies not readily visible with the naked eye, loupe, or slit lamp. Rule out intraocular foreign body with soft tissue x-ray or CT scan as indicated.

Treatment

Loose foreign bodies can often be removed with a moist cotton swab. Foreign bodies superficially embedded can be removed with the tip of a hypodermic needle or blunt spud. Anesthetize the cornea first with proparacaine or tetracaine solution, 0.5%. Instill ophthalmic antibiotic ointment after the foreign body has been successfully removed.

Disposition

The child should be seen again in 24 hours unless they have no symptoms or changes in vision. Referral to an ophthalmologist may be indicated for deep corneal foreign bodies or large foreign bodies within the visual axis.

TRAUMATIC LENS DISLOCATION & CATARACT FORMATION

Clinical Findings

Lens dislocation following blunt trauma to the eye may present with double vision in one eye (rarely both), blurred vision, and distortion. A tremor of the iris after rapid eye movements may also be present. The lens may be visualized by ophthalmoscopy or imaging with CT scan. History and physical examination are critical to diagnosis. Lens dislocation may be associated with medical disorders, such as Marfan syndrome, homocystinuria, or spherophakia. Lens dislocation becomes an emergency if the subluxed lens (anterior subluxation) obstructs aqueous flow leading to acute glaucoma. If the lens capsule is disrupted, the stroma of the lens may swell and become cloudy, also leading to acute glaucoma and development of cataracts. These may be present after lightning strike or electrical injury.

Treatment

Children with lens dislocation should be referred to an ophthalmologist for surgical repair, with emergent referral for increased IOP. There is no treatment for traumatic cataracts.

Disposition

Emergent referral to an ophthalmologist for dislocation associated with increased IOP; otherwise timely referral to ophthalmologist is sufficient.

EQUIPMENT & SUPPLIES

Basic Equipment

A number of specialized instruments have been devised for the investigation of eye disorders. Most emergency conditions can be diagnosed with the aid of a few relatively simple instruments. The following should be available in the emergency department:

- Handheld flashlight
- Slit lamp
- Ophthalmoscope (preferably with a blue filter lens)
- Visual acuity chart (Snellen and/or age-appropriate picture charts)
- Tonometer
- Pin hole and occluder
- Eye shield (plastic or metal) and tape

Basic Medications

Commonly used ophthalomic medications are listed in Table 32–3.

► Local Anesthetics

Proparacaine, 0.5%, or tetracaine, 0.5%, may be used. These medications have white caps on the bottles.

DYES

Fluorescein papers or drops should be available.

► Topical Antibacterial Agents

Antibacterial agents include a variety of antibiotics with different spectrums of coverage in liquid and ointment delivery vehicles (see Table 32–3).

COMMON TECHNIQUES FOR TREATMENT OF OCULAR DISORDERS

Eversion of the Upper Eyelid

The child is instructed to look down. Grasp the eyelashes at the outer margin of the eyelid with the thumb and forefinger of one hand, and gently and slowly draw the eyelid downward and outward. Using a cotton swab, press against the upper edge of the tarsus over the center of the eyelid while turning the eyelid margin rapidly outward and upward over the applicator. With the lashes thus held against the upper orbital rim, the exposed palpebral conjunctiva can be inspected closely. After the examination is completed and the foreign body removed (if possible), when the child looks up, the eyelid returns to its normal position (Figure 32–5).

► Eye Drops

Eye drops can be uncomfortable and are usually poorly tolerated by young children. As needed, they may be used in older children. The child should sit with both eyes open and looking up. Pull down slightly on the lower eyelid, and place two drops in the lower cul-de-sac. The child is then asked to look down while finger contact on the lower eyelid is maintained. Do not let the child squeeze the eye shut. Do not touch the eye or the eyelid with the applicator; likewise, do not instill eye drops with the dropper held far away from the eye.

For very young children, when drops are absolutely necessary, a different approach may be necessary; position the child supine, have an assistant hold child's head still, and place drops around the medial canthus. Even a child who refuses to open the eye will receive medication past the eyelids.

► Ointments

Ointments are instilled in the same manner as liquids. While the child is looking up, lift out the lower eyelid to trap the medication in the conjunctival sac. In the very young child who will not open the eyes, although not optimal, smearing the ointment on the eyelids and lashes may

Table 32–3. Commonly used ophthalmic medications.

Medication	Indication	Dosage, Forms, and Duration
Antimicrobials		
Bacitracin	Gram-positive organisms	Ophthalmic ointment: place ointment 4 times daily for 7-10 d
Bacitracin and polymyxin B (Polysporin)		
Chloramphenicol (Chloroptic)	Gram-positive and Gram-negative organisms	0.5% solution, 1% ointment: 1-2 drops or place ointment 3-6 times daily for 7-10 d
Ciprofloxacin (Ciloxan)	Gram-positive and Gram-negative organisms	0.3% solutions for conjunctivitis: 1-2 drops every 2 h for 2 d, then 1-2 drops every 4 h for 5 d
Norfloxacin (Chibroxin)		
Ofloxacin (Ocuflox)		For ulcer, 2 drops every 15 min for 6 h, then 2 drops every 30 min for the next 18 h; day 2, use 2 drops every h; days 3-14, use 2 drops every 4 h
Erythromycin (Ilotycin)	Gram-positive organisms, *Chlamydia*	0.5 % ointment 4 times a day for 5-7 d
Gentamicin (Genoptic, Garamycin)	Gram-positive and Gram-negative organisms; covers *Pseudomonas*	Gentamicin and tobramycin as 0.3% solution and 0.3% ointment
Tobramycin (Tobrex)		Neomycin, 1-2 drops every 2-4 h for 10 d; for ointment, use every 2-4 h for 7-10 d
Neomycin with bacitracin and polymyxin B (Neosporin)		
Polymyxin B and trimethoprim (Polytrim)	Gram-positive organisms	Ophthalmic solution: 1 drop every 3 h for 7-10 d
Sulfacetamide sodium (Bleph-10, Sulamyd)	Gram-positive and gram-negative organisms; does not cover *Pseudomonas*	10%, 15%, 30% solutions: 2 drops every 2-3 h for 7-10 d
		10% ointment; place ointment every 3-4 h for 7-10 d
Trifluridine (Viroptic)	Herpes	1% solution: 1 drop every 2 h while awake with maximum 9 drops/d; after reepithelialization, decrease to 1 drop every 4 h for 7 d
Mydriatics		
Atropine sulfate	Dilation, uveitis, cycloplegia	0.25-2% solution; lasts 2 wk
Cyclopentolate (Cyclogyl)	Dilation, cycloplegia	2-5% solution; lasts 48 h
Phenylephrine (Neosynephreine)[a]	Dilation, no cycloplegia	2.5-10% solution; lasts 2-3 h
Scopolamine (Hyoscine)	Dilation, cycloplegia	0.25% solution; lasts 7 d
Anesthetics[b]		
Proparacaine (Ophthetic Alcaine)	Local anesthesia	0.5% solution
Tetracaine (Pontocaine)	Local anesthesia	0.5% solution

[a]Cardiac patients should not use phenylephrine.
[b]Anesthetics should not be prescribed for unsupervised use.
Reproduced, with permission, from Stone CK, Humphries RL: *Current Diagnosis & Treatment Emergency Medicine*, 7th ed. New York: McGraw-Hill, 2011. Copyright © McGraw-Hill Education LLC.

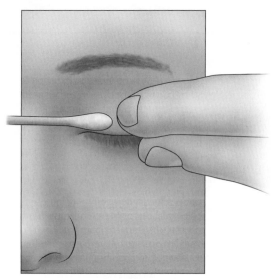

Twist cotton-tipped
swab upward

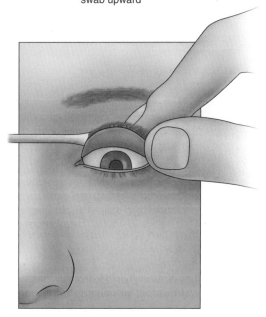

Look downward

▲ **Figure 32–5.** Technique of upper eyelid eversion.

provide some direct and indirect delivery of the medication into the conjunctiva.

▶ Warm Compresses

Use a clean towel or washcloth soaked in warm tap water well below the temperature that will burn the thin skin covering the eyelids. Warm compresses are usually applied to the area for 15 minutes, four times daily. The therapeutic rational is to increase blood flow to the affected area and decrease pain and inflammation.

Removal of Superficial Corneal Foreign Body

Main considerations are good illumination, magnification, anesthesia, proper positioning of the child, and sterile technique. The child's visual acuity should be recorded first. The child may be sitting or supine. A loupe should be used unless a slit lamp is available. Utilize a topical anesthetic, either proparacaine, 0.5%, or tetracaine, 0.5% drops. An assistant should direct a strong flashlight into the eye at an oblique angle. The examiner may then see the corneal foreign body and remove it with a moist cotton swab. If this attempt fails, the foreign body may be removed with a metal spud while the eyelids are held apart with the other hand to prevent blinking. Antibacterial ointment may be instilled after the foreign body has been removed.

Tonometry

Tonometry is the determination of IOP using a special instrument that measures the amount of corneal indentation produced by a given weight. Tonometry readings should be taken on a child with suspicion of increased IOP.

▶ Precautions

Tonometry should be done with great caution on children with corneal ulcers. It is extremely important to clean the tonometer before each use by carefully wiping the footplate with a cotton swab moistened with sterile solution (determine it is dry before using) and to sterilize the instrument. Corneal abrasions are rarely caused by tonometry. Epidemic keratoconjunctivitis can be spread by tonometry, and can be prevented if the tonometer is cleaned before each use and hand washing between patients is meticulously observed. Disposable covers are available for some tonometers.

▶ Technique

Anesthetic solution (tetracaine, 0.5%; or proparacaine, 0.5%) is instilled into each eye. The child lies supine and is asked to stare at a spot on the ceiling with both eyes or at a finger held directly in the line of gaze overhead. The eyelids are held open without applying pressure on the globe. The tonometer is then placed on the corneal surface of each eye and the scale reading taken from the tonometer. The IOP is determined by referring to a chart that converts the scale reading to millimeters of mercury for a Schiotz tonometer or by digital readout on the electronic device. Normal IOP is 12-20 mm Hg.

Interpretation of Abnormalities

If the IOP is 20 mm Hg or more, further investigation is indicated to determine if glaucoma is present.

Corneal Staining

Corneal staining consists of instillation of fluorescein into the conjunctival sac to outline irregularities of the corneal surface. Staining is indicated in corneal trauma or other corneal disorders (herpes simplex keratitis) when examination with a loupe or slit lamp in the absence of a stain has not been satisfactory.

Precautions

Because the corneal epithelium—the chief barrier to corneal infection—is usually interrupted when corneal staining is indicated, ensure that the dye used (particularly fluorescein) is sterile.

Equipment & Materials

Note: Fluorescein should be sterile. Fluorescein papers or sterile individual dropper units are safest. Fluorescein solution from a dropper bottle may be used, but there is substantial risk of contamination.

Technique

Individually wrapped fluorescein paper is wetted with sterile saline, a topical anesthetic, or touched to the wet conjunctiva so that a thin film of fluorescein spreads over the corneal surface. Any irregularity in the cornea is stained by the fluorescein and is thus more easily visualized using a light with a blue filter.

Normal & Abnormal Findings

If there is no superficial corneal irregularity, a uniform film of dye covers the cornea. If the corneal surface has been altered, the affected area absorbs more of the dye and will stain a deeper green.

Allman KJ, Smiddy WE, Banta J, et al: Ocular trauma and visual outcome secondary to paintball projectiles. *Am J Ophthalmol.* 2009;147: 239-242 [PMID:18835471].

Bord SP, Linden J: Trauma to the globe and orbit. *Emerg Med Clin North Am.* 2008:26:97-123 [PMID: 18249259].

Burger BM, Kelty PJ, Bowie EM: Ocular nail gun injuries: Epidemiology and visual outcomes. *J Trauma.* 2009;67: 1320-1322 [PMID: 20009684].

Moren Cross J, Griffin R, Owsley C, et al: Pediatric eye injuries related to consumer products in the United States, 1997-2006, *J AAPOS.* 2008;12:626-628 [PMID: 18848479].

Podbielski DW, Surkont M, Tehrani NN, et al: Pediatric eye injuries in a Canadian emergency department. *Can J Ophthalmol.* 2009;44:519-522 [PMID: 19789585].

Pokhrel PK, Loftus SA: Ocular emergencies. *Am Fam Physician.* 2007;76:829-836 [PMID: 17910297].

Pollard KA, Xiang H, Smith GA: Pediatric eye injuries treated in US emergency departments, 1990-2009. *Clin Pediatr.* 2012;51:374-381 [PMID: 22199176].

Soparkar CN, Patrinely JR: The eye examination in facial trauma for the plastic surgeon. *Plast Reconstr Surg.* 2007;120:49S-56S [PMID: 18090728].

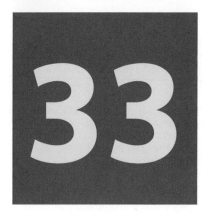

ENT & Oral Emergencies

Jason N. Collins, MD, FACEP

Sandy Y. Lee, BS

IMMEDIATE MANAGEMENT OF LIFE-THREATENING DISORDERS

OBSTRUCTION

Acute obstruction within the nasal and oropharyngeal region is a seconds-to-minutes emergency. Rapid assessment is imperative to evaluate the degree and level of obstruction, and plans for intervention must be determined concomitantly. Severe obstruction can be caused by foreign objects, swelling secondary to trauma or infection, masses, and burns. History and examination are usually revealing; a high degree of suspicion should be maintained for foreign body in the context of severe, abrupt symptoms in the absence of other historical clues.

CLINICAL FINDINGS

History

Acute onset of signs and symptoms of respiratory distress is common; the insidious change of a subacute process can create equally serious management problems, although clues from the historical progression can guide evaluation and management. Maintain a high degree of suspicion for foreign body presence and do not discount the parents' concern of foreign body, as this may be an important diagnostic key. Determine the chronology of symptom onset and suspected site (right nare, mouth, in the throat). Did the child admit to inserting or ingesting a foreign object? Was a specific event witnessed? Is the child making an effort to clear an obstruction (coughing or retching)? Is the child having noisy respiration with cry or exertion, and/or at rest? Has there been any color change, apnea, or inability to talk or cry? Have treatments or interventions been attempted prior to arrival that may have improved or possibly worsened the condition? Determine an accurate immunization history, if

there has been an antecedent illness or fever, and whether this illness has been slowly progressive or of abrupt onset with rapid change.

Recent history of a traumatic injury, burn, or caustic ingestion can refine the differential diagnosis. Situations may present with similar symptoms of respiratory distress and airway compromise. Management of maxillofacial and neck traumatic injuries is discussed in Chapter 24. See Chapter 9 for a discussion of airway emergencies.

Physical Examination

Is the child in distress currently? Do not delay airway protection and supportive interventions for the sake of a detailed history and examination. If possible, have the patient report the history or describe symptoms. This provides the physician with opportunity to evaluate quality and limitation of phonation.

Does the child appear toxic? Depressed mental status, cyanosis, and poor respiratory effort are ominous signs. Recognize tachypnea, increased work of breathing, stridor, and other upper airway noises, and the position the child spontaneously assumes. Specific history of trauma may not be available; evaluate for burns, lacerations, punctures, or swelling that might indicate an unwitnessed injury. Examine the external head and neck structures for swelling, erythema, limitation in range of motion, and frank meningismus. If the condition permits, visually inspect the nares and oropharynx and note tolerance of secretions, signs of unilateral versus diffuse edema, erythema, purulent discharge, or apparent foreign body.

Nasal foreign bodies are generally unilateral and visible on direct inspection. In the appropriate setting, a high suspicion for foreign body must be maintained even if a structure is not easily seen. Partial or complete nasal obstruction may be present; airway compromise may develop if an object becomes dislodged or a secondary process develops such as traumatic bleeding or edema. Laryngotracheal foreign bodies may be visible on examination but the primary signs will likely be distress, choking, gagging, coughing, increased work of breathing, stridor, and pain.

Respiratory compromise secondary to airway obstruction may often be diagnosed clinically and airway stabilization should not be deferred for laboratory or imaging results. The following diagnostic studies are useful adjuncts to guide management.

Laboratory Analysis

Blood analysis is generally not required; however, if vascular access is indicated, consider sending basic laboratory tests for evaluation. Blood gas analysis and other routine blood tests can be used to assess initial condition and response to treatment.

Diagnostic Imaging

Radio-opaque objects may be noted, but normal x-rays do not rule out the presence of foreign bodies. Soft tissue neck x-rays can demonstrate foreign bodies, masses, retropharyngeal swelling, soft tissue gas, and enlarged epiglottis (thumbprint sign), or airway narrowing (steeple sign). Chest x-ray may demonstrate postobstructive airway collapse, air trapping with hyperinflation, or developing pneumonia. Radiographic imaging may be acquired rapidly if stability of the patient permits. Consider portable x-ray to minimize disturbance of the child and avoid transport away from the emergency department.

Computed tomography (CT) scanning can provide a definitive diagnosis, the specific location of the obstruction, and may obviate the need for bronchoscopy. Unstable patients are not candidates for transport to the CT scanner. The physician must weigh the benefit of this modality versus the need to leave the controlled setting of the emergency department and concerns of ionizing radiation exposure.

Direct visualization, via upper endoscopy or bronchoscopy, is the best method to evaluate the airway and identify type of obstruction. It allows simultaneous diagnostic examination and intervention, such as retrieval of an object. Endoscopy or bronchoscopy should be performed only by an experienced operator and is usually carried out in the operating room under general anesthesia.

Pediatric airway ultrasound is noninvasive and imparts no ionizing radiation risks; however, reliability of this mode can be limited by patient cooperation and operator experience. This modality has been used successfully in adults to evaluate presence of epiglottitis. Pediatric normal anatomy can reliably be identified with ultrasound, but its routine use to determine diagnoses is not widely performed.

TREATMENT

Evaluation of the airway, breathing, and circulation (ABC) and initiation of life support protocols may be indicated.

Regardless of the cause, assessment of degree of respiratory distress determines management. Rapidly assess the condition to determine if immediate airway control is warranted and intubate if immediate decompensation is likely (see Chapter 9). Early consultation with an otolaryngologist (ENT), anesthesiologist, or intensivist is appropriate for patients who have high potential for decompensation but don't require immediate intubation.

Diagnosis-directed management should be started if historical clues, objective examination findings, and diagnostic test results are available to specify the cause. Utilize supportive treatments (albuterol, racemic epinephrine, steroids, antibiotics) as indicated.

Foreign bodies in the mouth, larynx, and tracheobronchial tree present the most concern for airway obstruction. Use back blows or the Heimlich maneuver if the obstruction is complete. Visible foreign bodies can be removed by direct grasp, but do not blindly sweep the oral cavity to avoid pushing the object farther posterior. Pharyngeal and laryngeal foreign bodies may be grasped and removed with MaGill forceps while attempting direct laryngoscopic intubation. Objects distal to the larynx generally require removal via bronchoscopy.

Heroic maneuvers may be necessary for complete obstruction caused by difficulty to remove objects and objects located distally. Needle or surgical cricothyroidotomy (above age 12) is used for objects above the larynx. For distal objects, intubate the trachea and gently push the object into the right mainstem bronchus. Subsequently, the endotracheal tube (ETT) can be withdrawn to ventilate the left lung.

DISPOSITION

Patients presenting with severe respiratory distress, even if intubation is avoided, may be candidates for intensive care unit (ICU) admission. Clinical judgment and consultation with a pediatric intensive care physician is critical to determine proper disposition location.

Anticipated difficult foreign body removal, failed attempts at removal, and the presence of high-risk foreign body (button batteries, magnet) necessitate urgent consultation with an otolaryngologist (ENT) for possible bronchoscopy.

Boudewyns A, Claes J, Van de Heyning P: Clinical practice: An approach to stridor in infants and children. *Eur J Pediatr.* 2010; 169:135-141 [PMID: 19763619].

D'Agostino J: Pediatric airway nightmares. *Emerg Med Clin N Am.* 2010;28(1):119-126 [PMID: 19945602].

Nentwich L, Ulrich AS: High risk chief complaints II: Disorders of the head and neck. *Emerg Med Clin North Am.* 2009;27(4): 713-746 [PMID: 19932402].

Oncel M, Sunam GS, Ceran S: Tracheobronchial aspiration of foreign bodies and rigid bronchoscopy in children. *Pediatr Int.* 2012;54(4):532-535 [PMID: 22414345].

Santillanes G, Gausche-Hill M: Pediatric airway management. *Emerg Med Clin N Am.* 2008;26(4):961-975 [PMID: 19059095].

Sodhi KS, Aiyappan SK, Saxena AK, et al: Utility of multidetector CT and virtual bronchoscopy in tracheobronchial obstruction in children. *Acta Paediatr.* 2010;99(7):1011-1015 [PMID: 20178519].

Veras TN, Hornburg G, Schner AM, et al: Use of virtual bronchoscopy in children with suspected foreign body aspiration. *J Bras Pneumol.* 2009;35(9):937-941 [PMID: 19820821].

MANAGEMENT OF SPECIFIC DISORDERS

DISORDERS OF THE EAR

External Ear Infections

▶ **Clinical Findings**

External infections can involve structures from the skin (cellulitis) to the level adjacent to (perichondritis) and involving (chondritis) the auricular cartilage. Surface features reveal warm, red, inflamed skin that is painful. Infection is commonly a result of direct local trauma such as ear piercing. Infection may extend to the ear from a distinct site of infection on the head or neck, or may be a direct extension from acute otitis externa.

▶ **Treatment**

Recommend local wound care at the site of any skin injury. Foreign bodies, including jewelry, should be removed. Systemic antibiotics are required and significant infections necessitate intravenous (IV) therapy. Common responsible organisms include *Streptococcal, Staphylococcal,* and *Pseudomonas* species. Antibiotic coverage should be directed at these bacteria. Incision and drainage may also be necessary; small abscesses are amenable to bedside drainage by the experienced emergency department physician. Deeper infections involving cartilage warrant otolaryngologist (ENT) or plastic surgery consultation for surgical drainage.

▶ **Disposition**

Mild infections can be appropriately managed with oral antibiotics and close follow-up. Moderate or severe skin infections, those with concomitant abscess formation, and infections involving the cartilage require admission for IV antibiotics and specialist consultation.

Acute Otitis Externa

Commonly known as swimmer's ear, acute otitis externa (AOE) is an inflammatory condition of the external auditory canal, typically secondary to a bacterial infection.

▶ **Clinical Findings**

Patients commonly report unilateral symptoms including pain or itching, swelling, drainage from the ear canal, and changes in hearing. Recent swimming may be the most likely risk factor in a patient, but ear canal moisture from any cause may promote microbe growth and subsequent infection.

External findings include erythema of the auricular and facial skin, canal drainage, and pain with palpation and movement of the external ear structures. Inspection of the canal with otoscope will likely cause pain. Edema and discharge are commonly present. Direct visualization of the tympanic membrane (TM) is important to confirm that it is intact and to discriminate otitis externa from otitis media, TM rupture, and conditions that may present with similar symptoms. Discharge from the ear canal may limit visualization. TM erythema is common. TM perforation is unlikely to be secondary to AOE, and other diagnoses must be considered. Although the condition is rare in children, pain out of proportion to clinical findings, or granulation tissue in the canal suggests more serious malignant otitis externa. Infection extends into deeper tissue and surrounding bone and may be associated with fever, vertigo, facial nerve palsy, and meningeal signs.

▶ **Treatment**

Guidelines recommend clearing of debris from the external canal is the first step in treatment. This can be accomplished through manual removal using an ear loop or swab; gentle irrigation is effective if an intact TM has been confirmed.

Topical otic formulations are the mainstay of treatment, preferentially treating the most common organisms: *Pseudomonas aeruginosa, Staphylococcus aureus,* and *Staphylococcus epidermidis.* Instillation of the medicated drops into a cleared canal is ideal to achieve optimal medication concentration throughout the canal. Recommended medications include antibiotics (ciprofloxacin, ofloxacin), acidifying solutions (acetic acid), steroids (hydrocortisone), or a combination of these. Preparations containing a steroid plus acetic acid may be used in mild cases; treatment combinations containing an antibiotic are warranted in moderate or severe conditions. Continue treatment for approximately 1 week.

Pain control is an important component of treating the infection. Oral antibiotics are indicated for treatment failures or if there are signs of complications or systemic illness on initial examination.

▶ **Disposition**

Otitis externa is unlikely to require adjunctive testing, ENT consultation from the emergency department, or hospital admission. However, if there are signs of severe disease or complications, consultation with an otolaryngologist is appropriate. Primary care physician follow-up for more severe cases should be recommended to verify resolution of symptoms; improvement should be noted within 2-3 days of starting treatment, otherwise treatment modification should be considered. Referral to otolaryngologist is appropriate in cases of unclear diagnosis, suspected TM perforation, and other treatment complications.

Bhattacharyya N, Kepnes LJ: Initial impact of the acute otitis externa clinical practice guideline on clinical care. *Otolaryngol Head Neck Surg.* 2011;145(3):414-417 [PMID: 21531870].

Burton MJ, Singer M, Rosenfeld RM: Extracts from The Cochrane Library: Interventions for acute otitis externa. *Otolaryngol Head Neck Surg.* 2010;143:8-11 [PMID: 20620612].

Kaushik V, Malik T, Saeed SR: Interventions for acute otitis externa. *Cochrane Database Syst Rev.* 2010;(1):CD004740 [PMID: 20091565].

Phillips JS, Jones SE: Hyperbaric oxygen as an adjuvant treatment for malignant otitis externa. *Cochrane Database Syst Rev.* 2013;5:CD004617 [PMID: 23728650].

Rosenfeld RM, Brown L, Cannon CR, et al: Clinical practice guideline: Acute otitis externa. *Otolaryngol Head Neck Surg.* 2006;134(suppl 4):S4-S23 [PMID: 16638473].

Wall GM, Stroman DW, Roland PS: Ciprofloxacin 0.3%/ dexamethasone 0.1% sterile otic suspension for the topical treatment of ear infections: A review of the literature. *Pediatr Infect Dis J.* 2009;28(2):141-144 [PMID: 19116600].

Acute Otitis Media

Acute otitis media (AOM) is defined by the presence of infection and inflammation of the middle ear, typically associated with rapid onset of symptoms, significant otalgia, and fever. Most common bacteria include *Streptococcus pneumoniae*, nontypeable *Haemophilus influenzae*, *Moraxella catarrhalis*, and group A *Streptococcus*. Due to the seven-valent pneumococcal conjugate vaccine (PCV7), there has been a decline in the vaccine-covered *S. pneumoniae* causing otitis media. Viruses cause approximately 20% of AOM and include respiratory syncytial virus, parainfluenza, rhinovirus, influenza virus, enterovirus, and adenovirus.

AOM is one of the most common reasons for a visit to the primary care physician and one of the most common diagnoses for which antibiotic treatment is prescribed. The illness may be present, though self-limiting and require only supportive care. Over the past several years, there has been controversy over the observation method (48-72 hours of no antibiotic treatment) versus immediate prescriptions for diagnosed AOM. Concerns center around increased antibacterial resistance secondary to inappropriate antibiotic use. The theory responsible for a physician's prescribing antibiotics is to prevent adverse events such as mastoiditis or deafness. Physicians must also consider the adverse and delayed effects of antibiotics. Based upon patient's age, rate of onset, chronology of symptoms, and physical examination, the emergency physician may decide to observe and provide pain relief for AOM before prescribing antibiotics.

Clinical Findings

Conventional, generally accepted criteria indicative of AOM include acute onset of symptoms, middle ear effusion (MEE), and middle-ear inflammation. Patients under 2 years may present with nonspecific signs and symptoms such as ear tugging, irritability, otorrhea, fever, cough, rhinorrhea, decreased appetite, and sleep disturbances. Older children may report ear pain; the presence of other clinical findings is variable and can include those listed above. To confirm the presence of MEE, a bulging TM should be seen. Other indicators of MEE include a pneumatic otoscopy examination revealing an immobile TM, cloudiness, edema, air behind the TM, and otorrhea. Middle-ear inflammation often leads to otalgia on examination and an erythematous TM. In a distraught patient, wait a few minutes before attempting otoscopic examination of the TM, as crying may increase blood flow and demonstrate erythema that is not due to inflammation. Distinguish between AOM and otitis media with effusion, as the latter is often due to viruses that do not require antibiotics.

Treatment

Treatment guidelines are based on age of the patient and clinical findings. The general management recommendations of the American Academy of Pediatrics include empiric treatment with antibiotics in patients aged 6 months-12 years who have AOM with otorrhea or unilateral or bilateral AOM with severe symptoms. Severe condition is indicated by uncertain plan for follow-up, presence of otalgia present for longer than 48 hours, temperature greater than 39°C (102.2 F), or toxic appearance. Children aged 6 months-2 years with bilateral AOM without otorrhea should receive empiric antibiotics; children older than 2 years may be treated empirically or treated supportively and observed. Patients aged 6 months-12 years diagnosed with unilateral AOM without otorrhea can be managed with a trial of observation or empiric antibiotic therapy.

Pain management is the initial consideration in the first 24 hours of presenting symptoms regardless of antibiotic use. Acetaminophen and ibuprofen should be the first-line treatments for children (aged > 6 months). Adjunctive treatment with topical medications like lidocaine or benzocaine drops may be used for temporary relief. Severe pain may warrant narcotics; use these agents with caution as they may cause respiratory depression and other adverse effects.

Amoxicillin is the recommended first-line antimicrobial. Dosage is 80-90 mg/kg/d divided twice daily. First-line alternatives include cefdinir 14 mg/kg/d, cefpodoxime 10 mg/kg/d, or cefuroxime 15 mg/kg twice daily. Those with a true allergic reaction to amoxicillin can be given 10 mg/kg/d of azithromycin on the first day and 5 mg/kg/d for the next 4 days, 50 mg/kg/d of erythromycin, or 6-10 mg/kg/d of TMP/SMX. For severe illness and wider coverage, treatment failure, or recurrence within 30 days of initial treatment with amoxicillin, give high-dose amoxicillin-clavulanate (90 mg/kg/d amoxicillin and 6.4 mg/kg/d of clavulanate) in two doses. Patients who cannot tolerate anything by mouth can be administered a single dose of 50-mg/kg IV ceftriaxone. Medications are usually given for 10 days in patients younger than 2 years; a 5- to 7-day course in older children. If patients fail initial antibiotic therapy, a 3-day course of IM ceftriaxone (50 mg/kg/d for 3 days) can be given. Failed treatment after broad-coverage antibiotics warrants consideration for tympanocentesis that can provide identification of the organism after Gram stain and culture. A workup to exclude other causes is necessary.

▶ Disposition

Initial outpatient treatment is generally appropriate for AOM. Failure to show improvement within 48-72 hours of an observation period or to initial antibiotic treatment warrants initiation of empiric antibiotics or an antibiotic change, respectively. A specific plan and mechanism to ensure follow-up is necessary, especially for additional observation. Consider the need for more extensive evaluation in the emergency department for the systemically ill or toxic-appearing child, even in the presence of diagnosis of AOM. Serious sequelae, such as mastoiditis or meningitis, can develop and must be worked up accordingly.

Fischer T, Singer AJ, Chale S: Observation option for acute otitis media in the emergency department. *Pediatr Emerg Care.* 2009;25(9):575-578 [PMID: 19755891].

Leibovitz E, Broides A, Greenberg D, et al: Current management of pediatric acute otitis media. *Expert Rev Anti Infec Ther.* 2010;8(2):151-161 [PMID: 20109045].

Lieberthal AS, Carroll AE, Chonmaitree T, et al: The diagnosis and management of acute otitis media. *Pediatrics.* 2013;131(3):e964-e999 [PMID: 23439909].

Stevanovic T, Komazec Z, Lemajic-Komazec S, et al: Acute otitis media: To follow-up or treat? *Int J Pediatr Otorhinolaryngol.* 2010;74(8):930-933 [PMID: 20599127].

Thornton K, Parrish F, Swords C: Topical vs. systemic treatments for acute otitis media. *Pediatr Nurs.* 2011;37(5):263-267 [PMID: 22132572].

Varrasso DA: Acute otitis media: Antimicrobial treatment or the observation option? *Curr Infect Dis Rep.* 2009;11(3):190-197 [PMID: 19366561].

Vouloumanou EK, Karageorgopoulos DE, Kazantzi MS, et al: Antibiotic versus placebo or watchful waiting for acute otitis media: A meta-analysis of randomized controlled trials. *J Antimicrob Chemother.* 2009;64(1):16-24 [PMID: 19454521].

Mastoiditis

Mastoiditis is a complication of and exists to some degree in most cases of AOM due to the anatomic relation of the compartments involved. Similar to AOM, the course may be silent and self-limiting. Serious illness can develop if the suppurative process does not resolve spontaneously or is inadequately treated (inappropriate duration or failure of treatment of antibiotics for AOM). Stage of the illness at time of presentation guides treatment. The clinical picture may range from relative mild and uncomplicated (acute coalescent) to serious illness with intracranial (meningitis, dural sinus thrombophlebitis) or extracranial disease (subperiosteal abscess, facial nerve palsy). Masked, or subacute, mastoiditis is an insidious complication and can progress to a state of severe illness with intracranial involvement despite apparent resolution of AOM. Maintain a high degree of suspicion in patients with prolonged illness.

▶ Clinical Findings

Historical clinical features that suggest mastoiditis include fever, ear pain, and recent diagnosis of AOM. Additionally, lethargy, irritability, and poor feeding may be indicators in younger children. Prolonged duration of illness relative to the expected course AOM suggests acute mastoiditis.

Ear pain, TM findings consistent with AOM, and swelling/sagging of the auditory canal may be noted. Classic features include displacement of the auricle, posterior-auricular erythema, swelling, fluctuance, and tenderness; however, these findings are not present in all patients. High fever, focal neurological findings, meningismus, lethargy, and mental status changes indicate a complicated course and suggest intracranial involvement.

As the patient may present for evaluation at any point within the spectrum of this disease, clinical judgment should guide the workup. Diagnosis can be made on clinical features alone and additional testing is not required. Laboratory tests may show leukocytosis or elevated inflammatory markers, although results are nonspecific. A clinical scenario suggestive of meningitis must be evaluated and treated accordingly as discussed in Chapter 41. A CT of the head and lumbar puncture may be appropriate in these cases. If imaging is required for confirmation of diagnosis or to rule out complications, a contrast-enhanced cranial or temporal bone CT is the test of choice.

▶ Treatment

Parenteral antibiotics are indicated in all cases and may be sufficient as a solo therapy. Common bacteria include *S. pneumoniae, Streptococcus pyogenes, S. aureus, P. aeruginosa,* and *H. influenzae*—broad-spectrum antibiotics are appropriate initially. Tympanocentesis or surgical management of abscess or other extracranial complications may be necessary and should be performed by an otolaryngologist.

▶ Disposition

Hospital admission for IV antibiotics is indicated. Consultation with an otolaryngologist should be made from the emergency department, especially if there is a known complicating condition. Consultation with a neurosurgeon and intervention may be required for intracranial complications.

Abdel-Aziz M, El-Hoshy H: Acute mastoiditis: A one year study in the pediatric hospital of Cairo university. *BMC Ear Nose Throat Disord.* 2010;10:1 [PMID: 20205885].

Holt GR, Gates GA: Masked mastoiditis. *Laryngoscope.* 1983;93(8): 1034-1037 [PMID: 6877011].

Lin HW, Shargorodsky J, Gopen Q: Clinical strategies for the management of acute mastoiditis in the pediatric population. *Clin Pediatr (Phila).* 2010;49(2):110-115 [PMID: 19734439].

Pang LH, Barakate MS, Havas TE: Mastoiditis in a paediatric population: A review of 11 years experience in management. *Int J Pediatr Otorhinolaryngol.* 2009;73(11):1520-1524 [PMID: 19758711].

van den Aardweg MT, Rovers MM, de Ru JA: A systematic review of diagnostic criteria for acute mastoiditis in children. *Otol Neurotol.* 2008;29(6):751-757 [PMID: 18617870].

Cerumen Impaction

▶ Clinical Findings

Cerumen (earwax) is composed of normal secretions and debris in the external auditory canal, and accumulation can lead to impaction. The presence of an impaction may cause symptoms directly or be an incidental finding noted upon inspection of the external auditory canal and tympanic membrane. The patient may report pain or fullness in the ear, dizziness, or hearing loss; symptoms may be subtle and nonspecific in infants and toddlers.

Home treatments for removal of earwax including cotton swabs, irrigation kits, and "ear candling" may have been attempted prior to presentation to the emergency department and can result in adverse effects such as TM perforation, burns, allergic reactions, direct trauma, and acute hearing loss. These home treatments are not well studied and their use is discouraged. The disease process as well as complications of home treatment should be identified and treated appropriately.

▶ Treatment

Removal of cerumen impaction in the emergency department should be considered in cases where the patient is experiencing significant symptoms or when visualization of the TM is needed to aid in diagnosis of another condition. Common and accepted methods of wax removal include manual removal, irrigation, and cerumenolytics.

Chemicals such as acetic acid, hydrogen peroxide, or mineral oil may be prescribed for home use with planned outpatient follow-up. Brief applications of a cerumenolytic for a short duration of treatment may soften wax and aid in removal. No agent is clearly superior. Agents can be combined with other therapies while the patient is in the emergency department.

Irrigation may be performed by the physician or nursing staff and is generally efficient and effective. Warm tap water or saline may be used. Do not attempt irrigation in patients with known TM perforation or prior ear surgery.

Manual removal should be performed by the physician and not delegated to untrained individuals. Curettes, spoons, forceps, and suction devices may be utilized to retrieve wax under direct visualization through an otoscope.

The canal and TM should be reexamined after the procedure to evaluate for signs of disease that correlate with the presenting complaint and identify any possible complications of the procedure.

▶ Disposition

Discharge home is appropriate. Recommend follow-up with primary care physician to confirm resolution, continue treatment, and to discuss options for prevention. Referral to an otolaryngologist is appropriate for patients with persistent symptoms after removal of wax, chronic impactions, or existence of contraindications that preclude wax removal.

Browning GG: Ear wax. *Clin Evid (Online).* 2008;1:504 [PMID: 19450340].

Mitka M: Cerumen removal guidelines wax practical. *JAMA.* 2008;300(13):1506 [PMID: 18827201].

Roland PS, Smith TL, Schwartz SR, et al: Clinical practice guideline: Cerumen impaction. *Otolaryngol Head Neck Surg.* 2008;139(3 suppl 2):S1-S21 [PMID: 18707628].

Ear Canal Foreign Bodies

▶ Clinical Findings

External ear is a common site for foreign bodies to be discovered. Commonly, witnessed or reported insertion, ear pain, discharge from the ear canal, or the sensation of a moving insect will be the presenting complaint. Objects may be incidentally noted on examination of the asymptomatic patient. Though typically not associated with severe symptoms, existence of dangerous objects (needles, button batteries) can present with complications such as trauma or burns.

▶ Treatment

Many objects are amenable to removal in the emergency department and a number of techniques are reported (see Chapter 3). The emergency department physician should be aware of and experienced with a variety of techniques as no single option will be successful in every patient. Instillation of topical analgesic solution (if the TM is intact) can facilitate ease of the procedure and will kill a live insect. Exercise caution to avoid pushing the object farther into the canal or damaging the TM or canal wall. Consider topical antibiotics if there has been trauma to the canal or if there are signs of otitis externa.

Disposition

Button batteries are dangerous and cause significant necrosis that warrants consultation with an otolaryngologist in the emergency department. Dangerous objects (pills, needles) that cannot be removed by the emergency physician also justify consultation. Discharge is appropriate after uncomplicated removal of foreign bodies. Some nontoxic, nondangerous objects (small beads, stones) may be left in the canal temporarily and referred to an otolaryngologist for outpatient evaluation. It is best to discuss this option with the consultant to confirm follow-up and ensure parent/patient understanding and agreement with the plan.

Heim SW, Maughan KL: Foreign bodies in the ear, nose, and throat. *Am Fam Physician.* 2007;76(8):1185-1189 [PMID: 17990843].

DISORDERS OF THE NOSE

Sinusitis

Clinical Findings

Sinusitis is characterized by infection and inflammatory changes of the mucosa in the paranasal sinuses. Similar changes occur in the nasal mucosa simultaneously and the infection is more accurately termed rhinosinusitis. Viral infection of the upper respiratory tract usually precedes the onset of bacterial infection. Historical clues of a typical upper respiratory infection (URI) can be key to discriminate bacterial from viral infection, and make the diagnosis of acute bacterial process that requires antibiotic treatment.

Symptoms of sinusitis are similar to viral URIs and include fever, nasal congestion and discharge, halitosis, cough, facial pain, and headache. Purulent-colored nasal discharge and sleep disturbance seem to be more likely associated with sinusitis versus URI, and presence of these findings may increase diagnostic accuracy. Recent guidelines suggest that if the symptoms are abrupt and severe early in the course of illness (days 1-3), abruptly worsen later in the course of illness (days 4-7), or persist and worsen after a longer time (days 10-14), an acute bacterial infection is likely present.

A general, thorough physical examination must be performed in infants and small children as the reported symptoms may be nonspecific and diagnostic clues can be gathered from examination. Purulent nasal discharge, periorbital edema or cellulitis, high fever, and facial tenderness may be noted on examination. Initial diagnosis of acute uncomplicated sinusitis is clinical and requires no adjunctive diagnostic tests; radiographic studies are not recommended.

Severe illness, toxic appearance, meningismus, mental status changes, or focal neurological deficits suggest complications of sinusitis and may be intracranial or intraorbital. These complications include meningitis, dural venous thrombosis, facial cellulitis, orbital cellulitis, and abscess formation. Contrast-enhanced CT imaging should be considered to evaluate for intracranial or orbital complications. Aspiration and culture of sinus fluid is the gold standard of diagnosis though this is not practical in the emergency and should be performed only by a specialist.

Treatment

Viral illnesses should be treated supportively. Antibiotics are indicated and should be initiated for an illness that is diagnosed as bacterial in origin. Common pathogens include *S. pneumoniae, H. influenzae,* and *M. catarrhalis,* and antimicrobial agents should target these agents. Recent guidelines suggest that amoxicillin-clavulanate should be the first-line empiric oral agent, and the course should be continued for 7-10 days depending on the severity of the illness. Standard dosing is appropriate for mild or moderate uncomplicated illness; high-dose regimen should be used for severe illness, risk of resistance, or for cases of treatment failure that may still be appropriate for outpatient management.

Penicillin allergy provides treatment challenges; acceptable oral agents for patients with non severe, non type 1-hypersensitivity reactions include a third-generation cephalosporin (eg, cedfdinr, cefpodoxime) combined with clindamycin. Levofloxacin may be used (if age appropriate) for patients who have severe penicillin allergy. Azithromycin has been commonly utilized in the past, though use of macrolides is discouraged due to a high risk of resistance.

IV ceftriaxone, cefotaxime, ampicillin-sulbactam, and levofloxacin are other options. Ceftriaxone may also be administered intramuscularly. Consider the severity of illness, treatment setting, failure of other recent treatments, or culture-guided treatment in patients that the bacterial pathogen has been identified.

Treatment adjuncts such as decongestants, nasal saline irrigation, and steroids are currently not well studied in pediatric patients and are not generally recommended for routine use.

Disposition

Initiation of antibiotic therapy and outpatient treatment is appropriate for uncomplicated illness. Toxic-appearing patients, cases of failed treatment and those with complicating factors (comorbid illness, meningitis, abscess formation, etc), should be admitted for IV antibiotics.

Chow AW, Benninger MS, Brook I, et al: IDSA clinical practice guideline for acute bacterial rhinosinusitis in children and adults. *Clin Infec Dis.* 2012;54(8):e72-e112 [PMID: 22438350].
Desrosiers M, Evans GA, Keith PK, et al: Canadian clinical practice guidelines for acute and chronic rhinosinusitis. *Allergy Asthma Clin Immunol.* 2011;7(1):2 [PMID: 21310056].

Shaikh N, Hoberman A, Kearney DH, (et al): Signs and symptoms that differentiate acute sinusitis from viral upper respiratory tract infection. *Pediatr Infect Dis J.* 2013;32:1061-1065 [PMID: 23694838].

Smith MJ: Evidence for the diagnosis and treatment of acute uncomplicated sinusitis in children: A systematic review. *Pediatrics.* 2013;132:e284 [PMID: 23796734].

Wald ER, Applegate KE, Bordley C, et al: Clinical practice guideline for the diagnosis and management of acute bacterial sinusitis in children aged 1 to 18 years. *Pediatrics.* 2013;132:e262 [PMID: 23796742].

Nasal Foreign Body

Nasal foreign body is a commonly encountered chief complaint in the emergency department. Small beads, toys, and organic matter/food are frequently discovered. Often times, children will present with a reported history of foreign object insertion. Parents or patients may report nasal discharge, other upper respiratory symptoms, or epistaxis. Nasal objects are usually not life-threatening though they may cause significant symptoms. Button batteries and magnets can cause significant morbidity and must be removed urgently. Sequelae of prolonged exposure to battery chemicals or pressure necrosis can be severe.

▶ Clinical Findings

Symptoms and signs such as unilateral nasal discharge, obstruction of a nare, foul odor from nose or mouth, or epistaxis may be the initial findings. Purulent discharge can be a sign of secondary infection, and black drainage material can suggest tissue necrosis. Foreign bodies are most often lodged in the anterior nasal cavity, and direct visualization confirms the diagnosis. Objects more posterior or those that are obscured by the turbinates make diagnosis and retrieval more challenging. A cooperative, well-positioned patient who is sitting or lying with the neck extended optimizes inspection. Headlamps provide direct hands free illumination but an otoscope with speculum is adequate. Additional diagnostic studies are not required to make the diagnosis and are generally not indicated.

▶ Treatment

Objects that are easily visualized are generally more amenable to removal. Gentle restraint may be required with smaller children; consider procedural sedation in appropriate patients. Instillation of a vasoconstrictor and topical or aerosolized analgesic (oxymetazoline, lidocaine, respectively) prior to the procedure can aid in removal and is necessary in patients in whom manual extraction is the method of choice.

A number of extraction techniques have been discussed in the literature. No one method is clearly superior to others; physicians should use the technique with which they are most familiar and have the necessary supplies readily available.

Contralateral nasal irrigation has been discussed as a method of removal but has not been well studied. The possibility of aspiration of the nasal wash or the foreign body is concerning and should preclude general use of this method.

Positive pressure technique, commonly referred to as the "parent's kiss," uses a forced puff of air delivered directly into the patient's mouth to force the object out of the nare. Thought to be less emotionally traumatic for the child, the parent will "kiss," creating a seal around the mouth and deliver a puff of air in force similar to a nose blow. An Ambu bag delivered breath can be similarly effective. A natural reflex causes the glottis to close forcing retrograde flow of air through the nares and hopefully decreases the risk of lung barotrauma.

Direct, manual extraction is the most commonly chosen method. A nasal speculum will facilitate visualization of objects that are more posterior and provide more room to operate. Commercial devices, such as the Katz extractor, utilize an inflatable balloon located at the end of a thin catheter that can be inserted into the nare past the object. The balloon is inflated and gentle traction is applied to pull the object out. Special suction tip catheters (Schuknecht) can attach directly to an object with a smooth surface. Forceps and hooks are used to directly grasp the object. Use caution when choosing a method and weigh the risks and benefits in each case.

▶ Disposition

Discharge is appropriate after successful removal. Poorly visualized objects, posterior objects, inadvertent posterior displacement, or unsuccessful extraction attempts warrant ENT consultation. Consultation is also indicated in the presence of complications such as local tissue damage or trauma.

Chinski A, Foltran F, Gregori D, et al: Nasal foreign bodies: The experience of the Buenos Aires pediatric otolaryngology clinic. *Pediatr Int.* 2011;53(1):90-93 [PMID: 20500553].

Cook S, Burton M, Glasziou P: Efficacy and safety of the "mother's kiss" technique: a systematic review of case reports and case series. *CMAJ.* 2012;184(17):E904-E912 [PMID: 23071371].

Kiger JR, Brenkert TE, Losek JD: Nasal foreign body removal in children. *Pediatr Emerg Care.* 2008;24(11):785-792 [PMID: 19018225].

Epistaxis

▶ Clinical Findings

Childhood nosebleeds are very common and prevalence increases with age. While most bleeds are mild and self-limiting, severe hemorrhage can develop. Initial evaluation should focus on assessment of the hemodynamic stability of the patient and to initiate general resuscitative measures as indicated. After initial stabilization, a more thorough evaluation is warranted. Determine the activity at onset, duration, location (bilateral or unilateral nare), and associated symptoms. Light-headedness, orthostasis, lethargy, chest pain, or dyspnea in the setting on epistaxis suggests hypovolemia or symptomatic anemia. Most bleeds are secondary to dry, crusting nasal mucosa and digital trauma. Recent upper respiratory illness, local surgery, and trauma can predispose to nasal bleeding. Children are less likely to be intentionally anticoagulated, and bleeding may be the only sign of accidental warfarin ingestion. It is also important to consider other general and childhood-specific systemic conditions that can predispose to bleeding (hypertension, foreign body, bleeding diathesis, or tumors). Epistaxis in children younger than 2 years should prompt consideration of non-accidental trauma.

Directly examine the nose to attempt identification of the bleeding site. Most bleeds originate in the anterior medial septal wall within the three-artery anastomotic zone known as Kiesselbach triangle. Examine both nares using a good light source and a nasal speculum. After hemostasis, the only indicator of previous site of bleeding may be a hyperemic or ulcerated area of the mucosa. Note any lesion, mass, or secondary markers of trauma such as septal hematoma or foreign body. The specific site of bleeding may be difficult to identify after hemostasis and nasal clearing; this may however indicate that that bleeding site is posterior.

Diagnostic Studies

Laboratory and imaging studies are not routinely indicated for mild, uncomplicated bleeding. Hemoglobin levels may not accurately reflect the degree of anemia in the acute setting. Utilize adjunctive studies as indicated by the clinical condition.

▶ Treatment

Most nosebleeds will respond to direct pressure placed at the site of bleeding. Have the child or parent pinch the anterior cartilaginous portion of the nose firmly between two fingers continuously for 15 minutes. Repeat if bleeding persists. After successful hemostasis, instruct the patient to clear the nasal cavity with a gentle blowing and inspect for a specific site/source of bleeding. Judicious use of vasoconstrictors such as oxymetazoline and phenylephrine is acceptable for additional hemostasis.

Chemical cautery with silver nitrate is effective, relatively straightforward, and well tolerated. Nasal mucosa can be anesthetized with topical lidocaine prior to the procedure to decrease discomfort and improve patient tolerance of the procedure. Brief exposure of silver nitrate to the mucosa at the identified bleeding site and in a small zone around this area creates a visible eschar. This technique is limited by the

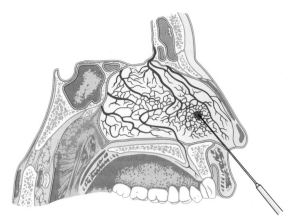

▲ **Figure 33–1.** Cauterization of epistaxis at the site of bleeding (Kiesselbach plexus). (Reproduced, with permission, from Stone CK, Humphries RL: *Current Diagnosis & Treatment Emergency Medicine*, 7th ed. New York: McGraw-Hill, 2011. Copyright © McGraw-Hill Education LLC.)

need for a relatively dry, hemostatic surface for appropriate cauterization (Figure 33–1).

Nasal packing is the classic standard for bleeding that is unresponsive to conservative measures. This is an invasive, uncomfortable procedure and may be best reserved for the otolaryngologist to perform. Chemical applications including fibrin glue and thrombin matrix sealants act quickly and may preclude the need for packing though may not be readily available. Commercial balloon products such as the Rhino Rocket (Shippert Medical Technologies Corporation, Centennial, CO) are commonly stocked in many emergency departments and use is similar to that in adult patients. These nasal tampons are invasive but generally better tolerated and require fewer procedural steps compared to traditional packing. Antibiotics are conventionally prescribed after nasal packing or tampon insertion. Preexisting acute sinusitis warrants treatment; empiric antibiotics may not be beneficial in prevention of post procedure infections.

Refractory bleeding may require surgical ligation or intra-arterial embolization. Consultation with an otolaryngologist is required to determine the best treatment option.

▶ Disposition

Patients with uncomplicated bleeding and successful hemostasis may be discharged home. Gentle application of ointment or nasal saline may aid in moisturizing the nasal mucosa. Children requiring resuscitation or those with complicating conditions (severe anemia, thrombocytopenia, significant trauma) should be admitted for further evaluation. Outpatient referral to an otolaryngologist is appropriate for packing removal and workup for chronic, recurrent epistaxis.

Calder N, Kang S, Fraser L, et al: A double-blind randomized controlled trial of management of recurrent nosebleeds in children. *Otolaryngol Head Neck Surg.* 2009;140:670-674 [PMID: 19393409].

Douglas R, Wormald PJ: Update on epistaxis. *Curr Opin Otolaryngol Head Neck Surg.* 2007;15(3):180-183 [PMID: 17483687].

Kasperek ZA, Pollock GF: Epistaxis: An overview. *Emerg Med Clin N Am.* 2013;31:443-454 [PMID: 23601481].

Qureishi A, Burton MJ: Interventions for recurrent idiopathic epistaxis (nosebleeds) in children. *Cochrane Database Syst* Rev. 2012;9:CD004461 [PMID: 22972071].

Rudmik L, Smith TL: Management of intractable spontaneous epistaxis. *Am J Rhinol Allergy.* 2012;26(1):55-60 [PMID: 22391084].

Weber RK: Nasal packing and stenting. *GMS Curr Top Otorhinolaryngol Head Neck Surg.* 2009;8:1 [PMID: 22073095].

DISORDERS OF THE OROPHARYNX

Peritonsillar Abscess & Peritonsillar Cellulitis

Peritonsillar abscess (PTA) is most common in adolescents and the most common deep space infection of the head and neck. It has been reported in children younger than 2 years. A history of recurrent tonsillitis or tonsillitis that has not improved with therapy is common. Abscess develops from the usual oral flora (both aerobic and anaerobic) in the theoretical peritonsillar space between the palatine tonsil and its capsule. Peritonsillar cellulitis is a similar frequently unilateral condition that may be difficult to discriminate on physical examination.

▶ Clinical Findings

Sore throat and fever are typical symptoms; more concerning symptoms include drooling, neck pain, dysphagia, odynophagia, and a "hot potato" (muffled or distorted) voice. Voice changes, stridor, dyspnea, and other signs of respiratory distress may indicate advanced swelling and related effect on the airway.

Physical examination reveals an erythematous posterior oropharynx with asymmetric swelling in the peritonsillar region. Swelling may extend into the soft palate. Classic description of PTA includes uvular deviation toward the opposite contralateral side of the abscess, which should heighten concern compared to cellulitis, although uvular deviation may be a normal variant of anatomy in the absence of other signs of infection (Figure 33–2). Trismus is an additional finding that may indicate abscess.

Diagnostic Studies

Diagnostic certainty and the need for abscess drainage are difficult as peritonsillar cellulitis may have a very similar clinical appearance. The presence of fluid in the peritonsillar space should be confirmed and has been traditionally

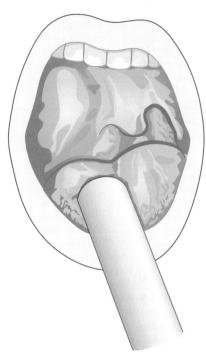

▲ **Figure 33–2.** Peritonsillar abscess. Note the classic findings unilateral asymmetric tonsillar pillar swelling and uvular swelling. (Reproduced, with permission, from Stone CK, Humphries RL: *Current Diagnosis & Treatment Emergency Medicine,* 7th ed. New York: McGraw-Hill, 2011. Copyright © McGraw-Hill Education LLC.)

determined by needle aspiration. This procedure is within the scope of emergency medicine practice, but many practitioners elect to consult with an otolaryngologist. Alternative diagnostic methods include contrast-enhanced CT scan of the neck and ultrasound of the oropharynx. Imaging may be preferred by the consultant or emergency physician to limit the unnecessary discomfort of a needle aspiration when abscess versus cellulitis is unclear. The treating physician should consider the risk of radiation with CT. Oropharynx-specific ultrasound availability varies by institution.

▶ Treatment

Drainage of abscess fluid (when present) should occur without delay. If needle aspiration reveals fluid, incision and drainage may be indicated to further open the abscess and eliminate loculated tissue spaces. Immediate tonsillectomy is uncommon but may be indicated at the consultant's discretion. After drainage and in the case of peritonsillar cellulitis, antibiotics should be provided as well as adequate analgesia. Clindamycin or a third-generation cephalosporin is generally preferred; the clinician may elect to provide the first dose intravenously in the emergency department. Dehydration is a concern in these patients, and initial IV hydration may be indicated. There has been no demonstrated benefit from the use of steroids in these infections.

▶ Complications

Airway involvement, if evident, should be addressed immediately. Aspiration of blood or pus may occur during drainage. Peritonsillar abscess and cellulitis can cause erosion to deeper tissues including the carotid sheath. Lemierre syndrome is a condition where deeper spread of infection occurs at the internal jugular vein and thrombophlebitis results. Septic spread of the infection from the vein may occur, particularly to the lungs.

▶ Disposition

After drainage is completed, the patient's tolerance of oral fluids and medications will determine disposition. If pain is controlled and the patient is tolerating oral intake, discharge home and close follow-up with otolaryngologist are appropriate. A delayed tonsillectomy is performed in many patients after the initial infection has improved. Antibiotics should be continued as an outpatient for 14 days, and precautions regarding dehydration should be given. Patients with complications, persisting pain not relieved in the emergency department, or who cannot tolerate oral intake should be admitted.

Tagliareni JM, Clarkson EI: Tonsillitis, peritonsillar and lateral pharyngeal abscesses. *Oral Maxillofac Surg Clin North Am.* 2012;24(2):197-204 [PMID: 22503067].

Retropharyngeal Abscess

Retropharyngeal abscess (RPA) forms in the potential retropharyngeal space. Preceding abscess formation, a recent pharyngitis or URI typically occurs and leads to retropharyngeal lymph node involvement. Rupture of purulent material from retropharyngeal nodes into the retropharyngeal space results in abscess. RPA is an emergency and occurs in children of all ages, most commonly 6 years or younger.

▶ Clinical Findings

Fever and sore throat are typical symptoms, as well as neck pain and dysphagia or odynophagia. Younger children may have decreased oral intake and associated fever without an immediately clear source. Progression of the condition leads to more dramatic symptoms including drooling, stiff neck, and respiratory distress. Stridor may be present from local spread of inflammation. Pharyngeal erythema may be absent depending on the timing of the antecedent infection and its source.

▶ Treatment

Stabilize the patient's airway if needed. If the patient is oxygenating well and not in respiratory distress, obtain anteroposterior (AP) and lateral neck radiographs as screening tests. The steeple sign on the AP view suggests croup and discriminates this cause of stridor from RPA. Figure 33–3 demonstrates radiographs with normal anatomy, RPA, and croup. See Chapter 41 for a detailed discussion of croup. The lateral view may demonstrate enlargement of the retropharyngeal space. If the patient is in respiratory distress, immediate consultation with otolaryngologist is needed. Contrast-enhanced CT of the neck will likely be more diagnostic than plain film and should be considered in cases where RPA is likely. It will discriminate from other causes of the painful neck and throat including peritonsillar abscess. Once RPA is confirmed, consult with an otolaryngologist. Airway involvement or other decompensation warrants urgent management in the operating room setting.

▶ Complications

Complications are most common in younger children where diagnosis often proves more difficult. A delay in or missed diagnosis of RPA may lead to necrotizing fasciitis or mediastinitis. Thrombophlebitis of the jugular vein, carotid artery involvement, airway involvement, and aspiration are potential complications.

▶ Disposition

Patients with RPA warrant admission to the hospital. The consulted specialist may opt to perform immediate surgery or may choose a 1-2 day trial of IV antibiotics followed by repeat clinical assessment and repeated diagnostic imaging. Initial abscess size may determine the operative or nonoperative approach.

Stoner MJ, Dulaurier M: Pediatric ENT emergencies. *Emerg Med Clin North Am.* 2013;31(3):795-808 [PMID: 23915604].
Virk JS, Pang J, Okhvat S, et al: Analysing lateral soft tissue neck radiographs. *Emerg Radiol.* 2012;19(3):255-260 [PMID: 22351123].

Epiglottitis

Epiglottitis is a potential airway emergency resulting from local inflammation of the epiglottis and surrounding tissues. The incidence of acute epiglottitis in children has decreased since the 1980s because of routine immunization for the most common responsible bacteria, *H. influenzae* type B (HiB). It is more commonly diagnosed in adults and in unvaccinated children. The disease may be rapidly progressive and should be treated as a true emergency.

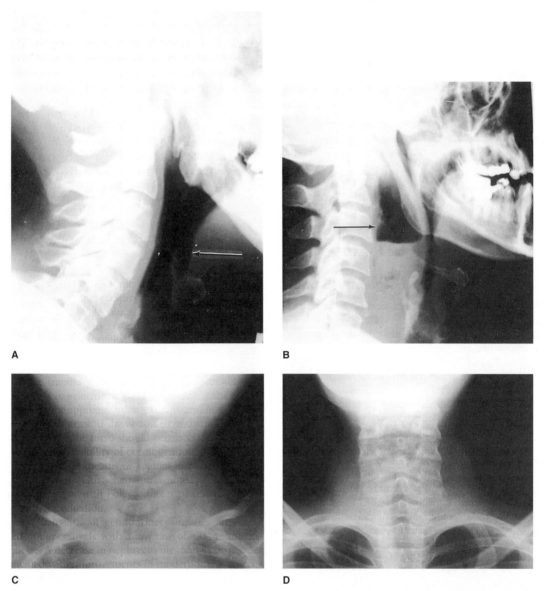

▲ **Figure 33–3.** Soft tissue neck radiographs. (**A**) Normal soft tissue lateral x-ray with no enlargement or distortion of the prevertebral tissues or epiglottis. (**B**) Retropharyngeal abscess—the airway is anteriorly displaced by swelling, and an air-fluid level is present. (**C** and **D**) AP views of an infant (C) and a 12-year-old (D) demonstrate the "steeple" sign indicative of croup. (A-D: Reproduced, with permission, from Stone CK, Humphries RL: *Current Diagnosis & Treatment Emergency Medicine,* 7th ed. New York: McGraw-Hill, 2011. Copyright © McGraw-Hill Education LLC.)

▶ **Clinical Findings**

Fever, sore throat, and fussiness or irritability are common findings. Difficulty breathing, dyspnea, and increased respiratory effort are frequently noted. Stridor is often present and concerning. The cause of stridor should be discriminated from other causes including croup, RPA, and obstructing foreign body. Anterior neck tenderness and sore throat are frequently present in the older child with a more reliable history and examination. Physical examination will commonly reveal pharyngeal inflammation, drooling, cervical lymphadenopathy, and a muffled voice. Patients usually appear toxic initially or soon after presentation. Classic presentation of the younger child is to sit in the "tripod" position, with chin hyperextended and body leaning forward, possibly to maximize the ease of breathing. The tongue may be protruding on examination. A detailed inspection of the oral cavity and oropharynx is not recommended as this may upset the patient (especially the younger child) and further compromise breathing. Patients younger than 5 years are particularly prone to airway collapse in epiglottitis.

▶ Treatment

History and clinical examination suspicious for epiglottitis should be followed by emergent surgical consultation with an otolaryngologist. A portable, lateral soft-tissue neck radiograph can be considered in the stable patient while awaiting the consultant. Distortion of normal anatomy including prevertebral swelling and the classic "thumbprint" sign (Figure 33–4) may be noted. While a positive radiographic finding may be helpful, the study has low sensitivity and specificity.

Diagnosis can be confirmed only by laryngoscopic demonstration of a red, swollen epiglottis and surrounding tissue. Given the high likelihood of airway compromise and possible further obstruction during direct laryngoscopy, patients suspected of having epiglottitis should have laryngoscopy performed in the controlled setting of the operating room by an otolaryngologist with anesthesiology and/or

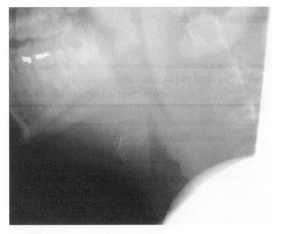

▲ **Figure 33–4.** Epiglottitis. Soft tissue lateral neck x-ray demonstrates an enlarged epiglottis with a "thumbprint" shape. (Reproduced, with permission, from Stone CK, Humphries RL: *Current Diagnosis & Treatment Emergency Medicine*, 7th ed. New York: McGraw-Hill, 2011. Copyright © McGraw-Hill Education LLC.)

pediatric surgery immediately available. Intubation in the operating room should proceed only in the presence of a surgeon or otolaryngologist. In the event of failed intubation, emergent cricothyroidotomy or tracheostomy will be required.

Patients with known or suspected epiglottitis should receive broad-spectrum IV antibiotics (ampicillin/sulbactam, cefotaxime, or ceftriaxone) to cover *S. pneumoniae*, *S. aureus*, *H. influenzae*, and β-hemolytic streptococci. Constant attention to airway stability should be maintained while the patient remains in the emergency department. If the consultant is delayed or unavailable, emergent endotracheal intubation may be required to secure the airway. Extreme caution should be exercised if intubation is attempted, and a surgeon present for backup if possible.

Patients with known or suspected epiglottitis should be treated and managed in the controlled setting of the operating room as described previously.

Hung TY, Li S, Chen PS, et al: Bedside ultrasonography as a safe and effective tool to diagnose acute epiglottitis. *Am J Emerg Med.* 2011;29(3):359.e1-e3 [PMID: 20674236].

Ko DR, Chung YE, Park I, et al: Use of bedside sonography for diagnosing acute epiglottitis in the emergency department: A preliminary study. *J Ultrasound Med.* 2012;31(1):19-22 [PMID: 22215764].

Postoperative Complications

Adenoidectomy and tonsillectomy procedures are primarily performed in pediatric patients for indications ranging from recurrent pharyngeal infections to airway obstruction secondary to enlarged tonsils. Although the procedures are routinely performed, they are not necessarily benign. Common perioperative complications that prompt presentation to the emergency department include bleeding, uncontrolled pain, dehydration, and airway compromise.

▶ Clinical Findings

Pain-control-related complications can be secondary to inadequate dosing or adverse effects from medications. Incorrect dosing and variable responses to narcotic medications can produce unwanted effects. Patients may present with somnolence or frank respiratory depression secondary to taking opioid medications. Underdosing or noncompliance with recommended regimens can lead to uncontrolled pain and dehydration secondary to poor oral intake.

History, vital signs, and physical examination findings can suggest dehydration. The patient may appear uncomfortable, have mild trismus and muffled voice but generally will not appear toxic, have meningeal signs or respiratory compromise. These signs are ominous and suggest a serious infection or imminent airway obstruction.

Bleeding can occur in the acute postoperative setting (first 24 hours) or be delayed. Late bleeding usually occurs between postoperative days 5-8. Incomplete hemostasis, premature separation of the eschar, and vascular injury can cause hemorrhage. Presentation may be secondary to perceived mild bleeding at the surgical site or due severe hemorrhage and resultant shock.

▶ Treatment

For patients who require improved pain control only, properly dosed oral or parenteral analgesia is appropriate. Continuation of oral pain medications and fluid intake are key to successful home treatment and should be demonstrated by the child prior to discharge.

Situations suggesting narcotic overdose warrant respiratory support and airway control as indicated by the severity of the condition. Consider naloxone for reversal of opioid effects.

Bleeding can respond to direct pressure, which should be attempted initially. Adjuncts to achieve hemostasis can be used (epinephrine, thrombin). Provide IV fluid resuscitation as needed, including the use of blood products. Intubation for airway protection may be required if the patient is choking, desaturating, or otherwise appears at risk for aspiration. Surgical management by an otolaryngologist is indicated for uncontrolled bleeding.

Laboratory studies and diagnostic imaging are generally not required. Hemoglobin measurement can identify anemia and/or relative significant change compared to pre-operative values. Through consultation with otolaryngologist and radiologist, arteriography can be considered in refractory bleeding to evaluate possible arterial injuries.

▶ Disposition

In the absence of bleeding, discharge is appropriate if the patient is able to tolerate oral fluids and pain control with oral medication. Consultation with an otolaryngologist (preferably the patient's surgeon) is warranted for all patients with postoperative bleeding. Patients who have mild conditions with easily achieved hemostasis and without apparent hemodynamic or airway compromise can be considered for discharge with close follow-up. Admit patients who have moderate or severe bleeding, hypotension, airway compromise, or severe pain.

Sore Throat

Sore throat is a common complaint in the emergency department and a comprehensive differential diagnosis is extensive. Conditions that affect structures from the mouth through the neck may relate to a patient's sense of throat pain, although true pharyngitis is a painful, inflammatory condition of the throat. Group A *Streptococcus* (GAS) is the most common bacterial cause of infectious pharyngitis in children and attracts much attention considering controversies in diagnostic strategies, potential overtreatment with promotion of resistant bacteria, and risk of latent complications (Table 33–1). See Chapter 41 for detailed discussions of pharyngitis, croup, and mononucleosis.

▶ Clinical Findings

As with most conditions that are proximal to the airway, initial assessment should focus on determining degree of and risk of respiratory compromise. Be prepared to aggressively stabilize the patient and secure the airway.

The spectrum of symptoms will overlap in different disease processes but historical clues and examination findings should help differentiate conditions and help guide further evaluation. It is imperative to verify the vaccination status of the child. Also, note the time and progression of symptom onset, fever, associated respiratory symptoms or difficulty breathing, and any other recent or recurrent illness.

▶ Treatment

See Table 33–1 for disease specific treatment.

▶ Disposition

Most cases of pharyngitis, croup, and mononucleosis are safe for discharge if the patient is well hydrated or tolerating oral fluids. Retropharyngeal abscess, peritonsillar abscess, and epiglottitis are emergency conditions requiring consultation in the emergency department.

Cirilli AR: Emergency evaluation and management of the sore throat. *Emerg Med Clin North Am.* 2013;31(2):501-515 [PMID: 23601485].

Le Marechal F, Martinot A, Duhamel A, et al: Streptococcal pharyngitis in children: A meta-analysis of clinical decision rules and their clinical variables. *BMJ Open.* 2013;3(3):e001482 [PMID: 23474784].

Luzuriaga K, Sullivan JL: Infectious mononucleosis. *NEJM.* 2010;363(15):1486 [PMID: 20505178].

Martin JM: Pharyngitis and streptococcal throat infections. *Pediatr Ann.* 2010;39(1):22-27 [PMID: 20151621].

Roggen I, van Berlaer G, Gordts F, et al: Centor criteria in children in a paediatric emergency department: For what it is worth. *BMJ Open.* 2013;3(4):e002712 [PMID: 23613571].

Shaikh N, Swaminathan N, Hooper EG: Accuracy and precision of the signs and symptoms of streptococcal pharyngitis in children: A systematic review. *J Pediatr.* 2012;160(3):487-493 [PMID: 22048053].

Shulman ST, Bisno AL, Clegg HW, et al: Clinical practice guideline for the diagnosis and management of group A streptococcal pharyngitis: 2012 update by the Infectious Diseases Society of America. *Clin In Infect Dis.* 2012;55(10):1279-1282 [PMID: 23091044].

Wessels MR: Streptococcal pharyngitis. *NEJM.* 2011;364:648-655 [PMID: 21323542].

Table 33–1. Diagnosis and treatment of sore throat.

Diagnosis	Diagnostic Clues	Treatment	Comment
Allergic reaction	Often history of recent food intake; may progress over 5-30 min, voice changes signify possible airway compromise	Epinephrine 1:1000, 0.01 mg/kg IM; Diphenhydramine 1-2 mg/kg IV; Methylprednisolone 2 mg/kg IV; H_2-blockers (ranitidine) 1.5 mg/kg IV	Consider prolonged observation in emergency department or hospital admission
Bacterial pharyngitis	Fever, sore throat without cough; bilateral tonsillar swelling with exudate; tender cervical lymphadenopathy, palatal petechiae	Amoxicillin 20 mg/kg twice daily for 10 d; Benzathine penicillin G 600,000 units IM (< 27 kg), 1.2 M units IM (> 27 kg)	Challenging to differentiate from viral cause on clinical grounds. Throat culture is test of choice group A *Streptococcus* (GAS) which is most common cause in children. GAS peaks in wintertime (temperate climates); associated with latent complications such as glomerulonephritis, rheumatic fever, peritonsillar abscess
Viral (nonspecific) pharyngitis	Fever, cough, rhinorrhea, oral ulcers, possible more gradual onset and protracted course	Supportive care with analgesics, antipyretics, hydration	Most common general cause of pharyngitis
Croup	Fever, rhinorrhea, "barking cough," relatively mild illness, may have stridor, "steeple sign" on x-ray	Dexamethasone 0.6 mg/kg PO or IM; racemic epinephrine for severe cases	Intubation, diagnostics, admission generally not required
Epiglottitis	Abrupt onset of fever, voice hoarseness, drooling, severe pain with swallowing; may preferentially conform to sniffing position soft tissue neck x-ray (enlarged epiglottis—"thumbprint" sign)	Secure airway immediately in unstable patients; maintain position of comfort with minimal stimulation in less urgent situations. Consultation with otolaryngologist and operating room intubation if stable; labs after airway secure; consider blood cultures and early IV antibiotics (ceftriaxone and vancomycin); all patients need admission	Decreased incidence secondary to *H. influenzae* vaccine; also associated with GAS, *S. aureus*.
Infectious mononucleosis	Malaise/fatigue, headache, pharyngitis, fever; enlarged and tender cervical lymph nodes; symptoms may be vague and variable in young children. CBC: peripheral lymphocytosis. Monospot: high specificity but insensitive; unreliable in young children (specific EBV serologic test required)	Supportive care; IV fluids, and admission for patients with severe swelling and dehydration. Steroids optional, not required	Hyperplasia of lymphoid tissue and edema can cause airway obstruction. Typically in adolescents (> 15 y)
Peritonsillar abscess	Fever, drooling, muffled voice, halitosis, trismus; progression of local bacterial cellulitis; unilateral soft palate swelling, deviated uvula Diagnosis often clinical but can be confirmed by needle aspiration, CT scan, or ultrasound	Antibiotics for polymicrobial coverage for 14 d, pain control; needle aspiration if experienced physician, cooperative child, uncomplicated case; I&D generally reserved for otolaryngologist	Most common deep space infection; discharge if tolerating PO intake, pain controlled, and no complicating conditions
Retropharyngeal abscess	Mainly affects children < 6 y; decreased oral intake, fever, neck pain/stiffness, and difficult swallowing; voice changes; stridor if severe; pain; lateral neck x-rays for screening; CT scan with IV contrast is test of choice if patient is stable for scan	Stabilize airway, ENT consultation, IV antibiotics are standard to cover anaerobes, GAS, MRSA/MSSA, surgery for large abscesses (usually > 2 cm)	Progression of illness may be insidious in young children; presentation may be at time of airway compromise. Severe complications include septic thrombophlebitis (Lemierre disease) and mediastinitis

DISORDERS OF THE MOUTH

Odontogenic Infections

▶ Clinical Findings

Odontogenic infections exist and can cause morbidity similar to that seen in adults. Dental pain associated with caries is less common in children and initial presentation to the emergency department may be because of facial cellulitis or abscess; evaluate for a possible odontogenic source of these infections. Symptoms include swelling of the gingiva, face, jaw or neck, as well as dentalgia, redness, and localized pain. Uncomplicated periapical and periodontal abscesses are seen in the gum near the affected tooth. Evaluate for signs of extension of infection into the face or deep spaces of neck; submandibular swelling, crepitus, and meningismus are ominous signs.

Diagnostic Studies

Laboratory tests and imaging studies are generally not required unless evaluating for a complication. CT of the face or neck is the test of choice for identifying abscess, signs of deep space infection, and post septal orbital involvement.

▶ Treatment

Dental pain and caries without signs of cellulitis or abscess can be treated supportively with pain control and referred to dental specialist. Consider empiric antibiotics for isolated, severe pain that is believed to be dental in origin as this may represent early infection. Periapical and periodontal abscesses can undergo incision and drainage in the emergency department. Oral amoxicillin is frequently prescribed to cover suspected infections, as they are usually polymicrobial with anaerobic predominance.

An oromaxillofacial specialist should be consulted for severe infections that have spread into regional structures and for face or neck deep space infections. IV antibiotics (ampicillin/sulbactam, clindamycin) should be started early.

▶ Disposition

Discharge patients with mild infections and including those requiring uncomplicated incision and drainage. Referral for dental evaluation is recommended. Admission and IV antibiotics are indicated for patients with face or deep space infections and abscess requiring operative management.

Hodgdon A: Dental and related infections. *Emerg Med Clin North Am.* 2013;31(2):465-480 [PMID: 23601483].

Nguyen DH, Martin JT: Common dental infections in the primary care setting. *Am Fam Physician.* 2008;77(5):797-802 [PMID: 18386594].

Rush DE, Abdel-Haq N, Zhu JF, et al: Clindamycin versus Unasyn in the treatment of facial cellulitis of odontogenic origin in children. *Clin Pediatr.* 2007;46(2):154-159 [PMID: 17325089].

Thikkurissy S, Rawlins JT, Kumar A, et al: Rapid treatment reduces hospitalization for pediatric patients with odontogenicbased cellulitis. *Am J Emerg Med.* 2010;28(6):668-672 [PMID: 20637381].

Dental Fracture, Subluxation, & Avulsion

Maxillofacial trauma is discussed in Chapter 24.

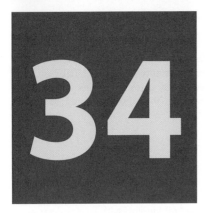

Pulmonary Emergencies

David A. Smith, MD

ACUTE RESPIRATORY FAILURE

Clinical Findings

▶ **Hypoxemic Respiratory Failure (arterial O_2 saturation < 90% while receiving an inspired O_2 fraction > 0.6)**

This represents a wide A-a gradient that is relatively resistant to supplemental oxygen. Frequently there are opacities on chest x-ray that represent fluid-filled aveoli. Common causes are pneumonia, pulmonary edema, and diffuse pneumonitis of various types, including aspiration, and diffuse lung injury due to sepsis, trauma, and shock. Cause is frequently multifactorial. Additional causes are atelectasis, tumor masses, and pleural disease.

▶ Hypercarbic Respiratory Failure (respiratory acidosis with pH < 7.30)

Patients with carbon dioxide (CO_2) retention are often stable and compensate for it. A compensating metabolic acidosis returns the pH to near normal. Acute respiratory acidosis is characterized by CO_2 retention above the patient's normal baseline and low pH on arterial or venous blood gas. Hypercarbia represents inadequate ventilation of the aveoli. A number of diseases that cause this condition do not show opacity of the lung tissue on chest x-ray. Common causes of CO_2 retention include drugs that suppress respiration, weakness of the muscles of respiration, and diseases of the lung that reduce its elasticity or obstruct the airways. Conditions outside the lungs such as obesity or distension of the abdomen may contribute. Depression of consciousness frequently leads to inadequate ventilation from depression of respiratory

drive or from airway obstruction by the tongue against the posterior pharynx.

Treatment

Upon diagnosis of respiratory failure, supplemental oxygen is not adequate treatment, and the patient requires positive pressure to support respiration. Hypoglycemia should be corrected and opiate toxicity should be reversed before initiating ventilator support. Obstruction such as inspissated secretions should be suctioned and cleared from the upper airways.

▶ Noninvasive Positive-Pressure Ventilation

Noninvasive positive-pressure ventilation (NIPPV) includes continuous positive airway pressure (CPAP) and bilevel positive airway pressure (BiPAP). CPAP is applied throughout the respiratory cycle of a spontaneously breathing patient and is physiologically identical to constant positive end-expiratory pressure (PEEP). Emergency medical system (EMS) providers commonly use CPAP. BiPAP combines CPAP with an inspiratory pressure. BiPAP can provide modes nearly identical with standard ICU ventilators, such as pressure, volume, and assist control. Patients who are cooperative and can manage and protect their airways are candidates for NPPV, which avoids complications that result from an endotracheal tube (ETT). Endotracheal intubation is necessary for the patient who is fully comatose or who is unable to manage the airway or secretions.

Expectation for recovery plays a role in the decision to use invasive versus noninvasive management. Patients with asthma or acute heart failure are candidates for noninvasive airway management since bronchodilators and diuretics may effect a rapid reversal of respiratory distress. Pneumonia and other causes of extensive airspace disease are difficult to manage noninvasively if the patient meets the criteria for hypoxic respiratory failure.

Disposition

Patients with respiratory failure will typically require intensive care unit (ICU) care. Underlying disease is the major determinant of patients managed noninvasively. Patients with stable vital signs may be treated on a medical ward with good support from respiratory therapy.

FURTHER DIAGNOSTIC EVALUATION

PULSE OXIMETRY

Pulse oximetry provides two advantages over conventional blood gases in the determination of arterial oxygenation: (1) the method is noninvasive obviating the difficulties of obtaining arterial or venous blood, and (2) the information is available continuously, permitting real-time evaluation of tissue oxygenation. There is a slight lag between respiration and tissue oxygenation as advocates of capnography would point out. Waveform monitoring verifies the reliability of the readings.

Arterial Blood Gas

Arterial blood gas (ABG) analysis is useful in the critically ill child with respiratory distress. Analysis of ABG will reveal the adequacy of oxygenation, status of ventilation, and acid-base balance. It plays a significant role in documenting and monitoring of the child with respiratory failure, especially during ventilator therapy.

Venous Blood Gas

Venous blood gas (VBG) can be used as an alternative to ABG. The advantage of VBG is avoidance of an arterial sample in the children. Blood returning from the venous pool will have a slightly higher partial pressure of carbon dioxide (PCO_2) than arterial blood (due to tissue metabolism). This depresses the pH slightly (Table 34–1). The bicarbonate levels correlate closely in most patients. The inability of a VBG to measure oxygenation is the major shortcoming in contrast to an ABG. However, if the VBG is analyzed in conjunction with pulse oximetry, this limitation is eliminated.

CAPNOGRAPHY

Capnography is the monitoring of the partial pressure of CO_2 in exhaled respiratory gases. It provides the clinician with

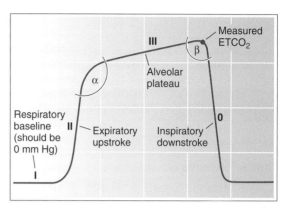

▲ **Figure 34–1.** Normal capnogram.

a real-time graphical representation of the CO_2 concentration in exhaled air. Display is a waveform (Figure 34–1) on the monitor with corresponding numerical measurement. Normal end-tidal carbon dioxide ($ETCO_2$) is 35-45 mm Hg. Capnography is used in intubated patients to identify obstructed or disconnected ETT; capnography detects these situations earlier than pulse oximetry. It can also be used in patients who are not intubated by using sidestream sampling.

Waveform Expiratory Segment

Phase I. Respiratory baseline—anatomical dead space, does not contain exhaled CO_2.

Phase II. Expiratory upstroke—anatomical progressing to alveolar dead space. Its slope is steep in a normal capnogram.

Phase III. Alveolar plateau—positive slope ending in the value of $ETCO_2$. This is an approximation of arterial CO_2.

α angle. Angle between phase II and phase III (ventilation-perfusion [V/Q] status of lung).

Waveform Inspiratory Segment

Phase 0. Inspiratory downstroke.

β angle. Angle between the alveolar plateau and the descending limb of the capnogram.

IMAGING

Plain film chest x-ray should be considered in most children with moderate respiratory distress. CT scanning has limited utility in children with nontraumatic respiratory distress.

Eipe N, Doherty DR: A review of pediatric capnography. *J Clin Monit Comput.* 2010;24:261-268 [PMID: 20635124].

Gregoretti C, Pelosi P, Chidini G, et al: Non-invasive ventilation in pediatric intensive care. *Minerva Pediatr.* 2010;62:437-458 [PMID: 20940679].

Table 34–1. Venous blood gas values versus arterial blood gas values.

PCO_2	Approximately 6 mm Hg higher in peripheral venous blood
pH	Approximately 0.03 pH units lower in venous blood
HCO_3^-	Correlates closely

Prabhakaran P: Acute respiratory distress syndrome. *Indian Pediatr.* 2010;47:861-868 [PMID: 21048239].

Timmons O: Infection in pediatric acute respiratory distress syndrome. *Semin Pediatr Infect Dis.* 2006;17:65-71 [PMID:16822468].

EMERGENCY TREATMENT OF SPECIFIC DISORDERS

ASTHMA

Clinical Findings

Diagnosis of acute asthma is usually straightforward with dyspnea, wheezing, and a history of prior episodes. Wheezing is a nearly universal physical finding but lung sounds may be diminished in parts of the chest due to mucus plugging, pneumothorax, or pneumonia. Wheezing may also be caused by illnesses, such as an aspirated foreign body or acute congestive heart failure.

Exacerbations of asthma may be triggered by viral respiratory infection, but may follow exposure to allergens in the environment. Significant fever greater than 38°C (100.4 °F) should prompt investigation for a complicating pneumonia. Anxiety and agitation are common in moderate to severe disease. Tachypnea correlates roughly with disease severity. Tachycardia is common due to the asthma but can be worsened by bronchodilators. Hypoxia is usually mild unless complications such as pneumonia are present.

Treatment

Risk factors for severe disease should be considered, including previous ICU admissions, intubation, repeated courses of oral corticosteroids, and rapidly progressive episodes. A more aggressive approach should be taken if risk factors are present. Diagnostic studies are not needed in most patients. Chest x-ray is usually not helpful except in severe disease or if there is fever or focal findings on physical examination. Supplemental oxygen should be provided if hypoxia is present. Thick and tenacious secretions tend to cause mucous plugging which contributes to impaired gas exchange and atelectasis. All patients should be appropriately rehydrated. Oral fluids are appropriate in patients who are mildly ill; however, those with moderate to severe illness require intravenous (IV) fluids. Normal saline boluses of 20 mL/kg are used, guided by signs of dehydration and clinical response.

Monitoring

Patients should be monitored with pulse oximetry, cardiac monitoring, and frequent determination of vital signs.

▶ Peak Expiratory Flow Rate Monitoring

Peak expiratory flow rate (PEFR) monitoring is used to gauge the effectiveness of treatment and to assist with disposition

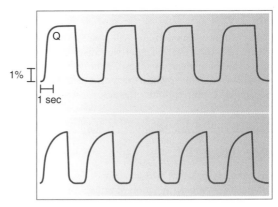

▲ **Figure 34–2.** Normal capnogram and "shark fin" capnogram in severe asthma.

of patients. PEFR monitoring can be accurately performed by most patients older than 5 years. The measurements are greatly affected by effort and technique, and patients may appear to improve as they learn to achieve better results. With this caveat in mind, the test can be useful in some patients with acute asthma.

▶ Waveform Capnography

Capnography can be useful in children with moderate to severe asthma to monitor during treatment. Severe or worsening asthma demonstrates a "shark fin" pattern on the capnogram with a wide angle and a steep slope to the alveolar plateau (Figure 34–2). However, capnography is less reliable in children than in adults who have asthma.

Asthma Scoring

Modified clinical asthma score ([CAS]; Woods and Downes) is a clinical scoring system for grading severity of an asthma exacerbation. Table 34–2 lists the criteria for the system. The scoring system is problematic because it is not effective in predicting children who required hospitalization more than 24 hours or patients who continued to have problems following discharge.

Medications

Medication in acute asthma is best applied in a stepwise approach based on severity of the disease on presentation. Albuterol is the standard therapy, and Table 34–3 presents the albuterol dose by body weight.

▶ Mild Episode

- Albuterol via small volume nebulizer (SVN) at a dose of 0.15 mg/kg (maximum 5 mg) for 20 minutes.
- Consider oral prednisone 2 mg/kg (maximum 60 mg) or dexamethasone 0.6 mg/kg (maximum dose 16 mg).

Table 34–2. Modified CAS (Woods and Downes) asthma score.

Score Points	SpO$_2$ by Pulse Oximetry	Wheezing	Accessory Muscle Use	Inspiratory Breath Sounds	CNS
0	95 + on room air	None/end-expiratory	None	Normal	Normal
1	< 95 on room air	Entire expiratory phase	Substernal, subcostal, intercostal, nasal flaring	Unequal	Altered mental status/agitated
2	< 95 with a simple mask	Expiration and inspiration	Supraclavicular, seesaw respiration	Decreased	Depressed

Mildly ill = less than 3.
Moderately ill = 3 to 4.
Severely ill = more than 5.

Moderate Episode

- Administer albuterol via SVN continuously for 1 hour. Patients should be evaluated by the respiratory therapist every 20 minutes.
- Combine albuterol with ipratropium (0.25 mg) if less than 20 kg; 0.5 mg if > 20 kg). Using a higher dose of ipratropium in a continuous SVN does not improve the outcome.
- Start IV fluids with a bolus of 20 cc/kg of normal saline.
- IV methylprednisolone (1-2 mg/kg, maximum 60 mg).

Severe Episode

- In addition to the above treatment for moderate episodes, add IV magnesium sulfate (75 mg/kg, maximum 2.5 g administered over 20 minutes).

Alternatives to Bronchodilators via Nebulizer

Subcutaneous Bronchodilators—Epinephrine or terbutaline (0.01 mL/kg of a 1-mg/mL solution) up to 0.4 mg (0.4 mL) may be administered intramuscularly or subcutaneously.

Metered-Dose Inhalers (MDIs)—MDIs are convenient devices to deliver medications directly to the lungs and when used properly compare favorably to medication delivery by nebulized aerosols. Dosage is one-quarter to one-third puff/kg

Table 34–3. Albuterol dose by body weight.

Body Weight	Dose
5-10 kg	10 mg/h
10-20 kg	15 mg/h
> 20 kg	20 mg/h

to a maximum of eight puffs every 20-30 minutes for as many as three doses.

Theophylline—Theophylline is rarely used in the treatment of asthma, not because it is ineffective in relieving bronchoconstriction, but because of the frequent occurrence of serious toxicity.

Leukotriene Receptor Antagonists—Leukotrienes are important mediators of symptoms in asthma. Montelukast (Singulair) and zafirlukast (Accolate) are leukotriene receptor antagonists. Zileuton (Zyflo CR) inhibits leukotriene formation. The drugs are not used in acute asthma but may be encountered in patients presenting with acute exacerbations. Therapy with these drugs should continue.

Disposition

Patients on no medications when they present respond more quickly and completely than those already on maximal therapy at home. Most patients who improve with treatment in the emergency department can be discharged home with close follow-up with their primary physician. When patients do not improve as expected, IV fluids should be provided. Patients considered not sufficiently improved after three SVN treatments and IV fluids will usually need to be admitted to the hospital. Patients who have responded poorly to maximal treatment or require any type of positive pressure ventilation should be treated in an ICU.

BRONCHIOLITIS

Bronchiolitis is a lower respiratory tract infection that occurs in children younger than 2 years. It is typically caused by a virus. Respiratory syncytial virus (RSV) infection is the usual etiology but both influenza and parainfluenza viruses may cause the same syndrome. Bronchiolitis demonstrates a strong seasonal predominance from November to April, with a peak in January and February. Bronchiolitis is a leading cause of hospitalization in infants and children younger than 2 years.

Clinical Findings

The virus causes inflammation of the small airways which partially or completely blocks the bronchioles. Lower respiratory symptoms typically include cough and wheezing. The illness is clinically similar to an exacerbation of asthma except that in children younger than 2 years, smooth muscle has not yet developed in the bronchioles. Wheezing is due to airway narrowing caused by inflammation and edema. The wheezing sound is somewhat coarser than that caused by asthma; however it is distinctly expiratory. Patients with bronchiolitis typically do not have a history of prior episodes nor an allergenic precipitant. Fever is variably present. Patients with underlying cardiac or respiratory disease such as bronchopulmonary dysplasia or congenital heart disease are prone to more severe illness.

Treatment

Treatment is supportive care with oxygen as needed. Consider fluid administration as needed to maintain hydration. A trial of a short-acting bronchodilator such as albuterol is reasonable. If a good clinical response is achieved, regular treatment with a bronchodilator every 4-6 hours would be appropriate. RSV testing is indicated to isolate or cohort patients especially if hospitalization is required. Corticosteroids are not useful and should be avoided.

Ribavirin has in vitro activity against RSV and is FDA approved for the treatment of RSV infection. It is an expensive drug and is not used in RSV infection unless the patient is severely ill and is admitted to the ICU. Studies of its efficacy demonstrate mixed results. Consultation with an infectious diseases specialist is recommended before its use.

Disposition

Bronchiolitis is frequently mild enough to allow outpatient management. Hypoxia is a significant concern and patients should be admitted to the hospital if hypoxic on room air. Other indications for admission include apnea episode, respiratory rate greater than 70 after treatment, infants requiring frequent suctioning, respiratory distress, dehydration, or the inability to maintain oral intake. Social circumstances should be considered in the disposition as well. Access to medical care in the event of deterioration is an important consideration.

BRONCHOPULMONARY DYSPLASIA

Bronchopulmonary dysplasia (BPD) is a consequence of early acute lung disease from prematurity and rarely occurs in infants born after 30 weeks' gestation. Infants with pulmonary disease from the neonatal period have BPD if they require supplemental oxygen after 28 days. Most will have persistently abnormal chest radiographs.

Clinical Findings

By definition, BPD is chronic which implies another type of acute illness or precipitant develops to cause pulmonary function to decline. This may be an episode of aspiration or an intercurrent infection such as pneumonia. The most frequent cause is viral infection such as rhinovirus or RSV. Exacerbations are clinically similar to those of patients with asthma except that these patients are more often hypoxic and have less wheezing.

Treatment

Support of respiration including oxygen therapy is the main therapy for patients with BPD during exacerbations. Short courses of inhaled bronchodilators and steroids may be used during exacerbations when wheezing is present. Antibiotics should be used if bacterial pneumonia is suspected.

Disposition

Patient may be a candidate for outpatient treatment if a caretaker who is familiar with the patient's history and condition can monitor the patient in the outpatient setting. A simple measure such as suctioning may resolve the distress but most patients with BPD and acute respiratory distress are admitted to the hospital. Caretakers of the patient and pediatric physician are usually familiar with the patient's disease and should be involved in the management when possible.

CYSTIC FIBROSIS

Cystic fibrosis (CF) is an autosomal recessive genetic disorder that affects the lungs, pancreas, liver, and intestine. It is characterized by abnormal transport of chloride and sodium across the epithelium, leading to thick, viscous secretions. The lungs are most affected by the clogging of the airways from a buildup of mucus along with a decreased mucociliary clearance that results in inflamation.

Clinical Findings

Patients with CF typically have persistent productive cough and an obstructive pattern of pulmonary dysfunction. Radiographs demonstrate hyperinflation, bronchiectasis, and bronchial wall thickening. With acute illness, the cough increases as does sputum production and respiratory distress. Cystic fibrosis is a multisystem disease, and patients may have chronic sinusitis and malabsorption.

Treatment

Patients with CF are usually followed closely by a team of specialty providers. Emergency department care should be carried out in consultation when possible with these providers.

Most exacerbations of respiratory distress in patient with CF are due to infection. *Staphylococcus aureus* is a common pathogen, and *Haemophilus influenzae* is a prevalent infection in childhood. *Pseudomonas aeruginosa* infection is a particular problem in adolescence and adulthood, and increasing resistance to antibiotics makes treating pseudomonal infections challenging. Antibiotic therapy may be guided by age and sputum bacterial isolates; however, in vitro sensitivities correlate poorly with clinical response. Antibiotics that are not effective against the primary organisms are nevertheless sometimes beneficial presumably due to some collateral effect. Usually, antibiotics started in the emergency department are based on the history of what has been effective in the past. The patient's CF team should be consulted.

Chest physiotherapy in CF has seen considerable evolution of contemporary methods. Percussion and postural drainage that was provided by respiratory therapists has been replaced by methods that can be self-administered. Methods include chest vests driven by compressed air and other devices. Chest physiotherapy will need to be continued when patients are admitted to the hospital. Nebulized saline is used daily by many patients. It is also useful in acute illness.

Dornase alfa (Pulmozyme) is a recombinant human deoxyribonuclease that cleaves DNA in mucus of CF patients and reduces viscosity in the lungs. This promotes improved clearance of secretions. In children older than 5 years, inhalation of 2.5 mg once daily via nebulizer is used.

There is no evidence that noninvasive ventilation increases sputum expectoration or improves lung function. In patients who are severely ill, BiPAP may be used as a bridge to more controlled endotracheal intubation.

Spontaneous pneumothorax is a well known complication of CF. Small pneumothoraces may be observed in the emergency department. Large pneumothoraces should be treated with chest tube drainage. Surgical or chemical pleurodesis is required for recurrent disease.

Disposition

Some patients will need hospitalization but the patient's CF team should be consulted to guide a disposition decision.

PNEUMONIA

Pneumonia is an inflammatory condition of the lung that affects the alveoli. It is usually caused by infection with viruses or bacteria and less commonly other microorganisms.

Clinical Findings

▶ Neonatal Pneumonia

Serious infection in the neonates including pneumonia may occur without fever. Hypothermia is common. Lethargy is typical as are depressed respirations and hypoxia. Apnea may also occur. Neonates may have tachycardia and poor perfusion, sometimes progressing to septic shock.

▶ Early-Onset Neonatal Pneumonia (≤ 3 days old)

Early-onset pneumonia is usually maternally acquired during labor or delivery. It presents with respiratory distress beginning at or soon after birth and is often part of generalized sepsis. Group B *Streptococcus* (GBS) causes most early-onset pneumonia.

▶ Late-Onset Neonatal Pneumonia (> 3 days old)

Late-onset pneumonia usually occurs in neonatal ICUs among infants who require prolonged endotracheal intubation resulting from lung disease. The organisms are usually acquired from the ICU environment including the ventilator and health care providers.

▶ Childhood Pneumonia

Most commonly identified bacterial pneumonia in children is caused by *Streptococcus pneumoniae*. The organism is usually identified from blood cultures, not from sputum.

Fever and cough are the usual symptoms of pneumonia. *Mycoplasma pneumoniae* in children is common although rarely identified during the acute phase of the disease. *Chlamydia trachomatis* may be acquired during delivery but typically causes illness in an infant between 2 weeks and 3 months old. The resulting pneumonia usually causes diffuse bilateral infiltrates. There may be conjunctivitis by the same organism.

Community-acquired MRSA may cause invasive disease including rapidly progressive pneumonia. Pneumonia associated with a parapneumonic effusion is typical of the illness especially if the effusion progresses rapidly. There is typically a focus of infection in another location usually the skin.

Cough may not be present initially as no cough receptors are present in the aveoli. Tachypnea (Table 34–4) with normal pediatric respiratory rates and increased work of breathing are the usual signs that discriminate pneumonia from the common respiratory viral infections of childhood. In addition there may be listlessness and poor appetite. Vomiting is more common in children younger than 5 years. A minimum of one blood culture should be obtained in a patient with pneumonia to aid in identification of the organism.

Table 34–4. Normal pediatric respiratory rates.

Age	Rate
Infant (birth-1 y)	< 40
Toddler (1-3 y)	< 30
Preschooler (3-6 y)	< 30
School-aged child (6-12 y)	Low 20s
Adolescent (12-18 y)	Upper teens

PEDIATRIC HIV INFECTION

Pneumocystis jirovecii pneumonia (PCP) is a common AIDS-defining condition in children. The symptoms are often insidious with onset of cough, dyspnea, poor feeding, diarrhea, and weight loss. Chest auscultation may be normal; however, rales, rhonchi, and hypoxemia are the usual clinical signs. The radiographic pattern is that of an atypical pneumonia with bilateral perihilar interstitial infiltrates that become diffuse as disease progresses.

Treatment

Most common organism of concern with a localized alveolar infiltrate (typical pneumonia) is *S. pneumoniae* because of the potential for severe illness. First-line empiric antibiotic therapy is high-dose amoxicillin 90 mg/kg/day twice daily for 7-10 days.

Levofloxacin is an alternative for infants younger than 6 months and doxycycline for children older than 8 years.

A macrolide (azithromycin) is appropriate in school-aged children and adolescents with atypical pneumonia treated for 5 days.

Disposition

Hospitalization is advised if the patient is significantly dehydrated or exhibits respiratory distress, has a toxic appearance, or has significant underlying conditions (cardiopulmonary disease, genetic syndromes, neurocognitive disorders). Hospitalization is indicated for outpatient treatment failures.

Before outpatient therapy is initiated, the following should be demonstrated by the patient in the emergency department.

- Absence of hypoxia O_2 saturation > 93 with pulse oximetry.
- Ability to tolerate oral intake including the first dose of oral antibiotics.
- Adequate social support including the means to obtain oral medication and reliable follow-up.

INTERSTITIAL LUNG DISEASE

Interstitial lung disease, known as interstitial pneumonitis, is a diverse group of rare illnesses that affect the pulmonary parenchyma and produce restrictive functional defects and impaired gas exchange. Most of the described illnesses in this group present from a subacute to chronic manner and require histopathology for diagnosis.

Clinical Findings

Lymphocytic interstitial pneumonia (LIP) is the most common interstitial lung disease in children. It occurs in 25-40% of children with perinatally acquired HIV and is an AIDS-defining illness in children. Findings include fever, cough, and dyspnea, with bibasilar pulmonary infiltrates from interstitial accumulations of lymphocytes and plasma cells.

Acute interstitial pneumonitis (Hamman-Rich syndrome) is an acute, severe, and rapidly progressive interstitial pneumonitis. The illness presents with abrupt onset of dyspnea, hypoxia, tachypnea and tachycardia, and fever.

Treatment

Patients with LIP require supportive care and immunosuppressives, most commonly corticosteroids. Cytotoxic therapy has been used but there is little evidence to support its use. Bronchodilators may be useful if significant wheezing is present.

Acute interstitial pneumonitis is difficult if not impossible to distinguish from a diffuse viral or bacterial pneumonia without histopathology. Antibiotics and respiratory isolation are indicated. Patients require supportive care including supplemental oxygen. Intravenous hydration may be necessary, but caution is advised as excessive fluids will worsen gas exchange especially oxygenation. Any potential offending agent or drug should be avoided. Bronchodilators can be used if there is evidence of reversible airway obstruction.

Disposition

Patients with either LIP or acute pneumonitis (Hamman-Rich syndrome) require admission to the hospital. Many are seriously ill and may require intubation and ICU care.

INFLUENZA

Influenza occurs in wintertime with outbreaks each year. Transmission from person to person occurs via respiratory secretions with coughing and sneezing. The incubation period is typical of other upper respiratory tract viruses, approximately 3 days.

Clinical Findings

Usual symptoms are abrupt onset of fever, cough, rhinitis, sore throat, and headache. Vomiting is common in small children as is high fever. Myalgia is a prominent symptom in adolescents. The pattern of illness is variable. It may cause bronchiolitis clinically indistinguishable from that caused by RSV or parainfluenza virus.

Rapid diagnostic test results have been shown to alter decision making in febrile infants without a focus of infection. A positive rapid influenza test reduces the amount of diagnostic testing, prescriptions for antibiotics, emergency department length of stay, and increases the number of prescriptions for antiviral therapy.

Bacterial pneumonia caused by streptococcal or staphylococcal organisms develops in approximately 2% of patients. Coinfection with *S. aureus* may be severe and rapidly fatal. Otitis media develops in approximately 30% of children.

Treatment

Influenza strains mutate from year to year which affects treatment especially immunization. Antiviral therapy shortens the duration of illness approximately 1 day if given within 48 hours, and 3 days if given within 12 hours. Treatment beyond the first 48 hours of symptom onset is not usually indicated unless the child is hospitalized or has preexisting respiratory illness such as asthma or CF. The duration of viral shedding is not reduced.

Neuraminidase inhibitors, oseltamivir and zanamivir, are active against influenza A and B, and nearly all strains are sensitive. Oseltamivir is given orally to children for 5 days in doses as follows.

- 2 weeks-11 months: 3 mg/kg PO twice daily
- > 1 year and < 15 kg: 30 mg PO twice daily
- > 1 year and 15-23 kg: 45 mg PO twice daily
- Children weighing 23-40 kg: 60 mg PO twice daily
- Children weighing > 40 kg: 75 mg PO twice daily

Zanamivir is a dry powder that is inhaled by children older than 7 years with a dose of two puffs every 12 hours for 5 days. The adamantanes to include amantadine and rimantadine are active against only influenza A and many strains are resistant. Coverage for bacterial coinfection should be included if there is a clinical suspicion for bacterial pneumonia particularly if there are alveolar infiltrates.

Disposition

Influenza is a self-limited disease in most healthy individuals. A precise diagnosis of acute infection with influenza requires acute and convalescent titers and cannot be established in the emergency department. Treatment is supportive. Individuals who are at high risk for severe disease should avoid contact with those with suspected disease. Household contacts and caregivers are priorities for immunization.

PULMONARY EMBOLISM

Pulmonary embolism is rare in children unless the patient has known risk factors. However, as the number of children surviving chronic illness increases, so will the incidence of thromboembolic disease. The presence of a central venous catheter is the most common risk factor encountered in children. Risk factors include recent surgical procedures, immobility congestive heart failure, and hypercoagulability from congenital disorders such as deficiency of antithrombin III, protein C, or protein S.

Clinical Findings

Presentation of pulmonary embolism in children is different from that in adults. Presenting signs include unexplained tachycardia and hypoxia. There may be increasing oxygen requirements in some with chronic illness. Patients who are verbal may have complaint of chest pain or dyspnea.

Of the modalities available for diagnosis (V/Q scanning, echocardiography, angiography), CT angiogram is the most useful for diagnostic accuracy, availability, and cost. MR angiography may have a role if it is available and has the advantage of not exposing the patient to radiation.

Treatment

Heparin or low-molecular-weight (LMW) heparins are appropriate treatments. Heparin is given with a loading dose of 75 U/kg IV followed by a maintenance infusion of 28 U/kg/h (aged < 1 year), 20 U/kg/h (aged > 1 year). Enoxaparin is dosed in infants younger than 2 months at 1.5 mg/kg/dose every 12 hours subcutaneously and for infants younger than 2 months at 1 mg/kg/dose each 12 hours subcutaneously.

Disposition

Although pulmonary embolism is an unusual diagnosis in children, it remains a potentially fatal disease. The treatments for pulmonary embolism also attend significant risk. Almost all children will have significant underlying disease. Hospitalization will be required.

PULMONARY EDEMA

Clinical Findings

Dyspnea, tachypnea, and hypoxia are the usual clinical manifestations resulting from heavy wet lungs as in pulmonary edema. Engorgement of the pulmonary veins and bronchospasm also play a role in pulmonary dysfunction. Wheezing, usually considered in the context of asthma, is the rule rather than the exception. Other symptoms include orthopnea, exercise intolerance, and fatigue. Cough is not a prominent symptom in mild disease but in severe disease patients may cough up a frothy pink fluid. In infants, prominent symptoms are restlessness, irritability, and poor feeding. Tachycardia is frequently a reflex response to hypoxia, but a primary arrhythmia may be present and may contribute to ineffective cardiac output. In adults, severe hypertension is usually the cause of outflow obstruction.

The brain natriuretic peptide (BNP) test is useful for determining a cardiogenic versus a noncardiogenic cause for pulmonary edema. Normal result (< 100 pg/mL) rules out a cardiac cause. Noncardiogenic pulmonary edema is pulmonary edema that results from an increase in the permeability of the vascular endothelium of the lung causing fluid to accumulate in the aveoli. This is due to a noninflammatory process such as hypoxia as in high-altitude pulmonary edema or an inflammatory process which is synonymous with ARDS. In either case radiographic appearance may be similar to pulmonary edema resulting from congestive heart failure.

Treatment

Supportive care will include supplemental oxygen as hypoxia is indicated. The upright posture should be maintained. Procedures that require recumbency such as insertion of a Foley catheter may need to be deferred.

Children with cardiogenic pulmonary edema are managed with vasodilators, diuretics, and inotropic agents (Table 34–5). Furosemide is the usual diuretic chosen unless the patient is known to be intolerant of it. The beneficial effect is noticeable well before any significant diuresis occurs, and the adverse effects of a single dose are trivial. Vasodilators are used to reduce cardiac afterload.

Table 34–5. Medications for acute pulmonary edema.

Medication	Dosage	Comments
Furosemide	1 mg/kg/dose PO or IV	
Dopamine	Starting dose 5-10 mcg/kg/min IV	Titrated to effect, maximum dose is 28 mcg/kg/min)
Dobutamine	Starting dose 5-10 mcg/kg/min IV	Titrated to effect, less vasoconstriction than with dopamine
Nitroglycerin	0.1-0.5 mcg/kg/min IV	Vasodilator
Nitroprusside	Nitroprusside 0.5-10 mcg/kg/min IV	More difficult to use than nitroglycerin
Alprostadil	0.03-0.1 mcg/kg/min IV	Prostaglandin E$_1$ (PGE$_1$)

Nitroglycerin is a more familiar drug and is easier to use than nitroprusside. Dobutamine or dopamine may be indicated for inotropic support.

Prostaglandin infusion may be indicated in patients with congenital heart disease who are dependent on a patient ductus arteriosus. Ductus dependent neonates typically become symptomatic within the first 2 weeks of life. Most are discovered shortly after birth but some may return to the emergency department with hypoxia, hypotension, poor peripheral perfusion, and acute pulmonary edema. The patency of ductus can be maintained with an infusion of prostaglandins. Prostaglandin E$_1$ (alprostadil) is the medication with an FDA-approved indication, but a similar dose of prostaglandin E$_2$ is equally effective and much cheaper. Half-life during IV infusion is less than 1 minute. Respiratory depression and apnea are common. Consultation with a pediatric cardiologist is essential.

Disposition

Acute pulmonary edema often improves dramatically with treatment if diuretics are used. Hospitalization is usually indicated. Patients who require BiPAP or continuous drips will require ICU care.

PERTUSSIS

Pertussis is caused by gram-negative coccobacillus *Bordetella pertussis* which is spread by respiratory droplets. The incubation period for pertussis is approximately 7-10 days, longer than the 1-3 days of most viral upper respiratory tract illnesses.

Clinical Findings

In adolescents and adults, pertussis is typically associated with respiratory illnesses with prolonged cough, longer than 3 weeks. Pertussis is classically divided into three stages.

▶ Catarrhal

Nasal congestion similar to a common cold with a mild cough lasts 1-2 weeks.

▶ Paroxysmal

More persistent and severe cough develops. The characteristic whoop and repetitive cough is primarily found in patients between 6 months and 5 years of age. Infants younger than 6 months may have respiratory depression or apnea. Serious complications may occur in this stage.

▶ Convalescent

Cough subsides but may persist for weeks to months.

Polymerase chain reaction (PCR) test is the most clinically useful test for diagnosis. Other tests such as culture and the ELISA test are useful for confirmation.

Treatment

With PCR testing, pertussis may be identified in the emergency department and specific therapy initiated. If PCR testing is not available immediately, presumptive therapy should be started if pertussis is strongly suspected. Macrolides are the treatment of choice for pertussis. Azithromycin is the usual choice with a dose of 10 mg/kg/day for 5 days in infants younger than 6 months and 10 mg/kg/day (maximum: 500 mg) on day 1, followed by 5 mg/kg/day (maximum: 250 mg) on days 2-5 for infants and children older than 6 months. Trimethoprim-sulfamethoxazole (TMP-SMZ) is a second-line choice, except in infants younger than 2 months in whom it is contraindicated.

Disposition

Children younger than 5 years and particularly younger than 6 months may need hospitalization. They should be admitted to a unit where the respiratory rate, heart rate, and oxygen saturation can be monitored. Infants younger than 3 months should be transferred to a center that has a pediatric intensive care unit (PICU) as clinical deterioration can occur without warning.

TUBERCULOSIS

Tuberculosis (TB) is caused by *Mycobacterium tuberculosis* that is spread from person to person through respiratory droplets. Infants and young children are more likely than older children to develop life-threatening forms of TB including disseminated TB or meningitis. Most TB infections are seen in children younger than 5 years and in children older than 10 years.

Clinical Findings

Symptoms of active TB pneumonia include a cough for greater than 3 weeks and fever greater than 2 weeks. Additional symptoms in children include listlessness, loss of appetite, and vomiting. TB may present with a pneumonic consolidation. Care must be taken not to confuse this with the usual pediatric pneumonia. Findings such as anemia, night sweats, and weight loss usually indicate a more indolent disease.

Treatment

Diagnosis of TB is not possible in the emergency department. Skin testing can be initiated but the tests must be read in 48 hours. Because TB pneumonia cannot be proven, routine treatment for pediatric pneumonia should be initiated in the emergency department. If tuberculosis pneumonia is suspected based on clinical findings, three steps are essential in care of the patient: (1) respiratory isolation, (2) definitive tests including skin testing, and (3) treatment with anti-TB medications. TB in young children can rapidly disseminate with serious sequelae including meningitis. Prompt initiation of therapy is critical.

The World Health Organization (WHO) publishes guidelines for the treatment of TB. First-line drugs are rifampin (RIF), isoniazid (INH), pyrazinamide (PZA), and ethambutol/ethionamide (ETH). Consultation with an infectious disease physician before initiating therapy in the emergency department is recommended.

Disposition

TB is a significant health issue as well as a serious illness for the affected patient. Children suspected of having active disease should be admitted to the hospital and treatment initiated. Follow-up should be ensured on low-risk patients who are discharged. The patient's social circumstances frequently pose difficulties for treatment compliance and disease containment.

ACUTE RESPIRATORY DISTRESS SYNDROME

Acute lung injury follows a direct pulmonary or systemic insult resulting in injury to the alveolar-capillary unit. It causes an acute onset of hypoxemia with poor lung compliance and high work of breathing. Acute respiratory distress syndrome (ARDS) is caused by a number of etiologies, typically infectious (pneumonia, sepsis) or aspiration. Treatment of the condition often requires aggressive and intensive therapy.

Clinical Findings

ARDS usually presents within 72 hours of a serious illness or injury. The disease can progress gradually or in fulminant fashion with diffuse lung edema leading to respiratory distress and hypoxemia. Patients often require intubation. They can be particularly difficult to oxygenate and often require advanced ventilation strategies.

Treatment

The treatment for ARDS is supportive with particular attention to ventilation. The underlying cause must be identified and treated.

Disposition

All children presenting with ARDS need to be admitted to a pediatric ICU.

Baraldi E, Filippone M: Chronic lung disease after premature birth. *N Engl J Med.* 2007;357:1946-1955 [PMID: 17989387].

Choi J, Lee GL: Common pediatric respiratory emergencies. *Emerg Med Clin North Am.* 2012;30:529-563 [PMID: 22487117].

Dawood FS, Fiore A, Kamimoto L, et al: Burden of seasonal influenza hospitalization in children, United States, 2003 to 2008. *J Pediatr.* 2010;157:808 [PMID: 20580018].

Dell S, Cernelc-Kohan M, Hagood JS: Diffuse and interstitial lung disease and childhood rheumatologic disorders. *Curr Opin Rheumatol.* 2012;24:530-540 [PMID: 22820514].

Flume PA, Van Devanter DR: State of progress in treating cystic fibrosis respiratory disease. *BMC Med.* 2012;10:88 [PMID: 22883684].

Goss CH, Ratjen F: Update in cystic fibrosis 2012. *Am J Respir Crit Care Med.* 2013;187:915-919 [PMID: 23634859].

Guibas GV, Makris M, Papadopoulos NG: Acute asthma exacerbations in childhood: Risk factors, prevention and treatment. *Expert Rev Respir Med.* 2012;6:629-638 [PMID: 23234449].

Iroh Tam PY: Approach to common bacterial infections: Community-acquired pneumonia. *Pediatr Clin North Am.* 2013;60: 437-453 [PMID: 23481110].

Miller EK, Bugna J, Libster R, et al: Human rhinoviruses in severe respiratory disease in very low birth weight infants. *Pediatrics.* 2012;129:e60-e67 [PMID: 22201153].

Monagle P: Diagnosis and management of deep venous thrombosis and pulmonary embolism in neonates and children. *Semin Thromb Hemost.* 2012;38:683-690 [PMID: 23034828].

Nagakumar P, Doull I: Current therapy for bronchiolitis. *Arch Dis Child.* 2012;97:827-830 [PMID: 22734014].

Perez-Velez CM: Pediatric tuberculosis: New guidelines and recommendations. *Curr Opin Pediatr.* 2012;24:319-328 [PMID: 22568943].

Prabhakaran P: Acute respiratory distress syndrome. *Indian Pediatr.* 2010;47:861-868 [PMID: 21048239].

Saleeb SF, Li WY, Warren SZ, et al: Effectiveness of screening for life-threatening chest pain in children. *Pediatrics.* 2011;128:e1062-8 [PMID: 21987702].

Silvennoinen H, Peltola V, Lehtinen P, et al: Clinical presentation of influenza in unselected children treated as outpatients. *Pediatr Infect Dis J.* 2009;28:372-375 [PMID: 19295464].

Snyder J, Fisher D: Pertussis in childhood. *Pediatr Rev.* 2012;33: 412-420 [PMID: 22939025].

Timmons O: Infection in pediatric acute respiratory distress syndrome. *Semin Pediatr Infect Dis.* 2006;17:65-71 [PMID:16822468].

World Health Organization. *Treatment of Tuberculosis: Guidelines.* Available at http://whqlibdoc.who.int/publications/2010/9789241547833_eng.pdf. Geneva, Switzerland, 2010. Accessed August 29, 2012.

Cardiac Emergencies

Douglas Patton, MD
Eric William Stern, MD

EMERGENCY MANAGEMENT OF CARDIAC DISORDERS

Cardiac emergencies in children are relatively common with congenital heart defects affecting approximately 1% of live births, not accounting for bicuspid aortic valve, which affects approximately 1% of children. In addition, children with structurally normal hearts may have electrophysiologic disturbances that manifest throughout childhood into adulthood, and may acquire heart diseases such as rheumatic fever and myocarditis. Because early in infancy the initial presentation of cardiac disease may be nonspecific, a wide differential should be entertained, including a concern for neonatal sepsis. A family history of sudden cardiac death and congenital heart disease should be obtained. Careful attention to the history and physical examination is essential for the clinician to recognize patterns of illness that may suggest a cardiac etiology for the patient's presentation.

Clinical Findings

In infants, the most serious congenital heart defects generally present during the first days to 2 weeks of life with cyanosis, congestive heart failure, audible murmurs, and feeding difficulties. In infants, pulmonary volume overload often manifests as wheezing on the lung examination. In children, rales are uncommonly heard acutely and if heard on auscultation represent a very late finding. The absence of an audible murmur most definitely does not rule out the presence of significant cardiac pathology. Later presentations of cardiac disease may manifest in children as palpitations, tachycardia, diaphoresis, tachypnea, hyperpnea, syncope, and, in older children, chest pain.

History and physical examination as well as age of the child may suggest cardiac disease to the clinician's differential diagnosis. Congenital heart defects may present during stereotyped times during infancy as outlined in Table 35–1.

In general, more severe cases of each abnormality will present earlier than milder forms of each disease.

Chest x-ray and electrocardiogram (ECG) are the most important basic studies in evaluating heart disease in children. Although the large cardiothymic silhouette in infants may confuse the diagnostic picture, cardiomegaly on chest radiographs in children should always raise the suspicion for underlying cardiac disease. Pulmonary vascular congestion and volume overload may be very difficult to discriminate from findings of bronchiolitis or other primary pulmonary infection in young children. ECG findings of chamber enlargement or axis deviation should be noted, and rhythm disturbances should be acknowledged and treated as the clinical situation demands.

Laboratory studies to consider include complete blood count (CBC) and metabolic panels, and blood, urine, and cerebrospinal fluid (CSF) cultures should be obtained if sepsis or meningitis is in the differential diagnosis. Because intercurrent respiratory infections may lead to increased pulmonary pressures and may precipitate the decompensation of previously compensated congenital heart conditions, the clinician may consider the testing of nasal secretions for common respiratory viruses. There are clinical situations where the troponin and brain natriuretic peptide (BNP) should be sent in consultation with a pediatric cardiologist; however, these studies are not routine in the evaluation of undifferentiated pediatric patients in the emergency department. The ultimate noninvasive study for the evaluation of heart disease in young children is two-dimensional echocardiography; however, as pediatric echocardiography is rarely available in most community emergency department settings, this remains a study usually confined to the pediatric specialty hospital setting.

Treatment

Pediatric patients with suspected heart disease, as with all patients seen by the emergency physician, require initial

Table 35–1. Congenital heart defects presenting during infancy.

Birth to 2 wk	Hypoplastic left heart syndrome Severe aortic coarctation Severe aortic stenosis Transposition of the great vessels Total anomalous pulmonary venous return Truncus arteriosus
1–4 wk	Ventricular septal defect Patent ductus arteriosus
6 wk to 6 mo	Coronary artery anomalies Truncus arteriosus
Older than 6 mo	Atrial septal defect Isolated valvular lesions Milder aortic coarctation

stabilization prior to transfer to pediatric specialty services. If the patient has a tenuous respiratory status or mentation and long transport times to definitive care, it may be prudent to electively intubate prior to transport. Initial support of oxygenation and ventilation may be accomplished by blow-by oxygenation, high-flow nasal cannula, or if available and indicated, bubble continuous positive airway pressure (CPAP). However, oxygen delivery devices such as the nasal cannula or oxygen mask may irritate the child and lead to increased respiratory effort.

In patients with hemodynamic compromise, intravenous (IV) access should be obtained, and if there is difficulty in establishing working IV access, it may be necessary to insert an umbilical catheter or intraosseous line. Rhythm disturbances leading to cardiovascular compromise or collapse should be treated. In some patients inotropic or pressor support may be indicated.

Disposition

Care of children with cardiac emergencies is best accomplished in a multidisciplinary manner, with early involvement of in-house or receiving facility pediatric intensive care physicians and cardiologists.

Hsu DT, Canter CE: Dilated cardiomyopathy and heart failure in children. *Heart Fail Clin.* 2010;6:415-432 [PMID: 20869643].

Rao PS: Diagnosis and management of cyanotic congenital heart disease: Part 1. *Indian J Pediatr.* 2009;76:57-70 [PMID: 19391004].

Rao PS: Diagnosis and management of cyanotic congenital heart disease: Part 2. *Indian J Pediatr.* 2009;76:297-308 [PMID: 19347670].

Yee L: Cardiac emergencies in the first year of life. *Emerg Med Clin North Am.* 2007;25:981-1008 [PMID: 17950133].

EMERGENCY MANAGEMENT OF SPECIFIC CARDIAC DISORDERS

CONGENITAL HEART DISEASE

Approximately 1% of live-born infants have congenital heart disease. Neonates with critical disease are symptomatic and identified shortly after birth. However, less critical patients are often not diagnosed until after they leave the hospital and present to the emergency department. There are a great number of congenital cardiac disorders and defects, and it is neither likely nor necessary for the emergency physician to have a rote memory of all. The emergency physician should be familiar with the basic patterns of pathophysiology possible with congenital cardiac conditions, and the physical, laboratory, and radiologic findings one might expect with each.

Clinical Findings

More severe manifestations of severe congenital cardiac defects present earlier in infancy. Severe congenital heart disease often presents at or shortly after birth with neonatal distress, cyanosis or heart failure, and respiratory failure. During the neonatorum and early infancy, cyanosis, apparent life-threatening events (ALTEs), failure to thrive, or distress with feedings, and respiratory failure are common presentations of congenital heart disease.

Congestive heart failure in infants may present with seemingly primary pulmonary symptoms such as cyanosis, tachypnea, hyperpnea, and wheezing, and such presentations in young infants should raise a suspicion for potential of congenital heart disease. Volume overload in infants often presents with wheezing in contrast to rales as a primary physical finding; however, absence of rales or a murmur on physical examination does not rule out significant cardiac pathology.

Congenital disorders may have right-to-left or left-to-right shunting. Classically, one might expect a patient with right-to-left shunting to present with cyanosis as a predominant symptom and similarly for a patient with left-to-right shunting to present with congestive heart failure. The hyperoxia test is a classically taught exercise that may help to discriminate pulmonary cyanosis from cardiac cyanosis. When confronted with a patient with significant cyanosis, application of 100% oxygen therapy may resolve the cyanosis, which increases the likelihood that the systemic deoxygenation is due to a primary pulmonary issue. If application of 100% oxygen des not improve the cyanosis, a cardiac cause for the cyanotic disorder is more likely. However, there is considerable overlap that is possible in presenting symptoms, and conditions such as anemia may blunt the appearance of cyanosis.

In addition to shunting, congenital cardiac conditions present with ductal-dependent or ductal-independent blood flow to the pulmonary or systemic circulation.

Table 35–2. Classification of ductal-related congenital heart disease.

Ductal-independent mixing lesions	Truncus arteriosus D transposition of the great vessels Total anomalous pulmonary venous return
Ductal-dependent pulmonary blood flow	Tetralogy of Fallot with pulmonary atresia Ebstein abnormality Critical pulmonary stenosis Heterotaxy
Ductal-dependent systemic blood flow	Hypoplastic left heart syndrome Interrupted aortic arch Critical aortic coarctation Critical aortic stenosis TVA with transposition

Ductal-dependent lesions commonly present with acute deterioration at the expected time of the closing of the ductus arteriosus. Examples of the classification are listed in Table 35–2.

For patients presenting with potential congenital cardiac disease, a full history and physical examination are the most important portions of the evaluation. Careful attention should be paid to determine the details of the patient's breathing and feeding behaviors. Complete vital signs should be obtained, including blood pressures in all extremities, as well as central and peripheral perfusion. Blood work should be obtained including CBC, complete metabolic panels, urine and blood cultures, as well as potentially troponin and BNP studies. Respiratory viral panels may be obtained to determine if intercurrent infectious illness is contributing to a decompensation of a previously compensated congenital heart condition.

Chest x-ray should be obtained and evaluated for signs of volume overload and cardiomegaly. Chest radiography should be interpreted with caution, as the cardiothymic silhouette in infants may mimic cardiomegaly, and volume overload and bronchiolitic lung markings can appear remarkably similar. In suspected cases of congenital heart disease, noninvasive 2D echocardiography is invaluable and the most accessible means to determine cardiac structure and function. If available, echocardiography should be obtained emergently in consultation with a pediatric cardiologist. After being stabilized, the patient with congenital heart disorder may need to undergo more advanced diagnostic studies such as cardiac catheterization or magnetic resonance imaging (MRI).

Treatment

Decompensated patients with congenital heart disorders require emergent stabilization in the emergency department contemporaneously with diagnostic evaluation. Cyanotic patients in extremis should receive oxygen, however patients not acutely decompensated with known standing congenital defects may be adversely affected by excess administration of oxygen. Patients with known cardiac defects who are at or near their baseline oxygenation status and not in extremis should not receive oxygen in excess of their baseline requirements.

The classic cyanotic crisis of tetralogy of Fallot provides a window into the treatment of cyanotic heart disease. Patients with a "tet spell" have an acute cyanotic crisis that often they are able to "break" on their own. In the emergency department, patients with refractory tet spells may initially be approached gently by medical professionals. Patients may be encouraged to stay in their caregiver's arms. Blow-by oxygen may be administered, and if the cyanosis does not improve, morphine may be administered subcutaneously. In rare cases of completely refractory tet spells, it may be necessary to obtain IV access and use of agents that increase the systemic vascular resistance and decrease the right-to-left shunting, such as phenylephrine, may be indicated.

Patients with congestive heart failure may require aggressive ventilatory support, such as high-flow nasal oxygen, bubble CPAP, and ultimately endotracheal intubation. Patients with cyanosis secondary to severe right-to-left shunting may not have resolution of the cyanosis with endotracheal intubation. Ductal-dependent lesions often present with decompensation early after birth at the time of closure of the ductus, and stabilization of the open ductus may improve the patient's clinical condition. In decompensated patients with suspected congenital heart defects in the first week of life that may be ductal dependent, rapid administration of prostaglandin E_1 (PGE_1) may be lifesaving, and the PGE_1 drip may act to stabilize the ductus until surgical palliation may be achieved. PGE can be administered at 0.05-0.1 mcg/kg/min IV. Most common side effect of PGE is apnea, which may necessitate endotracheal intubation and mechanical ventilation.

Disposition

In patients with decompensated congenital heart disease, early involvement of neonatal and pediatric intensive care physician as well as pediatric cardiologist are essential to guide treatment. In community centers, stabilization should be followed by rapid transport to a pediatric specialty hospital.

INFECTIOUS ENDOCARDITIS

Endocarditis, inflammation of the heart lining and valves, usually arises from tissue insult, whether from turbulent flow, direct trauma, or other process that leads to formation of a sterile thrombus. It is this clot that becomes colonized with bacteria, causing fibrin and platelet deposition and leading to vegetation growth.

Infective endocarditis (IE) most commonly presents in patients with structural heart disease, indwelling devices, or a history of injection drug use. Diabetes, kidney disease, congenital heart disease, and recent instrumentation are additional risk factors for IE.

Clinical Findings

IE should be considered in a patient with unexplained fever or signs of unexplained systemic illness such as night sweats. A thorough evaluation consists of a careful history, examination of skin, mucous membranes and extremities, and thorough cardiac auscultation.

Modified Duke criteria remain the diagnostic criteria of choice for suspected IE. Two major criteria are needed to diagnose IE, and the combination of one major and three minor criteria, or five minor criteria (Table 35–3).

Table 35–3. Duke criteria for infective endocarditis.

Major Criteria

Two blood cultures positive for infective endocarditis drawn > 12 h apart

- Viridans streptococci, *Streptococcus bovis*, HACEK group, *Staphylococcus aureus*
- Community-acquired enterococci with no focal infection
- Single positive blood culture for *Coxiella burnetii* or antiphase I IgG antibody titer > 1:800

Echocardiogram evidence of endocardial involvement

- Oscillating intracardiac mass on a valve or on supporting structures, in the path of regurgitant jets, or on implanted material, in the absence of an alternative anatomic explanation
- Myocardial abscess
- New partial dehiscence of prosthetic valve
- New onset valvular regurgitation (worsening or changing of preexisting murmur not sufficient)

Minor Criteria

- Predisposing heart condition or history of injection drug use
- Fever
- Vascular phenomena, major arterial emboli, septic pulmonary infarcts, mycotic aneurysm, intracranial hemorrhage, conjunctival hemorrhages, and Janeway lesions
- Immunologic phenomena: glomerulonephritis, Osler nodes, Roth spots, rheumatoid factor
- Microbiological evidence of a positive blood culture but does not meet a major criterion as noted above or serological evidence of active infection with organism consistent with infective endocarditis

Presence of one major and two or three minor criteria confirms the diagnosis of possible endocarditis (PE). Patients with PE should be treated as patients with IE until alternative diagnosis is confirmed, or if symptoms resolve within 4 days after the start of antibiotic therapy.

A patient with IE or PE should be evaluated further with comprehensive laboratory testing, including urinalysis (UA), cross-reactive protein (CRP), erythrocyte sedimentation rate (ESR), CBC, and three blood cultures drawn from three separate sites, preferably before antibiotic therapy is begun. ECG should be performed, especially if no baseline study is available, and echocardiography should take place as soon as it is available.

Treatment

Most patients with IE can be managed with antibiotic therapy alone; however, because most agents penetrate heart vegetations poorly, protracted therapies are usually necessary. IV formulations, tailored to blood culture sensitivities, are usually indicated in order to maintain effective titers. When prospective clinical data is limited, the combination of an aminoglycoside and a methicillin-resistant *Staphylococcus aureus* (MRSA)-active agent such as vancomycin forms a reasonable empiric first-line therapy until sensitivities are available.

Congestive heart failure, usually due to aortic valve dysfunction, occurs in more than 50% of IE patients. Approximately 50% of those patients will require surgery; therefore, early consultation with a cardiothoracic surgeon is advised. Medical management is required in these patients for optimal results. Intracardiac abscess is another common IE complication, and when related to the aortic valve, the conduction system can become involved, causing heart block. Accurate diagnosis usually requires transesophageal echocardiography (TEE). Surgical intervention is the only effective therapy.

Between 20 and 50% of IE patients will suffer embolic events, as vegetations grow and fragment; however, decision to begin anticoagulation therapy should be made in conjunction with a surgeon, as intervention is frequently required.

Disposition

Children presenting to the emergency department with a strong suspicion for IE require admission for additional diagnostic testing and treatment in consultation with infectious disease specialist and cardiologist.

KAWASAKI DISEASE

Kawasaki disease (KD) is an acute systemic vasculitis most commonly found in children aged 6 months to 5 years and remains the most common cause of acquired heart disease in children. No definitive cause of the disease has been identified, therefore KD remains a clinical diagnosis, and should be considered in a child with prolonged fever. KD affects multiple organ systems; however, the most feared complication of KD is coronary artery aneurysm (CAA), which can lead to fatal thrombosis. With treatment, the aneurysm formation rate in KD drops from approximately 20% to less than 5%. As a result, prompt diagnosis and management of the disease is vital.

Clinical Findings

In a child with fever for more than 5 days, diagnosis of KD can be made with four of the following five clinical features: bilateral conjunctival infection; a change in mucous membranes (red, fissured or infected lips, tongue, cheek); a change in the extremities (erythema or edema of feet, hands); a polymorphous rash; and cervical lymphadenopathy.

Incomplete KD diagnosis is made if there are two or three criteria present, and the triad of conjunctivitis, mucous membrane involvement, and rash may increase sensitivity to the disease. Serum ESR, CRP, and BNP should be drawn and patients with diagnosis of full or incomplete disease should receive a prompt echocardiogram. As with any acutely ill patient, abnormal vital signs should be addressed and volume status should be assessed and managed appropriately in the emergency department.

Treatment

After diagnosis of full or incomplete KD is made, the mainstay of treatment includes high-dose (2 g/kg) intravenous immunoglobulin (IVIG) given over 12 hours, with high-dose (80-100 mg/kg/day) aspirin divided into four doses. Addition of methylprednisolone may improve outcomes; however, its use is controversial, and therefore is reserved for patients whose symptoms fail to respond to initial treatment. Prompt ECG should be performed to provide a baseline for the necessary follow-up studies.

Disposition

Patients with KD should be admitted for administration of IVIG and observation.

MYOCARDITIS

Myocarditis, inflammation of the myocardium, is often viral and self-limiting. Etiologies range from protozoan (trypanosoma cruzii) to certain drug toxicities. Most infections resolve completely without therapy; however, evidence of chronic myocarditis appears in 10% of unrelated autopsies, which indicates that the disease is far more common than previously suspected. Up to 20% of sudden infant death syndrome

(SIDS) had evidence of myocarditis on postmortem endocardial biopsy.

Clinical Findings

Symptoms of viral myocarditis range from trivial to shock, depending upon the extent of myocyte infiltration of the cardiac muscle. Most patients experience prodromal symptoms typical of upper respiratory infection (URI) or gastrointestinal illness. As a result, 83% of myocarditis patients receive an alternative diagnosis on their first visit. As myocardial damage progresses, symptoms of cardiac stress may emerge, including shortness of breath, chest pain, reduced urine output, and other symptoms of heart failure.

The disease often takes an indolent course; however, progression can occasionally be exceedingly rapid. Initial studies should include ECG, although no criteria have proved sensitive or specific for the disease. In children, however, the presence of T-wave inversions, ST-segment elevations, or other signs of cardiac ischemia warrant further investigation. Troponin elevations are common, but by no means universal, and echocardiography is typically abnormal but nonspecific. Although endocardial biopsy is the gold standard, it continues to suffer from low sensitivity due to the patchy nature of the disease. Cardiac MRI is reported to be highly sensitive and specific, if available. The diagnosis of myocarditis remains a clinical one, and therapy should be initiated based on the patient's presentation.

Treatment

Initial treatment is typically symptom based. Patients presenting in acute heart failure should be stabilized immediately through afterload reduction, including diuresis and vasodilation. Routine use of steroids and other immune modulators is controversial, and the traditional administration of IVIG (2 g/kg in the first 24 hours), although likely safe, there is insufficient evidence at present to support its high cost. Interferon-beta shows promise, particularly against enteroviral and adenoviral illnesses but similarly lacks adequate trials in children to recommend it at this time. Digoxin should be used with caution, as it has the potential to increase inflammatory mediators.

Approximately 12-40% of patients with myocarditis will progress to dilated cardiomyopathy, with a higher percentage presenting in early, fulminant disease. If the patient fails the above therapies, a ventricular assist device may be necessary to maintain perfusion. Extracorporeal membrane oxygenation (ECMO) has been used with success.

Chronic active myocarditis is the persistence of symptoms for 3 months after resolution of the acute phase of the illness; however, most patients will completely resolve within 2 years. Among patients who continue to deteriorate, heart transplant may be the only long-term option, with a 15-year mortality rate of 50%.

Disposition

Children diagnosed with myocarditis should be admitted to the hospital, even with mild symptoms. Rapid progression to severe heart failure and/or hemodynamic collapse may occur. Consultation with a cardiologist is indicated in all patients and transfer to a facility with a pediatric intensive care unit (PICU) and cardiology care should occur if the services are not available locally.

ACUTE PERICARDITIS

Acute pericarditis is caused by various infectious and inflammatory mediators that produce pericardial irritation. Viral infections are a common cause of pericarditis. Other etiologies are bacterial or fungal infections, autoimmune disorders, trauma, uremia, malignancy, radiation, and drug effects.

Clinical Findings

Classic presentation in verbal patients consists of sharp or stabbing chest pain that may be pleuritic in nature, worsened by the recumbent position, and improved with sitting upright. Patients with acute uncomplicated pericarditis generally do not appear toxic or lethargic.

There is a stereotyped pattern of ECG changes in pericarditis; however, 50% of patients go through all four ECG pattern changes (Figure 35–1). The first stage consists of generalized concave upward ST-segment elevation accompanied by PR depression. This is followed by normalization of the ST-segments with flattening of the T waves. Later, the T waves may invert without Q-wave formation, before the ECG returns to normal. When interpreting pediatric ECGs, the clinician must remember the normal pediatric T-wave pattern. In all ECGs performed for pericarditis, the clinician should look for electrical alternans as an ominous sign of pericardial tamponade. The physician should document the presence or absence of other signs of cardiac tamponade, such as jugular venous distension. The presence or absence of a pericardial friction rub should be noted.

Pericarditis is a clinical diagnosis. Blood work, if sent, may demonstrate an increase in the white blood cell count and a concomitant increase in inflammatory markers. Acute uncomplicated pericarditis should not cause significant elevation of the serum troponin or BNP. In acute uncomplicated pericarditis, chest radiography should be normal. Cardiomegaly, a "bottle-shaped" cardiothymic silhouette should raise the clinician's suspicion for complications such as pericardial tamponade and congestive heart failure. Bedside echocardiography may demonstrate no effusion to

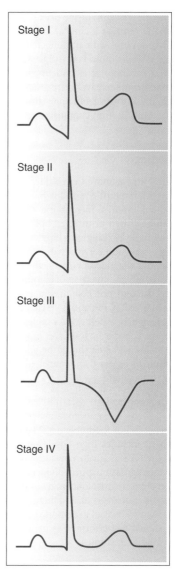

▲ **Figure 35–1.** Electrocardiogram findings in four stages of pericarditis.

a small pericardial effusion in acute uncomplicated pericarditis. The presence of a large effusion, right ventricular collapse, or other findings of tamponade indicate complicated disease and the need for emergent intervention.

Treatment

Nonsteroidal anti-inflammatory drugs (NSAIDS) are the mainstay of therapy. Most patients with even a small pericardial effusion should be admitted for observation. Patients at risk for tamponade should be stabilized in consultation with a thoracic surgeon. Patients with tamponade and cardiovascular collapse should undergo emergent thoracotomy or pericardiocentesis. Patients with tamponade or impending tamponade require pericardial drainage prior to transfer to a receiving facility for definitive care.

Disposition

Acute uncomplicated pericarditis can generally be managed as outpatient in healthy immunocompetent patients. Fever, trauma, subacute onset, immunocompromise, presence of oral anticoagulant therapy, significant effusion, tamponade, and NSAID treatment failure are indications for inpatient treatment.

ELECTROPHYSIOLOGIC DISORDERS

Arrhythmias are relatively common in children and may occur in the presence of known cardiac defects or may occur in a structurally normal heart. Common dysrhythmias seen in children presenting to emergency departments are sinus tachycardia (50%), SVT (13%), bradycardia (6%), and atrial fibrillation (4.6%).

Clinical Findings

Arrhythmias may present in infants as fussiness, crying, difficulty feeding, respiratory difficulty, or diaphoresis. In older children, a history of palpitations or chest pain may be obtained. Syncope in a pediatric patient is always concerning for a possible underlying electrophysiologic disorder. Family history of sudden cardiac death should be noted. Severe dysrhythmias may present as cardiovascular collapse, congestive heart failure, or hypotension. Postoperative patients with congenital heart defects may be at increased risk for arrhythmias. Patients may present in normal sinus rhythm after experiencing symptoms of an arrhythmia.

The ECG is the mainstay of diagnosis of any electrophysiological disturbance. In patients who arrive after the arrhythmia has abated, the ECG may reveal the presence of an underlying electrophysiologic disorder such as Wolf-Parkinson-White (WPW) syndrome. Patients may benefit from event or Holter monitoring in the inpatient or outpatient setting. In patients with tachydysrhythmias, the physician must first ascertain the electrical origin of the arrhythmia and whether it is narrow or wide complex. Wide complex tachycardias such as supraventricular tachycardia (SVT) with aberrancy or ventricular tachycardia (VT) are quite alarming, and VT may cause hemodynamic instability. Narrow complex tachydysrhythmias are more common in children and may be stable or unstable. Bradydysrhythmias are less common but may present with impaired perfusion. Electrophysiologic causes of syncope with associated ECG findings after the arrhythmia has abated are listed in (Table 35–4).

Table 35–4. Common electrophysiological causes of syncope.

Wolf-Parkinson-White syndrome	Delta wave: slurred upstroke of QRS complex Shortened PR interval
Hypertrophic obstructive cardiomyopathy	Left ventricular hypertrophy Possible strain pattern
Long QTc syndrome	Prolonged QTc interval (usually > 480-500 msec)
Brugada syndrome	Type 1: Precordial J point elevation with coved ST-segment and inverted T wave Type 2: Precordial "saddleback" ST-segment elevation Type 3: Precordial ST-segment elevation < 1 mm

Treatment

Unstable tachydysrhythmias require immediate electrical cardioversion. Significant bradydysrhythmias with impaired perfusion may require electrical pacing or pharmocologic management with adrenergic agents or atropine. Stable narrow complex tachydysrhythmias may be terminated with adenosine. In children less than 50 kg give 0.05-0.1 mg/kg one time dose. If the arrhythmia persists increase the dose by 0.05-0.2 mg/kg. Children more than 50 kg should receive the adult dose of 6 mg followed by 12 mg X 2 as needed to terminate the arrhythmia. Beta blockers and calcium channel blockers are effective in narrow complex tachycardias but should be avoided in patients with WPW syndrome. If adenosine fails to terminate narrow complex tachydysrhythmias, sedation and electrical cardioversion may be attempted.

Stable wide complex tachydysrhythmias may be treated pharmacologically with agents such as amiodarone. Serious electrophysiologic disorders such as Brugada syndrome must be recognized immediately by the emergency physician, and these patients should be admitted to the intensive care setting until an AICD can be placed, as the risk of sudden cardiac death is enormous. Early consultation with pediatric intensive care and cardiology teams is essential.

Disposition

Children with stable narrow complex tachycardias that are terminated with treatment in the emergency department can be safely discharged after a brief observation. Referral to a cardiologist for follow-up evaluation is important. Patients with unstable narrow complex, wide complex tachycardias (stable or unstable), and bradydysrhythmias should be admitted or transferred depending on availability of consultation with a cardiologist and intensive care services.

Baltimore R: New recommendations for the prevention of infective endocarditis. *Curr Opin Pediatr.* 2008;20:85-89 [PMID: 18197045].

Berger S, Dubin AM: Arrhythmogenic forms of heart failure in children. *Heart Fail Clin.* 2010;6:471-481 [PMID: 20869647].

Biondi EA: Focus on diagnosis: Cardiac arrhythmias in children. *Pediatr Rev.* 2010;31:375-379 [PMID: 20810702].

Dominguez SR, Anderson MS, Eladawy M, et al: Preventing coronary artery abnormalities: A need for earlier diagnosis and treatment of Kawasaki disease. *Pediatr Infect Dis J.* 2012;3:1217-1220 [PMID: 22760536].

Doniger SJ, Sharieff GQ: Pediatric dysrhythmias. *Pediatr Clin North Am.* 2006;53:85-105 [PMID: 16487786].

Durani Y, Giordano K, Goudie BW: Myocarditis and pericarditis in children. *Pediatr Clin North Am.* 2010;57:1281-1303 [PMID: 21111118].

Duro RP, Moura C, Leite-Moreira A: Anatomophysiologic basis of tetralogy of Fallot and its clinical implications. *Rev Port Cardiol.* 2010;29:591-630 [PMID: 20734579].

Fischer JW, Cho CS. Pediatric syncope: Cases from the emergency department. *Emerg Med Clin North Am.* 2010;28:501-516 [PMID: 20709241].

Hoyer A, Silberbach M: Infective endocarditis. *Pediatr Rev.* 2005;26:394-400 [PMID: 16264027].

Knirsch W, Nadal D: Infective endocarditis in congenital heart disease. *Eur J Pediatr.* 2011;170:1111-1127 [PMID: 21773669].

Levine MC, Klugman D, Teach SJ: Update on myocarditis in children. *Curr Opin Pediatr.* 2010;22:278-283 [PMID: 20414115].

Luca NJ, Yeung RS: Epidemiology and management of Kawasaki disease. *Drugs.* 2012;72(8):1029-1038 [PMID: 22621692].

May LJ, Patton DJ, Fruitman DS: The evolving approach to pediatric myocarditis: A review of the current literature. *Cardiol Young.* 2011;21:241-251 [PMID: 21272427].

McDonald JR: Acute infective endocarditis. *Infect Dis Clin North Am.* 2009;23:643-664 [PMID: 19665088].

National Institute for Health and Clinical Excellence (NICE): *Feverish Illness in Children: Assessment and Initial Management in Children Younger than 5 years.* Available at http://www.nice.org.uk/nicemedia/pdf/CG47Guidance.pdf. London, UK, 2007. Accessed August 14, 2013.

Payne L, Zeigler VL, Gilette PC: Acute cardiac arrhythmias following surgery for congenital heart disease: Mechanisms, diagnostic tools, and management. *Crit Care Nurs Clin North Am.* 2011:23:255-272. [PMID: 21624689].

Pierce D, Calkins BC, Thornton K: Infectious endocarditis: Diagnosis and treatment. *Am Fam Physician.* 2012;85:981-986 [PMID: 22612050].

Rowley AH, Shulman ST: Pathogenesis and management of Kawasaki disease. *Expert Rev Anti Infect Ther.* 2010;8:197-203 [PMID: 20109049].

Scuccimarri R: Kawasaki disease. *Pediatr Clin N Am.* 2012;59:425-445 [PMID: 22560578].

Sharkey AM and Sharma A: Tetralogy of Fallot: Anatomic variants and their impact on surgical management. *Semin Cardiothorac Vasc Anesth.* 2012;16:88-96 [PMID: 22275348].

Simpson KE, Canter CE: Acute myocarditis in children. *Expert Rev Cardiovasc Ther.* 2011;9:771-783 [PMID: 21714608].

Williams GD, Hammer GB: Cardiomyopathy in childhood. *Curr Opin Anaesthesiol.* 2011;24:289-300 [PMID: 21478741].

Zheng J, Yao Y, Han L, et al: Renal function and injury in infants and young children with congenital heart disease. *Pediatr Nephrol.* 2012;28:99-104 [PMID: 22923204].

Gastrointestinal Emergencies

Pamela J. Okada, MD, FAAP, FACEP
Robert K. Minkes, MD, PhD

▼ IMMEDIATE MANAGEMENT OF SERIOUS & LIFE-THREATENING PROBLEMS

Gastrointestinal (GI) emergencies in infants and children often present similarly. Key historical facts alert the emergency physician to these surgical conditions that require immediate interventions.

PERFORM A BRIEF EXAMINATION

Determine stability of the patient.

- Develop a general impression: Is the infant or child ill appearing?
- Determine general appearance, work of breathing, and circulation to the skin:
  - General appearance includes tone, interaction, consolability, ability to gaze upon a face, and quality of cry or speech.
  - Work of breathing includes airway—is it patent and maintainable? And breathing—quality of airflow, associated sounds, use of accessory muscles, nasal flaring, and presence of grunting respirations?
  - Circulation to the skin—is the skin pale, mottled, or cyanotic?
- Obtain vital signs including oxygen saturation and blood pressure.
- Assess the abdomen: assess for signs and symptoms of an acute abdomen:
  - Abdominal skin color—pink, gray, blue.
  - Appearance—scaphoid, protuberant.
  - Assess for tenderness, guarding, and rigidity.
- If instability is suspected, begin resuscitation immediately per standard PALS guidelines.
- Treat shock:
  - Apply 100% oxygen via nonrebreathing mask or if the airway is not maintainable, prepare for rapid sequence intubation.
  - Insert two peripheral intravenous (IV) lines if possible, or an interosseous (IO) line to initiate therapy while definitive IV access is obtained.
  - Give crystalloid fluid bolus at 20 mL/kg IV or IO rapidly and repeat up to 3-4 boluses unless rales, respiratory distress, or hepatomegaly develops.

- Obtain blood samples for point-of-care glucose, venous blood gas (VBG) or arterial blood gas (ABG), lactate, ionized calcium, a complete blood cell count (CBC) with differential, blood culture, serum electrolytes, tests of renal and liver function, amylase, lipase, type and crossmatch for packed red blood cells (PRBC), urine analysis (including dipstick chemical and microscopic analysis), and urine culture.
- Treat hypoglycemia with dextrose (0.5-1 g/kg IV or IO). Use $D_{25}W$ (2-4 mL/kg) in children and adolescents; $D_{10}W$ (5-10 mL/kg) in infants and young children.
- For fluid unresponsive shock, begin vasoactive drug therapy and titrate to correct poor perfusion or hypotension.
  - Normotensive: begin dopamine (5-20 mcg/kg per min IV/IO).
  - Hypotensive vasodilated (warm) shock: begin norepinephrine (0.1-2 mcg/kg per min IV/IO).
  - Hypotensive vasoconstricted (cold) shock: begin epinephrine (0.1-1 mcg/kg per min IV/IO).
- Transfuse with PRBC to maintain hemoglobin (Hb > 10 g/dL).
- Initiate antimicrobial emergency as soon as an intra-abdominal emergency is likely. Current recommendations for community-acquired infections in the pediatric patient are listed in Table 36–1.
- Insert a nasogastric (NG) tube in infants or children with persistent vomiting, especially if vomitus is feculent or bilious; this strongly suggests an intestinal obstruction.
- Consult surgery. Infants and children with abdominal pain or an abdominal emergency may require immediate surgical evaluation. Infants with bilious emesis, a rigid abdomen, or shock and a suspected acute abdominal process, consult surgery immediately.
- Keep the child nothing by mouth (NPO) pending surgical evaluation.

FURTHER EVALUATION OF INFANT OR CHILD WITH ABDOMINAL EMERGENCY

After stabilization, obtain a more complete history, and unless the patient requires immediate surgery, obtain further diagnostic tests as indicated. Diagnostic testing is tailored

Table 36–1. Agents and regimens that may be used for the initial empiric treatment of extra-biliary complicated intra-abdominal infection.

Regimen: Community-acquired infection in pediatric patients
Single agent: Ertapenem, meropenem, imipenem-cilastatin, ticarcillin-clavulanate, and piperacillin-tazobactam
Combination: Ceftriaxone or cefotaxime or cefepime, or ceftazidime plus metronidazole; gentamicin or tobramycin plus metronidazole or clindamycin, and with or without ampicillin

according to the patient's age, history, and signs and symptoms. Abdominal emergencies in the pediatric patient are, not surprising, age related (Table 36–2).

HISTORY

Vomiting is a common complaint in the pediatric patient. Determine frequency and timing in relation to feeding, the nature of vomit (projectile or not) and its content (food, blood, bile). Vomiting that occurs within 1 hour of feeding may indicate pyloric stenosis, gastroesophageal reflux, milk intolerance, or acute gastroenteritis in infants. Vomiting hours after feeding may suggest an intestinal obstruction such as incarcerated inguinal hernia, malrotation with volvulus, or Hirschsprung disease. Vomiting associated with episodic pain may indicate intussusception.

Vomit content may help identify the location of the obstruction or problem. Bilious emesis is indicative of an obstruction distal to the sphincter of Oddi. Bilious emesis in an infant is a surgical emergency and may indicate malrotation with midgut volvulus, intestinal duplication, or meconium ileus. Feculent vomitus occurs with lower intestinal obstruction as seen in small bowel obstruction.

In older children, vomiting is most commonly associated with gastroenteritis, but if associated with vague abdominal pain or more classic, right lower quadrant (RLQ) pain, it may be early presentation of appendicitis or intussusception due to a Meckel diverticulum, lymphoma, or Henoch-Schönlein purpura creating a lead point.

Diarrhea is another common pediatric complaint. Determining timing, nature, content, and frequency, may lead to the diagnosis. Onset may be acute or chronic (> 3 wk). Chronic diarrhea may be due to malabsorption, inflammatory bowel disease, cystic fibrosis, milk allergy autoimmune disorders, and a number of metabolic diseases. Content is also helpful. Watery, explosive diarrhea is common with viral infections such as rotavirus. Bloody diarrhea may result from bacterial infection caused by *Salmonella, Shigella, Campylobacter, Yersinia,* or *Escherichia coli* 0157H7. Bloody stools indicate a lower GI bleed and may be due to something as simple as an anal fissure or more ominous abdominal

Table 36–2. Disorders causing abdominal complaints (pain, vomiting, rectal bleeding) in the pediatric patient by age.

Age: Younger than 2 yrs	
Colic	Malrotation/volvulus
Gastroesophageal reflux	Intussusception
Acute gastroenteritis	Hypertrophic pyloric stenosis
Viral syndrome	Incarcerated hernia
Milk protein allergy	Hirschsprung disease
Necrotizing enterocolitis	Appendicitis
UTI	Tumors
Age: 2-5 yrs	
Acute gastroenteritis	Meckel Diverticulum
UTI	Intussusception
Appendicitis	Hepatitis
Constipation	Inflammatory bowel disease
Viral syndrome	Choledochal cyst
	Spontaneous peritonitis
Age: 6-12 yrs	
Acute gastroenteritis	Cholecystitis
Appendicitis	Pancreatitis
UTI	Testicular torsion
Functional abdominal pain	Ovarian torsion
Constipation	Renal calculi
Viral syndrome	Tumors
Inflammatory bowel disease	
Peptic ulcer disease	
Age: Older than 12 yrs	
Acute gastroenteritis	Appendicitis
Gastritis	Pelvic inflammatory disease
Colitis	UTI
Gastroesophageal reflux disease	Viral syndrome
Peptic ulcer disease	Ovarian cyst or torsion
Constipation	

Table 36–3. Extra-abdominal causes of referred abdominal pain in children.

Group A streptococcal pharyngitis
Pneumonia
Acquired heart disease (myocarditis, pericarditis)
Aortic aneurysm
Hemolytic uremic syndrome
Diabetic ketoacidosis
Sepsis
Collagen vascular disease (Systemic lupus erythematosus,
    Henoch-Schönlein purpura)
Toxic overdose

pathology such as intussusception associated with "currant jelly" stools or malrotation with volvulus and sloughing of necrotic intestinal tissue.

Pain is difficult to assess well in infants and young children. In infants, pain may present as irritability, fussiness, and crying. Causes of abdominal pain are age-dependent and associated with common symptom patterns. A careful history will often lead to the correct diagnosis. Fussiness and crying with or without back arching (Sandifer syndrome) may indicate gastroesophageal reflux. Crying that is episodic may be due to intussusception.

Careful history taking and examination are required because abdominal pain can be due to non-GI causes such as pneumonia, urinary tract infection (UTI), an incarcerated inguinal hernia, torsion of the testes, or ovarian cysts or torsion (Table 36–3).

Obtaining a pain history in older children and adolescents is feasible. Determine if the onset was acute or gradual, the location and quality, its ability to radiate, and associated symptoms to narrow the differential. Colicky pain may be due to nephrolithiasis, cholelithiasis, or intussusception. Severe midepigastric pain may be due to pancreatitis; RUQ pain may be due to hepatitis or gall bladder disease. Gradual steady RLQ pain may be due to intestinal obstruction or appendicitis. Pain radiating to the back may be indicative of nephrolithiasis or diskitis. Gradual steady RLQ pain may be due to appendicitis or intestinal obstruction. Pelvic inflammatory disease, tubo-ovarian abscess, Fitz-Hugh and Curtis perihepatitis, endometriosis, Mittelschmerz, ectopic pregnancy, ovarian cyst, or torsion are also sources of pain to be considered. Constipation and urinary retention also cause lower or vague abdominal pain.

PHYSICAL EXAMINATION

Inspection: When the patient is stabilized, a complete physical examination can be done with particular interest to the abdominal and genitourinary system. What is the nutritional state? Are there skin findings like bruising or petechiae? What is the shape of the abdomen? What color is the abdominal wall skin?

Auscultation: Listen for bowel sounds. Absent bowel sounds are typically associated with peritonitis, and high-pitched "tinkling" sounds are associated with intestinal obstruction. In gastroenteritis, bowel sounds may be hyperactive or hypoactive due to an ileus.

Palpation: Palpation of an infant or child's abdomen provides an abundance of information, but gaining the child's trust to get to that point of the examination takes time. A few "tricks of the trade" may help with this. For the infant, have the mother hold the swaddled infant in her arms and you unwrap the blanket to expose the abdomen. Another technique is to hold the infant in your nondominant hand, and while gently rocking the infant, examine the abdomen with the dominant hand. Finally, provide a pacifier dipped in "Sweet Ease," a natural sugar that is proven to be associated with statistically and clinically significant reductions in infant discomfort. To facilitate palpation of the "olive" in suspected pyloric stenosis, examine the infant held prone to allow the "olive" to fall forward in the abdominal cavity. For the older child, use distraction techniques (toys, age-appropriate books, electronic devices). Examine first with the stethoscope to distinguish between voluntary and involuntary guarding. Having the child flex the legs at the hips and knees may aid the examination.

A hard firm or rigid painful abdomen suggests intestinal perforation and peritonitis. Pain is worse with movement, and thus these children prefer to be still.

Palpation of abdominal organs: Feel for hepatosplenomegaly. A spleen or liver tip is normally 1-2 cm below the costal margin. Common abdominal masses include the "olive" palpated on the infant's right upper abdomen indicative of pyloric stenosis, and the "sausage-shaped" mass, found in the mid to upper right abdominal area in cases of intussusceptions. Abdominal tumors may also be appreciated. Hard but moldable masses in the left lower quadrant (LLQ) are commonly retained stool and consistent with constipation.

Examination of the hernia rings and male genitalia: Remove the diaper and look for inguinal or scrotal pathology. Abdominal pain in male infants and children require examination of the inguinal and genital system to rule out incarcerated inguinal hernia, hair tourniquet injuries, and torsion of the testicle. Lower abdominal pain in adolescent females deserves a complete genital and pelvic examination.

Percussion: Percussion helps distinguish between gas (tympanitic) and fluid (dull)-filled distension. It also aids in determining spleen, liver, and bladder size. Gentle percussion over the costovertebral angles may elicit pain in children with pyelonephritis, retrocecal appendicitis, or retroperitoneal abscess. In infants and children with peritoneal irritation, gentle percussion can elicit significant pain. Vigorous percussion and even testing for rebound tenderness is unnecessary.

ABDOMINAL SIGNS

Iliopsoas sign: Supine patient holds legs in extension; flex right leg at the thigh while pushing against the resistance of the examiner's hand. If pain is elicited in the abdominal or pelvic area, the sign is positive, and may indicate a retrocecal appendicitis, retrocecal abscess, hematomas, myositis, bursitis, tendonitis, cysticercosis, and pyomyositis.

Obturator sign: Supine patient, flex knee to 90 degrees, and rotate internally and externally. Increased abdominal pain and pelvic pain indicates a positive obturator sign.

Murphy's sign: Supine patient. Examiner palpates under the right lower anterior chest wall. As the patient takes a deep breath, the gall bladder descends onto the fingers, producing pain if the gallbladder is inflamed. Often the patient will stop breathing during inspiration while the gallbladder is being palpated.

Rovsing sign: Supine patient. Palpation of the LLQ elicits pain in the RLQ. A positive sign is seen in appendicitis.

Heel tap: Supine patient, elevate right leg 10-20 degrees, and firmly tap the bottom of the foot with the examiner's palm. A positive test elicits pain in the abdomen and is concerning for peritoneal irritation.

Markle sign: Supine patient, slowly palpate on the four areas of the abdomen. Pull suddenly away and if the patient experiences pain, this is rebound. A positive test indicates peritoneal irritation.

McBurney point: A point two-thirds the distance (from the umbilicus) on a line between the umbilicus and the right superior anterior iliac spine. Tenderness at this point suggests appendicitis.

LABORATORY EXAMINATION

Routine laboratory studies are not indicated in the evaluation of all infants or children with an abdominal complaint. Obtain laboratory studies in patients who are ill-appearing or in shock (Table 36–4). Urinalysis (dipstick, chemical, and microscopic analysis) and culture may provide the highest yield in well-appearing patients, even in those who present without a fever. Electrolyte, renal function, liver function, and glucose may be important if there is associated vomiting, diarrhea, or signs of dehydration. Point-of-care glucose testing is useful in infants because they have lower glycogen stores and are at risk for hypoglycemia with lack of adequate oral intake. Point-of-care glucose is useful because

Table 36–4. Helpful laboratory studies in the unstable pediatric patient with acute abdominal complaint.

Complete blood cell count (CBC) with differential
Blood culture
Electrolytes
Blood urea nitrogen
Serum creatinine
Amylase/ lipase
Glucose
Liver function tests (AST, ALT, bilirubin)
Prothrombin time/partial thromboplastin time
International normalized ratio (INR)
Fibrin split products
Fibrinogen
ABG or mixed VBG
Lactate
Urinalysis, urine culture
Urine pregnancy test
Stool studies
Type and crossmatched blood

abdominal pain, vomiting, and dehydration will often be the predominant symptoms in children presenting in diabetic ketoacidosis (DKA).

CBCs with differential may be helpful. Hemoconcentration may signify volume contraction and anemia may indicate acute blood loss. White blood cell count may be helpful if elevated (infection) or significantly decreased (viral suppression, sepsis, or DIC); however, normal counts do not rule out a surgical abdominal process.

Amylase and lipase may be elevated in children with pancreatitis. Elevated serum lipase levels are helpful in distinguishing peptic ulcer disease from pancreatitis. Serum amylase may be elevated in other disease processes such as obstruction, perforated viscous, renal failure, and ectopic pregnancy.

Liver function tests may be helpful in children and adolescents with RUQ tenderness, jaundice, or tea-colored urine.

Urinalysis will help identify UTI, urolithiasis, new-onset diabetes or DKA, renal disease, and pyuria seen in pelvic inflammatory disease.

Pregnancy test should be obtained for all adolescent girls of childbearing age.

RADIOLOGICAL STUDIES

Routine radiological studies are not indicated in the evaluation of all infants and children with an abdominal complaint. However, worrisome signs and symptoms coupled with a thorough history may not definitively identify the source of the problem; therefore, radiographic studies can aid in

Table 36–5. Helpful radiological studies.

Symptoms	Disease	Helpful Studies
Vomiting	Pyloric stenosis	Ultrasonography (US)
Vomiting, abdominal pain	Intussusception	Abdominal US, air contrast enema
Bilious emesis	Malrotation w volvulus	US, UGI
Constipation, distention	Hirschsprung disease	Barium enema
Pain		
Right upper	Cholecystitis	RUQ sonogram
	Biliary colic	RUQ sonogram
	Hepatitis	RUQ sonogram
	Right LL pneumonia	Chest radiograph 2 views
Epigastrium	Pancreatitis	US of pancreas, abdominal CT
	Peritonitis	Abdominal CT
	Abdominal aortic aneurysm	US, CT scan
Left upper	Splenic rupture	US, Abdominal CT
	Constipation	KUB abdominal radiograph
Flank	Pyelonephritis	Renal US (UA, Gram stain, and culture)
	Renal colic	Noncontrast (helical) CT scan, renal US
Lower abdomen	Appendicitis	US, CT scan
	Ovarian torsion	Pelvic sonogram
	Ectopic pregnancy	Pelvic sonogram
	Salpingitis	Pelvic sonogram
	Ovarian cyst	Pelvic sonogram
Diffuse or variable pain		
	Gastroenteritis	Stool studies (occult blood and culture)
	Intestinal obstruction	Supine and upright radiograph
	Constipation	KUB abdominal radiograph
	Intestinal perforation	Supine and upright radiograph, CT scan

narrowing the differential and tailoring care (Table 36–5). Because of the additive radiation risks associated with CT scans and the potential negative effects to growing cells, ultrasonography (US) is becoming the study of choice in pediatric patients.

ADDITIONAL MEASURES IN MANAGEMENT

- Perform serial examinations: Infants and children cannot articulate how they feel. Use serial examinations to help make a diagnosis or to determine if further interventions or tests are warranted.
- Withhold oral intake and provide resuscitative and maintenance IV fluids.
- Treat pain: Mild pain may be adequately treated with acetaminophen or ibuprofen. Treat moderate to severe pain with IV narcotics while monitoring vital signs and pulse oximetry. IV morphine or fentanyl are well tolerated in the pediatric population. Since the byproducts of morphine also have CNS depressant effects, repeated doses of morphine especially in the young child and infant, may be associated with respiratory depression. Be aware, be prepared, and be readily available if untoward side effects occur. Recent pediatric studies support the use of pain medication in children with suspected appendicitis. Use of narcotics did not affect surgical outcome, delay, or need for additional diagnostic studies.
- Control emesis: Nausea and vomiting are distressing to a child. Control emesis with an antiemetic such as ondansetron.
- Place an NG tube to low intermittent suction for infants and children with persistent vomiting, abdominal distension, and those who may have an intestinal obstruction.
- Surgical consultation: Immediate consultation with a surgeon is required in any infant with bilious emesis. Bilious emesis in an infant or child should be suspected to have malrotation with midgut volvulus until proven otherwise. Malrotation with volvulus is a life-threatening surgical emergency, and immediate consultation is necessary. Infants in shock, with a potential for having an abdominal catastrophe, also require immediate surgery consultation. For the majority of the infants and children who are stable, follow-up serial examinations and assimilate data from laboratory tests and radiographic tests. Once a surgical diagnosis is considered, obtain surgical consultation. Delays in consultation have the potential for worsening outcome and prognosis. Maintain nothing by mouth status pending surgical evaluation.
- Antibiotics: Consider IV antibiotics.

Solomkin JS, Mazuski JE, Bradley JS, et al: Diagnosis and management of complicated intra-abdominal infections in adults and children: Guidelines by the Surgical Infection Society and the Infectious Diseases Society of America. *Clin Infect Dis.* 2010;50(2)133-164 [PMID: 20034345].

MANAGEMENT OF SPECIFIC DISORDERS CAUSING ABDOMINAL COMPLAINTS IN THE PEDIATRIC PATIENT

COLIC

Clinical Findings

Infantile colic is excessive crying in a healthy infant for at least 3 hours a day, 3 days a week, for at least 3 weeks. It usually begins in the first weeks of life and ends approximately at 4-5 months of age. The crying may occur at any time of day, but tends to occur in the early evening hours. Infants may draw their knees to their stomachs, or even pass a large amount of gas.

It is unclear what may be the cause of these symptoms. It is important to rule out more serious symptoms of abdominal pain. However, many believe colic may be due to an increased sensitivity and inability to console oneself. Other causes include problems with the gut, such as allergy to cow's milk or gas, behavioral problems, either due to temperament of the infant or poor parent–infant interaction, or the extreme end of normal crying.

Diagnostic Studies

There is no specific test for diagnosis of colic. Colic is a clinical diagnosis and the history and physical examination are cornerstones in the evaluation of the crying infant. Studies have shown that afebrile crying infants in the first 4-6 months of life may benefit from a urine evaluation to rule out UTI as a cause of crying.

Treatment

Generally, the infant will outgrow these symptoms and the colicky crying may stop by 4-5 months of age. It is important to give the family general information about colic and reassurance. However, the family may be able to consider a few interventions that may improve the crying. Some suggest eliminating cows' milk protein from the diet. Breast-feeding mothers can eliminate cows' milk from their diet, and infants taking formula may benefit from a 1-week trial of hypoallergenic formula, such as protein hydrolysate. Behavioral interventions that may help include checking for hunger, preventing overstimulation of infant, and establishing a regular pattern during the day. It is important to remind parents that if they are feeling overwhelmed, they should ask for help from family and friends.

Cohen Silver J, Ratnapalan S: Management of infantile colic: A review. *Clin Pediatr (Phila)*. 2009;48:14 [PMID: 18832537].

Freedman SB, Al-Harthy N, Thull-Freedman J: The crying infant: Diagnostic testing and frequency of underlying disease. *Pediatrics*. 2009;123:841 [PMID: 19255012].

Savino F, Tarasco V: New treatments for infant colic. *Curr Opin Pediatr*. 2010;22:791 [PMID: 20859207].

Shelov SP, and Altmann TR: Caring for Your Baby and Young Child Birth to Age 5. *American Academy of Pediatrics*. United States of America: Bantam Books, 2009.

GASTROESOPHAGEAL REFLUX DISEASE

Clinical Findings

Gastroesophageal reflux (GER) is the movement of contents from the stomach into the esophagus. Occasionally, this may include vomiting. GER is a normal process, occurring several times a day, with very little or no symptoms at all. Gastroesophageal reflux disease (GERD) occurs when the reflux causes distressing symptoms or complications. Infants and children may present with cough, vomiting, and/or wheezing, whereas older children may present with complaint of chest or abdominal pain. However, symptoms and signs may be nonspecific.

Treatment

Parent education and reassurance are often sufficient for infants with suspected GERD who are healthy and growing well. Although use of thickened formulas does not decrease the frequency of reflux episodes, the appearance of overt vomiting may be less. Placing the child prone reduces the amount of reflux, but because of the concern for sudden infant death syndrome (SIDS), the child should be placed prone only with careful parental supervision. The child should be placed in the supine position when sleeping.

In older children and adolescents, lifestyle changes may include diet changes, weight loss, smaller meals, eliminating late-night eating, sleeping prone or on the left side, and/or elevation of the head of the bed. Histamine$_2$ receptor antagonists (H$_2$RA) are fast acting and may help in relieving immediate symptoms. However, proton pump inhibitors (PPIs) are preferred because they are able to maintain a higher intragastric pH for a longer period, inhibit gastric acid secretion after meals, and do not lose their effect with chronic use. H$_2$RAs may be used for occasional symptoms. If symptoms continue to occur, lifestyle changes with a trial of a PPI for a 2- to 4-week period may be beneficial. If the PPI helps in resolving symptoms, it may be used for up to 3 months. However, if symptoms persist, the child needs to be followed up by a pediatric gastroenterologist. PPIs are not approved for children younger than 1 year.

Blanco FC, Davenport KP, Kane TD: Pediatric gastroesophageal reflux. *Surg Clin North Am*. 2012;92:541 [PMID: 22595708].

Malcolm WF, Cotton CM: Metoclopramide, H2 blockers, and proton pump inhibitors: Pharmacotherapy for gastroesophageal reflux in neonates. *Clin Perinatol*. 2012;39:99 [PMID: 22341540].

Sullivan JS, Sundaram SS: Gastroesophageal reflux. *Pediatr Rev*. 2012;33:243 [PMID: 22659255].

Vandenplas Y, Rudolph CD, Di Lorenzo C, et al: Pediatric gastroesophageal reflux clinical practice guidelines: Joint recommendations of the North American Society for Pediatric Gastroenterology, Hepatology, and Nutrition (NASPGHAN) and the European Society for Pediatric Gastroenterology, Hepatology, and Nutrition (ESPGHAN). *J Pediatr Gastroenterol Nutr*. 2009;49:498 [PMID: 19745761].

ACUTE GASTROENTERITIS

Clinical Findings

Diarrhea is quite common in infants and children, especially those in developing countries. Poor water supplies and sanitary facilities correlate with increased contamination and spread of fecal-oral pathogens. However, the incidence of diarrhea in child care centers in the United States are increasing as well. Exposures for children in the United States include nosocomial diarrhea among hospitalized children and travel to endemic areas.

Acute gastroenteritis usually occurs for 3-7 days. It can be caused by viruses, bacteria, and parasites, but most cases are viral or bacterial. A major culprit of viral gastroenteritis is rotavirus. This virus causes a severe dehydrating diarrhea. It usually occurs in the fall to early spring. Although rotavirus tends to occur in younger children, Norwalk virus tends to cause diarrhea in children older than 6 years. It occurs in settings such as schools, camps, nursing homes, cruise ships, and restaurants. Adenovirus is the third most common organism to cause acute gastroenteritis. Symptoms tend to last longer than the other two viruses, and diarrhea may last for up to 5-12 days. These viruses produce watery diarrhea, which may be accompanied by vomiting and fever.

Bacterial diarrhea is characterized as secretory or inflammatory. During secretory diarrhea, the stool may be watery and often large in volume. The child may have complaints of nausea and vomiting. With inflammatory diarrhea, fever, myalgias, arthralgias, irritability, loss of appetite, and abdominal pain may accompany the diarrhea. The child frequently passes small amounts of mucous-like stool. The stool may also have leukocytes, red blood cells, and/or gross blood on examination.

Diagnostic Studies

Stool samples for bacterial cultures, ova and parasites, *Clostridium difficile* toxin, or rotavirus PCR are not routinely obtained but may be obtained if diarrhea is persistent or bloody.

Treatment

In immediate management of acute gastroenteritis, it is important to control fluid loss, dehydration, and electrolyte abnormalities. Most episodes of acute gastroenteritis are mild and can be taken care of at home with oral rehydration. For mild to moderate dehydration, oral rehydration is the preferred method with an isotonic or hypotonic carbohydrate solution including electrolytes. Small amounts (< 5 mL) of fluid may be given to the child every 5-10 minutes and increased if tolerated. In moderate to severe dehydration, or in patients where oral therapy is not possible, it is necessary to provide IV fluids. Patients who are severely dehydrated may also require hospitalization for continued IV hydration. IV rehydration initially begins with an isotonic solution, such as normal saline or lactated Ringer. Infusion rates of 20-40 mL/kg for the first 30 minutes for older children and up to 30 mL/kg over the first hour for infants may be administered with the remainder of the deficit provided depending on clinical observation. If tolerated, subsequent maintenance fluids can be given orally with IV fluids until the calculated deficit has been replenished. Full feedings may restart after rehydration.

Carter B, Seupaul R: Update: Antiemetics for vomiting associated with acute gastroenteritis in children. *Ann Emerg Med.* 2012;60:e5 [PMID: 22424648].

Churgay CA, Aftab Z: Gastroenteritis in children: Part 1, diagnosis. *Am Fam Physician.* 2012;85(11):1059-1062 [PMID: 22962877].

Churgay CA, Aftab Z: Gastroenteritis in children: Part 2, prevention and management. *Am Fam Physician.* 2012;85(11): 1066-1070 [PMID: 22962878].

MILK PROTEIN ALLERGY

Clinical Findings

Milk protein allergy can occur during the child's first year of life, with allergy to cow's milk protein the most common. It can occur in formula-fed and in breast-fed infants. Chronic diarrhea, blood in the stool, GERD, constipation, chronic vomiting, and/or colic are only a few symptoms that can be late reactions in children with milk protein allergy. Immediate symptoms include vomiting, hives, angioedema, wheezing, rhinitis, and dry cough. It is common for children with cow's milk protein allergy to have a positive family history for atopy.

Diagnostic Studies

In general, laboratory tests are seldom helpful. Confirmation of cow's milk allergy in a child is by means of elimination and challenge.

Treatment

If a milk protein allergy is suspected, elimination of cow's milk protein from the infant's diet can be tried for 2-4 weeks. During this period, infants may be fed extensively with hydrolyzed formula. Infants with allergy will usually have a decrease in vomiting episodes in the first 2 weeks and then have a recurrence if milk protein is added back into the diet. For infants who are breast-fed with moderate to severe symptoms, it is recommended that the mother eliminate cow's milk and eggs from her diet. If there is no improvement with the elimination diet after 4 weeks, the diet should be stopped. The child should follow-up with pediatrician to monitor symptoms. Referral to an allergist/immunologist may be required.

Caffarelli C, Baldi F, Bendandi B, et al.: Cow's milk protein allergy in children: A practical guide. *Itali J Pediatr.* 2010;36:5 [PMID: 20205781].

DeGreef E, Hauser B, Devreker T, et al: Diagnosis and management of cow's milk protein allergy in infants. *World J Pediatr.* 2012;8:19 [PMID: 22282379].

du Toit G, Meyer R, Shah N, et al: Identifying and managing cows' milk protein allergy. *Arch Dis Child Educ Pract Ed.* 2012;95:134 [PMID: 20688848].

Kattan JD, Cocco RR, Jarvinen KM: Milk and soy allergy. *Pediatr Clinic North Am.* 2011;58:407 [PMID: 21453810].

Kneepkens CM, Meijer Y: Clinical practice: Diagnosis and treatment of cow's milk allergy. *Eur J Pediatr.* 2009;168:891 [PMID: 19271238].

NECROTIZING ENTEROCOLITIS

Necrotizing enterocolitis (NEC) is primarily a disease of premature, very low birth-weight infants; however, it occasionally affects full-term infants. NEC is characterized by necrosis of the mucosal and submucosal layers of the GI tract.

The clinical presentation of a full-term infant with NEC can be subtle and resemble sepsis. Early signs include poor feeding, abdominal distension, vomiting, and jaundice. Late signs include abdominal tenderness, bilious emesis and grossly bloody stool, abdominal skin discoloration, hypotension, lethargy, respiratory distress, or apnea.

Diagnostic Studies

Laboratory studies are nonspecific. Stool may be occult or grossly bloody. Late in disease, respiratory and metabolic acidosis, neutropenia, thrombocytopenia, evidence of disseminated intravascular coagulopathy (DIC) may be evident.

Plain abdominal radiographs may show an ileus, persistent loop of bowel, pneumatosis intestinalis, or portal venous gas.

Hepatic US detects portal venous gas most clearly. Doppler US is helpful in evaluating mesenteric blood flow through the superior mesenteric artery in infants with a gasless abdomen on plain radiograph.

Treatment

Uncomplicated NEC is treated nonoperatively with antibiotics (Table 36–1), bowel rest and supportive care. Place an orogastric (OG) tube for low intermittent suction, administer broad-spectrum antibiotics, and allow no oral feeding for 10-14 days.

Late disease or shock states are treated with crystalloid, vasoactive agents, broad-spectrum antibiotics, and blood products. Assist ventilation for respiratory failure and provide nutritional support with total parenteral nutrition.

Consultation with a surgeon is needed immediately. Surgical intervention is necessary for evidence of perforation, intestinal necrosis, and clinical deterioration and progression of disease despite aggressive medical management. Relative surgical indications include refractory acidosis, oliguria, hypotension, persistent thrombocytopenia, portal venous gas, fixed dilated loop of bowel, erythema of the abdominal wall, and ventilator failure.

Surgical treatment includes laparotomy with resection and proximal colostomy or laparotomy with resection and primary anastomosis. Peritoneal drainage (PD), insertion of a Penrose drain into the peritoneal cavity is done at the bedside in the neonatal intensive care unit (NICU) and is a preferred option in the unstable premature infant. A recent Cochrane review showed no difference between PD and laparotomy regarding 28-day mortality, 90-day mortality, and number of infants needing total parenteral nutrition for more than 90 days. Further multicenter randomized clinical trials are needed to clearly identify benefits or complications of PD in the surgical treatment of NEC.

Dominguez KM, Moss RL: Necrotizing enterocolitis. *Clin Perinatol.* 2012;39:387 [PMID: 22682387].

Eicher C, Seitz G, Bevot A, et al: Surgical management of extremely low birth weight infants with neonatal bowel perforation: A single-center experience and a review of the literature. *Neonatology.* 2012:101:285 [PMID: 22286302].

Evennett N, Alexander N, Petrov M, Pierro A, Eaton S: A systematic review of serologic tests in the diagnosis of necrotizing enterocolitis. *J Pediatr Surg.* 2009;44(11):2192 [PMID: 19944232].

Neu J, Mihatsch W: Recent developments in necrotizing enterocolitis. *JPEN Parenter Enteral Nutr.* 2012;36:(1 suppl)30S [PMID: 22237874].

Neu J, Walker WA: Necrotizing enterocolitis. *N Engl J Med.* 2011;20;364(3):255 [PMID: 21247316].

Rao SC, Basani L, Simmer K, Samnakay N, Deshpande G: Peritoneal drainage versus laparotomy as initial surgical treatment for perforated necrotizing enterocolitis or spontaneous intestinal perforation in preterm low birth weight infants. *Cochrane Database Syst Rev.* 2011;15;(6):CD006182 [PMID: 216783540].

Schnabl KL, Van Aerde JE, Thomson AB, Clandinin MT: Necrotizing enterocolitis: A multifactorial disease with no cure. *World J Gastroenterol.* 2008;14:2142 [PMID: 18407587].

Song R, Subbarao GC, Maheshwari A: Haematological abnormalities in neonatal necrotizing enterocolitis. *J Matern Fetal Neonatal Med.* 2012;25(suppl 4):22 [PMID: 22958006].

Thompson AM, Bizzarro MJ: Necrotizing enterocolitis in newborns: Pathogenesis, prevention, and management. *Drugs.* 2008;68:1227 [PMID: 18547133].

MALROTATION WITH VOLVULUS

Malrotation occurs because of abnormal rotation and fixation of the midgut during gestation and may be complicated by a volvulus. This abnormal fixation allows peritoneal adhesion bands (Ladd bands) to compress the duodenum causing vomiting or obstruction, even without a volvulus. Because the small bowel is suspended on a narrow pedicle (containing the superior mesenteric artery), it is predisposed to twisting on itself, resulting in torsion of the midgut (volvulus). A volvulus results in varying degrees of bowel obstruction and vascular compromise and may be abrupt, intermittent, or gradual in onset. Small bowel necrosis can occur within a few hours of torsion. Thus, infants and children presenting with bilious emesis require prompt evaluation for malrotation and volvulus; this is a surgical emergency.

Clinical Findings

Malrotation usually presents in infants but may present at any age. Bilious emesis is usually the first sign and occurs in 77-100% of patients. Symptoms, however, may vary depending on the degree of obstruction or the presence of a volvulus. Infants present with feeding intolerance, bilious emesis, and abrupt onset of crying. Vague abdominal pain or vomiting is often seen in older children. Children with an acute volvulus often present with signs of an abdominal catastrophe and shock. Bilious emesis in an infant or child may indicate a true surgical emergency, and a high index of suspicion must be maintained to establish the diagnosis.

Physical examination findings in patients with early volvulus may be normal. Abdominal examination findings may be normal in 50-60% of infants. One-third of patients present with abdominal distension without tenderness. With time, intestinal ischemia progresses to necrosis and evidence of peritonitis develops. Late findings include fever, abdominal wall erythema and edema, peritonitis, profound dehydration, and shock.

Diagnostic Studies

Laboratory studies are not helpful in the diagnosis.

Plain radiographs of the abdomen may be normal. A limited upper gastrointestinal (UGI) contrast study is the most reliable method to diagnose malrotation with or without volvulus. Hallmark appearance of malrotation is failure of the duodenal-jejunal flexure (ligament of Treitz) to cross to the left of midline (Figure 36–1). In malrotation with volvulus, the duodenum is coiled giving a corkscrew appearance to the right of midline (Figure 36–2). Malrotation alone is important to diagnose because the infant is at risk to develop midgut volvulus later in life.

Treatment

Immediate resuscitation and surgical intervention is required for infants and children with malrotation and a volvulus. Resuscitate with crystalloid fluids, place an OG tube, and administer broad-spectrum antibiotics. The surgical procedure for correction of malrotation is the Ladd procedure which includes detorsion of the volvulus, division of the Ladd bands, and separation of the duodeno-jejunal

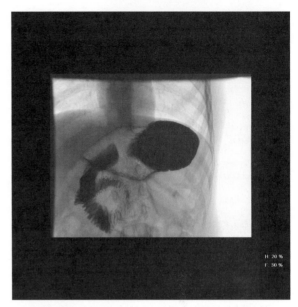

▲ **Figure 36–1.** Malrotation. Upper gastrointestinal study demonstrating duodenal-jejunal flexure fails to cross to the left of midline.

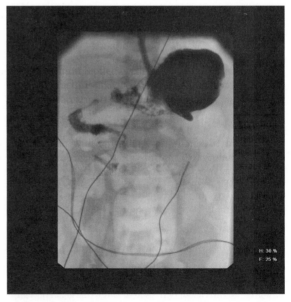

▲ **Figure 36–2.** Malrotation with volvulus. Upper gastrointestinal study demonstrating the corkscrew appearance of the coiled duodenum.

mesentery from the cecocolic mesentery. An appendectomy is done concomitantly because the colon is positioned in the LLQ during a Ladd procedure.

Applegate KE: Evidence-based diagnosis of malrotation and volvulus. *Pediatr Radiol.* 2009;39(suppl 2):S161 [PMID: 19308378].

Hagendoorn J, Vieira-Travassos D, van der Zee D: Laparoscopic treatment of intestinal malrotation in neonates and infants: Retrospective study. *Surg Endosc.* 2011;25:217 [PMID: 20559662].

Lampl B, Levin TL, Berdon WE, Cowles RA: Malrotation and midgut volvulus: A historical review and current controversies in diagnosis and management. *Pediatr Radiol.* 2009;39:359 [PMID: 19241073].

Laurence N, Pollock AN: Malrotation with midgut volvulus. *Pediatr Emerg Care.* 2012;28(1):87 [PMID: 22217896].

Lin YP, Lee J, Chao HC, et al: Risk factors for intestinal gangrene in children with small-bowel volvulus. *J Pediatr Gatroenterol Nutr.* 2011;53:417 [PMID: 21519283].

Sizemore AW, Rabbani KZ, Ladd A, Applegate KE: Diagnostic performance of the upper gastrointestinal series in the evaluation of children with clinically suspected malrotation. *Pediatr Radiol.* 2008;38:518 [PMID: 18265969].

Stanfill AB, Pearl RH, Kalvakuri K, et al: Laparoscopic Ladd's procedure: Treatment of choice for midgut malrotation in infants and children. *J Laparoendosc Adv Surg Tech A.* 2010;20:369 [PMID: 20218938].

Williams H: Green for Danger! Intestinal malrotation and volvulus. *Arch Dis Child Educ Pract Ed.* 2007;92:ep87 [PMID: 17517978].

HYPERTROPHIC PYLORIC STENOSIS

Hypertrophic pyloric stenosis (HPS) is the most common surgical cause of vomiting in infants. It is a result of hypertrophy of the circular musculature around the pylorus, leading to compression of the longitudinal mucosa and gastric outlet obstruction. Infants usually present with nonbilious projectile vomiting in the second to fourth weeks of life. It is more common in males.

Clinical Findings

HPS usually presents between 2 and 6 weeks of age with progressive or forceful nonbilious emesis. The emesis occurs within 30 minutes after a feed. The infant appears hungry and will feed vigorously. About half way through the feed, the infant will stop sucking and then play with the nipple. Because the feed cannot pass through the pylorus, reverse peristaltic waves may be seen on abdominal examination prior to vomiting. The infant will then vomit with force as if it is "hitting the wall." Early in the disease process, the infant may look well, with normal weight gain, and vital signs. As vomiting persists, the infant may present emaciated, dehydrated, and lethargic. The vomit may also be bloody from gastric irritation. Abdominal findings include abdominal distension, gastric peristaltic waves, and may have a palpable mass (olive) in the RUQ.

Diagnostic Studies

Classic electrolyte findings are hypochloremic, hypokalemic metabolic alkalosis. Infants may also have increased indirect bilirubin.

Plain radiographs might reveal a large dilated stomach and no air in the small bowel or colon. A UGI contrast study reveals a string sign, the beak sign, or double track sign. Currently, abdominal US is the imaging modality of choice. Muscles thickness of 4 mm or more and a channel length of 15 mm or more confirms HPS (Figure 36–3A and B).

Treatment

Treat electrolyte abnormalities; normalize acid-base status and fluid hydration. Decompress the stomach with an OG or NG tube to low intermittent suction as needed. Maintain NPO status. Surgical treatment is the Fredet-Ramstedt pyloromyotomy via an open or laparoscopic approach. Once repaired, refeeding begins within hours of postsurgical correction.

Haricharan RN, Aprahamian CJ, Morgan TL, et al: Smaller scars-what is the big deal: A survey of the perceived value of laparoscopic pyloromyotomy. *J Pediatr Surg.* 2008;43:92 [PMID: 18206463].

Hernanz-Schulman M: Pyloric stenosis: Role of imaging. *Pediatr Radiol.* 2009;39:S134 [PMID: 12637675].

Maheshwari P, Abograra A, Shamam O: Sonographic evaluation of gastrointestinal obstruction in infants: A pictorial essay. *J Pediatr Surg.* 2009;44:2037 [PMID: 19853770].

Panteli C: New insights into the pathogenesis of infantile pyloric stenosis. *Pediatr Surg Int.* 2009;25:1043 [PMID: 19760199].

Perger L, Fuchs JR, Komidar L, Mooney DP: Impact of surgical approach on outcome in 622 consecutive pyloromyotomies at a pediatric teaching institution. *J Pediatr Surg.* 2009;44:2119 [PMID: 19944219].

Ranells JD, Carver JD, Kirby RS: Infantile hypertrophic pyloric stenosis: Epidemiology, genetics, and clinical update. *Adv Pediatr.* 2011;58(1):195 [PMID: 21736982].

Sola JE, Neville HL: Laparoscopic vs open pyloromyotomy: A systematic review and meta-analysis. *J Pediatr Surg.* 2009;44:1631 [PMID: 19635317].

INTUSSUSCEPTION

Intussusception is the invagination of the proximal portion of bowel into an adjacent distal segment. Invagination of the ileum into the colon (ileocolic) is involved in 80-90%. The peak age of presentation is 5-9 months of age; however, intussusception occurs most often in infants and children between 3 months and 2 years of age. In this age group, no pathologic lead point can be found in 90% of cases. However, older children are more likely to have pathologic lead points such as a Meckel diverticulum, lymphoma, or vasculitis as seen in Henoch-Schönlein purpura. Association between older

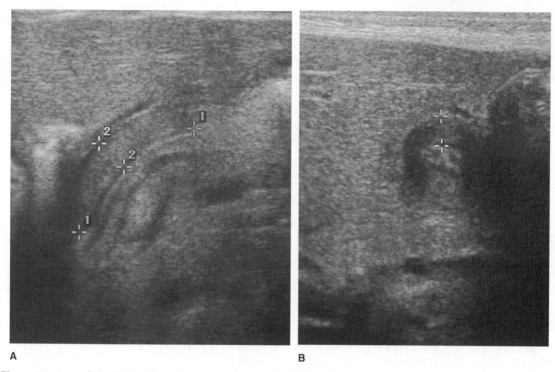

A **B**

▲ **Figure 36–3a and 3b.** US confirmation of pyloric stenosis. **(A)** Demonstrates a channel length of 17 mm on the long view and **(B)** transverse view demonstrates pyloric thickness of 4.2 mm.

rotavirus vaccines (RotaShield and Wyeth Lederle Vaccines) and intussusception led to the voluntary withdrawal in 1999. To date, current rotavirus vaccines have not been associated with intussusception. Also, adenovirus serotypes that typically cause respiratory symptoms have been identified in stool samples from children with intussusception. Small bowel intussusception is often identified by CT scan and is usually an incidental finding and self-limiting.

Clinical Findings

Classic clinical presentation is intermittent colicky abdominal pain, vomiting, and currant jelly stools. Most only present with two symptoms, the most common being colicky abdominal pain lasting 2 to 10 minutes, followed by general relief. The second most common symptom is vomiting. Vomit is initially clear and with progression becomes bilious or even feculent. Less commonly, infants may present with lethargy, pallor, and hypotension.

Intussusception should also be considered in the differential of altered mental status or lethargy in infants and young children. Profound lethargy with a palpable abdominal mass or occult blood in the stool may be the only clinical sign and symptom.

On examination, up to 30% of infants and children with intussusception have a normal examination. Occasionally, there may be emptiness in the RLQ with a soft sausage-shaped mass that is palpable in the RUQ extending along the transverse colon. Extensive involvement of bowel mass may be palpable only on rectal examination.

Diagnostic Studies

Laboratory tests are unhelpful and nonspecific. One study found that 43% of patients with intussusception had occult blood in their stool samples.

Plain abdominal radiographs may be helpful but if normal do not rule out intussusception (Figure 36–4). Barium enema is the "gold standard" study for the diagnosis. In many institutions, air contrast enema has replaced the barium study in the diagnosis and treatment (Figures 36–5 and 36–6).

US is currently the mainstay in diagnosis of intussusception (100% accuracy, 98-100% sensitivity, 88% specificity). Classic sonographic findings are the target or doughnut sign (Figure 36–7). US can also identify the presence of free intraperitoneal air or a lead point, if present.

Contrast enemas and CT scans are means of diagnosis if sonogram is not available.

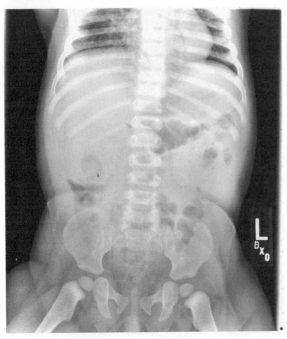

▲ **Figure 36–4.** Plain abdominal radiograph demonstrating paucity of air in the right upper quadrant suggestive of intussusception.

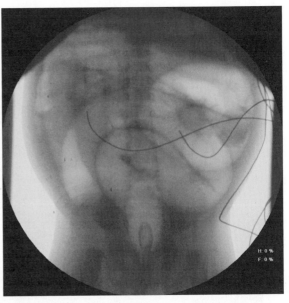

▲ **Figure 36–6.** Air contrast enema demonstrating inability to reduce mid-ascending colon intussusception.

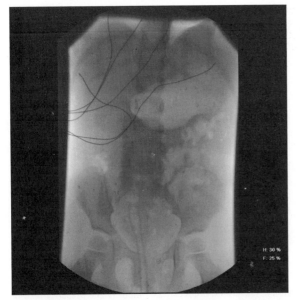

▲ **Figure 36–5.** Air contrast enema demonstrating ileocolic intussusception.

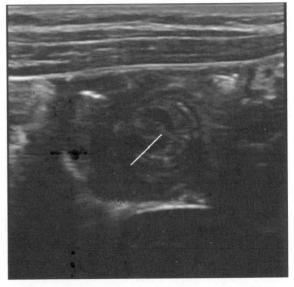

▲ **Figure 36–7.** Target lesion in intussusception. (Photo used with permission of Sonocloud.org.)

Treatment

Obtain consultation with a surgeon and support with IV fluid and bowel rest. Keep the child NPO and place an NG tube as indicated. Once intraperitoneal free air is excluded by US or plain radiograph, nonsurgical reduction by air contrast enema or barium enema can be done. This is successful in 60-90% of patients with a recurrence rate of 5-10%. Surgical intervention and antibiotics are indicated if there is evidence of hemodynamic instability, perforation, or peritonitis; or if hydrostatic reduction is unsuccessful. Laparotomy is performed to reduce the intussusception. A resection is required if the intussusception cannot be reduced, if there is necrotic tissue, or there is an anatomic lead point such as a Meckel diverticulum or intestinal duplication.

A serious but rare complication is perforation of the intestine during the air contrast enema. Free intraperitoneal air in an infant may cause respiratory embarrassment which requires immediate intervention. While supporting the ABC, prepare to decompress the abdomen. Locate the infraumbilical area, specifically, the linea alba. Using aseptic technique, place a 14- to 18-gauge angiocatheter 1-2 cm below the umbilicus entering just until free air is released. Remove the needle and slide the catheter into the space to allow continued release of air. This procedure is a time-saving maneuver until the infant can be safely intubated and taken to the operating room for laparotomy.

Following successful uncomplicated contrast enema reduction, children are typically observed for signs of bowel necrosis or recurrence of intussusceptions. However, recent literature suggests that postreduction fasting and hospitalization may not be necessary.

Adekunle-Ojo AO, Craig AM, Ma L, Caviness AC: Intussusception: Postreduction fasting is not necessary to prevent complications and recurrences in the emergency department observation unit. *Pediatr Emerg Care.* 2011;27:897 [PMID: 21960089].

Applegate KE: Intussusception in children: Evidence-based diagnosis and treatment. *Pediatr Radiol.* 2009;39:S140 [PMID: 19308373].

Bucher BT, Hall BL, Watern BW, Keller MS: Intussusception in children: Cost effectiveness of ultrasound vs diagnostic contrast enema. *J Pediatr Surg.* 2011;46:1099 [PMID: 21683206].

Committee on Infectious Diseases: American Academy of Pediatrics: Prevention of rotavirus disease; updated guidelines for use of rotavirus vaccine. *Pediatrics.* 2009;123:1412 [PMID: 19332437].

Gilmore AW, Reed M, Tenenbein M: Management of childhood intussusception after reduction by enema. *Am J Emerg Med.* 2011;29:1136 [PMID: 20980119].

Herwig K, Brenkert T, Losek JD: Enema-reduced intussusception management. Is hospitalization necessary? *Pediatr Emerg Care.* 2009;25:74 [PMID: 19194346].

Hryhorczuk AL, Strouse PJ: Validation of US as a first-line diagnostic test for assessment of pediatric ileocolic intussusception. *Pediatr Radiol.* 2009;39:1075 [PMID: 19657636].

Kleizen KJ, Hunck A, Wijnen MH, Draaisma JM: Neurological symptoms in children with intussusception. *Acta Paediatr.* 2009;98:1822 [PMID: 19673722].

Ko HS, Schenk JP, Troger J, Rohrschneider WK: Current radiological management of intussusception in children. *Eur Radiol.* 2007;17:2411 [PMID:17308922].

Morrison J, Lucas N, Gravel J: The role of abdominal radiography in the diagnosis of intussusception when interpreted by pediatric emergency physicians. *J Pediatr.* 2009;155:556 [PMID: 19560157].

Niramis R, Watanatittan S, Kruatrachue A, et al: Management of recurrent intussusception: nonoperative or operative reduction? *J Pediatr Surg.* 2010;45(11):2175 [PMID: 21034940].

Okimoto S, Hyodod S, Yamamoto M, et al: Association of viral isolates from stool samples with intussusception in children. *Int J Infect Dis.* 2011;15:e641 [PMID:21757385].

Waseem M, Rosenberg HK: Intussusception. *Pediatr Emerg Care.* 2008;24:793 [PMID: 19018227].

Weihmiller SN, Buonomo C, Bachur R: Risk stratification of children being evaluated for intussusception. *Pediatrics.* 2011; 127:e296 [PMID: 21242220].

MECKEL DIVERTICULUM

Meckel diverticulum is a congenital true diverticulum of the distal small intestine that may contain gastric or pancreatic tissue. The gastric tissue produces acid which causes ulceration and bleeding of the adjacent intestine. The most common clinical presentation includes lower GI bleeding, intestinal obstruction, and inflammatory complications such as diverticulitis. Bleeding can be tarry (melena) or bright red (hematochezia) and is usually painless, episodic, or sometimes, massive. Patients with vomiting, abdominal pain, bloody stools, or a palpable abdominal mass may have intussusception due to a Meckel diverticulum. Congenital bands from a Meckel to the mesentery or umbilicus may result in an internal hernia or localized volvulus, respectively, resulting in a closed loop bowel obstruction. Meckel diverticulitis (inflammation of a Meckel) can cause symptoms similar to that of acute appendicitis: vomiting, periumbilical, right or middle quadrant pain, or diffuse peritoneal irritation.

The "rule of twos" is a way to remember facts about Meckel diverticulum: occurs in 2% of the population, 2 types of heterotopic mucosa, located 2 ft from the ileocecal valve, approximately 2 in in length, 2 cm in diameter, and symptoms usually occur before the child is 2 years old.

Differential diagnosis for pediatric lower GI bleeding includes intestinal polyps, hemangiomas, or duplications, arteriovenous malformations, coagulopathy, inflammatory bowel disease, acute infectious gastroenteritis, pseudomembranous colitis, or Henoch-Schönlein purpura.

Diagnostic Studies

Laboratory studies are not specific; however, a complete blood cell count (CBC) and prothrombin time/partial

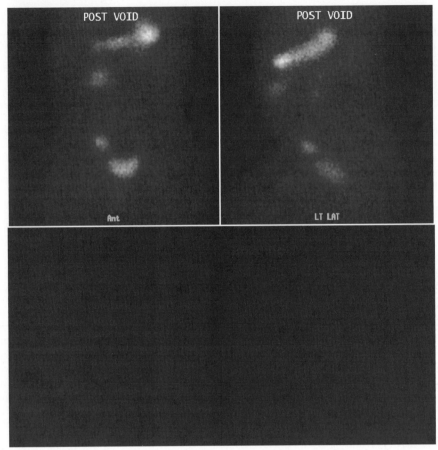

▲ **Figure 36–8.** Meckel scan demonstrating concentration of isotope in gastric mucosa of stomach and Meckel diverticulum.

thromboplastin time can help differentiate a coagulopathy as the cause of bleeding. A stool sample may be positive for occult blood and a CBC may show evidence of anemia.

A Meckel scan or technetium Tc 99m pertechnetate scintigraphy is the procedure of choice in children with GI bleeding suggestive a Meckel diverticulum. Tc 99m pertechnetate isotope concentrates in gastric mucosa of the stomach and Meckel diverticulum (Figure 36–8). The isotope collects in the bladder and is excreted. Fasting, NG suctioning, and bladder cathertization as well as using agents such as H_2 blockers, pentagastrin, or glucagon enhances the diagnostic yield of the scan.

Treatment

Support the ABC, obtain IV access, resuscitate with crystalloid, and consider PRBC for significant hemorrhage. Place an OG or NG tube to decompress the stomach and administer broad-spectrum antibiotics. Consult a pediatric surgeon.

Surgical interventions include laparoscopic or open excision of the diverticulum or small bowel resection. Many surgeons will also perform an appendectomy.

Kotecha M, Bellah R, Pena AH, Jaimes C, Mattei P: Multimodality imaging manifestations of the Meckel diverticulum in children. *Pediatr Radiol.* 2012;42(1):95 [PMID: 21984316].

Pepper VK, Stanfill AB, Pearl RH: Diagnosis and management of pediatric appendicitis, intussusception, and Meckel diverticulum. *Surg Clin North Am.* 2012;92(3):505 [PMID: 22595706].

Ruscher KA, Fisher JN, Hughes CD, et al: National trends in the surgical management of Meckel's diverticulum. *J Pediatr Surg.* 2011;46:893 [PMID: 21616248].

Thurley PD, Halliday KE, Somers JM, et al: Radiological features of Meckel's diverticulum and its complications. *Clin Radiol.* 2009;64(2):109 [PMID: 19103339].

Tseng YY, Yang YJ: Clinical and diagnostic relevance of Meckel's diverticulum in children. *Eur J Pediatr.* 2009;168(12):1519 [PMID: 19575216].

TESTICULAR TORSION

Acute testicular torsion must be rapidly diagnosed and treated to maximize testicular salvage. Frequently, children with testicular torsion present with abdominal pain and vomiting and are unable to localize their pain to the genitalia. Examination of the male genitalia is a vital part of the physical examination when a boy presents with abdominal pain. Typically, the pain presents with sudden onset. Nausea and vomiting are common. Early examination findings include a high-riding testis with transverse lie, diffuse tenderness, and absence of the cremasteric reflex. This presentation is classic for testicular torsion, and no further evaluation or imaging is needed before emergent surgery. With time, the scrotal skin appears erythematous, thickened, or swollen. Testicular salvage is related to duration of symptoms before exploration, good outcome is expected if less than 6 hours since the onset of symptoms. Beyond 48 hours of symptoms, salvage rate is poor.

Other causes of an acute scrotum are torsion of the testis appendix, epididymitis, orchitis, incarcerated inguinal hernia, hydrocele, varicocele, Henoch-Schönlein purpura (HSP), Kawasaki disease, scrotal cellulitis, scrotal arthropod bites, and testicular trauma (Table 36–6).

Diagnostic Studies

A urinalysis is not helpful in the diagnosis of testicular torsion; however, it may be helpful in exclusion of other processes that can cause scrotal pain such as UTI, epididymitis, STDs, urethritis, or trauma.

Color Doppler sonography is the "gold standard" for imaging the acute scrotum. Color Doppler imaging is easily accessible, noninvasive, and highly accurate. It allows visualization of arterial flow and testicular anatomy. The affected side will show decreased or absent flow to the affected side (Figure 36–9A and B).

Treatment

If testicular torsion is suspected, do not delay consultation with urologic or pediatric general surgeon. Emergency scrotal exploration is indicated. Detorsion of the affected side, evaluation for viability, and orchiopexy are indicated if viable. If clearly nonviable, the testis is removed. The contralateral testis is also explored to determine presence of the bell clapper deformity or abnormal fixation.

If definitive surgical care is not readily available, manual detorsion can be attempted to preserve testicular viability. Administer analgesia or procedural sedation. Manual detorsion can be done by twisting the affected testis in an outward manner, as in opening a book. Twist the left testis to the patient's left or the right testis to the patient's right until the pain is relieved. Success is evident if there is significant relief of pain and lengthening of the cord structures and improved arterial flow demonstrated on follow-up US.

Table 36–6. Differential diagnosis of testicular torsion.

Torsion of the testicular appendage	Point of tenderness at upper pole of testis; blue dot sign
Epididymitis or orchitis	History of dysuria, recent fever, new incontinence with pyuria or bacteruria, sexual activity, history of sudden increase in abdominal pressure as in lifting or trauma
Scrotal trauma, testicular rupture	History of direct blow or straddle injury, evidence of scrotal hematoma or ecchymosis
Intrascrotal tumors	Nontender enlargement of scrotum; abnormal serum beta-human chorionic gonadotropin and alpha fetoprotein levels
Incarcerated inguinal hernia	Mass that extends to the inguinal area; may or may not transilluminate
Hydroceles, spermatoceles	Mass usually transilluminates, does not extend to the upper scrotum and external inguinal ring
Varicocele	Onset near or after puberty; enlargement of the veins along the cord structures that increases with Valsalva or standing, decreases with laying supine
Henoch-Schönlein purpura	Prodrome of fever, headache, anorexia followed by purpuric rash of lower trunk, extremities, perineum, buttocks. Also associated with colicky abdominal pain, nausea and vomiting, joint swelling, renal disease
Scrotal cellulitis	Cremasteric reflexes are intact and testis is usually normal and nontender
Arthropod bites	Characteristic bite lesions on skin, local reaction, pain

Manual detorsion is a temporizing procedure. Surgical exploration is still indicated.

Color Doppler US is helpful in equivocal cases but should not delay surgical consultation. Similarly, pain medication and IV fluids are helpful in relieving painful symptoms; however, administration should not delay surgical consultation or manual detorsion.

Boettcher M, Bergholz R, Krebs TF, Wenke K, Aronson DC: Clinical predictors of testicular torsion in children. *Urology.* 2012;79(3):670 [PMID: 22386422].

Cubillos J, Palmer JS, Friedman SC, et al: Familial testicular torsion. *J Urol.* 2011;185(6 suppl):2469 [PMID: 21555017].

Lopez RN, Beasley SW: Testicular torsion: Potential pitfalls in its diagnosis and management. *J Paediatr Child Health.* 2012;48(2):E30 [PMID: 22017291].

Lyronis ID, Ploumis N, Vlahakis I, Charissis G: Acute scrotum-etiology, clinical presentation and seasonal variation. *Indian J Pediatr.* 2009;76(4):407 [PMID: 19205631].

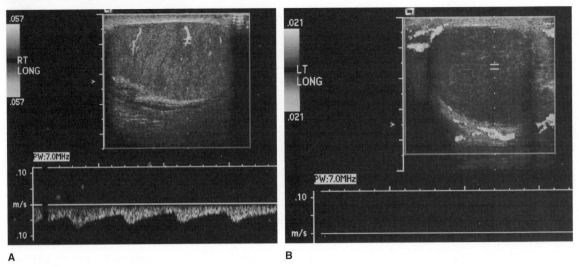

A   **B**

▲ **Figure 36–9.** Color Doppler sonography demonstrating absent flow on the left (**A**) compared to the right (**B**).

Rizvi SA, Ahmad I, Siddiqui MA, Zaheer S, Ahmad K: Role of color Doppler ultrasonography in evaluation of scrotal swellings: Pattern of disease in 120 patients with review of literature. *Urol J.* 2011;8(1):60 [PMID: 21404205].

PEDIATRIC INGUINAL HERNIA

An inguinal hernia is a type of ventral hernia where an abdominal structure such as bowel, omentum, or ovary protrudes through an abnormal opening of the abdominal wall. Pediatric inguinal hernias are common with an incidence ranging from 0.8 to 4.4%. The incidence is up to 10 times higher in boys than girls, and much higher in premature infants; 7-10% of infants born at less than 36 weeks' gestation have hernias. Right-sided hernias are more common in males due to the later descent of the right testis.

The exact molecular mechanism involved in the failure of closure of the processus vaginalis is unknown, but it is known that incomplete obliteration of the proximal processus vaginalis results in various types of inguinal hernias and hydroceles encountered in the pediatric population. Fusion of the distal processus with proximal patency results in an inguinal hernia. Fusion of the proximal processus with distal patency results in a noncommunicating scrotal hydrocele; and if the proximal portion of the processus retains a small opening, fluid can freely enter from the abdominal cavity to the scrotal sac resulting in a communicating hydrocele.

Clinical Findings

Pediatric inguinal hernia and hydrocele present as an asymptomatic bulge in the groin that becomes more apparent during crying or straining. The groin swelling usually resolves spontaneously with relaxation, sleep, or gentle manual pressure. For the infant, examination during crying will typically increase intra-abdominal pressure and cause a bulge in the groin. For the older child, having them blow bubbles or into an occluded straw will also increase intra-abdominal pressure. In females, the ovary may herniate and be at risk for torsion. A palpable ovary in an infant is almond-shaped and may not reduce easily if it is edematous.

The "silk purse" or "silk glove" sign is an alternative physical examination finding that is suggestive of an inguinal hernia. The sign is elicited by gently rolling the cord structures across the pubic tubercle. The feeling is similar to moving two pieces of silk on itself.

Differentiating between a hydrocele and hernia is often difficult. For most hydroceles, the swelling is confined to the scrotum outside the inguinal canal. Swelling above the scrotum is more suggestive of a hernia. However, a high hydrocele or hydrocele of the spermatic cord may extend into the inguinal canal. Transillumination may help distinguish between a sac filled with fluid versus one with bowel; however, bowel distended with air and fluid may also transilluminate especially in infants and is thus not reliable. The key in discrimination of a tense inguino-scrotal hydrocele from an incarcerated inguinal hernia is that typically the hydrocele causes no symptoms. An incarcerated hernia is usually tender and causes obstructive symptoms such as vomiting.

If a loop of bowel becomes incarcerated in a hernia, the infant or child presents with crying due to intense pain. Signs of bowel obstruction such as vomiting ensue. If the hernia is not reduced, strangulation with ischemia of the bowel occurs within 4-6 hours. Incarceration of omentum usually causes local discomfort without associated bowel symptoms.

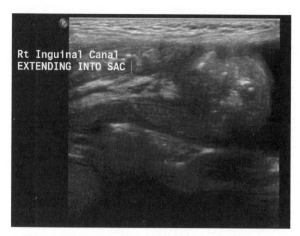

▲ **Figure 36–10.** Ultrasound of right inguinal hernia extending into scrotal sac.

Diagnostic Studies

Laboratory studies are neither indicated nor helpful. Radiologic studies are also not necessary. Some advocate US to distinguish between hydrocele and inguinal hernia (Figures 36–10 and 36–11). Ultrasonography is useful to document flow to an ovary that cannot be reduced.

Treatment

Incarcerated inguinal hernias can usually be manually reduced using a technique known as taxis. Provide the infant with pain medication or procedural sedation, and then apply gentle inferolateral pressure to the incarcerated hernia with some pressure above to straighten the inguinal canal. Most hernias can be reduced using this technique. Because of the possibility of reduction of ischemic bowel and a high rate of early recurrent incarceration, many

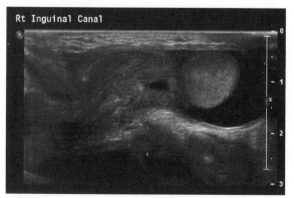

▲ **Figure 36–11.** Ultrasound of right incarcerated inguinal hernia with testicle.

children are admitted for observation and undergo surgery in 24-48 hours.

Manual reduction is contraindicated if there is clear evidence of peritonitis, bowel compromise, or hemodynamic instability. Consult a surgeon as soon as possible since these children should undergo emergent surgical intervention once resuscitated. Reduction of incarcerated omentum is often not possible because the omentum may be adherent within the hernia sac. Nonreducible omentum poses little immediate risk to the child. Similarly, a high hydrocele or hydrocele of the cord does not need to be reduced and attempts can cause unnecessary pain.

Patients with asymptomatic inguinal hernias can be referred to a pediatric surgeon for repair. Inguinal hernias will not spontaneously resolve. Repair should occur as soon as possible to reduce the future risk of incarceration, especially in the first year of life.

Brandt ML: Pediatric Hernias. *Surg Clin N Am*. 2008;88:27 [PMID: 18267160].

Clarke S: Pediatric inguinal hernia and hydrocele: An evidence-based review in the era of minimal access surgery. *J Laparoendosc Adv Surg Tech A*. 2010;20:305 [PMID: 20374016].

Deeba S, Purkayastha S, Paraskevas P, Athanasiou T, Darzi A, Zacharakis E: Laparoscopic approach to incarcerated and strangulated inguinal hernias. *JSLS*. 2009;13(3):327 [PMID: 19793471].

Gholoum S, Baird R, Laberge JM, Puligandia PS: Incarceration rates in pediatric inguinal hernia: Do not trust the coding. *J Pediatr Surg*. 2010;45:1007 [PMID: 20438943].

Lao OB, Fitzgibbons RJ Jr, Cusick RA: Pediatric inguinal hernias, hydroceles, and undescended testicles. *Surg Clin North Am*. 2012;92(3):487 [PMID: 22595705].

Lee SL, Gleason JM, Sydorak RM. A critical review of premature infants with inguinal hernias: Optimal timing of repair, incarceration risk, and postoperative apnea. *J Pediatr Surg*. 2011;46(1):217 [PMID: 21238671].

Merriman LS, Herrel L, Kirsch AJ: Inguinal and genital anomalies. *Pediatr Clin North Am*. 2012;59(4):769 [PMID: 22857828].

Okada T, Sasaki S, Honda S, et al: Irreducible indirect inguinal hernia containing uterus, ovaries, and Fallopian tubes. *Hernia*. 2012;16:471 [PMID: 21213003].

Yang C, Zhang H, Pu J, et al: Laparoscopic vs open herniorrhaphy in the management of pediatric inguinal hernia: A systemic review and meta-analysis. *J Pediatr Surg*. 2011;46(9):1824 [PMID: 21929997].

APPENDICITIS

Acute appendicitis is the most frequent surgical condition for which children present to the emergency department. In up to 33% of children with appendicitis, the appendix ruptures before surgery. The incidence of appendicitis is 1-2 cases per 10,000 cases in children aged 1-4 years; however, the rate of perforation is as high as 80-100%. This is in contrast to older children (aged 10-17 years) where appendicitis is more common (25 cases per 10,000) and perforation rate is much lower (10-20%). Despite its relatively high occurrence, the diagnosis of appendicitis in a child can be difficult with even the most experienced physicians.

Clinical Findings

Classically, children present with periumbilical pain, followed by anorexia, nausea, vomiting, RLQ pain, and fever. Unfortunately, the classic presentation occurs in less than 50% of children with appendicitis. Anorexia is frequently missing; dysuria or pyuria may be present suggesting a UTI; diarrhea or loose stools are a frequent finding, often misleading the physician to believe the child has acute gastroenteritis. The presence of fever in association with abdominal tenderness increases the likelihood of appendicitis by three-fold; the presence of rebound tenderness triples the odds of acute appendicitis.

Children often present earlier in their clinical course in comparison with adults and thus may present with mild or vague symptoms. The most common findings are RLQ pain, guarding, vomiting; peritoneal signs may be confirmed with percussion tenderness or rebound tenderness on examination.

In female adolescents, it may be difficult to distinguish appendicitis from torsion of the ovary or pelvic inflammatory disease.

Examination of a child in pain is often difficult and requires a physician who can engage and distract the child with conversation, books, or toys. Children who are fearful of the examination may state they feel pain even when they do not. Telling the child you are "listening to bubbles" in their stomach, allows you to approach the abdominal area. Using your stethoscope will allow you to palpate all four quadrants lightly to determine if involuntary guarding or rebound tenderness is present. Historically, rebound tenderness can be elicited by palpating the abdomen and removing the hand quickly from the abdominal wall. In children with peritonitis, this maneuver produces undue pain and stress. In children, peritoneal irritation can be elicited by gentle percussion, tapping the feet, or jiggling the bed and watching for the child's reaction to discomfort.

As with all causes of abdominal pain, a full examination including the oropharynx, lungs, and genitalia (including a pelvic examination in sexually active girls) needs to be done to exclude other causes of abdominal pain in children such as streptococcal pharyngitis, lower lobe pneumonia, or testicular torsion.

Diagnostic Studies

In a child with classic history and physical findings consistent with acute appendicitis, no further testing is necessary. However, as stated previously, children often do not present with classic symptoms. Unfortunately, no single laboratory test will diagnose appendicitis. A normal WBC in a child with RLQ pain does not exclude the diagnosis of appendicitis; a WBC above 13,000 per cubic millimeter (cmm) in children

10 years and older or 15,000 cmm in children younger than 10 years increased the likelihood of appendicitis (LR, 3.4; 95% CI, 1.9-6.3). However, WBC can be elevated in a number of conditions presenting with lower abdominal pain. C-reactive protein (CRP) and erythrocyte sedimentation rate (ESR) are inconsistent predictors of appendicitis. Newer inflammatory biomarkers such as interleukin 6 (IL-6), IL-8, and CD-64 have been associated with appendicitis compared with non-surgical causes of abdominal pain; however, discriminative accuracy currently limits clinical applicability. The presence of WBC, RBC, or bacteria in the urine must also be viewed with caution. These findings can also be present if the inflamed appendix is located adjacent to the ureter.

Plain abdominal radiographs, US, CT, and barium enema are available as imaging studies for children with abdominal pain suspicious for appendicitis.

Plain film abdominal series are nonspecific and of low yield. Occasionally (10%), appendicoliths are present indicating appendicitis. Barium enema is no longer used due to unnecessary radiation exposure, advent and availability of CT scans, and high missed rate due to failure of the inflamed appendix to fill with contrast.

US is considered the study of choice to determine etiology of abdominal pain in children because it is rapid, noninvasive, requires no contrast, and is without radiation exposure. Since most young children have less abdominal wall fat than adults, the appendix is usually visualized readily. Inflammation is determined by graded compression. An inflamed appendix is usually difficult to compress and greater than or equal to 6 mm in diameter (Figure 36–12). Periappendiceal fluid collection may be present with perforation but can be seen with inflammation only.

Abdominal CT scans are of greatest accuracy, have the ability to diagnose other intra-abdominal causes of pain, but it does come with its costs. It takes considerably more time to mobilize a patient ready for CT; cost of drinking contrast: some centers still require oral contrast and if the child is vomiting, this can present significant challenges; and finally, it exposes the child to significant radiation, adding to the child's lifetime risk of developing cancer. In the case of perforation with abscess formation, an abdominal CT can help identify the abscesses that can be drained percutaneously with an interval appendectomy performed several weeks later.

Treatment

Consult the pediatric surgeon immediately. Allow nothing by mouth, administer IV fluids, broad-spectrum antibiotics, and appropriate pain medications. Correct any fluid and electrolyte abnormalities, although in children this is rare. Laparoscopic appendectomy is the accepted treatment of uncomplicated appendicitis in children. Laparoscopic appendectomy is associated with reduced postoperative pain, earlier recovery, shortened length of stay, and decreased abdominal scarring.

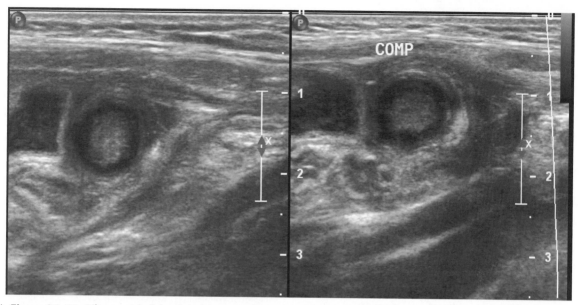

▲ **Figure 36–12.** Ultrasound of the right lower quadrant demonstrating a fecalith within a noncompressible appendix consistent with acute appendicitis.

Gasior AC, St Peter SD, Knott EM, Hall M, Ostlie DJ, Snyder CL: National trends in approach and outcomes with appendicitis in children. *J Pediatr Surg.* 2012;47:2264 [PMID: 23217886].

Bhatt M, Joseph L, Ducharme FM, et al: Prospective validation of the Pediatric Appendicitis Score in a Canadian Pediatric Emergency Department. *Acad Emerg Med.* 2009;16:591 [PMID: 19549016].

Bundy DG, Byerley JS, Liles EA, et al: Does this child have appendicitis? *JAMA.* 2007;298(4):438 [PMID: 17652298].

Hennelly KE, Bachur R: Appendicitis update. *Curr Opin Pediatr.* 2011;23:281 [PMID: 21467940].

Kharbanda AB, Cosme Y, Liu K, et al: Discriminative accuracy of novel and traditional biomarkers in children with suspected appendicitis adjusted for duration of abdominal pain. *Acad Emerg Med.* 2011;18:567 [PMID: 21676053].

Kulik DM, Uleryk EM, Maguire JL: Does this child have appendicitis? A systematic review of clinical prediction rules for children with acute abdominal pain. *J Clin Epid.* 2013;66:95 [PMID: 23177898].

Reed JL, Strait RT, Kachelmeyer AM, et al: Biomarkers to distinguish surgical etiologies in females with lower quadrant abdominal pain. *Acad Emerg Med.* 2011;18:686 [PMID: 21762231].

Sharwood LN, Babl FE: The efficacy and effect of opioid analgesia in undifferentiated abdominal pain in children: A review of four studies. *Pediatr Anes.* 2009;19:445 [PMID: 19453578].

CONSTIPATION

Constipation defined as a delay or difficulty in defecation, occurring for 2 or more weeks, is a common cause of abdominal pain in children. It is estimated that 3-10% of all visits to the pediatrician and up to 25% of referrals to the gastroenterologist are for constipation, and, not surprisingly, a common complaint presenting to the emergency department. Abdominal pain can be severe, causing the child to double over and cry, such that caregivers and providers have concerns of a surgical etiology for the pain.

Peak incidence occurs at the time of toilet training, but occurs from newborns to young adults. Little consensus exists as to the cause of constipation. Obesity, family history, low dietary fiber consumption, insufficient fluid intake, and low parental education have all been implicated. A recent systematic review showed that genetic predisposition could play a role in the development of childhood constipation, but no specific gene mutations have been identified. In less than 10% of children, constipation is secondary to organic disorders such as Hirschsprung disease, anorectal malformations, metabolic or neurologic disorders. In the majority, no organic etiology accounts for the problem, and is termed functional constipation.

Clinical Findings

Careful history and physical examination cannot be overemphasized. Abdominal pain is colicky in nature, localized to any quadrant, associated with infrequent and painful passage of hard stools, and sometimes associated with fecal incontinence mistaken as "diarrhea." Associated complaints include blood coating the stools, blood on toilet paper, nausea, vomiting, decreased appetite, weight loss, decreased activity, as well as urinary symptoms such as frequency and incontinence. Upon questioning, parents may report straining or behavior of the child associated with stool holding, such as rocking back and forth, rising to the toes, stiffening the buttocks and legs, often times in a corner or behind furniture.

Fever, abdominal distension, weight loss, dry skin, coarse hair, delayed growth and development in a child, or explosive bloody diarrhea in an infant possibly indicates an organic cause of constipation. Palpation of the abdomen often reveals palpable mobile masses in the lower quadrants. Anorectal examination may reveal a large amount of stool and stretching of the rectum. Assess sensation, tone, size, and presence of anal wink, as well as amount and consistency of stool within the rectal vault.

Diagnostic Studies

Constipation is a clinical and not a radiological diagnosis; however, there are times when a rectal examination may be too traumatizing for a child. For children with a history of sexual abuse, autism, developmental delay, or multiple rectal examinations, a plain abdominal radiograph may be helpful. Scoring systems have been developed to grade the stool burden on x-ray, and have been found to valid and correlate with presence of firm stool on rectal examination, but are subjective at times and dependent upon observer experience. US has been used to determine presence of "megarectum" seen in constipated children. In addition, infants with guaiac positive stool or explosive foul-smelling diarrhea following rectal examination or children with fever, distension, weight loss, or poor weight gain, may have an organic etiology to constipation and further testing is recommended. Testing such as rectal biopsy to diagnose Hirschsprung disease, sweat test to rule out cystic fibrosis, celiac disease antibodies, lead level, and thyroid function tests, calcium, vitamin D level, electrolytes, and glucose to rule out metabolic causes such as hypothyroidism, diabetes, and hypercalcemia or hypokalemia may be useful.

Treatment

Treatment of abdominal pain due to functional constipation in a child includes oral or rectal medications or combination of both. Rectal medications are faster but invasive. In the emergency department, it allows immediate relief of abdominal pain and reassessment to determine if further evaluation for other causes of pain is necessary. Rectal medications include saline water, phospho-soda, or milk with molasses enemas. Other methods of rectal disimpaction include glycerin suppositories for infants and bisacodyl suppositories for older children. Oral solutions include polyethylene glycol electrolyte solutions, mineral oil, magnesium citrate, magnesium hydroxide, sorbitol, lactulose, senna, or bisacodyl (Table 36–7).

When the impaction of stool is removed, maintenance therapy includes dietary changes: increase fluid intake, increase carbohydrates containing sorbitol such as pear,

prune, or apple juices to increase frequency and water content of the stool, and aim for a balanced diet containing whole grains, fruits and vegetables. Achieve regular toilet habits, specifically, unhurried toilet time after meals. Combine toilet time with a positive reward system, such as stickers. Medications in addition to behavior management are recommended. Mineral oil (lubricant), magnesium hydroxide, lactulose, polyethylene glycol (PEG) (osmotic laxative), or a combination have been used safely and successfully in children. Minimal data are available for infants and thus use is not currently recommended. PEG 3350 (1 g/kg/day) appears to be superior to other osmotic agents in taste and acceptance by children. Follow-up with primary care physician is warranted to monitor treatment effectiveness, need for consultation with a pediatric gastroenterologist, and need for further evaluation for organic causes of constipation.

Greenwald BJ: Clinical practice guidelines for pediatric constipation. *J Am Acad Nurse Pract.* 2010;22:332 [PMID: 20590953].

Hansen SE, Whitehill JL, Goto CS: Safety and efficacy of milk and molasses enemas compared with sodium phosphate enemas for the treatment of constipation in a pediatric emergency department. *Pediatr Emerg Care.* 2011;27(12):1118 [PMID: 22134228].

Miller MK, Dowd MD, Friesen CA, Walsh-Kelly CM: A randomized trial of enema versus polyethylene glycol 3350 for fecal disimpaction in children presenting to an emergency department. *Pediatr Emerg Care.* 2012;28(2):115 [PMID: 22270500].

North American Society for Pediatric Gastroenterology, Hepatology and Nutrition: Evaluation and treatment of constipation in children: Summary of updated recommendations of the North American Society for Pediatric Gastroenterology, Hepatology and Nutrition. *J Pediatr Gastroenterol Nutr.* 2006;43:405 [PMID: 16954970].

Peeters B, Benninga MA, Hennekam RC: Childhood constipation; an overview of genetic studies and associated syndromes. *Best Pract Res Clin Gastroenterol.* 2011;25:73 [PMID: 21382580].

Pijpers MA, Tabbers MM, Benninga MA, Berger MY: Currently recommended treatments of childhood constipation are not evidence based: A systematic literature review on the effect of laxative treatment and dietary measures. *Arch Dis Child.* 2009;94:117 [PMID: 18713795].

Walia R, Mahan L, Steffen R: Recent advances in chronic constipation. *Curr Opin Pediatr.* 2009;21:661 [PMID: 19606041].

PELVIC INFLAMMATORY DISEASE

Pelvic inflammatory disease (PID) is an acute infection of the upper female genital tract. Upper tract infections include endometriosis, salpingitis, tubo-ovarian abscess, perihepatitis, and/or peritonitis. Typically, acute PID is caused by ascending spread of microorganisms from the vagina and/or endocervix to the endometrium, fallopian tubes, and adjacent structures. *Neisseria gonorrhoeae* and/or *Chlamydia trachomatis* are the most common organisms causing PID. Aerobic and anaerobic organisms have also been implicated in causing PID.

Table 36–7. Medications used in the treatment of constipation.

Laxative	Dosage	Side Effects
Lactulose Osmotic	1-3 mL/kg/d in divided doses; available as 70% solution	Flatulence, cramps, hypernatremia, nontoxic megacolon in elderly
Sorbitol Osmotic	1-3 mL/kg/d in divided doses; available as 70% solution	Same as lactulose
Magnesium hydroxide Osmotic	1-3 mL/kg/d of 400 mg/5 mL; (400 mg/5 mL or 800 mg/5 mL) Liquid or tablets	Infants are susceptible to magnesium toxicity. Overdose can cause hypermagnesemia, hypophosphatemia, and secondary hypocalcaemia
Magnesium citrate Osmotic	< 6 yrs: 1-3 mL/kg/d 6-12 yrs: 100-150 mL/d > 12 yrs: 150-300 mL/d (16.17% magnesium) liquid	Infants are susceptible to magnesium toxicity. Overdose can cause hypermagnesemia, hypophosphatemia, and secondary hypocalcaemia
PEG 3350	Disimpaction: 1-1.5 g/kg/d for 3 days Maintenance: 1 g/kg/d	No data for infants
Phosphate enema Osmotic enema	< 2 years: do not use ≥ 2 years: 6 mL/kg up to 135 mL	Risk of trauma to rectal wall, abdominal distension or vomiting, may cause severe/lethal episodes of hypophosphatemia, hypocalcaemia with tetany; avoid in renal failure or Hirschsprung
Polyethylene glycol electrolyte solution Lavage	Disimpaction: 25 mL/kg/h (to 1000 mL/h) by NG tube until clear or 20 mL/kg/h for 4 h/d. Maintenance 5-10 mL/kg/d	Difficult to take, nausea, bloating, abdominal cramps, vomiting, anal irritation, aspiration, pneumonia, pulmonary edema, Mallory-Weiss tear. Long-term safety not well established. Requires hospitalization for NGT
Mineral oil Lubricant	< 1 yr: not recommended Disimpaction: 15-30 mL/yr of age, max 240 mL/d Maintenance: 1-3 mL/kg/d	Lipoid pneumonia if aspirated. Theoretically interferes with absorption of at soluble substances. Foreign body reaction in intestinal mucosa
Senna Stimulant	2-6 yr: 2.5-7.5 mL/d 6-12 yr: 5-15 mL/d (8.8 mg sennosides/5 mL syrup) Tablets and granules	Idiosyncratic hepatitis, melanosis coli, hypertrophic osteoarthropathy, analgesic nephropathy
Bisacodyl Stimulant	≥ 2 yr: 0.5-1 suppository 1-3 tablets per dose 5 mg tablets and 10 mg suppositories	Abdominal pain, diarrhea, hypokalemia, abnormal rectal mucosa, rarely proctitis. Case reports of urolithiasis
Glycerin suppositories		No reported side effects

Clinical Findings

Patient often has complaints of lower abdominal pain, vaginal discharge, and intermenstrual bleeding. With more severe disease, complaints of fever, malaise, nausea, and vomiting are present. Five percent present with RUQ abdominal pain and tenderness, known as Fitz-Hugh and Curtis syndrome.

Examination often reveals abdominal, adnexal tenderness, mucopurulent discharge from the vagina or cervical os and pain with movement of the cervix on pelvic examination.

Diagnostic Studies

ESR and CRP are elevated in severe disease. Elevated ESR (> 15 mm/hour) is found in 75% laparoscopy-confirmed PID patients. Similarly CRP has a sensitivity of 94% and specificity of 83% in patients with laparoscopy confirmed PID. WBC counts may be elevated; 60% patients with PID have leukocytosis. Wet mount of vaginal secretions provides a useful indicator of upper genital tract infection. Patients without mucopurulent cervicitis and/or inflammatory cells on wet mount carry an excellent negative predictive value for excluding acute PID.

Table 36–8. Criteria for the clinical diagnosis of pelvic inflammatory disease.

Minimal criteria (1 required)
   Cervical motion tenderness or
   Uterine tenderness or
   Adnexal tenderness
Additional criteria
   Oral temperature ≥ 38.3°C (101°F)
   Abnormal cervical or vaginal mucopurulent discharge
   Presence of abundant WBCs on saline microscopy of vaginal secretions
   Elevated erythrocyte sedimentation rate (ESR)
   Elevated C-reactive protein (CRP)
   Laboratory confirmation of cervical infection with *N. gonorrhoeae* or *C. trachomatis*
Most specific criteria
   Endometrial biopsy with histologic evidence of endometritis
   Transvaginal sonography or MRI showing thickened, fluid-filled tubes with or without free pelvic fluid or tubo-ovarian complex or Doppler studies suggesting pelvic infection (tubal hyperemia)
   Laparoscopy demonstrating acute PID

Adapted from the Centers for Disease Control and Prevention: Sexually Transmitted Diseases Treatment Guidelines, 2010. MMWR 2010; 59(RR-12): 63-67.

US is the first-line approach for the evaluation of lower abdominal pain in children. US is relatively noninvasive and widely available. Transvaginal sonography that is highly suggestive of PID includes thickened fluid-filled fallopian tubes with or without free pelvic fluid. CT and MRI have recently been used for evaluation of patients with PID; the sensitivity is over 95%. Table 36–8 delineates the criteria for the clinical diagnosis of PID.

Treatment

According to the CDC, it is important that empiric treatment be initiated as soon as the diagnosis of PID is made as to minimize long-term complications (Table 36–9).

Disposition

Most patients can be treated as outpatient. CDC indications for in-hospital management are need for surgical involvement, severe disease with nausea, vomiting or high fever, tubo-ovarian abscess, pregnancy, lack of response to oral therapy, and intolerance of oral therapy.

Pregnant adolescents with PID have a high incidence of miscarriage and preterm delivery. Patients with TOA are at risk of leaking or rupture of the abscess or severe sepsis, and thus it is recommended to treat with IV antibiotics until improved.

Since the data was lacking on management of adolescents, the CDC removed adolescence as a criteria for hospitalization. The decision to hospitalize adolescents can be based upon the same criteria for admission of older women. Some still recommend hospitalization for the adolescent since adolescence is a proxy for poor compliance and high-risk sexual activity.

Table 36–9. Centers for Disease Control and Prevention recommendations for the treatment of acute pelvic inflammatory disease.

Parenteral
Regimen A
Cefotetan 2 g IV every 12 h *or* cefoxitin 2g IV every 6 h
plus
Doxycycline 100 mg orally or IV every 12 h

Regimen B
Clindamycin 900 mg IV every 8 h
plus
Gentamicin loading dose IV or IM (2 mg/kg) followed by maintenance dose (1.5 mg/kg) every 8 hours. A single daily dose of 3-5 mg/kg IV can be substituted.

Alternative parenteral regimen
Ampicillin/sulbactam 3 g IV every 6 h
plus
Doxycycline 100 mg orally or IV every 12 h

Oral Treatment
Regimen 1
Ceftriaxone 250 mg IM in a single dose
plus
Doxycycline 100 mg orally twice a day for 14 d
with or *without*
Metronidazole 500 mg orally twice a day for 14 d

Regimen 2
Cefoxitin 2 g IM in a single dose and probenecid 1 g orally administered concomitantly
plus
Doxycycline 100 mg orally twice a day for 14 d
with or *without*
Metronidazole 500 mg orally twice a day for 14 d

Regimen 3
Other parenteral third-generation cephalosporin (ceftizoxime or cefotaxime) in a single dose
plus
Doxycycline 100 mg orally twice a day for 14 d
with or *without*
Metronidazole 500 mg orally twice a day for 14 d

Complications of Pelvic Inflammatory Disease

▶ Perihepatitis

Also known as Fitz-Hugh and Curtis (FHC) syndrome, perihepatitis is a serious complication of PID involving "violin string" adhesions between the liver capsule and the anterior abdominal wall. Patients present with severe RUQ abdominal pain and tenderness similar to cholecystitis. Pain can be pleuritic and radiate to the right shoulder. In addition, lower abdominal tenderness and evidence of PID is almost always present. Laboratory tests may be helpful in eliminating other causes of RUQ pain such as hepatitis; however, they are not characteristic in FHC. WBC count, ESR, and liver function tests may be elevated or normal. Radiographic studies such as US or CT may also be helpful in ruling out diseases such as cholecystitis, cholelithiasis, subphrenic abscess, pancreatitis, nephrolithiasis, and perforated ulcer. CT finding of perihepatitis typically present with hepatic capsular enhancement in the arterial phase. Definitive diagnosis can be made only by direct visualization of the liver by laparoscopy or laparotomy.

Treatment of FHC is the same as that for parenteral PID. Surgical exploration is rare but can be considered if symptoms do not resolve with appropriate antimicrobial therapy.

▶ Tubo-ovarian Abscess

Tubo-ovarian abscess (TOA) is a polymicrobial collection of bacteria and inflammatory cells that adhere to lower abdominal structures such as the fallopian tube, ovary, bowel, or omentum. Cultures obtained from TOA include aerobes and anaerobes such as *E. coli*, *Bacteroides fragilis*, and *Peptostreptococcus*. We know that *N. gonorrhoeae* is a significant causative bacterial agent, but it is rarely cultured from the abscess cavity.

Patients present with lower abdominal or pelvic pain, a mass, fever/chills (50%), vaginal discharge (28%), intermenstrual bleeding (21%), nausea (26%), and vomiting. On examination, the patient may have a palpable mass, abdominal tenderness, or evidence of peritonitis. Leukocytosis is present in 24% of women with TOA. However, it is important to know, that a patient without fever and leukocytosis may still very well have TOA.

Several imaging modalities are useful in diagnosis of TOA. CT scan, US, scintigraphy, and radionuclide scanning are available. CT and US are the most readily available. On CT with IV contrast, TOAs tend to have a thick enhancing abscess wall and are multilocular, with increased fluid density (95%). Commonly, there is an associated thickening of the meso-salpinx and infiltration into the pelvic fat, bowel thickening, and thickening of the utero-sacral ligaments. US may reveal complete obliteration of the normal architecture of one or both adnexas. Within the indistinguishable ovary and tube, there is often a cystic or multiseptated mass (Figure 36–13). Speckled fluid is also seen and this correlates with the purulent material within the abdomen. Laparoscopy is sometimes needed to establish the diagnosis.

Treatment is now with conservative medical management involving antimicrobial therapy with greater than 70% success rate. Laparoscopy or interventional radiology drainage is reserved for patients with poor response to antibiotics, especially if there is an abscess that needs to be drained. Patients with TOA mass 10 cm have a greater than 60% chance of requiring surgery, and those with a mass 4-6 cm have a less than 20% chance of surgery. Clinical deterioration or worsening peritonitis suggests rupture of the TOA and is an indication for laparoscopy. Laparoscopic treatment involves drainage and irrigation with sparing organs of fertility and intensive medical therapy. Antimicrobial therapy is the same as the parenteral treatment for PID. Hospitalization is usually required until adequate response to antibiotics is evident and to monitor for signs of rupture of TOA.

Percutaneous drainage of TOA is effectively done using US or CT guidance. Low-lying pelvic abscesses can be drained through a posterior colpotomy. Pelvic or abdominal abscesses can be drained using image-guided techniques via the abdominal, vaginal, rectal or gluteal wall. Success rate of minimally invasive drainage are very high but is dependent upon the location of the abscess, accessibility, and expertise.

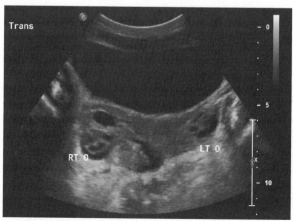 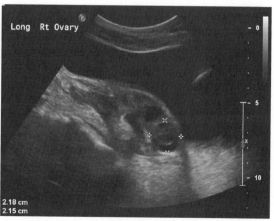

▲ **Figure 36–13.** (**A**) Ultrasound of para-ovarian mass surrounding right ovary. (**B**) Mass consistent with abscess formation.

Balamuth F, Zhao H, Mollen C: Toward improving the diagnosis and the treatment of adolescent pelvic inflammatory disease in emergency departments: Results of a brief educational intervention. *Pediatr Emerg Care.* 2010;26:85 [PMID: 20094001].

Centers for Disease Control and Prevention: Sexually transmitted diseases treatment guidelines, 2010. *MMWR.* 2010;59 (RR-12):63 [PMID: 21160459].

Haggerty CL, Ness RB: Diagnosis and treatment of pelvic inflammatory disease. *Womens Health.* 2008;4:383 [PMID: 19072503].

Sweet RL: Pelvic Inflammatory Disease: Current concepts of diagnosis and management. *Curr Infect Dis Rep.* 2012;14:194 [PMID: 22298157].

OVARIAN TORSION

Ovarian torsion is reported to account for 2.7% of all cases of acute abdominal pain in children, most commonly presenting during the perimenarchal or early adolescence. Fifteen percent of cases occur during infancy and childhood. Causes of adnexal torsion include benign cystic teratomas, hemorrhagic or follicular cysts, paratubular cysts, cystadenomas, and hydrosalpinx. Rarely (< 1%) is malignancy the cause of ovarian torsion in children.

Clinical Findings

Most common symptoms of ovarian torsion are pain, nausea, and vomiting. Pain is sudden, colicky, and persistent with some radiation of pain to the flank, groin, or back. Fever (20%) may be present and there may be a palpable mass on examination (20-36%). The pain may be out of proportion to the examination and be intermittent if the torsion is intermittent or evolving. Children may present with an incarcerated hernia which may contain an ovary that is torsed and infarcted. Thus, repair of inguinal hernias in females with a herniated ovary should be done timely to minimize the small risk of torsion and ovary loss.

Diagnostic Studies

There are no specific laboratory tests to diagnose ovarian torsion. However, the evaluation of abdominal pain in a female includes a urinalysis, pregnancy test, and CBC. If a tumor is suspected, serologic markers including alpha fetoprotein and beta HCG are recommended.

US with Doppler remains the most useful radiologic test to determine ovarian torsion. Common sonographic findings include an enlarged ovary echogenic mass with nonvisualization of the ipsilateral ovary, fluid in the cul-de-sac, coiling of the ovarian vessels or in true adnexal torsion, absent arterial and venous blood flow with Doppler. However, the presence of Doppler flow does not completely exclude torsion. Doppler US is operator dependent, and at times it is difficult to distinguish flow from background noise. There is also the entity of intermittent torsion and the ovary is not completely torsed at the time of the study.

When US is unavailable, computed tomography (CT) may be useful to find an ovarian mass or exclude other causes of abdominal pain in females. However, abdominal CT scans do expose the child to radiation that may have other unaccounted for long-term effects.

Treatment

Prompt diagnosis of ovarian torsion is key to optimizing survival and function of the ovary. Pain control, IV fluids, and immediate consultation with a gynecologic or pediatric surgeon are important in the emergency department. Surgical management includes laparoscopy and detorsion of the ovary. For the ovary with minimal edema or ischemia, cystectomy, tumorectomy, or cyst aspiration may be considered if the pathology can be identified. In patients with no obvious underlying ovarian pathology, oophoropexy (stabilization of the ovarian tissue) may be considered for both the involved and contralateral ovary but is not routinely performed. It is hypothesized that this procedure would reduce the risk of future torsion. For the ovary with significant edema or hemorrhage, the ovary can be detorsed alone. For the ovary with concerns for tumor, follow-up tumor markers and sonogram are obtained and, if abnormal, the ovary can be removed at another surgery. Girls who have torsion with functional cysts are prescribed combination oral contraceptives to suppress future cyst development that possibly predisposed them to torsion.

Balci O, Icen MS, Mahmoud AS, Capar M, Colakoglu MC: Management and outcomes of adnexal torsion: A 5 year experience. *Arch Gynecol Obstet.* 2011;284(3):643 [PMID: 20922399].

Chang YJ, Yan DC, Kong MS, et al: Adnexal torsion in children. *Pediatr Emerg Care.* 2008;24:534 [PMID: 18645541].

Galinier P, Carfagna L, Delsol M, et al: Ovarian torsion. Management and ovarian prognosis: A report of 45 cases. *J Pediatr Surg.* 2009;55:1759 [PMID: 19735822].

Guthrie BD, Adler MD, Powell EC: Incidence and trends of pediatric ovarian torsion hospitalizations in the United States, 2000-2006. *Pediatrics.* 2010;125(3):532 [PMID: 20123766].

Piper HG, Oltmann SC, Xu L, Adusumilli S, Fischer AC: Ovarian torsion: Diagnosis of inclusion mandates earlier intervention. *J Pediatr Surg.* 2012;47(11):2071 [PMID: 23164000].

Poonai N, Poonai C, Lim R, Lynch T: Pediatric ovarian torsion: Case series and review of the literature. *Can J Surg.* 2013;56(2):103 [PMID: 23351494].

Rossi BV, Ference EH, Zurakowski D, et al: The clinical presentation and surgical management of adnexal torsion in the pediatric and adolescent population. *J Pediatr Adolesc Gynecol.* 2012;25(2):109 [PMID: 22206683].

Tsafrir Z, Azem F, Hasson J, et al: Risk factors, symptoms, and treatment of ovarian torsion in children: The twelve-year experience of one center. *J Minim Invasive Gynecol.* 2012;19(1):29 [PMID: 22014543].

GALLBLADDER DISEASE: CHOLELITHIASIS & CHOLECYSTITIS

Gallbladder (GB) disease is an uncommon cause of abdominal pain in infants and children; however, over the past 30 years, the incidence is on the rise. This could be due to factors such as an increase in childhood diabetes and obesity and improved diagnostic capabilities using US. GB encompasses a host of disorders ranging from asymptomatic cholelithiasis to symptomatic cholelithiasis, cholecystitis, acalculous cholecystitis, choledocholithiasis, gallstone pancreatitis, ascending cholangitis, and gallbladder dysfunction such as biliary dyskinesia. The incidence of pediatric cholelithiasis ranges from 0.13 to 1.9%. Risk factors for pediatric GB disease include obesity, history of total parental nutrition with and without resection or dysfunction in infancy, antibiotic use, cystic fibrosis, biliary dyskinesia, congenital anomalies, systemic infection, and hemoglobinopathies such as sickle cell disease (SCD) and hereditary spherocytosis. Ceftriaxone use has also been associated with the development of gallstones in children. Ceftriaxone is concentrated in the bile after excretion and causes a reversible pseudolithiasis after a minimum of 4 days of antibiotic use.

The content of pediatric stones differs from adult stones; adult stones are mostly made of cholesterol. Pediatric stones are primarily of three types: black pigment associated with hemolytic diseases; cholesterol associated with obesity, female sex, estrogen/progesterone therapy, and genetic factors; or calcium carbonate which is associated with a prolonged neonatal intensive care unit stay or Down syndrome.

Clinical Findings

Clinically, children present with an array of findings. Abdominal pain may be one of the constitutional symptoms; however, infants may present with jaundice only; older children may present with vomiting alone. Children may present with intermittent RUQ pain, nausea, vomiting, jaundice, fatty food intolerance, acholic stools, and fever. Children with hemolytic disease, specifically SCD present with nonspecific abdominal pain mimicking sickle cell crisis pain. Murphy sign may be present; however, it is highly nonspecific.

Diagnostic Studies

A CBC, liver enzymes, lipase, urinalysis, and routine studies are helpful in eliminating certain disease entities considered in the differential. A WBC, liver function tests, and pancreatic evaluation even if normal, do not rule out gallbladder disease. If gallbladder disease is suspected and the child's abdomen is tender, imaging is indicated.

US is the best diagnostic tool for pediatric GB disease. US is 95% accurate in diagnosing cholelithiasis. Gallstones appear as echogenic foci within the gallbladder (Figure 36–14). Gallstones may also be accompanied by gallbladder sludge. Other findings include dilation of the gallbladder, pericholecystic fluid, wall hyperemia on Doppler, and a sonographic Murphy's sign (SMS). In severe cases, emphysema (bright echoes from intramural air), gangrene (thickened walls and sloughed membranes), or evidence of frank perforation (wall disruption) may be present.

The single most powerful indicator of gallbladder disease is the presence of the SMS, presence of maximum tenderness over the gallbladder identified during the US procedure.

US may also diagnose dilation of the common bile duct (CBD). In pediatric patients, the normal CBD diameter varies with age. Children younger than 13 years have a healthy CBD less than 3.3 mm, and children younger than 3 months have a CBD less than 1.2 mm.

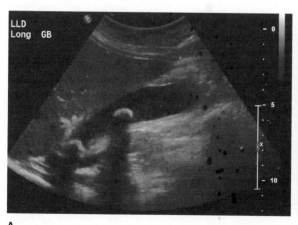
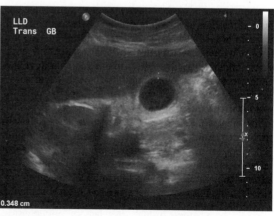

▲ **Figure 36–14.** **(A)** Longitudinal US view of gallbladder demonstrating single echogenic stone. **(B)** In the same patient, the transverse view demonstrates gallbladder wall thickening consistent with cholecystitis in addition to cholelithiasis.

Plain radiographs may reveal pigment stones but are generally not helpful. CT can identify stones, in addition to many other disease processes such as wall thickening, pericholecystic fluid and stranding, and biliary obstruction, but again at the cost of radiation exposure to the child. MRI is not readily available at most institutions and young children require procedural sedation.

Treatment

Treatment regimens are age-dependent and usually involve supportive care and pain control. Neonates and infants with cholelithiasis may require observation only, and symptoms usually resolve spontaneously. Symptomatic infants with calcified stones may benefit from cholecystectomy. Children with biliary colic without evidence of cholecystitis can be treated with pain medications, dietary changes, and outpatient follow-up for consultation with a pediatric surgeon. If there is US confirmation of cholecystitis, systemic illness, vomiting, or severe pain, these children require aggressive fluid resuscitation, pain medications, IV antibiotics, and prompt surgical evaluation. Laparoscopic cholecystectomy is currently the procedure of choice. Recent data show that this procedure is associated with less pain and fewer inpatient hospital days as compared to open cholecystectomy.

Patients with hemolytic disease, specifically SCD, who have symptomatic cholelithiasis or cholecystitis, require laparoscopic cholecystectomy. Prior to surgery, transfusion with packed red blood cells, aggressive fluid resuscitation, pain control, IV antibiotics, and oxygen are recommended.

Mehta S, Lopez ME, Chumpitazi BP, et al: Clinical characteristics and risk factors for symptomatic pediatric gallbladder disease. *Pediatrics*. 2012;129(1):e82 [PMID: 22157135].

Poffenberger CM, Gausche-Hill M, Ngai S, et al: Cholelithiasis and its complications in children and adolescents. *Pediatr Emerg Care*. 2012;28:68 [PMID: 22217893].

Tsung JW, Raio CC, Ramirez-Schrempp D, Blaivas M: Point-of-care ultrasound diagnosis of pediatric cholecystitis in the ED. *Am J Emerg Med*. 2012;28:338 [PMID: 20223393].

Wesdorp I, Bosman D, Graaff A, et al: Clinical presentations and predisposing factors of cholelithiasis and sludge in children. *J Pediatr Gastroenterol Nutr*. 2000;31(4):411 [PMID: 1045839].

URINARY TRACT INFECTION

Urinary tract infection (UTI) in infants and children commonly present to the emergency department as a febrile event without a source. In the older child, an UTI may present as abdominal pain with or without a fever. An emergency department physician's job is to identify the patient at risk for a UTI based upon history, risk factors, and physical examination. These are especially relevant since infants and young children present with vague nonspecific symptoms and are nonverbal.

Uncircumcised males younger than 60 days have a 21% incidence of UTI compared to a 5% incidence in females, and 2.3 percent in circumcised males. Beyond the 6-month period, females have a significant increased risk of UTI, compared to males. Most experts recommend obtaining urine samples in all febrile females 0-24 months of age to make the diagnosis.

Clinical Findings

Presentation of UTI is age-dependent. Young infants often present with vague and nonspecific symptoms such as poor feeding, crying, decreased urine output, lethargy, increased sleeping, vomiting, poor weight gain, or jaundice. Fever alone, is not necessary. A clinical pearl is that jaundice is significantly associated with UTI in infants especially, unconjugated hyperbilirubinemia outside 8 days of life.

Older infants present with fever as the main symptom of UTI. High fever [39°C (102.2°F) or greater] and occult UTI are highly associated, the positive likelihood ratio of 4 (95% CI, 1.2-13). Other nonspecific findings include vomiting, loose stools, and abdominal discomfort or pain. Even if there may be another potential source of fever, such as an upper respiratory syndrome, acute gastroenteritis, bronchiolitis, or otitis media, it does not entirely exclude the presence of UTI. Even febrile, respiratory syncytial virus-positive infants younger than 60 days still have a 5.4% risk of UTI compared to respiratory syncytial virus (RSV) negative infants (10% risk.)

Older children have complaints of dysuria, frequency, abdominal or flank pain, and fever. A word of caution, adolescent girls with urethritis from sexually transmitted diseases (STDs) often experience similar symptoms; therefore, laboratory testing for both UTI and STDs is necessary.

Diagnostic Studies

The gold standard for UTI diagnosis is the urine culture. Culture results are not available for 24-48 hours, so rapid screening using the urinalysis and/or microscopic analysis is used to identify pediatric patients likely to have UTI.

Urine dipstick gives rapid results primarily looking for the presence of leukocyte esterase (LE) or nitrites in the urine sample. LE is released when leukocytes are broken down and nitrites are the byproduct of nitrate metabolism by bacteria. The problem is that LE misses more than 20% of children with UTI and also gives a 10% false-positive result. Nitrites, too, have a high false-negative result, and greater than 50% children with UTI are missed on screening. This is because not all uropathogenic bacteria produce nitrites, urine samples may be dilute, and non–toilet-trained infants void frequently, reducing the time for nitrite conversion.

Urine microscopy showing the presence of bacteria reveals excellent sensitivity and specificity for UTI.

Urine culture is the gold standard for diagnosis of UTI. A positive urine culture is a single organism cultured from a specimen: suprapubic aspiration specimen, greater than 1000 colony-forming units (CFUs) per mL; catheter specimen, greater than 10,000 CFU/mL; or clean-catch, midstream sample, 100,000 CFU/mL. Common uropathogenic bacteria in children include *E. coli, Klebsiella, Proteus, Enterobacter, Citrobacter, Staphylococcus saprophyticus,* and *Enterococcus.*

Procalcitonin and C-reactive protein have been hypothesized to discriminate upper UTI from lower UTI. To date, there is limited pediatric data to support this hypothesis. Blood cultures are frequently the standard evaluation for fever without a source for infants. Positive blood cultures associated with UTI tend to be in the infants aged younger than 6 months. Lumbar puncture is also a known standard performed in neonates 30 days or younger with a UTI.

Treatment

Infants younger than 2-3 months, or children who appear toxic, unable to tolerate oral fluids, or dehydrated are best managed in the hospital with parenteral antibiotics. Recommended antibiotics include IV third-generation cephalosporin or aminoglycoside. Single daily dosing with aminoglycosides is safe and effective and usually involves a short course of 2-4 days of IV therapy followed by oral therapy for lower tract disease. For gentamicin single daily dosing is based on the following recommendations: 1 month to <5 years: 7.5 mg/kg/dose every 24 hours; 5-10 years: 6 mg/kg/dose every 24 hours; >10 years: 4.5 mg/kg/dose every 24 hours. The optimal duration of IV therapy for pyelonephritis is currently being studied, but traditionally occurs over 10-14 days.

Infants and children with uncomplicated UTIs can be managed as an outpatient. Due to increased rates of *E. coli* resistance, studies have found higher cure rates using cephalosporins such as cefixime, cefpodoxime, cefprozil, or cephalexin, and even amoxicillin/clavulanate and trimethoprim/sulfamethoxazole. Nitrofurantoin is not recommended for febrile UTI because therapeutic serum or renal concentrations are not achieved. Fluoroquinolones are generally not used in children due to the unsubstantiated concerns of injury to developing joints. Fluoroquinolone therapy is recommended by the American Academy of Pediatrics (AAP) for patients with UTIs caused by *Pseudomonas aeruginosa* or other multidrug-resistant gram-negative bacteria for which there is no effective alternative.

A recent Cochrane review comparing short duration (2-4 days) versus standard duration (7-14 days) of oral antibiotics in children with lower UTIs found no difference in positive urine cultures between therapies immediately after treatment. Short or long course in children with lower UTIs appear equally effective.

Follow-up assessment at 48-72 hours in all infants and children with UTIs is necessary to ensure appropriate response to antibiotics. Infants and children who remain febrile or symptomatic require US to evaluate for the presence of a renal abscess, obstruction, or pyelonephritis. Additionally, further diagnostic imaging (renal US, voiding cystourethrography, or radionuclide cystography) following a first time UTI is recommended by the AAP.

Beetz R: Evaluation and management of urinary tract infections in the neonate. *Curr Opin Pediatr.* 2012;24:205 [PMID: 22227782].

Bhat RG, Katy TA, Place FC: Pediatric urinary tract infections. *Emerg Med Clin N Am.* 2011;29:637 [PMID: 21782079].

Brady PW, Conway PH, Goudie A: Length of intravenous antibiotic therapy and treatment failure in infants with urinary tract infections. *Pediatrics.* 2010;126:196 [PMID: 20624812].

Ghaemi S, Fesharaki RJ, Kelishadi R: Late onset jaundice and urinary tract infection in neonates. *Indian J Pediatr.* 2007;74:139 [PMID: 17337825].

Hodson EM, Willis NS, Craig JC: Antibiotics for acute pyelonephritis in children. *Cochrane Database Syst Rev.* 2007;4:CD003772 [PMID: 17943796].

Kotoula A, Gardikis S, Tsalkidis A, et al: Comparative efficacies of procalcitonin and conventional inflammatory markers for prediction of renal parenchymal inflammation in pediatric first urinary tract infection. *Urology.* 2009;73:782 [PMID: 19152962].

Koyle MA, Elder JS, Skoog SJ, et al: Febrile urinary tract infection, vesicoureteral reflux, and renal scarring: Current controversies in approach to evaluation. *Pediatr Surg Int.* 2011;27:337 [PMID: 21305381].

Montini G, Tullus K, Hewitt I: Febrile urinary tract infections in children. *N Engl J Med.* 2011;365:239 [PMID: 21774712].

Shaikh N, Morone NE, Lopez J, et al: Does this child have a urinary tract infection? *JAMA.* 2007;298:2895 [PMID: 18159059].

Subcommittee on Urinary Tract Infection, SCoQlaM: Urinary tract infection: Clinical practice guideline for the diagnosis and management of the initial UTI in febrile infants and children 2 to 24 months. *Pediatrics.* 2011;128:595 [PMID: 21873693].

INFLAMMATORY BOWEL DISEASE

Crohn disease (CD) and ulcerative colitis (UC) are related but distinct types of inflammatory bowel disease (IBD) affecting children. Approximately 25% of newly diagnosed patients are diagnosed in childhood and adolescence with the mean age at diagnosis in the United States of 12.5 years. Risk factors are primarily related to genetic predisposition of the host. Up to 25% children have a positive family history of IBD. The specific causes of IBD are unknown, but the current theory is that a genetically susceptible host becomes exposed to an environmental trigger such as smoke, infection, or a medication, and this trigger enables luminal gut bacteria to cross the epithelial barrier leading to uncontrolled signaling among the gut immune cells. This result in recruitment and differentiation of T-cell lymphocytes, the exaggerated response leads to intestinal inflammation and damage.

Clinical Findings

CD and UC have similar clinical features: abdominal pain, diarrhea, weight loss, rectal bleeding, anemia, and evidence

Table 36–10. Differential diagnosis for abdominal pain and diarrhea in children.

Bloody diarrhea
Bacterial infection
Henoch-Schönlein purpura
Ischemic bowel
Radiation colitis
Hemolytic uremic syndrome
Rectal bleeding
Anal fissure, polyps, rectal ulcer syndrome
Meckel diverticulum
Perirectal disease (think Crohn disease)
Fissure
Streptococcal infection
Appendicitis
Intussusception
Mesenteric adenitis
Meckel diverticulum
Ovarian cyst
Lymphoma

Table 36–11. Commercially available serologic markers.

Serologic Marker	Crohn Disease	Ulcerative Colitis
ASCA (anti-Saccharomyces cerevisiae antibody) immunoglobulin A and G	40-56%	0-7%
ANCA (anti-neutrophil cytoplasmic antibody) histamine 1 protein, DNAse specified	18-24%	60- 80%
Anti-Omp C (outer membrane protein of E. coli)	25%	6%

Approximately 70% of children have anemia and ESR is elevated in 75% of children with moderate to severe disease. Stool studies to exclude infectious causes of diarrhea should be sent. Fecal markers, such as calprotectin (FC) and lactoferrin (FL), are noninvasive markers of gut inflammation and are elevated in children with IBD and normal in children with irritable bowel syndrome. Serologic markers that discriminate CD from UC were recently discovered; however, their use in children is limited since seroconversion depends on exposure and a mature immune system (Table 36–11).

A barium upper GI radiographic series may show stenosis, abnormal separation of bowel loops, and fistula formation in CD. CT scan often shows intestinal wall thickening, abscess formation, fistulas, or strictures. MRI has a 90% sensitivity and specificity for detecting CD in the small intestine and has the potential for discriminating CD from UC because mucosal and full-thickness wall inflammation enhance differently. MRI has also become the imaging modality of choice for perianal disease. Advantage is that most children with IBD receive multiple radiological examinations in a lifetime, and MRI offers a nonionizing option. Ultrasound is sensitive and specific in the detection of CD; however, US is highly dependent upon the experience of the operator.

Video capsule endoscopy (VCE) is a promising imaging technique that involves no radiation. The capsule is the size of a multivitamin and has the capability of imaging the small bowel. Within 24-48 hours, the capsule is passed in the stool. Images are transmitted and downloaded to a computer and read by a gastroenterologist. Negatives with VCE are that the child must be able to swallow it, it cannot be used in patients with strictures, and lesions that are seen cannot be biopsied.

Endoscopy with biopsy is the most sensitive and specific imaging modality available. It allows for direct visualization and biopsy. It is the most sensitive and specific for evaluation of the colon and ileum. Continuous inflammation is seen in the rectum and extends proximally into the colon in patients with UC. Endoscopic features of CD are the characteristic skip lesions: normal-appearing gut interspersed with inflamed mucosa. Strictures, exudates, and aphthous ulcers

of malnutrition. Children with CD present with abdominal pain, diarrhea, and weight loss. Some will present with melanotic or bloody stools, aphthous stomatitis, and perianal tags, fissures, fistulas, or abscesses. CD can affect the intestines from the mouth to the anus. Inflammation is transmural and characterized by skip lesions. Many will have poor appetite, fevers, and iron deficiency anemia, and are diagnosed while being evaluated for malnutrition and poor growth or delayed puberty. Arthralgias and arthritis are common in CD. Erythema nodosum occurs with CD and is characterized by tender, warm, red nodules or plaques on the extensor surfaces of the lower extremities.

Children with UC characteristically present with diarrhea, rectal bleeding, and abdominal pain. The diarrhea is insidious and usually without systemic features such as fever or weight loss (Table 36–10). One-third of the children present with hematochezia, abdominal cramping with fecal urgency, low-grade or intermittent fever, weight loss, anemia, and hypoalbuminemia. Pyoderma gangrenosum occurs rarely, but is associated with more extensive colonic involvement in patients with UC. UC involves primarily the mucosal layer of the colon, the inflammation is continuous, starting from the rectum and extending proximally. There are no skip lesions. Children are more likely to experience pancolitis.

Diagnostic Studies

Blood tests may be helpful in a child suspected of having IBD. WBC, total protein/albumin, ESR, CRP, aminotransferases, alkaline phosphatase, and bilirubin are classically abnormal.

may be present throughout the intestine. Inflammation of CD is full thickness.

Treatment

Current IBD medications include corticosteroids, 5-aminosalicylates (5-ASA), immunomodulators, biologic agents, antibiotics, and probiotics. Corticosteroids control moderate to severe symptoms and provide improvement in 80% of patients with IBD. Steroid dependency is a problem. Immunomodulators, such as azathioprine and 6-mercaptopurine, are tolerated well and provide remission in approximately 75% of patients. Methotrexate inhibits dihydrofolate reductase, an enzyme necessary for folic acid metabolism, and is effective at providing short-term symptom control and long-term remission in patients with CD.

Biologic therapy is used for induction and maintenance for children with moderate to severe disease. Infliximab is a monoclonal antibody directed against the cytokine TNF-α and works both for CD and UC. Infliximab is the only immunomodulator approved by the United States FDA for children with CD. Two anti-TNF agents, adalimumab and certolizumab, have been studied recently and found to be as effective as infliximab.

Nutritional therapy may provide some benefit in children with CD. Exclusive enteral nutrition from elemental or polymeric formulas has been associated with short-term remission in up to 80% children with CD. Enteral nutrition suppresses bowel inflammation and allows mucosal healing. After induction, medications such as immunomodulators are necessary to maintain remission.

Antibiotics are used to treat certain disease entities. Metronidazole and ciprofloxacin are used to treat perirectal fistulas, pouchitis following colectomy or ileoanal pouch procedures in UC patients. Rifaximin also reduces abdominal pain and diarrhea in children with IBD.

Probiotics are not helpful in children with CD, but in children with UC, probiotics may help maintain remission when added to standard regimens. Probiotics may also be helpful in the prevention and treatment of pouchitis.

Indications for surgery include uncontrolled GI bleeding, bowel perforation, stricture, obstruction, fulminant colitis, and dysplasia. UC surgery involves resection of the entire colon with ileal pouch-anal anastomosis. The procedure can be performed as a primary surgery or in stages. This technique avoids permanent ileostomy and preserves anorectal function. Long-term results are excellent. CD surgery involves segmental bowel resection, removing the terminal ileum and adjacent inflamed colon.

Long-term complications include toxic megacolon, colonic perforation, severe colitis, and colorectal cancer. Patients with early onset of CD have a lower final adult height compared with predicted mid-parental height. This is not seen in patients with UC. Bone development, osteopenia and osteoporosis, may also be affected in Crohn disease.

Austin GL, Shaheen NJ, Sandler RS: Positive and negative predictive values: Use of inflammatory bowel disease serologic markers. *Am J Gastroenterol.* 2006;101:413 [PMID: 16542272].

Bossuyt X: Serologic markers in inflammatory bowel disease. *Clin Chem.* 2006;52:171 [PMID: 16339302].

Horsthuis K, Bipat S, Bennink RJ, Stoker J: Inflammatory bowel disease diagnosed with US, MR, scintigraphy, and CT: Meta-analysis of prospective studies. *Radiology.* 2008;247:64 [PMID: 18372465].

Jose FA, Heyman MB: Extraintestinal manifestations of inflammatory bowel disease. *J Pediatr Gastroenterol Nutr.* 2008;46:124 [PMID: 18223370].

Shikhare G, Kugathasan S: Inflammatory bowel disease in children: Current trends. *J Gastroenterol.* 2010;45:673 [PMID: 20414789].

Szigethy E, McLafferty L, Goyal A: Inflammatory bowel disease. *Pediatr Clin N Am.* 2011;58:903 [PMID: 21855713].

PANCREATITIS

Acute pancreatitis is characterized by reversible inflammation within the parenchyma of the pancreas. Despite having multiple etiologies, the inflammation results from a cascade of events involving zymogen activation, cytokine production, intra- and extrapancreatic inflammation, leading to pancreatic ischemia and pancreatitis. The incidence of pediatric pancreatitis is increasing for reasons that are unclear and most likely multifactorial such as the changing trends in etiology, referral patterns, and in diagnosis.

Clinical Findings

The most common presenting symptom is abdominal pain (80-95%) located in the epigastric region. Back pain or radiation to the back is uncommon in children. Diffuse abdominal pain can occur in up to 20% of children. Other common symptoms include nausea and vomiting (40-80%), abdominal distension, fever, jaundice, ascites, and pleural effusion. Infants and nonverbal children often present with nonspecific and uncharacteristic complaints such as crying, irritability, abdominal distension, and fever. In this age group, they are less likely to present with abdominal pain, nausea, and have epigastric tenderness on examination.

The etiology of pancreatitis is very wide in children compared with adults. The most common causes of pancreatitis in children are biliary, medications (valproic acid, L-asparaginase, prednisone, and 6-mercaptopurine), idiopathic, multisystem disease (sepsis, hemolytic uremic syndrome, systemic lupus erythematosus), trauma (motor vehicle crashes, non-accidental trauma), infection (mumps, hepatitis A and E, rotavirus, mycoplasma pneumonia, adenovirus, enterovirus Coxsackie B4), and metabolic causes (DKA, hypertriglyceridemia, hypercalcemia).

Diagnostic Studies

Elevations in amylase and lipase levels are the most common tests to be abnormal in pancreatitis. The sensitivity of amylase in diagnosing pancreatitis ranges from 50 to 85% and lipase is 77%. Peak lipase levels are up to five times higher than amylase levels in children. However, amylase levels are not dispensable. In children, an elevated amylase level may be the only laboratory study that is abnormal. On the other hand, in infants and young toddlers, lipase levels are elevated in up to 100% of patients compared to amylase levels which are elevated in 40-60% in this population. This discrepancy may be due to developmental differences in gene expression of pancreatic enzymes. Laboratory biomarkers of pancreatitis not readily available for clinical use are serum cationic trypsinogen, and serum or urine trypsinogen activation peptide.

Elevations in amylase and lipase can be due to a myriad of disease processes, and the level of elevation does not correlate with severity of disease (Table 36–12).

CRP is a useful marker of disease activity. Routine blood tests to consider in a child with pancreatitis are plasma glucose, calcium, VBG, liver function tests, a CBC, and urea and creatinine.

US is currently the diagnostic imaging tool in the evaluation of pancreatitis. It affords no radiation, is noninvasive, and gives additional information of other more common causes of abdominal pain in children. US is superior to CT scan in detecting gallstones as a cause of pancreatitis. Diagnostic features of pancreatitis on US include pancreatic heterogeneity, edema, peripancreatic or peritoneal fluid collections. US may also show the presence of dilation of the common bile duct, pancreatic duct, and/or a pseudocyst.

CT scan is generally not recommended as the first study of choice in the evaluation of pancreatitis, unless the diagnosis is unclear. CT findings are similar to US findings. Later in the disease process, CT scan is helpful in identifying pancreatic necrosis.

There is limited information on the use of MRI and endoscopic US in the children due to accessibility, patient's size, need for general anesthesia. Endoscopic retrograde cholangiopancreatography (ERCP) and magnetic resonance cholangiopancreatography (MRCP) are not useful in the diagnosis of pancreatitis but have a role in investigation of associated biliary obstruction in children with recurrent or chronic pancreatitis.

Treatment

For most children, the acute treatment of pancreatitis is supportive and includes IV fluids, pain management, and pancreatic rest; however, newer recommendations advocate for early enteral feeding by nasojejunal tube when the associated ileus resolves. Patients with severe pancreatitis with evidence of shock, respiratory failure, or renal failure require intensive care management. Support the ABC and consider transfer to a tertiary center. Treat with aggressive fluid hydration, stress ulcer prophylaxis, broad-spectrum antibiotics, and glycemic control. In the acute setting, surgery is rarely required. Consultation with a pediatric surgeon may be necessary to treat any underlying cause of pancreatitis or for complications of pancreatitis specifically pancreatic pseudocyst. Asymptomatic pseudocysts regardless of size can often be managed medically. Symptomatic, infected, or bleeding pseudocysts may require drainage either surgically or by radiographic, endoscopic, or laparoscopic drainage.

Table 36–12. Additional reasons for elevated lipase or amylase in the pediatric patient.

Amylase	Lipase
Biliary tract disease	Pancreatic cancer
Intestinal obstruction or ischemia	Macrolipasemia
Mesenteric infarction	Renal insufficiency
Peptic ulcer	Acute cholecystitis
Appendicitis	Esophagitis
Ruptured ectopic pregnancy	Hypertriglyceridemia
Ovarian tumor	
Dissecting aortic aneurysm	
Salivary gland trauma	
Infection (mumps)	
Salivary gland obstruction	
Myocardial infarction	
Pulmonary embolism	
Pneumonia	
Drug use (opiate, phenylbutazone)	
Trauma (burns, cerebral trauma)	
Renal insufficiency	
Renal transplantation	
Macroamylasemia	

Bai HX, Lowe ME, Husain SZ: What have we learned about acute pancreatitis in children? *J Pediatr Gastroenterol Nutr.* 2011;52(3):262 [PMID: 21336157].

Bai HX, Ma MH, Orabi AI: Novel characterization of drug-associated pancreatitis in children. *J Pediatr Gastroenterol Nutr.* 2011;53(4):423 [PMID: 21681111].

Coffey MJ, Nightingale S, Ooi CY: Serum lipase as an early predictor of severity in pediatric acute pancreatitis. *J Pediatr Gastroenterol Nutr.* 2013;56(6):602 [PMID: 23403441].

Lowe ME, Greer JB: Pancreatitis in children and adolescents. *Curr Gastroenterol Rep.* 2008;10(2):128 [PMID: 18462598].

Morinville VD, Husain SZ, Bai H, et al: Definitions of pediatric pancreatitis and survey of present clinical practices. *J Pediatr Gastroenterol Nutr.* 2011;53(4):423 [PMID: 22357117].

Teh SH, Pham TH, Lee A, et al: Pancreatic pseudocyst in children: The impact of management strategies on outcome. *J Pediatr Surg.* 2006;41:1889 [PMID: 17101365].

Neurological Emergencies

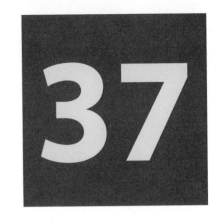

Nicholas Irwin, MD
Roger L. Humphries, MD

IMMEDIATE LIFE-THREATENING NEUROLOGICAL CONDITIONS

THE COMATOSE CHILD

GENERAL CONSIDERATIONS

A rapid and systemic approach to assessment and management of coma in the pediatric patient is of paramount importance guided by initial clinical evaluation. Careful monitoring and continuous reassessment are necessary. The initial assessment should be performed at the same time as initial basic medical therapy such as placement of monitoring devices and intravenous access.

Coma is characterized by decreased levels of arousal and may be graded by clinical findings. The Glasgow coma scale (GCS) is a common and easily used scale in the adult patient and may be adapted to pediatric use (Table 37–1).

The most common cause of coma in children is infectious, and rapid management of potential infectious causes is recommended (Table 37–2).

TREATMENT

Immediate treatment and management of an emergency should begin by assessing airway, breathing, and circulation (ABC). Blood glucose should be checked on a patient with abnormal mental status, especially in the pediatric patient. IV access should be obtained and initial broad laboratory evaluation in the undifferentiated comatose child should be obtained including complete blood cell count (CBC), complete metabolic profile, blood gas, urinalysis (UA), blood culture, toxicological screen, as well as a C-reactive protein (CRP) and erythrocyte sedimentation rate (ESR). Further laboratory analysis may be warranted determined by clinical considerations including sickle cell, amino acids, lumbar puncture, and urine electrolytes.

The use of imaging in the management of pediatric patients is a complex topic and should be considered on a case-by-case basis; general considerations include trauma, focal examination findings, signs of increased intracranial pressure (ICP), or an ill or toxic appearance. If trauma or increased ICP is suspected, emergent noncontrast computed tomography (CT) of the brain is indicated.

INTRACRANIAL HYPERTENSION

GENERAL CONSIDERATIONS

Intracranial hypertension is defined by elevated opening pressure on lumbar puncture, which is normally between 10 and 100 mm H_2O in children younger than 8 years and 60 and 200 mm H_2O in children older than 8 years or in adults. Intracranial hypertension is an endpoint to various infectious, traumatic, structural, and metabolic disorders (Table 37–3).

CLINICAL FINDINGS

History

Common historical findings in elevated intracranial hypertension include a history of trauma, a ventriculoperitoneal (VP) shunt, bleeding diathesis, morning vomiting, nocturnal headache, and developmental regression. These findings are often more vague in those with chronically elevated ICP. Typical symptoms include headaches, diplopia, nausea, and vomiting.

Physical Examination

Physical examination findings vary depending on chronicity and severity of disease and include abnormal fundoscopic examination, ataxia, seizures, pupillary asymmetry, cranial nerve VI palsy, and decreased level of consciousness. Some patients with VP shunt dysfunction and acutely elevated

Table 37–1. Pediatric Glasgow coma scale.

Eye opening response	
Spontaneous	4
To speech	3
To pain	2
None	1
Verbal response: Child (*Infant modification*)[a]	
Oriented (*Coos, babbles*)	5
Confused conversation (*Irritable cry, consolable*)	4
Inappropriate words (*Cries to pain*)	3
Incomprehensible sounds (*Moans to pain*)	2
None	1
Best upper limb motor response: Child (*Infant modification*)[b]	
Obeys commands (*Normal movements*)	6
Localizes pain (*Withdraws to touch*)	5
Withdraws to pain	4
Flexion to pain	3
Extension to pain	2
None	1

[a]The appropriate number from each section is added to total between 3 and 15. A score less than 8 usually indicates CNS depression requiring positive-pressure ventilation.
[b]If no modification is listed, the same response applies for both infants and children.
(Reproduced, with permission, from Hay WW, Levin MJ, Deterding RR, Abzug MJ, Sondheimer JM (eds): *Current Diagnosis & Treatment: Pediatrics*, 21st ed. McGraw-Hill, Inc., 2012. Copyright © McGraw-Hill Education LLC.)

ICP will have "sunset eyes" with paralysis of upward gaze (Parinaud phenomenon). Cushing triad, hypertension, bradycardia, and abnormal respirations, is a late finding and often incomplete. Decerebrate and decorticate posturing can indicate that brain herniation is occurring or is about to occur.

Transtentorial herniation is associated with ipsilateral pupillary dilation with or without contralateral hemiparesis. Foramen magnum herniation presents with decreased level of consciousness and aspects of Cushing triad.

Imaging

CT scanning is the imaging modality of choice in the acute setting but should never delay stabilization or initial steps in management if the diagnosis of intracranial hypertension is suspected. Magnetic resonance imaging (MRI) may be of value in chronic patients where emergent management is not necessary.

TREATMENT & DISPOSITION

Initial treatment should be oriented toward stabilization and management of ABC as indicated. A stepwise approach to management should be considered (Figure 37–1) and should be done in consultation with a neurosurgeon. Aggressive fluid resuscitation with maintenance of blood pressure greater than the fifth percentile for age is indicated. Patient disposition will vary depending on severity and chronicity and will be guided by input from neurosurgical consultants.

INFECTIOUS DISORDERS

BACTERIAL MENINGITIS

General Considerations

Meningitis is an infection involving the pia mater, arachnoid mater, and subarachnoid space. Untreated mortality for bacterail meningitis approaches 100%. Typical pathogens affecting infants and children include Group B *Streptococcus, Escherichia coli, Listeria monocytogenes, Haemophilus influenzae* type B, *Streptococcus pneumoniae, Neisseria meningitidis,* and *Staphylococcus aureus*; however, any pathogenic microbe may cause meningitis. Organisms often vary by age (ie < 30 days-*E coli* + group B *strep*, greater than 30 days *S. pneumonia, N. meningitidis*). The introduction of protein-conjugated polysaccharide vaccines has markedly reduced incidence of meningitis caused by *S. pneumoniae, H. influenzae* type B (Hib), and *N. meningitidis*.

Clinical Findings

▶ **Signs & Symptoms**

Presenting signs and symptoms will vary depending on the age of child, duration of illness, and host responsiveness to illness. Clinical features may be nonspecific and subtle, especially in younger children.

Typical findings in infants may include fever or hypothermia, lethargy, irritability, poor feeding, vomiting, diarrhea, respiratory distress, seizures, bulging fontanels, hypotonia, and coma. Older children likely present with fever, meningismus, headache, photophobia, nausea, vomiting, confusion, lethargy, and irritability.

Traditional physical examination findings associated with meningeal irritation include Kernig sign, in which the examiner flexes hips and extends at the knee producing pain in the back and legs, and Brudzinski sign, in which the examiner passively flexes the neck producing involuntary flexion at the hips. The findings may occur in up to 75% of older children, but are generally too insensitive and nonspecific to be of use, and are even less likely to be present in infants with meningitis.

Table 37–2. Common causes of coma.

Mechanism of Coma	Likely Cause	
	Newborn Infant	Older Child

Anoxia
    Asphyxia
    Respiratory obstruction
 	
    Severe anemia
	Birth asphyxia, HIE (hypoxic ischemic encephalopathy)
	Meconium aspiration, infection (especially respiratory syncytial virus)
	Hydrops fetalis
		Carbon monoxide (CO) poisoning
		Croup, tracheitis, epiglottitis
		
		Hemolysis, blood loss

Ischemia
    Cardiac
    shock
	Shunting lesions, hypoplastic left heart
	Asphyxia, sepsis
		Shunting lesions, aortic stenosis, myocarditis blood loss, infection

Head trauma (structural cause)	Birth contusion, hemorrhage, non-accidental trauma (NAT)	Falls, auto accidents, athletic injuries
Infection (most common cause in childhood)	Gram-negative meningitis, enterovirus, herpes encephalitis, sepsis	Bacterial meningitis, viral encephalitis, postinfectious encephalitis, sepsis, typhoid, malaria
Vascular (CVA or stroke, often of unknown cause)	Intraventricular hemorrhage, sinus thrombosis	Arterial or venous occlusion with congenital heart disease, head or neck trauma
Neoplasm (structural cause)	Rare this age. Choroid plexus papilloma with severe hydrocephalus	Brainstem glioma, increased pressure with posterior fossa tumors
Drugs (toxidrome)	Maternal sedatives; injected pudendal and paracervical analgesics	Overdose, salicylates, lithium, sedatives, psychotropic agents
Epilepsy	Constant minor motor seizures; electrical seizure without motor manifestations	Nonconvulsive or, absence status, postictal state; drugs given to stop seizures
Toxins (toxidrome)	Maternal sedatives or injections	Arsenic, alcohol, CO, pesticides, mushroom, lead
Hypoglycemia	Birth injury, diabetic progeny, toxemic progeny	Diabetes, "prediabetes," hypoglycemic agents
Increased intracranial pressure (metabolic or structural cause)	Anoxic brain damage, hydrocephalus, metabolic disorders (urea cycle; amino-, organic acidurias)	Toxic encephalopathy, Reye syndrome, head trauma, tumor of posterior fossa
Hepatic causes	Hepatic failure, inborn metabolic errors in bilirubin conjugation	Hepatic failure
Renal causes, hypertensive encephalopathy	Hypoplastic kidneys	Nephritis, acute (AGN) and chronic, uremia, uremic syndrome
Hypothermia, hyperthermia	Iatrogenic (head cooling)	Cold weather exposure, drowning; heat stroke
Hypercapnia	Congenital lung anomalies, bronchopulmonary dysplasia	Cystic fibrosis (hypercapnia, anoxia)

Electrolyte changes
    Hyper- or hyponatremia
    Hyper- or hypocalcemia
    Severe acidosis, lactic acidosis
	Iatrogenic ($NaHCO_3$ use), salt poisoning (formula errors)
	SIADH, adrenogenital syndrome, dialysis (iatrogenic) epti-
	cemia, metabolic errors, adrenogenital syndrome
		Diarrhea, dehydration
		Lactic acidosis
		Infection, diabetic coma, poisoning (eg, aspirin), hyperglycemic nonketotic coma

Purpuric	Disseminated intravascular coagulation (DIC)	DIC, leukemia, thrombotic thrombocytopenic purpura

AGN, acute glomerulonephritis; SIADH, syndrome of inappropriate antidiuretic hormone secretion.
(Modified and reproduced, with permission, from Lewis J, Moe PG: The unconscious child. In Conn H, Conn R (eds): *Current Diagnosis*, 5th ed. WB Saunders, 1977. Copyright Elsevier.)

Table 37–3. Pediatric illness commonly associated with increased intracranial pressure.

Diffuse processes
Trauma
Hypoxic ischemic
Near-drowning
Cardiorespiratory arrest
Infectious
Encephalitis
Meningitis
Metabolic
Reye syndrome
Liver failure
Inborn errors of metabolism
Toxic
Lead intoxication
Vitamin A overdose
Focal processes
Trauma
Hypoxic ischemic
Trauma
Stroke
Infectious
Abscess
Mass lesions
Tumors
Hematomas

(Reproduced, with permission, from Hay WW, Levin MJ, Deterding RR, Abzug MJ, Sondheimer JM (eds): *Current Diagnosis & Treatment: Pediatrics*, 21st ed. McGraw-Hill, Inc., 2012. Copyright © McGraw-Hill Education LLC.)

▶ Imaging

Imaging in suspected meningitis is indicated when patients have focal signs on examination suggestive of abscess, or are immunocompromised with an increased risk of invasive disease.

Elevated ICP is a relative contraindication to lumbar puncture due to the risk of cerebral herniation. Patients at increased risk for elevated ICP may benefit from imaging prior to lumbar puncture include those with a history of central nervous system (CNS) diseases, CNS shunts, space-occupying lesions, altered mental status, trauma, hydrocephalus, or papilledema on examination.

▶ Laboratory Findings

Lumbar puncture is of paramount importance for diagnosis and opening pressures should be recorded. Typical cerebrospinal fluid (CSF) studies include Gram stain and

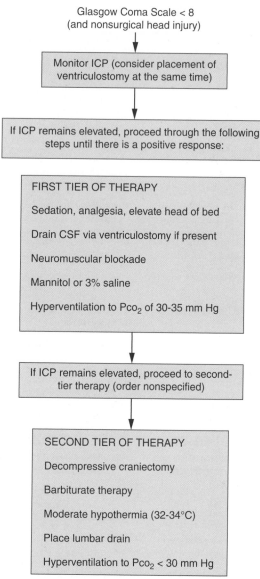

▲ **Figure 37–1.** Proposed treatment algorithm for intracranial hypertension in head injury. (Reproduced, with permission, from Hay WW, Levin MJ, Deterding RR, Abzug MJ, Sondheimer JM (eds): *Current Diagnosis & Treatment: Pediatrics*, 21st ed. McGraw-Hill, Inc., 2012. Copyright © McGraw-Hill Education LLC.)

culture, cell count with differential, protein, glucose, a viral culture, and herpes simplex virus polymerase chain reaction (HSV PCR) in neonates younger than 1 month. Further studies may be warranted depending on the clinical situation.

Table 37-4. CSF findings in meningitis.

Measure	Normal	Bacterial Meningitis	Viral Meningitis	Fungal Meningitis	Tuberculous Meningitis	Abscess
WBC/mL	0-5	> 1000	< 1000	100-500	100-500	10-1000
PMNs (%)	0-15	> 80	< 50	< 50	< 50	< 50
Lymphocytes (%)	> 50	< 50	> 50	> 80	Increased monocytes	Variable
Glucose	45-65	< 40	45-65	30-45	30-45	45-60
CSF–blood glucose ratio	0.6	< 0.4	0.6	< 0.4	< 0.4	0.6
Protein	20-45	> 150	50-100	100-500	100-500	> 50
Pressure	6-20	> 25-30	Variable	> 20	> 20	Variable

PMN, polymorphonuclear leukocytes; WBC, white blood cells.
(Reproduced, with permission, from Hay WW, Levin MJ, Deterding RR, Abzug MJ, Sondheimer JM (eds): *Current Diagnosis & Treatment: Pediatrics*, 21st ed. McGraw-Hill, Inc., 2012. Copyright © McGraw-Hill Education LLC.)

Blood cultures should always be drawn. A CRP and procalcitonin have been used in discrimination between viral and bacterial meningitis and thus may be useful, especially if antimicrobial therapy has been started prior to lumbar puncture (Table 37-4). In one study Procalcitonin > 10 mg/dL was 84% specific for bacterial meningitis. Similarly CRP > 10 mg/dL was 62% specific for bacterial meningitis.

Management

Bacterial meningitis is a true emergency and time to administration of appropriate antimicrobial therapy is of paramount importance. If a lumbar puncture cannot be obtained immediately; for example, in a patient in whom a CT scan is required, antimicrobial therapy should be started prior to lumbar puncture. This may decrease the yield on CSF, Gram stain and culture. However CSF glucose, protein, and cell count with differential should aid in the decision to continue antibiotics.

Administration of IV corticosteroids, particularly dexamethasone, is controversial. When given prior to or with initial antibiotic therapy, it has been shown to decrease hearing loss associated with HiB meningitis in children older than 6 months, and benefit has been suggested in *S. pneumoniae* meningitis. However, studies to evaluate its effectiveness among other types of bacterial meningitis have not demonstrated this benefit, and its empiric use in children remains controversial. In children older than 2 months, the dose of dexamethasone is 0.15 mg/kg, if the decision is made to administer.

Choice of empiric antibiotics will depend on the age of the patient with suspected meningitis. Infants less than 1 month of age are treated with ampicillin (87.5 mg/kg/dose q6h), gentamycin (under 7 days 2.5 mg/kg/dose q12h or 2.5 mg/kg/dose q8h) or cefotaxime (50 mg/kg/dose q6h), and acyclovir (20 mg/kg/dose q8h). Older infants and children are treated with vancomycin (15 mg/kg/dose q6h) in combination with a third generation cephalosporin such as cefotaxime or ceftriaxone (50 mg/kg/dose q12h).

Disposition

Children with suspected or proven meningitis may require care in an ICU setting if condition warrants it, as demonstrated by abnormal vital signs or clinical examination. Post-meningitis neurologic sequelae such as seizures, focal neurologic deficits, hearing or vision loss, and impaired congnitive function are common in pediatric patients especially infections caused by *S. pneumoniae*.

Alkholi UM, Al-monem NA, El-Azim AA. Serum Procalcitonin in Viral and Bacterial Meningits. *J Glob Infect Disease*. 2011;3:14-18 [PMID: 21572603].

BRAIN ABSCESS

General Considerations

Brain abscesses are rare in immunocompetent hosts in developed countries. Three mechanisms allow entry of abscess to the brain: direct extension (sinusitis, otitis media; odontogenic infections), hematogenous, and following penetrating cerebral trauma or neurosurgery. Incidence has decreased due to improved antibiotic coverage of middle ear infections. Hematogenous spread is frequently associated with multiple abscesses. Amebic and fungal etiologies are frequent in immunocompromised hosts.

Clinical Findings

Most common presentation is headache and vomiting secondary to increased ICP. Classic triad of fever, headache, and focal neurological findings is rare. Seizures may be present. If brain abscess is high on the differential, imaging (CT with contrast) should be obtained prior to lumbar puncture due to risk of cerebral herniation.

Treatment

Immediate parenteral antibiotic therapy is indicated. Antibiotic selection should be guided by suspected cause: hematogenous, postoperative, or direct extension. Immediate neurosurgical consultation is mandatory. Until culture results can direct specific therapy, common empiric antibiotic choices include ceftriaxone (50 mg/kg/dose q12h) or cefotaxime (50 mg/kg/dose q12h) and metronidazole (7.5 mg/kg/dose q6h). For patients with abscesses associated with cranial trauma, antistaphylococcal coverage, such as vancomycin (15 mg/kg/dose q6h) is a reasonable choice.

Felsenstein S, Williams B, Shingadia D, et al. Clinical and microbiologic features guiding treatment recommendations for brain abscesses in children. *Pediatr Infect Dis J.* 2013;32:129-35 [PMID: 23001027].

ENCEPHALITIS

General Considerations

Encephalitis is inflammation of the brain, often indicating direct invasion of the brain by pathogens. Noninfectious etiologies are often related to auto-immune conditions such as parainfectious immune-mediated encephalitis, lupus cerebritis, and other paraneoplastic syndromes (see Central Nervous System Demyelinating Disorders). Infectious encephalitis is discussed here.

The majority of infectious encephalitides is viral in nature and tends to occur in epidemic or seasonally. Enterovirus encephalitis is traditionally seen in the spring or summer; arthropodborne illnesses (West Nile virus, Eastern and Western equine encephalitides) are most common in the summer and fall, whereas respiratory mediated viruses are most common in the fall and winter.

Clinical Findings

▶ History & Physical Examination

The presentation of encephalitis may be a combination of altered mental status, seizure, behavior change, weakness, sensory, or motor changes without identifiable external causes such as trauma, stress, or intoxication. In contrast to meningitis, encephalitis often presents in younger children with subtle findings: weak suck, lethargy, irritability, and abnormal eye movements.

There is often a history of a viral prodrome or fever in the preceding 1-4 weeks. Causes of encephalitis include

immunosuppression, season, local epidemiology, and focal neurological deficits. Recurrent and/or polyphasic course is concerning for demyelinating disorders.

▶ Imaging

MRI is the imaging modality of choice for suspected encephalitis. Early imaging in the course of illness may provide a false negative. CT scanning is insensitive, but should be considered if concern for elevated ICP prior to lumbar puncture.

▶ Laboratory Findings

Lumbar puncture is the most important test. Results are nonspecific and early in the course of illness may be normal. Common findings include increased opening pressure, normal to elevated protein, normal glucose, and pleocytosis (often initially neutrophilic and later lymphocytic). Certain syndromes are associated with specific findings. In herpes simplex virus (HSV) encephalitis, a hemorrhagic pleocytosis may be present, whereas Epstein-Barr virus (HBV) infections are associated with atypical lymphocytes.

Viral polymerase chain reaction (PCR) is a specific, but not sensitive test, and is often normal initially. Turn-around time for results is often prohibitive whereas treatment should not be delayed. Parainfectious immune-mediated or demyelinating disorders can be ruled out if a positive PCR is obtained.

The most reliable test is pairing of acute and convalescent serum titers. A fourfold increase in immunoglobulin M (IgM) to a specific agent is considered diagnostic; however, these tests are of limited utility in the emergent setting.

▶ Management

Initial management should be aimed at stabilizing of symptoms such as seizures, hypotension, and agitation. Empiric acyclovir is indicated in a patient with suspected encephalitis. The dosage of acyclovir is 60 mg/kg/day dosed at 8-hour intervals. A full 21-day course is typically given regardless of HSV PCR results, because of the high false-negative rate. Empiric antimicrobial therapy for meningitis should also be considered prior to obtaining results of lumbar puncture and may be tailored appropriately.

Management of symptomatic intracranial hypertension is mandatory. Initial measures include head elevation, fluid restriction, and neurosurgical consultation or transfer to a center with pediatric critical care and neurosurgical specialists.

▶ Disposition

Disposition is variable depending on the severity of the disease but often ICU level care is indicated. Neurosurgical consultation may be warranted. Long-term outcomes are difficult to predict initially, as they are largely based on causative agents.

STATUS EPILEPTICUS

GENERAL CONSIDERATIONS

Status epilepticus (SE) is a neurological emergency defined as recurrent seizures, lasting more than 5 minutes or seizures that recur without interictal resumption of baseline CNS function. The definition is arbitrary, and a child who is actively seizing should be managed emergently due to significant risk for morbidity and mortality.

SE is classified into four groups for purposes of diagnosis and management.

- Generalized convulsive SE—most frequent type
- Nonconvulsive SE—includes absence or partial complex seizures
- Subtle SE—may occur as the endpoint of convulsive SE
- Simple partial SE—recurrent motor movements without loss of consciousness

Children who have seized and not returned to a neurological baseline may be in subclinical SE. SE may result as a complication of epilepsy or be secondary to an underlying illness, the most common cause of new-onset seizures presenting as SE in children is febrile SE.

CLINICAL FINDINGS

History & Physical Examination

History is paramount in the management of SE. History of epilepsy, recent illness, trauma, or congenital disorders will direct treatment and diagnostic evaluation. Signs and symptoms of SE may be obvious or very subtle. A careful physical examination for signs of nystagmus or repetitive movements is mandatory.

TREATMENT

Treatment should begin immediately and be performed concurrently with diagnostic management, and should include stabilization of the airway, IV access, as well as diagnosis and treatment of hypoglycemia (Table 37–5). (See Chapter 20.)

Bernardo WM, Aires FT, DeSa FP: Effectiveness of the association of dexamethasone with antibiotic therapy in pediatric patients with bacterial meningitis. *Rev Assoc Med Bras.* 2012;58(3):319-322.

Falchek S: Encephalitis in the pediatric population. *Pediatr Rev.* 2012;33(3):122-133 [PMID: 22383515].

Kim K: Acute bacterial meningitis in infants and children. *Lancet Infect Dis.* 2010;10(1):32-42 [PMID: 20129147].

Moorthy RK, Rajshekhar V: Management of brain abscess: An overview. *Neurosurg Focus.* 2008;24(6):E3 [PMID: 18518748].

Pitfield AF, Carroll A, Kissoon N: Emergency management of increased intracranial pressure. *Pediatr Emerg Care.* 2012;28(2):200-204 [PMID: 22307193].

Singh RK, Stephens S, Berl MM, et al: Prospective study of new-onset seizures presenting as status epilepticus in childhood. *Neurology.* 2010;74(8):636-642 [PMID: 20089940].

Table 37–5. Status epilepticus treatment.

1. ABC
   a. Airway: maintain oral airway; intubation may be necessary.
   b. Breathing: oxygen.
   c. Circulation: assess pulse, blood pressure; support with IV fluids, drugs. Monitor vital signs.
2. Start glucose-containing IV (unless patient is on ketogenic diet); evaluate serum glucose; electrolytes, HCO_3^-, CBC, BUN, anticonvulsant levels.
3. Consider arterial blood gases, pH.
4. Give IV glucose if serum glucose is low (5 ml/kg of D10 for infants or 2 ml/kg of D25 for children).
5. Begin IV drug therapy; goal is to control status epilepticus in 20-60 min.
   a. Diazepam, 0.3-0.5 mg/kg over 1-5 min (20 mg max); may repeat in 5-20 min; or lorazepam, 0.05-0.2 mg/kg (less effective with repeated doses, longer-acting than diazepam); or midazolam: IV, 0.1-0.2 mg/kg; intranasally, 0.2 mg/kg.
   b. Phenytoin, 10-20 mg/kg IV (not IM) over 5-20 min; (1000 mg maximum); monitor with blood pressure and ECG. Fosphenytoin may be given more rapidly in the same dosage and can be given IM; order 10-20 mg/kg of "phenytoin equivalent" (PE).
   c. Phenobarbital, 5-20 mg/kg (sometimes higher in newborns or refractory status in intubated patients).
6. If unable to establish IV—consider rectal valium (0.5 mg/kg/dose) or intramuscular midazolam (0.3 mg/kg/dose).
7. Correct metabolic perturbations (eg, low-sodium, acidosis). Administer fluids judiciously.
8. Other drug approaches in refractory status:
   a. Repeat phenytoin, phenobarbital (10 mg/kg). Monitor blood levels. Support respiration, blood pressure as necessary.
   b. Other medications: Valproate sodium, available as 100 mg/mL for IV use; give 15-30 mg/kg over 5-20 min.
   c. Levetiracetam may be helpful (20-40 mg/kg/dose IV).
   d. For patients who fail initial intervention, consider midazolam drip: 1-5 mcg/kg/min (even to 20 kg/min); pentobarbital coma; propofol and general anesthesia.
9. Consider underlying causes:
   a. Structural disorders or trauma: MRI or CT scan.
   b. Infection: lumbar puncture, blood culture, antibiotics.
   c. Metabolic disorders: consider lactic acidosis, toxins, and uremia if child is being treated with chronic AEDs, obtain medication levels. Toxin screen.
10. Initiate maintenance drug treatment with IV medications: phenytoin (10 mg/kg); phenobarbital (5 mg/kg); valproate IV 30 mg/kg; levetiracetam 20-30 mg/kg. Transition to oral medication when patient can safely take them.

BUN, blood urea nitrogen; CBC, complete blood count; CT, computed tomography; ECG, electrocardiogram; IM, intramuscularly; IV, intravenously; MRI, magnetic resonance imaging.
(Reproduced, with permission, from Hay WW, Levin MJ, Deterding RR, Abzug MJ, Sondheimer JM (eds): *Current Diagnosis & Treatment: Pediatrics*, 21st ed. McGraw-Hill, Inc., 2012. Copyright © McGraw-Hill Education LLC.)

NEUROLOGICAL COMPLAINTS, SYNDROMES, & SYMPTOMS PRESENTING TO EMERGENCY DEPARTMENT

SEIZURE

GENERAL CONSIDERATIONS

Seizures are the outward signs and symptoms associated with abnormal and excessive neuronal activity in the brain. Seizures may be classified into three categories: generalized, focal, and febrile. Generalized seizures originate at a given focal point and rapidly engage bilateral hemispheres. This can involve cortical or subcortical structures, but does not necessarily have to involve the entire cortex. Individual seizures may begin with localizing symptoms, but these locations are not consistent from one seizure to the next. Generalized seizures may be further categorized into tonic-clonic (gran mal), clonic, tonic, atonic (drop attacks), absence (petit mal), and myoclonic.

Focal seizures originate at one locus in a network within a single hemisphere. Onset of seizures is consistent between seizures and preferentially develops in a common manner. The seizure may remain ipsilateral or spread to the contralateral hemisphere. Seizure may be described by impairment of consciousness. A focal seizure without impairment of consciousness or awareness is a "simple partial seizure." A seizure that occurs with impairment of consciousness or awareness is a "complex partial seizure." Focal seizures that evolve to bilateral, convulsive seizures are "secondarily generalized."

Febrile seizures are those occurring within the context of fever (> 100.4°F) without any evidence of intracranial infection or other cause on history and physical. These may be further categorized into simple and complex febrile seizures. Simple febrile seizures are generalized, do not recur within the same illness, and last less than 15 minutes. Febrile seizures are complex if there are focal features, repeated seizures within the same illness, or last greater than 15 minutes. Febrile seizures are extremely common; 3-5% of all children aged 6 months to 5 years will have a febrile seizure.

Etiology of afebrile seizures is divided into four groups. Epilepsy is diagnosed in approximately 30% of children and may be idiopathic or familial. Isolated seizures account for approximately 25%, and have no known underlying cause. Seizures are the secondary manifestation of primary disease processes in approximately 25% of children (infectious, structural, metabolic, traumatic, or intracranial hemorrhages). Neonatal seizure is one that occurs in a child younger than 3 months and accounts for 15% of afebrile seizures (Table 37–6). Seizures may be

Table 37–6. Benign childhood epileptic syndromes.

Syndrome	Characteristics
Benign idiopathic neonatal convulsions (BINC)	So-called 5th day fits (97% have onset on 3rd-7th d of life); 6% of neonatal convulsions; clonic, multifocal, usually brief; occasional status epilepticus
Benign familial neonatal convulsions (BFNC)	Autosomal dominant; onset in 2-90 d; genes, *KCNQ2* or *KCNQ3*; clonic; 86% recover
Generalized tonic-clonic seizures (GTCS)	Age at onset, 3-11 y; may have family or personal history of febrile convulsions; 50% have 3/s spike-wave EEG; may have concurrent absence seizures
Childhood absence seizures	Incidence higher in girls than in boys; age at onset, 3-12 y (peak 6-7 y); 10-200 seizures per day; 3/s spike-wave EEG; up to 40% may develop GTCS
Juvenile absence seizures	Incidence higher in boys than in girls; age at onset, 10-12 y; uncommon; less frequent seizures; 3-4/s general spike-wave EEG; most have GTCS; some remit
Juvenile myoclonic epilepsy (Janz syndrome)	Age at onset, 12-18 y (average, 15 y); myoclonic jerks upper limbs, seldom fall; 4-6/s general spike-wave EEG; untreated, 90% have GTCS, mostly on waking; 20-30% have absence seizures; 25-40% are photosensitive; 10% remission rate (90% do not remit)
Benign epilepsy with centrotemporal spikes (BECTS); "rolandic epilepsy"	Age at onset 3-13 y (most at 4-10 y); 80% have brief, 2-5 min nocturnal (sleep) seizures only; usually simple partial seizures (face, tongue, cheek, hand) sensory or motor; occasionally have GTCS; bilateral independent spikes on EEG; may not need medication if seizures infrequent; remits at puberty
Benign epilepsy of childhood with occipital paroxysms (Panayiotopoulos syndrome)	6% of children with epilepsy; age at onset 3-6 y in 80% of patients (mean age, 5 y; range, 1-12 y); autonomic symptoms and visual aura may suggest migraine

EEG, electroencephalogram.
(Reproduced, with permission, from Hay WW, Levin MJ, Deterding RR, Abzug MJ, Sondheimer JM (eds): *Current Diagnosis & Treatment: Pediatrics*, 21st ed. McGraw-Hill, Inc., 2012. Copyright © McGraw-Hill Education LLC.)

secondary or related to hypoxic encephalopathy, congenital infection, drug withdrawal, or electrolyte abnormalities (Table 37–7).

CLINICAL FINDINGS

History & Physical Examination

Historical information is the most important aspect in determining the underlying etiology of the seizure. Detailed account of the episode and the period surrounding the episode should be sought. Attention should be paid to visual problems, headaches, developmental milestones, and school performance.

Physical examination should include level of consciousness, pupil responses, fundi, posture, gait, reflexes, head circumference, and a thorough neurological and skin examination.

Laboratory Findings

As in all emergency situations, initial treatment and diagnostic management should occur concurrently including evaluation and management of the ABC'. A rapid blood glucose should be obtained and hypoglycemia corrected. Further workup should be dictated by historical and physical findings.

History of fever, or signs or symptoms of infection should direct care. A child with headache and fever before the seizure, bulging fontanel, GCS less than 15, drowsiness, or decreased mental status preseizure should be treated as meningitis until proven otherwise. Workup of a simple febrile seizure without any concerning findings should be directed toward finding and treating the underlying cause of fever. No further workup other than measurement of blood glucose, and vital sign measurement is indicated in a child older than 1 year with a simple febrile seizure.

Laboratory workup in other afebrile patients may include a CBC, electrolytes, calcium, phosphorus, magnesium, blood urea nitrogen (BUN), creatinine, blood gas analysis, lactate, UA, and culture, blood culture, ECG, and toxic screen. Consideration should be given to obtaining organic acids, hemoglobin electrophoresis, lumbar puncture, and urine electrolytes. Children with history of epilepsy on antiepileptics should have a serum level checked if possible. Although meningitis is rare in otherwise well-appearing infants, lumbar puncture should be considered in children younger than 1 year with a febrile seizure or if the child appears ill, after a careful history and physical examination. A higher index of suspicion for meningitis is appropriate in infants and children already taking antibiotics as classic signs and symptoms may not be prominent.

Imaging

The physician's decision to obtain imaging again should be directed by history and physical and the concern for underlying etiology. General indications include focal findings, altered mental status, findings suggestive of trauma, or new-onset SE. Non contrast CT is the recommended imaging modality in emergent evaluations.

Emergent electroencephalogram (EEG) is not usually indicated after a simple afebrile or febrile seizure, but may be offered on an outpatient basis in follow-up.

TREATMENT

Antiepileptics are generally not indicated for the management of a first-time seizure. If there is concern that the patient may have experienced seizures in the past that have gone unrecognized, or undiagnosed, treatment with chronic antiepileptic drug therapy should be started in consultation with a neurologist.

Antipyretics may be given for febrile seizures, although there is limited evidence that they will reduce the risk of further seizure. In general, the treatment for the infant or child with a simple febrile seizure is the same as that for the patient who presents to the emergency department with fever in the absence of seizure.

DISPOSITION

The patient with a first afebrile seizure should be admitted for observation and further workup and management; if the patient is not at neurological baseline, there are any signs of increased ICP or meningismus, the child appears unwell, is younger than 12 months, the seizure is complex, or there are signs of aspiration. The decision for inpatient management should be guided by the patient's age, parental comfort level, and access to rapid follow-up with primary care physician or a pediatric neurologist. If there is concern for underlying pathology or parental anxiety, admission is a reasonable option.

Children older than 1 year with a simple afebrile seizure may be safely discharged home after a period of observation, providing there is close follow-up. Similarly, infants and children with simple febrile seizures who appear well after a short period of observation in the emergency department may be discharged home. The family should be educated that a second febrile seizure will occur in approximately 33% of children, but the lifetime risk of developing epilepsy remains low, approximately 2%. Antipyretics have not proven to decrease the incidence or severity of subsequent seizures, but a number of practitioners recommend scheduled antipyretics for the next 24 hours and early administration if fever develops thereafter.

PEDIATRIC MIGRAINE

GENERAL CONSIDERATIONS

Most migraine patients experience the first migraine attack during childhood or adolescence. Diagnosis of pediatric migraines can be challenging because of the wide variety

Table 37–7. Seizures by age at onset, pattern, and preferred treatment.

Seizure Type Epilepsy Syndrome	Age at Onset	Clinical Manifestations	Causative Factors	EEG Pattern	Other Diagnostic Studies	Treatment and Comments
Neonatal seizures	Birth–2 wk	Often subtle; sudden limpness or tonic posturing, brief apnea, cyanosis; odd cry; eyes rolling up; blinking or mouthing or chewing movements; nystagmus, twitchiness or clonic movements (focal, multifocal, or generalized). Some seizures are nonepileptic: decerebrate, or other posturings, release from forebrain inhibition. Poor response to drugs.	Neurologic insults (hypoxia/ischemia; intracranial hemorrhage) present more in first 3 d or after 8th day; metabolic disturbances alone between 3rd and 8th days; hypoglycemia, hypocalcemia, hyper- and hyponatremia. Drug withdrawal. Pyridoxine dependency. Other metabolic disorders. Structural CNS infections. Structural abnormalities.	May correlate poorly with clinical seizures. Focal spikes or slow rhythms; multifocal discharges. Electroclinical dissociation may occur: electrical seizure without clinical manifestations.	Lumbar puncture; CSF PCR for herpes, enterovirus; serum Ca^{2+}, PO_4^{3-}, serum and CSF glucose, Mg^{2+}; BUN, amino acid screen, blood ammonia, organic acid screen, TORCHS, other metabolic testing if suspected. Ultrasound or CT/MRI for suspected intracranial hemorrhage and structural abnormalities.	Benzodiazepines, phenobarbital, IV or IM; if seizures not controlled, add phenytoin IV. Recent experience with levetiracetam and topiramate. Treat underlying disorder. Seizures due to brain damage often resistant to anticonvulsants. When cause in doubt, stop protein feedings until enzyme deficiencies of urea cycle or amino acid metabolism ruled out.
Infantile spasms	3–18 mo, usually about 6 mo	Abrupt, usually but not always symmetrical adduction or flexion of limbs with flexion of head and trunk; or abduction and extensor movements (similar to Moro reflex). Occur in clusters typically upon awakening. Associated irritability and regression in development.	Symptomatic in approximately two-thirds. Acquired CNS injury in approximately one-third; biochemical, infectious, degenerative in approximately one-third; cryptogenic in approximately one-third. With early onset, pyridoxine dependency, inherited metabolic disorders. Tuberous sclerosis in 5–10%. TORCHS, homeobox gene mutations, *ARX*, and other genetic mutations.	Hypsarrhythmia (chaotic high-voltage slow waves or random spikes [90%]); other abnormalities in 10%. Rarely normal at onset. EEG normalization early in course usually correlates with reduction of seizures; not helpful prognostically regarding mental development.	Funduscopic and skin examination, amino and organic acid screen. Chromosomes, TORCHS screen, CT, or MRI scan should be done to (1) establish definite diagnosis, (2) aid in genetic counseling. Trial of pyridoxine. Occasionally, surgical resection of cortical malformation.	ACTH gel (40 IU/d 150 IU/ m^2/d) IM once daily. Vigabatrin, especially if tuberous sclerosis. B_6 (pyridoxine) trial. In resistant cases, topiramate, zonisamide, valproic acid, lamotrigine, ketogenic diet. Early treatment leads to improved outcome.
Febrile convulsions	3 mo–5 y (maximum 6–18 mo); most common childhood seizure (incidence 2%)	Usually generalized seizures, < 15 min; rarely focal in onset. May lead to status epilepticus. Recurrence risk of 2nd febrile seizure 30% (50% if < 1 y of age); recurrence risk is same after status epilepticus.	Nonneurologic febrile illness (temperature rises to 39°C or higher). Risk factors: positive family history, day care, slow development, prolonged neonatal hospitalization.	Normal interictal EEG, especially when obtained 8–10 d after seizure. Therefore, not useful unless complicating features.	Lumbar puncture in infants or whenever suspicion of meningitis exists.	Treat underlying illness, fever. Diazepam orally, 0.3–0.5 mg/kg, divided 3 times daily during illness may be considered. Diastat rectally for prolonged (> 5 min) seizure. Prophylaxis with phenobarbital or valproic acid rarely needed.

Syndrome	Age of Onset	Clinical Features	Cause	EEG	Diagnostic Studies	Treatment
Cryptogenic generalized epilepsies of early childhood (Lennox-Gastaut syndrome, Myoclonic astatic epilepsy [Doose syndrome] and Dravet syndrome)	Any time in childhood (usually 2-7 y)	Mixed seizures dependent on particular syndrome, including tonic, myoclonic (shock-like violent contractions of one or more muscle groups, singly or irregularly repetitive), atonic ("drop attacks") and atypical absence with episodes of absence status epilepticus.	Multiple causes, usually resulting in diffuse neuronal damage. History of infantile spasms; prenatal or perinatal brain damage; viral meningoencephalitis; CNS degenerative disorders; structural cerebral abnormalities (eg, migrational abnormalities). Doose syndrome. Dravet syndrome associated with SCN1A mutation.	Atypical slow (1-2.5 Hz) spike-wave complexes and bursts of high-voltage generalized spikes, often with diffusely slow background frequencies. Electrodecremental and fast spikes during sleep.	As dictated by index of suspicion: genetic testing; inherited metabolic disorders, neuronal ceroid lipofuscinosis, others. MRI scan, WBC lysosomal enzymes. Skin or conjunctival biopsy for electron microscopy; nerve conduction studies if degenerative disease suspected.	Difficult to treat. Topiramate, ethosuximide, felbamate, levetiracetam, zonisamide, valproate, clonazepam, rufinamide, clobazam (approval pending) ketogenic diet, vagus nerve stimulation. Avoid phenytoin, carbamazepine, oxcarbazepine, gabapentin. (Stiripentol used in Europe but not approved in the United States.)
Childhood absence epilepsy	3-12 y	Lapses of consciousness or vacant stares, lasting about 3-10 s, often in clusters. Automatisms of face and hands; clonic activity in 30-45%. Often confused with complex partial seizures but no aura or postictal confusion. Some risk for developing generalized tonic clonic seizures.	Unknown. Genetic component. Abnormal thalamocortical circuitry.	3/s bilaterally synchronous, symmetrical, high-voltage spikes and waves provoked by hyperventilation. EEG always abnormal. EEG normalization correlates closely with control of seizures.	Hyperventilation often provokes attacks. Imaging studies rarely of value.	Ethosuximide most effective and best tolerated; valproic acid. Lamotrigine, in resistant cases, zonisamide, topiramate, levetiracetam, acetazolamide, ketogenic diet.
Juvenile absence epilepsy	10-15 y	Absence seizures less frequent than in childhood absence epilepsy. May have greater risk of convulsive seizures.	Unknown (idiopathic), possibly genetic.	3-Hz spike wave and atypical generalized discharges.	Not always triggered by hyperventilation.	Same as childhood absence epilepsy but may be more difficult to treat successfully.

(Continued)

Table 37–7. Seizures by age at onset, pattern, and preferred treatment. (*Continued*)

Seizure Type Epilepsy Syndrome	Age at Onset	Clinical Manifestations	Causative Factors	EEG Pattern	Other Diagnostic Studies	Treatment and Comments
Simple partial or focal seizures (motor/sensory/jacksonian)	Any age	Seizure may involve any part of body; may spread in fixed pattern (jacksonian march), becoming generalized. In children, epileptogenic focus often "shifts," and epileptic manifestations may change concomitantly.	Often unknown; birth trauma, inflammatory process, vascular accidents, meningoencephalitis, malformations of cortical development (dysplasia), etc. If seizures are coupled with new or progressive neurologic deficits, a structural lesion (eg, brain tumor) is likely. If epilepsia partialis continua (simple partial status epilepticus), Rasmussen syndrome is likely.	EEG may be normal; focal spikes or slow waves in appropriate cortical region; "rolandic spikes" (centrotemporal spikes) are typical. Possibly genetic.	MRI, repeat if seizures poorly controlled or progressive.	Oxcarbazepine, carbamazepine; lamotrigine, gabapentin, topiramate, levetiracetam, zonisamide, lacosamide, and phenytoin. Valproic acid useful adjunct. If medications fail, surgery may be an option.
Complex partial seizures	Any age	Aura progressing to larger event, aura and seizure stereotyped for each patient and related to part of brain seizure originates, eg, temporal lobe seizures may have a sensation of fear, déjà vu; epigastric discomfort, odd smell or taste (usually unpleasant). Seizure may consist of vague stare; facial, tongue, or swallowing movements and throaty sounds; or various complex automatisms. Usually brief, 15-90 s, followed by confusion or sleep.	As above. Temporal lobes especially sensitive to hypoxia; seizure may be a sequela of birth trauma, febrile convulsions, viral encephalitis, especially herpes. Malformations of cortical development (dysplasia) common in medication-resistant patients. Remediable causes are small cryptic tumors or vascular malformations. May be genetic.	As above.	MRI; PCR of CSF in acute febrile situation for herpes or enteroviral encephalitis. SPECT, PET scan, video-EEG monitoring when epilepsy surgery considered.	As above.

	Age	Clinical Features	Genetics	EEG	Imaging	Treatment
Benign epilepsy of childhood with centrotemporal spikes (BECTS/rolandic epilepsy)	5-16 y	Simple partial seizures of face, tongue, hand. With or without secondary generalization. Usually nocturnal. Similar seizure patterns may be observed in patients with focal cortical lesions. Almost always remits by puberty.	Seizure history or abnormal EEG findings in relatives of 40% of affected probands and 18-20% of parents and siblings, suggesting transmission by a single autosomal dominant gene, possibly with age-dependent penetrance.	Centrotemporal spikes or sharp waves ("rolandic discharges") appearing paroxysmally against a normal EEG background.	Seldom need CT or MRI scan.	Often no medication is necessary, especially if seizure is exclusively nocturnal and infrequent. Oxcarbazepine, carbamazepine or others. (See complex partial seizures.)
Juvenile myoclonic epilepsy (of Janz)	Late childhood and adolescence, peaking at 13 y	Mild myoclonic jerks of neck and shoulder flexor muscles after awakening. Usually generalized tonic-clonic seizures as well. Often absence seizures. Intelligence usually normal. Rarely resolves but usually remits on medications.	40% of relatives have myoclonias, especially in females; 15% have the abnormal EEG pattern with clinical attacks.	Interictal EEG shows variety of spike-and-wave sequences or 4- to 6-Hz multispike-and-wave complexes ("fast spikes").	If course is unfavorable, differentiate from progressive myoclonic syndromes by appropriate studies (eg, biopsies [muscles, liver, etc]). Imaging may not be necessary.	Lamotrigine, valproic acid, topiramate, levetiracetam, zonisamide.
Generalized tonic-clonic seizures (grand mal) (GTCS)	Any age	Loss of consciousness; tonic-clonic movements, often preceded by vague aura or cry. Incontinence in 15%. Postictal confusion and somnolence. Often mixed with or masking other seizure patterns.	Often unknown. Genetic component. May be seen with metabolic disturbances, trauma, infection, intoxication, degenerative disorders, brain tumors.	Bilaterally synchronous, symmetrical multiple high-voltage spikes, spikes waves (eg, 3/s). EEG often normal in those < 4 y. Focal spikes may become "secondarily generalized."	Imaging; metabolic and infectious evaluation may be appropriate.	Levitiracetam; topiramate, lamotrigine, zonisamide, valproic acid, felbamate. Combinations may be necessary. Carbamazepine, oxcarbazepine or valproic acid; phenytoin may also be effective.

ACTH, adrenocorticotropic hormone; BUN, blood urea nitrogen; CNS, central nervous system; CSF, cerebrospinal fluid; CT, computed tomography; EEG, electroencephalogram; IM, intramuscularly; IV, intravenously; MRI, magnetic resonance imaging; PCR, polymerase chain reaction; PET, positron emission tomography; SPECT, single-photon emission tomography; TORCHS, toxoplasmosis, other infections, rubella, cytomegalovirus, herpes simplex, and syphilis; WBC, white blood cell.

Table 37–8. Classification of pediatric migraine.

Migraine Type	Incidence	Key Features
Migraine without aura (formerly common migraine)	Most common migraine type 60-85% of cases	Intense disabling headache, often bilateral especially if younger than 15 pulsing or throbbing pain, exacerbated by activity, light or sound
Migraine with aura (formerly classic migraine)	15-30% of children with migraine report visual disturbances	Binocular visual impairment with scotomata (77%) Visual distortion or hallucinations (16%) Monocular visual impairment or scotomata (7%)
Childhood "periodic syndromes" (common precursors of migraine) Benign Paroxysmal Vertigo Cyclic Vomiting Syndrome Abdominal Migraine	Relatively uncommon compared to other two categories	Onset occurs in young children, abrupt onset of ataxia or unsteadiness Pattern of cyclic (occur every 2-4 wk for 1-2 d at a time) Vomiting with symptom free periods Chronic episodic, vague or dull midline or upper abdominal pain.

of presentations; however, correct and timely diagnosis is essential to avoid serious and needless suffering of patients. Pediatric patients are more likely to present with transient neurological, autonomic, gastrointestinal, or visual symptoms rather than the "classic" migraine headache characterized in adults. As in adults, the key to diagnosis is the episodic and recurrent nature of the symptoms, which are separated by symptom-free periods. Migraines increase in prevalence throughout childhood, and by 15 years of age the prevalence of migraine headache is 8-23%. It is extremely important to consider other conditions (mitochondrial or metabolic disorders, epilepsy syndromes, vascular disorders, congenital malformations) with episodic symptoms that overlap those of migraine so that patients receive the correct treatment, and other serious or life-threatening diagnoses can be treated urgently or emergently. Classification of pediatric migraine is listed in Table 37–8.

DIAGNOSTIC TESTING

Laboratory testing is not usually indicated in migraine patients. If imaging is a consideration for patients with new-onset headache, it is better to obtain an MRI as it is a more sensitive test to identify serious causes of headache and avoids the ionizing radiation associated with CT.

TREATMENT OF PEDIATRIC MIGRAINE

Pediatric patients with migraine symptoms are treated in a similar manner to adult migraine patients. For children younger than 12 years, NSAIDs or nonopiate medications such as ibuprofen (7.5-10 mg/kg) or acetaminophen (15 mg/kg) are often very safe and effective to control symptoms and should

be administered initially if not use prior to presentation to the emergency department. Nasal, oral, or subcutaneous triptans (serotonin 1B/1D receptor antagonists) have been studied in children and adolescents although none has been FDA approved for use in children and adolescents. Intranasal sumatriptan (5 and 20 mg), zolmitriptan (5 mg), oral rizatriptan (5 and 10 mg), and almotriptan (6.25, 12.5, and 25 mg) tablets have shown efficacy and safety in children 12-17 years of age. Key principles in the treatment of pediatric migraine include: (1) Initiate treatment for the headache at the earliest time possible (within 20-30 min of headache onset), (2) Keep medications on hand in locations where the child is most likely to be at the onset of the headache (school), (3) Use appropriate doses of abortive medications and do not "baby" the headache, (4) Avoid analgesic overuse ($\geq$ 3 doses of medication/week) to prevent "rebound" headaches.

DISPOSITION

For patients with frequent migraine headaches, preventative therapy should be considered. In general pediatric migraine patients improve with treatment in the emergency department and can be discharged home if symptoms have resolved or significantly improved. Patients with severe symptoms that do not abate with treatment in the emergency department should be admitted for treatment and further evaluation of status migrainosus. Outpatient follow-up with a primary care physician or pediatric neurologist is recommended for all patients.

Lewis DW: Pediatric migraine. *Neurol Clin.* 2009;27:481-501 [PMID: 19289227].

CENTRAL NERVOUS SYSTEM DEMYELINATING DISORDERS

GENERAL CONSIDERATIONS

CNS demyelinating disorders are autoimmune in etiology and classified as monophasic and relapsing disorders. Monophasic disorders include acute disseminated encephalomyelitis (ADEM), clinically isolated syndrome (CIS), and neuromyelitis optica ([NMO], Devic syndrome). ADEM is characterized by encephalopathy: behavior change or altered level of consciousness, with multifocal neurological involvement. CIS is characterized by the first neurological episode that lasts at least 24 hours and is caused by inflammation or demyelination in one or more sites in the CNS. It may be monofocal (isolated optic neuritis) or polyfocal but does not include encephalitis. NMO is an autoimmune inflammatory disorder that affects the optic nerve and spinal cord. Unlike multiple sclerosis (MS), it is believed to be mediated by antibodies called NMO-IgG or NMO antibodies. MRI lesions are found over three or more vertebral segments with a positive NMO IgG titer revealing the optic neuritis and transverse myelitis.

Relapsing diseases are characterized by recurrent or new symptoms after the initial presentation. Symptoms include recurrent ADEM, a repeat neurological episode meeting the criteria for ADEM, greater than 3 months after the initial episode, with no new findings on MRI. Multiphasic ADEM is recurrent ADEM with new MRI findings. MS is a disease in which the body's immune system attacks the myelin surrounding nerve cells believed to be mediated by the immune system's T cells. Pediatric MS is two or more demyelinating events (the first is a clinically isolated syndrome) occurring at different sites at least 4 weeks apart.

Signs and symptoms demyelination vary greatly depending on the site of the lesion and range from cognitive dysfunction, upper motor neuron signs, vision changes, and cerebellar signs, to pain and fatigue.

ACUTE DISSEMINATED ENCEPHALOMYELITIS

Clinical Findings

ADEM is more common in children than in adults, with the mean age at presentation of 5-8 years. The incidence is 0.4/100,000 per year among persons younger than 20 years. Symptoms often begin 2-4 weeks after a viral illness or vaccination. A prodrome of fever, malaise, headache, nausea, and vomiting may be observed before the rapid onset of encephalopathy and multifocal neurological deficits. Seizures and ataxia are common. Severity is widely variable and ranges from subtle to comatose.

The main diagnostic studies include lumbar puncture and imaging. CSF analysis will demonstrate a pleocytosis. If ADEM is suspected, MRI should be obtained, as CT is insensitive. MRI with and without contrast will demonstrate many large lesions involving the central white matter and cortical gray-white junction of the cerebral hemispheres, cerebellum, brainstem, and spinal cord.

Treatment

Treatment should initially involve stabilizing measures. When diagnosis of ADEM is made, immunotherapy is indicated and should begin in consultation with a neurologist. Therapy may include plasmapheresis, intravenous immunoglobin (IVIG), or high-dose corticosteroids.

Disposition

Generally, ICU level care is indicated for careful observation. Full neurological recovery occurs in 60-90% of patients. Residual neurological deficits, behavioral and cognitive impairment, and recurrent disease occur.

NEUROMYELITIS OPTICA

Clinical Findings

Neuromyelitis optica (NMO) is a characterized by findings of both optic neuritis and transverse myelitis. Optic neuritis presents with ocular pain and loss of vision, either unilaterally or bilaterally. Transverse myelitis involves severe symmetric paraplegia with sensory loss and bladder dysfunction. In contrast to ADEM, NMO is more common in adults, with median age 14 years in children. The course is typically relapsing. CSF analysis will demonstrate pleocytosis (in contrast to MS), and MRI of the brain will demonstrate optic neuritis only. MRI imaging of the spine will demonstrate segmental demyelination.

Treatment

Treatment will initially be principally supportive, with careful attention to respiratory status as spinal cord involvement may be located near the brainstem and be associated with respiratory failure. Immunotherapy with IV corticosteroids is indicated in consultation with a neurologist.

Disposition

Because of risk of respiratory failure, admit to an ICU setting; unfortunately, 80-90% of patients will experience a relapse after initial recovery.

MULTIPLE SCLEROSIS

Clinical Findings

Multiple sclerosis (MS) is a relatively rare condition in the pediatric population, with 2-5% of patients presenting younger than 18 years. Findings vary depending on the site of demyelination. Symptoms include Lhermitte sign, an electrical sensation in descending spine when the neck is flexed, and Uhthoff phenomenon, a transient increase in symptoms when core body temperature rises. Visual, sensory, motor, brainstem, or cerebellar deficits are seen in children with MS presentation. Initial episode is known as a clinically isolated syndrome, and diagnosis is made only after repeated symptoms appear separated in time and space. There may be associated encephalopathic symptoms, especially in children. A family history of MS is often present.

Laboratory analysis may aid if diagnosis is not clear; however, imaging and clinical findings are key. CSF analysis may demonstrate oligoclonal bands, may have elevated protein, and typically a normal cell count. Imaging modality of choice is MRI, which will demonstrate focal or confluent changes in white matter in 95% of patients.

Treatment

Supportive therapy only is generally indicated in the emergent setting.

Disposition

Severity of the symptoms indicates if outpatient management is needed. Clinical course evolves over decades, with the median time to death 30 years from onset, with death attributable to MS in 66% of patients.

VENTRICULOPERITONEAL SHUNT MALFUNCTION

GENERAL CONSIDERATIONS

Ventriculoperitoneal (VP) shunts are devices used for management of hydrocephalus and consist of three parts: (1) The proximal end resides in a ventricle, is radio-opaque, and has perforations to allow for drainage of the CSF; (2) Distal to this a valve is present that allows for only unidirectional CSF flow, controls the pressure that CSF will flow out of the valve, and often contains a CSF reservoir for sampling; (3) The distal end is usually placed in the peritoneal cavity to allow for drainage of CSF.

Malfunction may occur secondary to obstruction or infection. Obstruction most commonly occurs proximally due to choroid or debris, but may occur distally due to migration, infection or tube kinking. Infection is most likely to occur early after placement and generally occurs within the first few weeks. Late occurrence of infection is rare unless skin over tubing is broken. (See Chapter 49.)

CLINICAL FINDINGS

Signs & Symptoms

Signs and symptoms of VP shunt malfunction are variable depending on severity and age. Findings range from headache, malaise, change in personality, decreased school performance, vomiting, neck pain, nerve palsy, bulging fontanelle, change in head circumference, and Cushing triad.

Infected VP shunt may present with fever, pain or redness along tubing site, peritoneal signs, or meningeal signs.

Imaging

Imaging is the initial diagnostic step. Generally this consists of a shunt series, a series of plain x-rays to look for shunt continuity, and imaging of the brain to look for presence or change in hydrocephalus. Either a CT scan or MRI may be obtained. Rapid MRI is a feasible choice in some centers, as higher speed, lower resolution imaging is adequate for evaluation of hydrocephalus without the risk of ionizing radiation. Certain externally programmable CSF shunts may be affected by MRI and may require reprogramming after the study. In addition, the position of the shunt should be determined radiographically prior to and after MRI in order to ensure changes have not been made.

Laboratory Findings

CSF may be drawn and ICP recorded by sampling at the reservoir; this is typically done in consultation with a neurosurgeon. (See Chapters 3 and 49.)

Treatment

Treatment of suspected or proven VP shunt malfunction should be performed in consultation with a neurosurgeon. Operative intervention may be necessary. Typical measures to decrease ICP such as head elevation and treatment of pain are indicated. If infection is a concern, empiric therapy should be initiated and guided by time course of shunt placement. Typical empiric regimens include vancomycin and a third-generation cephalosporin.

Disposition

Disposition will be dictated by time course and severity of symptoms. Intermittent symptoms may require further evaluation or imaging and admission for observation.

STROKE

GENERAL CONSIDERATIONS

Stroke, loss of brain function associated with a disturbance to cerebral blood supply, is a relatively rare condition in children. The associated morbidity and mortality, however, are significant. The most common etiology and presentation of stroke in the pediatric population is different from a typical adult population. Approximately 50% of strokes in children are ischemic, compared with 80-85% in adults. In children, 50% with an acute focal neurological finding have a previously identified risk factor such as cardiac disease or sickle cell disease.

CLINICAL FINDINGS

History & Physical Examination

Similar to other neurological syndromes, presentations vary by age. Older children will present with syndromes similar to adults, but children younger than 3 years present with nonspecific symptoms such as seizures, lethargy, deterioration of general conditions, and sleepiness. Most common focal neurological finding is hemiplegia. Hemorrhagic strokes in children present with headache (76%), change in mental status (52%), and vomiting (48%).

Cavernous venous sinus thrombosis may be suspected based on a compatible history and often presents with non-specific and vague complaints including seizures, fatigue, headache, and signs and symptoms of increased ICP. Common underlying etiologies include dehydration, sickle cell anemia, leukemia, sinusitis, and mastoiditis.

Physical examination should be thorough with careful examination of integumentary system looking for signs of trauma, infection, congenital abnormalities, including neurocutaneous syndromes.

Laboratory Findings

Basic metabolic profile, CBC and PT, PTT, factor V Leiden, and antithrombin III should be obtained. Studies of protein electrophoresis, assays for protein C/S, various clotting mutations, as well as tests for clotting function may be considered. Lumbar puncture is indicated if subarachnoid hemorrhage is suspected and imaging shows no signs of increased ICP. Additional studies to be considered are ECG, echocardiography, fibrinogen, ESR, liver function testing, and toxicologic screening.

Imaging

CT is the initial imaging modality of choice and is sensitive for acute hemorrhagic stroke. Ischemic stroke will not be evident before 6 hours and often takes longer to be radiographically abnormal. MRI is considered the more sensitive and versatile imaging technique and can identify abnormalities within hours of onset. In specific patients, ultrasound or angiography may be clinically useful. In addition, angiography, standard or MRI may be of use.

TREATMENT

Supportive therapies such as control of fever, maintenance of oxygenation, control of hypertension in hemorrhagic strokes, and normalization of serum glucose levels are recommended. Dehydration and anemia should be corrected, particularly in sickle cell patients. Sickle cell patients with acute stroke should be hydrated and treated with a simple or partial exchange transfusion to obtain a hemoglobin SS fraction of less than 30% and a hemoglobin level not greater than 10 g/dL.

Thrombolytic therapy may be considered in cavernous venous sinus thrombosis, but is not currently recommended for acute ischemic stroke in pediatric patients. Secondary prevention with low-molecular-weight heparin or unfractionated heparin should be considered.

DISPOSITION

Admission to the hospital is indicated for all stroke patients, and ICU level care may be warranted. Consultation with a neurologist or neurosurgeon is recommended.

GUILLAIN-BARRÉ SYNDROME

GENERAL CONSIDERATIONS

Guillain-Barré syndrome (GBS) is a postinfectious polyneuropathy that usually follows a nonspecific viral illness by 10 days. Incidence is 0.5-2 cases per 100,000/year. All age groups are affected, but uncommon in children younger than 3 years.

CLINICAL FINDINGS

Signs & Symptoms

Onset may be gradual over the course of days or sudden over 12-24 hours. Classic symptoms include symmetric weakness that starts in the lower limbs and ascends with or without sensory symptoms. As in most neurological diseases, signs and symptoms vary by age. Younger children often present with nonspecific symptoms such as feeding intolerance, lethargy, respiratory distress, or decreased responsiveness. Hyporeflexia or areflexia is usually present. Cranial nerves are involved in 50% of patients, with the seventh cranial nerve (CN VII) most commonly affected. Autonomic dysfunction and urinary retention are observed. Respiratory impairment results when respiratory muscles become involved. Fever is absent at the time of onset. Miller-Fisher syndrome, a subtype of Guillain-Barré, is characterized by ophthalmoplegia, ataxia, and areflexia without motor weakness of the extremities.

Laboratory Findings

CSF analysis classically shows elevated protein without pleocytosis and a normal glucose. Elevated CSF protein levels may be normal initially and take 7 days to develop. Acute and convalescent serum with viral and mycoplasmal titers may be useful. *Campylobacter jejuni* isolates in stool cultures have been associated with GBS. Other tests may be indicated as EMG, and ECG (as automonic dysfunction may occur with tachycardia or bradycardia) assesses for associated or predisposing conditions (HIV disease, gammopathies) or to evaluate the possibility of alternative diagnoses (systemic lupus erythematosus, structural lesions, MS, encephalitis, meningitis, epidural abscess, heavy metal intoxication).

Imaging

MRI is the imaging modality of choice to exclude other demyelinating diseases, and if GBS is suspected, imaging of the spinal cord as well as the brain is recommended. An MRI should be obtained rapidly as other causes (such as compressive myelopathy) and comorbid conditions such as ADEM and acute transverse myelitis may present similarly.

TREATMENT

In the emergent setting supportive care is the mainstay of treatment. Careful monitoring for respiratory failure is critical. Vital capacity may be monitored and trended. Severe values are those less than 20 mL/kg. Immunotherapy is indicated in consultation with a neurologist. Plasmapheresis is the gold standard; plasma exchange, and IVIG are also commonly used.

DISPOSITION

Admission the ICU is warranted. Symptoms plateau at 2-4 weeks without therapy and recovery begins. Prognosis is excellent in children with full recovery in 90-95% of children aged 3-12 months.

GENETIC DISORDERS OF NEUROMUSCULAR SYSTEM

GENERAL CONSIDERATIONS

This is heterogenous group of disorders, with various pathophysiological mechanisms affecting neuromuscular function. Genetic deficits may disrupt neuromuscular function by affecting the muscle itself, the neuromuscular junction, or the upper or motor neuron (Table 37–9).

CLINICAL FINDINGS

Symptoms & Signs

Clues to neonatal disease include poor feeding, hypotonia, limb weakness, ptosis, and respiratory insufficiency. Older children present with delays in motor milestones, weakness (often greater proximally than distally), ptosis, fatigue, and respiratory insufficiency.

Diagnostic Findings

Basic laboratory workup should be obtained in the emergency department, including creatinine kinase, CBC, and comprehensive metabolic panel. Imaging is typically not diagnostically useful in the emergent setting. While not part of the emergency department evaluation, many diagnoses are made either in the hospital or as an outpatient with muscle biopsy, EMG, and genetic testing.

TREATMENT & DISPOSITION

Supportive cardiorespiratory management is indicated, as well as inpatient admission for further testing and monitoring. Underlying etiologies guide further treatment. Corticosteroids may be effective in slowing the rate of muscle deterioration in the patient with muscular dystrophy, but the effect is not realized without weeks of therapy.

TICK PARALYSIS

GENERAL CONSIDERATIONS

Tick paralysis is far more common in children than adults, which has been reported with all types of ticks. The most commonly reported ticks in North America are hard body ticks, particularly the *Dermacentor* genus. The underlying mechanism is a neurotoxin release while the tick is engorging when attached to the host.

CLINICAL FINDINGS

Classically presents as an acute symmetric ascending flaccid paralysis evolving over hours to days. A prodrome of paresthesias, myalgias, restlessness, irritability, and fatigue is common. Diminished deep tendon reflex may be absent on examination. A thorough history and physical are paramount to making the diagnosis. Generally if the paralysis is not improving, the tick should still be present, and at minimum, evidence or history of a tick bite should be sought.

TREATMENT

Treatment involves removal of the offending tick. Symptoms should improve over the course of hours with complete resolution in approximately 24 hours.

BELL'S PALSY

GENERAL CONSIDERATIONS

Bell's palsy is the acute idiopathic paralysis of the seventh cranial nerve (CN VII [facial nerve]). It is the most common cause of facial nerve palsy in children, although more common in adults. Bell's palsy is a diagnosis of exclusion and

Table 37–9. Muscular dystrophies, myopathies, myotonias, and anterior horn diseases of childhood.

Disease	Genetic Pattern	Age at Onset	Early Manifestation	Involved Muscles	Reflexes	Muscle Biopsy Findings	Other Diagnostic Tests	Treatment	Prognosis
Muscular dystrophies									
Duchenne muscular dystrophy (pseudohypertrophic infantile)	X-linked recessive; Xp21; 30-50% have no family history and are spontaneous mutations.	2-6 y; rarely in infancy.	Clumsiness, easy fatigability on walking, running, and climbing stairs. Walking on toes; waddling gait with excessive lumbar lordosis. Motor delays. Positive Gowers maneuver.	Proximal (pelvic and shoulder girdle) muscles; pseudohypertrophy of gastrocnemius, triceps brachii, and vastus lateralis. Second decade, progressive scoliosis, cardiomyopathy and respiratory weakness develop.	Knee jerks +/- or 0; ankle jerks + to ++	Areas of degeneration and regeneration, variation in fiber size, inflammatory changes, proliferation of connective tissue. Immunostaining for dystrophin absent.	Myopathic EMG. CK levels can be up to 50-100x normal, but decrease with increasing disease severity, reflecting replacement of muscle with fat/connective tissue. Genetic testing will show deletion 60% of time, while 5-15% are duplications, and 20-30% are point mutations, intronic deletions, or repeats.	Corticosteroids may prolong extend independent ambulation by 2.5 y if started between age 4 and 8 y; management is largely supportive. Close pulmonary and cardiac follow-up should be maintained due to risk of cardiorespiratory failure in 2nd-3rd decade of life. Osteoporosis should be treated with calcium and vitamin D.	Patients are wheelchair-bound by ~12 y old. Death from cardiorespiratory causes usually occurs by the early 20s.
Limb-girdle muscular dystrophy	Autosomal dominant, autosomal recessive, and X-linked forms.	Variable; early childhood to adulthood.	Weakness, with distribution according to type. Waddling gait, difficulty climbing stairs. Excessive lumbar lordosis.	Slowly progressive, symmetric proximal muscle involvement; characteristically involves shoulder and pelvic muscles.	Usually present	Necrosis and fiber splitting, increased endomysial connective tissue and inflammation, absent immunostaining for various DGC proteins by subtype.	Myopathic EMG. CK often > 5000 IU/L. MRI of the legs may show selective involvement (eg, peroneal muscles in Miyoshi myopathy).	Physical therapy. Echocardiogram to screen for cardiomyopathy. PFTs to screen to respiratory weakness. No curative treatment available.	Variable by subtype.
Congenital myopathies									
Myotubular myopathy	X-linked recessive; Xq27.	Neonatal period.	Floppy infant; severe hypotonia and respiratory insufficiency.	Ptosis, ophthalmoplegia; severe symmetric distal and proximal weakness.	+ to –	Small rounded myotube-like myofibers. Patchy central clearing with radial spokes.	Normal to mildly elevated CK. Myopathic EMG with fibrillations and complex repetitive discharges.	No curative treatment. Respiratory, nutritional support. Liver and peritoneal hemorrhage reported in cases.	Generally death before 5 mo of age.

(Continued)

Table 37–9. Muscular dystrophies, myopathies, myotonias, and anterior horn diseases of childhood. (*Continued*)

Disease	Genetic Pattern	Age at Onset	Early Manifestation	Involved Muscles	Reflexes	Muscle Biopsy Findings	Other Diagnostic Tests	Treatment	Prognosis
Central core myopathy	Most autosomal dominant, some autosomal recessive, 19q13, RYR1.	Infancy to adulthood.	Reduced fetal movements; hypotonia; ankle contractures.	Nonprogressive proximal weakness of legs more than arms, mild facial weakness, normal eye movements.	+ to –	Variable myofiber size; oxidative staining shows central cores absent of mitochondrial activity.	High CK, mild myopathic changes on EMG, muscle MRI shows increased T1 signal.	Physical therapy. Respiratory follow-up required. Avoid inhalational anesthetics and succinylcholine due to risk of malignancy hyperthermia.	Weakness is nonprogressive. Life expectancy normal.
Metabolic myopathies									
Pompe disease	Autosomal recessive; 17q23.	Classic infantile presentation: present by 6 mo of age. Juvenile: 2-18 y.	Severe hypotonia, hepatomegaly, cardiomyopathy, hypoventilation. Proximal muscle weakness.	Proximal more than distal muscles, bulbar and respiratory muscles. Recurrent respiratory infections; nocturnal hypoventilation.	0	Cytoplasmic lysosomal vacuoles stain positive with acid phosphatase.	High CK in infants (< 10 x normal). Mildly high CK in teens.	Enzyme replacement therapy with alglucosidase alfa (myozyme). Respiratory and nutritional support. Monitor cardiomyopathy. As above.	Significant but variable with treatment, with improved survival, cardiorespiratory status, and motor skills. Variable, some become nonambulatory and most require ventilatory support.
Ion channel disorders									
Hyperkalemic periodic paralysis	Autosomal dominant 17q35.	Childhood, usually by 1st decade.	Episodic flaccid weakness, precipitated by rest after exercise, stress, fasting, or cold.	Proximal and symmetric muscles, distal muscles may be involved if exercised.	Normal, may be 0 with episode	Hyperkalemic periodic paralysis.	CK normal to 300 IU/L; attacks associated with high serum K^+; NCS shows increased CMAP amplitude after 5 min exercise.	Many attacks are brief and do not need treatment; treat acute attack with carbohydrates; if needed, chronic treatment with acetazolamide.	Attacks may be more frequent with increasing age.
Congenital muscular dystrophies (CMD)									
CMD with CNS involvement: includes laminin α_2 (merosin) deficiency, Ullrich CMD.	Autosomal recessive, autosomal dominant.	Birth–1st mo.	Hypotonia, generalized weakness. Contractures proximally and lax hypermobility distally.	Generalized and respiratory muscle weakness.	0 to +	Laminin α_2 deficiency: absent/reduced laminin α_2 staining. Ullrich CMD: reduced/absent COLVI.	CK normal to 10 x normal. Laminin α_2 deficiency: mild neuropathy. Skin changes in Ullrich CMD: follicular hyperkeratosis.	Most never walk or lose ability to walk early. Respiratory support required early.	Variable: death by 1st-2nd decade secondary to respiratory failure.

Myotonic disorders

Myotonic dystrophy type 1 (DM1)	Autosomal dominant, expanded CTG triple repeat on chromosome 19q13.	Congenital presentation. Typical teen to adult onset (2nd-4th decade).	Decreased fetal movement, respiratory insufficiency, difficulties in feeding, sucking, and swallowing. Complaints of difficulty opening jars, releasing objects, manipulating small objects.	Generalized weakness; facial and pharyngeal involvement prominent; mental retardation. Distal more than proximal weakness; involved hands and feet. Slow release of hand grip or eyelid closure (myotonia); cataracts; insulin resistance, cardiac conduction defects.	Decreased to 0 + to ++	Mild myopathic changes, centralized nuclei, variation in fiber size, ring fibers.	Usually normal CK. Electrical myotonia on EMG. Cataracts on slit lamp examination. Reduced testosterone levels. ECG shows conduction defects, like ventricular arrhythmias. Insulin resistance. Sleep study shows hypercapnia and hypoventilation.	No curative treatment. Patients should avoid medications that predispose to arrhythmia such as quinine, amitriptyline, and digoxin. Should be closely followed by pulmonologist with sleep studies, by cardiologist for risk of arrhythmia, by endocrinologist for insulin resistance, and by ophthalmologist for cataracts. May have GI hypomotility with constipation and pseudo-obstruction.	Reduced survival to age 65; mean survival to 60 y. 50% patients are wheelchair bound before death.

Spinal muscular atrophy

SMA type 1 (Werdnig-Hoffman)	Autosomal recessive, rare cohorts with autosomal dominant or X-linked inheritance, 5q.	1st 6 mo of life.	Hypotonia, "floppy" infant, with alert look, fasciculations may be noted of tongue.	Severe progressive, symmetric proximal and respiratory muscle weakness; face spared.	0	Large areas of grouped muscle fiber atrophy, most larger fibers are type I.	EMG shows fibrillation and fasciculation potentials, large amplitude motor unit potentials. Normal to mildly elevated CK.	No curative treatments. Respiratory and nutritional support. Clinical trials underway with sodium phenylbutyrate, valproic acid, and riluzole.	No independent sitting or standing. Life expectancy < 2 y without respiratory or nutritional support
SMA type 2		1st 18 mo.	Motor delays.	Progressive symmetric proximal muscles, mild to moderate respiratory weakness, limited cough and secretion control.	0 to +	As above.	EMG also shows fibrillation potentials and large amplitude motor unit potentials, but fasciculations not as common as in SMA type 1; tremor of fingers.	No curative treatments. Mild to moderate respiratory weakness, sleep-disordered breathing, and limited cough and secretion control require close follow-up with pulmonologist.	Will achieve independent sitting but not standing. 75% alive at 25 y old.

(Continued)

Table 37–9. Muscular dystrophies, myopathies, myotonias, and anterior horn diseases of childhood. (*Continued*)

Disease	Genetic Pattern	Age at Onset	Early Manifestation	Involved Muscles	Reflexes	Muscle Biopsy Findings	Other Diagnostic Tests	Treatment	Prognosis
SMA type 3 (Kugelberg-Welander)		Recognized after 18 mo of age.	Motor delays, difficulty with climbing stairs, may achieve independent walking but may lose this.	Progressive symmetric proximal muscle weakness, +/– tremor of hands.	0 to +	As above.	EMG similar to SMA type 2.	No curative treatments.	Independent ambulation may be achieved, but this skill may be lost. Normal life expectancy.

ASA, acetylsalicylic acid; CK, creatine kinase; CPT, carnitine palmityl transferase; CSF, cerebrospinal fluid; CT, computed tomography; ECG, electrocardiogram; EMG, electromyogram; MRI, magnetic resonance imaging; PCR, polymerase chain reaction; SIDS, sudden infant death syndrome.

(Reproduced, with permission, from Hay WW, Levin MJ, Deterding RR, Abzug MJ, Sondheimer JM (eds): *Current Diagnosis & Treatment: Pediatrics*, 21st ed. McGraw-Hill, Inc., 2012. Copyright © McGraw-Hill Education LLC.)

evaluation for more serious causes is crucial. Its etiology is considered to be secondary to an inflammatory condition leading to swelling of the facial nerve as it exits through the temporal bone.

CLINICAL FINDINGS

Bell's palsy presents with a rapid onset of unilateral facial nerve palsy over the course of 24 hours. A history of recent infection, signs and symptoms of malignancy should be sought.

Physical examination will demonstrate a drooping face on the affected side with difficultly blinking, lacrimating, and salivating. Muscles of the upper face, forehead, and brow are typically involved, in contrast to facial weakness associated with an acute stroke of the motor cortex. There is shared bilateral upper motor neuron control of these muscles and the loss of an upper motor neuron associated with a stroke will leave some contralateral function. Bell's palsy, a lower motor neuron disease, affects these muscles equally. On attempted eye closure the globe will roll upward and inward, which is normal. Determination of child's ability to close the eyelids spontaneously is important for treatment.

Thorough examination for untreated otitis media and mastoiditis is warranted. Vesicular lesions should raise concern for Ramsey-Hunt syndrome, a reactivation of varicella-zoster virus involving CN VII, which requires specific treatment.

TREATMENT & DISPOSITION

No specific treatment of Bell's palsy has been studied in children, although corticosteroids have shown some benefit in adults. A course of prednisone (1-2 mg/kg/day) over 7-10 days is recommended. Addition of an antiviral (valacyclovir) has been suggested with steroid use because of the possible link between Bell's palsy and HSV and varicella as etiologic agents. Most children with Bell's palsy will recover spontaneously. Patients who are unable to close their eyes should be provided with appropriate means to avoid corneal abrasions, including artificial tears, sunglasses, and protective dressing at night.

BOTULISM

GENERAL CONSIDERATIONS

Botulism is a potentially fatal disease with five types of presentation: food-borne, infantile, wound, hidden, and iatrogenic. In the pediatric population, most patients are classified as "infantile botulism" which occurs in infants aged 1 week to 12 months (median age 10 weeks). Disease is caused by ingestion of *Clostridium botulinum* spores (usually from soil or honey) that colonize in the gastrointestinal tract and produce botulinum toxin after an incubation period of 3-30 days. Botulinum toxin is a potent protein neurotoxin that blocks acetylcholine release at the neuromuscular junction.

CLINICAL FINDINGS

Patients with infantile botulism present without fever in an insidious fashion with nonspecific symptoms of constipation initially, followed by poor feeding, weak cry, and listlessness but also with unusual findings of hypotonia, hyporeflexia combined with respiratory difficulty. Infantile botulism presents with a symmetric descending flaccid paralysis. Characteristically, the weakness starts in the muscles supplied by the cranial nerves.

TREATMENT

Patients with infantile botulism are treated supportively with diligent attention to the airway and breathing. Antibiotics are not recommended. Treatment with human botulinum immune globulin (Baby BIG-IV) in a single IV dose of 50 mg/kg is recommended because it is effective in reducing the length of hospitalization (from a mean of 5.7 to 2.6 weeks), the length of ICU admission, and the number of complications. Patients with infant botulism have a low mortality as long as ventilation and other supportive measures are carefully instituted as necessary in the course of the illness.

SYDENHAM CHOREA

CLINICAL FINDINGS

Chorea is an involuntary movement that involves multiple body areas in an unpredictable frequency in an asymmetrical and asynchronous pattern. Sydenham chorea is an acute onset movement disorder that occurs as a complication of rheumatic fever. Although symptoms are usually bilateral, approximately 25% of patients have unilateral symptoms. Psychiatric symptoms may accompany the movement disorder, most likely the result of an autoimmune response that triggers unknown changes in the motor control areas of the brain.

LABORATORY STUDIES

Leukocytosis, elevated ESR, and CRP are common. Patients may have a positive Group A β-hemolytic streptococcus culture although it is not a diagnostic requirement. The antistreptolysin O or anti-DNase titers are often elevated. Imaging including standard CT and MRI of the head do not show structural abnormalities.

TREATMENT

Treatment of Sydenham chorea is not standardized but includes dopamine antagonists and immunomodulators. Haloperidol, prednisone, sodium valproate, IVIG, and plasma exchange have been used with varying degrees of success. The condition is self-limited and usually lasts from weeks to months. Fortunately, more than 50% of patients will be improved at 6 months, and 89% will be improved after 2 years.

Agrawal S, Peake D, Whitehouse W: Management of children with Guillain-Barre syndrome. *Arch Dis Child Educ Pract Ed.* 2007;92(6):161 [PMID: 18032711].

Berg A, Berkovic S, Brodie M: Revised terminology and concepts for organization of seizures and epilepsies: Report of the ILAE Commission on Classification and Terminology, 2005–2009. *Epilepsia.* 2010;51(4):676-685 [PMID: 20196795].

Compston A, Coles A: Multiple sclerosis. *Lancet Infect Dis.* 2008;25(372):1502-1517 [PMID: 18970977].

Frim D, Gupta N. Hydrocephalus. In: Frim D, Gupta N, eds: *Pediatric Neurosurgery.* Landes Bioscience; 2006:117-129.

Hahn J, Pohl D, Rensel M, Rao S: Differential diagnosis and evaluation in pediatric multiple sclerosis. *Neurology.* 2007;68(suppl 2): S13-S22.

Karande S: Febrile seizures: A review for family physicians. *Ind J Med Sci.* 2007;61(3):161-172 [PMID: 17337819].

Kinali M, Beeson D, Pitt MC, et al: Congenital myasthenic syndromes in childhood: Diagnostic and management challenges. *J Neuroimmunol.* 2008;201-202(0):6-12 [PMID: 18707767].

Krupp L, Banwell B, Tenenbaum S: Consensus definitions proposed for pediatric multiple sclerosis and related disorders. *Neurology.* 2007;68(S7-12) [PMID: 17438241].

Lollis SS, Mamourian AC, Vaccaro TJ, et al: Programmable CSF shunt valves: Radiographic identification and interpretation. *Am J Neuroradiol.* 2010;31:1343-1346 [PMID: 20150313].

Lotze T, Northrop J, Hutton G, et al: Spectrum of pediatric neuromyelitis optica. *Pediatrics.* 2008;122(5);e1039-e1047.

Ness JM, Chabas D, Sadovnick A, et al: *Neurology.* 2007;68(suppl 2):S37-S45.

Pavlou E, Gkampeta A, Arampatzi M: Facial nerve palsy in childhood. *Brain Dev.* 2011;33:644-650 [PMID: 21144684].

Roach ES, Golomb MR, Adams R, et al: Management of stroke in infants and children: A scientific statement from a Special Writing Group of the American Heart Association Stroke Council and the Council on Cardiovascular Disease in the Young. *Stroke.* 2008;39(9):2644-2691 [PMID: 18635845].

Tenembaum S, Chitnis T, Ness J, et al: Acute disseminated encephalomyelitis. *Neurology.* 2007;68(16 suppl 2):23-36 [PMID: 17438235].

Tsze DS, Valente JH: Pediatric stroke: A review. *Emerg Med Int.* 2011;2011:1-10 [PMID: 22254140]

Wingerchuk D, Lennon V, Lucchinetti C, et al: The spectrum of neuromyelitis optica. *Lancet Neurol.* 2007;6(9):805-815 [PMID: 17706564].

Wolf DS, Singer HS: Pediatric movement disorders. *Curr Opin Neurol.* 2008;21:491-496 [PMID: 18607212].

Wolf V, Lupo P, Lotze T: Pediatric acute transverse myelitis overview and differential diagnosis. *J Child Neurol.* 2012;27(11);1426-1436.

Worster A, Keim S, Sahsi R, et al: Do either corticosteroids or antiviral agents reduce the risk of long-term facial paresis in patients with new-onset Bell's palsy? *J Emerg Med.* 2010;38: 518-523 [PMID: 19846267].

Renal & Genitourinary Emergencies

38

Scott A. McAninch, MD, FACEP

Scott A. Letbetter, MD

Scott A. McAninch, MD, FACEP

Scott A. Letbetter, MD

▼ **IMMEDIATE MANAGEMENT OF LIFE-THREATENING CONDITIONS**

OLIGURIA/ANURIA & ACUTE KIDNEY INJURY

Anuria or oliguria is characterized as decreased urine output (< 1 mL/kg/hr in infants, < 0.5 mL/kg/hr in children) due to a decrease in glomerular filtration rate (GFR), resulting in varying degrees of acute kidney injury (AKI), also known as acute renal failure. AKI may be nonoliguric, where urine output is normal or increased. Decreased GFR in AKI results in changes in body fluid composition, blood pressure, and regulation of electrolytes and nitrogenous waste. Complications include hyperkalemia, uremia with neurologic sequelae, severe hypertension with fluid overload, pulmonary edema, and hypertensive encephalopathy.

AKI is categorized by the underlying etiology: prerenal, renal (intrinsic), postrenal in origin. Prerenal causes are conditions that result in inadequate renal perfusion. Renal causes are due to many etiologies that result in intrinsic injury to the components of the nephron. Insult to the glomerulus, renal tubules, interstitium, and renal vasculature may be due to prolonged hypoperfusion from a prerenal cause, sepsis, or nephrotoxins. Postrenal causes are typically due to a urinary tract obstruction distal to the kidneys, which may be congenital or acquired. AKI due to postrenal causes generally requires bilateral urinary tract obstruction, or obstruction to a known or undiagnosed solitary kidney. Neurogenic bladder and medications may cause urinary retention and AKI. Table 38–1 lists causes of AKI.

Clinical Findings

The clinician should attempt to identify the cause of the AKI, and uncover and treat life-threatening complications. A meticulous history of chronic medical conditions, recent illnesses, medications, intravenous (IV) contrast exposure should be obtained to elicit specific etiologies of AKI. Patients may present with decreased or no urine output, or be referred for evaluation of abnormal creatinine or urinalysis (UA) results.

Patients with prerenal causes of AKI often appear dehydrated with signs of intravascular depletion and poor perfusion. History of streptococcal pharyngitis or skin infection may be present in poststreptococcal glomerulonephritis (GN). Bloody diarrhea should prompt consideration of hemolytic uremic syndrome (HUS). Rash with joint pains or abdominal pain may be present in Henoch-Schönlein purpura (HSP). Hypertension may be accompanied by a headache or dizziness. Fever, hypotension, and tachycardia are seen with accompanying sepsis syndromes. Edema may be periorbital, scrotal/labial, dependent, or appear as anasarca. Lung examination may reveal signs of pulmonary edema. The abdomen should be palpated for masses, representing tumors. Flank pain or masses may be present in pyelonephritis, hydronephrosis, and renal vein thrombosis.

Laboratory tests should be directed to identify any life-threatening complications of AKI and the underlying etiology. Decreased GFR is the laboratory hallmark of AKI. GFR is more reliable to detect AKI in its early stages, as creatinine results may be normal initially. However, GFR measurements may not be available in the acute care setting. Therefore, the creatinine level is used in the acute care setting to estimate GFR. Comparison to previous creatinine levels is valuable in assessing changes in GFR. Of note, the use of the dietary supplement creatinine may cause a falsely elevated serum creatinine. The range of normal serum creatinine values vary by age:

- Newborn: 0.3-1.0 mg/dL
- Infant: 0.2-0.4 mg/dL
- Child: 0.3-0.7 mg/dL
- Adolescent: 0.5-1.0 mg/dL

Table 38–1. Causes of acute kidney injury in children.

Prerenal causes

Hypovolemia

- Gastrointestinal losses, urinary losses (diabetes mellitus), skin losses (burns), traumatic hemorrhage, gastrointestinal bleed
- Decreased effective circulation from congestive heart failure (CHF), nephrotic syndrome, cirrhosis, sepsis
- Decreased arterial pressure due to low cardiac output

Intrarenal (intrinsic) causes

Glomerular disease

- Glomerulonephritis (GN) (poststreptococcal, Henoch-Schönlein purpura nephritis, immunoglobulin A nephropathy, systemic lupus erythematosus nephritis)
- Nephrotic syndrome

Acute tubular necrosis (ATN)

- Due to prolonged hypoperfusion from prerenal AKI
- Nephrotoxins: aminoglycosides, acyclovir, IV contrast, hemoglobinuria, myoglobinuria, ethylene glycol, uric acid from tumor lysis syndrome
- Interstitial nephritis due to medications (NSAIDs, beta-lactam antibiotics, sulfonadmides, thiazide diuretics) and pyelonephritis

Renal vasculature

- Hemolytic uremic syndrome (HUS)
- Thrombosis of the renal artery or vein

Postrenal causes

- Congenital obstructions (posterior urethral valves)
- Acquired obstructions from renal stones, urinary blood clots, extrinsic compression (abdominal lymphoma, rhabdomyosarcoma, renal tumor)
- Neurogenic bladder, medication causing bladder spasm

Complete blood cell count (CBC), electrolytes (potassium, calcium, phosphate), blood urea nitrogen (BUN), creatinine, and UA should be obtained. The CBC may demonstrate microangiopathic hemolytic anemia with thrombocytosis in HUS. Hemolysis may occur due to a number of conditions and result in acute tubular necrosis (ATN). Eosinophilia may be seen in interstitial nephritis. Hyperkalemia, hyponatremia, hypocalcemia, and hyperphosphatemia may be present in AKI. The BUN:creatinine ratio is often greater than 20:1 in prerenal disease, although the BUN may be disproportionally elevated in GI bleeds.

The UA may be helpful to determine causes of AKI. The UA is usually normal in prerenal causes. Pyuria with bacteriuria is suggestive of a urinary tract infection (UTI), which may cause intrinsic AKI. The presence of red blood cell (RBC) casts is indicative of glomerular disease. Isolated proteinuria is seen in nephrotic syndrome. A urine dipstick test positive for blood and negative for RBCs is suggestive of hemoglobinuria or myoglobinuria, which may cause ATN.

If GN is suspected, rapid streptococcal pharyngeal tests, serum streptococcal antigens (streptozyme test or ASO titer), and compliment (C3, C4) levels may be useful. C3 levels are low in poststreptococcal GN. Urine sodium may be ordered to assess the fractional excretion of sodium (FENa). Sodium and water reabsorption is generally well maintained in prerenal causes of AKI. FENa less than 1% is consistent with prerenal causes of AKI. FENa greater than 2% is associated with ATN. FENa of 1-2% is nondiagnostic of an etiology. Additional laboratory tests may be ordered based upon clinical suspicion of the underlying cause.

ECG may demonstrate elevated T-wave amplitude, prolonged PR-interval, flattened P waves, prolongation of QRS, and ventricular dysrhythmias. Chest x-ray may indicate pulmonary edema in congestive heart failure (CHF). Renal ultrasound (US) may demonstrate hydronephrosis in postrenal obstructions, and Doppler US may reveal renal vein thrombosis. Noncontrast computed tomography (CT) scan of the abdomen and pelvis may reveal urinary calculus and urinary tract obstruction.

Treatment

Hypotension due to sepsis should be treated promptly with intravenous fluid (IVF) resuscitation and antibiotics. Hemorrhagic shock should be treated with IVF resuscitation and packed red blood cells (PRBCs), as soon as available, at 10 mL/kg. Hypotension due to a suspected prerenal etiology of AKI should receive fluid resuscitation with crystalloid fluid boluses of 20 mL/kg to reduce the risk of developing ATN due to prolonged hypovolemia. If no urine output is noted after an IV fluid challenge, a urinary catheter should be employed to assess for bladder obstruction.

Patients who are euvolemic with AKI should be maintained at normal maintenance intake levels. Patients with mild hypervolemia may be treated with fluid intake restriction. Patients with severe fluid overload in the setting of oliguria may receive a trail dose of furosemide 2 mg/kg IV to convert oliguric AKI to nonoliguric AKI. If urine output increases within 2 hours of diuretic, a maintenance IV drip may be started at 0.1mg/kg/hr. If there is no increase in urine output, discontinue use of the diuretic.

Hyperkalemia should be treated in the standard manner. Hypertension causing encephalopathy should be treated with IV antihypertensives, such as nicardipine or nitroprusside with a goal of reducing mean arterial pressure by 10-20% over minutes to hours. Hypertension due to increased vascular tone may be treated with oral antihypertensives, such as nifedipine. Angiotensin-converting enzyme (ACE) inhibitors should be avoided in the acute setting.

Renal replacement therapy (RRT) by means of hemodialysis, peritoneal dialysis, or continuous RRT (CRRT) is indicated for volume overload that is unresponsive to diuretic a challenge, persistent hyperkalemia despite medical treatment, uremia (BUN 80-100 mg/dL), persistent metabolic acidosis, and CHF not responsive to diuretics.

Specific treatment of AKI depends on the underlying etiology. In patients with prerenal etiologies, treatment of the underlying condition, to include adequate intravascular rehydration, often leads to resolution of the AKI. However, prolonged decreased renal perfusion may lead to a concurrent ATN. In renal causes of AKI, the suspected underlying cause should be treated accordingly. Offending medications should be discontinued. Postrenal patients may require relief of the urinary obstruction, allowing for increased GFR. Urine output volume from urinary catheterization should be noted.

Disposition

Well-appearing patients with only mild prerenal dehydration or mild pyelonephritis, and without significant renal insufficiency, hypertension, or electrolyte disorders may be discharged home with close primary care follow-up. Otherwise, consultation with the pediatric nephrologist is recommended for other causes. Hospitalization is indicated for patients with anuria or severe oliguria, moderate to severe renal insufficiency, unstable vital signs, hypertension causing end organ damage, electrolyte disorders (hyperkalemia), and patients requiring dialysis. Further treatment and disposition is related to the underlying etiology of the AKI.

Goldstein S: Advances in pediatric renal replacement therapy for acute kidney injury. *Semin Dial.* 2011;24:187-191 [PMID: 21517986].

Goldstein SL: Continuous renal replacement therapy: Mechanism of clearance, fluid removal, indications and outcomes. *Curr Opin Pediatr.* 2011;23:181-185 [PMID: 21178623].

Walters S, Porter C, Brophy PD: Dialysis and pediatric acute kidney injury: Choice of renal support modality. *Pediatr Nephrol.* 2009;24:37-48 [PMID: 18483748].

▼ EMERGENCY MANAGEMENT OF SPECIFIC DISORDERS

DISEASES OF THE MALE GENITOURINARY SYSTEM

TESTICULAR TORSION

Testicular torsion is a true urological emergency because delays in diagnosis and treatment could result in loss of spermatogenesis and necrosis of the testicle. The incidence of torsion has a bimodal distribution, a small increase in the neonatal period and a larger one during adolescent years. About 65% of cases occur in boys aged 12-18 years. Ischemia to the testicle may cause infarction within 4 hours. If the symptoms have been ongoing for less than 6 hours, salvage of the testicle is near 100%. The salvage rate becomes worse after 6 hours and is essentially zero when the torsion has been ongoing for 24 hours or longer.

Clinical Findings

The patient often has complaint of sudden onset of severe pain to the testicle or lower abdomen. Pain is typically constant, but may be intermittent if the testicle is torsing and detorsing. Nausea and vomiting may be present. On examination, the affected testicle may be extremely sensitive to touch, swollen, and erythematous. It may be higher due to the shortening of the spermatic cord and have a horizontal lie. The cremasteric reflex is almost always absent in torsion patients, but unfortunately is normally absent in many children without torsion. The newborn with testicular torsion will typically not be in distress, but careful examination will reveal an enlarged, fixed, and discolored hemiscrotum. After 24 hours of life, the neonate with torsion usually presents with uncontrollable crying and careful examination will reveal a swollen, erythematous testicle. Patients with an undescended testicle and acute abdominal pain warrant consideration of intra-abdominal testicular torsion.

The patient with acute scrotal pain should be considered for testicular torsion until proven otherwise. Diagnosis is often made from a characteristic history and physical examination. If the diagnosis is unclear, a Doppler US of the testicle may reveal reduced testicular blood flow to the affected side. A normal US may be seen in children with intermittent testicular torsion. US may be less reliable to detect blood flow in smaller, prepubertal testes. Alternatively, radionuclide scintigraphy with 99m technetium-pertechnetate scan will demonstrate good sensitivity and slightly less specificity for testicular torsion. Limited blood flow on the scan is not able to discriminate testicular torsion from other anatomical conditions of the testes.

Treatment

Prompt consultation with a urologist should obtained as soon as the diagnosis of testicular torsion is clinically suspected. Do not delay consultation for confirmatory studies. The patient should be NPO and receive adequate parenteral analgesia.

While waiting for urology consultation or transfer to the operating room, manual detorsion may be attempted. In most patients testicles tend to torse in a medial to lateral direction. However, in one-third of patients the testicles torse lateral to medial. Manual detorsion is performed by holding the testicle between the thumb and index finger of one hand and the other hand should gently hold the spermatic cord. The testicle is rotated in an outward direction, so that the anterior surface is rotated laterally, as in opening a book (Figure 38–1). The spermatic cord may be twisted up to 720 degrees, so more than one turn may be required. If pain increases with manual detorsion or the testicle cannot be rotated further, stop the procedure immediately as a less common lateral to medial torsion may be present. Instead,

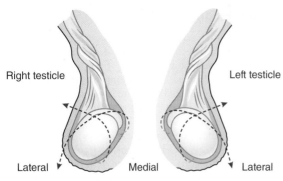

Right testicle   Left testicle

Lateral   Medial   Lateral

▲ **Figure 38–1.** Manual detorsion of testicular torsion. The testicle is rotated in an outward direction, so that the anterior surface is rotated laterally, as in opening a book. (Reproduced, with permission, from Reichman EF, Simon RR: *Emergency Medicine Procedures*. New York, McGraw-Hill; 2004. Copyright © McGraw-Hill Education LLC.)

turn in the opposite direction by rotating the anterior surface medially. Successful manual detorsion is evidenced by sudden relief of pain, normal positioning, and normal testicular perfusion by Doppler US. After a successful manual detorsion, the urologist should be consulted for admission and orchiopexy to prevent future episodes of torsion.

Disposition

Admission is indicated for patients with testicular torsion for definitive treatment.

TORSION OF THE TESTICULAR APPENDAGES

The appendix testis (92%) or appendix epididymis (8%) may undergo a torsion mechanism, resulting in moderate pain localized to the affected side. Cyanosis to the appendage may result in the "blue dot" sign on the scrotal sac in up to 25% of patients. Discrimination of torsion of the appendage from torsion of the testicle may require Doppler US. US should reveal normal testicular flow and the torsed appendage will be visualized as an area of low echogenicity. The affected appendage typically undergoes autoamputation within 1 week without significant sequelae. Pain control, scrotal support, and close follow-up with primary care are indicated. Surgical excision of the appendage may be indicated for persistent pain.

EPIDIDYMITIS

Inflammation of the epididymis is the most common cause of scrotal pain. It may be due to infections or strenuous physical activity and trauma. Sexually active patients commonly have sexually transmitted infections (STIs) with *Chlamydia trachomatis*, *Neisseria gonorrhoeae*, or from

common uropathogens, such as *Escherichia coli* and viruses. Nonsexually active and prepubertal patients often have noninfectious etiologies, but infection may occur with *Mycoplasma pneumoniae* and viruses.

Clinical Findings

Patient may have complaint of dysuria, mild testicular pain, and fever. Urethral discharge may be present with STIs. On examination, tenderness to palpation of the posterior aspect of the testicle is present. More diffuse testicular pain suggests orchitis or an alternative cause, such as testicular torsion. Scrotal edema may be present. Cremasteric reflex should be present, but may be normally absent in many patients. The patient may experience relief of pain with elevation of the affected testicle (positive Prehn sign); however, the test is unreliable to rule out other causes of pain, such as testicular torsion.

UA may demonstrate evidence of infection with pyuria and bacteriuria or results may be normal. Urine culture is recommended with evidence of UTI in all children younger than 2 years, even with a normal UA. Patients with urethral discharge or suspicion for STIs should prompt testing for *N. gonorrhoeae* and *C. trachomatis*.

Doppler US of the testicle or nuclear scan will demonstrate normal or increased blood flow to the epididymis of the affected testicle without evidence of decreased perfusion as seen in testicular torsion. Scrotal abscess may be visualized with US.

Treatment

In patients with suspected sexually transmitted disease (STD), the patient should receive treatment for both *N. gonorrhoeae* and *C. trachomatis* in the emergency department with culture results pending. Table 38–2 lists treatment recommendations for STDs. Advise the patient to discuss STD testing with any sexual partners. Evidence of UTI (pyuria, bacteriuria) in the nonsexually active patient should prompt treatment for UTI with antibiotics, such as SMZ-TMP or cephalexin, for 10 days. Treatment for noninfectious patients includes rest, decreased athletic activity, scrotal support, ice, and NSAIDs.

Disposition

Well-appearing patients with no evidence of sepsis or alternative conditions, such as testicular torsion, may be discharged with close follow-up with the pediatric urologist.

ORCHITIS

Orchitis is inflammation of the testicle which is more commonly seen in postpubertal males. Viral causes include

Table 38–2. Treatment of sexually transmitted disease in children and adolescents.

Treatment of *N. gonorrhoeae* urethritis	
< 45 kg with uncomplicated urethritis	Ceftriaxone 125 mg IM
< 45 kg with urethritis and bacteremia	Ceftriaxone 50 mg/kg IM/IV (max 1 g) daily for 7 d
≥ 45 mg with uncomplicated urethritis	Ceftriaxone 250 mg IM in a single dose, or cefixime 400 mg PO in a single dose, or azithromycin 2 g PO in a single dose[a]
≥ 45 kg with urethritis and bacteremia	Ceftriaxone 50 mg/kg IM/IV daily for 7 d
Treatment of *C. trachomatis* urethritis	
< 45 kg	Erythromycin base 50 mg/kg/d, by mouth, divided 4 times daily for 14 d
≥ 45 kg, younger than 8 y	Azithromycin 1 g by mouth in a single dose
≥ 45 kg, and 8 y or older	Azithromycin 1 g by mouth in a single dose, or doxycycline 100 mg by mouth twice daily for 7 d

[a]Azithromycin is given to patients with a cephalosporin allergy.

mumps, EBV, Coxsackie virus, and West Nile virus. Up to 38% of postpubertal males with mumps will develop orchitis. Bacterial etiologies include *N. gonorrhoeae, C. trachomatis, Brucella, E. coli, Enterococcus faecalis,* and *Neisseria meningitidis* may be causes in infants. Orchitis may occur after receiving the measles, mumps, rubella (MMR) vaccine.

Clinical Findings

Patients may have complaints of dysuria, scrotal pain, and fever. Physical examination usually reveals a tender, swollen scrotum. The testicles should have a normal vertical orientation. UA may reveal pyuria and bacteriuria. A urine culture should be ordered for UTI and in all children younger than 2 years. Concern for testicular torsion or a scrotal abscess warrants Doppler US of the testicle. A concurrent infection of the epididymis (epididymo-orchitis) may be identified.

Treatment

Patients who are sexually active should be treated for *N. gonorrhoeae* and *C. trachomatis* (Table 38–2). Patients who are well-appearing with bacterial orchitis due to suspected enteric organisms may be treated with SMZ-TMP or

cephalexin for 10 days and discharged with close follow-up with a urologist. Treatment for viral orchitis is symptomatic, and includes rest, support of the inflamed testicle, ice packs, and pain control.

Disposition

Infants with bacterial orchitis should be considered for inpatient treatment and evaluation for concurrent infections. Admission is appropriate for ill-appearing patients, those with scrotal abscesses, and patients who have failed outpatient therapy.

HYDROCELE

A hydrocele is an accumulation of fluid within the tunica vaginalis. It is the most common cause of painless scrotal mass in children. A communicating hydrocele has a patent connection between the peritoneum and scrotum through the processus vaginalis, which failed to obliterate during development. A hydrocele is considered noncommunicating if the processus vaginalis has closed. The type of fluid depends on the type of hydrocele. In a communicating hydrocele the fluid is peritoneal fluid, while fluid in the noncommunicating type is from the mesothelial lining of the tunica vaginalis. Communicating hydroceles may increase the risk of testicular torsion. Most hydroceles reabsorb by 12-18 months of age. Inflammatory conditions, such as testicular torsion, epididymitis, orchitis, and tumors, may cause a reactive hydrocele.

Clinical Findings

In most cases of hydrocele, patients present with a painless scrotal mass, usually right sided. Transillumination with a light source demonstrates a cystic fluid collection, although bowel may transilluminate. In a communicating hydrocele, the swelling may increase with Valsalva maneuver or may be reducible. Noncommunicating hydroceles are not reducible and do not change shape with an increase in intra-abdominal pressure. Palpation of the entire testis and surface should be performed to assess for other conditions, such as testicular torsion and infection. Doppler US of the testicle may be indicated to identify a condition causing a reactive hydrocele.

Treatment

Surgical repair may be needed for communicating hydrocele and swelling that causes damage to the skin. Elective surgical repair may be indicated for communicating hydroceles and those that persist beyond the first year of life.

Disposition

Patients with asymptomatic hydroceles may be discharged with close follow-up with urologist.

VARICOCELE

Varicocele is a complex of prominent varicosities described as a "bag of worms" in the scrotal sac due to dilation of the spermatic veins. Incomplete drainage of the veins may be due to incompetent venous valves or by increased venous pressure from renal vein obstruction or other extrinsic compression. Varicoceles are usually subacute in timing of symptoms, and found on the left side due to the angle at which the spermatic vein enters the left renal vein, although some are bilateral. Right-sided varicoceles may be due to pathologic dilation of the pampiniform plexus. Causes such as IVC thrombosis, right renal vein thrombosis and external compression of the IVC by abdominal and retroperitoneal masses, and lymphadenopathy should be considered.

Clinical Findings

Patient should be evaluated in the standing position. Higher grade varicoceles may be identified visually. Otherwise, palpation of the scrotum or spermatic cord reveals a varicocele with a bag of worms texture, which may be more prominent with Valsalva. Idiopathic varicoceles are identified while the patient is in the standing position only. If the varicocele persists while the patient is in the supine position, has a sudden onset, or right-sided in location, a pathologic cause of the varicocele should be considered. A Doppler US may reveal vascular thrombosis and abdominal masses as a cause.

Treatment & Disposition

Patients with idiopathic varicoceles may be referred for outpatient follow-up with a urologist. Outpatient operative repair may be indicated for symptomatic varicoceles.

SPERMATOCELE

A spermatocele is a fluid-filled cyst located at the head of the epididymis. It is typically painless, but some patients may have discomfort.

Clinical Findings

On examination, a small mass may be palpated with minimal to no pain to palpation. Transillumination of the swelling should show a fluid-filled cyst. Testicular tumors should not transilluminate. If the diagnosis is not clear, Doppler US of the testicle should be considered to evaluate for other entities, such as testicular tumor.

Disposition

Patients may be discharged with follow-up to urologist. Elective surgery may be indicated for symptomatic spermatoceles.

TESTICULAR TUMORS

Testicular tumors are uncommon in young children, but are the most common solid tumor in adolescent males. Risk factors of testicular cancer include family history of testicular cancer, cancer in the other testicle, and cryptorchidism.

Clinical Findings

Typical presentation of the tumor is a painless, firm scrotal mass on one hemiscrotum. Of note, pain may be present with germ cell tumors, as they cause hemorrhage and infarction. On examination, the painless, fixed mass will not transilluminate, unless a concurrent reactive hydrocele is present. Gynecomastia may be seen in a small number of patients with testicular germ cell and Leydig cell tumors. Scrotal US is indicated for diagnosis. MRI may be helpful to evaluate further if US is unable to discriminate benign lesion from malignant lesion.

Treatment & Disposition

Well-appearing patients may be discharged with close follow-up to urologist for further testing and definitive treatment.

PRIAPISM

Priapism is prolonged, involuntary erection of the penis without sexual stimulation. Priapism is categorized as either low flow (ischemic) or high flow (nonischemic). Causes of priapism are listed in Table 38–3.

Low-flow priapism is a urologic emergency caused by reduced venous outflow of deoxygenated blood from the corpora cavernosa, leading to a compartment syndrome and penile ischemia. Sickle cell disease is the most common cause in children. Recurrent, or stuttering, priapism is a type of low-flow priapism, usually seen in males with sickle cell disease, characterized by clustered episodes of priapism,

Table 38–3. Causes of priapism in children.

Ischemic (low flow) priapism
Hematologic: Sickle cell disease, leukemia, thalassemia
Medications: Antidepressants, antipsychotics, anticoagulants, antihypertensives
Recreational drugs: Cocaine, ethanol, marijuana
Spinal cord injury
Malaria
Black widow spider bite
Nonischemic (high flow) priapism
Straddle injuries
Penile injection of medications, such as papaverine, phentolamine
Penetrating injuries to the penis
Urologic procedures

with varying times in between episodes, approximately 2–3 times per week for several weeks duration. In low-flow priapism, microscopic damage of penile tissue has been noted with as little as 4-6 hours of sustained erection, leading to fibrosis of the corporal body with possible erectile dysfunction and rarely, impotence.

High-flow priapism is usually secondary to extravasation of blood into the corpora cavernosa from AV fistula in the corpora, often due to trauma to the penis or perineum, and penile procedures. Priapism may not occur until up to 72 hours after the injury. High-flow priapism does not result in ischemic injury as the blood is well oxygenated. However, some patients have long-term erectile dysfunction.

Clinical Findings

Priapism is a clinical diagnosis. History and physical examination should focus on duration of erection and possible underlying causes of priapism, attempting to discriminate low-flow from high-flow types. Low-flow priapism is typically painful, whereas high-flow priapism is generally painless. Patients should be asked about medical history of sickle cell disease, leukemia, medication use (including accidental ingestion), and illicit drug use. There may be a history of trauma to the penis or perineum, especially a saddle injury, resulting in high-flow priapism. On examination, there is swelling of the dorsal corpora cavernosa and flaccidity to the ventral corpus spongiosum. Fullness of bladder is associated with urinary obstruction. Compression of the perineum in children with high-flow priapism may lead to detumescence (reversal of erection), known as the piesis sign.

If history and physical are unable to discriminate low-flow from high-flow priapism, blood from the cavernosa may be aspirated for arterial blood gas analysis. Ischemic, low-flow blood will have a darker red (venous) appearance, and blood gas analysis will demonstrate a low pH and O_2, with elevated CO_2. Nonischemic, high-flow blood will appear brighter red, and normal results for blood gases are expected. Additionally, Doppler US of the penis may be used to discriminate low-flow from high-flow states, demonstrating decreased or no blood flow through the cavernosal arteries in low-flow priapism, and an AV fistula in high-flow priapism.

Treatment

The primary objective of treatment is rapid detumescence to prevent long-term complications. Early consultation with a pediatric urologist is warranted for treatment guidance. The patient should be NPO in preparation for possible procedural sedation or operative intervention. Pain control and relief of urinary obstruction, should occur promptly. Parenteral analgesics and dorsal penile nerve block using a long-acting anesthetic without epinephrine may be indicated. Treatment of underlying conditions, such as sickle cell disease, to include IVFs, supplemental oxygen, and consideration of exchange transfusion, is paramount.

Treatment for suspected low-flow priapism of greater than 4 hours duration includes cavernosal blood aspiration, with or without irrigation, followed by intercavernosal injection of an α-agonist, phenylephrine. Application of heat to the penile shaft with protection of the overlying skin may help to relieve the venous blood obstruction while preparing for the procedure. After adequate analgesia is obtained, aspiration of blood from the cavernosa may be attempted. A 19- or 21-gauge needle is inserted at the 3- or 9-o'clock position of the midshaft of the penis (Figure 38–2). Blood

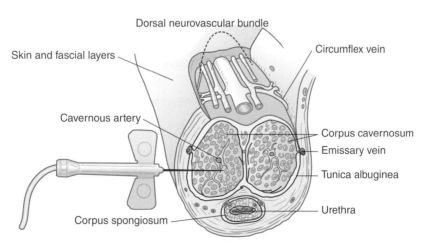

▲ **Figure 38–2.** Penile aspiration technique. A 19- or 21-gauge needle is inserted at the 3- or 9-o'clock position of the midshaft of the penis and the blood may drain or be gently aspirated. (Reproduced, with permission, from Reichman EF, Simon RR: *Emergency Medicine Procedures*. New York: McGraw-Hill, 2004. Copyright © McGraw-Hill Education LLC.)

may drain spontaneously or be gently aspirated and submitted for blood gas analysis. Irrigation with normal saline may be attempted after aspiration, especially if there is difficulty with aspiration. Irrigation may be performed on only one side of the penis, as there is vascular communication between the two corporal bodies. If detumescence is achieved with aspiration with or without irrigation, the needle may be removed. As the needle is removed, pressure should be applied to the area in which the needle resided to prevent hematoma formation. If detumescence has not been achieved, intercavernosal injection of an α-agonist, phenylephrine, should be performed. The phenylephrine solution is obtained by mixing 1 ampule of phenylephrine (1 mL:1000 mcg) with 9 mL of normal saline. Inject 0.3-0.5 mL of the diluted phenylephrine solution every 10-15 minutes until detumescence is obtained up to a maximum of 1 hour. The patient should be monitored for cardiovascular side effects of phenylephrine. Low-flow priapism that is refractory to treatment warrants consultation with a pediatric urologist for consideration of a penile venous shunt procedure. In high-flow priapism, the patient should be evaluated and treated for coexisting trauma.

Disposition

Patients with low-flow priapism should be admitted for exacerbations of underlying diseases, such as sickle cell anemia or leukemia, inability to obtain detumescence, or procedural complications. Patients with low-flow priapism in whom the erection has completely resolved and without complications from underlying medical conditions, that are controlled may be discharged home with close follow-up with pediatric urologist. High-flow priapism often resolves spontaneously, but may be treated by selective embolization. Consultation with a pediatric urologist is indicated for decisions regarding early intervention versus observation with close outpatient follow-up. Patients should be made aware of the possible complication of long-term impotence.

PHIMOSIS

Phimosis is a condition in the uncircumcised male where the distal foreskin is unable to be retracted fully to expose the glans penis. Phimosis may be physiologic or due to pathologic conditions. Phimosis is physiologic at birth, but the foreskin is freely mobile in most males older than 4 years. By early adolescence, less than 2% of patients have physiologic phimosis. Pathologic causes of phimosis may result from poor hygiene, swelling due to infection, such as balanoposthitis, trauma, contact dermatitis from irritants, excessive soap use or condoms. Complications of phimosis include urinary obstruction, UTIs, and significant swelling may result in ischemia to the glans penis.

Clinical Findings

Phimosis is a clinical diagnosis. The patient may report painful urination, blood in the urine, a narrowed urinary stream or ballooning of the foreskin during urination. Physical examination may reveal inflammation of the foreskin and glans penis due to balanoposthitis or contact dermatitis. The glans should be evaluated for signs of ischemia. Penile adhesions may mimic phimosis. Decreased urinary output and suprapubic tenderness suggest urinary retention.

UA may reveal hematuria and evidence of UTI. BUN and creatinine should be checked in suspected urinary obstruction. Renal US should be considered to assess for severity of urinary obstruction.

Treatment

Topical corticosteroids may be used to resolve phimosis in order to avert circumcision. Betamethasone 0.05% may be applied twice daily for 21 days or twice daily for 30 days. Corticosteroids should be avoided if infection is suspected. Associated balanoposthitis should be treated accordingly. Bladder outlet obstruction may be relieved by gentle dilation of the prepuce (foreskin) with forceps or passage of a urinary catheter. Signs of ischemia to the glans penis may warrant a dorsal slit procedure to relieve pressure. Urology consultation should be obtained for significant infection, urinary obstruction, or signs of ischemia to the penis.

Disposition

Patients with mild swelling, minor infection, or inflammation, who are able to urinate without difficulty may be discharged with follow-up in 2-3 days to a urologist. Instructions for care of the uncircumcised penis should be provided, including gentle retraction and replacement of foreskin with good hygiene measures. Patients using topical steroid creams should be monitored for development of infections and skin integrity.

PARAPHIMOSIS

Paraphimosis is a true urologic emergency in which foreskin of the uncircumcised or partially circumcised penis is retracted and fixed behind the glans penis. The retracted foreskin develops a tight phimotic ring, which causes venous and lymphatic congestion distally to the glans penis, leading to soft tissue damage and gangrene. Paraphimosis may be caused by not replacing the retracted foreskin after cleaning or medical examination, self-manipulation, and penile piercing. Sexually active males may incur the condition with erection or sexual intercourse. Circumcision status should be verified, as hair or thread tourniquet syndrome may mimic a paraphimosis in the fully circumcised child.

Clinical Findings

The constricting phimotic ring of foreskin just proximal to the coronal sulcus should be identified. Absence of a phimotic ring in the uncircumcised child with penile swelling should prompt consideration of other conditions, such as insect bites and allergic reaction. The healthy salmon color of the glans may develop a black discoloration when tissue becomes necrotic. The glans penis may be tense with edema. Erythema may be present with infection, such as balanoposthitis. Suprapubic pain and distention should prompt consideration of urinary outlet obstruction.

Treatment

Goal of treatment is to restore circulation to the distal penis by reduction of the constricting phimotic ring of the prepuce distally over the glans penis. The patient should be made NPO for possible procedural sedation or operative procedures. Analgesia may be provided by topical medication, regional anesthesia (dorsal penile nerve block) using a long-term anesthetic without epinephrine and parenteral narcotics. Topical anesthetics, such as lidocaine 2% without epinephrine, placed inside the fingertip of a glove may be applied to the distal penis.

Paraphimosis with minimal swelling of the glans penis may require only quick manual reduction of the phimotic ring. When moderate to severe edema of the glans penis is present, it may be necessary to decreasing swelling of the glans prior to manual reduction. Decreasing swelling by compression of the swollen glans penis may be attempted by squeezing the distal penis with a gloved hand for 5-10 minutes. More than one person may be required to assist due to expected muscle fatigue. Alternatively, compression of the distal penis may be achieved by application of circumferential compression dressing first placed on the distal glans and moving proximally to the phimotic band. Leave in place for 5 minutes to compress the edema then remove the dressing. Also, ice water may be placed in the finger of a glove, which is then tied off, invaginated, and placed over the glans for 2- to 3-minute intervals. Additionally, an osmotic agent, such as granulated sugar or dextrose 50%, may be applied directly to the edematous glans penis and foreskin and covered with a bandage or finger of a glove may diminish swelling. However, the osmotic method may require up to 1-4 hours to reduce swelling.

After decreasing swelling of the glans penis, the clinician attempts manual reduction by placing the thumbs on the distal glans penis and fingers behind the phimotic ring of the prepuce (Figure 38–3). The examiner's thumbs push inward on the penis while the fingers pull the phimotic ring distally over the glans penis. If manual reduction is unsuccessful, more advanced techniques may be required. Consultation with a pediatric urologist is warranted for more invasive techniques.

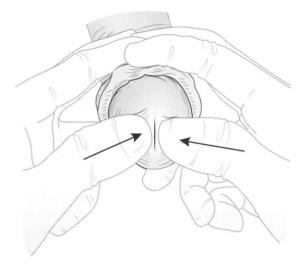

▲ **Figure 38–3.** Manual reduction of paraphimosis. The thumbs are placed on the distal glans penis with the fingers behind the phimotic ring. The thumbs push inward on the penis while the fingers pull the phimotic ring distally over the glans. (Reproduced, with permission, from Reichman EF, Simon RR: *Emergency Medicine Procedures.* New York: McGraw-Hill, 2004. Copyright © McGraw-Hill Education LLC.)

Dorsal band traction with Babcock clamps, which do not crush tissue, may be attempted. Several Babcock clamps are placed on the phimotic ring, with one clamp edge just proximal to the phimotic ring and the other clamp just distal to the ring. The clamps are pulled in a distal direction simultaneously to pull the ring distally over the glans (Figure 38–4). A more invasive method to relieve penile swelling is needle decompression, in which an 18- or 21-gauge needle is used to puncture the swollen foreskin at depths of 3-5 mm, followed by gentle squeezing of the foreskin to allow fluid drainage (Figure 38–5). Approximately 8-12 puncture holes are required. Additionally, the phimotic ring may be incised using the dorsal slit procedure, allowing reduction of the prepuce over the glans (Figure 38–6). Patients with evidence of infection or penile ischemia should receive IV fluid resuscitation, parenteral antibiotics, and consultation with a urologist for admission.

Disposition

Admission is recommended in cases that do not respond to minimally invasive techniques of reduction, procedural complications, such as bleeding, and any signs of infection or ischemia to the penis. Discharge with close outpatient follow-up to pediatric urologist if reduction is successful,

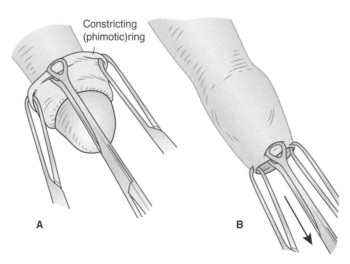

Constricting
(phimotic) ring

A   B

▲ **Figure 38–4.** Babcock clamp reduction of paraphimosis. (A) Clamps are placed on the phimotic ring, with one clamp edge just proximal to the phimotic ring and the other clamp just distal to the ring. (**B**) The clamps are pulled in a distal direction simultaneously to pull the ring distally over the glans. (Reproduced, with permission, from Reichman EF, Simon RR: *Emergency Medicine Procedures.* New York: McGraw-Hill, 2004. Copyright © McGraw-Hill Education LLC.)

no signs of infection or ischemia, and patient is able to urinate without difficulty. Instructions on care of the foreskin should be provided to include gentle retraction and replacement of foreskin with good hygiene measures. Circumcision may be advised in the future to prevent recurrence.

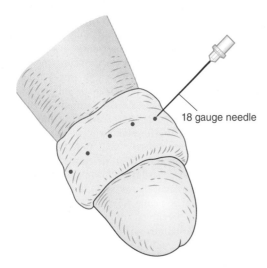

18 gauge needle

▲ **Figure 38–5.** Needle decompression technique. Use an 18- or 21-gauge needle to puncture the swollen foreskin at depths of 3-5 mm, followed by gentle squeezing of the foreskin to allow fluid drainage. (Reproduced, with permission, from Reichman EF, Simon RR: *Emergency Medicine Procedures.* New York: McGraw-Hill, 2004. Copyright © McGraw-Hill Education LLC.)

BALANOPOSTHITIS

Balanoposthitis is inflammation of the glans penis and foreskin in uncircumcised males. Balanitis is inflammation of the glans penis only. Posthitis is inflammation of the foreskin (prepuce). The inflammation is usually due to infection, but may be due to trauma or contact dermatitis. Common infectious causes include *Candida albicans*, Group A β-hemolytic *Streptococcus*, and *Staphylococcus aureus*. *N. gonorrhoeae* and *C. trachomatis* may be present in sexually active patients.

Clinical Findings

Children often have complaints of genital itching, penile pain, and dysuria. On examination, the glans penis and prepuce may have erythema and edema suggestive of cellulitis. A concurrent streptococcal infection (pharyngitis or impetigo) may be present, suggesting that organism as the cause of penile infection. Candidal infections may have mild erythema, satellite lesions, fissures, and whitish discharge around the penile skin. Urethral discharge should prompt consideration of STIs, such as *N. gonorrhoeae* and *C. trachomatis*. Chronic inflammation may cause phimosis, meatal stenosis, and rarely urinary outlet obstruction.

Cultures and potassium hydroxide (KOH) wet prep may help to identify the offending organism. Urethral discharge suspicious of STI may be sent for appropriate cultures. A blood glucose may be considered to assess for occult diabetes mellitus in patients with recurrent candidal infections.

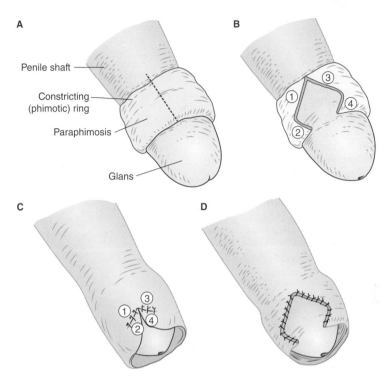

▲ **Figure 38–6.** Dorsal slit to relieve paraphimosis. (**A**) The incision line. (**B**) The foreskin will open after the incision is made. The numbers represent the edges of the incision. (**C**) The foreskin has been reduced and the edges sewn edge 1 with 2 and edge 3 with 4. A small gap should remain in the midline that is free of sutures. (**D**) Alternatively, a simple running stitch can close the edges. (Reproduced, with permission, from Reichman EF, Simon RR: *Emergency Medicine Procedures.* New York: McGraw-Hill, 2004. Copyright © McGraw-Hill Education LLC.)

Treatment

Candidal infections may be treated with a topical antifungal, such as clotrimazole 1% twice daily or miconazole 2% twice daily for 4 weeks. Bacterial cellulitis should be treated with 7-10 days of oral antibiotics effective against *S. aureus* (MRSA) and Group A *Streptococcus*. Suspected STIs should be treated as outlined in Table 38–2. Contact dermatitis may be treated with avoidance of possible irritants, hydrocortisone 1% cream twice daily, sitz baths twice daily, and emphasis on good hygiene and frequent diaper changes.

Disposition

Admission should be considered for patients with significant cellulitis and significant phimosis with urinary outlet obstruction. Otherwise, patients may be discharged with outpatient follow-up to urologist. Recurrent balanoposthitis may warrant outpatient circumcision.

HAIR TOURNIQUET SYNDROME

Disruption of blood flow to tissue by external compression, such as from hair and synthetic materials, or by auto manipulation may lead to a tourniquet syndrome with soft tissue injury and necrosis. Up to 33% of hair or synthetic material tourniquet syndrome cases involve the external genitalia. The median age of incidence is 2 years, but may occur in a wide range of ages. Tourniquet syndrome of the penis is typically due to external compression from hair or synthetic material such as threads, clothing, wires, and penile rings. The penis may be twisted or wrapped to prevent enuresis. Complications of penile tourniquet syndrome include soft tissue injury, neurovascular bundle damage, and thrombosis leading to ischemia, and urethral transection.

Clinical Findings

Infants may present with uncontrollable crying only. A thorough physical examination of the infant, including the genitalia and all digits, is paramount to detect tourniquet syndromes. The offended tissue may appear edematous, erythematous, and strangulated. Hair, string or the constricting material may be grossly apparent, or may be hidden by swelling or re-epithelialization. Examination should identify other conditions with similar presentations, such as paraphimosis, balanoposthitis, trauma, insect bites, abscesses, or allergic reactions.

Treatment

Pain control may be obtained through local anesthesia, such as a penile block, or parenteral medications. The patient may require procedural sedation and should be kept NPO. Superficial hair or thread may be removed carefully by acquiring the loose end of the string/hair and unwrapping circumferentially or inserting a blunt probe under the string and cutting the fiber with scissors or scalpel. Incisions should be made at the 3- or 9-o'clock positions of the penis with the cutting surface oriented perpendicular to the skin to avoid dorsally positioned neurovascular bundles.

Depilatory (hair removal) creams may be applied for hair tourniquets, but will not work on synthetic fibers. Local skin irritation may occur with depilatory creams. Deeply embedded hair or thread is usually surrounded by significant edema and may have signs of ischemia. Consultation with a urologist should be sought expeditiously as operative intervention may be required for removal. Reperfusion should be apparent within minutes of release of constriction, but may not be restored completely for days. Suspected penile urethral injury may be assessed by retrograde urethrogram. Doppler US of the penis may be used to evaluate for injuries and occlusions of the penile blood vasculature.

Disposition

Consultation with a urologist should be sought for signs of penile ischemia, concerns for urethral injury, neurovascular injury, and incomplete removal of the offending material. Patients with uncomplicated removal of the constricting material, no signs of ischemia, and who are able to urinate spontaneously may be considered for outpatient follow-up in 24 hours with a pediatric urologist. Patient and family should evaluate the penis periodically for verification of good perfusion.

ZIPPER INJURIES

Zipper injuries to the penis most commonly involve the uncircumcised foreskin, and occasionally affect the redundant tissue of the circumcised penis, the urethra, or glans penis. A zipper is composed of interlocking dentitions, or teeth, aligned by a fastener comprising an inner face plate, outer faceplate, and median bar. The fastener holds together the dentitions. Disruption of the fastener will cause the dentitions to fall apart.

Treatment

If the penis is entrapped within the interlocking dentitions, but not the fastener, carefully cut the cloth between the individual teeth, then pull the teeth apart, allowing liberation of the trapped tissue (Figure 38–7). If the penis is entrapped within the zipper fastener, penile tissue may be more difficult

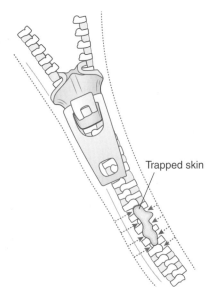

Trapped skin

▲ **Figure 38–7.** Penile skin entrapped in the interlocking dentitions only. Cut the cloth between the teeth (red lines) to free the entrapped skin. (Reproduced, with permission, from Reichman EF, Simon RR: *Emergency Medicine Procedures*. New York: McGraw-Hill, 2004. Copyright © McGraw-Hill Education LLC.)

to liberate. Dorsal penile block using local anesthetic without epinephrine should be considered. Procedural sedation may be required for younger children. An alternative method is application of a lubricant, such as mineral oil, to the entrapped tissue for 15 minutes, followed by gentle traction to free the penile tissue. Another method is to carefully cut the median bar of the fastener, causing the zipper mechanism to fall apart (Figure 38–8). Wire cutter, bone cutter, or a mini hacksaw may be used to cut the median bar. Alternatively, the thin blade of a flat-head screwdriver may be placed between the faceplates on the side of the fastener in which the penile tissue is not entrapped. The screwdriver is then rotated toward the median bar to widen the gap between the faceplates and release the entrapped tissue. Consultation with a urologist is indicated if initial attempts at disengagement of entrapped tissue are unsuccessful, and for complications, such as significant soft tissue injury or urethral injury.

Disposition

Patients who are able to void and have no significant complications after zipper removal may be discharged with follow-up in 2 days to primary care physician or urologist. Superficial abrasions may be treated with topical triple antibiotic ointment. Patients should be encouraged to wear underpants.

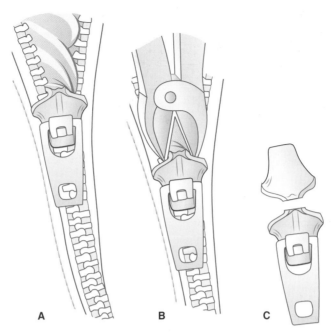

▲ **Figure 38–8.** Penile skin entrapped in slider and dentitions. (A) Penile skin trapped between the sliding piece and the zipper dentitions. (**B**) The median bar is cut. (**C**) The front and back plates of the sliding piece separate and the skin is released. (Reproduced, with permission, from Reichman EF, Simon RR: *Emergency Medicine Procedures*. New York: McGraw-Hill, 2004. Copyright © McGraw-Hill Education LLC.)

CIRCUMCISION COMPLICATIONS

Most common complications of circumcision are hemorrhage and infection. Bleeding typically responds to direct pressure or a circumferential pressure dressing for 10 minutes. Care must be taken to avoid causing penile ischemia and urinary retention with application of pressure dressings. After bleeding is controlled, silver nitrate may be applied. Consultation with a urologist is warranted for more severe bleeding. Patient should be examined for signs of generalized bleeding indicative of underlying bleeding disorders.

Localized infection should be treated with topical antibiotics. More significant local infections and the presence of systemic symptoms should raise concern for coexistent bacteremia or serious bacterial infection. Meatal stenosis may occur if a small Plastibell device was placed. Patient will have a high-velocity urine stream and pain with urination. Outpatient follow-up with urologist for possible meatotomy is warranted. Skin bridges are adhesions that develop between the glans penis and shaft. Gentle retraction may be applied periodically at home to manually lyse the adhesions, followed by application of a petroleum or antibiotic ointment. Outpatient follow-up with a urologist is appropriate for possible surgical lysis of the adhesions. Excess remnant foreskin may lead to phimosis and should be treated accordingly.

Badawy H, Soliman A, Ouf A, et al: Progressive hair coil tourniquet syndrome: Multicenter experience with 25 cases. *J Pediatr Surg*. 2010;45:1514-1518 [PMID: 20638535].

Centers for Disease Control and Prevention: Update to CDC's Sexually transmitted diseases treatment guidelines, 2010: oral cephalosporins no longer a recommended treatment for gonococcal infections. *MMWR*. 2012;61:590-594 [PMID: 22874837].

Lieberman L, Kirby M, Ozolins L, et al: Initial presentation of unscreened children with sickle cell disease: The Toronto experience. *Pediatr Blood Cancer*. 2009;53:397-400 [PMID: 19405139].

Montague DK, Jarrow K, Broderick GA, et al: American Urological Association guideline on the management of priapism. *J Urol*. 2003;170:1318-1324 [PMID: 14501756].

O'Gorman A, Ratnapalan S: Hair tourniquet management. *Pediatr Emerg Care*. 2011;27:203-204 [PMID: 21378520].

Palmer LS, Palmer JS: The efficacy of topical betamethasone for treating phimosis: A comparison of two treatment regimens. *Urology*. 2008;72:68-71 [PMID: 18455770].

Raman SR, Kate V, Ananthakrishnan N: Coital paraphimosis causing penile necrosis. *Emerg Med J*. 2008;25:454 [PMID: 18573970].

Raveenthiran V: Release of zipper-entrapped foreskin: A novel nonsurgical technique. *Pediatr Emerg Care*. 2007;23:463-464 [PMID: 17666927].

Srinivasan A, Cinman N, Feber KM, et al: History and physical examination findings predictive of testicular torsion: An attempt to promote clinical diagnosis by house staff. *J Pediatr Urol*. 2011;7:470-474 [PMID: 21454130].

Vorilhon P, Martin C, Pereira B, et al: Assessment of topical steroid treatment for childhood phimosis: Review of the literature. *Arch Pediatr.* 2011;18:426-431 [PMID: 21354771].

Weiss HA, Larke N, Halperin D, et al: Complications of circumcision in male neonates, infants and children: A systematic review. *BMC Urol.* 2010;10:2-13 [PMID: 20158883].

Workowski KA, Berman S: Centers for Disease Control and Prevention: Sexually transmitted diseases treatment guidelines, 2010. *Morb Mortal Wkly Rep.* 2010;59:1-110 [PMID: 21160459].

OTHER GENITOURINARY DISEASES

URINARY TRACT INFECTION

Urinary tract infection (UTI) is infection of the lower urinary tract (cystitis) or upper urinary tract (pyelonephritis). Risk factors for UTI in the pediatric population are listed in Table 38–4. Most UTIs ascend from the periurethral skin through the urethra to bladder, but neonates may have seeding of the urinary tract from bacteremia. Gram-negative bacteria are the cause of 90% of UTIs. *E. coli* is the most common organism in all age groups and is responsible for approximately 80-85% of UTIs. Other gram-negative organisms include *Klebsiella, Proteus,* and *Enterobacter.* Gram-positive bacteria are less common causes and include *Enterococcus, Staphylococcus saprophyticus* (especially in adolescent females), and Group B *Streptococcus* (prominent in neonates). *Trichomonas vaginalis* may cause UTI in sexually active patients. Infections from urinary tract instrumentation or indwelling catheters may be due to *C. albicans* and *Pseudomonas aeruginosa*. Viruses, such as adenovirus, may cause hemorrhagic cystitis in immunocompromised children. Sepsis is a known complication of UTI, and untreated pyelonephritis may cause renal scarring with subsequent hypertension and chronic renal insufficiency.

Clinical Findings

Symptoms of UTI in children younger than 2 years are often nonspecific, such as fever, irritability, vomiting, and jaundice. Children older than 2 years with cystitis may have complaint of localized suprapubic pain and dysuria. Table 38–5 demonstrates differential diagnosis for dysuria in children. Pyelonephritis should be suspected with flank pain and systemic symptoms, such as fever and chills. New-onset bedwetting or urinary incontinence may occur in the toilet-trained child. A confidential history regarding sexual activity may increase suspicion for concurrent STDs or pregnancy.

Physical examination should identify contributing conditions, such as circumcision status, the presence of phimosis and urethral strictures in males, urethral foreign bodies (toilet paper), and labial adhesions. Testicular examination should assess for evidence of epididymo-orchitis. Abdominal examination and flank examination may reveal masses with hydronephrosis or neoplasms (neuroblastoma, teratoma, Wilms tumor). Urethral and vaginal discharge or skin manifestations of STI, such as painful vesicles, may prompt testing for STDs.

Urine culture is the gold standard for diagnosing UTI. If urine culture results are available, the presence of UTI is determined by the bacterial colony count, which is relative to method of urine collection (Table 38–6). In the acute care setting, urine culture results are not commonly available. Therefore, UTI is diagnosed presumptively in the acute setting by patient evaluation and UTI screening tests, such as the urine dipstick test and the UA. Statistical reliability of the dipstick method and UA in evaluation of UTI vary widely relative to patient populations studied. Table 38–7 lists the sensitivities, specificities, and likelihood ratios (LR) among various tests in diagnosing UTI in children.

The dipstick method analyzes for the presence of leukocyte esterase (LE) and nitrite. LE is present is some WBCs. A positive LE result is a relatively good indicator of UTI but may be false positive in other conditions, such as streptococcal

Table 38–4. Higher risk patients for obtaining urinalysis and urine culture.

Girls and uncircumcised boys < 2 y with at least 1 risk factor for UTI
- History of UTI
- Temperature > 39°C (102.2° F)
- Fever without apparent source
- Ill appearance
- Suprapubic tenderness
- Fever > 24 hrs

Circumcised boys < 2 y with suprapubic tenderness and at least two risk factors for UTI
- History of UTI
- Temperature > 39°C (102.2° F)
- Fever without apparent source
- Ill appearance
- Fever > 24 hrs

Girls and uncircumcised boys > 2 y with following urinary symptoms
- Abdominal pain back
- Pain, dysuria
- Polyuria
- High fever
- New-onset urinary incontinence

Circumcised boys > 2 y with multiple urinary symptoms
- Abdominal pain
- Back pain
- Dysuria
- Polyuria
- High fever
- New-onset urinary incontinence

Febrile infants and children with abnormalities of the urinary tract
- VUR
- Posterior urethral valves
- Family history of urinary tract infection (UTI)

Table 38–5. Causes of dysuria in children.

Condition	History and Physical Examination	Diagnostic Studies
Stevens-Johnson syndrome	Target lesion rash, oral ulcerations, conjunctivitis	Presumptive diagnosis by clinical examination in acute setting
Reactive arthritis/Reiter syndrome	Conjunctivitis, arthritis, and urethritis. More common in males	Diagnosis by physical examination
Behçet syndrome	Arthritis, conjunctivitis, and oral and genital ulcerations	Diagnosis by physical examination
Varicella	Fever, crops of vesicles begin centrally and extend to genitals	Diagnosis by physical examination, or positive viral culture
Urinary tract infection (UTI)	Dysuria, frequency, suprapubic or flank pain	UA with positive nitrite, leukocyte esterase, pyuria, and bacteriuria. Organisms present on urine culture
Bacterial urethritis	Dysuria, discharge	UA shows LE and pyuria, positive gonorrhea, and chlamydia tests
Chemical urethritis	Dysuria, use of detergents, bubble baths, perfumed soaps. Examination normal or mild erythema to urethra	UA normal, or LE positive and pyuria. UC normal
Genital herpes	Painful vesicles or ulcerations, from auto-inoculation from oral ulcers or from sexual abuse	Positive viral culture of lesion
Balanoposthitis	Erythema to glans penis and/or prepuce	UA may be normal, have isolated hematuria, or shows associated UTI on UA
Urolithiasis	Dysuria, hematuria, flank pain, history of hypercalciuria	UA shows hematuria and RBCs
Labial adhesions	Adhesions to labia minora	UA normal
Local trauma	Due to self-exploration, masturbation or sexual abuse. Examination normal or urethral irritation, hymen tears, ecchymosis	UA normal or hematuria with trauma. May have evidence of STDs in sexual abuse
Vaginal pinworms	Anal and vaginal itching, worse at night. Pinworms may be seen on adhesive tape	Pin worms or bean-shaped eggs seen with microscopy
Vulvovaginitis	Vaginal erythema. May have discharge. Foreign body, such as toilet paper, may be present	Clue cells with *Gardnerella vaginalis*. Yeast or pseudohyphae with Candida
Vulvar/virginal/Lipschütz ulcers	Adolescent females. One or more painful ulcers, each > 1 cm. Fever, headache, malaise. May be of viral origin	Tests negative for HSV. Monospot negative
Psychogenic dysuria	Recurrent complaints of dysuria	UA and UC normal, STD tests normal. No GU abnormalities or positive alternative diagnoses

Table 38–6. Urine culture results based upon method of collection.

Suprapubic aspiration: single urinary pathogen*
≥ 1000 CFU/mL (pediatrics UTI)
Catheterized urine: ≥ 50,000 CFU/mL catheter *or*
          ≥ 10,000 and < 50,000 CFU/mL from catheter with positive UA screening results
Clean catch urine: > 100,000 CFU/mL

Lactobacillus spp., Staphylococcus epidermidis, Corynebacterium spp. are not considered clinically relevant urinary organisms in the 2- to 24-month-old child.

infections and Kawasaki disease. LE has a reported sensitivity of 94% in patients with a high pretest probability of UTI.

Nitrite is produced when nitrates in the urine are reduced by gram-negative bacteria (except *P. aeruginosa* and *Acinetobacter*). A positive nitrite result is highly specific for UTI caused by gram-negative bacteria. A negative nitrite result is not helpful (low sensitivity) in assessing for UTI, as it will provide a false-negative result in gram-positive UTIs and in patients with frequent urination, as nitrate will not be reduced to nitrite unless urine has been in the bladder for at least 4 hours.

Combined positive results for LE and nitrite are highly specific for UTI. The UA detects the presence of WBCs

Table 38–7. Diagnostic tests for urinary tract infection.

Test Dipstick	Sensitivity (%)	Specificity (%)	Positive LR[a]	Negative LR[b]	References
Leukocyte esterase	84	78	4	0.2	1
Nitrite	50	98	25	0.5	1
Nitrite or LE	88	93	13	0.1	1
Nitrite and LE	72	96	18	0.3	1
Microscopy (uncentrifuged)					
Pyuria (> 10/mm³) (all ages)	77	89	7	0.4	1
Pyuria (> 10/mm³) (< 2 years)	90	95	18	0.1	1, 2
Bacteriuria (Gram-stained)	93	95	19	0.1	1
Overall (P + B) = enhanced	85	99.9	85	0.1	1
Overall (P or B)	95	89	9	0.1	1
Microscopy (centrifuged)					
Pyuria (> 5/HPF)	67	79	3	0.4	1
Bacteriuria	81	83	5	0.2	3
Overall (P + B)	66	99	7	0.4	2

Reproduced, with permission, from: Palazzi DL, Campbell JR: Acute cystitis in children more than 2 years and adolescents. In: *UpToDate*, Basow, DS (ed). UpToDate: Waltham, MA, 2012. Copyright © 2012 UpToDate, Inc. For more information visit www.uptodate.com.

[a]Positive Likelihood ratio: The positive likelihood ratio is the probability that a child with a UTI will have a positive test divided by the probability that a child without a UTI will have a positive test (true-positive rate/false-positive rate). The higher the positive likelihood ratio, the better the test.

[b]Negative likelihood ratio: The negative likelihood ratio is the probability that a child with a UTI will have a negative test divided by the probability that a child without a UTI will have a negative test (false-negative rate/true-negative rate). The lower the negative likelihood ratio, the better the test (a perfect test has a negative likelihood ratio of zero).

Gorelick MH, Shaw KN: Screening tests for urinary tract infection in children: A meta-analysis. *Pediatrics* 1999. [PMID:10545580].

Huicho L, Campos-Sanchez M, Alamo C: Metaanalysis of urine screening tests for determining the risk of urinary tract infection in children. *Pediatr Infect Dis J.* 2002.

Finnell SM, Carroll AE, Downs SM: Subcommittee on Urinary Tract Infection: Technical Report:Diagnosis and Management of an Initial UTI in Febrile Infants and Young Children. *Pediatrics.* 2011.

(pyuria) and bacteria (bacteriuria). UA may be performed using the standard centrifuged or uncentrifuged UA methods, either through microscopy or automated analysis. Gram-stain results may help to guide initial antibiotic therapy. The uncentrifuged method is preferred over the centrifuged method especially in young children, due to higher sensitivities, specificities, and LRs for UTI. The presence of both bacteriuria and pyuria is 99.9% specific for UTI.

Importantly, up to 12% of children younger than 2 years with UTIs will have normal UA results. Therefore, urine cultures should generally be ordered in the emergency department for patients regardless of dipstick and UA results. Urine culture may be deferred in low-risk patients older than 2 years with normal dipstick results and alternative diagnosis for the presenting symptoms.

Patients who are able to void on command may have urine collected by the midstream clean catch method. Patients who are not toilet-trained or unable to provide a clean catch specimen should have urine collected by either urethral catheterization or US-guided suprapubic aspiration (SPA). Samples from bladder catheterization are very reliable in UTI, demonstrating a sensitivity of 95% and specificity of 99%. SPA is a relatively uncomplicated procedure and may be considered when a catheterized specimen cannot be obtained (labial adhesions, severe phimosis). Bag collection method is not recommended due to an 85% false-positive culture rate. Urine samples should be tested within 1 hour of collection if unrefrigerated and no longer than 4 hours after collection if refrigerated.

WBC, CRP, and ESR will not discriminate lower and upper lower tract infections and are not generally required in the well-appearing patient. Patients with suspected renal insufficiency or urinary tract calculus should be evaluated for elevated BUN and creatinine. Blood cultures are positive in up to 9% of children younger than 2 months with UTI; however, management is generally unchanged as the same organism is found in blood and urine. Blood culture is recommended for children younger than 2 months and for all ill-appearing patients.

About 1% of children less than 29 days old with UTI may have coexisting bacterial meningitis; therefore, CSF workup should be considered even if UTI is discovered in the febrile neonate. Of note, approximately 10% of infants with UTI will have a coexisting sterile CSF pleocytosis.

Treatment & Disposition

Antibiotics should be administered in the emergency department expeditiously to reduce risk of renal scarring and subsequent renal insufficiency and hypertension. Urine cultures should be obtained before administering antibiotics to allow for identification of offending organisms. When previous urine culture results are available in the acute setting, known antibiotic sensitivities may help guide treatment if the same organism is suspected. Otherwise, antibiotics should generally be directed against the most likely organisms, such as *E. coli*.

Antibiotic options for first-time UTIs in children greater than 29 days are listed in Tables 38–8 and 38–9. Second- or third-generation cephalosporins are first option for outpatient antibiotic treatment of UTIs due to *E. coli* and gram-negative bacteria. A third-generation cephalosporin is a reasonable first choice for a parenteral antibiotic. Local antibiotic resistance patterns should further guide initial antibiotic selection. *Enterococcus* should be treated with amoxicillin or nitrofurantoin. *S. saprophyticus* may be treated with TMP-SMX or nitrofurantoin. Nitrofurantoin is not recommended for suspected pyelonephritis and prostatitis due to its poor tissue penetration. Fluoroquinolones are reserved for use in known *Pseudomonas* and multidrug resistant gram-negative infections in children older than 1 year when indicated by culture sensitivities.

Disposition

Children younger than 29 days with UTI should receive parenteral antibiotics in the emergency department and

Table 38–8. Parenteral antibiotics for urinary tract infection.

Ceftriaxone	50 mg/kg IV/IM q24hr
Cefotaxime	150 mg/kg/d IV/IM divided q8hr
Ceftazidime	150 mg/kg/d IV divided q8hr
Gentamicin	7.5 mg/kg/d IV/IM divided q8hr
Tobramycin	5 mg/kg/d IV/IM divided q8hr
Piperacillin	300 mg/kg/d IV divided q6hr

Table 38–9. Oral antibiotics for urinary tract infection.

Amoxicillin w/ or w/o clavulanic acid	45 mg/kg/d divided twice daily
Trimethoprim(TMP)/ sulfamethoxazole (SMX)	8 mg/kg/d divided twice daily
Cefixime	8 mg/kg/d, divided twice daily
Cefpodoxime	10 mg/kg/d, divided twice daily
Cefprozil	30 mg/kg/d, divided twice daily
Cefuroxime	20-30 mg/kg/d, divided twice daily
Cephalexin	50-100 mg/kg/d, divided four times daily
Nitrofurantoin	5-7 mg/kg/d, divided four times daily

admitted to the hospital. Ampicillin plus cefotaxime or gentamicin are reasonable antibiotic choices in this age group:

Ampicillin 50 mg/kg IV/IO/IM ≤ 7 d every 8 hr, 8-28 d give every 6 hr

plus-

Cefotaxime 50 mg/kg IV/IO/IM, ≤ 7d every 12 hr, 8-28 d give every 8 hr

or

Gentamicin 2.5 mg/kg IV/IO/IM every 12-18 hr.

All children up to 29 days of life who are ill-appearing, show signs of sepsis, have complicated underlying medical conditions (uncontrolled diabetes mellitus), are unable to tolerate oral medications, or have failed outpatient treatment should receive parenteral antibiotics, adequate rehydration, and hospital admission. Admitted patients remaining in the emergency department who are awaiting an inpatient bed or transfer should be closely monitored closely for worsening overall appearance and hemodynamic instability.

Children aged 29 days-2 years with UTI, who are well-appearing and tolerating oral medications, may receive a dose of parenteral antibiotics (rocephin 50 mg/kg IV/ IM) or oral antibiotics while in the emergency department and be discharged home with outpatient follow-up in 24 hours. Oral antibiotics should be continued for 7-14 days. Well-appearing children 2 years and older with UTI may be treated with oral antibiotics for 7 days. All discharged patients should have outpatient follow-up in 1-2 days for reevaluation, urine culture results, and consideration of outpatient screening for underlying genitourinary abnormalities (vesico-ureteral reflex [VUR], posterior urethral valves [PUV]).

Discharged patients should drink a large amount of fluids during the course of antibiotic treatment to maintain good urine output. Bladder pain and dysuria may be treated with phenazopyridine (< 12 years, 4 mg/kg/three times a day; > 12 years, 100 mg/kg/three times a day) for up to 48 hours.

Warm water baths for 20-30 minutes as needed may provide some relief from dysuria.

HEMATURIA

Hematuria is the presence of RBCs in the urine. Microscopic hematuria is defined as five or more RBCs per high-power field (HPF). Macroscopic or gross hematuria is blood in the urine able to be seen by the naked eye. RBCs may enter the urinary tract at various locations. Common etiologies of hematuria in children are listed in Table 38–10. Hematuria due to trauma is discussed Chapter 27. Of note, a number of pigments may cause a red discoloration of the urine: beets, vegetable dyes, phenolphthalein (ingredient in many laxatives), and benign urate crystals produced most commonly by neonates. *Serratia marcescens* is a fecal bacterium that may produce red discoloration in a child's diaper.

Table 38–10. Diagnostic clues to causes of hematuria.

Diagnosis	Clinical Findings	Diagnostic Studies
Cystitis, pyelonephritis, epididymitis	Dysuria, urinary frequency, fever	Urine dipstick with positive Leukocyte Esterase, nitrites. UA with positive pyuria, bacteriuria
Meatal stenosis	Small caliber meatal opening. Possibly due to small Plastibell from circumcision, or chronic phimosis may be present	Diagnosis by clinical findings
Glomerulonephritis (GN)	Recent streptococcal infection, edema, hypertension	UA with hematuria, red cell casts, dysmorphic RBCs, proteinuria
Sickle cell disease or sickle cell trait	Intermittent hematuria. May be painful (disease) or painless (trait)	UA has evidence of RBC and isosthenuria. Hemoglobin electrophoresis is abnormal
Trauma, exercise	History or physical examination evidence of genital or abdominopelvic trauma, recent genitourinary instrumentation, or excessive exercise	UA will show blood and RBCs. See Chapter 27 for trauma evaluation
Renal or bladder tumor	Painless hematuria, palpable abdominal or flank masses	US or CT scan reveals tumors
Urethral foreign body or manipulation	Pain and urethral irritation may be present. Foreign body, such as toilet paper may be seen	Proximally located foreign bodies may require imaging for localization and retrieval
Urolithiasis	Hematuria usually associated with pain. Stones in the bladder may be painless but may cause intermittent urinary obstruction	CT scan may have evidence of the stone. US and IV pyelogram may be alternatives to CT
Henoch-Schönlein purpura (HSP) nephritis	Rash, joint pains, abdominal pain	UA demonstrates hematuria possibly and proteinuria
Hemolytic uremic syndrome (HUS)	Typically has prodrome of diarrhea, which is often bloody	UA shows hematuria. CBC with hemolytic anemia
IgA nephropathy	URI 1-3 d before hematuria. Not genetically linked	Isolated hematuria. Renal biopsy is definitive
SLE nephritis	Fever, malaise, joint pains. Malar rash in 1/3. Red-colored urine, edema, and hypertension in renal disease	UA shows hematuria, proteinuria. CBC with neutropenia, hemolytic anemia. ANA elevated
Hypercalciuria	Asymptomatic hematuria, unless associated with nephrolithiasis	Hematuria. Elevated urine calcium level
Alport syndrome	Family history of AKI with deafness. May have edema, hypertension	UA shows hematuria. May lead to AKI with elevated BUN/creatinine
Renal vein or artery thrombosis	Flank pain or mass, hematuria. May be associated with trauma, severe dehydration, hypercoagulable state, and nephrotic syndromes. May have associated pulmonary embolism	Hematuria on UA. Proteinuria present in nephrotic syndrome. Renal vein and artery thrombosis demonstrated on Doppler US or CT scan with IV contrast

Clinical Findings

History should be focused on identification of the underlying etiology of hematuria. Dysuria, suprapubic or flank pain may indicate UTI or a renal stone. A history of trauma, urinary instrumentation, urethral foreign bodies, or excessive exercise should be noted. Family history of hematuria may prompt consideration of hereditary disorders, such as systemic lupus erythematosus nephritis, immunoglobulin A nephropathy, and Alport syndrome. Medication use, especially aspirin and anticoagulants, may cause hematuria. Recent streptococcal pharyngitis or skin infections may be suggestive of poststreptococcal GN. Bloody diarrhea is associated with HUS.

On examination, hypertension may be present. Edema may be present in the face, mimicking an allergic reaction, in the scrotum and labia, or be dependent in location. Examination of the genitals may reveal trauma, irritation, or a urethral foreign body. Ensure that the bleeding is not from the vagina or rectum.

Hematuria is demonstrated on the UA as great as 5 RBC/HPF. A positive blood result on the urine dipstick is roughly equivalent to 2-5 RBCs/HPF on UA. UA may reveal evidence of UTI with WBC, bacteriuria, nitrites, or leukocyte esterase. Urine culture should be ordered for suspected UTI. The UA may help to distinguish a glomerular versus non-glomerular cause of hematuria. RBC casts and dysmorphic RBCs (acanthocytes) are associated with glomerular disease. Concerns for glomerular etiologies may prompt assessment for evidence of streptococcal disease, such as a streptococcal throat culture and the streptozyme test or ASO titer. A UA showing positive blood, but no RBCs, may be due to the presence of hemoglobin or myoglobin in the urine. Of note, substances that mimic hematuria, such urinary pigments, should test negative for blood on urine dipstick or UA. Further testing will be guided by suspected etiologies.

Noncontrast CT scan/urogram will identify urinary stones greater than 1 mm, urinary obstructions, and abdominal masses. Renal US may identify hydronephrosis from urinary tract obstruction.

Treatment

Treatment is guided by the underlying cause of the hematuria. UTIs should be treated with antibiotics as detailed below in this chapter. GN treatment should be guided by consultation with a nephrologist.

Disposition

Patients with AKI, significant hematuria or proteinuria, hypertension, electrolyte disorders, or volume overload should be considered for consultation with a pediatric nephrologist or urologist and admission. Patients suitable for discharge should be well-appearing, well-hydrated, and have reliable outpatient follow-up.

UROLITHIASIS

Stones, or calculi, may form in the kidneys, ureters, and bladder. Most urinary stones are composed of calcium oxalate or phosphate. Struvite, uric acid, and cysteine are less common types of stones. Risk factors for urolithiasis include previous personal or family history of urinary stones, malabsorption syndromes with increased intake of oxalate, structural urinary tract abnormalities, history of recurrent UTIs (especially *Proteus* and *Klebsiella*), and medication use (loop diuretics, sulfadiazine, indinavir).

Clinical Findings

Gross hematuria is initial complaint in up to 50% of children. Older children often have complaint of flank pain, often radiating to the lower back or groin. Young children may have less-specific symptoms, such as dysuria (from a concurrent UTI), vomiting, and diffuse abdominal pain. A subset of pediatric patients will have hematuria without flank or abdominal pain.

Children with recurrent UTIs and hematuria should be considered for a struvite-producing stone caused by *Proteus, Klebsiella,* or *Pseudomonas* infection. Fever may be present with a concurrent pyelonephritis. Hypertension may be present with pain; however, persistent hypertension after pain control should prompt consideration of other conditions.

Characteristically, costovertebral angle tenderness is present. Abdominal examination should assess for intra-abdominal emergencies, such as appendicitis and intussusception. Significant groin and testicular pain should assess for testicular torsion, testicular infection, and hernia. An extensive abdominal examination should be performed to try to distinguish the pain and rule out a palpable mass or other pathology.

UA may reveal RBCs and blood. Up to 15% of children with urolithiasis have no hematuria. Crystals may be seen in the sediment to give clues to the etiology of the calculi. A creatinine should also be drawn if there are concerns for renal dysfunction.

The noncontrast CT scan of the abdomen and pelvis, or CT urogram, is the most sensitive imaging modality to detect renal calculi in children. It is able to localize small stones as small as 1 mm in diameter and may identify both renal and ureteral stones, including radiolucent (uric acid) stones, and identify associated hydronephrosis and hydroureter. In addition, it may identify alternative intra-abdominal or pelvic sources of symptoms. Radiation exposure from CT scan is a concern in children. CT urogram should be considered in suspected first-time urinary stones, history of complicated urinary stones, and concern for significant urinary obstruction or infection.

The renal US and abdominal radiograph are alternative imaging modalities. Renal US may identify intrarenal stones greater than 5 mm, including radiolucent (uric acid) stones, hydronephrosis, and hydroureter. Renal US avoids radiation exposure from a CT urogram. Negative aspects of the US are that it may be difficult to identify stones less than 5 mm and stones in the ureter. Abdominal x-ray is able to identify most urinary stones, but they cannot be discriminated from other radiopaque findings, such as phlebolits. Further, plain radiograph is unable to detect signs of urinary obstruction.

Treatment

Goals of treatment in the acute setting are control of pain, ensure ample hydration, and treatment of coexisting infections. Analgesia with parenteral opioids and NSAIDs are often required for pain control. Patients with evidence of UTI should be treated with antibiotics after obtaining urine culture. Stones less than 5 mm in diameter generally pass spontaneously in children.

Disposition

Admission should be considered for patients with renal stones and coexisting infection, renal insufficiency, significant urinary obstruction, as well as patients with a solitary kidney. Patients who are well-appearing, adequately hydrated with good pain control may be discharged with close outpatient follow-up with a urologist. A urine strainer should be provided to the patient and used to obtain expelled urinary stones for analysis at outpatient follow-up. Patients should be encouraged to maintain adequate oral fluid intake and avoid dehydrating substances.

INCARCERATED HERNIA

Herniation of abdominal contents, such as bowel, mesentery, and the hernia sac into the inguinal region may occur at any age, but is more common in children younger than 1 year, with a peak incidence during the first month of life. It occurs more commonly in children that are premature, in males, and is more often right sided. Hernias are bilateral in 10% of full-term cases and 50% of premature cases.

A direct inguinal hernia protrudes through a weak point in the fascia of Hesselbach triangle in the abdominal wall. An indirect inguinal hernia passes through the patent processus vaginalis, which failed, in infancy to obliterate into the scrotal sac. Hernias may be mobile, moving with relative ease in and out of the abdominal cavity, and thus reducible with manual pressure. Mobile hernias may be asymptomatic or symptomatic with pain. Irreducible hernias, known as incarcerated hernias, may become strangulated, wherein the hernia contents experience vascular compromise. Differential diagnosis includes testicular torsion, epididymo-orchitis, hydrocele, tumor, and appendicitis.

Clinical Findings

Patient with an easily reducible, asymptomatic hernia may present with a nonpainful mass, which may be absent on examination, and is nonreproducible with attempts to increase intra-abdominal pressure. Child with a symptomatic hernia may have complaints of scrotal or abdominal pain, vomiting, and fever. Infants may present with nonspecific symptoms, such as uncontrollable crying or difficultly feeding. It is important to examine the genitalia of infants with nonspecific symptoms, such as crying, and the genitalia of older children with abdominal pain.

On examination, the nonincarcerated hernia has a nontender mass that is easily reducible with manual reduction. Patients with irreducible incarcerated hernias are usually in distress with a painful mass of the scrotum or labia majora. The presence of erythema or bluish discoloration may suggest vascular compromise. Bowel sounds may also be present in the scrotum. Patients with bowel obstruction may have vomiting and abdominal distention. Female patients often present with a painful mass to the labia majora. Reproductive organs, including the fallopian tube and ovary, may be contained in the hernia sac and ovarian torsion may occur in such cases. Hydroceles may mimic inguinal hernias in males, and both hydroceles and gas-filled bowel will transilluminate with direct light.

Indirect inguinal hernias are often diagnosed clinically, but if testicular torsion is suspected, a Doppler US of the testicle is recommended. Abdominal x-ray may demonstrate bowel obstruction.

Treatment

Patients with suspected strangulated hernias, who are toxic-appearing, with signs of peritonitis from bowel necrosis should receive IV fluid resuscitation, parenteral antibiotics, and immediate consultation with a pediatric surgeon.

The nontoxic patient with incarcerated hernia should have manual reduction performed expeditiously in the emergency department. The patient should receive adequate analgesia and sedation, as needed. Place the patient in the Trendelenburg position at 20 degrees, and apply ice to the hernia to reduce swelling and facilitate reduction. Placing the patient in frog-leg position may also be helpful. One method of manual reduction involves applying gentle pressure on the distal end of the hernia sac with one hand, while the other hand feeds the proximal hernia sac, and bowel contents and gas contained within, back through the fascial deficit. Too much pressure on the distal end will cause ballooning of the proximal sac around the external ring. Steady pressure for 5-10 minutes may be required for reduction. A second method is to apply gentle traction on the distal end of the hernia sac with one hand, and the other hand is placed just around the external ring pulling the skin upward and laterally, better aligning the internal and external rings, allowing the distal hernia sac to be gently walked back into the fascial deficit. If initial attempts at manual reduction are unsuccessful, immediate consultation with a pediatric surgeon is indicated.

Disposition

Well-appearing patients with easily reducible, nonincarcerated hernias may be discharged with follow-up with a pediatric surgeon for consideration of definitive repair. Patients with incarcerated hernias that have been manually reduced in the emergency department should have consultation with a surgeon for disposition and timing of elective repair. Discharged patients may wear support devices such as a jock strap and avoid precipitants to increase intra-abdominal pressure, such as exercise and straining with bowel movement.

Bradley JS, Jackson MA; and the Committee on Infectious Diseases: The use of systemic and topical fluoroquinolones. *Pediatrics*. 2011;128:e1034-e1045 [PMID: 21949152].

Cincinati Children's Hospital Medical Center: *Evidence-based care guideline for medical management of first urinary tract infection in children 12 years of age or less.* Cincinnati, OH: 2006. Available at http://www.cincinnatichildrens.org/ass ets/0/78/1067/2709/2777/2793/9199/c2dda8f2-f122–4cc4– 9385-f02035d4f322. pdf. Accessed August 21, 2013.

Finnell SM, Carroll AE, Downs SM, et al: Technical report-Diagnosis and management of an initial UTI in febrile infants and young children. *Pediatrics*. 2011;129:e749-e770 [PMID: 21873694].

Fogazzi GB, Edefonti A, Garigali G, et al: Urine erythrocyte morphology in patients with microscopic haematuria caused by a glomerulopathy. *Pediatr Nephrol*. 2008;23:1093-1100 [PMID: 18324420].

Goldman RD: Cranberry juice for urinary tract infection in children. *Can Fam Physician*. 2012;58:398-401 [PMID: 22499815].

Greenfield SP, Williot P, Kaplan D: Gross hematuria in children: A ten-year review. *Urology*. 2007;69:166-169 [PMID: 17270642].

Hodson EM, WIlis NS, Craig JC: Antibiotics for acute pyelonephritis in children. *Cochrane Database Sys Rev*. 2007;(4):CD003772 [PMID: 17943796].

Hom J: Are oral antibiotics equivalent to intravenous antibiotics for the initial management of pyelonephritis in children? *Paediatr Child Health*. 15:150-2, 2010. [PMID: 21358894].

Huppert JS, Biro F, Lan D, et al: Urinary symptoms in adolescent females. *J Adolesc Health*. 2007;40:418-424 [PMID: 17448399].

Ismaili K, Wissing KM, Lolin K, et al: Characteristics of first urinary tract infection with fever in children: A prospective clinical and imaging study. *Pediatr Infect Dis J*. 2011;30; 371-374 [PMID: 21502928].

Kalorin CM, Zabinkski A, Okpareke I, et al: Pediatric urinary stone disease—does age matter? *J Urol*. 2009;181: 2267-2271 [PMID: 19296968].

Levy I, Comarsca J, Davidovits M: Urinary tract infection in preterm infants: The protective role of breast feeding. *Pediatr Nephr*. 2009;24:527-531 [PMID: 18936982].

Osifo OD, Ovueni ME: Inguinal hernia in Nigerian female children: Beware of ovary and fallopian tube as contents. *Hernia*. 2009;12:149-153 [PMID: 18998195].

Persaud AC, Stevenson MD, McMahon DR, et al: Pediatric urolithiasis: Clinical predictors in the emergency department. *Pediatrics*. 2009;124:888-894 [PMID: 19661055].

Schnadower D, Kupperman N, Macias CG, et al: Febrile infants with urinary tract infections at very low risk for adverse events and bacteremia. *Pediatrics*. 2010;126:1074-1083 [PMID: 21098155].

Shaikh N, Morone NE, Lopez J: Does this child have a urinary tract infection? *JAMA*. 2007;298:2895-2904 [PMID: 18159059].

Shaikh N, Morone NE, Bost JE, et al: Prevalence of urinary tract infection in childhood: A meta-analysis. *Pediatr Infect Dis J*. 2008;27:302-308 [PMID: 18316994].

Springhart WP, Marguet CG, Sur RL, et al: Forced versus minimal intravenous hydration in the management of acute renal colic: A randomized trial. *J Endourol*. 2006;20:713-716 [PMID: 17094744].

Subcommitee on Urinary Tract Infection, Steering Committee on Quality Improvement and Management, Roberts KB: Urinary tract infection: Clinical practice guideline for the diagnosis and management of the initial UTI in febrile infants and children 2 to 24 months. *Pediatrics*. 2011;128:595-610 [PMID: 21873693].

Tebruegge M, Pantazidou A, Clifford V, et al: The age-related risk of co-existing meningitis in children with urinary tract infection. *PLoS One*. 2011;6:e26576 [PMID: 22096488].

RENAL DISORDERS

POSTSTREPTOCOCCAL GLOMERULONEPHRITIS

Glomerulonephritis (GN) is damage to the glomerulus resulting in a nephritic syndrome, which is characterized by varying degrees of hematuria, proteinuria, edema, hypertension, and AKI. The most common cause of GN in children is Group A β-hemolytic *Streptococcus* (GAS). Strains of GAS that cause pharyngitis and skin infections are nephritogenic, leading to complement activation and immune complex formation, resulting in inflammation and damage to the glomerular basement membrane. GN typically develops 2 weeks after streptococcal pharyngitis and 3-6 weeks after streptococcal skin infection. It may occur sporadically or as an epidemic. Other causes of pediatric GN include immunoglobulin A nephropathy, HSP nephritis, systemic lupus erythematosus nephritis, toxin induced (mercury, lead, hydrocarbons), membranoproliferative GN, and hereditary nephritis.

Clinical Findings

Patients aged 2-12 years may have complaint of recent upper respiratory tract infection or skin infection. Brown or red-colored urine is often the first symptom of GN and is found in 30-50% of patients. Generalized weakness and malaise is common. Two-thirds of patients have either facial swelling from periorbital edema or tight-fighting clothes from more generalized edema. The edema is caused by salt and water retention or acute kidney injury. More advanced cases may present with dyspnea on exertion representative of pulmonary edema. Hypertension may cause headache, dizziness, or altered mental status from hypertensive encephalopathy.

Diagnosis of poststreptococcal GN (PSGN) is made by the presence of nephritis with evidence of recent streptococcal infection. Clinical findings of nephritis may range from isolated microscopic hematuria to the full-blown nephritic syndrome with hematuria, proteinuria, edema, hypertension, and AKI. UA reveals hematuria, possibly reported as dysmorphic RBCs. RBC casts are present in up to 85% of patients. Mild proteinuria is often present, and up to 15% of patients may have nephrotic syndrome range proteinuria. Hyaline casts may be present. Urine cultures should be sent for possible UTI as a cause of hematuria. Serum chemistries should be assessed for elevated BUN, creatinine, hyperkalemia, and hyponatremia. ECG may show signs of hyperkalemia. Chest x-ray may reveal signs of CHF.

Assessment of streptococcal infection may be performed by streptococcal cultures or by serum antibody testing. Streptococcal pharyngeal and skin cultures are positive in 25% of cases after onset of GN symptoms. The streptozyme test measures different streptococcal antibodies and is positive in 95% of cases of streptococcal pharyngitis and 80% of streptococcal skin infections. Anti-streptolysin O (ASO) titers, anti-DNase B, and anti-nicotinamide-adenine dinucleotidease are elevated after pharyngeal infections. Anti-DNAase B and anti-hyaluronidase are elevated in response to skin infections.

Treatment

Salt and water intake should be restricted. Volume overload and hypertension typically respond well to loop diuretics (furosemide 1 mg/kg IV, maximum 40 mg). Persistent hypertension may require more aggressive treatment with parenteral antihypertensives. A nephrologist should be consulted early in severe AKI. Dialysis may be indicated for uremia, hyperkalemia, and CHF unresponsive to medical therapy. Patients with underlying GAS infections should be treated with appropriate antibiotics. Additionally, close contacts of the patient should be evaluated for evidence of streptococcal disease with a skin evaluation and oropharyngeal cultures and treated with appropriate antibiotics to eliminate the suspected nephritogenic strain of GAS.

Disposition

Disposition should be made in consultation with a nephrologist. Generally, patients with mild hematuria, no hypertension or renal impairments may follow-up with a nephrologist for consideration of outpatient renal biopsy. All other patients should be considered for admission. Most patients with PSGN have complete resolution of urinary symptoms without sequelae after antibiotic treatment for the underlying streptococcal infection.

HEMOLYTIC UREMIC SYNDROME

Hemolytic uremic syndrome (HUS) is characterized by the simultaneous occurrence of acute renal injury, microangiopathic hemolytic anemia, and thrombocytopenia. HUS is the most common cause of AKI in young children. About 90% of cases, termed "typical" HUS, are caused by Shiga toxin–associated disease presenting with a prodrome of diarrhea, which is often bloody, prior to onset of HUS. E. coli subtype 0157:H7 is the most common organism known to produce Shiga toxin. Typical HUS may occur with an epidemic incidence, as the Shiga toxin–associated bacteria may be acquired by patients from ingestion of undercooked beef, contaminated fruits and vegetables, as well as exposure to animals, especially cattle.

The remaining 10% of cases, termed "atypical," of HUS are not associated with Shiga toxin and do not present with a prodrome of diarrhea. Atypical HUS is often a complication of S. pneumococcus infection, HIV, pregnancy, genetic predispositions, or drug induced (cyclosporine, tacrolimus, cisplatin). Complications of HUS include chronic renal insufficiency, hypertension, CHF, ischemic colitis with intestinal perforation, intussusception, bowel perforation, pancreatitis with glucose intolerance, and central nervous system complications.

Clinical Findings

Typical cases of HUS present with a prodrome of watery diarrhea, often becoming bloody by day 5, followed by the abrupt onset of HUS symptoms of renal injury, hemolytic anemia, and thrombocytopenia. Symptoms of dark-colored urine, decreased urine output, and edema are suggestive of renal impairment. Hypertension is present in up to 50% of patients. Patients may have complaint of dyspnea and have abnormal lung sounds in CHF. Up to 33% of patients may develop neurologic symptoms such as seizures and focal neurologic deficits. The patient may have been previously treated with antibiotics or antimotility agents for diarrhea, both of which increase the risk of HUS in E. coli 0157:H7 infections. A dietary history, travel history and recent exposure to farm animals or petting zoo trips, or to other human contacts with diarrheal disease may elicit exposure to *E. coli* 0157:H7. In patients with atypical HUS, signs of infections from invasive disease with *S. pneumoniae*, such as pneumonia, empyema, or meningitis, may be present without diarrhea.

CBC and peripheral blood smear may reveal leukocytosis, thrombocytopenia, and hemolytic anemia with fragmented RBCs, such as schistocytes, helmet cells, and burr cells. BUN and creatinine may be elevated with renal insufficiency. Electrolytes should be obtained early to assess for hyperkalemia, metabolic acidosis, and hyponatremia. Hyperbilirubinemia may be present due to hemolytic anemia. Prothrombin time/partial thromboplastin time (PT/PTT) will be normal in HUS, thus discriminating it from TTP/DIC. Coombs test will be negative. UA may demonstrate RBCs and proteinuria. Stool cultures with specific tests for *E. coli* 0157:H7 may be obtained. Fecal leukocytes may be absent in one-half of cases of *E. coli* 0157:H7.

ECG may show signs of hyperkalemia. Chest x-ray may show volume overload, or free air under diaphragm with intestinal perforation, and pneumonia may be present with invasive pneumococcal disease. Severe abdominal pain may warrant abdominal US or CT scan to assess for GI complications. Noncontrast CT of the head is indicated in patients with aseptic meningitis syndrome (AMS) to assess for cerebral edema, intracranial hemorrhage.

Treatment

Treatment of HUS in the acute setting is supportive. Hypotension may be treated with IV crystalloid replacement with 20 cc/kg bolus. Patients should be monitored for development of pulmonary edema. Hyperkalemia should be treated in the standard manner. Patients with hemoglobin less than 6 g/dL should be slowly transfused PRBC to a goal of hemoglobin of 7-8 g/dL.

Generally, platelet transfusions are not recommended due to concerns about transfusion-related platelet consumption seen in TTP, which is a similar disorder. However, significant thrombocytopenia (< 20,000) or need for invasive procedures, such as dialysis catheter placement, may warrant platelet transfusion and should be discussed with a hematologist. Hypertension should be treated by oral fluid restriction and antihypertensive medications, such as calcium channel blockers. Nifedipine orally is a reasonable first option. ACE inhibitors are typically avoided in the acute phase as they reduce renal perfusion.

Acute renal injury warrants consultation with a nephrologist, as dialysis may be indicated initially for significant uremia, hyperkalemia, or CHF. Seizures should be treated with benzodiazepine or phenytoin. Contributing condition such as malignant hypertension or symptomatic hyponatremia should be corrected accordingly. Children with severe CNS symptoms may benefit from eculizumab and plasma exchange therapy. Antibiotics and antimotility agents should be avoided in typical diarrhea-associated HUS. Patients with atypical HUS, without diarrhea, due to invasive pneumococcal disease warrant antibiotic treatment against *S. pneumoniae*. Patients with atypical HUS may benefit from plasma exchange therapy.

Disposition

Patients with HUS should be admitted to the hospital. Intensive care should be considered for patients with significant renal manifestations, CHF, neurologic symptoms, and sepsis. Most patients with HUS have complete resolution of hemolytic and renal manifestations, although 5-25% of patients may develop chronic renal insufficiency or hypertension. Public health authorities should be notified of cases of infection with *E. coli* 0157:H7 for purposes of identifying potential sources.

NEPHROTIC SYNDROME

Nephrotic syndrome is the presence of significant amounts of protein in the urine due to increased permeability of the glomerulus. It is characterized clinically by proteinuria (> 50 mg/kg/day), hypoalbuminemia (< 3 g/dL), hyperlipidemia, and peripheral edema. Primary nephrotic syndrome, or idiopathic nephrotic syndrome (INS), is due to diseases limited to the kidney and is responsible for approximately 90% of cases. It typically occurs in patients younger than 6 years. About 85% of cases of INS are due to minimal change disease (MCD), 8% membranoproliferative GN (MPGN), 7% focal segmental glomerulosclerosis (FSGS), 2% mesangial proliferation, 2% proliferative GN, 2% focal and global glomerulosclerosis, and 2% membranous glomerulonephropathy.

Secondary nephrotic syndrome accounts for the remaining 10% of cases and is due to renal effects of systemic conditions, such as HSP, poststreptococcal GN, diabetes mellitus, systemic lupus erythematosus, and Alport syndrome. Up to 2% of patients experience thrombotic complications, such as renal vein thrombosis and pulmonary embolism, due to thrombocytosis, hyperfibrinogenemia, hemoconcentration, and urinary loss of antithrombotic proteins. Also, children with nephrotic syndrome are at increased risk of bacterial infections with encapsulating organisms, such as peritonitis and pneumonia, due to loss of opsonizing proteins, decreased levels of immunoglobulins, and possible concurrent steroid use.

Clinical Findings

The patient may initially complain of periorbital edema, which may mimic an allergic reaction. The edema typically progresses to the body, including the scrotum and vulva, causing weight gain, and complaints of tight-fitting clothes.

Decreased urine output with dark-colored or foamy urine suggests renal injury. Signs of intravascular depletion, in the midst of peripheral edema, may be manifested by hypotension, tachycardia, and poor perfusion. Hypertension may be present in some cases of nephrotic syndrome, especially with underlying GN. Pulmonary edema or pleural effusions may present with dyspnea and abnormal lung sounds. Chest pain or dyspnea should also raise consideration for pulmonary embolism. Decreased appetite, nausea, and vomiting may represent edema to the intestines. Significant abdominal pain may be present with ascites or peritonitis. Renal vein thrombosis may cause flank pain and scrotal edema in males.

UA will demonstrate proteinuria, usually 3 + or 4 + on urine dipstick. The presence of urinary RBCs, with or without RBC casts, may represent a GN as an underlying cause. Hemoglobin and hematocrit are often elevated due to hemoconcentration. Acute renal injury is unusual in primary nephrotic syndrome, so BUN and creatinine are typically normal. Elevated BUN and creatinine and microscopic or gross hematuria may be seen with secondary causes of nephrotic syndrome and renal vein thrombosis. Hyperkalemia may be present due to renal injury, and hyponatremia may be present due to hypertriglyceridemia. Total serum protein and albumin are characteristically decreased. Lipid panel, if available, may demonstrate elevated total cholesterol, LDL, and triglycerides.

Chest x-ray may reveal pulmonary edema or pleural effusions. Abdominal radiographs may reveal ascites. Abdominal US with Doppler may demonstrate compromised renal vein blood flow in renal vein thrombosis. CT scan of the chest with IV contrast or ventilation-perfusion (V/Q) scan should be considered for suspected pulmonary embolism.

Treatment

Hypotension should be corrected with IV crystalloid solution, despite presence of extravascular edema. Mild dehydration may be treated with oral intake of sodium-deficient fluid or IV hydration with D5Ü normal saline. Once intravascular hydration is adequate, peripheral edema may be managed with loop diuretics, such as furosemide 1 mg/kg IV. However, diuresis may be difficult in the setting of significant hypoalbuminemia (albumin < 1.5 g/dL). In such cases, a 25% albumin solution (1 g/kg IV) over 24 hours may be given concurrent with loop diuretics in consultation with a pediatric nephrologist or intensivist. Watch for signs of developing pulmonary edema.

The specific underlying cause of the nephrotic syndrome, if known, will guide further treatment. Underlying causes of INS are defined as being responsive to treatment with corticosteroids or steroid resistant. MCD, which is the most common cause of INS, and mesangial proliferation nephritis are generally steroid responsive within 8 weeks of treatment.

MCD is suspected in patients who are younger than 6 years, with no hypertension, no hematuria, no renal insufficiency, and normal compliment levels. If MCD is suspected as a cause, prednisone 2 mg/kg/day by mouth divided twice a day for 6 weeks, followed by 1.5 mg/kg every other day for 6 weeks may be prescribed in consultation with a pediatric nephrologist. Recurrent cases of steroid responsive INS may be treated with repeat courses of oral corticosteroids in consultation with a nephrologist. If the patient has a known steroid-resistant cause of nephrotic syndrome, immunosuppressants, such as cyclosporin, may be recommended by the nephrologist. Fever or signs of secondary infection should prompt evaluation for suspected sources, including paracentesis for peritonitis with ascites. Thrombotic complications, such as renal vein thrombosis and pulmonary embolism, should be treated with heparin or thrombolytics, as indicated, in consultation with the admitting physician.

Disposition

Hospital admission is indicated in patients with hypotension, renal insufficiency, significant edema, respiratory complications, evidence of infection, or thrombotic complications. Patients with only mild edema, who are otherwise well-appearing, may be discharged with close outpatient follow-up with a pediatric nephrologist for trending of urine protein levels. The patient and family should be advised on the importance of a low-sodium diet. Some patients may have recurrent episodes of nephrotic syndrome.

Banerjee R, Hersh AL, Newland J, et al: Streptococcus pneumoniae-associated hemolytic uremic syndrome among children in North America. *Pediatr Infect Dis J.* 2011;30:736-739 [PMID: 21772230].

Blyth CC, Robertson PW, Rosenberg AR: Post-streptococcal glomerulonephritis in Sydney: A 16-year retrospective review. *K Paediatr Child Health.* 2007;43:446-450 [PMID: 17535174].

El Bakkali L, Rodrigues Pereira R, et al: Nephrotic syndrome in the Netherlands: A population-based cohort study and a review of the literature. *Pediatr Nephrol.* 2011;26:1241-1246 [PMID: 21533870].

Gipson DS, Massengill SF, Yao L, et al: Management of childhood onset nephrotic syndrome. *Pediatrics.* 2009;124:747-757 [PMID: 19651590].

Kerlin BA, Blatt NB, Fuh B, et al: Epidemiology and risk factors for thromboembolic complications of childhood nephrotic syndrome: A Midwest Pediatric Nephrology Consortium (MWPNC) study. *J Pediatr.* 2009;155:105-110 [PMID: 19394032].

Lapeyraque AL, Malina M, Fremeaux-Boppel T, et al: Eculizumab in severe Shiga-toxin-associated HUS. *N Engl J Med.* 2011;364:2561-2563 [PMID: 21612462].

Michael M, Elliott EJ, Craig JC, et al: Interventions for hemolytic uremic syndrome and thrombotic thrombocytopenic purpura: A systematic review of randomized controlled trials. *Am J Kidney Dis.* 2009;53:259-272 [PMID: 18950913].

Rodriguez-Iturbe B, Musser JM: The current state of poststrepto-coccal glomerulonephritis. *J Am Soc Nephr.* 2008;19:1855-1864 [PMID: 18667731].

Smith KE, Wilker PR, Reiter PL, et al: Antibiotic treatment of Escherichia coli 0157infection and the risk of hemolytic ure-mic syndrome, Minnesota. *Pediatr Infect Dis J.* 2012;31:37-41 [PMID: 21892124].

Trachtman H, Austin C, Lewinski M, et al: Renal and neurological involvement in typical Shiga toxin-associated HUS. *Nat Rev Nephrol.* 2012;8:658-669 [PMID: 22986362].

Waters AM, Kerecuk L, Luk D, et al. Hemolytic uremic syndrome asso-ciated with invasive pneumococcal disease: The United Kingdom experience. *J Pediatr.* 2007;151:140-144 [PMID: 17643764].

Wong CS, Mooney JC, Brandt JR, et al: Risk factors for the hemo-lytic uremic syndrome in children infected with Escherichia coli 0157:H7: A multivariable analysis. *Clin Infect Dis.* 2012;55: 33-41 [PMID: 22431799].

Zaffanello M, Franchini M: Thromboembolism in childhood nephrotic syndrome: A rare but serious complication. *Hematology.* 2007;12:69-73 [PMID: 17364996].

Gynecologic Emergencies

Kenneth Yen, MD, MS

Jendi Haug, MD

PEDIATRIC & ADOLESCENT GYNECOLOGY

NORMAL DEVELOPMENT

An important aspect of the pediatric and adolescent gynecologic examination is an understanding of the various stages of development and when each would typically occur. The Tanner stages, known as sexual maturity ratings, classify the progression of boys and girls through pubertal development. Table 39–1 presents the classification of sexual maturity ratings in girls.

Normal age of onset of puberty in girls is considered to be between 8 and 13 years of age. Puberty involves thelarche, (onset of breast development), pubarche, (onset of pubic hair development), and menarche (onset of menses). The sequence of puberty progression usually begins with thelarche, then pubarche, followed by menarche. Thelarche occurs about 1 year earlier in non-Hispanic African American and Hispanic American girls. The trend toward earlier age of puberty onset in girls has continued over the past several decades and, as a result, there is uncertainty about the current range of normal. Obesity decreases the age of onset by approximately 0.5 years.

EXAMINATION

Gynecologic examination of the female pediatric patient is a procedure that some physicians are uncomfortable performing. This may be due to the fact that some of the examination involves a nulliparous patient who may also be prepubertal. It can be a challenging situation caused by anxiety of the parent and patient. It is best to develop a strategy for approaching the examination beforehand in order to improve success.

Genital anatomy of the prepubertal girl differs from that of the adult woman. The pediatric vulva is more susceptible to irritants and trauma due to its inherent anatomy and lack of estrogenization. Prior to puberty, the pediatric vulva is hairless and has very little subcutaneous fat. The labia minora lack pigmentation and have an atrophic appearance. The distance from the vestibule to the anus is shorter, which places the vulva at an increased risk of irritation. The vagina is proportionally smaller in length and diameter and has very little distensibility. The vaginal mucosa will be red, thin, and moist. The vestibule and vagina are not glycogenated or estrogenized, and the glans clitoris may appear relatively more prominent due to the flat appearance of the labia in the prepubertal patient. The cervix is either flush with the vaginal vault or protrudes slightly. The hymen is a vascularized mucous membrane that separates the vestibule from the vagina. It is originally solid, but begins to open during the fetal period. There is great physiologic variability in thickness, size, and shape. There is no distensibility prior to puberty.

A speculum examination is not generally indicated in most children. It is usually reserved for those that are sexually active or in the setting of sedation required for vaginal foreign body or surgical repair of traumatic injuries. Examination of the child is best performed by placing her in the supine frog-leg position (butterfly position), or in the prone knee-chest position. The frog-leg position involves having the child lie on her back with feet together and knees spread wide apart. The prone knee-chest position is performed with the chest on the bed with the head turned to one side, and an assistant holding the buttocks apart. As always, appropriate gowning and covering should be provided. Examination can be improved if the child can perform a Valsalva maneuver while in these positions. For optimal visualization, the physician should gently grasp the posterior labia between the thumb and forefinger and provide a moderate amount of traction of the skin away from the introitus, avoiding rough or painful movements. Involving parents and having them assist with comforting the child in concert with communicating sensitivity to the family and patient are pivotal aspects of the physician's approach.

Table 39–1. Classification of sexual maturity ratings in girls.

Tanner stage	Pubic hair	Breasts
1	Preadolescent	Preadolescent
2	Sparse, lightly pigmented, straight, medial border of labia	Breast and papilla elevated as small mound; diameter of areola increased.
3	Darker, beginning to curl, increased amount	Breast and areola enlarged, no contour separation.
4	Coarse, curly, abundant, but less than in adult	Areola and papilla form secondary mound.
5	Adult feminine triangle, spread to medial surface of thighs	Mature, nipple projects, areola part of general breast contour.

Bordini B, Rosenfield RL: Normal pubertal development: part I: The endocrine basis of puberty. *Pediatr Rev.* 2011;32(6):223-229 [PMID: 21632873].

Van Eyk N, Allen L, Giesbrecht E, et al: Pediatric vulvovaginal disorders: A diagnostic approach and review of the literature. *J Obstet Gynaecol Can.* 2009;31(9):850-862 [PMID: 19941710].

VAGINAL DISORDERS

The section following discusses vulvovaginitis, both infectious and inflammatory causes, labial adhesions, vaginal foreign body, and Bartholin gland cyst/abscess. Sexually transmitted causes of vaginitis are discussed in detail.

VULVOVAGINITIS

General Considerations

Vulvovaginitis is the most common gynecologic problem in the pediatric patient. It manifests as inflammation from irritation of the vulva and most distal portion of the vaginal vault. Children are at an increased risk of vulvovaginitis compared with adults. This is due to the close proximity of the anus to the vestibule, lack of the fat pads, lack of pubic hair, thin, atrophic nonestrogenized vaginal mucosa, thin vulvar skin, and alkaline vaginal pH.

When taking the patient's history, it is important to focus on underlying medical disorders such as diabetes, specific hygiene habits, possible irritants, and concern for possible sexual abuse.

In younger girls, the most common cause of inflammatory vulvovaginitis is inadequate vaginal hygiene as they take over responsibility for bathing and post-void or bowel movement hygiene. Local irritation from perfumed soaps or detergents can cause vulvovaginitis as well as constrictive, non-cotton clothing, or prolonged time in wet undergarments.

Infectious causes of vulvovaginitis include multiple different types of organisms. A vaginal infection can result from a preceding bacterial upper respiratory tract infection (URTI) from *Haemophilus*, *Streptococcus*, or *Staphylococcus* species. Bacteria are transmitted from the child's nose or mouth to the genitalia. The patient and family should be instructed on proper hygiene. Group A β-hemolytic *streptococcus* is the most common isolated agent.

Candidal infections in younger pediatric patients are uncommon. In one study of prepubertal girls with vaginitis, *Candida* was not identified in any patients. However, it can be seen in diabetic patients and in adolescents with some frequency.

Shigella and *Yersinia* vulvovaginitis can present in the pediatric patient as a chronic infection.

Enterobius vermicularis, known as pinworms, can also cause vulvovaginitis.

Gardnerella vaginitis is also known as bacterial vaginosis (BV). Although it the most common cause of vaginal discharge in childbearing-age women, it is not usually associated with vaginal discharge in prepubertal girls. Data on its association with sexual abuse is conflicting. *Gardnerella* infection results from the overgrowth of bacteria that can be a normal part of the vaginal flora.

 ESSENTIALS OF DIAGNOSIS

▶ Pruritus.

▶ Tenderness.

▶ Dysuria.

▶ Erythema of vulva.

▶ Discharge (vaginitis).

▶ Bleeding (less common).

Clinical Findings

Transmitted URTI: History of URTI in the last several weeks may be present.

 Candida

Symptoms include pruritus and discharge, which can be curd-like or watery. Patients may have complaint of dysuria and vaginal irritation or pain.

▶ ***Shigella***

It is passed from the intestinal tract to the vulva and involves whitish-yellowish discharge.

▶ Pinworms

Patients have complaint of pruritus and irritation, especially at night. The pruritus is oftentimes perianal, but can be vulvar.

▶ *Gardnerella*

Symptoms include white or gray discharge with a fishy odor.

Laboratory Tests & Special Examinations

No specific laboratory tests are usually required for patients that present without discharge. A thorough physical examination that demonstrates vulvovaginitis is required. If there is vaginal discharge present, a sample can be obtained through the hymen and into the vagina while the patient is in one of the above positions. Avoid touching the sensitive edges of the hymen.

For patient with group A *Streptococcus, Staphylococcus,* or *Haemophilus*-suspected infection, cultures should be obtained if the infection is persistent or purulent.

In the setting of possible *Candida* vaginitis, diagnosis can be made by obtaining a sample of the discharge and viewing on a wet mount or KOH-prepped slide. Spores and *pseudo-hyphae* will be observed on the slide under microscope view.

Families can make the diagnosis of pinworms with the "scotch tape" test, which involves placing a piece of adhesive tape against the perianal region at night or in the early morning to recover the parasite.

For BV, clue cells, which are epithelial cells with *coccobacilli* surrounding the membrane, are found on wet saline mount. (see Sexually Transmitted Diseases, Bacterial Vaginosis).

Treatment & Disposition

Anticipatory guidance and education regarding hygiene and avoidance of irritants is important in order to treat the inflammatory variants of vulvovaginitis and prevent future occurrences. For more serious inflammation, topical estrogen or topical steroids may help with healing.

If a transmitted URTI is suspected, antimicrobial therapy should be directed by the culture and sensitivity.

Treatment for *Candida* infections is local application of antifungal cream.

Vaginal cultures will identify a possible enteric pathogen, such as *Shigella* or *Yersinia*, which can be treated with trimethoprim-sulfamethoxazole (TMP-SMX).

The treatment of choice for pinworm infections is albendazole or mebendazole.

When *Gardnerella* is identified on saline prep, treatment with metronidazole or clindamycin is appropriate.

LABIAL ADHESIONS

Labial adhesions typically occur in prepubescent girls aged 1-6 years. The adhesions are an acquired condition. They

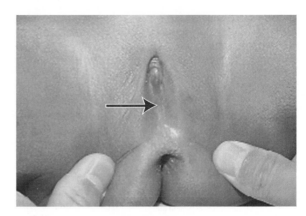

▲ **Figure 39–1.** Labial adhesion. (Reproduced, with permission, from Shah BR, Lucchesi M (eds): *Atlas of Pediatric Emergency Medicine*, 1st ed. McGraw-Hill, Inc., 2006. Copyright © McGraw-Hill Education LLC.)

can be partial or complete and may or may not affect the urine stream. With complete adhesions, as shown in Figure 39–1, the introitus is not seen, which may be interpreted by parents as absence of the vagina. It may also appear that there is no urethral opening through which the child can urinate. A thin line of central raphe (arrow) where the labia are fused is seen. Visualization of a midline raphe excludes the diagnosis of imperforate hymen.

 ESSENTIALS OF DIAGNOSIS

▶ Evaluate for any signs of urinary retention.
▶ May be confused with imperforate hymen, ambiguous genitalia, congenital absence of the vagina.

Treatment & Disposition

Conservative therapy includes watchful waiting if urination is unaffected. Hygiene measures, sitz baths, emollients to the adhesion, avoidance of irritants, can be employed for conservative management. If symptomatic, local estrogen cream can be applied directly to the adhesion twice daily with care to avoid trauma to the site. Breast buds can be a side effect of the cream.

VAGINAL FOREIGN BODIES

When a prepubertal child presents with complaint of bloody and purulent, possibly foul-smelling vaginal discharge, foreign body must be suspected. Initially, the foreign body will cause irritation, which can progress to infection. The most common cause is retained toilet paper, but hair adornments and small toys are also found.

ESSENTIALS OF DIAGNOSIS

▸ Recurrent discharge.

▸ Discharge resistant to treatment with topical or antibiotics.

▸ Foul-smelling.

▸ Vaginal bleeding.

Treatment & Disposition

In order to remove the foreign body, a topical anesthetic, such as topical lidocaine jelly, must first be applied to the vaginal area. Irrigation of the vagina can remove some objects as well as toilet paper. A Calgiswab can also be used to remove toilet paper. If irrigation is unsuccessful, it may become necessary to remove the foreign object with the aid of sedation and a speculum examination.

BARTHOLIN GLAND CYST & ABSCESS

The Bartholin glands are located at the 4- and 8-o'clock positions of the labia minora. They can become enlarged as a result of a blockage of the ducts. If a cyst forms, the patient is at risk for infection of these focal collections of fluid. They are exquisitely painful.

ESSENTIALS OF DIAGNOSIS

▸ Location at 4- and 8-o'clock position of the vaginal orifice.

▸ Exquisitely painful.

Laboratory Tests & Special Examinations

If concern for methicillin-resistant *Staphylococcus aureus* (MRSA) infection, a culture of the cyst/abscess material may be obtained at the time of incision and drainage.

Treatment & Disposition

Modalities for treatment of the cysts include placement of a Word catheter, marsupialization, application of silver nitrate to the abscess cavity, curettage and suture, and surgical excision. Placement of a Word catheter after incision and drainage is the most frequently employed technique for emergency department management. The advantages of the Word catheter include simplicity and ease of placement.

The catheter remains in place for 4 weeks. The cavity can also be filled with iodoform packing gauze in order to promote appropriate epithelialization if a Word catheter or Foley catheter is unavailable. Pain management with analgesics or sedation may be required for the procedure. If recurrent, the cyst must be marsupialized. Antibiotic treatment should be guided toward specific MRSA concerns or culture results. Appropriate antibiotic choices are clindamycin, cefoxitin, and amoxicillin-clavulanate.

Kushnir VA, Mosquera C: Novel technique for management of Bartholin gland cysts and abscesses. *J Emerg Med.* 2009;36(4):388 [PMID: 19038518].

Van Eyk N, Allen L, Giesbrecht E, et al: Pediatric vulvovaginal disorders: A diagnostic approach and review of the literature. *J Obstet Gynaecol Can.* 2009;31(9):850 [PMID: 19941710].

ABNORMAL VAGINAL BLEEDING

Occurrence of vaginal bleeding in a child represents possible diagnoses that range from normal menses, trauma, threatened abortion, abuse, precocious puberty, to urethral prolapse. Vaginal bleeding can be due to vaginal foreign body or vulvovaginitis. The first step in a patient presenting with complaint of genitourinary (GU) blood is to determine that the complaint of bleeding actually represents blood. Several foods and medications can cause discoloration of stool or urine, and when found on a child's undergarments, might be concerning for genital bleeding. The second step is to determine the actual source within the GU region, possibly ruling out either hematuria or hematochezia. Blood found in the undergarments of a child can mean a number of diagnoses are possible, including pathology of the gastrointestinal (GI) tract or urinary tract, unrelated to the genital system. If vaginal bleeding is found, it is important for the emergency department physician to determine if the patient requires immediate intervention or whether further evaluation can occur as an outpatient with primary care or gynecologic, endocrinologic, forensic or surgical subspecialty involvement.

If the patient presents in hemorrhagic shock due to vaginal bleeding, it is critical to primarily and promptly stabilize the patient. If the patient is an adolescent postmenarche female, ascertaining the presence of pregnancy is of utmost importance. A patient that is extremis with hemorrhagic shock likely will require transfusion with type O negative infusion while waiting crossmatching by the blood bank. Management of airway, controlling source of bleeding, and dealing with the patient's hemodynamics take precedence. The following discussion will involve those patients that are hemodynamically stable and are not presenting in hemorrhagic shock.

Table 39–2 lists the differential diagnosis for vaginal bleeding for the premenarche and postmenarche patient.

Table 39–2. Differential diagnosis of abnormal vaginal bleeding.

Premenarche	Postmenarche
Menarche	**Pregnancy**
Vulvovaginitis	Implantation
Vaginal foreign body	Ectopic
Neonatal maternal estrogen withdrawal	Threatened, missed, spontaneous abortion
Urethral prolapse	Retained products of conception
Trauma, straddle injury	Placenta accreta
Abuse	**Hematologic**
Precocious puberty	Thrombocytopenic
Medications (see postmenarche)	von Willebrand disease
Lichen sclerosus	Factor deficiencies
Neoplasm	Coagulation defects
	Platelet dysfunction
	Endocrine
	Thyroid disorders
	Hyperprolactinemia
	Polycystic ovary syndrome (PCOS)
	Adrenal disorders
	Ovarian failure
	Infectious
	Cervicitis
	Pelvic inflammatory disease (PID)
	Reproductive tract pathology
	Fibroid
	Myoma
	Cervical dysplasia
	Endometriosis
	Neoplasm
	Medication
	Hormonal contraceptives
	Antipsychotics
	Platelet inhibitors
	Anticoagulants
	Trauma
	Abuse
	Laceration
	Foreign body
	Postop or post-procedure
	Other
	Stress
	Excessive exercise
	Eating disorders
	Systemic disease
	Intrauterine device

PRECOCIOUS PUBERTY

Precocious puberty is the onset of secondary sexual characteristics at an age that is greater than 2.5 standard deviations below the mean age of pubertal onset for the population. The mean age is often before 8 years in girls. However, in non-Hispanic African American or Mexican American girls, thelarche is normal at 7 years of age. Normal menarche generally occurs about 2.5 years after the onset of breast development. This is usually when a girl is at Tanner stage 4 or 5 for breast development. Above 90% of cases of precocious pubertal development are idiopathic in girls. Typically, precocious puberty initially presents with early thelarche or pubarche, but not with isolated vaginal bleeding.

General Considerations

Precocious puberty can be divided into two subtypes: central and peripheral. Central precocious puberty is due to the premature activation of the hypothalamopituitary-gonadal (H-P-G) axis. Peripheral puberty results from the production of sex steroids independent of the H-P-G axis. Central is the most common form, and is more frequently seen in girls. Central is also more common between 4 and 8 years of age. Ovarian causes are the most frequent cause of the peripheral form in girls. Peripheral precocious puberty can be caused by sex steroid–secreting tumors, congenital adrenal hyperplasia (CAH), McCune-Albright syndrome, and exogenous exposure to estrogens or androgens.

 ESSENTIALS OF DIAGNOSIS

▶ Painless vaginal bleeding.
▶ Tanner stage of breast development greater than expected for age.
▶ Estrogenized hymen.

Clinical Findings

Patient with vaginal bleeding suspected to have precocious puberty as the etiology may have other signs of advanced development such as breast buds, pubic hair, and advanced growth. Vaginal bleeding in the absence of breast development is not likely to be hormonally mediated.

Treatment & Disposition

Concern for central nervous system (CNS) malignancy, infection, or trauma in the patient with vaginal bleeding warrants imaging. CNS imaging with CT and/or MRI may help determine the cause of the central form of precocious puberty.

If the patient is stable in the emergency department, and causes of vaginal bleeding such as vulvovaginitis, trauma, urethral prolapse, abuse, or vaginal foreign body have been ruled out, consultation with a pediatric endocrinologist is warranted to determine if the patient has precocious puberty and cause of the abnormality.

URETHRAL PROLAPSE

Urethral prolapse results from the extrusion of urethral mucosa outward through the urethral meatus. This tissue is more friable and susceptible to injury than the epithelium and can bleed with minimal irritation. It can progress to tissue necrosis if left untreated. It is theorized that weaker smooth muscle attachments within the vaginal wall that uphold the urethra may prolapse when exposed to increased intra-abdominal pressure. It is more common in African American females.

 ESSENTIAL DIAGNOSIS

▶ Young African American female.

▶ Constipation history or chronic cough.

▶ Vaginal bleeding.

▶ Urinary tract symptoms: hematuria, dysuria.

▶ Blood staining the undergarments.

▶ Vaginal mass.

Clinical Findings

On examination, a reddish-violaceous doughnut-shaped mass will be seen with a central dimple to indicate the introitus (Figure 39–2).

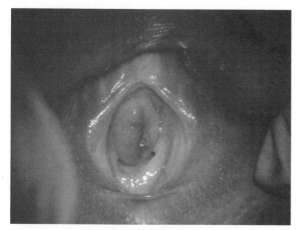

▲ **Figure 39–2.** Urethral prolapse. A urethral prolapse seen in a dark-skinned child. (Photo contributor: Cincinnati Children's Hospital Medical Center. Reproduced, with permission, from Knoop KJ, Stack LB, Storrow AB, Thurman RJ (eds): The Atlas of Emergency Medicine, 3rd ed. McGraw-Hill, Inc., 2010. Copyright © McGraw-Hill Education LLC.)

Treatment & Disposition

Treatment consists of sitz baths, analgesics, and voiding in the bathtub to alleviate symptoms. Also, estrogen cream applied to the prolapse for the 2 weeks has been shown to help. Most importantly, treatment of the cause of the persistent Valsalva maneuvers, from stool softeners and dietary changes in constipation to β-agonists for cough-variant asthma, must be performed. If no improvement with conservative treatment is shown, surgery can be performed to excise the tissue.

NEONATAL VAGINAL BLEEDING DUE TO MATERNAL ESTROGEN WITHDRAWAL

Parents of the neonate may present to the emergency department with complaint of vaginal bleeding in the infant that is concerning and distressful. While in utero, the female fetus is exposed to maternal estrogens. When withdrawal of the hormone occurs during the birthing process, the uterus of the neonate can slough the vascularized membrane similar to the process of withdrawal bleeding with the menstrual cycle, without the preceding ovulation.

 ESSENTIAL DIAGNOSIS

▶ Neonate.

▶ Painless vaginal bleeding.

▶ Otherwise normal physical examination.

Clinical Findings

Vaginal bleeding may be preceded by clear or whitish discharge that becomes more pink and then blood-tinged. This typically occurs during the first weeks of life and does not last longer than several days.

Treatment & Disposition

The family needs to be reassured that vaginal bleeding in female infants can be normal and no therapy is needed.

POSTMENARCHE ABNORMAL VAGINAL BLEEDING

General Considerations

In the first 2-3 years following menarche, menses frequently are irregular.

In the first year after menarche, evaluation should be considered for an unusual degree of menstrual irregularity. Evaluation could be considered for the following complaints: missing a period for greater than 90 days, bleeding more frequently than every 21 days, bleeding for greater than 7 days at time, bleeding that requires changing of tampon or pad every 1-2 hours.

Range of the normal menstrual cycle can vary from 21 to 35 days. Normal menstrual flow lasts from 3 to 7 days. Average amount of blood loss with each cycle is 30-40 mL. Greater than 80 mL of blood loss is pathologic and may lead to anemia. A menstrual period lasting longer than 10 days is considered pathologic.

Types of abnormal vaginal bleeding:

Menorrhagia: Heavy or prolonged vaginal bleeding that occurs at regular cycles.

Metrorrhagia: Acyclic or irregular vaginal bleeding.

Menometrorrhagia: Heavy vaginal bleeding occurring at irregular intervals.

Polymenorrhea: Frequent vaginal bleeding occurring more often than every 21 days.

In patient with abnormal bleeding, pregnancy must be the first condition that is considered. Ectopic pregnancy, threatened or spontaneous abortion can present with unusual vaginal bleeding. It cannot be overstated that it is imperative to test for pregnancy in this population from the outset.

Most common cause of abnormal vaginal bleeding in this population is dysfunctional uterine bleeding (DUB). DUB is the result of anovulatory bleeding that is excessive in amount and frequency. True DUB implies bleeding that is not due to underlying abnormalities or systemic conditions. It is caused by chronic anovulation and immaturity of the H-P-G axis. DUB is the most common cause of frequent or prolonged menses in young adolescents. However, this is a diagnosis of exclusion.

The differential diagnosis of DUB includes anovulation from sports participation, stress, eating disorders, polycystic ovary syndrome (PCOS), nutritional disturbance, hyperprolactinemia, other endocrinopathies, sexual abuse, neoplasms, and bleeding diathesis such as von Willebrand disease.

For menorrhagia patients, concern for uterine pathology or bleeding disorder should be addressed. The most common bleeding disorders are thrombocytopenia from idiopathic thrombocytopenic purpura (ITP) or chemotherapy and von Willebrand disease.

Superimposed intercycle bleeding should be concerning for cervicitis, endometritis, or pelvic inflammatory disease (PID) from *Chlamydia* or *Neisseria* infections. Endometriosis can also present in this manner.

Inquire about current medications, (prescription, over-the-counter, herbal/medicinal) that could be linked to bleeding.

Laboratory workup in a female patient presenting with complaint of abnormal vaginal bleeding includes the following: Complete blood count (CBC), complete metabolic profile (CMP), coagulation panel (prothrombin time [PT], partial thromboplastin time [PTT], INR), and urine

β-human chorionic gonadotropin (β-HCG). If the urine β-HCG returns positive, indicating pregnancy, the reasonable next step would be a quantitative serum β-HCG level, Rh blood typing, and a gynecologic ultrasound (US).

ESSENTIAL DIAGNOSIS

▶ Rule out pregnancy immediately.

▶ Detailed menstrual history.

▶ Family history of similar menstrual complaints.

▶ Evaluate for sexually transmitted infections (STIs).

▶ Evaluate for signs or symptoms of an underlying bleeding disorder.

▶ CBC and reticulocyte count.

Clinical Findings

Pregnancy should be the first concern and must be the first diagnostic test.

Patients with abnormal vaginal bleeding can present with signs of significant blood loss such as fatigue, pallor, and history of syncope or other mental status changes. Evaluate vital signs for tachycardia, hypotension, or orthostatic changes that would be concerning for hemodynamic instability.

Focus the physical examination on findings of underlying conditions that might be the cause of the abnormal bleeding. Look for signs of acne, hirsutism, and acanthosis nigricans in PCOS; evidence of epistaxis or gingival bleeding, bruising or petechiae for bleeding disorders; and thyroid nodules or thyromegaly in thyroid disorders. A pelvic examination and/or pelvic US can be performed to identify reproductive tract abnormalities or evaluate for a sexually transmitted infection or PID.

Patients' report of blood loss can be unreliable. Hemoglobin and reticulocyte counts can help objectify these reports and monitor symptoms.

Workup of patients is guided by history and physical examination, although a CBC with a reticulocyte count can be useful to determine the extent of bleeding. Findings can range from normal hemoglobin and reticulocyte count to a normal hemoglobin level with an elevated reticulocyte count to both a significantly low hemoglobin count with a microcytic anemia related to iron deficiency and elevated reticulocyte count.

Platelets would be abnormal in patients with immune thrombocytopenia (ITP). If any concern for a sexually transmitted infection is elicited with the history and examination, *Chlamydia* and gonorrhea screens can be ordered. Also, for severe bleeding or a family history that is concerning for excessive menstrual bleeding, the von Willebrand panel and coagulation studies can be added to the workup. For thyroid concerns, a free T4 and TSH should be drawn. Concerns for PCOS, based on examination findings, can be addressed as an outpatient with laboratory results of testosterone, free testosterone, and Dehydroepiandrosterone Sulfate (DHEA-S).

Treatment & Disposition

Pregnant patients should be referred or transferred to the appropriate facility for management under the care of an obstetrics specialist after stabilization has occurred.

Patients presenting with complaint of abnormal vaginal bleeding should receive iron supplementation.

NSAIDs can be used for both symptomatic analgesic purposes and treatment in patients with DUB. NSAIDs counteract prostaglandin synthesis in the uterine lining as well as increase thromboxane A_2 levels. Blood loss is reduced via vasoconstriction and platelet aggregation as a result of their action.

The goal of therapy after pregnancy is ruled out is to stop the vaginal bleeding. Estrogen is used to stop the bleeding and support the endometrium. A progestin is given concurrently to create a secretory endometrium. If not given in combination, bleeding will recur when the estrogen is discontinued. Randomized, controlled trials have shown that combination oral contraceptives decrease the amount of blood loss during menses.

Mild bleeding—Slightly prolonged or more frequent menses without anemia

Observation with iron and NSAIDs

If choose to treat, 1 combo pill for 21 d, then 1 wk of placebo

Moderate bleeding—Menses > 7 d, cycle < 3 wk; Hb 10-11 g/dL

1 combo pill twice daily until bleeding stops; then 1 pill d for 21 d; then 1wk of placebo

Severe bleeding with moderate anemia—Hb 8-10 g/dL

Consider admission.

Prescribe following medication schedule

1 combo pill 4×/d for 2-4 d, antiemetic 2 h prior to pill

1 combo pill 3×/d for 3 d, antiemetic

1 combo pill 2×/d for 2 wk, +/− antiemetic

Severe bleeding with severe anemia—Hb < 7 g/dL

Admit

Consider transfusion with PRBCs

IV conjugated estrogens 25 mg q4h × 2-3 doses for severe acute hemorrhage

or

1 combo pill q4h until bleeding slows, antiemetic 2 h prior to pill,

then

1 combo pill 4×/d for 2-4 d, antiemetic

1 combo pill 3×/d for 3 d, antiemetic

1 combo pill 2×/d for 2 wk, +/− antiemetic

(h, hour; Hb, hemoglobin; IV, intravenous; mg, milligram; q, every; wk, week)

(Combo pill, combination oral contraceptive pill containing both an estrogen and progesterone)

Patients determined to have von Willebrand disease or ITP or other bleeding disorders should be referred to a hematologist for further care.

Long-term follow-up is important for these patients.

VAGINAL BLEEDING IN THE PREGNANT ADOLESCENT

General Considerations

When an adolescent presents with vaginal bleeding, determine if she is pregnant. If so, determine if the pregnancy is intrauterine (IUP) or is not.

The differential diagnosis of vaginal bleeding in early pregnancy includes spontaneous abortion, missed abortion, threatened abortion, ectopic pregnancy, as well as nonobstetric causes, such as sexual activity. The cervix is very friable during pregnancy and postcoital bleeding is not uncommon. However, it should not be associated with abdominal or back pain.

If the patient presents with hemodynamic instability, ruptured ectopic pregnancy is at the top of the differential list. It is unusual for a spontaneous abortion to present as shock in patients.

PID is a possibility during the first trimester, but is less likely than in a nonpregnant patient.

Definitions of abortion types:

Threatened abortion: Vaginal bleeding with no cervical dilation/effacement. Bleeding may occur for days or weeks and is self-limited.

Inevitable abortion: Open cervical os but no passage of tissues yet.

Incomplete abortion: Only part of the tissues have passed through the cervical os. The os may be closed again. Main signs and symptoms occur when all or part of the placenta is retained in the uterus.

Missed abortion: Retention of dead tissue in utero for several weeks. May terminate spontaneously.

Complete abortion: Any spontaneous abortion when resolution of symptoms and total expulsion of tissue occur. Cervical os is empty and the uterus is empty.

Ectopic pregnancy is pregnancy that occurs outside the uterus cavity. The most common risk factor is a previous history of PID.

ESSENTIAL DIAGNOSIS

▶ Vaginal bleeding.

▶ Abdominal cramping.

▶ Low back pain.

▶ Verify with a β-HCG (urine and serum quantitative) and pelvic US.

▶ Rule out ectopic pregnancy.

Clinical Findings

See section Life-Threatening Gynecologic/Obstetric Causes of Pelvic Pain.

In a pregnant patient with vaginal bleeding, a pelvic examination should be performed with special attention to the cervical os. If tissue is visualized, it should be removed as it will often help decrease or cease bleeding. After speculum examination, digital examination of the internal os should be performed to determine if it is open or closed. The remainder of the pelvic examination should evaluate for cervical motion tenderness, adnexal masses or fullness, or adnexal pain.

Serum or urine qualitative β-HCG levels confirm the presence of a pregnancy. Serum quantitative β-HCG levels can also be drawn. The "rule of 10s" is helpful to recall appropriate β-HCG levels during the course of pregnancy: 100 mIU/mL at missed menses, 100,000 mIU/mL at 10 weeks, and 10, 000 mIU/mL at term. The level dictates what should be seen on US. The rate of rise of the level, which can be followed by an obstetrician, can help determine if there is abnormal pregnancy, such as ectopic pregnancy or missed abortion.

Pelvic US should be performed to determine the absence or presence of an IUP in a patient who has a positive β-HCG level. A uterine pregnancy is usually not recognized on abdominal US until 5-6 weeks of gestation. If not visualized on transabdominal US, pregnancy can be confirmed with the transvaginal US view, if available.

Landmarks of an IUP on US are the gestational sac and yolk sac. The gestational sac is visualized at 4-5 weeks of gestation, whereas the yolk sac is apparent after 5 weeks. The fetal pole and heart motion can be seen at 6 weeks.

Discriminatory zone with an IUP verified on transvaginal US is a β-HCG level greater than 1500 mIU/mL, and a level greater than 6500 mIU/mL for transabdominal US. If no IUP is visualized with either modality at the above levels, an ectopic or complete spontaneous abortion should be considered. Rh (D) blood typing should also be obtained.

Treatment & Disposition

▶ Unstable Patient

Manage the patient as a patient presenting with hemorrhagic shock. Stabilize the airway, provide oxygen, establish IV access, and start IV replacement with either normal saline or type O negative blood. Obtain a β-HCG level, CBC, and type and cross. Perform a pelvic examination to evaluate the source of bleeding and decrease bleeding with the removal of tissue at the cervical os. Uterine massage may also be helpful in a patient who is past the first trimester. The patient will need to be transferred quickly to a facility that provides obstetric care.

▶ Spontaneous Abortion

See section Life-Threatening Gynecologic/Obstetric Causes of Pelvic Pain.

Conservative management is an option if the patient is stable and reliable for follow-up with an obstetrician. In the case of threatened abortion, there remains the possibility of a normal pregnancy and therefore watchful waiting is appropriate, especially in these patients.

Most spontaneous abortions will complete without medical intervention. Rarely is there a need for emergent dilation and curettage in these patients. Adolescent pregnant patients will need intensive monitoring after leaving the emergency department and will have to see an obstetrician the following day. It may be more appropriate to arrange transfer to the appropriate facility rather than having the patient sent home if there concerns regarding patient follow-up.

▶ Ectopic Pregnancy

See section, Life-Threatening Gynecologic/Obstetric Causes of Pelvic Pain.

The obstetrician should be immediately consulted for a patient suspected of having an ectopic pregnancy. Dilation and curettage (D&C) is often used by the specialist as a diagnostic method in patients with a low or abnormally rising β-HCG level and no evidence of IUP on pelvic US. Options for treatment include expectant management, surgery, or medical management with methotrexate as determined by the obstetrician. Adolescents are not usually candidates for expectant management. Any unstable patient with signs of an ectopic pregnancy is taken immediately to the operating room.

Benjamins LJ: Practice guideline: Evaluation and management of abnormal vaginal bleeding in adolescents. *J Pediatr Health Care.* 2009;23(3):189-193 [PMID: 19401253].

Bordini B, Rosenfield RL: Normal pubertal development: part II: Clinical aspects of puberty. *Pediatr Rev.* 2011;32(7):281-292 [PMID: 21724902].

Gray SH, Emans SJ: Abnormal vaginal bleeding in adolescents. *Pediatr Rev.* 2007;28(5):175-182 [PMID: 17473122].

Hamman AK, Wang NE, Chona S: The pregnant adolescent with vaginal bleeding: Etiology, diagnosis, and management. *Pediatr Emerg Care.* 2006;22(10):761-767 [PMID: 17047481].

Van Eyk N, Allen L, Giesbrecht E, et al: Pediatric vulvovaginal disorders: A diagnostic approach and review of the literature. *J Obstet Gynaecol Can.* 2009;31(9):850-862 [PMID: 19941710].

PELVIC PAIN

GENERAL CONSIDERATIONS

A number of conditions can cause pelvic pain (Table 39–3). Pelvic pain most often is the result of gastrointestinal and urinary systems in prepubertal girls. As adolescent females, approach puberty, begin menstruation, and advance to young adulthood, the differential expands and includes

Table 39–3. Pelvic pain differential diagnosis.

Life-threatening gynecologic conditions
    Ovarian torsion

Life-threatening obstetrical conditions
    Ectopic pregnancy
    Placental abruption
    Incomplete abortion
    Septic abortion
    Uterine rupture

Common gynecologic conditions
    Ruptured ovarian cyst
    Dysmenorrhea
    Mittelschmerz
    Sexual transmitted infections (STIs)
    Pelvic inflammatory disease (Salpingitis, Salpingitis with tubo-ovarian abscess)
    Endometriosis

Other gynecologic conditions
    Imperforate hymen
    Endometritis
    Ovarian tumors (germ cell tumors, dermoid cyst)
    Vaginal foreign bodies
    Chemical irritants
    Sexual assault/sexual abuse

Other nongynecologic conditions
    UTI (pyelonephritis, cystitis)
    Appendicitis
    Nephrolithiasis/ureterolithiasis
    Inguinal hernia
    Constipation
    Somatization

more gynecologic and possible obstetric causes of pelvic pain. Gastrointestinal and urologic causes of pelvic pain are discussed in Chapters 36 and 38. Differential diagnosis and approach to the adolescent female with pelvic pain with emphasis on gynecologic conditions are discussed here.

The first goal of evaluation of the adolescent female with pelvic pain is to identify life-threatening conditions that require emergency interventions. After this has been done, identifying other causes of pelvic pain can be attempted.

CLINICAL FINDINGS

History

Pain characteristics, related symptoms, menstrual status, and sexual history will help differentiate among the likely causes and guide further evaluation and management. For menstrual status, identify if patient is premenarchal or postmenarchal. For postmenarchal patient, determine the timing of pelvic pain in relation to the last menstrual period. For adolescents, questions regarding sexual history should be posed when the patient's parent or guardian is not present. Knowledge of specific state and federal laws pertaining to teenager's confidentiality is important.

Physical Examination

Physical examination should include attention to vital signs. Fever and signs of shock should be acknowledged and managed. Examination of the abdomen is indicated, and a pelvic examination, including speculum examination, is indicated in all sexually active adolescent females. Although vaginal bimanual examination is preferred, a rectal bimanual examination may be substituted for virginal patients.

Laboratory

It is preferred that pregnancy test be performed on all postmenarchal adolescents with pelvic pain. It may also be done in some premenstrual girls with unclear history or clinical picture. Urine pregnancy tests are extremely sensitive. If test is positive in the presence of significant pelvic pain and/or vaginal bleeding, quantitative β-HCG and Rh(D) blood typing should be performed. The Rh(D) status is important especially in patients who have spontaneous abortion, ectopic pregnancy, or placental abruption to determine the need for anti–D immunoglobulin.

An additional test for adolescent with pelvic pain is the urine dipstick. If positive, more extensive urinalysis and urine culture should usually be performed.

CBC should be considered in patients with acute pelvic pain who have vaginal bleeding to look for thrombocytopenia and anemia. An elevation on the white blood cell count (WBC) (left shift), erythrocyte sedimentation rate (ESR),

C-reactive protein (CRP) may be useful in patients with PID or appendicitis.

If the patient is sexually active and/or there is sufficient clinical suspicion, tests for possible STD should be performed. During the pelvic examination, cervical cultures for *Chlamydia trachomatis*, *Neisseria gonorrhea*, *Trichomonas*, and BV should be obtained. If there are concerns, serology for HSV and syphilis are test options. Urine nucleic acid amplification tests (NAATs) for *C. trachomatis* and *N. gonorrhea* may be of use.

Imaging

Standard radiographs, US (standard and transvaginal, bedside or complete), CT of abdomen and pelvis, and laparoscopy are mainstays of imaging. Decision about when to use each depends on suspected diagnosis, clinical expertise, and local availability as discussed in the following specific sections.

Treatment & Disposition

Treatment depends on specific cause of pelvic pain. See specific etiology.

LIFE-THREATENING GYNECOLOGIC/ OBSTETRIC CAUSES OF PELVIC PAIN

OVARIAN TORSION

ESSENTIALS OF DIAGNOSIS

▶ Single or recurrent moderate unilateral pelvic pain.
▶ Negative pregnancy test.
▶ Pelvic mass.
▶ Pelvic US.

General Considerations

Ovarian (adnexal) torsion refers to twisting of the adnexa upon its pedicle. It is an infrequent but significant cause of acute abdominal pain in adolescents and young women.

Clinical Findings

Torsion of ovary is associated with a history of sharp intermittent attacks of severe unilateral pain in the lower abdomen that may be associated with nausea and vomiting. Puberty represent one of the periods of time when it is more likely. Formation of ovarian cysts may predispose to torsion, and therefore torsion has higher incidence in adolescents than prepubertal girls. The symptoms may be gradual, or occur suddenly. The physical examination may be unreliable in adolescents. They may be less accustomed, less cooperative, and/or less able to tolerate the examination. It is especially true for those who have not had a prior pelvic examination. Getting an adequate examination may not be possible. US is usually the diagnostic method of choice with Doppler.

Treatment & Disposition

Urgent gynecologic consultation is required. Ovarian torsion presents a significant risk to future fertility and prompt surgical intervention can prevent necrosis and loss of the ovary. Laparoscopic surgery is frequently required. Laparotomy is indicated if diagnosis is confirmed or if patient's condition deteriorates.

ECTOPIC PREGNANCY

ESSENTIALS OF DIAGNOSIS

▶ Unilateral pelvic pain in early pregnancy.
▶ Vaginal bleeding (variable).
▶ Risk factor assessment (history of STDs).
▶ Unilateral adnexal tenderness or mass.
▶ Uterine size smaller than expected for gestational dates.
▶ Quantitative β-HCG and pelvic US.

General Considerations

Ectopic pregnancy is the leading cause of pregnancy-related death in the first trimester. Diagnosis is often difficult, especially in adolescents who may not be forthright concerning their risk factors for pregnancy or sexual activity. Given appropriate time to discuss privately with the patient without parents/caregivers around is a best practice and always obtain a urine pregnancy test. Incidence is increased in those with a prior history of PID or sexually transmitted diseases (STDs), tubal surgery, prior ectopic pregnancy, endometriosis, and use of intrauterine device (IUD).

Clinical Findings

Patients usually present with vaginal bleeding and crampy lower abdomen/pelvic pain approximately 6-8 weeks after last menstrual period. There is a positive pregnancy test. Later presentation is possible if the fetus is not within the fallopian tubes. Rupture may bring initial temporary relief of pain; however, massive intraperitoneal hemorrhage may ensue with high risk of maternal mortality. Abdominal US of the right upper quadrant (RUQ) can be very useful in the unstable pregnant patient. If fluid is seen in Morison space between the liver and the right kidney, it is very likely that the patient has a ruptured ectopic pregnancy and a gynecologist should be called immediately and arrangements made to take the patient to the operating room immediately for control of hemorrhage. Transvaginal US is useful to confirm the IUP or to confirm the absence. It is also useful to visualize secondary signs of an ectopic such as free fluid in the pelvis or an extrauterine cystic structure that might represent an ectopic pregnancy. Patients with an ectopic pregnancy may span the range from minimally symptomatic to decompensated hemorrhagic shock.

Treatment & Disposition

As all pregnant patients who present with vaginal bleeding, adolescents should first be assessed for hemodynamic stability. They often present in shock and require immediate shock management. For stable patients, if ectopic pregnancy is found early before there is damage to the fallopian tubes, medical treatment is an option. Consultation with obstetrician and/or gynecologist is recommended. Use of IV or IM or oral methotrexate has been shown to be effective. Multiple protocols have been reported for use of methotrexate. If methotrexate is used, repeating testing of quantitative β-HCG levels is often done. Prior to treatment, β-HCG, blood type, CBC, and renal and liver function tests are drawn and transvaginal US is performed. Rh(D) immunoglobulin should be administered if the patient is Rh(D)-negative (RhoGAM 300 mcg IM). Surgery, however, is safer and more likely to be successful than medicine.

PLACENTAL ABRUPTION

ESSENTIALS OF DIAGNOSIS

▶ Vaginal bleeding.

▶ Abdominal and/or back pain.

▶ Uterine contractions.

▶ Treat shock and acute disseminated intravascular coagulation (DIC).

General Considerations

Placental abruption occurs during the second or third trimester of pregnancy. Peak incidence is 24-26 weeks' gestation although placental abruption may occur at any time.

Clinical Findings

Acute placental abruption classically presents with vaginal bleeding, abdominal and or back pain, and uterine contractions. If abruption is severe (≥ 50% placental separation),

fetus and mother are at risk. Acute DIC develops because blood is exposed to large amounts of tissue factor over a brief period of time. The exposure leads to massive generation of thrombin, resulting in the acute triggering of coagulation. This can lead to a profound systematic bleeding diathesis in the mother and due to widespread intravascular fibrin deposition, tissue ischemic injury, and microangiopathic hemolytic anemia.

Treatment & Disposition

Treat and manage shock and DIC. Consultation with an obstetrician is required.

SPONTANEOUS (COMPLETE, MISSED, INCOMPLETE, OR THREATENED) ABORTION

ESSENTIALS OF DIAGNOSIS

▶ Vaginal bleeding in early pregnancy.

▶ Pelvic and back pain common.

▶ Exclude ectopic pregnancy.

▶ Quantitative β-HCG and pelvic US.

General Considerations

Definitions

Spontaneous abortion: Estimated 20% of pregnancies terminate in abortion. One-half occur before 8 weeks' gestation and one-fourth before 16 weeks' gestation. Many go unnoticed and unrecognized. This is a common cause for visit to the emergency department.

Complete abortion: Fetal demise and all products of conception are spontaneously expulsed.

Missed abortion: Fetal demise and failed expulsion of the products of conception from the uterus, with a closed cervix. If the condition lasts longer than 4-6 weeks, the patient is increased risk for infection and DIC.

Incomplete abortion: Incomplete expulsion of the products of conception. There is retained products of conception. The cervix is open.

Threatened abortion: Gestation has not reached the stage of viability (< 20 weeks). Patient may have pelvic pain and some vaginal bleeding, or any of the above symptoms. US may show a gestational sac and evidence of fetal cardiac activity.

Clinical Findings

Most patients have signs and symptoms of possible pregnancy. They have or are sexually active, have a period of amenorrhea or abnormal period, and may have nausea and vomiting. Urine pregnancy tests are positive. They will develop uterine cramps and vaginal bleeding and can pass fetal or placental tissue. Pelvic examination should be performed on all patients with suspected abortion and pregnant patients with vaginal bleeding less than 20 weeks' gestation. For patient greater than 20 weeks' gestation, pelvic examination should be performed by obstetrician if available because of the increase risk of placenta previa.

In the first trimester of pregnancy, a β-HCG level that does not double within 48 hours suggests fetal demise or abnormal pregnancy. Real-time US, using abdominal or vaginal probes, can be diagnostic, demonstrating a fetus without heartbeat or movement or evidence of expulsion of all products of conception and a clean uterine stripe. US will also aid in ruling out ectopic pregnancy and retained products of conception. Pathologic examination of the expelled uterine tissue can confirm passage of products of conception.

Treatment & Disposition

Blood typing and Rh(D) antibody screening are required in all patients with abortion of any type. If patients are Rh-negative, give RH_0(D) immunoglobulin (RhoGAM 300 mcg IM) within 72 hours after an event in which fetal maternal transfusion may occur including an abortion.

Patients with incomplete abortion, will need consultation with gynecologic/obstetric physician. The gynecologist will likely need to perform suction curettage or dilation and curettage. It is important to identify patients who are hypovolemic and/or anemic and treat accordingly. These patients should generally be admitted to the hospital for further care and monitoring. It is important to watch for signs of infection (septic abortion), shock, and DIC. Patients with missed abortion may need the above management if signs of infection, DIC, or products are retained more than 4 weeks. Outpatient management of missed abortion is possible if the patient has close follow-up, and consideration is made that the patient is an adolescent and has your faith of close follow up.

Patients with threatened abortion should be advised to rest and avoid coitus. Discharge should include pain medications, clear next-day follow-up instructions, and indications to return to the emergency department if the following occur: passage of fetal tissue, severe vaginal bleeding (more than one pad per hour), significant abdominal or pelvic pain, fever.

Patient with likely complete abortion typically will have normal vital signs and stable hematocrit, and if vaginal bleeding is still present, it is clearly decreasing and cervical os is closed. US may be used to confirm a clean uterine stripe. If products of conception are brought in, it can be confirmed by pathology. Again, referral to obstetrician and gynecologist is recommended.

For these conditions, emotional support should be provided.

SEPTIC ABORTION

 ESSENTIALS OF DIAGNOSIS

▸ History of abortion procedure.
▸ Pelvic pain.
▸ Systemic signs of infection.
▸ Tender uterus.
▸ Profuse, malodorous vaginal discharge.

General Considerations

Septic abortion is a rare complication after some obstetric-gynecologic procedures. Septic abortion may occur as a result of nonsterile nontherapeutic abortion. The usual cause of sepsis is incomplete evacuation of the products of conception. Infection is usually due to mixed aerobic and anaerobic bacteria (bacteroides, group B streptococci, Enterobacteriaceae, and *C. trachomatis*) and is rapidly progressive, extending quickly through the myometrium and involving adnexa and pelvic peritoneum. Septic pelvic thrombophlebitis with or without signs pulmonary embolism is a complication.

Clinical Findings

Symptoms and signs are consistent with history of recent pregnancy and induced abortion, followed by pelvic pain, and symptoms of infection. Nonjudgmental questioning in a private setting may be necessary to obtain history of nontherapeutic abortion. Clinical findings include signs of infection (fever and leukocytosis), diffuse pelvic tenderness, profuse foul vaginal discharge. Septic shock may be present. US or CT may show retained intrauterine material, uterine emphysema, or intraperitoneal air from uterine perforation.

Treatment & Disposition

Treat septic shock. Hospitalize patient and consult with obstetrician or gynecologist. Blood cultures and uterine cultures should be done. Consider CBC, hepatic and renal panels, electrolyte panels, prothrombin time (PT), partial thromboplastin time (PTT), platelet count, and DIC screening tests. Start antibiotics for aerobic and anaerobic organisms. Suggested regimens include doxycycline 100 mg IV every 12 hours and either cefoxitin 2.0 g every 6-8 hours IV or piperacillin/tazobactam 4.5 mg every 8 hours or ampicillin/sulbactam 3 g IV daily. An alternative regimen consists of clindamycin 900 mg IV every 8 hours, plus ceftriaxone 1 g IV daily.

UTERINE RUPTURE

ESSENTIALS OF DIAGNOSIS

▶ Prior caesarean delivery (C-section) or uterine surgery.

▶ Active labor or blunt trauma.

▶ Pregnant.

▶ Vaginal bleeding.

▶ Shock.

General Considerations

Uterine rupture occurs usually during labor in women who have had a C-section or prior uterine surgery. It can also be the result of blunt trauma during pregnancy. Rupture of an unscarred uterus during pregnancy is rare.

Clinical Findings

Signs and symptoms occur typically in labor. These include nonreassuring fetal heart rate tracings or fetal death, uterine tenderness, peritoneal irritation, vaginal bleeding, loss of fetal station, and shock.

Treatment & Disposition

Treat shock accordingly. Consultation with a gynecologist or general surgeon is necessary. Hysterectomy will likely need to be performed.

COMMON/OTHER GYNECOLOGIC CAUSES OF PELVIC PAIN

RUPTURED OVARIAN CYST

ESSENTIALS OF DIAGNOSIS

▶ Sudden severe unilateral pelvic pain.

▶ No signs of sepsis or infection.

▶ Negative pregnancy test.

▶ Unilateral adnexal tenderness without mass.

▶ US to confirm diagnosis.

General Considerations

Pain often begins during strenuous physical exercise or sexual intercourse. Blood from the ruptured cyst will irritate the peritoneum or stretch ovarian cortex causing pain.

Clinical Findings

Ovarian cyst that ruptures can cause sudden, severe, unilateral pelvic pain without fever, and gastrointestinal, urinary, or vaginal symptoms. Symptoms and pain typically occur preceding a menstrual period. Tenderness may be found over affected ovary and there is no adnexal mass. Pregnancy test should be done to exclude ectopic pregnancy. US will show the ovarian cyst or free pelvic fluid.

Treatment & Disposition

In general, pain control with analgesics is given. The patient should be observed and may require admission for pain control. Surgery is not typically required unless significant hemoperitoneum resulting from the rupture of a hemorrhagic corpus luteum cyst with hemodynamic instability.

DYSMENORRHEA

ESSENTIALS OF DIAGNOSIS

▶ Painful, crampy abdominal pain with menstruation.

▶ Negative pregnancy test.

▶ No evidence of pelvic infection.

General Considerations

Menstrual pain (dysmenorrhea) affects many if not most females in the United States, some of whom experience severe pain sufficient to affect daily activities. It is the most common gynecologic cause of pelvic pain during adolescence. The causes of dysmenorrhea can be divided into primary cause or secondary (acquired) causes (underlying pelvic pathology, such as endometriosis discussed as follows). Primary or idiopathic dysmenorrhea is attributed to production of excessive quantities of prostaglandins by the endometrium with subsequent uterine tone.

Clinical Findings

Dysmenorrhea is usually crampy and intermittent. Nausea, vomiting, diarrhea, headache, dizziness, or back pain may accompany the crampy abdominal pain. The symptoms and pain usually appear a few hours before menstruation and may continue for several days.

Treatment & Disposition

Both types can be managed with ibuprofen or naproxen, which are prostaglandin inhibitors. Local application of heat to the lower abdomen reportedly lessens pain.

MITTELSCHMERZ

ESSENTIALS OF DIAGNOSIS

▶ Recurrent midcycle abdomen or pelvic pain.

▶ Negative pregnancy test.

▶ No fever.

General Considerations

Mittelschmerz (Ger. *mittel*, middle + *schmerz*, pain) is midcycle pain, associated with ovulation. Pain is caused by normal follicular enlargement just prior to ovulation or to normal follicular bleeding at ovulation.

Clinical Findings

Patients have midcycle recurrent pain that lasts from a few hours to 2 days. Pain is typically mild to moderate and unilateral. Patients have normal menstrual periods and commonly have some midcycle spotting due to estrogen surge. There is no fever and no abnormal discharge or bleeding. Examination may reveal unilateral lower abdomen tenderness over the ovulating ovary.

Treatment & Disposition

Pain control and reassurance are usually all that are required.

ENDOMETRIOSIS

ESSENTIALS OF DIAGNOSIS

▶ Recurrent crampy pelvic, flank, or abdominal pain with menses.

▶ Negative pregnancy test.

General Considerations

Endometrial tissue found outside the uterus in ectopic locations can cause pelvic pain. In general, more common in adult women, but detection of endometriosis in adolescents is increasing and should be included in the differential of pelvic pain.

Clinical Findings

Patient will have complaint of crampy pelvic pain associated with menstruation. Symptoms may occur gradually or suddenly if bleeding is present. It has been known to cause painful defecation and dyspareunia, depending on location.

Treatment & Disposition

Refer to gynecologist for further evaluation. Control pain with analgesics. Patients may require laparoscopy for definitive diagnosis.

IMPERFORATE HYMEN

ESSENTIALS OF DIAGNOSIS

▶ Cyclical lower abdominal/pelvic pain.

▶ Primary amenorrhea and secondary sexual characteristics.

▶ Midline tender mass.

▶ Bulging bluish membrane at the introitus.

General Considerations

Imperforate hymen is the most frequent cause of vaginal outflow obstruction, occurring in 0.1% of female infants. The exact cause is unclear, but the result is persistence of intact hymenal membrane causing the obstruction. Obstruction may cause accumulation of products proximally which may cause a bulge. In the adolescent if the material behind the membrane are menstrual products, the resulting mass effect in the vagina and uterus are referred as hematocolpos and hematometrocolpos respectively. It may be an incidental finding in the prepubertal infant or child, but in an adolescent it is a cause of primary amenorrhea.

Clinical Findings

In an adolescent with this condition, cyclic lower abdominal pain may be reported. Back pain and urinary retention can occur. A midline tender mass may be appreciated in adolescent female with imperforate hymen. The hymenal membrane and the retained material may bulge out and a distended bluish membrane at the introitus can be observed.

Treatment & Disposition

In the adolescent, surgery is most often required. A hymenotomy is necessary to allow drainage of any contents and will help eliminate the pain and discomfort. It will also decrease the risk of secondary endometriosis.

COMMON NON-GYNECOLOGIC CAUSES OF PELVIC PAIN

NEPHROLITHIASIS

ESSENTIALS OF DIAGNOSIS

▸ Intense paroxysmal colicky flank pain.

▸ Hematuria.

▸ US or CT to confirm.

▸ Pain control.

General Considerations

Kidney stones are an increasingly recognized cause of pelvic pain in adolescents (see Chapter 38).

Clinical Findings

Patients present with intense, paroxysmal flank pain, which may radiate to the lower abdomen and groin. Pain is usually unilateral and colicky and causes patients to writhe about because they are unable to find a comfortable position. Nausea, vomiting, and urinary symptoms (hematuria, dysuria) may accompany the pain.

Treatment & Disposition

Diagnosis of nephrolithiasis is initially suspected by clinical presentation and urinalysis. It is confirmed by imaging such as US or CT or by visualized passage of the stone.

URINARY TRACT INFECTION (CYSTITIS, PYELONEPHRITIS)

ESSENTIALS OF DIAGNOSIS

▸ Common and frequent cause of pelvic pain.

▸ Suprapubic pain.

▸ Dysuria, increase urinary frequency, urgency, or hesitancy.

▸ Urinalysis and urine culture.

General Considerations

Urinary tract infections (UTIs) are relatively common. Females are more likely to develop them because of anatomy. In the adolescent female, UTIs can occur spontaneously or can occur in relation to first-time sexual activity or recent, frequent, prolonged sexual activity in women with low baseline of activity. The term "honeymoon cystitis" is frequently used to describe this phenomenon.

Clinical Findings

Cystitis can cause suprapubic pain and dysuria. Fever, increase urinary frequency, and urination hesitancy or urgency may be present.

Pyelonephritis frequently presents with fever, vomiting, flank and upper back pain, rigors.

Rapid urine dipstick and/or microscopic urinalysis will give diagnosis.

Treatment & Disposition

Multiple treatment regimens are available. The mainstay are antibiotics (see Chapter 38). Outpatient management is appropriate for most patients with UTIs. Pyelonephritis may need IV antibiotics and admission.

APPENDICITIS

ESSENTIAL OF DIAGNOSIS

▸ Have high index of suspicion for pelvic pain.

▸ Examine the abdomen as well.

▸ Initials diffuse periumbilical pain which later localizes to right lower quadrant.

▸ Consider use of Pediatric Appendicitis Score.

▸ US or CT of the abdomen are common imaging modalities for diagnosis.

General Considerations

Acute appendicitis is the most common cause of emergent abdominal surgery in children. Incidence increases with age and peaks in adolescence. It is rare in children younger than 2 years and most common in individuals 10-30 years (see Chapter 26).

Clinical Findings

Initial periumbilical pain which later localizes to the right lower quadrant (RLQ) is the classic history. Fever, vomiting, and anorexia are common associated symptoms. Obstruction of the appendix usually by stool leads to swelling and inflammation, and then to thrombosis, necrosis, and if untreated perforation. Diagnosis can be difficult. The Pediatric Appendicitis Score (PAS) is a recently develop and validated clinical prediction tool that can be used to guide workup. PAS uses a 10-point scale with 1 point for migration of pain to RLQ, 1 for anorexia, 1 for nausea/vomiting, 2 for RLQ tenderness, 2 for cough/percussion tenderness, 1 for fever, 1 for leukocytosis (> 10,000), and 1 for neutrophilia. A PAS score of 6 and above shows a high probability of appendicitis with varying sensitivity and specificity depending on population applied. Other clinical scoring systems have been developed with varying utility (Alvarado score, low risk for appendicitis score, Lintula score, etc). US and/or CT with or without contrast are common diagnostic tools to identify appendicitis. US of acutely inflamed appendix shows a noncompressible, thickened appendix. CT scanning remains the gold standard to diagnose appendicitis but does have drawbacks of large dose of ionizing radiation and cost. An individual with classic signs and symptoms may forgo these imaging modalities and go directly for an appendectomy. Regional, local, and specific physician factors and experience play a role in the preferred imaging modality and decision for surgery.

Treatment & Disposition

Definitive finding of appendicitis and consultation with surgeon, indicate emergency appendectomy. With equivocal findings, consultation with surgeon is often indicated and may involve a period of observation and repeated examinations. Exploratory laparotomy or laparoscopy is often indicated when diagnosis of appendicitis cannot be excluded after a period of observation. Preoperative or intraoperative dose of antibiotics is recommended for all patients to prevent postoperative complications. Antibiotic choices include piperacillin/tazobactam, cefoxitin, ampicillin/sulbactam, cefotetan or gentamicin and metronidazole are used. Complications include ileus, abscess formation, intestinal obstruction, peritonitis, sepsis, and shock.

Bhatt M, Joseph L, Ducharme FM, et al: Prospective validation of the pediatric appendicitis score in a Canadian pediatric emergency department. *Acad Emerg Med.* 2009;16(7):591-596 [PMID: 19549016].

Damle LF, Gomez-Lobo V: Pelvic pain in adolescents. *J Pediatr Adolesc Gynecol.* 2011;24(3):172-175 [PMID: 21751453].

Goldman RD, Carter S, Stephens D, et al: Prospective validation of the pediatric appendicitis score. *J Pediatr.* 2008;153(2):278-282 [PMID: 18534219].

Hatcher-Ross K: Sensitivity and specificity of the Pediatric Appendicitis Score. *J Pediatr.* 2009;154(2):308 [PMID: 19150684].

Kirkham YA, Kives S: Ovarian cysts in adolescents: Medical and surgical management. *Adolesc Med State Art Rev.* 2012;23(1):178-191, xii [PMID: 22764562].

Kruszka PS, Kruszka SJ: Evaluation of acute pelvic pain in women. *Am Fam Physician.* 2010;82(2):141-147 [PMID: 20642266].

Thompson, G: Clinical scoring systems in the management of suspected appendicitis in children. In: Lander A, ed. *Appendicitis: A Collection of Essays From Around the World.* InTech; 2012. Available at http://www.intechopen.com/books/appendicitis-a-collection-of-essaysfrom-around-the-world/clinical-scoring-systems-in-the-management-of-suspected-appendicitis-in-children.

Tucker R, Platt M: Obstetric and gynecological emergencies and rape. In: Stone CK, Humphries RL, eds: *Current Diagnosis & Treatment Emergency Medicine.* 7th ed. New York: McGraw-Hill; 2011.

Vichnin M: Ectopic pregnancy in adolescents. *Curr Opin Obstet Gynecol.* 2008;20(5):475-478 [PMID: 18797271].

SEXUALLY TRANSMITTED DISEASES

ESSENTIALS OF DIAGNOSIS

► High index of suspicion.
► Adolescent needs to talk privately with physician.
► Presenting clinical syndromes often guide diagnosis and treatment.
► Presumptive treatment can be justified.

General Considerations

In 2013, the Centers for Disease Control (CDC) published estimates that 20 million new cases of sexually transmitted infections (STIs) occur annually in the United States. Sexually transmitted diseases (STDs) cost the US health system $16 billion every year. Adolescents and young adults are the most commonly affected. Undiagnosed and untested STDs can lead to serious long-term health consequences, especially for adolescent girls and young women, resulting in infertility. STDs in younger children result from sexual abuse (see Chapter 6). The adolescent needs time to discuss confidentially with the physician and allow the physician time to screen for STD risk factors.

Exceptions to the provision of confidentiality for health services include, suspected physical or sexual abuse, risk for harm to self or others, and STDs may be reported confidentially to the health departments. In the United States, 50 states and the District of Columbia allow minors to consent to STD services; 11 states require that a minor be a required age to consent (12 or 14 years); 31 states include HIV in package of STD services to which a minor may consent; and 18 states allow physicians to inform parents that a minor is seeking or receiving STI services. It is important to know the laws and statutes of your state.

Clinical Findings

See clinical findings for specific STDs listed below.

Treatment & Disposition

Specific STDs are listed in Table 39-4. CDC treatment guidelines (2010) recommend single-dose therapy for STDs

Table 39–4. Sexually transmitted diseases.

STDs caused by bacteria.
 Gonorrhea
 Chlamydia
 Syphilis
 Bacterial vaginosis (BV)
 Chancroid
 Granuloma inguinale
 Lymphogranuloma venereum
 Pelvic inflammatory disease (PID)

STDs caused by viruses
 Herpes
 Hepatitis
 HIV

STDs caused by protozoan
 Trichomonas

STDs caused by fungi
 Vulvovaginal candidiasis

STDs caused by parasites
 Pubic lice
 Scabies

when possible (Table 39–5). One-time dosing option is likely a better choice for adolescents presenting to the emergency department because follow-up and ability to obtain medication may be difficult for individuals.

STDs CAUSED BY BACTERIA

1. Gonorrhea

ESSENTIALS OF DIAGNOSIS

▶ Yellowish vaginal discharge.

▶ Cervix is edematous and friable.

▶ Vaginal/cervical swab for culture or NAATs.

▶ Treat presumptively in patient younger than 26 years.

▶ General Considerations

Gonorrhea is the second most prevalent bacterial STD in the United States. In 2010, 309,341 new gonorrheal infections were reported (100.8 cases per 100,000 population). Gonorrhea rates continue to be highest among adolescents and young adults. Among females in 2010, 15-19-year-olds and 20-24-year-olds had the highest rates of gonorrhea. Infections include cervicitis, urethritis, proctitis, pharyngitis,

ophthalmia, systemic infection, arthritis, tenosynovitis, perihepatitis, and dermatitis. In addition, gonorrhea is a cause of PID. Humans are the natural reservoir. Gonococci are present in the secretions of infected mucous membranes.

▶ Clinical Findings

Symptoms and Signs

In uncomplicated gonococcal cervicitis, 23-57% of females are symptomatic, presenting with vaginal discharge and dysuria. The cervix may be edematous and friable with a yellowish mucopurulent discharge. Urethritis and pyuria may also be present. Other symptoms include abnormal menstrual periods and dyspareunia. Approximately 15% of females with endocervical gonorrhea have signs of involvement of the upper genital tract. Complications include PID and other disseminated disease causing arthritis and dermatitis.

Laboratory Findings

Cervical swab from females should be sent for NAATs or Gram stain and culture. The physician should obtain specimens from the rectum or pharynx when clinically indicated. Gram stain and culture will show gram-negative intracellular diplococcic. Urine NAATs are very sensitive (PCR [83% sensitivity], ligase chain reaction [LCR] [99% sensitivity]).

▶ Treatment & Disposition

Patients diagnosed with gonorrhea should be treated for *Chlamydia* as well. Because *Chlamydia* testing with NAATs is more sensitive, the CDC suggests that treatment for coinfection is not always necessary (see Table 39–5).

Patients should be advised to abstain from sexual intercourse until both patient and partner have completed a course of treatment. Treatment for PID or other disseminated disease may require hospitalization (see Table 39–5). Quinolones should no longer be used to treat gonorrhea due to high levels of quinolone resistance in the United States.

2. *Chlamydia*

ESSENTIALS OF DIAGNOSIS

▶ Vaginal discharge.

▶ Cervix is edematous and friable.

▶ Cervical swabs of os for DFA or NAATs.

▶ Treat presumptively in patient younger than 26 years.

▶ General Considerations

Chlamydia trachomatis is the most common bacterial cause of STDs in the United States. In 2010, more than 1.3 million

Table 39–5. STD treatment guidelines for adults and adolescents.

Disease	Recommended Regimens	Dose/Route	Alternative Regimens
Chlamydia Uncomplicated infections in adults/adolescents[a]	Azithromycin *or* Doxycycline[b]	1 g po 100 mg po bid × 7 d	Erythromycin base 500 mg po qid × 7 d *or* Erythromycin ethylsuccinate 800 mg po qid × 7 d *or* Ofloxacin[c] 300 mg po bid × 7 d *or* Levofloxacin 500 mg po qd × 7 d
Pregnant women[d]	Amoxicillin *or* Azithromycin	500 mg po tid × 7 d 1 g po	Erythromycin base 250 mg po qid × 14 d *or* Erythromycin ethylsuccinate 800 mg po qid × 7 d *or* Erythromycin ethylsuccinate 400 mg po qid × 14 d Erythromycin base 500 mg po qid × 7 d
Gonorrhea[e] Uncomplicated infections in adults/adolescents	Ceftriaxone plus a *Chlamydia* recommended regimen listed above	250 mg IM	Ceftizoxime 500 mg IM *or* Cefotaxime 500 mg IM *or* Cefoxitin 2 g IM *plus* probenecid 1 g po *or* Spectinomycin[h] 2 g IM *plus* a *Chlamydia* recommended regimen Cefixime[f] 400 mg po *plus* a *Chlamydia* recommended regimen and test cure in 1 wk
Pregnant women	Ceftriaxone *plus* a *Chlamydia* recommended regimen listed above	250 mg IM	Spectinomycin[h] 2 g IM *plus* a *Chlamydia* recommended regimen Cefixime[f] 400 mg po *plus* a *Chlamydia* recommended regimen and test cure in 1 wk
Pelvic inflammatory disease[g]	Parenteral[i] Cefotetan *or* Cefoxitin *plus* Doxycycline[b] *or* Clindamycin *plus* Gentamicin Oral treatment Ceftriaxone *or* Cefoxitin with Probenecid *plus* Doxycycline[b] ± Metronidazole	2 g IV q12h 2 g IV q6h 100 mg po or q12h 900 mg IV q8h 2 mg/kg IV or IM followed by 1.5 mg/kg IV or IM q8h 250 mg IM 2 g IM 1 g po 100 mg po bid × 14 d 500 mg bid × 14 d	Parenteral Ampicillin/sulbactam 3 g IV q6h *plus* doxycycline[b] 100 mg po 12 h If parenteral cephalosporin therapy is not feasible, use of fluoroquinolones (levofloxacin 500 mg orally once daily) or ofloxacin (400 mg bid for 14 d) with or without metronidazole (500 mg orally bid for 14 d) may be considered if the community prevalence and individual risk of gonorrhea is low. Tests for gonorrhea must be performed prior to instituting therapy and the patient managed as follows: If NAAT test is positive, parenteral cephalosporin is recommended. If culture for gonorrhea is positive, treatment should be based on results of antimicrobial susceptibility. If isolate is quinolone-resistant or antimicrobial susceptibility cannot be assessed, parenteral cephalosporin is recommended.
Cervicitis[j]	Azithromycin *or* Doxycycline[b]	1 g po 100 mg po bid × 7 d	
Nongonococcal urethritis[j]	Azithromycin *or* Doxycycline[b]	1 g po 100 mg po bid × 7 d	Erythromycin base 500 mg po qid × 7 d *or* Erythromycin ethylsuccinate 800 mg po qid × 7 d *or* Ofloxacin[c] 300 mg po bid × 7 d *or* Levofloxacin[c] 500 mg po qd × 7 d

(Continued)

Table 39–5. STD treatment guidelines for adults and adolescents. (*Continued*)

Disease	Recommended Regimens	Dose/Route	Alternative Regimens
Epididymitis	Ceftriaxone *plus*	250 mg IM	For males at risk for both enteric organisms and sexually transmitted pathogens (MSM who report insertive anal intercourse)
	Doxycycline	100 mg po bid × 10 d	
	For acute epididymitis most likely caused by enteric organisms or with negative gonococcal culture *or* NAAT		Ceftriaxone 250 mg IM + doxycycline 100 mg po bid × 10 d
	Ofloxacin[c] *or*	300 mg orally bid for 10 d	
	Levofloxacin	500 mg orally once daily for 10 d	
Trichomoniasis	Metronidazole *or*	2 g po	Metronidazole 500 mg po bid × 7 d or for failure
	Tinidazole	2 g po	Tinidazole or metronidazole 2 g po × 5 d
Vulvovaginal candidiasis	Butoconazole cream[k]	2%, 5 g intravaginally × 3 d	Fluconazole 150 mg po once
	Butoconazole 2% cream (SR)[k]	Single application	
	Clotrimazole cream[k]	1%, 5 g intravaginally × 7-14 d	
	Clotrimazole[a] cream[k]	2% cream 5 g intravaginally × 3 d	
	Miconazole cream[k]	2% 5 g intravaginally × 7 d	
		4% tg intravaginally × 3 d	
	Miconazole vaginal suppository[k]	100 mg intravaginally × 7 d	
		200 mg intravaginally × 3 d	
		1200 mg intravaginally × 1	
	Nystatin	100,000 units intravaginal tablet × 14 d	
	Tioconazole cream[k]	6.5% 5 g intravaginally once	
	Terconazole cream[k]	0.4% 5 g intravaginally × 7 d	
		0.8% 5 g intravaginally × 3 d	
	Terconazole vaginal suppository[k]	80 mg intravaginally × 3 d	
Bacterial vaginosis (BV)			
Adults/adolescents	Metronidazole *or*	500 mg po bid × 7 d	Clindamycin 300 mg po bid × 7 d *or*
	Clindamycin cream[k] *or*	2%, one applicator full (5 g) intravaginally at bedtime × 7 d	Clindamycin ovules 100 g intravaginally qhs × 3 d
			Tinidazole 2 g po qd × 3 d
			Or
	Metronidazole gel	0.75%, one applicator full (5 g) intravaginally, bid × 5 d	Tinidazole 1 g po day × 5 d
Pregnant women	Metronidazole	250 mg po tid × 7 d *or*	
		500 mg bid × 7 d	
	Clindamycin	300 mg po bid × 7 d	
Chancroid	Azithromycin *or*	1 g po	Erythromycin base 500 mg po tid × 7 d
	Ceftriaxone *or*	250 mg IM	
	Ciprofloxacin[c]	500 mg po bid × 3 d	
Lymphogranuloma venereum	Doxycycline[b]	100 mg po bid × 21 d	Erythromycin base 500 mg po qid × 21 d
			Azithromycin 1 g po q wk × 3 wk

(Continued)

Table 39–5. STD treatment guidelines for adults and adolescents. (*Continued*)

Disease	Recommended Regimens	Dose/Route	Alternative Regimens
Human papillomavirus			
External genital/perianal warts	Patient applied: Podofilox[l] 0.5% solution or gel *or* imiquimod 5% cream *or* Sinecathechins 15% ointment Physician administered: Cryotherapy *or* Podophyllin resin 10-25% in tincture of benzoin *or* Trichloroacetic acid (TCA) *or* Bichloroacetic acid (BCA) 80-90% *or* Surgical removal		Intralesional interferon *or* laser surgery
Vaginal warts	Cryotherapy or TCA *or* BCA 80-90% *or* surgical removal		
Urethral meatus warts	Cryotherapy or podophyllin[12] 10-25% in tincture of benzoin		
Anal warts	Cryotherapy or TCA *or* BCA 80-90% *or* surgical removal		
Herpes simplex virus[m]			
First clinical episode of herpes	Acyclovir[n] *or* Acyclovir[n] *or* Famciclovir[n] *or* Valacyclovir[n]	400 mg po tid × 7-10 d 200 mg po 5 × qd × 7-10 d 250 mg po tid × 7-10 d 1 g po bid × 7-10 d	
Episodic therapy for recurrent episodes	Acyclovir[m] *or* Acyclovir[m] *or* Acyclovir[m] *or* Famciclovir[m,n] *or* Famciclovir[m,n] *or* Valacyclovir[m,n] *or* Valacyclovir[m,n]	400 mg po tid × 5 d 800 mg po bid × 5 d 800 mg po tid × 2 d 125 mg po bid × 5 d 1000 mg po bid × 1 d *or* 500 mg × 1, then 250 mg bid × 2 d 500 mg po bid × 3 d 1 g po qd × 5 d	
Suppressive therapy	Acyclovir[m] *or* Famciclovir[n] *or* Valacyclovir[n] *or* Valacyclovir[n]	400 mg po bid 250 mg po bid 500 mg po qd 1 g po qd	

(*Continued*)

Table 39–5. STD treatment guidelines for adults and adolescents. (*Continued*)

Disease	Recommended Regimens	Dose/Route	Alternative Regimens
Syphilis			
Primary, secondary, and early latent	Benzathine penicillin G	2.4 million units IM	Doxycycline[b] 100 mg po bid × 2 wk *or* Tetracycline[b] 500 mg po qid × 2 wk
Late latent and unknown duration	Benzathine penicillin G	7.2 million units, administered as 3 doses of 2.4 million units IM, at 1 wk intervals	Doxycycline[b] 100 mg po bid × 4 wk *or* Tetracycline[b] 500 mg po qid × 4 wk
Neurosyphilis[o]	Aqueous crystalline penicillin G	18-24 million units daily, administered as 3-4 million units IV q4h × 10-14 d	Procaine penicillin G, 2.4 million units IM qd × 10-14 d plus Probenecid 500 mg po qid × 10-14 d Ceftriaxone 2 g IM *or* IV qd × 10-14 d (penicillin-allergic patient)
Pregnant women[o]			
Primary, secondary, and early latent[p]	Benzathine penicillin G	2.4 million units IM	None
Late latent and unknown duration	Benzathine penicillin G	7.2 million units, administered as 3 doses of 2.4 million units IM, at 1 wk intervals	None
Neurosyphilis[p]	Aqueous crystalline penicillin G	18-24 million units daily, administered as 3-4 million units IV q4h × 10-14 d	Procaine penicillin G, 2.4 million units IM qd × 10-14 d plus Probenecid 500 mg po qid × 10-14 d or desensitization if penicillin
Congenital syphilis	Procaine penicillin G	50,000 U/kg IM daily for 10-14 d	Aqueous crystalline penicillin G 100,000-150,000 U/kg/d in doses of 50,000 U/kg IV q12h for 7 d then q8h for 3-7 d
Children: early (primary)	Benzathine penicillin G	50,000 U/kg IM once (max. 2.4 million units)	
Children: late latent or > 1 y late	Benzathine penicillin G	50,000 U/kg IM for 3 doses at 1 wk intervals, to max. total dose of 7.2 million units	
HIV with syphillis infection			
Primary, secondary, and early latent	Benzathine penicillin G	2.4 million units IM	The efficacy of nonpenicillin regimens in HIV-infected persons has not been well studied
Late latent and unknown duration[p]	Benzathine penicillin G	7.2 million units, administered as 3 doses of 2.4 million units IM, at 1-wk intervals	None
Neurosyphilis[p]	Aqueous crystalline penicillin G	18-24 million units daily, administered as 3-4 million units IV q4h × 10-14 d	Procaine penicillin G, 2.4 million units IM qd × 10-14 d plus Probenecid 500 mg po qid × 10-14 d
Pediculosis pubis "crab lice"	Permethrin cream rinse	1% applied to affected areas, rinsed after 10 min	Malathion 0.5% lotion applied for 8-12 h and washed off or Ivermectin 0.25 mg/kg po repeated in 2 wk
	Pyrethrins with piperonyl butoxide	Apply to affected area, wash after 10 min	

(*Continued*)

Table 39–5. STD treatment guidelines for adults and adolescents. (*Continued*)

Disease	Recommended Regimens	Dose/Route	Alternative Regimens
Scabies[q]	Permethrin cream	5% applied to entire body below neck, washed off after 8-14 h	Lindane 1% 1-oz lotion or 30 g cream applied thinly to entire body below neck, washed off after 8 h[b,q]
	Ivermectin	0.2 mg/kg po repeated in 2 wk	

CDC STD treatment guidelines. Reproduced, with permission, from South-Paul J, Matheny S, Lewis E (eds): *Current Diagnosis & Treatment in Family Medicine*, 3rd ed. McGraw-Hill, Inc., 2011. Copyright © McGraw-Hill Education LLC.

bid, twice a day; d, day; h, hours; IM, intramuscularly; IV, intravenously; po, orally; q, every; qd, every day; qid, four times a day; SR, sustained release; tid, three times a day; wk, week.

[a]Screen adolescents and women younger than 25 years annually, especially if new or multiple partners.

[b]Contraindicated for pregnant and nursing women.

[c]Contraindicated for pregnant and nursing women, and children younger than 18 years.

[d]Test-of-cure follow-up recommended because the regimens are not highly efficacious (amoxicillin and erythromycin).

[e]Cotreatment for *Chlamydia* infection is indicated.

[f]Not recommended for pharyngeal gonococcal infection.

[g]If risk of gonorrhea is low and pretreatment gonorrhea testing is available; if nucleic acid amplification test is positive, treat with cephalosporin, or if culture is positive, treat according to susceptibility.

[h]For patients who cannot tolerate cephalosporins or quinolones; not recommended for pharyngeal gonococcal infection.

[i]Discontinue 24 hours after patient improves clinically and continue with oral therapy for a total course of 14 days.

[j]Testing for gonorrhea and *Chlamydia* is recommended because a specific diagnosis may improve compliance and partner management and these infections are reportable.

[k]Might weaken latex condoms and diaphragms because oil-based.

[l]Contraindicated during pregnancy.

[m]Counseling especially about natural history, asymptomatic shedding, and sexual transmission is an essential component of herpes management.

[n]Safety in pregnancy has not been established.

[o]Patients allergic to penicillin should be treated with penicillin after desensitization.

[p]Some recommend a second dose of 2.4 million units of benzathine penicillin G administered 1 week after the initial dose.

[q]Bedding and clothing should be decontaminated (machine washed, machine dried, or dry cleaned) or removed from body contact for more than 72 hours.

[r]Note a recent change by the CDC to no longer recommend cefixime due to resistance; there are incidences where it can be used if ceftriaxone not available but recommend a test of the cure 1 week after treatment.

cases in adolescents and young adults were reported. The number of *Chlamydia* infections was more than three times the number of gonorrhea cases. *C. trachomatis* is an obligate intracellular bacterium that replicates within the cytoplasm of host cells. Destruction of *Chlamydia*-infected cells is mediated by host immune responses. It is the likely cause of PID.

▶ **Clinical Findings**

Symptoms and Signs

Clinical infection in females manifests as dysuria, urethritis, vaginal discharge, cervicitis, irregular vaginal bleeding, perihepatitis, and PID. The presence of mucopurulent cervicitis is a sign of *Chlamydia* infection or gonorrhea. *Chlamydia* infection is asymptomatic in 75% of females.

Laboratory Findings

NAAT (polymerase chain reaction [PCR] or ligase chain reaction [LCR]) is the most sensitive (92-99%) test to detect

Chlamydia. Enzyme-linked immunosorbent assay (ELISA) or direct fluorescent antibody (DFA) tests are less sensitive, but may be the only testing option in some centers. Culture is mandated for sexual abuse cases in most states.

A cervical swab should be obtained by inserting the swab in the cervical os and rotating it 360 degrees and sending for ELISA, DFA test, or NAAT. NAAT can be used to check urine and is currently used more for screening.

▶ **Treatment & Disposition**

Patients diagnosed with *Chlamydia* should be treated for gonorrhea as well. Adolescents and young women who are sexually active may be presumptively treated especially if cultures, NAATs, DFAs may be delayed. Many patients are managed and treated presumptively based on historical complaints, physical signs, local incidence, and practice patterns. A single dose of Azithromycin 1 g once is easiest and is the treatment of choice (see Table 39–5 for drug options).

3. Syphilis

▶ Chancre (painless, indurated, nonpurulent ulcer with a clean base).

▶ Nontender, firm adenopathy.

▶ Primary: chancre on sex organs.

▶ Secondary: fever, rashes on palms and soles and condylomata lata, generalized illness.

▶ Tertiary: infection of brain, blood vessels.

▶ General Considerations

Syphilis is caused by infection from *Treponema pallidum*. The national rate of syphilis has increased after reaching an all-time low in 2000. It remains more common in men; however, women have an increasing and significant rate,

▶ Clinical Findings

Symptoms and Signs

Primary syphilis usually presents as a solitary chancre. The chancre is painless, indurated, nonpurulent ulcer with a clean base and associated nontender, firm adenopathy. The chancre appears an average 21 days after exposure and resolves spontaneously in 4-8 weeks. Because it is painless, it may go undetected. Chancres occur at locations of inoculation (on the genitalia, anus, or oropharynx).

Secondary syphilis occurs 4-10 weeks after the chancre appears. Patient experience generalized malaise, adenopathy, and a nonpruritic maculopapular rash that often includes the palms and soles. Secondary syphilis resolves in 1-3 months, but can recur. Verrucous lesions known as *condylomata lata* may develop on the genitalia. These tend to occur in about one-third of patients and appear as painless, mucosal, warty erosions.

Tertiary syphilis is the chronic phase. Lesions develop on bone, viscera, aorta (aortitis), and CNS (neurosyphilis).

Laboratory Findings

If the patient has a suspect primary lesion, is high risk, has been in contact with someone with syphilis, or may have secondary syphilis, a nontreponemal serum screen—either RPR or VDRL—should be performed. If the nontreponemal test is positive, a specific treponemal test, a fluorescent treponemal antibody, absorbed (FTA-ABS) or microhemagglutination-*T. pallidum* (MHA-TP) test, is performed to confirm diagnosis. Darkfield microscopy can be used to detect spirochetes in scrapings of the chancre base. Darkfield

examinations and DFA tests of lesion exudate or tissue are the definitive methods for diagnosing early syphilis.

Syphilis, by law, must be reported to state health departments, and all sexual contacts need to be evaluated. Patients also need to be evaluated for other STDs, especially HIV, because HIV-infected patients have increased rates of failure with some syphilis treatment regimens.

▶ Treatment & Disposition

Benzathine penicillin G 2.4 million units IM × 1 is probably easiest and the recommended treatment (see Table 39–5 for other treatment recommendations). Refer patients to their primary physician or gynecologist as patients should be reexamined clinically and serologically with nontreponemal tests (RPR or VDRL) at 6 and 12 months after treatment. If signs or symptoms persist or recur, or patients do not have a fourfold decrease in the nontreponemal test titer, they should be considered to have either failed treatment or became reinfected and will need retreatment.

4. Bacterial Vaginosis

▶ Gray-white vaginal discharge.

▶ Fishy odor.

▶ "Clue cells" on microscopic examination.

▶ General Considerations

Bacterial vaginosis (BV) is a polymicrobial infection of the vagina caused by an imbalance of the normal bacterial flora. Although BV is presented here in the STD section, it should be noted that the infection can occur in individuals who have not had sex. The altered flora has a decreased number of hydrogen peroxide–producing lactobacilli and increased concentrations of *Mycoplasma hominis* and anaerobes, such as *Gardnerella vaginalis* and *Bacteroides*. Little progress has been made on specific causes. BV is associated with having multiple sex partners, but one-third of adolescents with BV are not sexually active. Douching is a risk factor.

▶ Clinical Findings

Symptoms and Signs

The most common symptom is a foul-smelling, gray-white vaginal discharge. Patients may report vaginal itching or dysuria. A fishy odor may be noted and is often times more noticeable after intercourse or during menses, when the high pH of blood or semen volatilizes the amines.

Laboratory Findings

BV is diagnosed by clinical criteria, which include (1) presence of gray-white discharge, (2) fishy (amine) odor before or after the addition of 10% KOH (whiff test), (3) pH of vaginal fluid greater than 4.5 determined with narrow-range pH paper, and (4) presence of "clue cells" (epithelial cells of the vagina that have a distinctive stippled appearance noted) on microscopic wet mount examination (slide with a few saline drops placed over the vaginal discharge). Diagnosis requires three of the four criteria to be met, although many female patients who meet the criteria have no discharge or other symptoms.

▶ Treatment & Disposition

Female patients who have symptomatic disease should receive treatment to relieve vaginal symptoms and signs of infection. Metronidazole 500 mg po × 7 days is likely the best option (see Table 39–5 for treatment regimens). It should be noted that current recommended treatment options have been associated with high rates of recurrence. In addition to antibiotic treatment, non-antibiotic efforts to maintain a healthy bacterial vaginal flora are being evaluated.

5. Chancroid

ESSENTIALS OF DIAGNOSIS

▶ Tropics or subtropics travel.

▶ Painful ulcer, in combination with

▶ Suppurative inguinal adenopathy.

▶ General Considerations

Chancroid is caused by the bacteria *Haemophilus ducreyi*. It is relatively rare outside the tropics and subtropics, but is endemic in some urban areas. A detailed history, including travel, may be useful in identification of the infection.

▶ Clinical Findings

Symptoms and Signs

Lesions appear 1-21 days after exposure. Lesion begins as a papule that erodes after 24-48 hours into a painful ulcer (unlike syphilis). The ulcer has ragged, sharply demarcated edges and a yellow-gray purulent base. Lesions may occur anywhere on the genitals; 50% have tender, fluctuant adenopathy. A painful ulcer in combination with suppurative inguinal adenopathy is usually a chancroid. Syphilis has a painless ulcer and nontender nonsuppurative adenopathy. HSV vesicles are painful ulcers and nonsuppurative

adenopathy. Ulcers in HSV are also multiple, smaller, and shallower than chancroid ulcers

Laboratory Findings

Gram stain shows gram-negative cocci arranged in a boxcar formation. Bacterial culture needs special collections and may not be available except in larger academic centers. PCR testing may improve laboratory diagnosis in areas where such testing is available.

▶ Treatment & Disposition

Symptoms improve within 3 days after therapy. One regimen is single dose of azithromycin 1 g po (see Table 39–5 for other regimens). All sexual contacts need to be examined and given treatment, even if asymptomatic.

6. Pelvic Inflammatory Disease

ESSENTIALS OF DIAGNOSIS

▶ Cervical motion and adnexal tenderness.

▶ Fever > 38.3°C (>101°F).

▶ Mucopurulent vaginal and cervical discharge.

▶ WBC on wet mount.

▶ Elevated WBC, ESR, and CRP.

▶ Laboratory evidence of *C. trachomatis* or *N. gonorrhoeae*.

▶ Treat empirically.

▶ General Considerations

More than 1 million females develop pelvic inflammatory disease (PID) annually; 60,000 are hospitalized, and more than 150,000 females are evaluated in outpatient settings. The incidence is highest in the adolescent population. Predisposing risk factors include multiple sex partners, younger age of initiating sexual intercourse, prior history of PID, and lack of condom use.

PID is a polymicrobial infection. It is most commonly caused by *C. trachomatis* and *N. Gonorrhoeae*. Other causes include anaerobic bacteria that reside in the vagina and genital mycoplasmas. PID is an infection of the upper genital tract in females and includes endometritis, salpingitis, tuboovarian abscess, and pelvic peritonitis.

Scarring of the fallopian tubes is major sequelae of PID. After one episode of PID, 17% of patients become infertile, 17% develop chronic pelvic pain, and 10% will have an ectopic pregnancy. Infertility rates increase with each episode of PID; three episodes of PID result in 73% infertility.

Duration of symptoms appears to be the largest determinant of infertility.

Fitz Hugh-Curtis syndrome is inflammation of the liver capsule (perihepatitis) from hematogenous or lymphatic spread of organisms from the fallopian tubes. This results in right upper quadrant pain and elevation of liver function tests.

▶ Clinical Findings

Symptoms and Signs

Adolescents with PID may present with bilateral lower abdominal pain, nausea, vomiting, and fever. Recent onset of pain that worsens during coitus or with movement may be the single presenting symptom. Diagnosis is usually made clinically. Common presentation to the emergency department is an adolescent or young adult female with a classic antalgic shuffling walk. Onset of pain during or shortly after menses is particularly suggestive. Approximately 50% of patients will have a history of fever. On pelvic examination, the findings of purulent endocervical discharge and/or acute cervical motion and adnexal tenderness with bimanual examinations are strongly suggestive of diagnosis. Additional symptoms include abnormal vaginal bleeding, dysmenorrhea, vaginal discharge, and GI symptoms.

Laboratory Findings

Laboratory findings include elevated WBC with a left shift and elevated acute phase reactants (ESR or CRP). A positive test for *N. gonorrhoeae* or *C. trachomatis* is supportive, although in 25% of patients neither bacterium is detected. Liver function tests may be elevated if there is perihepatitis (Fitz Hugh-Curtis syndrome).

Diagnostic Studies

Laparoscopy is the gold standard for detection of salpingitis. Laparoscapy is used to confirm diagnosis or to discriminate PID from ectopic pregnancy, ovarian cysts, and adnexal torsion. Pelvic US is used for detection of tubo-ovarian abscesses, which are found in about 20% of adolescents with PID. Transvaginal US is more sensitive than abdominal US.

▶ Treatment & Disposition

Objectives of PID treatment are to achieve a clinical cure and prevent long-term sequelae. PID patients are frequently managed at the outpatient level, although some physicians assert that adolescents with PID should be hospitalized because of the rate of complications. Hospitalization is recommended for the following: severe systemic symptoms and toxicity, signs of peritonitis, inability to take fluids, pregnancy, nonresponse or intolerance of oral antimicrobial therapy, and tubo-ovarian abscess. In addition, if the physician determines that the patient will not adhere to treatment, hospitalization is warranted. Surgical drainage may be required to ensure adequate treatment of tubo-ovarian abscesses. One regimen for outpatient management includes ceftriaxone 250 mg IM in a single dose plus doxycycline 100 mg orally twice a day for 14 days with metronidazole 500 mg orally twice a day for 14 days.

Treatment regimens outlined in Table 39–5 are broad-spectrum to cover the numerous microorganisms associated with PID. Treatment regimens should be effective against *N. gonorrhoeae* and *C. trachomatis* because negative endocervical screening tests do not rule out upper reproductive tract infection with these organisms. Outpatient treatment is reserved for compliant patients who have classic signs of PID with no systemic symptoms. Patients with PID who receive outpatient treatment should be reexamined within 24-48 hours, to detect persistent disease or treatment failure. Patients should have substantial improvement within 48-72 hours. An adolescent should be reexamined 7-10 days after the completion of therapy to ensure resolution of the PID.

STDs CAUSED BY VIRUSES

7. Herpes Simplex Virus

 ESSENTIALS OF DIAGNOSIS

▶ Initial vesicles.

▶ Painful shallow ulcers that recur.

▶ HSV culture.

▶ Antiviral medication within the first 5 days.

▶ General Considerations

Herpes simplex virus (HSV) is the most common cause of visible genital ulcers. It is a lifelong and incurable disease. Herpes simplex virus type 1 (HSV-1) and type 2 (HSV-2) infect humans primarily. HSV-1 is commonly associated with infections of the face, including the eyes, pharynx, and mouth. HSV-2 is commonly associated with anogenital infections. However, each serotype is capable of infecting either region. HSV-1 infections are frequently established in children by 5 years of age; lower socioeconomic groups have higher infection rates. HSV-2 is an STD and the prevalence of infection in the United States increases during adolescence and reaches rates of 20-40% in 40-year-olds.

▶ Clinical Findings

Symptoms and Signs

Symptomatic initial HSV infection causes vesicles of the vulva, vagina, cervix, penis, rectum, or urethra, which are quickly followed by shallow, painful ulcerations. Atypical presentation of HSV infection includes vulvar erythema and fissures. Initial infection can be severe, lasting up to 3 weeks, and associated with fever and malaise, as well as localized tender adenopathy. The pain and dysuria can be extremely uncomfortable.

Symptoms tend to be more severe in females. Recurrence in the genital area with HSV-2 is likely (65-90%). Approximately 40% of individuals infected with HSV-2 experience up to or more than six episodes per year. Prodromal pain in the genital, buttock, or pelvic region is common prior to recurrences. Recurrent genital herpes is of shorter duration (5-7 days), with fewer lesions and usually no systemic symptoms. Commonly, there is decreased frequency and severity of episodes over time. First-episode genital herpes infection caused by HSV-1 is usually the consequence of oral-genital sex. Primary HSV-1 infection is as severe as HSV-2 infection, and treatment is the same. Recurrence of HSV-1 is less than 50% in patients, and frequency of recurrences is much less than in patients with prior HSV-2 infection.

Laboratory Findings

Diagnosis of genital HSV infection is often made presumptively. Viral cultures have been the gold standard and provide results in a few days. Culture is obtained by unroofing an active vesicle and swabbing the base of the lesion. DFA testing can provide results within hours. DFA can also determine serotype, which is important for prognosis. NAAT of viral DNA is currently a more common diagnostic method.

Differential Diagnosis

Genital HSV infections must be discriminated from other ulcerative STD lesions, including syphilis, chancroid, and lymphogranuloma venereum. Other non-STDs include herpes zoster, Behçet syndrome, or lichen sclerosis.

Complications

Complications, usually with the first episode of genital HSV infection, include viral meningitis, urinary retention, transmission to neonate, and pharyngitis.

▶ Treatment & Disposition

Antiviral drugs administered within the first 5 days of primary infection decrease duration and severity of HSV infection (see Table 39–5). The effect of antivirals on the severity or duration of recurrent episodes is limited. For best results, therapy should be started with the prodrome or during the first episode. Patients should have a prescription drug at home to initiate treatment if needed. If recurrences are frequent and cause significant physical or emotional

discomfort, patients may elect to take antiviral prophylaxis on a daily basis to reduce frequency (70-80% decrease) and duration of recurrences. Treatment of first or subsequent episodes will not prevent future episodes, but frequency and severity decrease in many individuals over time.

8. Human Papillomavirus

▶ Verrucous lesions on genital mucosal surface.

▶ Very high current rates of infection among sexually active females.

▶ Prevention and HPV vaccine.

▶ Referral to physicians for annual cervical screening and PAP test.

▶ General Considerations

Condylomata acuminata, or genital warts, are caused by human papillomavirus (HPV), which is associated with cervical dysplasia and cervical cancer. HPV is transmitted sexually. Twenty million people (9 million aged 15-24 years) are infected annually with HPV. In females younger than 25 years, prevalence is 28-46%. In the United States adolescent females having sexual intercourse have HPV infections(~32-50%); however, only 1% have visible lesions. Males (30-60%) whose partners have HPV have evidence of condylomata on examination. An estimated 1 million new cases of genital warts occur every year in the United States.

Although there are almost 100 serotypes of HPV, types 6 and 11 cause approximately 90% of genital warts, and HPV types 16 and 18 cause more than 70% of cervical dysplasia and cervical cancer. The infection is more common in individuals with multiple partners and in those who initiate sexual intercourse at an early age.

A sexually active adolescent should be referred to a gynecologist for annual cervical screening including Pap test.

▶ Clinical Findings

Symptoms and Signs

HPV presents as single or clusters of verrucous lesions on genital mucosal surfaces. Lesions can be internal or external. They do not usually cause discomfort.

Laboratory Findings

External, visible lesions have unique characteristics and diagnosis is typically straightforward. *Condylomata acuminata* can be discriminated from *condylomata lata* (syphilis), skin tags, and *molluscum contagiosum* by application of 5% acetic acid solution. Internal and cervical lesions require a speculum examination, often a Pap test which looks for atypical cervical cells, and possible HPV testing to identify high-risk serotypes. Acetowhitening can be used to indicate the extent of cervical infection. This is not performed in the emergency department.

Differential Diagnosis

Differential diagnosis includes skin tags, *molluscum contagiosum*, seborrheic keratosis, and syphilis.

Prevention

Use of condoms significantly reduces, but does not eliminate, risk of transmission to uninfected partners. There are two currently used HPV vaccines marketed in the United States, which are more than 93% effective in preventing HPV-6 and HPV-11–related genital warts and HPV-16 and HPV-18–related cervical dysplasia. CDC and partners, including the American Academy of Pediatrics, recommend HPV vaccination of both girls and boys at ages 11 or 12 years and suggest that physicians strongly recommend HPV vaccination for children and adolescents who have not yet been fully vaccinated.

▶ Treatment & Disposition

External vaginal or vulvar lesions can be treated topically with medications such as podofilox prescribed by the gynecologist. The emergency department physician could refer patients to gynecologist for other types of wart-removing treatments (cryotherapy, trichloracetic acid, surgical removal, electrocautery, or laser excision). The sexually active adolescent should also be referred to begin annual cervical screen, PAP test, and/or HPV testing.

STDs Caused by Protozoan

9. *Trichomonas Vaginalis*

ESSENTIALS OF DIAGNOSIS

- ▶ Vaginal itching.
- ▶ Green-gray malodorous frothy discharge.
- ▶ Dysuria.

▶ General Considerations

Trichomoniasis is caused by *T. vaginalis*, a flagellated protozoan that infects 2.3 million (3.1%) women aged 14-49 years in the United States.

▶ Clinical Findings

Symptoms and Signs

Fifty percent of females with trichomoniasis develop a symptomatic vaginitis with vaginal itching, a green-gray malodorous frothy discharge, and dysuria. Occasionally postcoital bleeding and dyspareunia may be present. The vulva may be erythematous and the cervix friable. Many females have no symptoms.

Laboratory Findings

Mixing the discharge with normal saline facilitates detection of the flagellated protozoan on microscopic examination (wet preparation). The infection may be detected by the pathologist when reviewing the Pap test. Culture and PCR testing are indicated when diagnosis is unclear. PCR tests are sensitive but expensive and not readily available.

▶ Treatment & Disposition

One oral dose of metronidazole 2 g is a recommended regimen (see Table 39–5).

STDS CAUSED BY FUNGI

10. Vulvovaginal Candidiasis

ESSENTIALS OF DIAGNOSIS

- ▶ White, cottage cheese-like vaginal discharge without odor.
- ▶ Vulvar edema, redness, pain, and itching.
- ▶ Dysuria.

▶ General Considerations

Vulvovaginal candidiasis is usually caused by *Candida albicans* in 85-90% of cases. Most females will have at least one episode of vulvovaginal candidiasis in their lifetime, and about one-half will have multiple episodes. Recent use of antibiotics, diabetes, pregnancy, and HIV predispose to these infections. Other risk factors include vaginal intercourse, especially with a new sexual partner, use of oral contraceptives, and use of spermicide. Disease is usually caused by unrestrained growth of *Candida* that colonizes the vagina or is present in the GI tract, and is only rarely an STD. Most occur in women 15-30 years of age. Vulvovaginal candidiasis does occur in prepubertal girls.

Clinical Findings

Symptoms and Signs

Patients will have pruritus and a white, cottage cheese-like vaginal discharge without odor. The itching is more common midcycle and shortly after menses. Other symptoms include vaginal soreness, vulvar burning, vulvar edema and redness, dyspareunia, and dysuria (especially after intercourse).

Laboratory Findings

The diagnosis is usually made by visualizing yeast or pseudohyphae with 10% KOH (90% sensitive) or Gram stain (77% sensitive) in the vaginal discharge. Fungal culture can be used if symptoms and microscopy are not definitive or if disease is unresponsive or recurrent. However, culture is not very specific as colonization is common in asymptomatic females. Vaginal pH is normal with yeast infections.

Complications

Complication of vulvovaginal candidiasis is recurrent infection. Most females with recurrent infection have no apparent predisposing or underlying conditions.

Treatment & Disposition

Short-course topical treatments effectively treat uncomplicated vaginal yeast infections (see Table 39–5). The topically applied azole drugs are more effective than nystatin. Treatment with azoles results in relief of symptoms and negative cultures in 80-90% of patients who complete therapy. Oral fluconazole as a one-time dose is an effective oral medication. Persistent or recurrent yeast infections are relatively common. Recurrent disease is usually due to *C. albicans* and should be treated for 14 days with oral azoles.

STDs CAUSED BY PARASITES

11. PUBIC LICE

ESSENTIALS OF DIAGNOSIS

▶ Nits on hair shaft.

▶ Itching and detection of insects.

▶ Topical treatment.

General Considerations

Pthirus pubis, the pubic or crab louse, lives in pubic hair. The louse or the nits can be transmitted by close contact from person to person. Patients present with complaint of itching and they may report having seen the insect. Pubic louse can infect any hairy body part including the eyebrows, eyelashes, beard, axilla, perianal area, rarely the scalp. It can be transferred by towels and bedding.

Clinical Findings

Examination of the pubic hair may reveal the louse crawling around or attached to the hair. Closer inspection may reveal the nit or sac of eggs, which is a gelatinous material (1-2 mm) stuck to the hair shaft.

Treatment & Disposition

Treatment is with permethrin or lindane (see Table 39–5). Bedding and clothing should be decontaminated (either machine-washed or machine-dried using the heat cycle, or dry-cleaned) or removed from body contact for at least 72 hours. Fumigation of living areas is not necessary.

12. Scabies

ESSENTIALS OF DIAGNOSIS

▶ Classic burrows between fingers and toes.

▶ Severe itching.

General Considerations

Scabies is caused by *Sarcoptes scabiei* mite. It is smaller than the louse. Scabies can be sexually transmitted by close skin-to-skin contact and can be found in the pubic region, groin, lower abdomen, or upper thighs. The rash is intensely pruritic, especially at night, erythematous, and scaly.

Clinical Findings

Classic burrow created by the organism laying eggs and traveling just below the skin surface and often in the space between the fingers and toes. Intense pruritus is noted.

Treatment & Disposition

Patients should be given scabicides such as lindane and permethrin (see Table 39–5). When treating with lotion or shampoo, the entire area needs to be covered for the time specified by the manufacturer. One treatment usually clears the infestation, although a second treatment 7 days later may be necessary. Bed sheets and clothes must be washed in hot water. Sexual and close personal or household contacts within the preceding month should be examined and treated.

Ballard R. Klebsiella granulomatis (Donovanosis, Granuloma Inguinale). In: Mandel G, Bennett JE, Dolin R, ed. *Principles and Practice of Infectious Diseases*. 7th ed. Philadelphia, PA: Elsevier Churchill Livingstone; 2010.

Centers for Disease Control: Bacterial vaginosis (BV). *Sexually Transmitted Diseases (STDs)*. Also available at http://www.cdc.gov/std/bv/default.htm. Accessed August 29, 2012.

Centers for Disease Control: Chlamydia. *Sexually Transmitted Diseases (STDs)*. Also available at http://www.cdc.gov/std/chlamydia/default.htm. Accessed August 29, 2012.

Centers for Disease Control: Gonorrhea. *Sexually Transmitted Diseases (STDs)*. Also available at http://www.cdc.gov/std/gonorrhea/. Accessed August 29, 2012.

Centers for Disease Control: HIV/AIDS & STDs. *Sexually Transmitted Diseases (STDs)*. Also available at http://www.cdc.gov/std/hiv/default.htm. Accessed August 29, 2012.

Centers for Disease Control: Human papillomavirus (HPV). *Sexually Transmitted Diseases (STDs)*. Also available at http://www.cdc.gov/std/hpv/default.htm. Accessed August 29, 2012.

Centers for Disease Control: Other STDs. *Sexually Transmitted Diseases (STDs)*. Also available at http://www.cdc.gov/std/general/other.htm. Accessed August 29, 2012.

Centers for Disease Control: Syphilis. *Sexually Transmitted Diseases (STDs)*. Also available at http://www.cdc.gov/std/syphilis/default.htm. Accessed August 29, 2012.)

Centers for Disease Control: Trichomoniasis. *Sexually Transmitted Diseases (STDs)*. Also available at http://www.cdc.gov/std/trichomonas/default.htm. Accessed August 29, 2012.

Chakraborty R, Luck S: Syphilis is on the increase: The implications for child health. *Arch Dis Child*. 2008;93(2):105-109 [PMID: 18208988].

Fethers KA, Fairley CK, Hocking JS, et al: Sexual risk factors and bacterial vaginosis: A systematic review and meta-analysis. *Clin infect Dis*. 2008;47(11):1426-1435 [PMID: 18947329].

Forhan SE, Gottlieb SL, Sternberg MR, et al: Prevalence of sexually transmitted infections among female adolescents aged 14 to 19 in the United States. *Pediatrics*. 2009;124(6):1505-1512 [PMID: 19933728].

Haamid F, Holland-Hall C: Overview of sexually transmitted infections in adolescents. *Adolesc Med State Art Rev*. 2012;23(1):73-94 [PMID: 22764556].

Jasper JM: Vulvovaginitis in the prepubertal child. *Clin Pediatr Emerg Med*. 2009;10(1):10-13 (PMID)

Nyirjesy P: Vulvovaginal candidiasis and bacterial vaginosis. *Infect Dis Clin North Am*. 2008;22(4):637-652, vi [PMID: 18954756].

South-Paul JE, Matheny SC, Lewis EL: *Current Diagnosis & Treatment in Family Medicine*, 3rd ed. New York: McGraw-Hill/Medical; 2011.

Wendel KA, Workowski KA: Trichomoniasis: Challenges to appropriate management. *Clin infect Dis*. 2007;44 (Suppl 3):S123-129 [PMID: 17342665].

White JA: Manifestations and management of lymphogranuloma venereum. *Curr Opin Infect Dis*. 2009;22(1):57-66 [PMID: 19532081].

Workowski KA, Berman S: Sexually transmitted diseases treatment guidelines, 2010. *MMWR Recomm Rep*. 2010;59(RR-12):1-110 [PMID: 21160459].

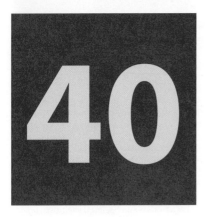

Hematologic & Oncologic Emergencies

Michelle Eckerle, MD

Richard M. Ruddy, MD

▼ HEMATOLOGIC EMERGENCIES

DISORDERS OF RED BLOOD CELLS

SEVERE ANEMIA

Hemoglobin (Hb) and hematocrit for a child will vary depending on the age of the child, which is of key importance in the diagnosis of anemia. Table 40–1 lists average Hb values by age. In the neonatal period, Hb levels are elevated due to polycythemia of the fetus, with average Hb of 17 mg/dL at birth. Equilibration occurs over the first 2 months, leading to a physiologic nadir of about 11 mg/dL at 2 months of age. Hb levels normalize by approximately 6 months of age and remain so until adolescence, with an average level of 12-13 mg/dL. In adolescence, Hb levels diverge between boys and girls due to differences in hormones and onset of menses in girls.

Severe anemia may be due to acute or chronic disorders. The child with acute blood loss leading to anemia may present with signs of hypovolemic shock, including tachycardia, delayed capillary refill, cool extremities, mental status changes, respiratory distress, and in advanced cases, hypotension. However, children generally tolerate severe anemia from a chronic cause and may remain asymptomatic to Hb levels of 5-6 g/dL. Chronic severe anemia is most commonly due to iron deficiency, but can also be due to deficiencies of folate, vitamin B_{12}, copper or vitamin E, or to inherited hemoglobinopathies. Presentation may include symptoms of lethargy, fatigue or poor feeding, and physical findings of pallor, mild tachycardia, and systolic murmur, without signs of hypovolemic shock. Children should be carefully examined for signs of heart failure, including hepatomegaly and cardiomegaly. Iron deficiency is most commonly due to nutritional deficiency in children younger than 3 years; older children require gastrointestinal evaluation to identify sources of possible occult blood loss. Possible causes of anemia can be identified by measurement of the mean corpuscular volume (MCV) on the complete blood cell count (CBC). Table 40–2 outlines causes of anemia based on low, normal, and high MCV.

AUTOIMMUNE HEMOLYTIC ANEMIA

Autoimmune hemolytic anemia (AIHA) is most common in young children and often presents acutely, with a precipitous drop in Hb and signs of hemolysis including jaundice, splenomegaly, and signs of heart failure if severe anemia. Diagnosis is aided by a positive Coombs test, as the disease is most commonly mediated by immunoglobulin G (IgG) and less frequently by immunoglobulin M (IgM). Patients require aggressive management and corticosteroid therapy initiated (prednisone 2-4 mg/kg/day). Alternative treatment includes intravenous immunoglobulin (IVIG). Response to therapy is expected within hours to days. Transfusion should not be administered except in the case of life-threatening anemia, manifested by poor perfusion, hypoxemia, or lactic acidosis.

HEMOGLOBINOPATHIES—SICKLE CELL DISEASE

The most commonly encountered inherited hemoglobinopathy in the emergency department setting is sickle cell disease (SCD). The disorder encompasses genotypic variants which lead to greater than 50% hemoglobin S and subsequent hemolytic anemia. Severity of disease varies by genotype, with (HbSS) the most severe variant. Less common than HbSS are sickle beta-thalassemia (Hb S-βthal) and Hemoglobin SC disease (HbSC). The most common clinical manifestations presenting to the emergency department include fever, infection, acute pain/vaso-occlusive crisis, acute chest syndrome, aplastic crisis, priapism, splenic sequestration, and stroke. Stroke is discussed in a later section.

Table 40–1. Pediatric hemogram.

Age	Lower Limits (−2 SD) of Hemoglobin (Hb) Concentrations (g/dL)
Birth	14.5
2 wk	12.5
1 mo	11.0
2-6 mo	10.0
0.5-2 y	10.5
2-6 y	11.0
6-12 y	11.5
Males 12-18 y	14.0
Females 12-18 y	12.3

Age	Normal reticulocyte counts (% and absolute)
Birth	3-7% (100-500x10^3/mm^3)
1 wk-2 mo	0.1-1% (10-50x10^3/mm^3)
>12 mo	1-2% (50-100 x10^3/mm^3)

Age	Normal MCV (fl) values
Birth	98-116
> 1 mo to ≤ 9 y	70 + age in years-96
> 9 y to adults	80-96

Table 40–2. Differential diagnosis of anemia.

Type of Anemia	MCV	Clinical Diagnoses
Microcytic	< 70	**Disturbance of Hb synthesis:** Iron deficiency, thalassemia, chronic inflammation, sideroblastic (hereditary), drugs/toxins (isoniazid, lead).
Normocytic	70-96	**Hemolytic:** Autoimmune, hemoglobinopathy, enzyme deficiency, membrane defect, microangiopathy. **Nonhemolytic:** Chronic inflammation, acute blood loss, splenic sequestration, chronic renal failure, transient erythroblastopenia of childhood.
Macrocytic	> 96	**Megaloblastic (disturbance of Hb synthesis):** Vitamin B$_{12}$ or folate deficiency, purine or pyrimidine deficiency, drugs (methotrexate, anticonvulsants). **Nonmegaloblastic:** Aplastic anemia, Diamond-Blackfan anemia, hypothyroidism, liver disease, dyserythropoietic anemia.

Infection in Patients With Sickle Cell Disease

Patients with sickle cell disease (SCD) are at higher risk for infection by encapsulated bacteria due to functional asplenia, which often occurs by 18 months of age. Use of penicillin prophylaxis and routine pneumococcal vaccination have decreased the risk. Recent studies have cited an incidence of 1% of positive blood cultures among febrile patients with SCD, which is 2-3 times higher than in immunized healthy children. In addition, children without SCD have a lower risk of clinical sepsis from these pathogens. Patients presenting to the emergency department with fever should have a careful physical examination to detect the etiology of infection. CBC, reticulocyte count, blood culture, chest radiograph, and/or oxygen saturation should be performed, as well as tests indicated from history or on examination. Risk factors for invasive disease include temperature greater than 40°C, ill appearance on examination or signs of poor perfusion and shock, white blood cell count (WBC) greater than 30,000/μL or less than 5000/μL, Hb less than 5 g/dL, infiltrate on chest radiograph, and prior history of pneumococcal sepsis. Children with one or more risk factors should receive intravenous (IV) antibiotics and be admitted for observation after appropriate stabilization in the emergency department. Infants younger than 6-12 months are typically admitted for observation, even in the absence of risk factors for invasive disease. Well-appearing children without pain, respiratory distress, or risk factors as listed above can receive a dose of long-acting IV antibiotic, usually ceftriaxone 50 mg/kg, and be discharged home for outpatient follow-up.

Pain in Sickle Cell Disease

Pain crises are characteristic of SCD and represent occlusion of the microvasculature by sickled red blood cells (RBCs). Infants may present with dactylitis of the hands or feet, characterized by pain and swelling over the dorsal surfaces of the hands and feet. Older children may localize pain to other bony sites, including humerus, femur, or vertebrae. Differentiating pain with fever from osteomyelitis can be difficult, especially if pain is localized to a single site. Young children may complain of abdominal pain, which must be discriminated from splenic sequestration, cholelithiasis, or other clinical causes of abdominal pain by means of examination, laboratory studies, and imaging.

Table 40–3. Management of acute pain in opioid-naïve children with sickle cell disease.

1. Rapid clinical assessment.

2. If pain severe and nonopioids not effective, give opioids:

   Oral regimen: oral morphine 0.4 mg/kg PO, or slow release morphine 1 mg/kg (rounded up to nearest 5 mg) every 12 hrs, with oral morphine 0.3 mg/kg every 3 hr as necessary.

   IV regimen: morphine 0.1 mg/kg repeated every 20 min until pain controlled, then 0.05-0.1 mg/kg every 2-4 hr. Consider patient-controlled analgesic (PCA) pump.

3. Give adjuvant nonopioid analgesic: acetaminophen 10-15 mg/kg every 4-6 hr, ibuprofen 10-15 mg/kg every 6-8 hr.

4. Monitor pain, sedation, vital signs, respiratory rate, oxygen saturation: every 15 min until pain controlled, then every 30 min.

5. For severe respiratory depression/sedation, give naloxone 10 mcg/kg IV, increase to 100 mcg/kg if no response.

6. If requiring > 1 dose of IV opioid medication, consider inpatient management.

Home therapy for pain crises typically consists of acetaminophen or nonsteroidal anti-inflammatory drugs (NSAIDs); however, patients often present to the emergency department because these medications have proved ineffective. Acetaminophen and NSAIDs are generally considered adequate for mild to moderate pain. Table 40–3 lists recommendations for management of SC pain in children. Patients presenting with pain crisis should have CBC, reticulocyte count, and measurement of serum electrolytes and serum creatinine, as well as any other investigations indicated by physical examination. Acute pain crisis can be accompanied by an episode of acute anemia and transfusion may be required. Adequate hydration is important, and children who cannot take fluids by mouth should be started on IV maintenance fluids, used with care when the Hb is less than 7 g/dL. Supplemental oxygen is not indicated if the child has oxygen saturations at baseline or greater than 95%. Children who require admission for pain control should have incentive spirometry ordered, if age-appropriate, to reduce the risk of acute chest syndrome.

▶ Priapism

Priapism is localized vaso-occlusion within the corpora cavernosa, resulting in unwanted and sustained erection. Diagnosis is made by physical examination and CBC should be obtained for these patients. Initial treatment involves hydration, pain control, administering opioids if indicated, and urologic consultation in the emergency department for consideration of aspiration of the corpora. If erection persists, the child should receive transfusion of packed red blood cells (PRBCs) to achieve Hb of 9-10 g/dL, and exchange transfusion should be considered if these measures are unsuccessful.

▶ Splenic Sequestration

Splenic sequestration is one of the earliest occurring life-threatening complications in children with SCD. Average age at first presentation is 1.4 years, and patients with a first episode have greater than 50% risk for recurrence. Splenic sequestration typically occurs before 6 years of age in patients with HbSS disease, but may occur in patients with HbSC or Hb Sβ-thal disease. Splenic sequestration is defined as a decrease in Hb of at least 2 g/dL below baseline with acute enlargement of the spleen, often accompanied by increased reticulocyte count and thrombocytopenia. Depending on the age of patient, left upper quadrant (LUQ) pain may be a complaint. Patients diagnosed with splenic sequestration are at risk of cardiovascular collapse from acute anemia and hypovolemia. Immediate administration of normal saline boluses at 20 mL/kg to normalize heart rate and blood pressure is indicated. Transfusion of PRBC (5-10 mL/kg) is often required in severe cases.

▶ Aplastic Crisis

Aplastic crisis in patients with SCD presents with severe anemia. However, in contrast to splenic sequestration, this manifestation represents a temporary failure of production, usually associated with concurrent infection with parvovirus B19. While splenic sequestration is typically seen in younger patients, aplastic crises are more often seen in older patients. Children present with fever, pallor and tachycardia, and are found on CBC to have decreased Hb accompanied by low reticulocyte count. Occasionally, mild neutropenia and thrombocytopenia are seen as well. These children should be admitted for monitoring and blood transfusion, if indicated, until the peripheral blood shows evidence of marrow recovery.

Brousse V, Elie C, Benkerrou M, et al: Acute splenic sequestration crisis in sickle cell disease: Cohort study of 190 paediatric patients. *Br J Haematol.* 2012;156:643-646 [PMID: 22224796].

De Montalembert M: Current strategies for the management of children with sickle cell disease. *Exp Rev Hematol.* 2009;2(4):455(9) [PMID: 21082949].

Kavanagh PL, Sprinz PG, Vinci SR: Management of children with sickle cell disease: A comprehensive review of the literature. *Pediatrics.* 2011;128:e1552 [PMID: 22123880].

Narang S, Fernandez ID, Chin N, et al: Bacteremia in children with sickle hemoglobinopathies. *J Pediatr Hematol Oncol.* 2012;34:1 [PMID: 22215095].

Rees DC, Olujohungbe AD, Parker NE, et al: Guidelines for the management of the acute painful crisis in sickle cell disease. *Br J Haematol.* 2010;120(5):744-752 [PMID:2614024].

Rogovik AL, Friedman JN, Persaud J, et al: Bacterial blood cultures in children with sickle cell disease. *Am J Emerg Med.* 2010;28:511-514 [PMID: 20466235].

WHITE BLOOD CELL DISORDERS

The most common emergency involving white blood cells (WBCs) is neutropenia. Neutropenia can be a presentation of hematologic malignancy, secondary to therapy for malignancy, due to congenital neutrophil defects or due to another cause. The former is discussed in the section on oncologic emergencies. Neutropenia can also be due to congenital causes. It is defined as an absolute neutrophil count (ANC) of less than 1500 cells/μL. An ANC less than 500 cells/μL places the patient at increased risk for life-threatening infection. Published reports suggest that risk of infection increases significantly with an ANC less than 250 cells/μL. The duration and depth of neutropenia, as well as function of the cells, contribute to risk of infection.

NEUTROPENIA WITHOUT MALIGNANCY

Neutropenia without malignancy can be classified as acquired or inherited. Acquired causes of neutropenia include suppression secondary to viral infections, drug induced, or autoimmune. Viral and drug induced causes may be suspected from the history or concurrent symptoms. Autoimmune neutropenia is typically a self-limited event and patients recover over several weeks. The diagnosis is made in most patients by establishing the presence of anti-neutrophil antibodies. Corticosteroids and granulocyte-colony stimulating factor (G-CSF) are sometimes used for treatment in consultation with a pediatric hematologist.

Inherited causes of neutropenia include congenital, cyclic, and neutropenia as part of a marrow failure syndrome. Patients with cyclic neutropenia have periodic episodes of severe neutropenia, typically lasting 3-21 days. Patients most commonly manifest with oral ulcers, sinusitis, otitis media, lymphadenitis, cellulitis, or pharyngitis. Unlike children with malignancies, overwhelming infection is relatively uncommon in children with congenital or cyclic neutropenia, even if the ANC is less than 500/μL. Patients presenting with neutropenia should have a thorough physical examination to ascertain treatable causes of infection. The perianal area should be inspected, but digital rectal examination should not be performed due to increased risk of Gram-negative sepsis when neutropenic. Patients who appear well when viral suppression is the likely cause of neutropenia can usually be safely observed without antibiotics, with close clinical follow-up. Patients who appear ill, have evidence of a bacterial infection, or there is suspicion of other risk factors, should be monitored on appropriate antibiotics in the hospital. Broad-spectrum antibiotic coverage should include therapy for *Staphylococcus aureus* as well as coverage for Gram-negative organisms.

Ammann RA, Tissing WJE, Phillips B: Rationalizing the approach to children with fever in neutropenia. *Curr Opin Infect Dis.* 2012;25:258-265 [PMID: 22395759].

Segal GB, Halterman JS: Neutropenia in pediatric practice. *Pediatr Rev.* 2008;29:12.
Teuffel O, Sung L: Advances in management of low-risk febrile neutropenia. *Curr Opin Pediatr.* 2012;24:40-45 [PMID: 22037219].

PLATELET & BLEEDING DISORDERS

IMMUNE THROMBOCYTOPENIC PURPURA

Immune thrombocytopenic purpura, also known as Idiopathic thrombocytopenic purpura (ITP) is a condition arising from the production of autoantibodies against platelet antigens. Antiplatelet glycoprotein antibodies cause thrombocytopenia through two mechanisms: (1) reducing the survival of circulating platelets, and (2) inhibiting the production of new platelets by bone marrow megakaryocytes.

The condition can be acute or chronic. Chronic ITP is defined as having a platelet count $<150 \times 10^9$/L for longer than 6 months. The initial presentation is typically an otherwise well-appearing child with acute onset of petechiae, purpura, and/or bruising. The average age at presentation is 5.7 years, with 70% of children between ages 1 and 10 years. In two-thirds of cases, the symptoms are preceded by a viral illness, with an average interval of 2 weeks between infectious symptoms and development of thrombocytopenia. However, fever and infectious symptoms are not a characteristic of ITP. In addition, children with ITP do not have constitutional symptoms of weight loss, fatigue, or joint pain. One quarter of children will present with mild epistaxis. CBC shows isolated thrombocytopenia with no abnormality of other cell lines.

Spontaneous bleeding in children with ITP is rare but has been observed (~ 1% of patients). Children with platelet count less than 10,000 are at higher risk. Initial labs include CBC, prothrombin time (PT), partial thromboplastin time (PTT), and type and screen. Children with signs or symptoms of severe life-threatening hemorrhage should be treated emergently. Treatment for these patients involves IV methylprednisolone (30 mg/kg, maximum dose 1 g) over 20-30 minutes plus a platelet transfusion with two- to threefold increase in the volume of transfused platelets. After receiving steroids and platelets, an IVIG infusion should commence (1 g/kg), which may increase survival of donor platelets. When bleeding is controlled, the child should be admitted for subsequent IVIG and methylprednisolone infusions as indicated.

Many children will recover with expectant management alone. In the absence of spontaneous bleeding or life-threatening hemorrhage, medical treatment is considered for patients with platelet counts $< 20 \times 10^9$/L. Children with findings of isolated thrombocytopenia can safely be treated with plasma-based therapies. Controversy exists as to whether bone marrow biopsy is indicated prior to initiating steroid therapy in children without spontaneous bleeding. Consultation with a pediatric hematologist is recommended. Corticosteroid treatment most often is administered as oral prednisone at 1-2 mg/kg in divided doses and continued for a period of weeks. IVIG is administered as a single infusion of 0.8-1 g/kg with subsequent doses given based on clinical assessment or platelet counts. IV anti-D has also been used in treatment of ITP. Therapy is used for patients who are rhesus (D) positive, and is given as a single dose of 75 mcg/kg. The most commonly seen adverse effect from this therapy is a transient decrease in Hb due to hemolysis by infused RBC alloantibodies, typically evident within 1 week after the infusion and resolving by 3 weeks after the infusion. Therefore, use Rho(D) immune globulin with caution in patients with Hb < 10 g/dL at presentation.

Children with spontaneous bleeding from thrombocytopenia should be stabilized and admitted. In addition, most children with platelet count < 20×10^9/L will be admitted for consultation with the pediatric hematologist and observation, given the small but present risk of spontaneous bleeding. Incidence rates for intracranial hemorrhage are variable but range from 0.17 to 0.9%. Most children will recover spontaneously, with two-thirds reaching complete remission (platelet count > 150×10^9/L without ongoing platelet enhancing therapy) within 6 months of diagnosis.

Blanchette V, Bolton-Maggs P: Childhood immune thrombocytopenic purpura: Diagnosis and management. *Hematol Oncol Clin North Am.* 2010;24:249-273 [PMID: 20113906].

HEMORRHAGIC DISEASE OF THE NEWBORN

Bleeding due to vitamin K deficiency is a rare cause of hemorrhage or bleeding in the neonate. Vitamin K is necessary for the synthesis of prothrombin and factors VII, IX, and X. The incidence has dramatically decreased since the advent of vitamin K injections at birth. Infants who are breast-fed are at higher risk because maternal stores of vitamin K are often inadequate.

Bleeding due to vitamin K deficiency is rarely seen in the first 24 hours of life. It is often secondary to maternal medications taken while pregnancy which interfere with vitamin K metabolism. Classical vitamin K deficiency bleeding occurs between 2 and 7 days of age. Late presentation of disease occurs between 8 days and 6 months of age. Late-onset disease occurs most often in exclusively breast-fed infants, and association is identified between presentation of the disease and hepatobiliary dysfunction in the infants. Infants presenting with jaundice after 2-3 weeks of age, as an indicator of cholestasis, should receive an assessment of vitamin K status. Compromised intestinal absorption of vitamin K can contribute to the disease, even if maternal breast milk provides adequate amounts. Infants receiving broad-spectrum antibiotics, with diarrhea and breast-feeding are at additional risk.

One-half of infants presenting with late-onset hemorrhagic disease (> 1 wk of age) present with intracranial hemorrhage.

If vitamin K deficiency bleeding is suspected, CBC, coagulation studies, and fibrinogen levels should be obtained. Vitamin K deficiency is most likely in infants younger than 6 months of age with spontaneous bleeding, bruising, or intracranial hemorrhage, with PT greater than twice the normal value and no history of inherited coagulopathy or disseminated intravascular coagulation (DIC). Confirmatory tests include the protein induced by vitamin K antigen (PIVKA-II) that should be ordered as soon as possible, even after reversal of bleeding.

Treatment for infants with non–life-threatening bleeding is vitamin K at a dose of 250-300 mcg/kg administered IV. The standard neonatal dose of 1-2 mg given as a subcutaneous injection is often adequate to correct mild to moderate bleeding, with effect typically seen within an hour. For severe or life-threatening bleeding, FFP at a dose of 10-15 mL/kg should be administered.

Shearer MJ: Vitamin K deficiency bleeding (VKDB) in early infancy. *Blood Rev.* 2009;23:49-59 [PMID: 18804903].

INHERITED BLEEDING DISORDERS

The emergency provider will encounter children with acute bleeding as a consequence of an inherited bleeding disorder. Most commonly, this is seen in patients with hemophilia, although serious bleeding can also be seen in severe cases of von Willebrand disease. In children with hemophilia, bleeding is seen less frequently now than in earlier years due to prophylactic factor replacement. Patients with hemophilia A receive replacement and treatment with factor VIII and hemophilia B with factor IX. Children with bleeding disorders may present with clinically evident bleeding, such as hemarthrosis. In these patients, the provider must first establish the severity of the child's underlying condition. Patients with hemophilia may have severe (< 1% of factor levels before therapy), moderate (1-5% of factor level), and mild (6-25% of factor level). A patient with severe hemophilia is more likely to bleed without trauma and to experience joint bleeds. A patient with mild hemophilia is more likely to require significant trauma to sustain a clinically significant bleed. In most patients, the family is aware of when a bleed requires intervention; many patients will manage minor bleeding episodes at home. Episodes of bleeding into joint spaces or muscle, or other more rare instances, such as intra-abdominal bleeding or gross hematuria, should be discussed with a hematologist to determine optimal duration and timing of therapy. Arthrocentesis is rarely indicated. Table 40–4 lists replacement products indicated for specific common factor deficiencies. Although dosing should be individualized for each patient and for each product employed, dose required to raise factor VIII

Table 40–4. Factor deficiencies and replacement therapy.

Factor Deficiency	Replacement Therapy
Factor VIII	Factor VIII concentrates (recombinant and plasma derived
Factor IX	Prothrombin complex concentrates
	Factor IX concentrates (recombinant and plasma derived)
von Willebrand disease	DDAVP
	Certain factor VIII concentrates high in vWF

concentration by a specified amount can be estimated using the following formula:

$$\text{Dose of factor VIII (IU)} = \text{Weight (kg)} \times (\text{desired \% increase}) \times 0.5$$
$$\text{Dose of factor IX (plasma derived factor IX)} = \text{Weight (kg)} \times (\text{desired \% increase})$$
$$\text{Dose of IX} = \text{Weight (kg)} \times \text{desired increase} \times 1.2$$

Patients with factor VIII levels of greater than 5%, who have mild bleeding may not always require factor replacement. Desmopressin (DDAVP) causes endothelial storage sites to release von Willebrand factor (vWF) that is capable of carrying additional amounts of factor VIII in the plasma. The IV dose of desmopressin is 0.3 mcg/kg (maximum dose 20 mcg) over 30 minutes. The concentrated intranasal form is an antidiuretic agent and fluid restriction may be needed during use. For children older than 5 years, a single spray in a single nostril (150 mcg) is adequate. For adolescents and adults, the dose is a single spray in each nostril (300-mcg total dose). This will increase factor levels by 2-3.

Patients may develop inhibitors or autoantibodies against the replacement factor. Inhibitors not only interfere with the effectiveness of factor replacement therapy, but also may cause anaphylaxis to factor administration in patients with factor IX deficiency. The use of factor replacement is guided by the concentration of inhibitor (measured in Bethesda Inhibitor Assay [BIA] units) and by the type of response the patient has to factor replacement. Consultation with a hematologist is recommended in the care of patients with hemophilia.

Concern for potential intracranial bleeding presents a special challenge to the clinician. Relatively minor trauma can precipitate intracranial bleeding in a child with hemophilia, and children with severe hemophilia may have spontaneous intracranial bleeding. If intracranial bleeding is suspected, it is imperative that the emergency department provider treat the patient first with the appropriate replacement product, prior to obtaining any confirmatory testing such as CT scan. Most children can be discharged to home after factor replacement. Indications for hospital admission include bleeding that involves the CNS, neck, pharynx, retroperitoneum; potential compartment syndrome, patients who require several doses of factor or inability to control pain.

TRANSFUSION REACTIONS

Transfusion reactions, although rare, can be life-threatening and the emergency department provider must remain vigilant for signs of reaction. Although transfusion reactions are typically thought of in the context of RBC transfusions, they occur infrequently with ABO-mismatched platelets. Transfusion reaction should be suspected if the patient develops acute onset of dyspnea, fever, chills, abdominal/back pain, or hypotension while receiving blood products. The patient may also be noted to develop hemoglobinuria. Severe cases can progress to DIC and acute renal failure. An acute transfusion reaction occurs within 24 hours of a transfusion and is an antibody-mediated response caused by preexisting antibodies attached to the RBCs and causing hemolysis. Delayed transfusion reaction occurs more than 24 hours after transfusion, and may be due either to preexisting antibody or production of a new antibody.

Management of an acute transfusion reaction begins by stopping the transfusion and rapidly verifying that the correct patient has received the correct blood product. In addition, a sample from the transfused product should be returned to the blood bank to verify the original type and screening results. The direct antiglobulin test (DAT) will be positive in the setting of a hemolytic transfusion reaction; a negative test, however, does not rule out the reaction as antibody-bound red cells may be rapidly cleared from the circulation.

The management of transfusion reactions focuses on providing appropriate supportive care to maintain normal blood pressure and urine output, as well as appropriate treatment of DIC and renal failure if present. It should be noted that patients may also have nonhemolytic transfusion reactions, which tend to be less severe but may manifest with fever, urticaria, chills, and headache. In this case the clinician should look for signs of hemolysis, and, if none are found, decide whether to proceed with the transfusion using antihistamines and antipyretics to treat the symptoms of this nonhemolytic reaction.

DISSEMINATED INTRAVASCULAR COAGULATION

Disseminated intravascular coagulation (DIC) arises from systemic activation of the coagulation cascade, resulting in formation of intravascular fibrin and thrombosis of small and midsize blood vessels. Subsequent consumption of clotting factors and platelets can then lead to bleeding. DIC can arise due to a number of causes, including sepsis, trauma, head injury, malignancies, reactions to toxins, hemolytic transfusion reactions, and others. DIC due specifically to sepsis may manifest clinically with purpura fulminans (PF), hemorrhagic infarction of the skin in association with DIC. PF presents as erythematous macules which progress to areas of blue-black central necrosis, with subsequent hemorrhage into the dermis causing pain and sometimes vesicle or bulla formation. Unless there is rapid recognition and reversal of the underlying condition, lesions progress to full-thickness skin necrosis often requiring debridement or leading to amputation. Treatment is directed at the root cause of the condition. Causative conditions must be aggressively managed as appropriate with antibiotics, circulatory support with volume and inotropic support, ventilation, and blood product replacement. If needed these include platelet transfusions (10 mL/kg) and FFP (15 mL/kg) to correct severe thrombocytopenia and/or abnormal clotting functions. Goals include fibrinogen above 150 mg/dL, platelets between 30 and 50×10^9/L until resolution of all clinical and laboratory signs of coagulopathy.

Chalmers E, Cooper P, Forman K, et al: Purpura fulminans: Recognition, diagnosis and management. *Arch Dis Child.* 2011;96:1066-1071 [PMID: 21233082].

DISORDERS OF HYPERCOAGULATION & THROMBOSIS

VENOUS THROMBOEMBOLISM/PULMONARY EMBOLISM

Incidence of venous thromboembolism (VTE) appears to be rising in children. This is thought to be due to longer life expectancy of children with chronic medical conditions (who are therefore at increased risk for VTE events), increased frequency of interventions that place children at risk (such as central venous catheters [CVCs]), increased recognition of the condition, or a combination of factors. In addition to CVCs, risk factors include malignancy, especially during treatment with L-asparaginase and corticosteroids, and increased by the presence of dehydration or infection, as well as inherited thrombophilic conditions, and congenital venous abnormalities. Prevalence estimates in the United States range from 0.6 to 1.1 per 10,000 for VTE. Children who experience a first episode of VTE have an overall risk of recurrence of 5-10%, but individual risk is higher for children with predisposing conditions. The presence of a central venous access device is major risk factor for children with VTE, present in more than 50% of cases. Approximately 70% of children with VTE will have an underlying chronic medical condition and a higher percentage will have an acute predisposing event such as trauma or surgery. Idiopathic VTE is relatively rare, comprising approximately 5% of cases. Approximately 14% of children will experience recurrence of VTE, and these children have the same risk for morbidity and mortality as accompanied their first episode. Children may present with pain and extremity swelling, or the finding may be asymptomatic, incidentally discovered on imaging studies. If VTE is suspected, the imaging study of choice will depend on the anatomic location. For suspected thrombosis of the central veins, a combination of Doppler ultrasound (US) of the jugular vein and venography of the subclavian and central veins is suggested. Compression Doppler US is suggested for suspected VTE of the lower extremities. Magnetic resonance venography (MRV) may be an alternative imaging modality; however, the procedure may not be available in the ED setting, sedation may be required for some patients, and utility may depend in part on the local experience with performing and interpreting pediatric studies.

Pulmonary embolism (PE) is an equally rare event in children, with an estimated incidence of 0.86-5.7 per 10,000 hospital admissions (see Chapter 34). Less than 5% of cases are idiopathic, with the majority of patients having an identifiable risk factor and approximately 50% having radiographic evidence of VTE. As with VTE, common risk factors are immobilization, presence of a central venous catheter, and recent surgery. The D-dimer assay measures one of the fibrin degradation products and has been used in adults to assist in "ruling out" the diagnosis of PE. There is not sufficient evidence in pediatrics that a normal D-dimer is adequate to rule out PE. For children in whom PE is suspected, the diagnosis is made by ventilation perfusion scanning. Computed tomography angiography is also used but there is no pediatric data describing testing characteristics for this imaging modality. Mortality rates up to 10% have been published.

Anticoagulation therapy for children with confirmed VTE should be initiated as soon as any contraindications have been resolved and after initial diagnostic laboratory tests have been obtained. Treatment options in the emergency department include unfractionated heparin (UFH) and low-molecular-weight heparin (LMWH). UFH has a short half-life and is easily reversible with protamine sulfate. It is therefore the preferred method of anticoagulation for children who have risk factors for severe bleeding, such as children with multisystem trauma, or who may imminently require surgical intervention. Therapeutic monitoring of UFH follows antifactor Xa levels that correlate to the appropriate pediatric activated partial thromboplastin time (aPTT) reference range. Adult reference ranges for aPTT are not applicable to younger pediatric patients due to baseline hemostatic differences. Heparin-induced thrombocytopenia is rare in children but is more likely to be seen with use of UFH as compared with LMWH, with a reported incidence of 2.4%. LMWH is also used for treatment of VTE, but pharmacokinetics are not as predictable in children as in adults, and antifactor Xa levels should be monitored.

Children older than 1 year with confirmed VTE should have a bolus dose of UFH 75-100 U/kg administered, followed by initiation of an infusion of 20 U/kg/hr. Older children require a lower dose, with suggested infusion rate of 18 U/kg/hr. For anticoagulation with LMWH, the most experience in pediatric patients is with enoxaparin, and should be initiated at a dose of 1 mg/kg twice daily, with neonates requiring higher doses of 1.5-1.7 mg/kg. Inferior vena cava filters for VTE are considered in patients with a contraindication to anticoagulation or who have infrarenal thrombi. Duration of anticoagulation is related to the presence of predisposing conditions or risk factors and should be decided in consultation with a pediatric hematologist.

STROKE

Stroke is an uncommon event in the pediatric population, with an incidence of approximately 2.5 per 100,000 per year, with hemorrhagic strokes more common than ischemic. Current understanding of pediatric stroke holds that children with stroke have a combination of risk factors that predispose them to initial stroke and to recurrence. Most common risk factors for ischemic stroke are SCD and congenital heart disease. Approximately 50% of children with stroke have at least one risk factor, such as primary or secondary hypercoagulable state (Table 40–5). Stroke most commonly presents with hemiparesis. Older children are more likely to have accompanying headache, and children younger than 4 years are more likely to have seizures.

When stroke is suspected in a child, emergent non contrast CT of the head should be ordered. CT will be diagnostic for hemorrhagic stroke; however, signs of ischemic stroke may not be present for 12-24 hours after the stroke. Diagnosis of ischemic stroke is suspected based on history and physical examination. CT imaging can demonstrate larger mature acute ischemic strokes and exclude hemorrhage. However, magnetic resonance imaging (MRI) identifies early and small infarcts and is therefore required to exclude ischemic stroke. Diffusion-weighted MRI can demonstrate acute ischemic stroke within minutes of onset and magnetic resonance angiography (MRA) can confirm vascular occlusion and suggest arteriopathy as an underlying cause. Management is based on whether the cause is hemorrhagic or ischemic.

Table 40–5. Risk factors for pediatric stroke.

Primary hypercoagulable states
- Protein C and S deficiency, antithrombin deficiency, anticardiolipin antibodies and lupus anticoagulant, disorders of fibrinogen or plasminogen activator inhibitor

Secondary hypercoagulable states
- Malignancy, oral contraceptive use, pregnancy, nephrotic syndrome, polycythemia vera

Sickle cell anemia

Cerebral vasculitis
- Infectious, necrotizing, hypersensitivity, associated with collagen vascular disease

For both types of stroke, initial emergency department care is focused on stabilization of the patient, including optimization of respiratory effort, controlling of seizures, managing increased intracranial pressure (ICP), correction of hypoxemia and hypotension, or slow correction of hypertension if present, and maintenance of euglycemia. Hemorrhagic stroke requires emergent consultation with a neurosurgeon to determine if surgical evacuation is indicated. Surgical intervention is typically reserved for patients with impending herniation or embolization of arteriovenous malformation, if present. For acute stroke in the setting of SCD, treatment includes hydration and exchange transfusion to reduce sickle Hb to less than 30% of total Hb. For patients with ischemic stroke, intravascular thrombolysis can be considered in consultation with a specialized stroke team; however, it should be noted that this therapy has not been studied in pediatric patients. If considered, it should be noted that in adults, increased risk of intracerebral hemorrhage is seen if IV thrombolysis is administered more 3 hours after initial event. In ischemic stroke, prophylactic use of antiepileptics in the absence of clinical or electroencephalographic seizures is not indicated. There is no proven role for therapeutic hypothermia in those with neurologic progression.

Ischemic stroke can present due to cervicocephalic arterial dissection. This can occur as a result of trauma or infection, or in a child with a predisposing condition such as Ehlers-Danlos, Marfan syndrome, or coarctation of the aorta. It is best detected on arteriography or MRI. Treatment is immediate anticoagulation with UFH or LMWH followed by long course anticoagulation with warfarin, LMWH, or an antiplatelet agent.

Cerebral venous sinus thrombosis (CVST) can present with a variety of conditions including seizures, signs of increased ICP, or headache. Subdural effusion or hematoma, subarachnoid hemorrhage, intracranial hemorrhage, and infarction have also been described. Infection is also a well-known cause of septic venous thrombosis in older children, associated with infections such as otitis media and meningitis. Between one- and two-thirds of children with a CVST are found to have a hypercoagulable disorder, the majority of which are inherited rather than acquired. Treatment in the initial phase is supportive, with control of epileptic activity, control of ICP, hydration, and antibiotics, if appropriate. Special attention should be paid to evaluation of vision and visual fields in these children, as the CVST may be an acute presentation of a chronic process and patients may have had long-standing increased ICP. Diagnosis is made with CT venogram or MRI venogram. Patients who are unconscious or mechanically ventilated should have continuous EEG monitoring given the high incidence of seizures in these patients. As with ischemic stroke patients, thrombolytic therapy should be considered in consultation with a specialized stroke team, and for patients with CVST it is reasonable to consider anticoagulation with IV UFH or subcutaneous LMWH, regardless of associated secondary hemorrhage.

Kenet G, Strauss T, Kaplinsky C, Paret G: Hemostasis and thrombosis in critically ill children. *Semin Thromb Hemost.* 2008;34:451-458 [PMID: 18956285].

Kerlin BA: Current and future management of pediatric venous thromboembolism. *Am J Hematol.* 2012;87:S68-S74 [PMID:22367975].

Macartney CA, Chan AKC: Thrombosis in children. *Semin Thromb Hemost.* 2011;37:763-771 [PMID: 22187399].

Roach ES, Golomb MR, Adams R, et al: Management of stroke in infants and children: A scientific statement from a special writing group of the American Heart Association Stroke Council and the Council on Cardiovascular Disease in the Young. *Stroke.* 2008;39:2644-2691 [PMID: 18635845].

▼ ONCOLOGIC EMERGENCIES

HEMATOLOGIC MALIGNANCIES

Hematologic malignancies are the most common cause of childhood cancer, accounting for 25-30% of cancer diagnoses. Leukemia is categorized as lymphoid (lymphoblastic, lymphocytic) or myeloid (myelogenous, myelocytic, myeloblastic, acute nonlymphoblastic). Acute lymphoblastic leukemia (ALL) is the most common diagnosis in younger children with peak incidence of 2-5 years. Children presenting with hematologic malignancies range from well-appearing to critically ill.

Symptoms of leukemia can be vague and nonspecific; however, the diagnosis should be considered in a child who presents with unexplained persistent fever, weight loss, fatigue, or bone pain. On physical examination, the child may be tired or ill-appearing, have pallor, unexplained bleeding or bruising, hepatomegaly and/or splenomegaly, lymphadenopathy. Less frequently, leukemia or lymphoma may present with a mediastinal mass, resulting in symptoms of superior vena cava (SVC) syndrome such as facial swelling, venous congestion, or respiratory or circulatory compromise. A child with acute myelogenous leukemia (AML) may present with gingival hyperplasia or extramedullary collections of blast cells called chloromas, appearing as discrete bluish areas in the subcutaneous tissues.

The diagnosis of leukemia is made by the presence of blast forms on CBC or suggested by suppression of at least two hematologic cell lines. Other disease processes, such as viral infections or aplastic anemia, can present with suppression of hematologic cell lines, and therefore the diagnosis should be considered in the context of the clinical presentation. Definitive diagnosis is made by bone marrow aspiration and examination. When a diagnosis is suggested by CBC, further studies should be obtained, as listed in Table 40-6.

LYMPHOMA

Lymphoma is the third most common pediatric malignancy. The most common type, Hodgkin lymphoma, is seen in adolescents (15-19 years). The remaining types are grouped

Table 40–6. Checklist for known or suspected new diagnosis of acute leukemia.

History and careful physical examination.
Measure accurate height and weight.
Place peripheral IV line(s) for supportive care (unless mediastinal mass suspected, then consider chest radiography first).
Laboratory evaluation • CBC with manual differential; Peripheral smear. • Critical chemistries: uric acid, creatinine, potassium, phosphorus, calcium. • Coagulation profile: prothrombin time (PT), partial thromboplastin time (PTT), fibrinogen; Type and screen. • If febrile, blood culture (aerobic, anaerobic, and fungal).
Obtain chest radiograph.
Start hydration at 125 mL/m²/h unless fluid load contraindicated. • Order alkalinized fluids (D5¼NS with 30 mEq/L sodium bicarbonate). • Start available fluid (D5½NS) and run until alkalinized fluid available. • Do not give potassium.
Start allopurinol.
If febrile, start empirical broad-spectrum antibiotic (ceftazidime 50 mg/kg IV).
Order and initiate blood products as indicated • If bleeding, give platelets, FFP, or cryoprecipitate. • If severely anemic, start slow transfusion of PRBC.

as non-Hodgkin lymphoma (NHL), including Burkitt lymphoma, precursor T- or B-cell lymphoblastic lymphoma, diffuse large B-cell lymphoma, and anaplastic large cell lymphoma. Lymphomas are uncommonly diagnosed in children younger than 5 years.

Lymphoma may be suspected in patients presenting with painless lymphadenopathy enlarging over a period of days to months, unresponsive to antibiotics, and accompanied by symptoms that include fever, night sweats, weight loss, and physical findings of abdominal mass or pleural effusion. History of difficulty breathing, wheezing, or orthopnea should prompt investigations for mediastinal mass (Figure 40–1), which are common in Hodgkin and non-Hodgkin lymphoma. It is important to note that lack of associated symptoms does not rule out lymphoma.

Solid Tumors

Central nervous system (CNS) tumors are the most common solid organ tumors in children. As with all malignancies, there can be a wide spectrum of symptoms on presentation. The most common complaint at presentation is headache, but children may also present with seizures, vomiting, or other signs of increased ICP. Tumors may manifest symptoms

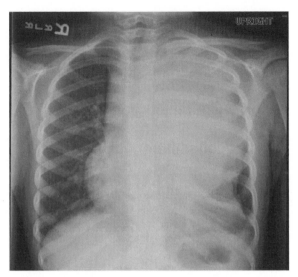

▲ **Figure 40–1.** Mediastinal mass on initial diagnosis of acute lymphoblastic leukemia (ALL).

from the location and tissue impacted, such as eye findings, diabetes insipidus when suprasellar, other endocrine disorders when located in the pituitary, for example. Only a small number of children who present with isolated complaint of headache will have an intracranial mass, and the practitioners may be challenged to determine if neuroimaging is indicated.

When an intracranial mass is identified, initial emergency department care should focus on identification and treatment of increased ICP. Children at risk of herniation may have all or part of Cushing triad (hypertension, bradycardia, altered respirations), mental status changes, or findings suggestive of cranial nerve palsy. Vital sign abnormalities indicate increased ICP leading to herniation, and these patients should be aggressively managed. Initial focus is on securing airway using CNS protective preparation, breathing, and circulation, with measures taken to decrease ICP. The head of the bed should be elevated and 3% normal saline bolus in the initial amount of 5 mL/kg administered. Methylprednisolone 2 mg/kg IV is indicated for a mass identified on neuroimaging which is causing edema and signs of herniation. Emergent consultation with a neurosurgeon is indicated.

Solid tumors encountered less frequently include abdominal masses such as Wilms tumor, neuroblastoma, and bone and soft tissue tumors. These tumors are most commonly diagnosed in children younger than 5 years. Wilms tumor presents as a painless abdominal mass. Neuroblastoma may present similarly, or may be accompanied by symptoms due to catecholamine release from the tumor, including hypertension and tachycardia. Metastases are present in 50% of children; the most common sites are bone, bone marrow, and liver. Children with neuroblastoma rarely present

with opsoclonus-myoclonus, with abnormal eye movement, ataxia, and myoclonic jerks.

Bone and soft tissue tumors comprise approximately 12% of childhood malignancies. They most frequently present as unilateral bone pain and/or swelling without a history of trauma. Tumor should be suspected in children who present with pain that awakens them, pain that does not improve with rest, or progressively worsens over time. In addition, diagnosis should be considered with pathologic fractures, in which a patient sustains a fracture after apparently minor injuries or in a bone that is not frequently fractured. For osteosarcoma, plain radiographs are indicated as the initial diagnostic test. Soft tissue tumors such as rhabdomyosarcoma require CT or MRI to characterize the mass.

Arndt CAS, Rose PS, Folpe AL, Laack NN: Common musculoskeletal tumors of childhood and adolescence. *Mayo Clin Proc.* 2012;87:5,475-487 [PMID: 22560526].

Kaatsch P: Epidemiology of childhood cancer. *Cancer Treatment Rev.* 2010;36:277-285 [PMID: 20231056].

Nazemi KJ, Malempati S: Emergency department presentation of childhood cancer. *Emerg Med Clin N Am.* 2009;27:477-495 [PMID: 19646649].

EMERGENCIES ASSOCIATED WITH PRESENTATION OF MALIGNANCY

Hyperleukocytosis

Hyperleukocytosis is defined as WBC count at presentation greater than 100,000/µL. It occurs most commonly in acute leukemia; in 9-13% with acute nonlymphoblastic leukemia and in most with chronic myelogenous leukemia. It may be detected on CBC or patients may present with symptoms of leukostasis. Most commonly affected are the respiratory and central nervous systems. Respiratory symptoms result from increased blood viscosity that cause sludging of the pulmonary vasculature as well as increased oxygen requirement of excessive numbers of leukocytes. Patients may have complaint of exertional dyspnea or exhibit respiratory distress. Neurologic manifestations range from mild to severe, including headache, confusion, and coma or intracranial hemorrhage.

Hyperleukocytosis is treated with leukapheresis, a type of apheresis in which blood is withdrawn from the patient, leukocytes removed, and the filtered blood transfused back to the patient. It is considered when the total WBC is greater than 100,000/µL or patient is symptomatic. A pediatric oncologist and pediatric intensivist should be emergently consulted to advise if leukapheresis should be initiated and to discuss initiation of chemotherapy. Initial emergency department management includes hydration with attention to fluid balance and monitoring for signs of respiratory distress. RBC transfusion should be avoided unless absolutely necessary due to increased risk for hyperviscosity and attendant complications.

Tumor Lysis Syndrome

Tumor lysis syndrome can occur prior to or after the initiation of therapy for malignancy. Cancers with a high tumor burden are most at risk for this syndrome. In pediatric patients, lymphoma and leukemia are the malignancies with the highest incidence. The most common predisposing factor for the syndrome is dehydration, hence the inclusion of aggressive hydration in pediatric protocols for induction chemotherapy for malignancies such as Burkitt lymphoma, traditionally associated with a high tumor burden. The syndrome is a result of lysing of cancer cells and the release of potassium, phosphorus, and nucleic acids, which are metabolized to uric acid. Laboratory abnormalities include hyperkalemia, hyperphosphatemia, hyperuricemia, and hypocalcemia. Clinical findings include increased creatinine level, seizures, cardiac arrhythmias, and death.

Treatment of tumor lysis syndrome begins with hydration. Patients should initially receive IV fluids at a rate of 2500-3000 mL/m^2 per day. Alkalization has not been shown to add significant benefit. If, after hydration, patients have suboptimal urine output, use of a loop diuretic, such as furosemide, is recommended, with a goal of urine output at 2 mL/kg/h. Additional emergency treatment is focused on managing electrolyte abnormalities with potential to cause serious complications or death. Hyperkalemia can lead to cardiac dysrhythmias and death. Initial treatments include polystyrene sulfonate, administered to function as a potassium binder, glucose with insulin, or β-agonists, and calcium gluconate. Hypocalcaemia may lead to dysrhythmias, and should be managed with calcium at the lowest possible doses, because of the risk of calcium phosphate crystallization and subsequent renal injury. Asymptomatic hypocalcaemia does not require treatment. Patients with evidence of kidney injury and elevated creatinine, suboptimal urine output, or refractory hyperkalemia should be considered for hemodialysis. Patients diagnosed with tumor lysis syndrome will be admitted under care of a pediatric oncologist. Subsequent treatment with allopurinol and rasburicase to reduce levels of uric acid is recommended.

Howard SC, Jones DP, Pui CH: The tumor lysis syndrome. *N Engl J Med.* 2011;364:19 [PMID: 21561350].

SUPERIOR VENA CAVA SYNDROME/SUPERIOR MEDIASTINAL SYNDROME

Superior vena cava (SVC) syndrome presents due to compression of the SVC from tumors arising from the mediastinum or lymph nodes. Patients with SVC syndrome may present with significant facial and neck swelling, plethora, cyanosis, and jugular venous distension. Significant edema can result in compression of the larynx or pharyngeal lumen, causing stridor, dyspnea, or dysphagia. SVC syndrome with tracheal compression is known as superior mediastinal syndrome. In pediatric patients, malignancies associated with the condition include non-Hodgkin lymphoma, Hodgkin disease, acute lymphoblastic leukemia, neuroblastoma, Ewing sarcoma, malignant teratoma, thyroid cancer, rhabdomyosarcoma, and primitive neuroectodermal tumors (PNET). Initial imaging by chest radiograph may show widening of the anterior mediastinum and displacement or compression of the trachea. Patients may also have associated pleural or pericardial effusion. Pleurocentesis may offer symptomatic relief, but should be undertaken cautiously in patients with suspected T-cell lymphoma, as removal of large volumes may cause cardiovascular decompensation. Emergent imaging by CT to characterize extent of compression is indicated, but with precaution in patients in whom compression may be worsened by being sedated and supine. If there has been no previous diagnosis of malignancy, consultation with a pediatric oncologist is advised prior to initiating treatment.

HYPERCALCEMIA

Hypercalcemia is an uncommon oncologic emergency in children, seen in approximately 1% of pediatric malignant disease. Pre-B cell ALL is the most common associated malignancy. In children, it is most often mediated by either secretion of parathyroid hormone-related peptide (PTHrP), direct osteolytic effect by the tumor on bone, or both. Initial presentation can be nonspecific, and symptoms depend on whether the hypercalcemia has developed acutely or chronically. Initial symptoms may include constipation, lethargy, or abdominal pain, but may progress to shortened QT interval on electrocardiogram (ECG) or arrhythmia, acute renal failure, seizures, coma, or death. Diagnosis is made by obtaining an ionized calcium level. Total serum calcium is not as reliable due to the relationship between serum albumin and calcium.

Management of hypercalcemia begins with IV fluids. Patients should receive normal saline at 2-3 L/m^2/day, if cardiovascular status permits. When the patient has clinically reached a euvolemic state, thiazide diuretics are administered to facilitate calcium excretion. Bisphosphonates are also used to bind calcium, and are used with increased frequency in pediatric patients, although data is limited. These should be used with caution if renal insufficiency is present, but may be useful in patients who are acutely symptomatic with life-threatening complications such as arrhythmias or seizures. In patients with ALL presenting with hypercalcemia, the mainstay of treatment is induction chemotherapy and may alone be sufficient for treatment. For a small number of cancer patients, hypercalcemia can be attributed to overproduction of vitamin D. This is most often seen in the setting of lymphoma. For these patients, steroids may be helpful for management of the hypercalcemia.

Sargent JTS, Smith OP: Haematological emergencies managing hypercalcaemia in adults and children with haematological disorders. *Brit J Haematol.* 2010;149:465-477 [PMID: 20377591].

FEVER & NEUTROPENIA

Chemotherapy as treatment of malignancy often results in periods of immunosuppression evidenced by low WBCs. Patients are at increased risk for infection, sepsis, and death. Early recognition and timely, aggressive treatment is imperative to prevent deterioration (Figure 40–2). In addition, a small but measurable number of newly diagnosed cancer patients present with fever and concurrently have serious bacterial illness.

The generally accepted definition of fever in cancer patients is temperature of 38.3°C (101°F) or two measurements of 38°. Rectal temperatures are not advised in these patients due to theoretical risk of harm to mucosal integrity, subsequent translocation of gastrointestinal flora with abnormal immune protection. In the setting of drug-induced neutropenia, neutropenia is defined at an absolute neutrophil count less than 500/μL or 1000/μL with a further expected decline.

An identified source for infection is found in 10-30% of patients with fever and neutropenia. However, of those patients, 85-90% of infections are due to gram-positive or gram-negative bacteria. Therefore, broad-spectrum empiric antimicrobial coverage is indicated. Pathogens to consider include flora from mucosal surfaces or from gastrointestinal translocation. In addition, methicillin-resistant *S. aureus* (MRSA) and vancomycin-resistant enterococcus (VRE) should be considered. Viral infections can result in severe disease in this patient population as well. Fungal pathogens

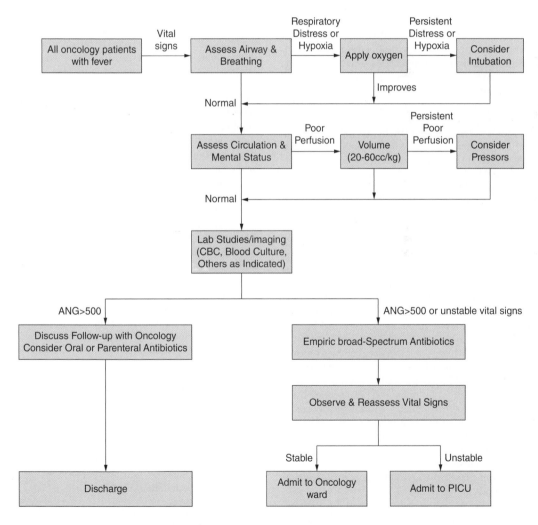

▲ **Figure 40–2.** General approach to the febrile pediatric oncology patient. CBC, complete blood count; PICU, pediatric intensive care unit.

are more likely if the child has had prolonged neutropenia, relapsed disease, or has received high-dose or prolonged treatment with steroids. *Pneumocystis jirovecii*, a protozoan, is an important pathogen for those who have prolonged immunosuppression, postbone marrow transplant, and when immunologic deficiency is from active human immunodeficiency virus (HIV).

Characteristics have been identified for children who are at increased risk for serious complications including sepsis and death when presenting with fever and neutropenia. Risk factors include history of relapsed leukemia, poorly controlled solid malignancies, patient receiving cytarabine as part of their chemotherapeutic regimen, and age younger than 1 year. In addition, children who present with clinical findings of pneumonitis, severe mucositis, shock, dehydration, hypotension, or respiratory distress are more likely to have poor outcomes. Factors that may place patients at lower risk include temperature less than 39°C, monocyte counts greater than 1000/μL, lack of medical comorbidity, anticipated short duration of neutropenia (< 7 days), or malignancies other than AML. However, current evidence-based guidelines do not exist regarding stratification and treatment of children as high- or low-risk, and most children with fever and neutropenia are admitted on broad-spectrum antibiotics pending culture results and increase in neutrophil count.

Initial management should be undertaken in consultation with the patient's primary care oncologist, if possible. Initial treatment is directed toward cardiopulmonary assessment with careful attention to signs of compensated shock. Respiratory support is provided with supplemental oxygen and assisted ventilation, if indicated, and cardiovascular support by means of IV fluids and vasoactive medications to treat hypotension or poor perfusion. If transfusion of PRBC is required, either as part of resuscitation or indicated by low Hb on CBC, cells should be irradiated and leukocyte reduced. If these products are not available, transfusion should be delayed in an otherwise stable patient pending transfer to definitive care at another facility. RBC transfusion in patients with fever and neutropenia should be considered for Hb less than 7 g/dL. However, if the patient is symptomatic with tachycardia, tachypnea, or hypotension, or has thrombocytopenia with a source of bleeding identified, transfusion should be considered at levels greater than 7 g/dL. General guidelines for transfusion platelets are listed in Table 40–7. Laboratory studies including cultures of blood (from each lumen of the central line, if applicable), urine, and any other relevant areas should be obtained and broad-spectrum antibiotic coverage initiated. Since it is important to establish end-organ involvement if sepsis is suspected, serum chemistries and stat results of blood gases are very beneficial.

Antibiotic choice will vary based upon institutional and provider practice patterns. Commonly employed regimens include monotherapy with broad-spectrum β-lactam

Table 40–7. Platelet transfusion guidelines.

Suggested Transfusion Level (cells/mm³)	Condition
< 10	Asymptomatic
< 20	Minor bleeding
< 100	Major bleeding (hemoptysis, GI or CNS bleed)
< 50	CNS tumor
< 10-20	Diagnostic LP
< 50-100	Surgical procedure

antibiotics with antipseudomonal coverage, such as cephalosporins (ceftazidime, cefepime) or carbapenems (imipenem, meropenem). Additional considerations include risk for *Streptococcus viridans*, a pathogen associated with treatment with high-dose cytarabine and associated with significant antibiotic resistance. Vancomycin should be added in these patients, as well as for patients with a history of exposure or infection with MRSA, a central line, and any signs of infection, including induration, erythema, or tenderness of the overlying skin. Use of antivirals and antifungals is not routinely indicated in the emergency department and decisions regarding their use can be made in consultation with the patient's oncologist.

It is important to note that administration of antibiotics can precipitate clinical deterioration in a patient with fever and neutropenia, due to lysis of bacteria and subsequent inflammatory response. This makes vigilant monitoring key with aggressive fluid replacement in response to persistent evidence of ongoing Systemic Inflammatory Response, unless the child has problems with handling parental fluid therapy. Patients are also at risk for allergic reaction to medications or transfusion of blood products. Patients receiving antibiotics should be closely monitored during administration and for a period of time afterward prior to transfer from the ED.

REFERENCES

Behl D, Wahner Hendrickson A, Moynihan TJ: Oncologic emergencies. *Crit Care Clin.* 2010;26:181-205 [PMID: 19944281].

Meckler G, Lindemulder S: Fever and neutropenia in pediatric patients with cancer. *Emerg Med Clin N Am.* 2009;27:525-544 [PMID: 19646652].

Meyer S, Reinhard H, Gottschling S: Pulmonary dysfunction in pediatric oncology patients. *Pediatric Hematol Oncol.* 2004;21:175-195 [PMID: 15160517].

Sadowitz PD, Amanullah S, Souid AK: Hematologic emergencies in the pediatric emergency room. *Emerg Med Clin N Am.* 2002;20:1 [PMID: 11826633].

Infectious Diseases

41

Ian D. Kane, MD

Cristina M. Estrada, MD

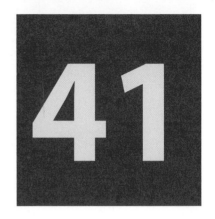

SEPTIC SHOCK

ESSENTIALS OF DIAGNOSIS

▶ Evidence of poor end-organ perfusion (altered mental status).

▶ Hypotension.

▶ Prolonged capillary refill.

▶ Abnormal oxygen saturation) with an infectious source.

Initial management is focused on ABCs (see Chapter 10).

General Considerations

Systemic inflammatory response syndrome (SIRS) may be provoked by a number of infectious and noninfectious causes. It occurs when at least two of the following criteria are met: fever greater than 38.5°C or less than 36°C; tachycardia or bradycardia for age; tachypnea for age, or leukocytosis or leukopenia (Table 41–1). Sepsis occurs when SIRS is caused by an infectious agent. Septic shock falls at the extreme end of this continuum and results when end-organ perfusion becomes compromised. Failure to correct this imbalance of nutrient delivery with nutrient demand leads to end-organ dysfunction and ultimately end-organ damage. Younger children and those with impaired immune systems are at increased risk of sepsis and rapid progression to shock.

Clinical Findings

Most children are classified as having "cold" shock, which occurs with low cardiac output in the setting of high systemic vascular resistance. Signs of cold shock include tachycardia, delayed capillary refill, cool and mottled extremities, and weak peripheral pulses. Unlike adults, children have the ability to increase their heart rate greatly to compensate for poor cardiac output; hypotension may be a late finding of shock. Some children will have "warm" shock, which occurs with high cardiac output and decreased systemic vascular resistance. These children may have flash capillary refill, widened pulse pressure, bounding pulses, and warm extremities. However, in each case, perfusion is not adequate, and evidence of end-organ dysfunction will manifest. Decreased perfusion to the brain leads to irritability and lethargy in infants and younger children, and to altered mental status in older children. Similarly, poor kidney perfusion leads to decreased urine output. During the later stages of fluid resuscitation, evidence of volume overload such as rales, hepatomegaly, peripheral edema may develop.

Laboratory Tests/Radiographs

Because tissue perfusion is compromised, a full comprehensive metabolic profile (CMP) with coagulation studies is recommended so that liver and kidney function may be established. Complete blood (cell) count (CBC) with differential may show leukocytosis with neutrophilic predominance in bacterial infections, though infants may have leukopenia in this situation. An initial blood gas with a lactate is important for assessing the degree of hypoperfusion as well as the patient's respiratory status. Glucose levels should be monitored frequently, particularly in infants. Inflammatory markers such as erythrocyte sedimentation rate (ESR), C-reactive protein (CRP), and procalcitonin are invariably elevated but may be of value as a baseline. Comprehensive viral and bacterial cultures from the blood, urine, and cerebrospinal fluid (CSF) are helpful for guiding long-term management including duration of antibiotic therapy but should not delay antibiotic administration. A chest x-ray (CXR) is of value when a

Table 41–1. Normal pediatric vital signs.

Age	Heart Rate (per min)	Systolic Blood Pressure (mm Hg)	Respiratory Rate (per min)
Newborn	100-170	50-80	30-60
1-12 mo	80-140	70-100	25-40
1-3 yr	80-130	80-110	25-35
3-5 yr	75-120	80-110	20-30
6-12 yr	70-110	80-120	18-30
≥ 13 yr	60-100	90-120	12-20

respiratory source is suspected or to check for cardiomegaly or signs of fluid overload. A random serum cortisol level can assess for adrenal insufficiency.

Treatment

Initial management includes a survey of airway, breathing, and circulation (ABCs). Supplemental oxygen should be provided and preparations made for intubation among patients unable to protect their airway. The patient should be placed onto continuous monitoring including pulse oximetry and IV access should be obtained. In true emergent situations, if conventional access cannot be obtained within 90 seconds, an intraosseous line should be placed. If sedation is needed, ketamine is a preferred agent due to its lack of hemodynamic effects. Etiomidate has been associated with adrenocortical depression and should be avoided if possible in patients with septic shock. Preparations should be made for admission to the pediatric intensive care unit (ICU) after the patient is stabilized.

Rapid restoration of circulating volume is essential for successful shock management. Up to three 20 cc/kg normal saline (NS) boluses should be administered, and the patient's pulse, capillary refill, mental status, urine output, and blood pressure should be monitored closely. Additional fluids may be given as NS, packed red blood cells (PRBC), or albumin. Volume overload is generally of secondary concern provided that congenital heart, lung, or kidney disease is not suspected.

If the patient does not have adequate response to 60 cc/kg or more of fluid administration, inotropic and vasopressor support with a dopamine infusion is indicated. Resistant cold shock may require the addition of epinephrine whereas warm shock may respond to norepinephrine. Peripheral arterial access as well as central access is necessary in these cases for continued monitoring. Persistent shock despite maximal support is often treated with empiric hydrocortisone for absolute or relative adrenocortical insufficiency.

Early administration of broad-spectrum antiobiotic therapy is vital and choice of agent is based on the patient age

and risk factors. Infants aged younger than 1 month should receive vancomycin or ampicillin, and gentamicin or cefotaxime, and acyclovir. Children older than 1 month should receive vancomycin and cefotaxime or ceftriaxone. Children with immunosuppression should receive antipseudomonal coverage with a fourth-generation cephalosporin such as cefepime. Anaerobic coverage with clindamycin or metronidazole should be considered for children with a suspected intra-abdominal source of infection.

Aneja RK, Varughese-Aneja R, Vetterly, et al: Antibiotic therapy in neonatal and pediatric septic shock. *Curr Infect Dis Rep.* 2011;13(5):433 [PMID: 21732046].

Fisher JD, Nelson DG, Beyersdorf H, et al: Clinical spectrum of shock in the pediatric emergency department. *Pediatr Emerg Care.* 2010;26(9):622 [PMID: 20805778].

Simpson JN, Teach SJ: Pediatric rapid fluid resuscitation. *Curr Opin Pediatr.* 2011;23(3):286 [PMID: 21508842].

Yager P, Noviski N: Shock. *Pediatr Rev.* 2010;31(8):311 [PMID: 20679096].

EMERGENCY TREATMENT OF SPECIFIC DISORDERS

FEVER (0-60 DAYS OF AGE)

 ESSENTIALS OF DIAGNOSIS

▶ Temperature > 38°C or < 36°C.

▶ Lethargy.

▶ Poor feeding.

▶ Jaundice.

▶ Seizures.

▶ Apnea.

▶ Tachycardia.

Treat with empiric antibiotics.

General Considerations

Fever in infants younger than 2 months is a common presentation for emergency department physicians. Of primary concern are infants who present with fever due to a serious bacterial infection (SBI), including bacteremia, urinary tract infection (UTI), omphalitis, and meningitis. However, since the widespread implementation of the *Hemophilus influenzae* type B virus (HIB), pneumococcal, and meningococcal vaccines, incidence of SBI, specifically meningitis, has fallen dramatically among febrile infants. Typical pathogens include group B *Streptococcus* (GBS), *Eshericia coli*, and *Listeria*, although *Listeria* remains rare. The most common SBI in this group is UTI. Despite the fact that invasive disease is rare, the devastating consequences

Table 41–2. Management of well-appearing neonates < 90 days of age.

Criteria	Rochester	Philadelphia	Boston
Age	< 60 d	29-60 d	28-89 d
Temperature	>38°C	>38.2°C	>38°C
Low-risk laboratory values	5,000/μL < WBC < 15,000/μL UA< 10 WBC/HPF Absolute band count < 1500/μL < 5 WBC/HPF in stool if diarrhea	WBC < 15,000/μL UA < 10 WBC/HPF Band:neutrophil ratio < 0.2 Stool with few/no bacteria CXR: no infiltrate Urine Gram stain negative CSF Gram stain negative CSF < 8 WBC/μL	WBC < 20,000/μL UA < 10 WBC/HPF CXR: no infiltrate CSF < 10 WBC/μL
Disposition if low risk	Discharge home with follow-up No antibiotics	Discharge home with follow-up No antibiotics	Discharge home with follow-up Empiric antibiotics

of a missed SBI in this age group demand conservative treatment, and until recently, it was recommended that infants younger than 60 days remain hospitalized on parenteral antibiotics until cultures were finalized. Clinical decision rules such as the Rochester, Boston, and Philadelphia criteria stratify high-and low-risk infants (Table 41–2). The decision rules were developed so that a cohort of "low-risk" infants, defined as healthy term infants with normal blood, urine, and CSF studies, could be managed as outpatients or as inpatients without antibiotics. Clinical history includes birth history—gestational age, maternal labs, history of maternal fever or chorioamnionitis, previous antibiotic use, sick contacts, and maternal HSV infection. A mother with known negative GBS status does not lower the risk of SBI in her child.

Clinical Findings

Fever, a rectal temperature above 38°C, may be the only presenting symptom. However, hypothermia below 36°C is equivalent to fever in this age group. Physical examination includes assessment of airway, breathing, and circulation (ABCs), as these infants are prone to apnea, cyanosis, and shock due to sepsis. Overall clinical impression is critical, as the clinical decision rules apply only to "well-appearing" infants. Lethargy, poor feeding, unexplained jaundice, petechial rash, grunting, and tachypnea are concerning findings; however, these may be absent even in ill infants.

Laboratory Tests/Radiographs

Most commonly used clinical decision rules are a combination of laboratory values, including CBC with differential, urinalysis, catheterized urine culture, blood culture, and CSF studies (Gram stain, protein, glucose, and CSF culture). All infants younger than 28 days should have a complete "septic workup," which consists of blood, urine, and CSF cultures, in addition to the CBC or other ancillary testing. Herpes simplex virus polymerase chain reaction (HSV PCR) from the CSF should be considered in all infants younger than 3 weeks and those with a potential exposure. During times of endemic infection, typically the summer, enteroviral PCR may also be sent from the CSF. Additional viral studies such as rapid influenza or respiratory syncytial virus (RSV) antigen testing may be considered; however, a positive result does not preclude the need for further studies, particularly among infants younger than 1 month. Pertussis direct fluorescent antibody (DFA) is indicated for infants with characteristic staccato cough or known exposure. Stool studies (Gram stain, stool leukocytes, and stool culture) may be added if diarrhea is a prominent feature and a CXR should be performed if there are focal findings on the respiratory examination.

Treatment

Ill-appearing infants should have all cultures drawn immediately so that broad-spectrum empiric antibiotics (ampicillin in combination with cefotaxime or gentamicin) may be started. Well-appearing infants (0-60 days) because of their immature immune systems, unvaccinated status, and inability to demonstrate reliable physical examination findings of serious illness may be treated conservatively in the emergency department with antibiotics and admission while blood, urine, and CSF cultures are pending. If HSV studies are sent, acyclovir should also be initiated.

Evidence suggests that it is appropriate to treat low-risk febrile infants aged 30-60 days expectantly provided there is reliable follow-up within 12-24 hours. In these children a blood culture, urine culture, CBC with differential, and urinalysis are essential; CSF studies may be deferred. Alternatively, CSF studies may be obtained and the patient discharged with close follow-up. Consideration may be given to using a long-acting IM cephalosporin such as ceftriaxone to provide the patient with 24 hours of antibiotic coverage after emergency department discharge.

Baker MD, Bell LM, Avner JR: The efficacy of routine outpatient management without antibiotics of fever in selected infants. *Pediatrics.* 1999;103(3):627-631 [PMID: 10049967].

Baskin MN, O'Rourke EJ, Fleisher GR: Outpatient treatment of febrile infants 28 to 89 days of age with intramuscular administration of ceftriaxone. *J Pediatr.* 1992;120(1):22-27 [PMID:1731019].

Ferguson CC, Roosevelt G, Bajaj L: Practice patterns of pediatric emergency medicine physicians caring for young febrile infants. *Clin Pediatr.* 2010;49(4):350-354 [PMID: 19564450].

Huppler AR, Eickhoff JC, Wald ER: Performance of low-risk criteria in the evaluation of young infants with fever: Review of the literature. *Pediatrics.* 2010;125(2):223-233 [PMID: 20083517].

Jaskiewicz JA, McCarthy CA, Richardson AC, et al: Febrile infants at low risk for serious bacterial infection: An appraisal of the Rochester criteria and implications for management. Febrile Infant Collaborative Study Group. *Pediatrics.* 1994;94(3): 390-396 [PMID: 8065869].

Meehan WP, Fleeger E, Bachur RG: Adherence to guidelines for managing the well-appearing febrile infant: Assessment using a case-based, interactive survey. *Pediatr Emerg Care.* 2010;26(12):875-880 [PMID: 21088637].

Morley EJ, Lapoint JM, Roy LW, et al: Rates of positive blood, urine, and cerebrospinal fluid cultures in children younger than 60 days during the vaccination era. *Pediatr Emerg Care.* 2012;28(2):125-130 [PMID: 22270498].

FEVER 60 DAYS-36 MONTHS

ESSENTIALS OF DIAGNOSIS

▶ Fever >39°C.

▶ Altered mental status.

▶ Tachycardia.

▶ Tachypnea.

▶ Lethargy.

Empiric antibiotics are usually unnecessary in the well-appearing infant. Consider occult UTI.

General Considerations

Children aged 2-36 months with fever are at less risk of SBI, and children in this group with bacteremia are less likely to develop complications such as osteomyelitis or septic arthritis. Meningitis, however rare, remains of concern due to the potential for neurologic sequelae. Rather than rely heavily on clinical prediction rules, the physician has greater latitude to tailor the diagnostic workup based on the patient presentation.

Although most fevers are viral in origin, the most common bacterial pathogen causing bacteremia and meningitis is *S. pneumoniae. E. coli* and other gram-negative bacteria are the causative agents of UTIs, the most common cause of SBI in this group. Among well-appearing children, the history and physical examination should address potential occult sources of bacterial infection.

Clinical Findings

Fever in this age group is defined as greater than 39°C; however, infants aged 2-3 months are held to a more conservative standard of greater than 38°C, particularly those who are not vaccinated. Ill-appearing children with fever and sepsis may be hypotensive, tachycardic, lethargic, or have altered mental status. Pneumonia is suggested by tachypnea, rales, oxygen saturation less than 95%, and respiratory distress, whereas history of trauma and unwillingness to move an extremity suggests osteomyelitis or septic arthritis. Children with UTI may have complaint of vomiting or diarrhea in addition to dysuria and abdominal pain. The skin should be examined carefully for signs of abscess or cellulitis, and the potential for otitis media (OM) should be evaluated.

Laboratory Tests/Radiographs

Infants aged 2-3 months should have a screening CBC with differential, blood culture, and catheterized urinalysis with culture. Procalcitonin is a relatively new inflammatory marker that has superior sensitivity and specificity for identifying SBIs among children without a clear source. However, little data exists as to its efficacy, as one study revealed that there was no impact on antibiotic usage in children aged 1-36 months who presented with fever without a source. CSF studies and CXR are considered at the physician discretion. Viral studies such as rapid influenza, RSV antigen, and pertussis DFA may also be ordered. Rapid *Streptococcus* antigen testing should be considered for children older than 2 years with a known exposure.

Treatment

As with infants, a full septic evaluation including blood, urine, and CSF cultures is indicated for ill-appearing children and or those with vital sign instability. Well-appearing infants aged 2-3 months require a CBC with differential, blood culture, urinalysis, and urine culture. CSF studies may be deferred as long as careful follow-up is ensured. Management of these children may include observation with no antibiotics in the hospital or discharged with a long-acting IM antibiotic.

Children aged 3-36 months may be managed less conservatively; however, the possibility of an occult UTI must be considered. A catheterized urinalysis with culture should be performed on all females younger than 24 months, uncircumcised males younger than 12 months, and circumcised males younger than 6 months. Unvaccinated and undervaccinated children should have a CBC with differential and a blood culture obtained. In children, a WBC count greater than 25,000 cells/mm³ has been associated with increased risk of pneumonia, and CXR should be considered. Well-appearing children with an abnormal urinalysis may be treated empirically for UTI and discharged provided that a urine culture is obtained.

Andreola B, Bressan S, Callegaro S, et al: Procalcitonin and C-reactive protein as diagnostic markers of severe bacterial infections in febrile infants and children in the emergency department. *Pediatr Infect Dis J.* 2007;26(8):672-677 [PMID: 17848876].

Bressan S, Berlese P, Mion T, et al: Bacteremia in feverish children presenting to the emergency department: A retrospective study and literature review. *Acta Paediatr.* 2012;101(3):271-277 [PMID: 21950707].

Colvin JM, Jaffe DM, Muenzer JT: Evaluation of the precision of emergency department diagnoses in young children with fever. *Clin Pediatr.* 2012;51(1):51-57 [PMID: 21868591].

Ishimine P: Fever without source in children 0 to 36 months of age. *Pediatr Clin North Am.* 2006;53(2):167-194 [PMID: 16574521].

Mansano S, Benoit B, Girodias J, et al: Impact of procalcitonin on the management of children aged 1-36 months presenting with fever without source: A randomized controlled trial. *Am J Emerg Med.* 2010;28:647-653 [PMID: 20637377].

Wilkinson M, Bulloch B, Smith M: Prevalence of occult bacteremia in children aged 3 to 36 months presenting to the emergency department with fever in the postpneumococcal conjugate vaccine era. *Acad Emerg Med.* 2009;16(3):220-225 [PMID:19133844].

FEVER (> 3 YEARS), FEBRILE NEUTROPENIA & LINE INFECTIONS

 ESSENTIALS OF DIAGNOSIS

▶ Fever > 39°C.

▶ Tachycardia.

▶ Irritability.

History of immunosuppression demands more conservative management.

General Considerations

Fever greater than 39°C in children older than 3 years is generally viral in origin, and children with SBIs typically have signs and symptoms that help identify source of infection. Among vaccinated children in this age group, the rates of SBI are exceedingly low (< 1%). However, a careful history often uncovers specific risk factors that make an older child with fever more likely to have an SBI. Children in this age group are often able to describe their symptoms, rendering routine screening tests unnecessary in most.

Relatively common SBIs of childhood include pneumonia, osteomyelitis, UTIs, and meningitis. *Staphylococcus* and *Pneumococcus* species are the most common etiologic agents of non-urologic bacterial infections. A careful history and physical examination is paramount in determining how to proceed with a diagnostic workup. Details that raise the potential for serious disease include history of delayed or missing immunizations, recent travel to areas of known endemic disease, chronic steroid use, medically complex children with indwelling lines or hardware, and underlying medical conditions such as sickle cell anemia, neutropenia (ANC < 500/μL), and other immunodeficiency syndromes.

Clinical Findings

Isolated fever greater than 39°C in the absence of other identifying features is rare in this cohort of children. The clinician must recognize that immunosuppression including chronic steroid use and neutropenia may mask the usual signs and symptoms of infection such as swelling, erythema, and pus formation.

Laboratory Tests/Radiographs

Routine laboratory tests are not necessary for children in this age group. Specific laboratory testing should be directed toward the suspected source of infection. An exception is the evaluation of children at risk for neutropenia, in whom a CBC with differential and a blood culture are recommended. Children with fever and a central line also need blood cultures drawn from each catheter lumen as well as peripherally.

Treatment

Management is determined by the source of infection. Most children with fever and viral infection need supportive care only. Ill-appearing children should have appropriate cultures drawn before broad-spectrum antibiotics are initiated.

Children with febrile neutropenia, usually secondary to recent chemotherapy, are at very high risk of invasive bacterial disease and must be managed conservatively in the emergency department in consultation with an oncologist. Initial assessment should focus on mental status and vital sign abnormalities because progression to septic shock can be rapid in these patients. For stable patients who are suspected to be neutropenic, a CBC with differential and blood cultures should be drawn. Broad-spectrum antibiotics, typically a fourth-generation cephalosporin (cefepime), should be started to provide coverage against *Staphylococcus*, *Streptococcus*, and gram-negative bacteria, such as *Pseudomonas*. Children with suspected line or skin infection require empiric vancomycin for methicillin-resistant *Staphylococcus aureus* (MRSA). For selected children, in consultation with their hematologist, antibiotics may be held until neutropenia is confirmed by CBC. Most of these children require admission, though some may be discharged on an oral antibiotic regimen such as ciprofloxacin and amoxicillin-clavulanate with close follow-up.

Children with fever and an indwelling central line including peripherally inserted central catheters (PICCs) are assumed to have a line infection until proven otherwise. Blood cultures should be drawn from each lumen of the line as well as from a peripheral line prior to the initiation of empiric antibiotics, usually vancomycin, with gram-negative coverage in specific patients. Many children will require admission for intravenous (IV) antibiotics and line removal.

Avner JR: Acute fever. *Pediatr Rev.* 2009;30(1):5-13 [PMID: 19118137].

Hakim H, Flynn PM, Srivastava DK, et al: Risk prediction in pediatric cancer patients with fever and neutropenia. *Pediatr Infect Dis J.* 2010;29(1):53-59 [PMID: 19996816].

Santolaya ME, Farfaj MJ, Maza DL, et al: Diagnosis of bacteremia in febrile neutropenia with cancer: Microbiologic and molecular approach. *Pediatr Infect Dis J.* 2011;30(11):957-961 [PMID: 21768922].

Sherman JM, Sood SK: Current challenges in the diagnosis and management of fever. *Curr Opin Pediatr.* 2012;24(3):400-406 [PMID: 22323720].

▼ ORGAN SYSTEMS

NEUROLOGY

MENINGITIS

ESSENTIALS OF DIAGNOSIS

▶ Fever.

▶ Headache.

▶ Vomiting.

▶ Nuchal rigidity.

▶ Altered mental status.

▶ Seizure.

Prompt administration of antibiotics is critical for suspected bacterial meningitis.

General Considerations

Meningitis is infection and inflammation of the tissues surrounding the brain and spinal cord. Since the widespread use of vaccines against HIB, meningococcus, and pneumococcus, the incidence of bacterial meningitis has decreased dramatically among children older than 3 months. Bacterial meningitis in children aged 0-3 months is most commonly due to GBS and gram-negative bacteria, whereas older children tend to be infected by *S. pneumoniae* and *Neisseria meningitidis.* Viruses, particularly enteroviruses, are responsible for the majority of meningitis cases among older children and adolescents and the infections are generally self-limited. Mycobacteria, fungi, and *Rickettsia* are rare causes of pediatric meningitis. A history of penetrating head trauma or indwelling hardware such as a ventriculoperitoneal shunt (VPS) or cochlear implants are risk factors for the development of meningitis. Among healthy children, infection usually reaches the central nervous system (CNS) through hematogenous spread following ear, sinus, or upper respiratory infection (URI). Detailed history is paramount, including immunization status and history of potential risk factors such as head trauma, VPS, recent sinus or ear infection, or immunosuppression.

Clinical Findings

Inflammation of the meninges causes fever, headache, vomiting, and lethargy. Severe inflammation can lead to seizures, obtundation, and signs of increased intracranial pressure (ICP) such as hypertension, bradycardia, and irregular respirations. Florid bacterial meningitis may be indistinguishable from septic shock. Children with meningitis classically have nuchal rigidity, although this finding is often difficult to elicit in younger patients. Infants with meningitis may have a bulging fontanel, jaundice, and a history of poor feeding and irritability. Petechiae and purpura are associated with meningococcal disease. Viral meningitis presents more nonspecifically with headache, low-grade fever, vomiting, diarrhea.

Laboratory Tests/Radiographs

CSF studies including culture, Gram stain, protein, glucose, and cell counts are the cornerstone for the diagnosis of meningitis (Table 41–3). HSV PCR is recommended for all infants younger than 3 weeks. Enteroviral PCR from the CSF is useful when viral meningitis is suspected. A blood culture, CBC with differential, and comprehensive metabolic panel (CMP) should also be obtained. Children with meningeal inflammation are at increased risk of SIADH and urine output, serum sodium, urine sodium, and urine osmolality should be monitored closely. Coagulation studies, D-dimer, and fibrinogen are useful if meningococcal infection is suspected or if the patient has a petechial rash. A head CT is necessary for the evaluation of children with suspected increased ICP. Children with intracranial shunts need a plain film shunt series to determine if there is shunt discontinuity.

Treatment

Meningitis must be approached with a focused evaluation of airway, breathing, and circulation (ABCs) as these patients are at risk for progression to septic shock. For stable patients, prompt administration of antibiotics following lumbar puncture is essential. Lumbar puncture

Table 41–3. CSF parameters among neonates and children and those with viral or bacterial meningitis.

	Neonate	Child	Viral Meningitis	Bacterial Meningitis
WBC (per mm³)	< 30	< 10	10-1000	150-10,000
Protein (mg/dL)	50-150	5-40	40-100	> 100
Glucose (mg/dL)	> 30	40-80	> 30	< 30

may be deferred pending head CT if there is suspicion for increased ICP (focal neurologic defects, papilledema, or seizures) or if lumbar puncture will significantly delay antibiotic administration. Empiric antibiotics for suspected meningitis should treat the common pathogens for a child's age. Children younger than 1 month are treated with ampicillin, gentamicin or cefotaxime, and acyclovir. Those older than 1 month should receive vancomycin in combination with a third-generation cephalosporin such as cefotaxime or ceftriaxone. When gram-negative bacteria are seen on the CSF Gram stain, double gram-negative coverage with amikacin or gentamicin is indicated. Addition of 2-4 days of dexamethasone, started within 1 hour of antibiotic administration, is shown to reduce the risk of hearing loss in children with HIB meningitis. However, studies to evaluate its effectiveness among other types of bacterial meningitis have not shown this benefit, and its empiric use in children is controversial.

Children with a VPS and a fever present a diagnostic challenge in the emergency department due to concern for meningitis particularly if they are otherwise well-appearing without an obvious source of infection. These children often receive a shunt series and a CBC with differential. Fever above 38°C, WBC count of greater than 15,000/uL, and intracranial shunt less than 90 days from placement or revision are known risk factors for meningitis and should prompt a full laboratory evaluation including CSF analysis. Among equivocal cases, CSF evaluation and consultation with neurosurgeon is advised.

Brayer AF, Humiston SG: Invasive meningococcal disease in childhood. *Pediatr Rev.* 2011;32(4):152-160 [PMID: 21460092].

Curtis S, Stobart K, Vandermeer B, et al: Clinical features suggestive of meningitis in children: A systematic review of prospective data. *Pediatrics.* 2010;126:952-960 [PMID: 20974781].

Mann K, Jackson MA: Meningitis. *Pediatr Rev.* 2008;29(12):417-429 [PMID: 19047432].

Rogers EA, Kimia A, Madsen JR, et al: Predictors of ventricular shunt infection among children presenting to a pediatric emergency department. *Pediatr Emerg Care.* 2012;28(5):405-409 [PMID:22531186].

Sinvanandan S, Soraisham AS, Swarnam K: Choice and duration of antimicrobial therapy for neonatal sepsis and meningitis. *Int J Pediatr.* 2011; vol 2011, ID number 712150:1-9 [PMID: 22164179].

HEAD, EARS, EYES, NOSE, THROAT

PERITONSILLAR & RETROPHARYNGEAL ABSCESSES

 ESSENTIALS OF DIAGNOSIS

▶ Fever.

▶ Neck pain.

▶ Trismus.

▶ Stridor.

▶ Muffled voice.

IV antibiotics and surgical drainage are mainstays of therapy for peritonsillar and retropharyngeal abscesses infections.

General Considerations

Common deep neck space infections in children include peritonsillar and retropharyngeal abscesses. Peritonsillar infections comprise the majority of deep neck infections and progress from cellulitis to a pus-containing abscess. Infections in this region are usually polymicrobial, with GAS, *Staphylococcus*, and anaerobes most commonly identified. Retropharyngeal abscesses occur when a retropharyngeal lymph node becomes infected; subsequent rupture and drainage of the node is contained in the retropharyngeal space. Rarely, infection spreads to the retropharyngeal space from direct extension of sinusitis, tonsillitis, pharyngitis, or a dental abscess. Children older than 9 years rarely develop retropharyngeal infections because the lymph nodes atrophy before puberty. Poor dentition, oral trauma, and preceding pharyngitis or URI are important risk factors to consider.

Clinical Findings

Regardless of type of infection, compromise of airway may cause patients to present with fever, stridor, tachypnea, and muffled voice. Patients often have severe pain with neck movement, sore throat, and inability to swallow secondary to pain. Peritonsillar abscesses are usually unilateral, and swelling of the posterior oropharynx often displaces the uvula to the opposite side of the infection. Tender cervical adenopathy is commonly found. Early retropharyngeal abscesses may present nonspecifically if the involved lymph node has not yet ruptured.

Laboratory Tests/Radiographs

A CBC with differential is recommended and the peripheral white blood cell count (WBC) is typically greater than

12,000 cells/μL. A blood culture may be obtained in severe cases. Rapid streptococcal antigen testing with confirmatory culture is recommended due to the prevalence of GAS. For children with stable airway, evaluation begins with a lateral neck radiograph, though neck CT with contrast or MRI may be preferable if clinical suspicion is high. On a lateral neck radiograph, a retropharyngeal abscess is associated with widening of the retropharyngeal space greater than 7 mm at C2 or 14 mm at C6. A contrasted neck CT may demonstrate contrast rim enhancement if abscess is present in the peritonsillar or retropharyngeal space.

Treatment

Management of abscesses in children depends on the level of airway obstruction. Sedation should be avoided if possible in these patients and intubation, if necessary, should be performed by experienced personnel (anesthesiologists, emergency medicine physicians), due to the risk of airway edema and obstructed visual landmarks. For stable children with confirmed peritonsillar or retropharyngeal abscess, the decision to proceed directly to surgery for drainage or needle aspiration remains controversial. Management of these children in consultation with an otolaryngologist is recommended; in some centers children are managed with prompt surgical drainage although others employ a trial of empiric antibiotics first. IV clindamycin or amoxicillin-clavulonic acid are frequently used antibiotics and have the advantage of easy transition to oral therapy. Some centers also broaden coverage with a cephalosporin such as cefuroxime.

Chang L, Chi H, Chiu NC, et al: Deep neck infections in different age groups of children. *J Microbiol Immunol Infect.* 2010;43(1):47-52 [PMID: 20434123].

Grisaru-Soen G, Komisar O, Aizenstein O, et al: Retropharyngeal and parapharyngeal abscess in children: Epidemiology, clinical features, and treatment. *Int J Pediatr Otorhinolaryngol.* 2010:74:1016-1020 [PMID: 20598378].

Millar KR, Johnson DW, Drummond D, et al: Suspected peritonsillar abscess in children. *Pediatr Emerg Care.* 2007;23(7):431-438 [PMID: 17666922].

Page NC, Bauer EM, Lieu JE: Clinical features and treatment of retropharyngeal abscess in children. *Otolaryngol Head Neck Surg.* 2008;138(3):300-306 [PMID: 18312875].

DENTAL ABSCESS

 ESSENTIALS OF DIAGNOSIS

▶ Tooth pain.

▶ Erythema *plus* lymphadenopathy.

Abscess must be addressed early as infection may spread to contiguous structures in the face and neck.

General Considerations

Complications arising from poor dentition are not uncommon among children. Untreated caries may progress to deep seated abscesses with the potential to spread contiguously to the face or the jaw, resulting in cellulitis or osteomyelitis. Further spread through the deep fascial layers of the face may reproduce the symptoms of a retropharyngeal or peritonsillar abscess. In medically complex children, including those with indwelling hardware or prosthetic valves, dental infections can lead to hematogenous spread of bacteria. Most dental infections are polymicrobial, with *Streptococcus* species and anaerobic organisms most commonly isolated.

Clinical Findings

Primary presenting symptom is pain and tooth sensitivity at the site of abscess. The gums surrounding the affected tooth are often inflamed, with or without visible purulence. Fever, foul odor, and lymphadenopathy may be present. Spread of the infection to the deeper tissue layers causes trismus, and soft tissue involvement of the face may result in superficial swelling, erythema, and tenderness.

Laboratory Tests/Radiographs

Routine laboratory tests are not required for diagnosis in most patients. A CBC with differential may be obtained for febrile children, with an elevated WBC most commonly seen. A blood culture is recommended only in ill-appearing children or those with an identifiable risk factor such as repaired congenital heart disease or a prosthetic heart valve. CT of the face and neck with contrast is the preferred modality for the assessment of advanced infections if required.

Treatment

Well-appearing children with poor dentition and tooth pain may be managed supportively with pain control as long as prompt follow-up with a dentist can be arranged. Children with concern for abscess should be evaluated by an oral maxillofacial surgeon or dentist. Because of the potential for spread along the fascial planes of the face and neck, surgical exploration of an abscess should be performed in consultation with an oral maxillofacial surgeon. Febrile children and those with concern for facial cellulitis should receive IV antibiotics, typically ampicillin-sulbactam. Extraction of the infected tooth may be performed inpatient or following hospital discharge.

Hodfdon A: Dental and related infections: *Emerg Med Clin North Am.* 2013;31 (2):465-480 [PMID: 23601483].

Lin YT, Lu PW: Retrospective study of pediatric facial cellulitis of odontogenic origin. *Pediatr Infect Dis J.* 2006;25:339-342 [PMID: 16567986].

PHARYNGITIS

ESSENTIALS OF DIAGNOSIS

▸ Pharyngeal exudates.

▸ Scarlitiniform rash.

▸ Palatal petechiae.

▸ Anterior cervical adenopathy.

If suggestive of GAS infection, antibiotic treatment of GAS pharyngitis lessens the risk of acute rheumatic fever.

General Considerations

Infectious pharyngitis is usually viral in origin, although bacterial pharyngitis accounts for roughly one-third of all cases. GAS pharyngitis is more common in children aged 5-15 years and viral causes predominate in younger children. Pharyngitis in children is generally a self-limited process though it may compromise a child's ability to maintain hydration. GAS pharyngitis is typically benign but in rare cases can lead to suppurative complications such as retropharyngeal or peritonsillar abscesses. Antibiotic treatment of GAS pharyngitis lowers the risk of acute rheumatic fever, a disease hypothesized to occur when molecular mimicry between certain GAS antigens and host cells leads to an autoimmune attack against tissues in the heart, joints, nervous system, and skin. Clinical manifestations of acute rheumatic fever include carditis, arthritis, chorea, subcutaneous nodules, and erythema marginatum. Rapid streptococcal antigen testing has emerged as an efficient means of identifying children with GAS; however, up to 20% of healthy children are asymptomatic GAS carriers and do not require treatment. A thorough history including sexual history and vaccination status is important for uncovering less common causes of pharyngitis such as gonococcus and diphtheria.

Clinical Findings

Children with pharyngitis have complaints of sore throat or pain with swallowing. Viral pharyngitis is often seen with other upper respiratory symptoms such as cough, congestion, conjunctivitis. Fever is common with both viral and bacterial causes of pharyngitis. Findings suggestive of bacterial pharyngitis include a scarlatiniform rash, palatal petechiae, pharyngeal exudates, and tender anterior cervical lymph nodes. Pharyngitis due to Epstein-Barr virus (EBV) infection (mononucleosis) presents with pharyngeal exudates but frequently involves the posterior cervical lymph nodes. Streptococcal pharyngitis is uncommon in children younger than 3 years but may present as "streptococcosis," a nonspecific symptom complex comprising fevers, adenopathy, and nasal drainage.

Laboratory Tests/Radiographs

Rapid streptococcal antigen testing is highly sensitive (85%) and specific (96%) for the presence of GAS. Confirmatory throat culture should be sent from every rapid test that is negative. In addition to cultures and rapid streptococcal tests, a number of clinical criteria aid in the diagnosis of GAS pharyngitis. The most well known are the Centor criteria. The modified Centor score gives one point each to temperature higher than 38°C, swollen tender anterior cervical nodes, tonsillar swelling or exudates, absence of upper respiratory tract symptoms (cough, coryza), and age between 3 and 15 years. If the patient is older than 45 years, a point is subtracted. If the score is 1 or less, no further testing or treatment is warranted. For score of 2-3, further testing may be indicated, such as cultures or rapid streptococcal tests. For score of 4 or higher, no further testing is required and all patients may receive antibiotics for GAS pharyngitis

Additional laboratory tests such as blood culture or CBC with differential are needed only in severe cases or if complications such as abscess are suspected.

Treatment

GAS testing should be reserved for children with a reasonable pretest probability of disease to avoid overtreatment of asymptomatic carriers. A number of clinical decision rules have been developed, but no rule has gained widespread acceptance; therefore testing is recommended for children without evidence of a viral infection who have symptoms suggestive of GAS pharyngitis. Because the sensitivity of rapid testing is not 100%, the clinician may choose to treat empirically without testing for children with a very high pretest probability of disease. GAS remains sensitive to penicillin and amoxicillin, penicillin V, or intramuscular (IM) benzathine penicillin. There has been as increased use of steroids in treatment of pharyngitis. Pain is thought to be caused by inflammation of the lining of the posterior oral pharynx. Corticosteroids, which inhibit the transcription of proinflammatory mediators, may prove useful in decreasing sore throat pain. Studies show that corticosteroids compared with placebo are more likely to relieve symptoms of sore throat pain at 24 hours. The physician must be thoughtful in using steroids and consider risk/benefit for each patient, for example patient with diabetes, peptic ulcer disease, immunocompromised states, and avascular necrosis.

Baltimore R: Re-evaluation of antibiotic treatment of streptococcal pharyngitis. *Curr Opin Pediatr*. 2010;22:77-82 [PMID: 19996970].

Shah R, Bansal A, Singhi SC: Approach to a child with sore throat. *Indian J Pediatr*. 2011;78(10):1268-1272 [PMID: 21660400].

Shaikh N, Swaminathan N, Hooper EG: Accuracy and precision of the signs and symptoms of streptococcal pharyngitis in children: A systematic review. *J Pediatr.* 2012;160:487-493 [PMID: 22048053].

Welch J, Cooper D: Do corticosteroids benefit patients with sore throat? *Ann Emerg Med.* 2014;63(6):711-712 [PMID: 23927959].

BACTERIAL TRACHEITIS

 ESSENTIALS OF DIAGNOSIS

► Stridor.

► Fever.

► Cough.

► Lack of response to inhaled epinephrine.

► High risk of airway compromise requiring intubation.

General Considerations

Bacterial tracheitis is a rare but potentially life-threatening infection that often follows a viral URI. It is hypothesized that virus-induced mucosal damage of the larynx allows bacteria to penetrate this region. Edema and inflammation of the trachea lead rapidly to airway compromise, and studies demonstrate that children with bacterial tracheitis require intubation ($\geq$ 75%). In the emergency department, bacterial tracheitis often presents when patients with suspected laryngotracheobronchitis (croup) do not respond to glucocorticoids and inhaled epinephrine. Common bacterial isolates include *S. aureus*, *S. pneumoniae*, GAS, *H. influenzae*, and *Moraxella catarrhalis*.

Clinical Findings

Children with bacterial tracheitis present with worsening inspiratory or expiratory stridor due to progressive airway obstruction. Cough and fever may be present. Children present clinically similar to those with laryngotracheobronchitis; however, they are far more likely to be toxic-appearing or refractory to common therapies for croup. Aphonia is an ominous sign of vocal cord involvement. Symptoms of a preceding URI may also be present.

Laboratory Tests/Radiographs

Bacterial tracheitis is a clinical diagnosis and routine laboratory tests are generally not required. Elevations in the peripheral WBC count, ESR, and CRP have not shown to correlate with disease severity. Gram stain and culture of tracheal exudates may be helpful to guide long-term antibiotic

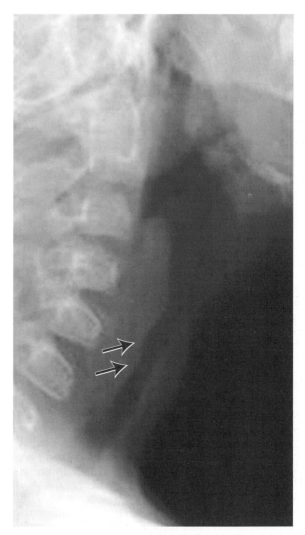

▲ **Figure 41–1.** Patient with bacterial tracheitis. Note presence of irregular tracheal margins as shown by the arrows. (Reproduced, with permission, from W. McAlister, Washington University School of Medicine, St. Louis, MO.)

therapy. Blood cultures are most infrequently positive and should be drawn only if there is concern for sepsis. Lateral neck films are recommended and may show narrowing of the subglottic region or irregularities of the tracheal mucosa (Figure 41–1).

Treatment

Primary management of bacterial tracheitis begins with an assessment of the child's airway. If there is concern for progressive obstruction, intubation is recommended by experienced personnel because of the potential for severe tracheal edema. Consultation with an otolaryngologist should be obtained immediately for endoscopy and debridement of tracheal exudates. Broad-spectrum parenteral antibiotics should be initiated; typically an antistaphlococcal agent such as clindamycin or vancomycin is used in combination with a third-generation cephalosporin. Children with tracheostomies should receive an anti-pseudomonal agent such as cefepime or a quinolone. Glucocorticoids have not been shown to benefit patients with bacterial tracheitis. Because of potential for rapid airway compromise, even children who are not intubated should be admitted to the ICU for monitoring.

Miranda AD, Valdez TA, Pereira KD: Bacterial tracheitis a varied entity. *Pediatr Emerg Care.* 2011;27:950 [PMID: 21975496].

Shargorodsky J, Whittemore KR, Lee GS: Bacterial tracheitis: A therapeutic approach. *Laryngoscope.* 2011;120:2498 [PMID: 21225825].

Tebruegge M, Pantazidou A, Thornburn K, et al: Bacterial tracheitis: A multicentre perspective. *Scand J Infect Dis.* 2009;41(8):548 [PMID: 19401934].

OTITIS MEDIA

 ESSENTIALS OF DIAGNOSIS

Based on the 2013 American Academy of Pediatrics (AAP) guidelines, diagnosis of OM is established by the following criteria:

▶ Moderate to severe bulging of the tympanic membrane (TM).

▶ New onset of otorrhea.

▶ Mild bulging of the TM plus recent onset of ear pain.

▶ Intense erythema of the TM.

Acute OM should not be diagnosed in patients without evidence of middle ear effusion on pneumatic otoscopsy and/or tympanometry. Antibiotic treatment is recommended for children younger than 2 years.

General Considerations

Otitis media (OM) remains the most commonly diagnosed pediatric illness and is the most frequent indication for antibiotic treatment. An acute URI causes Eustachian tube dysfunction and impaired mucociliary clearance, allowing bacteria to ascend into and grow within the middle ear. Infection is generally self-limited, but mastoiditis, meningitis, cavernous sinus thrombosis, and brain abscess are extremely uncommon sequelae of advanced or untreated infections. *S. pneumoniae,* non-typeable *H. influenzae,* and *M. catarrhalis* are most commonly implicated bacterial causes of acute OM. Risk factors for development of OM include age 6-18 months, day care attendance, smoke exposure, and pacifier use.

Clinical Findings

OM presents with a bulging tympanic membrane that overlies cloudy middle ear fluid. The mobility of the TM is reduced on pneumatoscopy. Erythema is often observed around or on the TM; however, this is a nonspecific finding that can be caused by crying or fever. Fluid-filled bullae on the TM are seen with bullous myringitis. Otalgia is apparent in older children although younger infants may be more irritable and fussy. Fever is generally present but is not required for diagnosis. Children with OM may have symptoms of an underlying viral URI such as cough, sore throat, and rhinorrhea. When fluid is seen behind the TM, but signs of infection are absent, serous OM should be suspected.

Laboratory Tests/Radiographs

No routine laboratory tests or radiographs are required for the diagnosis of OM. When complications such as mastoiditis are suspected, imaging with a head CT is recommended.

Treatment

Many studies have addressed treatment algorithms for OM. Children younger than 6 months as well as those with moderate or severe illness, defined as a temperature greater than 39°C or moderate or severe otalgia, should be treated with antibiotics (Table 41–4). Watchful waiting is an option for children 6 months to 2 years if the diagnosis is in question and the child appears mildly ill. Children older than 2 years require treatment only for severe illness. The use of a "safety script," given to parents to fill in the next 24-72 hours if the child fails to improve, is an option for children older than 6 months with mild to moderate illness.

Gould JM, Matz PS: Otitis media. *Pediatr Rev.* 2010;31(3):102-116 [PMID: 20194902].

Hoberman A, Paradise JL, Rockette HE, Shaikh S, et al: Treatment of acute otitis media in children under 2 years of age. *N Engl J Med.* 2011;364:105-115 [PMID: 21226576].

Johnson NC, Holger JS: Pediatric acute otitis media: The case for delayed antibiotic treatment. *J Emerg Med.* 2007;32(3):279-284 [PMID: 17394992].

Lieberthal A, Carroll A, Chonmaitree T, et al: The diagnosis and management of acute otitis media. *Pediatrics.* 2013;131; e964-991 [PMID: 23439909].

Pelton SJ, Leibovitz E: Recent advances in otitis media. *Pediatr Infect Dis J.* 2009;28:S133-S137 [PMID: 19918136].

Shaikh N, Hoberman A, Kaleida PH, et al: Otoscopic signs of otitis media. *Pediatr Inf Dis J.* 2011;30:822-826 [PMID: 21844828].

Vergison A: Microbiology of otitis media: A moving target. *Vaccine.* 2008;265:G5-G10 [PMID: 19094935].

Table 41–4. Treatment of acute otitis media.

Antibiotic	Dose	Maximum Daily Dose	Duration (days)
Amoxicillin	80-90 mg/kg div BID	3 g	7-10
Amoxicillin-clavulanic acid	80-90 mg/kg amoxicillin component div BID	3 g	7-10
Cefdinir	14 mg/kg div BID	600 mg	7-10
Cefpodoxime	10 mg/kg QD	800 mg	7-10
Azithromycin	10 mg/kg QD × 1 d then 5 mg/kg QD × 4 d	500 mg	5
Trimethoprim-sulfamethoxazole (TMP-SMZ)	10 mg/kg TMP component div BID	320 mg	7-10

MASTOIDITIS

 ESSENTIALS OF DIAGNOSIS

▶ Antecedent OM.
▶ Posterior auricular swelling.
▶ Erythema.
▶ Tenderness.
▶ Protrusion of auricle.

IV antibiotics and consultation with otolaryngologist are recommended.

General Considerations

A feared complication of OM, acute mastoiditis is now an uncommon presentation in the pediatric emergency department. Mastoiditis occurs when infected fluid from the middle ear spreads to and proliferates within the mastoid air cells of the temporal bone. Normally the fluid drains via the Eustachian tube; however, if the route is obstructed due to inflammation, accumulation will occur in the mastoid air cells. In severe cases, an abscess can form and spread further into the brain, meninges, and temporal bone. Despite the implementation of the pneumococcal vaccine, *S. pneumoniae* is the most common etiologic agent of acute mastoiditis, although GAS, *S. aureus*, and *H. influenzae* are also encountered. Risk factors include age younger than 2 years and history of recurrent OM.

Clinical Findings

Classic acute mastoiditis is suspected when there is posterior auricular tenderness, redness, and swelling in the setting of acute OM. Swelling behind the ear often causes the auricle to be displaced outward relative to the other side. Fever, otalgia, and irritability are common but less specific signs of

infection. In many patients, the TM may be ruptured with resultant otorrhea. High-spiking "picket fence" fevers are associated with increased risk of sigmoid sinus thrombophlebitis. Meningeal signs, facial nerve palsy, and dizziness and vertigo are uncommon but indicate further spread of infection.

Laboratory Tests/Radiographs

Laboratory tests are not required for diagnosis of mastoiditis; however a CBC with differential is typically obtained and may show leukocytosis with a neutrophilic predominance. Inflammatory markers such as ESR and CRP are helpful for monitoring response to therapy. Blood cultures are routinely drawn but are rarely positive. Cultures from the middle ear or mastoid bone should be sent when possible to guide antimicrobial therapy. Lumbar puncture with CSF studies should be performed if there are meningeal signs on examination.

Contrast CT scan with IV contrast is recommended for visualization of the mastoid air cells and positive findings include rim-enhancing fluid collections, cortical bone erosion, and mastoid air cell coalescence. Opacification of the mastoid air cells is not diagnostic of mastoiditis as it is commonly seen with uncomplicated cases of OM. MRI should be obtained when there is concern for intracranial abscess or sigmoid sinus thrombosis.

Treatment

Patients with confirmed acute mastoiditis may require admission, IV antibiotics, and referral to an otolaryngologist for drainage of the purulent middle ear fluid. Drainage may consist of simple myringotomy with or without tube placement or mastoidectomy. Empiric antibiotic therapy typically consists of an antipseudomonal cephalosporin such as cefipime (50 mg/kg q8h) or ceftazidine (100-150 mg/kg/d divided every 8 hours) in combination with an antistaphlococcal agent such as vancomycin (20 mg/kg divided every 8 hours). Patients in whom diagnosis is in doubt should be admitted for observation for 24 hours on IV antibiotics in consultation with an otolaryngologist.

Aardweg MT, Rovers MM, Ru JA, et al: A systematic review of diagnostic criteria for acute mastoiditis in children. *Otol Neurotol.* 2008;29(6):751-757 [PMID: 18617870].

Choi SS, Lander L: Pediatric acute mastoiditis in the post-pneumococcal conjugate vaccine era. *Laryngoscope.* 2011;121:1072-1080 [PMID: 21520127].

Lin HW, Shargorodsky J, Gopen Q: Clinical strategies for the management of acute mastoiditis in the pediatric population. *Clin Pediatr.* 2010;49(2):110-115 [PMID: 19734439].

Tamir S, Shwartz Y, Peleg U, et al: Shifting trends: Mastoiditis from a surgical to a medical disease. *Am J Otolaryngol.* 2010;31(6):467-471 [PMID: 20015791].

SINUSITIS

ESSENTIALS OF DIAGNOSIS

▶ Worsening viral URI symptoms after 7-10 days of illnesses.

▶ Persistent mucopurulent nasal drainage with fever.

Uncomplicated cases can be managed with outpatient antibiotics.

General Considerations

Acute bacterial sinusitis complicating a URI is thought to occur in 5-10% of patients. In children, the maxillary and ethmoid sinuses are present at birth and are continuous with the mucosa of the nose via their drainage at the middle meatus, just below the middle turbinate. Viral infection of the nasal mucosa and paranasal sinuses causes inflammation and may obstruct drainage from the sinuses. Negative pressure develops, causing bacteria from the nasal mucosa to be drawn up into the sinuses. At the same time, virus-induced damage to the mucociliary apparatus prevents infected material from being properly cleared from the sinuses. Common pathogens include *S. pneumoniae*, *H. influenzae*, and *M. catarrhalis*. Risk factors for the development of acute bacterial sinusitis include exposure to smoke, day care attendance, allergic rhinitis, and gastroesophageal reflux. In young children, recurrent or chronic sinusitis should prompt the clinician to consider possibility of underlying immunodeficiency. Left untreated, bacterial sinusitis has the potential to spread to surrounding tissues, causing periorbital and orbital cellulitis, osteomyelitis, brain abscesses, and meningitis.

Clinical Findings

The physician may have difficulty discriminating signs and symptoms of a viral URI from those of acute bacterial sinusitis. Fever, mucopurulent nasal drainage, congestion, headache, and erythema of the nasal turbinates are commonly seen in both infections. Sinus tenderness and swelling are classic but uncommon signs of sinusitis. Disease that has spread to involve the orbits may present with the periorbital swelling, pain, and proptosis. Frontal sinus osteomyelitis (Pott's puffy tumor) presents with prominent forehead swelling. Despite the lack of specific physical signs, a careful history is often adequate for the diagnosis of sinusitis. Worsening URI symptoms with persistent fever after 7-10 days of illness are highly suggestive of sinusitis, since most routine URIs present with fever that resolves as respiratory symptoms become more prominent. Children with severe acute bacterial sinusitis have fevers greater than 39°C for 3 or more days in addition to thick yellow nasal discharge.

Laboratory Tests/Radiographs

Acute bacterial sinusitis may be diagnosed clinically and routine laboratory tests, and imaging are not recommended. CT findings in uncomplicated sinusitis include sinus opacification, air fluid levels, and mucosal thickening greater than 4 mm; however, the findings are not sufficiently specific for bacterial sinusitis and indiscriminate use of CT imaging leads to overdiagnosis. A CT scan with IV contrast is the preferred imaging modality for children with suspected complications such as orbital cellulitis. Patients presenting with meningeal or focal neurologic signs suggestive of intracranial spread should be evaluated with lumbar puncture, CSF studies, and an MRI of the brain.

Treatment

Most children with acute bacterial sinusitis can be managed outpatient with an antibiotic such as high-dose amoxicillin or amoxicillin-clavulanic acid. If patients do not improve within 72 hours, the antibiotic should be changed to a third-generation cephalosporin (cefdinir). Antibiotic treatment dosage is between 10 and 14 days, or for at least 7 days after symptom resolution. Irrigation with nasal saline may be considered as an adjunctive agent, but intranasal steroids are generally not recommended unless there is marked nasal polyposis or edema on examination.

Brook I: Acute sinusitis in children. *Pediatr Clin North Am.* 2013;60(2):409-424 [PMID: 23481108].

Revai K, Dobbs L, Patal JA, et al: Incidence of acute otitis media and sinusitis complicating upper respiratory tract infection. *Pediatrics.* 2007;119:e1408-1412 [PMID: 17545367].

Revai K, Mamidi D, Chonmaitree T: Association of nasopharyngeal bacterial colonization during upper respiratory tract infection and the development of acute otitis media. *Clin Infect Dis.* 2007;46:e34-37 [PMID: 18205533].

Wald ER: Acute otitis media and acute bacterial sinusitis. *Clin Infect Dis.* 2011;52(S4):S277-S283 [PMID: 21460285].

PERIORBITAL & ORBITAL CELLULITIS

ESSENTIALS OF DIAGNOSIS

► Eyelid swelling.

► Pain.

► Erythema.

► Ophthalmoplegia (orbital cellulitis only).

► Proptosis (orbital cellulitis only).

► Pain with extraocular movements (orbital cellulitis only).

Admission and IV antibiotics required for suspected orbital cellulitis.

General Considerations

Periorbital and orbital cellulitis may present similarly but have different pathogenic mechanisms and risk of complications (Table 41–5). Anatomically, the orbit is surrounded by the sinuses, and the orbital septum is an extension of the orbital rim periosteum that extends through the upper and lower eyelids, separating the orbit into preseptal and postseptal compartments. Periorbital cellulitis, also known as preseptal cellulitis, is far more common and involves infection of the anterior portion of the eyelid. It is most often caused by trauma to the eye, including insect bites, eczema, and impetigo. Periorbital cellulitis is most often caused by *Staphylococcus* (including MRSA) and *Streptococcus* species, and is generally a mild disease with low risk for complications.

Table 41–5. Orbital versus periorbital cellulitis.

	Orbital cellulitis	Periorbital Cellulitis
Age	> 5 yr	< 5 yr
Cause	Sinusitis, surgery	Local skin trauma, sinusitis
Presentation	Opthalmoplegia, proptosis, diplopia, fever	Eye pain, erythema, swelling
Diagnosis	Contrast CT/MRI	History or contrast CT
Treatment	Vancomycin plus third-generation cephalosporin or ampicillin-sulbactam	Clindamycin or TMP-SMX plus amoxicillin or third-generation cephalosporin
Complications	Subperiosteal/orbital abscess, thrombophlebitis	Rare

Orbital cellulitis, in contrast, is nearly always caused by spread of bacteria from existing sinus disease through small fenestrations in the sinus bones or via the valveless system of veins which traverse the sinuses. Infection within the orbit can develop into subperiosteal or orbital abscesses, and since the orbital veins are connected to deeper intracranial structures such as the cavernous sinus, complications of orbital cellulitis include thrombophlebitis, brain abscess, meningitis, and vision loss. Causative organisms of orbital cellulitis include *Staphylococcus* species, *Streptococcus* species, *H. influenzae*, and anaerobes. Risk factors for orbital cellulitis include recurrent bacterial sinusitis, recent ophthalmologic surgery, and dental abscesses.

Clinical Findings

Ocular pain, swelling and erythema of the eyelid, and conjunctival irritation are commonly seen with periorbital and orbital cellulitis. Fever may be encountered in both conditions but is more common with orbital cellulitis. Hallmark features that suggest orbital cellulitis are opthalmoplegia, proptosis, and pain with extraocular eye movement. Loss of visual acuity and sluggish light reflex are seen in severe cases of orbital cellulitis, and intracranial spread may manifest as headache, cranial nerve palsies, and meningeal signs. When signs of orbital cellulitis are present bilaterally, cavernous sinus thrombosis should be suspected.

Laboratory Tests/Radiographs

A CBC with differential and blood culture is obtained in cases of suspected periorbital or orbital cellulitis. A peripheral ANC of greater than 10,000 cells/μL has been used to predict increased risk of orbital abscess. When surgical intervention is indicated, cultures of purulent material from the orbit should be sent for Gram stain and culture. Because it is difficult to discriminate orbital from periorbital cellulitis based on clinical symptoms alone, adjunctive radiography plays a large role in diagnosis. CT scan of the orbits and sinuses with IV contrast is preferred unless intracranial complications are suspected in which case an MRI should be obtained. Common CT findings of orbital cellulitis include inflammation of the extraocular muscles, fat stranding, abscess formation, and sinus disease. In contrast, inflammation of periorbital cellulitis is confined to the eyelids only.

Treatment

Patients with signs and symptoms concerning for orbital cellulitis should undergo a CT scan with contrast of the orbits to assess for abscess and extension of disease. IV antibiotics should be initiated immediately; empiric antibiotics should include coverage against MRSA with vancomycin or clindamycin in combination with a third-cephalosporin or ampicillin/sulbactam. Patients in whom the diagnosis of orbital cellulitis is equivocal may be admitted and placed on IV antibiotics; failure to improve over the next 24-48 hours is suggestive of orbital abscess. Consultation with an opthalmologist and otolaryngologist is required for potential surgical management of orbital cellulitis. Indications for surgery include abscess greater than 10 mm, worsening neurologic symptoms, and failure to respond to antibiotics.

Well-appearing patients (> 1 year) with symptoms of periorbital cellulitis only may be managed on outpatient basis if appropriate follow-up is arranged. Patients (< 1 year) should be admitted and monitored until response to antibiotics is documented. Outpatient antibiotic regimens include clindamycin monotherapy or trimethoprim-sulfamethoxazole (TMP-SMZ) in combination with amoxicillin-clavulanic acid.

Bedwell J, Bauman NM: Management of pediatric orbital cellulitis and abscess. *Curr Opin Otolaryngol Head Neck Surg.* 2011;19:467-473 [PMID: 21844410].

Hauser A, Fogarasi S: Periobital and orbital cellulitis. *Pediatr Rev.* 2010;31(6):242-249 [PMID: 20516236].

Mahalingam-Dhingra A, Lander L, Preciado DA, et al: Orbital and periorbital infections. *Arch Otolaryngol Head Neck Surg.* 2011;137(8):769-773 [PMID: 21844410].

Rudloe TF, Harper MB, Prabhu SP, et al: Acute periorbital infections: Who needs emergent imaging? *Pediatrics.* 2010;125:3719-3726 [PMID: 20194288].

Seltz LB, Smith J, Durairaj VD: Microbiology and antibiotic management of orbital cellulitis. *Pediatrics.* 2011;127:e566-572 [PMID: 21321025].

EPIGLOTTITIS

 ESSENTIALS OF DIAGNOSIS

▶ Tripod position.

▶ Drooling.

▶ Fever.

▶ Stridor.

Epiglottis is an emergency requiring a secure airway and IV antibiotics.

General Considerations

True bacterial epiglottitis has become a rare entity since the introduction of the HIB vaccine three decades ago. However, epiglottis is a life-threatening infection because of the risk of rapid airway compromise. Unvaccinated children or those on delayed immunization schedules are at risk of disease caused by HIB; vaccinated children may develop epiglottitis from *S. pneumoniae, Staphylococcus,* or viral sources. Infection of the supraglottic structures including the epiglottis often develops in the setting of existing virally-mediated mucosal damage. Swelling can develop, leading to a rapid reduction in the diameter of the airway.

Clinical Findings

Symptoms of epiglottitis often develop over 12-24 hours and include dysphagia, drooling, a tripod sitting position, and fever. Children with epiglottitis are frequently toxic-appearing and in obvious respiratory distress. Stridor is common and its presentation can be confused with laryngo-tracheobronchitis (croup). An erythematous and edematous epiglottis may be observed in cooperative children.

Laboratory Tests/Radiographs

Laboratory studies are of minimal use in emergent management of suspected acute epiglottitis. CBC with differential may show leukocytosis; blood cultures are frequently positive and may guide antibiotic therapy. Lateral neck radiograph may show the classic "thumb-print sign" of the edematous epiglottis but is not required for diagnosis.

Treatment

Airway management is of primary importance in the treatment of epiglottitis. Even in children who appear stable, placement of artificial airway is indicated since additional airway compromise is likely. Intubation should occur if possible in the operating room by experienced personnel. Examination of the oropharynx should be deferred if there is potential to distress the child further. In an emergent situation in which intubation is unsuccessful, tracheostomy or cricothyroidectomy is indicated. Empiric IV antibiotics include an antistaphylococcal agent such as vancomycin or clindamycin in combination with a third-generation cephalosporin (ceftriaxone). Glucocorticoids are not generally recommended in the initial management of acute epiglottitis.

Shah R, Stocks C: Epiglottitis in the United States: National trends, variances, prognosis, and management. *Laryngoscope.* 2010;120:1256-1262 [PMID: 20513048].

Tibballs J, Watson T: Symptoms and signs differentiating croup and epiglottitis. *J Paediatr Child Health.* 2011;47(3):77-82 [PMID: 21091577].

LYMPH

LYMPHADENITIS

ESSENTIALS OF DIAGNOSIS

Lymph node that is—
► Tender.
► Painful.
► Erythematous.

Acute unilateral lymphadenitis usually bacterial in origin and treated with oral antibiotics.

General Considerations

The lymphatic system consists of a series of channels which drain into lymph nodes, collections of immune cells which process antigens and create populations of lymphocytes and antibodies specific to that antigen. A wide variety of stimuli can cause the immune cells of the lymph node to multiply, resulting in enlargement of the node. Lymphadenopathy caused by an infection is known as lymphadenitis and is common in children. Cervical lymphadenitis is the most common location and is classified as unilateral or bilateral and acute or subacute/chronic. Bilateral acute cervical lymphadenitis is typically the result of a viral URI, whereas acute unilateral cervical lymphadenitis is often caused by a bacterial infection. Common bacterial causes of lymphadenitis include *S. aureus*, GAS, and anaerobes. A thorough history is vital in the diagnosis of lymphadenitis because the differential diagnosis is broad. Etiologic clues in the history include immunization status, trauma or antecedent infection in the area drained by the affected node, exposure to kittens (cat scratch disease) or rabbits (tularemia), recent dental work (anaerobes), and history of pharyngitis (GAS or mononucleosis). Subacute or chronic presentations of lymphadenitis increase possibility of indolent infectious agents such as mycobacteria or noninfectious causes such as malignancy.

Clinical Findings

Viral lymphadenitis results in bilateral cervical nodes which are enlarged (> 1 cm), mildly tender, mobile, and nonerythematous. Unilateral lymphadenitis caused by bacteria may be grossly enlarged (> 3 cm), tender, erythematous, and potentially fluctuant. Fever may or may not be present. The physical examination should focus on the area drained by the infected node(s), as symptoms of a superficial skin infection, URI, periodontal disease, or pharyngitis may provide clues to the diagnosis. Subacute or chronic lymph nodes may present with enlargement without signs of acute infection.

Laboratory Tests/Radiographs

Laboratory tests are not required in the workup of lymphadenitis if source of infection is readily apparent. CBC with differential may demonstrate leukocytosis with bacterial infection or atypical cells with mononucleosis. Blood culture is not required unless the patient appears toxic. Inflammatory markers may be obtained if a prolonged course is suspected so that response to treatment may be followed. If the lymph node is drained, Gram stain and culture of the fluid should be sent. Other laboratory tests as rapid streptococcal antigen, viral serologies, and tuberculin skin testing depend on the clinical history. Ultrasound of the node may be useful if surgical intervention is planned.

Treatment

Lymphadenitis due to viral URIs is self-limited and generally resolves in 2-4 weeks. In cases of suspected acute bacterial lymphadenitis, empiric antibiotics usually include cephalexin (in areas where community-acquired MRSA [CA-MRSA] is rare) or clindamycin. TMP-SMX may be selected if GAS is not suspected. Because periodontal disease is associated with anaerobic lymphadenitis, patients should be started on clindamycin or amoxicillin-clavulanic acid. Fluctuant nodes should be drained as well as those that fail to improve 48-72 hours after the initiation of antibiotics. Most children can be managed with oral antibiotics, but those who are ill-appearing or immunocompromised should be started on IV clindamycin or vancomycin. Suspected cat scratch disease is self-limited but may be treated with azithromycin. Subacute or chronic lymphadenitis is best managed in conjunction with consultation with infectious disease physician.

Leung AC, Davies HD: Cervical lymphadenitis: Etiology, diagnosis, and management. *Curr Infect Dis:* 2009;11(3):183-189 [PMID: 19366560].

Rosado FG, Stratton CW, Mosse CA: Clinicopathologic correlation of epidemiologic and histopathologic features of pediatric bacterial lymphadenitis. *Arch Pathol Lab Med.* 2011;135: 1490-1493 [PMID: 22032579].

CARDIAC

ENDOCARDITIS

ESSENTIALS OF DIAGNOSIS

► Preexisting heart disease.
► Fever.
► Bacteremia.

Manage with admission and IV antibiotics after blood cultures are obtained (see Chapter 35).

General Considerations

Endocarditis develops when turbulent blood flow or direct trauma causes damage to the endocardium, resulting in exposed fibronectin. Transient bacteremia, a common and generally subclinical occurrence, then seeds the exposed area with bacteria that grow into a nidus of infection. Gram-positive cocci including *S. aureus* and *Streptococcus* bind well to fibronectin and are the primary causative agents of endocarditis. Children with congenital heart disease make up the majority of those with endocarditis. Indwelling central venous catheters have the potential to damage the endocardium directly and are another important risk factor for endocarditis. A known bacterial illness or recent dental procedures raise the risk of bacteremia and subsequent endocarditis in susceptible patients. Complications of endocarditis may develop due to the deposition of circulating immune complexes as well as septic microemboli.

Clinical Findings

Endocarditis typically presents nonspecifically with fever, malaise, myalgias, and weight loss. A heart murmur can represent new valvular disease but is of limited use because children with fever and a high output state often have an innocent flow murmur. Hematuria may be seen secondary to glomuleronephritis from immune complex deposition in the kidney. Septic emboli can result in symptoms of osteomyelitis, pneumonia, neurologic symptoms. Rare findings of endocarditis in children include Osler nodes, Janeway lesions, splinter hemorrhages, and Roth spots. Occasionally endocarditis may present acutely as fulminant disease characterized by high fevers and an overall toxic appearance.

Laboratory Tests/Radiographs

Blood cultures are essential for diagnosis of endocarditis and should be obtained prior to the initiation of antibiotics when feasible. Three blood cultures of adequate volume should be collected prior to antibiotic initiation. Echocardiography should be performed to evaluate for vegetations, valvular damage, and overall cardiac function. Urinalysis is recommended if glomerulonephritis is suspected.

Treatment

Diagnosis of endocarditis remains difficult; management of suspected cases should involve consultation with a cardiologist. Broad-spectrum IV antibiotics with activity against the usual pathogens should be initiated and vancomycin is recommended. An aminoglycoside such as gentamicin is often added for its synergistic effect. Surgical therapy may be indicated if bacteremia persists following 2 weeks of therapy.

Antibiotic prophylaxis for endocarditis should be considered for patients deemed as high risk who require dental, oral,

respiratory tract or esophageal procedures. These include children who have unrepaired cyanotic congenital heart disease, including palliative shunts and conduits, repaired congenital heart defects with prosthetic heart valves, device, whether placed by surgery or by catheter intervention, during the first 6 months after the procedure, repaired congenital heart disease with residual defects at the site or adjacent to the site of the prosthetic device, or previous epidose if infective endocarditis.

American Heart Association (AHA) guidelines (2007) recommend the following pediatric dosing for endocarditis prophylaxis:

- Amoxicillin 50 mg/kg to a maximum dose of 2 g
- Azithromycin or clarithromycin 15 mg/kg to a maximum dose of 500 mg
- Clindamycin 20 mg/kg to a maximum dose of 600 mg
- Cephalexin 50 mg/kg to a maximum dose of 2 g

  Equivalent pediatric doses for IM or IV therapy as follows:

- Ampicillin 50 mg/kg to a maximum dose of 2 g
- Cefazolin or ceftriaxone 50 mg/kg to a maximum dose of 1 g
- Clindamycin 20 mg/kg to a maximum dose of 600 mg
- Vancomycin 15 mg/kg to a maximum dose of 1 g

Day MD, Gauvreau K, Schulman S, et al: Characteristics of children hospitalized with infective endocarditis. *Circulation.* 2009;119:865-870 [PMID: 19188508].

Pasquali S, He X, Mohamad ZMS, et al: Trends in endocarditis hospitalizations at US children's hospitals: Impact of the 2007 American Heart Association Antibiotic Prophylaxis Guidelines. *Am Heart J.* 2012;163(5):894-899 [PMID: 22607869].

Rosenthal LB, Feja KN, Levasseur SM, et al: The changing epidemiology of pediatric endocarditis at a children's hospital over seven decades. *Pediatr Cardiol.* 2010;31:813-820 [PMID: 20414646].

Wei HH, Wu KG, Sy LB, et al: Infectious endocarditis in pediatric patients: Analysis of 19 cases presenting at a medical center. *J Microbiol Immunol Infect.* 2010;43(5):430-437 [PMID: 21075710].

MYOCARDITIS

 ESSENTIALS OF DIAGNOSIS

► Shortness of breath.
► Recent URI infection
► Cardiomegaly.
► ECG changes.

Supportive care in severe cases include inotropes, diuretics, and afterload reduction.

General Considerations

Myocarditis is an uncommon and underdiagnosed condition in children that can result in life-threatening complications. Most common etiology in children is viral, although toxic and autoimmune phenomena are possible. Enteroviruses such as cocksackie virus, adenovirus, influenza, and parainfluenza are commonly identified pathogens. Direct injury to the myocardium induces a cytokine response that recruits macrophages, NK cells, and T cells to the inflamed site. The acute phase, which lasts 1-2 weeks, is followed by the second phase in which activated T cells indiscriminately attack the inciting agent as well as neighboring myocytes. Damage to the myocardium decreases ventricular function and may progress to congestive heart failure. The final phase involves healing and fibrosis of the damaged myocardium. Myocarditis is fatal in approximately 10% of patients and progresses to dilated cardiomyopathy in 33% of patients.

Clinical Findings

Although fulminant myocarditis may present acutely with signs of shock and cardiovascular collapse, most children with myocarditis have nonspecific complaints and are frequently misdiagnosed at their first physician encounter. Shortness of breath, vomiting, poor feeding, and history of recent URI are seen. Examination findings include tachypnea, tachycardia, abnormal lung sounds, and hepatomegaly. Chest pain in children, in contrast to adults, is rare. Hypotension, arrhythmias, a new heart murmur, and a gallop rhythm are late findings of ventricular compromise.

Laboratory Tests/Radiographs

Myocarditis is a clinical diagnosis; however, specific laboratory values provide corroborating evidence if the diagnosis is in doubt. Aspartate aminotransferase (AST) is a sensitive marker for myocarditis and is elevated in 85% of patients; however, specificity is low. Likewise, ESR and CRP may be elevated during the acute stage of illness. A CBC with differential may show a lymphocyte predominance reflecting a viral infection. Specific viral studies including rapid PCR swab and viral cultures fail to identify the causative agent in most patients. Cardiac enzymes, specifically troponins T, I, and CK-MB may be elevated due to myocardial cell necrosis. brain naturetic protein (BNP) will be elevated if in heart failure. CXR is abnormal in the majority of cases of myocarditis, with the most frequent finding being cardiomegaly. An ECG is typically abnormal and most often shows sinus tachycardia, nonspecific ST-T wave changes, or ventricular hypertrophy. Echocardiography is the mainstay of diagnosis. Most common findings are regional wall motion abnormalities, regurgitant valves, and other signs of ventricular dysfunction.

Endomyocardial biopsy remains the gold standard for diagnosis but is performed infrequently due to the patchy nature of myocarditis and invasiveness of the procedure.

Treatment

Clinical suspicion of myocarditis should prompt initial evaluation with an ECG and CXR, since most patients will have abnormal ECG or CXR. If suspicion persists, consultation with a cardiologist is warranted for an echocardiogram. Clinical presentation dictates the level of support required; minimally symptomatic children may require observation and cardiologist follow-up whereas children with signs of ventricular dysfunction and congestive heart failure often need admission to an ICU. Emergency department management of severe or fulminant cases of myocarditis should be directed at reestablishing adequate perfusion via addition of inotropes such as dopamine, dobutamine, and milrinone. Administration of excess volume must be carefully monitored as it may exacerbate signs of heart failure and pulmonary congestion; diuretics are often required. Adjunctive therapies such as steroids, IVIG, and β-blockers are controversial and should be used in consultation with the cardiologist.

Durani Y, Egan M, Baffa, et al: Pediatric myocarditis: Presenting clinical characteristics. *Am J Emerg Med.* 2009;27:942-947 [PMID: 19857412].

Durani Y, Giordano K, Goudie BW: Myocarditis and pericarditis in children. *Pediatr Clin North Am.* 2010;57:1281-1303 [PMID: 21111118].

Freedman SB, Haladyn JK, Floh A, et al: Pediatric myocarditis: Emergency department clinical findings and diagnostic evaluation. *Pediatrics.* 2008;120(6):1278-1285 [PMID: 18055677].

Levine MC, Klugman D, Teach SH: Update on myocarditis in children. *Curr Opin Pediatr.* 2010;22:278-283 [PMID: 20414115].

May LJ, Patton DJ, Fruitman DS: The evolving approach to paediatric myocarditis: A review of the current literature. *Cardiol Young.* 2011;21:241-251 [PMID: 21272427].

RESPIRATORY

UPPER RESPIRATORY INFECTIONS

ESSENTIALS OF DIAGNOSIS

▶ Cough.

▶ Congestion.

▶ Rhinorrhea.

▶ Fever.

▶ Sore throat.

Generally self-limited and respond well to supportive care.

General Considerations

Upper respiratory infections (URIs) are extremely common and most are benign. Young children have an average of 6-10 discrete episodes per year, each lasting up to 2 weeks. Direct virus-induced damage to the respiratory mucosa of the nasopharynx plays a minor role in the pathophysiology of URIs; the immune response produces most symptoms. A variety of ubiquitous viruses cause most infections including rhinoviruses, parainfluenza, coronavirus, adenovirus, RSV, and influenza. Of these, infections due to influenza are at highest risk resulting in complications such as encephalitis, myocarditis, and superimposed bacterial infections such as pneumonia and tracheitis. Special attention must be paid to medically complex children and those with chronic illnesses such as asthma, cystic fibrosis, and cardiac disease. Complications of URIs include acute OM, sinusitis, pneumonia, and asthma exacerbations. URIs tend to demonstrate seasonality, with rhinoviruses presenting in late fall, followed by parainfluenza viruses, then RSV, influenza, and coronavirus in the winter months. Adenovirus has a year-round distribution of infection. Transmission of these viruses occurs through spread of droplets and direct contact and is augmented by the close quarters of day care, making these children at greatest risk for repeated infections.

Clinical Findings

Most URIs caused by viruses other than influenza present with signs of nasopharyngeal mucosal inflammation including cough, sore throat, fever, rhinorrhea, and nasal congestion. Symptoms peak on day 3 of illness and resolve in 7-10 days, with cough often the most persistent symptom. Failure to improve over this time frame should prompt an investigation into potential signs of bacterial superinfection such as a bulging tympanic membrane OM, thick mucopurluent drainage (sinusitis), or tachypnea, fever, and focal crackles (pneumonia).

Influenza presents acutely with myalgias, malaise, headache, and high fever which precede development of prominent respiratory symptoms, although some children may have a mild presentation which is clinically indistinguishable from a typical URI. Children with influenza infections generally show improvement in symptoms within 1 week of illness. CNS complications such as Guillian-Barre syndrome, acute cerebellar ataxia, and acute disseminated encephalitis manifest as ascending weakness, poor coordination, and altered mental status.

Laboratory Tests/Radiographs

Although a thorough search into the precise viral etiology of most URIs is not necessary, rapid antigen detection kits have been developed for influenza and RSV. PCR testing is more sensitive than the rapid antigen tests but takes at least 6 hours for results to be available. Viral culture is rarely indicated except for epidemiologic reasons. Radiographs play little role in diagnosis but are useful if superimposed pneumonia is suspected.

Treatment

Most children respond well to supportive care, including hydration, nasal suction with saline, fever control with acetaminophen and ibuprofen, and humidified air. Over-the-counter cough and cold preparations should not be used by children younger than 6 years and have not been shown to be of benefit to older children. Persistent cough is treated symptomatically with cool liquids and honey for children older than 1 year. Proper anticipatory guidance describing the epidemiology and natural course of most URIs is helpful for families. Antibiotics do not play a role unless bacterial superinfection is suspected. Healthy children with influenza may be treated with an antiviral agent such as oseltamivir provided they are diagnosed within 48 hours of disease onset. Children who are hospitalized or at risk for serious complications from influenza are also offered antiviral therapy.

Brownlee JW, Turner R: New developments in the epidemiology and clinical spectrum of rhinovirus infections. *Curr Opin Pediatr.* 2008;20:67-71 [PMID: 18197042].

Chung EY, Chiang VW: Influenza vaccination, diagnosis, and treatment in children. *Pediatr Emer Care.* 2011;27:760-772 [PMID: 21822091].

BRONCHIOLITIS

ESSENTIALS OF DIAGNOSIS

► Wheezing.

► Tachypnea.

► Retractions.

► Hypoxia.

Supportive care is mainstay of treatment for most uncomplicated cases.

General Considerations

Bronchiolitis involves inflammation of the small airways of the lower respiratory tract and is classically caused by RSV, though many viruses are capable of producing the same clinical presentation. Direct viral damage to the respiratory mucosa of the bronchioles induces an immune response characterized by edema, cell necrosis, and lymphocytic infiltrates that lead to airway obstruction. Small airway obstruction produces classic signs of wheezing and respiratory distress, although unlike asthma, airway hyper-responsiveness is not a key component. Young children, particularly those younger than 1 year, are at the greatest risk of developing clinically relevant disease. Although most children with bronchiolitis recover uneventfully, former preterm infants, those with congenital heart disease, and those with chronic lung disease are more likely to require hospitalization. A monoclonal antibody to RSV, pavil-zumab, is available as prophylaxis for children at greatest risk for disease and is typically given at monthly intervals over the winter season when the risk for RSV infection is greatest. RSV bronchiolitis has been shown to predict an increased risk for reactive airway disease and asthma for children as old as 11 years.

Clinical Findings

Bronchiolitis in its early stages is indistinguishable from URI and is characterized by fever, cough, congestion, and rhinorrhea. Illness typically peaks in severity on day 3-4 as wheezing and tachypnea become more prominent. In young infants, apnea may be a presenting feature. Respiratory distress in younger infants manifests as retractions, poor feeding, and grunting in severe cases. Examination of the lungs, aside from diffuse wheezing, may demonstrate crackles and a prolonged expiratory phase. Hypoxia is common in patients with bronchiolitis due to obstruction-related V/Q mismatch in the small airways. Concurrent OM may also be found.

Laboratory Tests/Radiographs

Bronchiolitis is a clinical diagnosis and ancillary studies are rarely helpful in evaluation of nontoxic-appearing children older than 2 months. A venous blood gas in severe cases may show hypoxia and hypercarbia. A CBC with differential is not typically indicated unless bacterial superinfection such as pneumonia is suspected. Routine rapid viral testing for RSV is unnecessary. CXR is rarely useful for diagnosis as shifting patterns of atelectasis are common but may be mistaken for infiltrates. Routine use of CXR for children with bronchiolitis leads to increased antibiotic use without changing clinical outcomes.

Treatment

Most children with mild cases of bronchiolitis may be managed expectantly with supportive care. Clinical presentation including history of known risk factors, degree of respiratory distress, and day of illness onset may be used to determine disposition and treatment. Hypoxia with oxygen saturations less than 90-92% is an indication for supplemental oxygen and continuous pulse oximetry. Hypertonic nasal saline and suctioning are useful adjuncts for the clearance of secretions.

Corticosteroids and routine bronchodilator therapy are not indicated; however, a trial of bronchodilators (albuterol and/or epinephrine) may be attempted if there is clinical history of atopy or family history of asthma. Antibiotics are infrequently useful unless there are clear signs of bacterial superinfection. Infants and children with severe respiratory distress frequently require positive pressure ventilation with CPAP or high-flow nasal airway respiratory support. Failure to improve after these interventions is an indication for intubation and monitoring in the ICU.

Corneli HM, Zorc JJ, Holubkov R, et al: Bronchiolitis: Clinical characteristics associated with hospitalization and length of stay. *Pediatr Emerg Care.* 2012;28(2):99-103 [PMID: 22270499].

Petruzella FD, Gorelick MH: Current therapies in bronchiolitis. *Pediatr Emerg Care.* 2010;26(4)302-311 [PMID: 20386418].

Schuh S: Update on management of bronchiolitis. *Curr Opin Pediatr.* 2011;23:110-114 [PMID: 21157348].

Stockman LJ, Curns AT, Anderson LJ, et al: Respiratory syncytial virus-associated hospitalizations among infants and young children in the United States, 1997-2006. *Pediatr Inf Dis J.* 2012;31:5-9 [PMID: 21817948].

Wagner T: Bronchiolitis. *Pediatr Rev.* 2009;30(10):386-395 [PMID: 19797481].

CROUP

 ESSENTIALS OF DIAGNOSIS

▶ Hoarse voice.

▶ Barky cough.

▶ Stridor.

Treat with dexamethasone and nebulized epinephrine.

General Considerations

Croup refers to laryngotracheobronchitis and is common among children aged 6-36 months. It affects boys slightly more often than girls and tends to occur in the late fall and winter months. Viral damage to the mucosal surfaces of the larynx, trachea, and large bronchioles induces an immune response consisting of edema and cellular infiltration which leads to airway narrowing. Subglottic region is particularly sensitive to airway swelling because it is constrained within a relatively fixed cartilaginous ring. Classic croup is caused by parainfluenza viruses which exhibit tropism for the mucosal epithelium of the trachea and larynx. Viruses such as adenovirus, influenza, RSV, and metapneumovirus can produce an identical clinical presentation. Risk factors for the development of croup include reflux, asthma, or family history of croup.

Clinical Findings

Inspiratory stridor with agitation, barky cough, and hoarseness present suddenly, often at night, and may be preceded by nonspecific signs of URI such as cough, rhinorrhea, and fever. Severe presentations are characterized by retractions and stridor at rest; increasingly quiet cough, biphasic stridor, and decreased level of consciousness are signs of impending respiratory failure.

Laboratory Tests/Radiographs

Routine laboratory tests and radiographs are not indicated for straightforward presentations of croup. CBC with differential may show leukocytosis with neutrophil predominance if there is bacterial superinfection. AP radiographs classically show the "steeple sign" of subglottic narrowing. Swelling of the epiglottis or retropharyngeal space suggests alternative explanation for clinical stridor.

Treatment

Children with croup are classified as having mild, moderate, or severe symptoms. Up to 85% of children have mild symptoms, whereas only 1% is classified as severe. Children with cough, no stridor, and minimal respiratory distress are managed with a dose of dexamethasone (0.6 mg/kg PO or IV, maximum 10 mg) and return to the emergency department if symptoms reoccur. Children with inspiratory stridor with agitation, prominent barky cough, and moderate retractions should be given nebulized racemic epinephrine and dexamethasone and observed in the emergency department for 2-4 hours. If symptoms improve as evidenced by minimal stridor and retractions, the child may be discharged with strict return precautions.

In children with severe symptoms of croup a rapid assessment of respiratory status should be undertaken. Children with signs of impending respiratory failure should be intubated with an endotracheal tube that is 0.5-1 mm smaller than what would typically be used. Severely affected children who do not require intubation should be managed in a way that limits agitation of the child. Dexamethasone and nebulized epinephrine (racemic epinephrine or standard L-epinephrine) should be provided. L-epinephrine is given as 5 mL of a 1:1000 solution (racemic epinephrine is given as 0.5 mL of 2.25% solution in 2.5 mL of NS) and delivered via nebulization. Supplemental oxygen, delivered via blow-by technique, should be provided if oxygen saturation is less than 92%. Children should be observed for 2-4 hours following treatment with nebulized epinephrine. Reccurrence of stridor at rest or moderate retractions within this time period should prompt readministration of epinephrine and admission to the hospital. Adjunctive treatment with heliox may promote laminar flow within the airways.

Bjornson CL, Johnson DW: Croup. *Lancet.* 2008;371:329-339 [PMID: 18295000].

Cherry JD: Croup. *N Engl J Med.* 2008;358:384-391 [PMID: 18216359].

PNEUMONIA

ESSENTIALS OF DIAGNOSIS

▶ Tachypnea.

▶ Fever.

▶ Hypoxia.

▶ Infiltrate on CXR.

Severe presentations require supplemental oxygen, antibiotics, and admission.

General Considerations

Pneumonia is a frequent diagnosis in children and significant cause of morbidity worldwide. Infection usually develops following virus-induced mucosal damage to the upper respiratory tract which allows pathogenic bacteria and viruses to spread to the lower respiratory tract. Invasion of the pulmonary parenchyma initiates an immune response characterized by lymphocytes, necrotic cell debris, and tissue edema. Obstruction of the small airways of the lung results in reduced compliance, airway collapse, and hypoxia via V/Q mismatch. Viral causes of pneumonia predominate in children younger than 5 years, whereas those older than 5 years are at risk of streptococcal and mycoplasma pneumonia (Table 41–6). Despite the widespread implementation of the pneumococcal vaccine, streptococcal pneumonia remains the most common etiologic agent of bacterial pneumonia beyond the first month of life. Pneumonia in neonates younger than 1 month is unique. There is a high significance of maternally transmitted bacteria such as GBS, gram-negative (*E. coli*), and *Listeria*. Up to 10% of older children with bacterial pneumonia subsequently develop a parapneumonic effusion as the inflamed pleura leaks fluid into the pleural space. Bacteria spread and proliferate within this fluid, further enhancing the cycle of inflammation and fluid leakage. Recent reports suggest that increasing rates of effusion may be due to antibiotic overuse, CA-MRSA, and changes in pneumococcal serotype prevalence since the pneumococcal vaccine was developed. Untreated, parapneumonic effusion can progress to empyema and lung abscess. Children at greatest risk for the development of bacterial pneumonia include those with preexisting heart and lung disease, immunodeficiency syndromes, and gastroesophageal reflux. Medically complex children including those

Table 41–6. Comparison of viral, bacterial, and atypical pneumonia.

	Viral	Bacterial	Atypical
Age (years)	< 5	> 5	> 5
Radiographic infiltrates	Interstitial	Lobar	Peribronchial
Pathogens	RSV, influenza, parainfluenza, adenovirus	S. pneumoniae, S. aureus, GAS	M. pneumoniae, C. pneumoniae
Clinical findings	Rhinorrhea, wheezing	Focal crackles/decreased breath sounds, tachypnea, fever	Pharyngitis, cough, headache, wheezing
Onset	Gradual	Abrupt	Gradual
Complications	Bacterial superinfection, SIADH	Pleural effusion, empyema, SIADH	Hemolysis, arthritits/arthralgias, meningoencephalitis (rare)
Treatment	Supportive	< 5 yr old: Ampicillin/amoxicillin > 5 yr old: third-generation cephalosporin	Azithromycin

with cerebral palsy, tracheostomies, and impaired levels of consciousness are at risk for aspiration pneumonia with anaerobic oral bacteria.

Clinical Findings

Tachypnea is the most sensitive indicator of pneumonia in children. Fever, cough, and rhinorrhea are common but may be seen with URIs as well. With bacterial pneumonia, the pulmonary examination reveals focally decreased breath sounds, tactile fremitus, and dullness to percussion indicating consolidation. Viral pneumonia is associated with diffuse auscultatory findings including wheezing. Crackles or rales may be heard with viral or bacterial infections. Severe respiratory distress is manifested by overall ill appearance, hypoxia, grunting, severe retractions, and nasal flaring. Young infants may display poor feeding due to tachypnea. Chronic symptoms of fever, night sweats, weight loss, and travel history should raise suspicion for tuberculosis.

Laboratory Tests/Radiographs

CBC with differential and blood culture are routinely obtained for patients admitted to the hospital. Leukocytosis greater than 15,000 cells/µL with neutrophil predominance suggests a bacterial infection, and blood culture is positive in up to 10% of those with pneumonia and in 30% of those with a parapneumonic effusion or empyema. Sputum cultures are reliable only in children older than 5 years. Basic metabolic profile (BMP) may demonstrate mild to moderate hyponatremia as a consequence of SIADH. Inflammatory markers are helpful when a prolonged course of treatment is anticipated. Viral studies including PCR and culture are not indicated unless they will change the management of

the patient. Culture and Gram stain should be sent if pleural fluid is obtained via thoracentesis. A tuberculin skin test should be sent if there is concern for tuberculosis.

Classic CXR findings of pneumonia vary according to the etiologic agent of disease but are not particularly specific. Bacterial pneumonia is associated with lobar consolidation whereas mycoplasma and viral infections show diffuse bilateral infiltrates. Pleural effusion blunts the costophrenic angle; lateral decubitus films with the affected side down are helpful in determining if the fluid is mobile or loculated. Ultrasound is the preferred imaging modality when a large effusion is present, whereas CT with contrast is best if a lung abscess is suspected.

Treatment

Most children older than 5 years with pneumonia may be managed as outpatients. Younger well-appearing children with classic localizing signs on examination may be diagnosed clinically with bacterial pneumonia and treated with a 7-10-day course of an oral antibiotic such as high-dose amoxicillin (60-90 mg/kg/d divided twice a day). A third-generation cephalosporin such as ceftriaxone (or oral cefdinir) may be used in children younger than 1 year if there is concern for gram-negative bacteria such as M. catarrhalis or K. pneumoniae. Children older than 5 years with mild disease not requiring hospitalization should be treated empirically with a 5-day course of a macrolide such as azithromycin to cover against mycoplasma.

Children with significant respiratory distress, supplemental oxygen requirement, chronic underlying medical conditions, and infants younger than 6 months should be admitted to the hospital. Empiric antibiotics include IV ampicillin or a third-generation cephalosporin in combination with a macrolide such as azithromycin. Severe cases of pneumonia should be treated empirically with a third-generation cephalosporin and vancomycin. Cases of suspected aspiration pneumonia should be managed with amoxicillin-clavulanic acid or clindamycin to cover against oral anaerobic bacteria. A clinically significant pleural effusion should be managed in consultation with the surgery service.

Alak A, Seabrook JA, Rieder MJ: Variations in the management of pneumonia in pediatric emergency departments: Compliance with the guidelines. *CJEM.* 2010;12(6):514-519 [PMID: 21073778].

Choi J, Lee G: Thoracic emergencies common pediatric respiratory emergencies. *Emerg Med Clin North Am.* 2012;30(2): 529-563 [PMID: 22487117].

Massimiliano D, Canciani M, Korppi M: Community-acquired pneumonia in children: What's old? What's new? *Acta Paediatrica.* 2010;99(11):1602-1608 [PMID: 20573146].

McBride SC: Management of parapneumonic effusions in pediatrics: current practice. *J Hosp Med.* 2008;3(3):263-270 [PMID: 18570324].

Ruuskanen O, Lahti E, Jennings LC, et al: Viral pneumonia. *Lancet.* 2011;377(9773):1264-1275 [PMID: 21435708].

PERTUSSIS

 ESSENTIALS OF DIAGNOSIS

▶ Coughing paroxysms > 2 weeks duration.

▶ Cyanosis.

▶ Apnea.

Treat patient and contacts with 5-7-day course of azithromycin.

General Considerations

A disease earlier thought to be on the decline, pertussis has been increasing since the early 1980s. Reasons for the resurgence include alternative immunization schedules, waning immunity among adults, and improved methods of detection. Pertussis is caused by a gram-negative bacillus, *Bordatella pertussis*, which is efficiently transmitted by aerosolized respiratory droplets. The bacteria exhibits tropism for the ciliated respiratory epithelial cells of the nasopharynx and upper respiratory tract and produces cytotoxins that destroy these cells, leading to the classic paroxysmal cough. Pertussis can reinfect older previously immunized adults and children, but most severely affects unimmunized infants younger than 2 months and those younger than 6 months who are not fully vaccinated. Pertussis infections progress through three phases: (1) catarrhal phase that resembles a URI and lasts 1-2 weeks; (2) paroxysmal phase characterized by coughing paroxysms that persists 2-6 weeks; and (3) convalescent phase that lasts up to several months. Infants may not have noticeable signs or symptoms prior to entering the paroxysmal phase. Unfortunately, pertussis is spread most efficiently during the catarrhal phase when symptoms are usually nonspecific. Risk factors for pertussis infection include age younger than 2 months, family members with cough, and preexisting lung disease.

Clinical Findings

Early symptoms of pertussis may be absent in infants or resemble a URI, including mild cough, rhinorrhea, and congestion. Patients tend to present to the emergency department in the paroxysmal phase with by paroxysms of cough that may be followed by an inspiratory gasp which gives rise to the name "whooping" cough. Young infants may present with apnea, cyanosis, and poor feeding during coughing paroxysms but may be clinically well-appearing between episodes. Posttussive emesis is common. Lung examination may reveal bilateral rhonchi or focal findings in cases of bacterial superinfection. Patients in the convalescent phase have a mild cough that gradually resolves. Vaccinated children with pertussis may progress through the same clinical stages but are usually less severely affected.

Laboratory Tests/Radiographs

Although pertussis may be diagnosed clinically, diagnostic testing is indicated for epidemiologic purposes and to determine if prophylaxis for close contacts is necessary. PCR testing has replaced DFA as the preferred rapid testing modality; however, a nasopharyngeal culture should be obtained to confirm the diagnosis. CBC with differential classically demonstrates marked lymphocytosis, though this finding is nonspecific. CXR is not usually required unless pneumonia is suspected on physical examination; typically the CXR is normal or shows only atelectasis or mild perihilar infiltrates.

Treatment

Children with significant respiratory distress, history of cyanotic or apneic episodes, those younger than 3 months, and children unable to maintain adequate intake due to coughing should be admitted to the hospital and placed on droplet precautions. Treatment with a 5-7-day course of a macrolide such as azithromycin is sufficient to reduce duration of illness and decrease infectivity. However, the mainstay of treatment is supportive care with cardiorespiratory monitoring for young infants, and enteral or parenteral nutrition for patients unable to tolerate adequate intake. Prophylaxis should be offered to all close contacts and consists of a

5-7-day treatment course of a macrolide or TMP-SMX for those with a macrolide allergy.

Mackey JE, Wojcik S, Long R, et al: Predicting pertussis in a pediatric emergency department population. *Clin Pediatr.* 2007;46:437-440 [PMID: 17556741].

Marconi GP, Ross LA, Nager AL: An upsurge in pertussis. *Pediatr Emer Care.* 2012;28:215-291 [PMID: 22344207].

GASTROINTESTINAL

GASTROENTERITIS

 ESSENTIALS OF DIAGNOSIS

▶ Diarrhea.

▶ Vomiting.

▶ Abdominal pain.

Treatment is supportive and antibiotics are generally not indicated.

General Considerations

Gastroenteritis is exceedingly common among children, with the average child having up to five episodes per year before 5 years of age. In the emergency department this translates to nearly 10% of all patient encounters. Gastroenteritis develops when a pathogen infects the cells lining the small intestine. The destruction of this cell layer disrupts the villous architecture that is responsible for nutrient absorption. Nutrients and other osmotically active substances remain in the intestine and fluid passes across the damaged villous layer into the lumen, leading to loose, frequent stools. Most infections in children are caused by viruses, although bacteria and parasites also cause disease. Rotavirus, once the cause of roughly 50% of all cases of childhood gastroenteritis, has declined rapidly since the introduction of the rotavirus vaccine in 2006. However, a range of other viruses including adenovirus, astrovirus, and calcivirus are frequently found. Bacterial gastroenteritis is more common among children younger than 5 years and may be caused by *E. coli*, *Shigella*, *Salmonella*, and *Campylobacter*. *Giardia* is the most common cause of parasitic gastroenteritis in developed countries. *E. coli* and *Shigella* species are associated with the development of hemolytic uremic syndrome (HUS), a potentially life-threatening complication of infectious diarrhea that occurs when toxin-mediated endothelial damage leads to intravascular hemolysis and kidney damage. *Clostridium difficile* is an important cause of antibiotic-associated diarrhea which develops after the natural bacterial flora of the gut is disrupted, allowing pathogenic bacteria to proliferate. Children younger than 1 year have coloizations rates of *C. difficle* of 14-37%, and therefore *C. difficle* is not considered a pathogen in this age group. Most cases of gastroenteritis are self-limited and last 3-7 days; however, it is a frequent cause of morbidity among very young children, the immunosuppressed, and those with chronic medical conditions.

Clinical Findings

Acute gastroenteritis is associated with loose stools or diarrhea (clinically defined as greater than 3 stools/24 hr in older children) that represents a change from a child's baseline stooling pattern. Vomiting and abdominal pain are common but fever is not. Other nonspecific symptoms such as headache, anorexia, cough, and myalgias may be reported. Frank blood or mucus in the stool is associated with a bacterial etiology; hemoccult positive stool does not differential between bacterial and viral causes. Signs of dehydration may be present, including poor urine output, tachycardia, delayed capillary refill, decreased skin turgor, and acute weight loss. In severe cases, dehydration can progress to shock with altered mental status, lethargy, and cool extremities.

Laboratory Tests/Radiographs

Children with suspected viral gastroenteritis may be managed without routine laboratory tests. Children with signs of moderate dehydration including those who require IV rehydration may have a BMP obtained. Decreased bicarbonate less than 17 mEq/L is the most sensitive indicator of moderate or severe dehydration, though hyper- or hyponatremia may also be seen. Elevated BUN suggests prerenal dehydration, though a concurrent rise in creatinine should raise suspicion for HUS. If bacterial gastroenteritis is a consideration, stool studies including culture and leukocytes should be collected. *C. difficle* testing is not recommended for children younger than 1 year. A CBC with differential and a blood culture, particularly if the patient is febrile. Stool pH less than 6 and stool-reducing substances suggest viral gastroenteritis but are not confirmatory. Rapid stool tests for rotavirus are available; however, testing for other viral sources of infection is uncommon unless required for epidemiologic purposes. Stool for ova and parasites should be obtained when patient history suggests potential exposure to *Giardia*.

Treatment

Patient level of dehydration should be assessed immediately and documented carefully as treatments are initiated. For most children gastroenteritis may be managed supportively with oral rehydration therapy. Feeding with a regular diet should be attempted, and breast-feeding infants should continue to feed. Children who fail oral rehydration or who present with severe dehydration should receive IV rehydration and be admitted. Antiemetic agents have been shown to be of benefit in some children with gastroenteritis but their widespread use is controversial. Antidiarrheal and antimotility agents are not indicated in children, and antibiotics are unnecessary in most patients with bacterial gastroenteritis unless there are signs of septicemia. *C. difficile*, when determined pathogenic, and *Giardia* may be treated with metronidazole. Limited studies of probiotics suggest they may be a useful adjunct for decreasing duration of diarrhea in children.

Dennehy PH: Viral gastroenteritis in children. *Pediatr Infect Dis J.* 2011;30(1):63-64 [PMID: 21173676].

Freedman SB, Gouin S, Bhatt M, et al: Prospective assessment of practice pattern variations in the treatment of pediatric gastroenteritis. *Pediatrics.* 2011;127(2):e287-295 [PMID: 21262881].

Schutze GE, Willoughby RE: Committee on infectious diseases policy statement. *Clostridium difficile* infection in infants and children. *Pediatrics.* 2013;131:196-200 [PMID: 23277317].

Szajewska H, Dziechciarz P: Gastrointestinal infections in the pediatric population. *Curr Opin Gastroenterol.* 2010;26(1): 36-44 [PMID: 19887936].

Wiegering V, Kaiser J, Tappe D, et al: Gastroenteritis in childhood: A retrospective study of 650 hospitalized pediatric patients. *Int J Infect Dis.* 2011;15:e401-e407 [PMID: 21489842].

HEPATITIS

ESSENTIALS OF DIAGNOSIS

▶ Mildly elevated transaminases.

▶ Jaundice.

▶ Malaise.

Typical treatment is supportive and chronic infection is common.

General Considerations

Infectious viral hepatitis is uncommon as an acute illness because it is often subclinical or only mildly symptomatic. In children it is caused by hepatitis A virus (HAV), hepatitis B virus (HBV), hepatitis C virus (HCV), or hepatitis E virus (HEV) (Table 41–7). Hepatitis D virus (HDD) is seen rarely in adults as a coinfection with HBV and HEV is rare in developed countries. HAV and HEV are transmitted via the fecal-oral route whereas HBV and HCV are blood-borne pathogens. In each case these viruses infect hepatocytes, causing direct cell damage as well as inducing a pathologic immune response. HAV is less prevalent since the implementation of the vaccine in the early 2000s but outbreaks can occur among day care attendees. HBV in children is

Table 41–7. Review of viral hepatitis in children.

	Hepatitis A	Hepatitis B	Hepatitis C	Hepatitis E
Transmission	Fecal-oral	Bloodborne	Bloodborne	Fecal-oral
Vertical transmission rate	N/A	30-90%	2-5%	N/A
Clinical presentation	Jaundice, fever, nausea, vomiting	Jaundice, malaise, RUQ pain	Usually subclinical	Jaundice, malaise, anorexia, nausea, vomiting
Laboratory markers	Conjugated bilirubinemia, transaminitis	Conjugated bilirubinemia, transaminitis	Acute: labs usually normal Chronic: mild transaminitis	Conjugated bilirubinemia, transaminitis
Diagnosis	IgM anti-HAV	HbsAg, HBV PCR, IgM anti-Hbc	Anti-HCV antibodies, HCV PCR	IgM anti-HEV, HEV PCR (neither commercially available)
Treatment	Supportive	Acute: supportive Chronic: interferon, lamivudine	Acute: supportive Chronic: pegylated interferon, ribavirin	Supportive
Complications	Acute liver failure (rare)	Chronic hepatitis (90% if perinatal transmission), polyarteritis nodosa, nephropathy, cirrhosis, HCC	Chronic hepatitis (50%), cirrhosis, HCC	Acute liver failure (rare unless patient is pregnant)

typically transmitted vertically; infants born to mothers with known disease are treated with the vaccine and hepatitis B immunoglobulin (HBIG) within 12 hours of birth. HBV progresses to chronic infection in as many as 90% of children who acquire it perinatally, compared to 5-10% who contract it postnatally. Children with chronic HBV often develop liver fibrosis but rarely cirrhosis or hepatocellular carcinoma. HCV is also primarily transmitted vertically from mother to child; however, no effective means of infant prophylaxis has been developed, although only 5% of at-risk infants will acquire the virus and 50% of those will clear the infection by 3 years of age. Chronic infection with HCV leads to cirrhosis and hepatocellular carcinoma (HCC), complications that are rare in children.

Clinical Findings

HAV may be misdiagnosed as viral gastroenteritis because it often presents acutely with fever, malaise, abdominal pain, vomiting, and diarrhea. Jaundice may occur after week 1 of illness and rash, and arthritis may also be seen. HBV is often subclinical but can present with nausea, jaundice, and mild right upper quadrant pain. HCV rarely presents with clinical symptoms.

Laboratory Tests/Radiographs

Children with acute HAV, HBV, and HCV may have elevated transaminases as well as a conjugated hyperbilirubinemia, but these do not always correlate with the severity of infection. Evidence of impaired liver function such as prolonged prothrombin time or decreased albumin is seen only in rare cases of fulminant hepatic failure. Diagnostic testing for HAV is rarely required but can be done by measuring the serum level of IgM antibodies to the virus. Serum HBV studies include hepatitis B surface antigen (HBsAg), anti-HBsAG, hepatitis B e antigen (HBeAg), and anti-hepatitis B core antigen (HBcAg) . Acute hepatitis B infection is characterized by positive HBsAg, IgM anti-HBcAg, HBeAg, and HBV DNA via PCR. Chronic HCV can be diagnosed with a positive anti-HCV antibody although in the acute setting HCV PCR assays are available.

Treatment

HAV, HBV, and HCV are managed supportively in the acute setting with careful attention to hydration status. Postexposure prophylaxis consisting of HAV immune globulin should be offered to unvaccinated children in close contact with a confirmed case of HAV. Rarely HAV infection can present as fulminant liver failure requiring intensive monitoring and potentially transplant. Treatment of chronic HBV and HCV infection requires consultation with a gastroenterologist or infectious disease specialist and may involve interferon, ribavirin, and nucleoside reverse transcriptase inhibitors.

Clemente MG, Schwarz K: Hepatitis: General principles. *Pediatr Rev.* 2011;32(8):333-340 [PMID: 21807874].

Jeong SH, Lee HS: Hepatitis A: Clinical manifestations and management. *Intervirology.* 2010;53(1):15-19 [PMID: 20068336].

Jhaveri R: Diagnosis and management of hepatitis C virus-infected children. *Pediatr Infect Dis J.* 2011;30(11):983-985 [PMID: 21997662].

Yeung LT, Roberts EA: Current issues in the management of paediatric viral hepatitis. *Liver Int.* 2009;30(1):5-18 [PMID: 19840256].

MUSCULOSKELETAL

OSTEOMYELITIS

 ESSENTIALS OF DIAGNOSIS

▶ Fever.

▶ Bony pain.

▶ Limited movement.

▶ Limp.

General Considerations

Cases of osteomyelitis make up about 1% of pediatric hospital admissions and in children osteomyelitis typically result from hematogenous spread of bacteria, although trauma or extension from a soft tissue infection are potential causes. The metaphyseal region of the long bones is most commonly affected in children because sluggish blood flow in this area can become a nidus of infection during otherwise transient and subclinical bacteremia. In children younger than 2 years, vascular channels allow bacteria to spread from the metaphysis across the physis into the joint space, resulting in concomitant septic arthritis. Minor trauma to a bone can cause a small hematoma in the metaphyseal region capable of harboring bacteria. As the infection spreads, a subperiosteal abscess can develop, leading to periosteal elevation. *S. aureus* is responsible for 70-90% of hematogenous osteomyelitis, due in large part to virulence factors that aid in adhesion to bone as well as proteolytic enzymes that help penetrate the bone surface. CA-MRSA has become a common cause of osteomyelitis and is associated with a greater risk of complications such as pyomyositis, abscess, and deep venous thrombosis. Other important pathogens include *S. pyogenes, S. pneumoniae,* and GBS in infants. *Kingella kingae,* a gram-negative bacillus more commonly associated with septic arthritis, is an increasingly recognized cause of osteomyelitis in children younger than 3 years. Risk factors for the development of osteomyelitis include sickle cell disease (SCD), having implanted hardware or an indwelling catheter, and neurovascular disease.

Clinical Findings

Osteomyelitis may present acutely with fever, malaise, and local bony tenderness. Conversely, among some children it presents more indolently as a limp with or without a fever. Younger children may not be able to localize the specific site of infection, instead presenting with irritability and decreased movement of the affected extremity. Pain with passive movement of the joint is uncommon unless there is concomitant septic arthritis. Erythema, warmth, and swelling over the site of infection are late findings.

Laboratory Tests/Radiographs

CBC with differential, ESR, CRP, and blood culture are recommended if osteomyelitis is a diagnostic consideration. Elevated inflammatory markers are extremely sensitive for osteomyelitis and are important for trending response to treatment. Elevated WBC count with neutrophilia is seen in fewer than 50% of children with osteomyelitis. Blood cultures are positive in up to 50% of patients with hematogenous osteomyelitis and ideally two blood cultures should be obtained prior to the initiation of antibiotics. If surgical drainage or debridement is performed, antibiotics should be withheld if possible until appropriate blood and tissue cultures are sent.

Plain films of the affected areas are commonly obtained upon initial evaluation of children with suspected osteomyelitis, but hallmark periosteal elevation may be seen only after 10-14 days of illness. Despite the need for sedation in young children, MRI with contrast has become the imaging modality of choice because it demonstrates marrow edema early in the course of disease and best characterizes surrounding edema, abscess, or myositis. Bone scan may be used to guide a subsequent MRI if the affected area cannot be determined from physical examination.

Treatment

Suspected cases of osteomyelitis should be managed in consultation with an orthopedist in case surgical drainage is indicated. Once appropriate cultures have been obtained, empiric IV antibiotics may be started. Because of the prevalence of CA-MRSA, vancomycin or clindamycin is recommended as initial treatment, with nafcillin, oxacillin, or cefazolin is acceptable if the rate of MRSA among community staphylococcal isolates is less than 10%. Septic and ill-appearing children should be treated empirically with vancomycin due to the association between severe disease and MRSA. When infection with *Kingella* is suspected, a first-generation cephalosporin should be added because vancomycin and clindamycin have little activity

against most gram-negative bacteria. Children with osteomyelitis should be admitted for IV therapy; transition to oral therapy is possible after pathogen identified and clinical improvement has been documented.

Conrad DA: Acute hematogenous osteromyelitis. *Pediatr Rev.* 2010;31(11):464-471 [PMID: 21041424].

Harik NS, Smeltzer MS: Management of acute hematogenous osteomyelitis in children. *Expert Rev Anti Infect Ther.* 2010;8(2):175-181 [PMID: 20109047].

Jackson MA, Newland JG: Staphylococcal infections in the era of MRSA. *Pediatr Rev.* 2011;32(12):522-532 [PMID: 22135422].

Thomsen I, Creech CB: Advances in the diagnosis and management of pediatric osteomyelitis. *Curr Infect Dis Rep.* 2011;13:451-460 [PMID: 21789499].

SEPTIC ARTHRITIS

 ESSENTIALS OF DIAGNOSIS

▸ Fever.

▸ Pain with passive movement of the joint.

▸ Warmth.

▸ Swelling.

▸ Refusal to bear weight.

General Considerations

Similar to osteomyelitis, septic arthritis develops most commonly in children as a result of hematogenous spread during a subclinical episode of transient bacteremia. Joints of the lower extremities, particularly hip and knee, are most frequently affected. The vascular nature of the synovial membrane and the high blood flow it receives makes it a nidus for infection. Septic arthritis can also result from direct inoculation via trauma or from contiguous spread from osteomyelitis through vascular channels in the growth plates that are present until 2 years of age. Inflammation within the joint space causes swelling, destruction of the synovium, and impairs cartilage synthesis. Bacterial pathogens predominate over viral or fungal pathogens, and the most commonly identified are *S. aureus* (including MRSA), *Streptococcus*, and *K kingae*. Because of improvements in detection methods, *Kingella* is increasingly recognized as a common cause of septic arthritis in children younger than 3 years. It can be a part of the normal oral flora of children and transient bacteremia due to *Kingella* following a URI leads to joint infection. Infants younger than 3 months are at risk for arthritis from *Staphylococcus*, GBS, and gram-negative bacteria, whereas adolescents are at risk for *N. gonorrheae* arthritis. *Salmonella* must be considered in children with SCD. Complications of septic arthritis include joint laxity, avascular necrosis, and limb-length discrepancy if the growth plate is affected.

Clinical Findings

Presentation of septic arthritis varies according to the joint affected but in general involves fever, pain with movement of the joint, limp, and refusal to bear weight. Swelling and erythema over the joint are sometimes found but can be subtle, particularly in children with hip arthritis. Infants present more nonspecifically with irritability, fever, and lack of movement of the involved extremity. Infants with hip arthritis often hold the leg flexed, abducted, and externally rotated. In contrast to osteomyelitis, passive range of motion of the joint in septic arthritis often causes pain. Among sexually active patients, the presence of a rash suggests gonococcal arthritis.

Laboratory Tests/Radiographs

Initial laboratory tests include CBC with differential, ESR, CRP, and a blood culture. Elevated WBC count, ESR, and CRP are common but may be more helpful for ruling out the possibility of a septic joint. When drainage or debridement is performed, cultures of the synovial fluid should be sent; in combination with blood cultures, a bacterial pathogen can be identified in more than 50% of cases of septic arthritis. Synovial fluid should also be sent for cell count, and Gram stain and a synovial WBC count greater than 50,000 cells/μL is suggestive of bacterial arthritis. Because *Kingella* is extremely difficult to culture, synovial fluid for PCR for *Kingella* should be sent if clinical suspicion is high. Gonococcal cultures and nucleic acid amplification tests (NAATs) should be sent if suspected.

Radiographs of the affected joint are commonly nondiagnostic but may demonstrate joint space widening, swelling, or signs of concomitant osteomyelitis. Ultrasound is used, particularly for the hip, to identify an effusion but cannot be used to determine if the fluid is infected. MRI with contrast is the most sensitive imaging modality and is helpful if osteomyelitis is also suspected.

Treatment

Diagnosis of a septic joint may be difficult in children and is often done in consultation with an orthopedist. The Kocher criteria listed below assist with diagnosis:

WBC > 12,000 cells/μL.

ESR > 40 mm/h.

Fever.

Non-weight-bearing status.

If 3 or 4 of the criteria are met there is a high predictive value for septic arthritis. However in equivocal cases a high index of suspicion should be maintained due to the serious complications of untreated septic arthritis. Successful therapy begins with prompt surgical drainage and irrigation through an open or percutaneous approach. Empiric IV antiobiotics should be started as soon as cultures have been drawn; for most children an antistaphylcoccal agent such as vancomycin or clindamycin is necessary because of the high prevalence of CA-MRSA. Nafcillin or oxacillin may be used in geographical areas where isolates of staphylococcal species are greater than 90% methicillin-sensitive *S. aureus* (MSSA). Cefazolin should be added empirically for children in whom *Kingella* is a consideration. Infants younger than 3 months should have additional Gram-negative coverage with gentamicin or a third-generation cephalosporin. Suspected cases of gonococcus or salmonella should also be treated with a third-generation cephalosporin. Duration of therapy ranges from 2 to 4 weeks, with transition to an appropriate oral agent when clinical improvement is documented.

Hariharan P, Karbrhel C: Sensitivity of erythrocyte sedimentation rate and c-reactive protein for the exclusion of septic arthritis in emergency department patients. *J Emerg Med.* 2011;40(4):428-431 [PMID: 20655163].

Joshy S, Choudry Q, Akbar N, et al: Comparison of bacteriologically proven septic arthritis of the hip and knee in children, a preliminary study. *J Pediatr Orthop.* 2010;30(2):208-211 [PMID: 20179572].

Saadi MM, Zamil FA, Bokhary NA, et al: Acute septic arthritis in children. *Pediatr Int.* 2009;51(3):377-380 [PMID: 19500280].

Young TP, Mass L, Thorp AW, et al: Etiology of septic arthritis in children: An update for the new millennium. *Am J Emerg Med.* 2010;29(8):899-902 [PMID: 20674219].

SKIN

ABSCESS AND CELLULITIS

 ESSENTIALS OF DIAGNOSIS

▶ Erythema.

▶ Warmth.

▶ Tenderness.

▶ Fluctuance.

Incision and drainage is vital for abscess treatment; many children can be treated safely with oral antibiotics.

General Considerations

Rise of CA-MRSA has led to an increase in the number of skin infections seen in the pediatric emergency department, the most common of which are cellulitis and abscesses.

In each case, bacteria seed an area via hematogenous spread or from overlying trauma to the skin. Cellulitis can develop from an existing abscess or vice versa. An abscess that involves a hair follicle is known as a furuncle and a collection of furuncles is a carbuncle. Cellulitis and abscesses typically develop in the deep dermis and subcutaneous fat; erysipelas, a similar skin infection, involves the upper dermis and lymphatic tissue. Cellulitis and erysipelas are most often caused by streptococci, particularly GAS, and *S. aureus*. Infection due to *H. influenzae* type B and *S. pneumoniae* occur far less frequently since advent of their vaccines. *S. aureus* including MRSA is by far the most prevalent etiologic agent of abscesses in children because of its ability to produce toxins that destroy tissue and leukocytes. CA-MRSA was not seen prior to the 1990s but has become an ever-increasing cause of soft tissue infections in children and adults. Attempts to eradicate MRSA colonization with nasal mupirocin, bleach baths, and chlorhexidine washes have met with mixed results. Risk factors for the development of cellulitis and abscess include positive family history of skin infections or condition such as eczema or tinea that compromises the natural protective barrier of the skin.

Clinical Findings

Hallmarks of cellulitis include spreading skin erythema, warmth, and tenderness. Because the infection is more superficial, erythema seen with erysipelas is clearly demarcated from the surrounding skin and may be slightly raised. Cellulitis is a more indolent process with indistinct borders. Abscess presents as a painful, erythematous swelling of the skin which may be fluctuant if the fluid collection is near the skin surface. The area surrounding the abscess may be indurated and the center may drain spontaneously. Systemic signs such as fever and chills are uncommon with abscesses and cellulitis but can be seen with erysipelas. An important exception is seen in the neonate with omphalitis—erythema and purulence surrounding the umbilical stump, which is frequently associated with lethargy, fevers, and sepsis.

Laboratory Tests/Radiographs

Routine laboratory tests are unnecessary in the evaluation of uncomplicated skin infections. Blood culture with CBC is not recommended unless the patient is toxic, has had an unusual exposure such as an animal bite, or has a serious underlying comorbidity. Purulent abscess material should be cultured if possible to assist with antibiotic therapy if there is concern for treatment failure with standard antibiotics. Inflammatory markers may be drawn in more severe cases if an extended inpatient hospital course is anticipated.

Bedside ultrasound has emerged as an important tool for evaluating skin infections in the pediatric emergency department. Cellulitis appears as cobblestoning and fat-stranding in the deep dermis whereas an abscess will show a well-demarcated hyperechoic fluid collection. Bedside ultrasound is recommended for routine evaluation of skin infections because it can demonstrate fluid collections that may not be apparent on examination and can guide incision and drainage.

Treatment

Children with cellulitis who lack signs of rapid spread or systemic disease may be managed as outpatient with oral antibiotics. Empiric therapy to cover against *S. aureus* and GAS is required and includes clindamycin monotherapy or a combination of amoxicillin and TMP-SMZ. Monotherapy with TMP-SMZ is not recommended for the treatment of suspected cellulitis because it has little coverage against GAS. Cellulitis associated with a dog bite should be treated with amoxicillin-clavulanic acid. The skin border of the cellulitis should be marked and next-day follow-up should be arranged. Infants with omphalitis should be admitted to the hospital for a full septic evaluation and started on IV vancomycin with gentamicin or a third-generation cephalosporin for gram-negative coverage. Children with cellulitis who appear toxic, have failed outpatient therapy, or have signs of rapid spread should be admitted with IV antibiotics.

The mainstay of therapy for abscess is incision and drainage; studies show that antibiotics do not improve outcomes for uncomplicated drained abscesses less than 5 cm. Empiric choices for abscess coverage should cover against MRSA, and knowledge of the local resistance patterns is vital. Clindamycin or TMP-SMZ is commonly used and both are available in oral formulations. Children with more complicated disease including those who have failed outpatient therapy should be admitted and started on IV antibiotic such as vancomycin or clindamycin until response to treatment can be documented.

Animal and human bites are a common problem. The predominant pathogens in animal bite wounds are the oral flora of the biting animal and human skin flora. Common pathogens include *Pasteurella* species, staphylococci, streptococci, and anaerobic bacteria. Cat bites can transmit *Bartonella henselae*, organism responsible for cat scratch disease.

Prophylactic antibiotics reduce the rate of infection due to some animal bites, especially cat bites. Prophylaxis should be administered in certain wounds: deep puncture wounds, crush injuries, wounds on the hands, face, genitalia, or near joints wounds requiring closure and in any immunocompromised patient. Amoxicillin-clavulanate is recommended or clindamycin plus TMP-SMZ in penicillin-allergic patients.

Elliot DJ, Zaoutis TE, Troxel AB, et al: Empiric antimicrobial therapy for pediatric skin and soft-tissue infections in the era of methicillin resistant *Staphylococcus aureus*. *Pediatrics*. 2009;123(6):e959-966 [PMID: 19470525].

Kam AJ, Leal J, Freedman SB: Pediatric cellulitis: Success of emergency department short-course intravenous antibiotics. *Pediatr Emerg Care.* 2010;26:171-176 [PMID: 20179663].

Khangura A, Wallace J, Kissoon N, et al: Management of cellulitis in a pediatric emergency department. *Pediatr Emerg Care.* 2007;23(11):805-811 [PMID: 18007211].

Kilbane BJ, Reynolds SL: Emergency department management of community-acquired methicillin-resistant *Staphylococcus aureus. Pediatr Emerg Care.* 2008;24(2):109-114 [PMID: 18277849].

Odell CA: Community-associated methicillin-resistant *Staphylococcus aureus* (CA-MRSA) skin infections. *Curr Opin Pediatr.* 2010;22(3):273-277 [PMID: 20386450].

Ramirez-Schrempp D, Dorfman D, Baker WE: Ultrasound soft tissue applications in the pediatric emergency department: To drain or not to drain? *Pediatr Emerg Care.* 2009;25:44-48 [PMID: 19148015].

Stryjewski ME, Chambers HF: Skin and soft-tissue infections caused by community-acquired methicillin-resistant *Staphylococcus aureus. Clin Infect Dis.* 2008;46:S368-377 [PMID: 18462092].

NECROTIZING FASCIITIS

ESSENTIALS OF DIAGNOSIS

▶ Pain out of proportion to skin findings.

▶ Warmth.

▶ Erythema.

▶ Fevers.

▶ Tachycardia.

▶ Signs of shock.

Surgical emergency treated with prompt debridement and broad-spectrum IV antibiotics.

General Considerations

Necrotizing fasciitis is a rare soft tissue infection in children with devastating consequences. In adults the infection is usually polymicrobial but in children GAS is the most common etiologic agent, although CA-MRSA has been reported. Bacterial invasion occurs during clinical or subclinical skin trauma, in association with a skin infection such as varicella, or from hematogenous spread. GAS adheres to deep subcutaneous tissues and spreads rapidly along fascial planes by producing toxins that destroy tissue and cause widespread activation of T cells. The resulting cytokine milieu incites more damage and leads to symptoms of shock. In contrast to adults, most children who develop necrotizing fasciitis are previously healthy, although a history of recent trauma or skin infection may be elicited.

Clinical Findings

Because the subcutaneous tissues are affected first, often the outward clinical signs of necrotizing fasciitis belie the severity of the disease. *Pain out of proportion* to the skin examination is classically seen, with the development of decreased sensation occurring later as nerve fibers are destroyed. The skin above the infection appears erythematous and warm without well-defined borders. Rapid spread of tenderness and erythema up to 1-2 cm/hr is possible. In late stages signs of frank necrosis including dark discoloration, crepitus, and skin breakdown are seen and fever, tachycardia, and altered mental status may develop quickly. Compartment syndrome manifested by swelling, pain, and poor perfusion of the affected area is a potential complication.

Laboratory Tests/Radiographs

Laboratory tests are a useful adjunct but are not required for diagnosis. CBC with differential may show leukocytosis and inflammatory markers such as ESR and CRP are typically elevated. Serum CK is indicated to assess for myositis. Blood cultures are positive in greater than 50% of cases of GAS necrotizing fasciitis. Definitive diagnosis is achieved from histopathologic examination and culture of debrided tissue; bacteria spreading along fascial planes, thrombosis of blood vessels, and widespread inflammatory cell infiltration are commonly seen. Radiography does not play a role in diagnosis of necrotizing fasciitis, particularly if it will delay surgical intervention. Plain films, MRI, or noncontrast CT may show gas in the subcutaneous tissues, but this finding is not adequately sensitive to be clinically useful. Ultrasound may be used to evaluate for the presence of a deep abscess.

Treatment

Suspected cases of necrotizing fasciitis must be managed aggressively with immediate consultation with orthopedic or general surgeon. Children with signs of shock on initial examination should be managed accordingly with fluids, hemodynamic support, and ICU admission. Tissue compartment pressures should be followed frequently if an extremity is involved. Antibiotic therapy should be directed at potential sources including GAS, CA-MRSA, and anaerobes. Piperacillin/tazobactam or ampicillin/sulbactam and an antistaphylococcal agent such as vancomycin are recommended, with clindamycin added to decrease the synthesis of destructive exotoxins. Although not widely studied in children, IVIG has shown promise as an adjunctive therapy in adults because it can neutralize the toxins and antigens produced by GAS.

Bilgol-Kologlu M, Yildiz RV, Alper B, et al: Necrotizing fasciitis in children: Diagnostic and therapeutic aspects. *J Pediatr Surg.* 2007;42:1892-1897 [PMID: 18022442].

Jamal N, Teach SJ: Necrotizing fasciitis. *Pediatr Emerg Care.* 2011;27(12):1195-1199 [PMID: 22158285].

Minodier P, Bidet P, Rallu F, et al: Clinical and microbiologic characteristics of group A streptococcal necrotizing fasciitis in children. *Pediatr Infect Dis J.* 2009;28(6):541-543 [PMID: 19504739].

HERPESVIRUS INFECTIONS

ESSENTIALS OF DIAGNOSIS

▶ Fever.

▶ Rash.

▶ Malaise.

Wide spectrum of presentations is possible. Antiviral therapy is generally unnecessary as most infections are self-limited.

General Considerations

Herpesviruses are ubiquitous DNA viruses that cause pathology in children, ranging from asymptomatic infection to shock and death. Herpesviruses include herpes simplex (HSV-1, HSV-2), varicella-zoster (VZV), Epstein-Barr virus (EBV), cytomegalovirus (CMV), human herpes virus 6 (HHV-6), and human herpes virus 8 (HHV-8). Among children the most clinically important infections are caused by HSV, VZV, EBV, and HHV-6.

HSV-1 causes most orofacial and CNS illness, and HSV-2 is associated with anogenital disease among sexually active adolescents and adults. HSV-1 infection is ubiquitous, with 25% of children infected by 7 years of age, and more than 50% by 18 years. HSV-2 infection rates increase in the adolescent years, with nearly 33% of adults affected by 40 years of age. The virus is spread by contact with active lesions or through saliva or respiratory droplets. Initial infection of the skin or mucous membranes is followed by a chronic latent stage during which the virus persists within sensory ganglion cells. Reactivation of the virus occurs in response to external stressors such as illness, sunlight, menstruation.

Incidence of primary VZV infection (chicken pox) has decreased dramatically since the introduction of the VZV vaccine in 1995. Earlier, VZV was a ubiquitous childhood infection, with greater than 95% of young adults showing evidence of prior infection. VZV now occurs most in unvaccinated children. Complications include skin and soft tissue bacterial superinfection, pneumonia, and rarely encephalitis. In adults latent VZV resides in neuronal ganglia but can reactivate, causing a painful skin eruption known as zoster or shingles.

Infection due to EBV is common, with a 90-95% seroprevalance rate among adults, with 50% of children infected by 5 years of age. The virus infects epithelial or B cells and has a lytic and latent phase. Spread of the disease occurs most commonly through saliva. Infection in children is often asymptomatic or mild and nonspecific; however, among older children and adolescents it causes mononucleosis. EBV can transform affected cells and primarily in adults has been linked with malignancies such as lymphoma and nasopharyngeal carcinoma.

HHV-6 causes roseola infantum in children, also known as exanthem subitum or Sixth disease. In adults the seroprevalence rate approaches 90%, with most infections occurring before 2 years of age. The virus exhibits tropism for T cells but can infect a number of cell types. Transmission occurs from infected respiratory secretions. Complications of HHV-6 infection include febrile seizures or rarely meningoencephalitis.

Clinical Findings

Cutaneous HSV infection presents as grouped vesicles on an erythematous base which rupture and become shallow ulcerations. Initial infection is often subclinical; reactivation may be preceded by burning at the site, fever, malaise, and lymphadenopathy. Eczema herpeticum develops following superinfection with HSV and presents as rapidly spreading painful vesicular lesions over existing eczematous skin. Herpetic gingivostomatitis is common in children and can be associated with significant pain, drooling, and anorexia. Infection of the lips can also occur, and bacterial superinfection of these lesions presents with honey-colored crusting. Genital herpes should prompt evaluation for sexual abuse in young children; skin manifestations are similar to those seen with oral infections. Vesicular lesions on the cornea with purulent conjunctivitis are seen with herpetic keratoconjunctivitis. HSV infections have the potential to spread systemically in the very young and immonocompromised. Infants with HSV meningitis may present with seizures, diffuse skin lesions, and septic shock.

Chicken pox (VSV) classically presents with a prodrome of fever and malaise followed by a rash that progresses from macular to papular to vesicular lesions on an erythematous base. Usually the rash appears in different stages as it spreads across the body. The vesicles become pustular and crust over within a week. Secondary bacterial skin infection may occur. Other complications are uncommon in healthy children but neurologic symptoms such as ataxia, altered mental status, and meningeal signs are possible.

EBV infections are usually subclinical in younger children and present nonspecifically with signs of a URI or viral gastroenteritis. Susceptible children older than 10 years are at highest risk of developing infectious mononucleosis, which presents with sore throat, malaise, fever, and lymphadenopathy. Examination of the throat may reveal palatal petechiae and an exudative pharyngitis. Patients treated with penicillin for treatment of presumed GAS pharyngitis develop a diffuse morbilliform rash in up to 95% of cases. Splenomegaly is found in up to 50% of patients.

Roseola infantum (HHV-6) presents with a 3-day fever up to 40°C which resolves and is followed by a diffuse blanching maculopapular rash on the torso. Rash spreads to the extremities over 1-2 days. Lymphadenopathy, irritability, and anorexia are common but nonspecific signs of infection. Febrile seizures are seen in a minority of children with roseola infantum due to the high fevers seen during acute infection.

Laboratory Tests/Radiographs

HSV infection may be confirmed by viral culture of vesicular fluid, but in practice rapid diagnostic tests are more commonly employed. Scrapings from the base of the suspected lesion should be sent for DFA for HSV; this has replaced the Tzanck smear as the preferred rapid test. PCR for HSV is used to detect the virus in blood or CSF samples.

VZV infections may also be detected via PCR, DFA, or viral culture. Serologic testing of IgG to VZV may be of value if vaccine failure is suspected.

Infectious mononucleosis is suggested by lymphocytosis on peripheral CBC and greater than 10% atypical lymphocytes. The monospot test for heterophile antibodies produced by activated B cells is 85% sensitive and 94% specific when applied to adolescents with symptoms of infection. However, younger children have a positive monospot in fewer than 50% of cases, and older children may not develop the antibodies until the second week of illness. Serologies consisting of IgG and IgM to EBV proteins are used to diagnose primary infection versus remote exposure to the virus.

Diagnosis of roseola infantum is clinical and confirmatory testing is with serologies, DFA, or PCR. These must be interpreted with caution since most children are exposed to HHV-6 and latent HHV-6 DNA can be recovered from asymptomatic children.

Treatment

Most cutaneous HSV infections in healthy children may be managed supportively, although oral acyclovir shortens duration of illness if initiated within 72 hours of symptom onset. It can be used for immune competent children who are unable to drink or have significant symptoms. Genital herpes is treated with a 7-10-day course of acyclovir, and suppressive therapy is offered for patients with frequent recurrences. Neonatal herpes and HSV meningitis should be managed aggressively with IV acyclovir. Severe cases of eczema herpeticum in young children are treated initially with IV acyclovir. Suspected herpetic keratoconjunctivitis should be managed in consultation with an ophthalmologist and treatment involves ophthalmic antiviral drops.

Chicken pox is managed supportively with pain control and measures to limit the risk of secondary bacterial infection. Acyclovir is less effective against VZV compared to HSV and consequently is not recommended for the routine treatment of otherwise healthy children. Because children older than 12 years are at risk of severe infection, oral acyclovir is recommended for this age group. Immunosuppressed patients should be admitted and treated with IV acyclovir because of the risk of severe disseminated disease. Neonates exposed to VZV should be given prophylaxis with varicella immune globulin; infants with suspected VZV infection should be treated with IV acyclovir.

Adolescents with suspected mononucleosis should undergo a rapid streptococcal antigen test due to the overlap in symptomatology. Infectious mononucleosis is managed supportively with pain control and relative rest. Corticosteroids are not recommended in routine cases but may be considered if there is concern that pharyngeal edema or lymphadenopathy may produce airway compromise. Antivirals have not been shown to be useful for the treatment of mononucleosis. Owing to splenomegaly and concern for rupture, it is recommended that patients avoid contact sports for at least 3 weeks after symptom onset.

Roseola infantum is treated supportively with fever control. Antiviral therapy with gangiclovir or foscarnet may be considered if there is concern for severe disease in an immunocompromised patient.

Agut H: Deciphering the clinical impact of acute human herpesvirus 6 (HHV-6) infections. *J Clin Virol.* 2011;52(3):164-171 [PMID: 21782505].

Chayavichitsilp P, Buckwater JV, Krakowski AC, et al: Herpes simplex. *Pediatr Rev.* 2009;30(4):119-229 [PMID: 19339385].

Dohno S, Maeda A, Ishiura Y, et al: Diagnosis of infectious mononucleosis caused by Epstein-Barr virus in infants. *Pediatr Int.* 2010;52(4):536-540 [PMID: 20113421].

Gershon AA: Varicella-zoster virus infections. *Pediatr Rev.* 2008;29(1):5-10 [PMID: 18166616].

Jen M, Chang MW: Eczema herpetium and eczema vaccinatum in children. *Pediatr Ann.* 2010;39(10):658-664 [PMID: 20954612].

Luzuriaga K, Sullivan JL: Infectious mononucleosis. *N Engl J Med.* 2010;362(21):1993-2000 [PMID: 20505178].

Whitley RJ: Therapy of herpes virus infections in children. *Adv Exp Med Biol.* 2008;609:216-232 [PMID: 18193668].

PARVOVIRUS

 ESSENTIALS OF DIAGNOSIS

▶ Slapped-cheeks rash.

▶ Fever.

▶ Coryza.

▶ Malaise.

▶ Arthritis.

Treatment is supportive unless patient is at risk for severe anemia.

General Considerations

Parvovirus is a ubiquitous DNA virus that in children is most often associated with erythema infectiosum (Fifth disease). The virus exhibits tropism for erythroid progenitor cells and can cause severe aplastic anemia in children with underlying conditions such as HIV, sickle cell anemia, hereditary spherocytosis, and thalassemia. Transmission of the virus occurs primarily through respiratory droplets, but it can also be transmitted vertically from mother to fetus. Fetal infection with parvovirus causes anemia and, in severe cases, eventually high-output heart failure and hydrops fetalis. The virus is highly infectious, with an rate of 50% among susceptible household contacts. Antibodies against parvovirus are protective but are thought to play a role in the pathogenesis of the classic rash associated with erythema infectiosum.

Clinical Findings

Children with parvovirus infection can remain asymptomatic or have only mild nonspecific upper respiratory symptoms of fever, coryza, malaise, and headache. Children develop a rash 2-5 days into the illness. The rash is erythematous, with a malar distribution across the cheeks and circumoral pallor. The "slapped cheeks" rash spreads to the trunk and extremities and has a lacy or reticulated appearance. It may persist for several weeks and becomes more prominent in response to temperature changes, sunlight, or stress. A small number of children may have complaint of joint pain, most commonly the knees or ankles. Children who develop aplastic anemia present with fatigue, pallor, and tachycardia.

Laboratory Tests/Radiographs

Diagnosis of parvovirus in otherwise healthy children may be made clinically. IgM antibodies may be detected after 10 days of illness and persist for up to 5 months. Viral DNA PCR testing is available for children with aplastic crises or those who are immunosuppressed since they may not produce an effective antibody response. Children with suspected aplastic crisis should have a CBC with differential and a reticulocyte count performed to document the level of anemia and confirm the absence of reticulocytosis.

Treatment

Erythema infectiosum is managed supportively with antipyretics for fever and anti-inflammatories for joint pain. Parents should be reassured that the child is no longer infectious after rash develops. Children with suspected aplastic crisis should be managed with consultation with a hematologist and an oncologist, as these patients need close monitoring and frequently require blood transfusions.

Immunosuppressed patients with severe infection may be treated with IVIG.

Mandel ED: Erythema infectiosum: Recognizing the many faces of fifth disease. *JAAPA.* 2009;22(6):42-46 [PMID: 19601449].
Servey JT, Reamy BV, Hodge JH: Clinical presentation of parvovirus B19 infection. *Am Fam Physician.* 2007;74(3):373-376 [PMID: 17304869].

MEASLES

ESSENTIALS OF DIAGNOSIS

▸ Cough.

▸ Coryza.

▸ Conjunctivitis.

▸ Koplik spots.

▸ History of international travel.

Alert public health authorities and consider adjunctive treatment with vitamin A in severe cases.

General Considerations

Although considered to be near eradication, measles continues to be a significant childhood cause of global morbidity and mortality. Across the world measles caused over 160,000 deaths in 2008. Sporadic outbreaks in developed countries are common due to inadequate immunization levels and imported international cases. The measles vaccine was developed in the 1960s and is currently given as a two-stage immunization beginning at 6-15 months. The virus is a highly contagious RNA virus spread primarily through respiratory droplets. The virus replicates in endothelial cells of the upper respiratory tract before spreading to local lymph nodes. Viremia develops after this stage, leading to disseminated disease across multiple organ systems, including the gastrointestinal tract, skin, liver, and kidneys. Complications of measles infection are pneumonia, encephalitis, and acute demyelinating encephalomyelitis. Children at risk of contracting measles include those who are inadequately immunized, are immunosuppressed, history of travel to known endemic areas.

Clinical Findings

Measles infection begins with a prodromal phase characterized by cough, conjunctivitis, and coryza. Fever, malaise, cough, and anorexia are also common. Koplik spots, tiny white lesions on an erythematous base, may be seen on the buccal mucosa and are specific to measles infection. On day 2 or 3 after prodromal symptoms appear the patient develops a blanching maculopapular rash that begins on the face and spreads caudally over the next 5 days to involve the torso and extremities. Clinical improvement is usually apparent within 48 hours after the rash begins, although cough may persist for several weeks. Similar but less severe presentation is possible in children with inadequate response to the vaccine.

Laboratory Tests/Radiographs

Measles is diagnosed clinically but for public health purposes confirmatory testing is advised. IgM against the measles virus is typically used for diagnosis; antibody levels become apparent 3-4 days after rash appears. Additional routine laboratory tests are not necessary in uncomplicated cases; a CBC with differential may show leukopenia or lymphopenia. CXR may be indicated if viral or superimposed bacterial pneumonia is suspected.

Treatment

Management of measles is primarily supportive. A 2-day course of vitamin A is recommended for children in developing countries or for those with signs of severe infection. Vitamin A plays a role in immune modulation. Public health authorities should be notified to prevent the spread of disease among susceptible contacts.

Machaira M, Papaevangelou: Current measles outbreaks: Can we do better for infants at risk? *Pediatr Infect Dis J.* 2012;31(7): 756-758 [PMID: 22695190].

Moss WJ, Griffin DE: Measles. *Lancet.* 2012;379(9811):153-164 [PMID: 21855993].

Mulholland EK, Griffiths UK: Measles in the 21st century. *N Engl J Med.* 2012;366(19):1755-1757 [PMID: 22571199].

Sugarman DE, Barskey AE, Delea MG, et al: Measles outbreak in a highly vaccinated population, San Diego, 2008: Role of the intentionally undervaccinated. *Pediatrics.* 2010;125(4):747-755 [PMID: 20308208].

SCABIES

 ESSENTIALS OF DIAGNOSIS

► Pruritic erythematous papular rash.

► History of exposure to scabies.

► Serpiginous skin burrows uncommon in children.

Treat with topical permethrin or oral ivermectin (see Chapter 47).

General Considerations

Scabies is a common skin eruption in children caused by the parasitic mite *Sarcoptes scabiei*. The adult female secretes a substance which dissolves the stratum corneum and burrows into the skin. The female lays eggs under the skin as she burrows and lives for about 1 month. The characteristic skin reaction develops as a result of a hypersensitivity reaction to the secretions and feces of the mite. Most scabies infections involve fewer than 15 active adult females per host. Spread occurs through direct contact, although transmission via contaminated clothing or bedding possible. Scabies outbreaks can occur in health care settings; however, most children acquire the parasite at home or school. Severe crusted or Norwegian scabies is possible in immunocompromised children and those with Down syndrome and occurs due to unchecked mite proliferation.

Clinical Findings

Rash associated with scabies typically develops 3-6 weeks after initial infection and 2-3 days after reinfection because of immune sensitization. Although the classic rash consists of serpiginous brown burrows with erythematous papules on the wrists, elbow, and finger webbing, in children the rash is highly variable. It may be found on the head, neck, palms, soles, or fingers and is characteristically pruritic, especially at night. The lesions may be papular, vesicular, or a combination of the two. In children the pathognomonic burrows are usually obscured by excoriations. Eczematization and signs of bacterial superinfection may be found. Crusted scabies presents as an erythematous patch of scaly skin that can involve the nails.

Laboratory Tests/Radiographs

Skin scrapings of infected skin may be examined under light microscopy for evidence of mites, eggs, or feces. Adhesive tape can be applied to the skin of children who do not tolerate skin scraping. However, these methods frequently do not show evidence of infection because in most patients the total number of active mites is low.

Treatment

Treatment of choice for children older than 2 months is 5% permethrin cream, applied to the skin and washed off after 8-12 hours, with retreatment in 1 week. Lindane preparations have fallen out of favor because of potential neurotoxicity. Oral therapy consisting of a single 200 μg/kg dose of ivermectin followed by second dose in 2 weeks has gained favor as an alternative for children older than 5 years. Treatment should be offered to all household and intimate contacts. Parents should be instructed to have the child's clothes and bed linens washed at 60°C; nonwashable items should be sprayed with insecticide or placed in a sealed plastic bag for 3 days. Severe pruritis may be treated with topical corticosteroids or oral antihistamines.

Bouvresse S, Chosidow O: Scabies in healthcare settings. *Curr Opin Infect Dis.* 2010;23(2):111-118 [PMID: 20075729].

Currie BJ, McCarthy JS: Permethrin and ivermectin for scabies. *N Engl J Med.* 2010;362(8):717-725 [PMID: 20181973].

Karthikeyan K: Scabies in children. *Arch Dis Child Educ Pract Ed.* 2007;92(3):ep65-ep69 [PMID: 17517973].

LICE

ESSENTIALS OF DIAGNOSIS

► Often asymptomatic.

► Pruritis.

► Nits on hair shafts.

► Live lice on the scalp.

Treat with a topical pediculocide such as permethrin or malathion.

General Considerations

Head lice, caused by the human parasite *Pediculus capitis*, affects up to 25% of elementary school students. The insect is up to 4 mm in length and survives on the scalp by grasping hairs and feeding on blood. Females lay eggs known as nits that are cemented to the base of the hair shaft and hatch after 1 week. Adult lice live up to 1 month and can survive for 2 days without a human host. Spread of infection is by direct contact and from shared combs, headphones, bedsheets, hats, and towels.

Clinical Findings

Most lice infections are asymptomatic but cause significant stress for the child and parents. Some children have complaint of scalp pruritis, and lymphadenopathy may be seen. Evaluation of the scalp with a fine comb may demonstrate live lice, but more commonly nits are identified. Nits may persist on the hair shaft for months after infection, and nits found greater than 1 cm from the scalp may not represent active disease. Secondary bacterial infection of the scalp may be seen caused by severe pruritis.

Laboratory Tests/Radiographs

Routine laboratory tests are not indicated for determination of lice infection unless a severe secondary bacterial infection is suspected.

Treatment

Over-the-counter and prescription pediculicides are available to treat head lice. Permethrin and malathion are topical lice neurotoxins with a good safety profile in children. Permethrin, available as a 1% over-the-counter preparation or in 5% prescription strength, is applied to the scalp, rinsed off 10 minutes later, and repeated 7-10 days. Malathion is left on the scalp overnight and repeated in a week if necessary. Formerly another neurotoxin, lindane, was used but is now a second line therapy due to its side effect profile. Newer alternative therapies include benzyl alcohol lotion and oral ivermectin or TMP-SMZ. Families should be counseled to limit transmission of lice by washing all of the child's clothing and bed linens greater than 50°C or with a drying cycle longer than 40 minutes. Items that cannot be washed should be sealed for 2 weeks in a plastic bag to interrupt the life cycle of the lice. Close household contacts of the child may also be treated with a topical pediculicide.

Diamantis SA, Morrell DS, Burkhart CN: Treatment of head lice. *Dermatol Ther.* 2009;22(4):273-278 [PMID: 19580574].

Frankowski BL, Bocchini JA: Head lice. *Pediatrics.* 2010;126(2): 392-403 [PMID: 20660553].

Tebruegge M, Pantazidou A, Curtis N: What's bugging you? An update on the treatment of head lice infestation. *Arch Dis Child Educ Clin Pract Ed.* 2011;96(1):2-8 [PMID: 20688849].

RENAL

URINARY TRACT INFECTION

ESSENTIALS OF DIAGNOSIS

► Dysuria.

► Urgency.

► Frequency.

► Positive nitrites and leukocyte esterase on urinalysis.

► Fever greater than 39°C is suggestive of renal involvement.

Oral antibiotics for uncomplicated cases. IV antibiotics for infants and children with signs of severe systemic infection.

General Considerations

UTIs including pyelonephritis are the most common SBIs in infants and children. Up to 8% of girls and 2% of boys will have a UTI during the first 8 years of life. Infection occurs when bacteria adhere and ascend the urinary mucosa, causing inflammation of the urethra, bladder, ureters, and ultimately renal parenchyma. *E. coli* causes greater than 80% of pediatric UTIs and has specialized fimbrae which allow

Table 41–8. Prevalence of UTI among children with fever > 38°C

Age (months)	Gender	Prevalence (%)
0-3	Female	7.5
	Male (uncircumcised)	20.1
	Male (circumcised)	2.4
3-6	Female	5.7
	Male	3.3
6-12	Female	8.3
	Male	1.7
12-24	Female	2.1
	Male	<1

it to adhere to uroepithelium. Other common pathogens include gram-negative bacteria such as *Klebsiella, Proteus, Citrobacter,* and *Enterobacter.* Gram-positive bacteria rarely cause UTI; however, *S. saprophyticus* is common among sexually active teenage females and young adults. Age, race, gender, and history of abnormal urogenital anatomy are important risk factors to consider. Infants and children are at highest risk for UTI; in females, up to age 2 years, and in circumcised males, to age 6 months. Uncircumcised males are at highest risk for UTI in the first 6 months of life, though they remain at increased risk until 12 months (Table 41–8). For reasons that are unclear, white children have almost twice the risk of UTI compared to African American and Hispanic children. Anatomic or neurologic abnormalities such as neurogenic bladder, obstruction due to posterior urethral valves, or vesicoureteral reflux prevent urine from being eliminated efficiently and predispose to infection. Among otherwise healthy children chronic constipation is a major contributor to UTI risk because stool in the colon compresses the adjacent bladder, leading to increased postvoid residual volumes.

Clinical Findings

UTI among infants presents nonspecifically with fever, vomiting, poor feeding, failure to thrive, jaundice, irritability. Older children present with urinary urgency, dysuria, and urinary frequency. Children previously toilet trained may develop nocturia or daytime incontinence, and parents may report malodorous urine. Fever may be absent or low-grade in children with uncomplicated cystitis in which the inflammation is confined to the bladder only. Fever greater than 39°C has been associated with increased risk of UTI, specifically pyelonephritis. Additional symptoms of renal parenchymal involvement include back or flank pain and chills.

On examination children with UTI may have suprapubic or abdominal tenderness, and associated nausea, vomiting, and diarrhea are reported.

Laboratory Tests/Radiographs

Urinalysis followed by a confirmatory urine culture is required for diagnosis of a UTI. Suprapubic aspiration is the gold standard; however, in practice urine is typically collected via catheterization from infants, and from a clean catch specimen among toilet-trained children. Bag specimens are not recommended because of the high rate of contamination. Standard urinalysis values used to diagnose UTI include nitrites, leukocyte esterase, pyuria, and Gram stain. Leukocyte esterase has a sensitivity of 70-80% and specificity of 70-85%; nitrite has a sensitivity of 30-40% and a specificity of 95-99%. Nitrites are frequently missed on urinalysis because the urine must remain in the bladder for several hours before levels become detectable. Pyuria, defined as greater than 5WBC per HPF, has a sensitivity of 74% and a specificity of 86% for UTI. The presence of squamous cells along with WBCs on urine microscopy suggests skin contamination. Sensitivity and specificity of bacteria on Gram stain of urine are 90-100%. Additional laboratory testing is not required for the diagnosis of most uncomplicated UTIs in children. CBC may show peripheral leukocytosis and inflammatory markers may be elevated. Blood cultures are drawn for infants younger than 2 months and may be positive in as great as 10% of cases. Radiography is not generally needed for the acute diagnosis of UTI but renal ultrasound may be used if there are symptoms suggestive of a renal abscess.

Treatment

In the acute setting infants younger than 2 months with a UTI should be managed with admission and IV antibiotics, typically ampicillin and gentamicin to cover against *E. coli* and *Enterococcus* species. Children older than 2 months may be managed initially with oral antibiotics if they do not have symptoms of upper urinary tract involvement. Initial therapy with a third-generation cephalosporin such as cefdinir or cefixime is recommended; TMP-SMZ or amoxicillin-clavulanic acid are alternatives but must be used in caution because of increasing resistance among *E. coli* strains. Nitrofurantion may be used among older children for cystitis but does not achieve therapeutic serum levels needed for the treatment of pyelonephritis. Treatment courses of 3-5 days are usually sufficient for lower tract disease, whereas 7-10 days of antibiotics are recommended for patients with pyelonephritis. IV antibiotics and admission may be reserved for children who are ill-appearing, immunosuppressed, cannot tolerate oral antibiotics, or have a significant underlying medical condition. Appropriate IV antibiotics include a third-generation cephalosporin or an aminoglycoside; children with a history of pseudomonal UTI should be treated with a fourth-generation cephalosporin (cefepime). Children who have failed an outpatient antibiotic regimen and those with a history of bladder instrumentation may need additional *Enterococcus* coverage with IV ampicillin. Imaging to rule out renal abscess should be perfomed on children who fail to improve after 24-48 hours of appropriate antibiotic therapy.

Proper long-term management of pediatric UTI remains controversial. Recent studies have begun to challenge the maxim that recurrent UTIs lead to scarring and long-term morbidity in children, including hypertension, proteinuria, and end-stage renal disease. Improvements in prenatal imaging suggest that some of the renal scarring previously attributed to recurrent pyelonephritis was instead due to congenital malformations. Additionally, the benefits of prophylactic antibiotics for children with UTIs secondary to vesicoureteral reflux have been questioned. Current recommendations for children 2-24 months of age with a febrile UTI include a renal ultrasound to assess for signs of hydronephrosis, with a voiding cystourethrogram reserved for children with a second febrile UTI or hydronephrosis on the initial ultrasound.

Ammenti A, Cataldi L, Chimenz R, et al: Febrile urinary tract infections in young children: Recommendations for the diagnosis, treatment and follow-up. *Acta Paediatr.* 2012;101(5): 451-457 [PMID: 22122295]

Beetz R, Westenfelder M: Antimicrobial therapy of urinary tract infections in children. *Int J Antimicrob Agents.* 2011;38:42-50 [PMID: 22036250].

Bhat RG, Katy TA, Place FC: Pediatric urinary tract infections. *Emerg Clin N Amer.* 2011 29(3):637-653 [PMID: 21782079].

Feld L, Mattoo TK: Urinary tract infections and vesicoureteral reflux in infants and children. *Pediatr Rev.* 2010;31(11):451-463 [PMID: 21041423].

Mattoo TK: Are prophylactic antibiotics indicated after a urinary tract infection? *Curr Opin Pediatr.* 2010;21(2):203-206 [PMID: 19663037].

Montini G, Tullus K, Hewitt I: Febrile urinary tract infections in children. *N Engl J Med.* 2011;365:239-250 [PMID: 21774712].

Saadeh SA, Mattoo TK: Managing urinary tract infections. *Pediatr Nephrol.* 2011;26(11):1967-1976 [PMID: 21409431].

Shaikh N, Morone NE, Bost JE, et al: Prevalence of urinary tract infection in childhood: A meta-analysis. *Pediatr Infect Dis J.* 2008;27(4):302-308 [PMID: 18316994].

Subcommittee on Urinary tract Infection, Steering Committee on Quality Improvement and Management: Urinary tract infection: Clinical practice guideline for the diagnosis and management of the initial UTI in febrile infants and children 2 to24 months. *Pediatrics.* 2011;128(3):595-608 [PMID: 21873693].

Williams GJ, Hodson EH, Isaacs D, et al: Diagnosis and management of urinary tract infection in children. *J Pediatr Child Health.* 2010;48(4):296-301 [PMID: 21199053].

GENITOURINARY

SEXUALLY TRANSMITTED INFECTIONS

 ESSENTIALS OF DIAGNOSIS

▶ Varies depending on the etiologic agent.

▶ Gonorrhea and *Chlamydia* infections associated with dysuria and discharge.

▶ Fever and chills suggestive of PID in women.

Treat *N. gonorrheae* and *Chlamydia* with antibiotics and consider other STIs.

General Considerations

Sexually transmitted infections (STIs) are common among adolescents, with a prevalence of up to 25% in females 14-19 years of age. Preadolescent children with suspected STI are assumed to be victims of child sexual abuse until proven otherwise (see Chapter 6). Genital warts caused by human papilloma virus (HPV) make up most STIs followed by *Chlamydia trachomatis*, *Trichomonas vaginalis*, herpes simplex virus (HSV-1, HSV-2), and *N. gonorrheae* (Table 41–9). HPV types 6 and 11 cause the majority of genital warts infections and are included in the quadrivalent three-stage HPV vaccine series now recommended for males and females beginning at 11 years of age. HSV-1 is typically transmitted in childhood by non-sexual contact but has emerged as an increasing cause of genital herpes, whereas HSV-2 is transmitted sexually. Teenagers at greatest risk of STI include those with young age at first intercourse, multiple partners, and those with inconsistent condom use. In contrast to other illnesses, teenage patients may be seen and treated in the emergency room for STI complaints without parental consent. Gathering an appropriate sexual history may be difficult due to the sensitive nature of the complaints and should be approached in a nonjudgmental manner alone with the patient if possible. Complications arising from STIs include pelvic inflammatory disease (PID) and disseminated gonococcal disease; specifically PID is associated with chronic pelvic pain, infertility, and ectopic pregnancy.

Clinical Findings

HPV infections are frequently asymptomatic, with the majority of infected females clearing the virus within 1 year. Genital warts (*condylomata acuminata*) may be asymptomatic or associated with pruritis, bleeding, and pain. Lesions are usually skin-colored with a verrucous surface. Similarappearing flat lesions with a characteristic velvety surface should raise suspicion for condyloma lata, a rash associated

Table 41–9. Sexually transmitted diseases among adolescents.

	HPV	Chlamydia	Trichomonas	Herpes	Gonorrhea
Prevalence (age 14-19 years)	24.5% (females)	3.2% (females) 0.7% (males)	2% (females)	HSV-1: 39% HSV-2: 1.6%	0.6% (females) 0.3% (males)
Clinical presentation	Condylomata acuminata	Asymptomatic (60-80% females, 40% males), cervicitis, urethritis	Vaginal discharge, pruritis, dysuria	Genital ulcers, fever, lymphadenopathy	Asymptomatic (50% females, 10% males), cervicitis, urethritis, epididymitis
Diagnosis	Clinical or HPV RNA/DNA	NAAT of urine, cervical, or vaginal swab	Wet prep of vaginal discharge	HSV PCR or DFA	NAAT of urine, cervical, or vaginal swab
Treatment	Observation; podophyllotoxin, tricholoroacetic acid	Azithromycin or doxycycline	Metronidazole	Acyclovir or valacyclovir	Third-generation cephalosporin
Complications	Cervical cancer, anal cancer	PID (30%), perihepatitis, tubo-ovarian abscess	Urethritis, cystitis	Recurrence, aseptic meningitis, encephalitis	PID (10-40%), perihepatitis, tubo-ovarian abscess, DGI (< 3%)

with secondary syphilis. *C. acuminata* are commonly located on the cervix, vulva, labia, or anus in females and along the penile shaft in males.

Chlamydia infection is frequently asymptomatic in males and females. Symptoms are nonspecific and include watery or mucopurulent vaginal discharge, vaginal bleeding, and dysuria. Examination of the cervix is usually normal but may reveal a friable surface with a mucopurulent discharge. Associated cervical motion tenderness, lower abdominal pain, fever, and chills are suggestive of infection that has ascended the genitourinary tract and developed into PID. Among men *Chlamydia* infection may present with dysuria and a thin or mucoid urethral discharge.

Gonococcal infection among women most often presents as cervicitis, with mucopurulent vaginal discharge, dysuria, and an inflamed, friable cervix. Signs of PID caused by gonorrhea are similar to those caused by *Chlamydia* and may include signs of perihepatitis such as pleuritic RUQ pain. Rarely, disseminated gonococcal infection (DGI) occurs. Symptoms included fever, chills, tenosynovitis, polyarthralgias, a scattered vesiculopustular rash, and arthritis of the knees, wrists, or ankles.

Trichomonas infection is generally asymptomatic in males but has the potential to cause severe pain and discomfort in some females. Symptoms include thin, purulent, and malodorous vaginal discharge, dysuria, urgency, frequency, vaginal pruritis, and dyspareunia. Examination of the cervix reveals erythema and edema, with the classic punctate hemorrhages associated with a "strawberry cervix" seen in a minority of cases.

HSV infection may be asymptomatic or present with a painful vesicular or ulcerated genital rash and tender inguinal lymphadenopathy. Systemic signs such as fever, malaise, and headache may also be present. Recurrent infections are generally less severe, are not associated with prominent systemic symptoms, and are sometimes preceded by pain or paresthesias along the distribution of the rash.

Laboratory Tests/Radiographs

Suspicion of one STI should prompt the physician to search for other STIs in the patient. Unless otherwise contraindicated, patients should have a urinalysis, urine culture, and urine pregnancy test performed. High-risk adolescents and suspected victims of child abuse should be screened for HIV, syphilis, and HBV and HCV.

HPV infection is typically diagnosed clinically and biopsy is generally unnecessary. The application of 5% acetic acid will cause HPV lesions to turn white. RNA testing for HPV is available and is usually performed in conjuction with a pap smear to assess for cervical cancer risk in older women.

The mainstay of diagnosis of *Chlamydia* infections is NAAT of urine, endocervical swab, or a urethral swab. Culture, antigen testing, and serologies are also available but do not match the sensitivity or specificity of NAAT, which approaches 90% and 99% respectively.

Likewise *N. gonorrheae* is best identified via NAAT from the urine, endocervical swab, or urethral swab. Gram stain and microscopy of urethral discharge may be perfomed in men with purulent urethral exudates; females may have other commensal gram-negative diplococci in their cervical secretions. Suspected disseminated gonococcal infection should be diagnosed with cultures submitted on Thayer-Martin media from the skin, urogenital tract, rectum, and synovial fluid (if there is joint involvement). Blood cultures should also be sent in these cases. Patients with moderate to severe signs of PID should have a pelvic ultrasound or CT performed to assess for the presence of a tubo-ovarian abscess.

Trichomonas is most easily diagnosed by visualizing motile trichomonads on a wet prep of the vaginal discharge. Care must be taken to view the specimen within 20 minutes of collection to maximize sensitivity, which is 60%. Culture should be sent on all patients with suspected infection and a negative wet prep. New rapid RNA testing kits may be available in some centers.

The gold standard for genital HSV infection remains viral culture, but the sensitivity is low unless the rash is diagnosed before the vesicles have drained. HSV PCR or DFA testing of swabs of the rash is the recommended modality in cases where there are no classic vesicular lesions. Serologies are not generally helpful in the acute setting because IgG levels remain elevated for life after infection and elevated IgM levels do not distinguish between a primary or recurrent infection.

Treatment

Genital warts frequently spontaneously regress and treatment of the lesions is best accomplished in the outpatient setting. Recurrent applications of podophyllin or trichloroacetic acid are used for smaller lesions and surgical excision is possible for larger warts. The HPV vaccine is not currently recommended for the prevention of recurrent HPV infection.

Chlamydia is treated with a one-time dose of azithromycin or a 7-day course of doxycycline, with azithromycin preferred due to increased compliance. Empiric treatment for gonorrhea is indicated if NAAT results are not available and treatment of the patient's sexual partner should be considered if allowed by state regulations.

A single dose of an IM or IV third-generation cephalosporin such as ceftriaxone is effective for the treatment of uncomplicated gonococcal infection. Flouroquinolones have fallen out of favor due to increased resistance patterns. The physician may add azithromycin or doxycycline to prevent the development of further resistance and as empiric treatment for chlaymdia. Disseminated gonococcal infection should be treated with IV ceftriaxone and admission. Patients with joint involvement may also require surgical drainage. Females with suspected PID are generally admitted unless symptoms are mild. Empiric inpatient treatment of PID is directed against *Neisseria* and *Chlaymdia* and includes an IV second-generation cephalosporin such as cefoxitin or cefotetan in combination with doxycycline. If a tubo-ovarian abscess is suspected, anaerobic coverage with clindamycin or metronidazole should be added.

Metronidazole is the preferred treatment for *Trichomonas* infection and may be given as a single dose or 7-day course. Male partners should be treated as well and the patient should avoid intercourse for 1 week after completion of the antibiotic course.

Primary genital HSV infections should be treated with acyclovir, valacyclovir, or famcyclovir for 7-10 days. Admission and parenteral therapy is generally not indicated unless there are concerns for disseminated disease or if the patient has an underlying immunodeficiency. Recurrent HSV infection may be suppressed with chronic antiviral therapy or treated episodically during flares with a short antiviral course.

Centers for Disease Control: *2010 Sexually Transmitted Diseases Prevalence.* Atlanta, GA; 2011. Also available at http://www.cdc.gov/std/stats10/natprointro.htm. Accessed August 15, 2012.

Cernik C, Gallina K, Brodell RT: The treatment of herpes simplex infections: An evidence-based review. *Arch Intern Med.* 2008;168(11):1137 [PMID: 1854182].

Chandran L, Boykan R: Chlamydia infections in children and adolescents. *Pediatr Rev.* 2009;30(7):243 [PMID: 19570922].

Forcier M, Musacchio N: An overview of human papillomavirus infection for the dermatologist: Disease, diagnosis, management, and prevention. *Dermatol Ther.* 2010;23(5):458 [PMID: 20868401].

Holder NA: Gonococcal infections. *Pediatr Rev.* 2008;29(7):228 [PMID: 18593752].

Huppert JS: Trichomoniasis in teens: An update. *Curr Opin Obstet Gynecol.* 2009;21(5):371 [PMID: 19491679].

Lewin LC: Sexually transmitted infections in preadolescent children. *J Pediatr Health Care.* 2007;21(3):153 [PMID: 17478304].

Soper DE. Pelvic inflammatory disease. *Obstet Gynecol.* 2010;116:419 ([PMID: 20664404].

Tarr ME, Gilliam ML: Sexually transmitted infections in adolescent women. *Clin Obstet Gynecol.* 2008;51(2):306 [PMID: 18463461].

Thornsberry L, English JC: Evidence-based treatment and prevention of external genital warts in female pediatric and adolescent patients. *J Pediatr Adolesc Gynecol.* 2012;25(2):150 [PMID: 22530225].

TICK-BORNE ILLNESSES

ROCKY MOUNTAIN SPOTTED FEVER AND EHRLICHIOSIS

 ESSENTIALS OF DIAGNOSIS

▶ Fever.

▶ Rash.

▶ Headache during the summer months.

Treat with doxycycline.

Table 41–10. Comparison of RMSF and *Ehrlichia* infections.

	RMSF	Ehrlichiosis
Etiologic agent	*R. rickettssii*	*E. chaffeensis, A. phagocytophilum*
Tick vector	Dog tick, wood tick	Lone Star tick, *I. scapularis*
Cell type affected	Endothelial cells	Leukocytes
Clinical presentation	Fever, rash, nausea, headache	Fever, myalgia, headache
Rash	90%	50%
Laboratory values	Thrombocytopenia, hyponatremia, transaminitis	Leukopenia, thrombocytopenia, transaminitis, hyponatremia
Complications	Shock, coma, renal failure, seizures	Seizures, renal failure, heart failure
Mortality	3%	1-3%
Treatment	Doxycycline	Doxycycline

General Considerations

Rocky Mountain spotted fever (RMSF) and ehrlichiosis are tick-borne illnesses caused by obligate intracellular bacteria commonly encountered in the summer months (Table 41–10). Each has a geographic distribution, with increased prevalence in the south central and southeastern United States. RMSF, caused by the gram-negative bacteria *R. rickettssii*, has tropism for human endothelial cells and manifestations of infection range from mild to life-threatening. Directly mediated damage to endothelial surfaces as well as the immune response to the bacteria cause the majority of RMSF symptoms and complications. RMSF is transmitted by the bite of a wood tick or dog tick, with symptoms occurring within 2 weeks of exposure to the bacteria. Risk factors for RMSF infection include male gender, age 5-9 years, and exposure to ticks or woods known to contain ticks. Ehrlichiosis is most commonly caused by *Ehrlichia chaffeensis* or *Anaplasma phagocytophillum*, closely related bacterial species that differ in their tropism for monocytes and granulocytes, respectively. Transmission occurs through several tick species including the Lone Star tick and *Ixodes scapularis*, which also transmits Lyme disease.

Clinical Findings

RMSF presents initially with fever, headache, malaise, nausea, and myalgias. A known tick bite is reported in fewer than 50% of patients. In 90% of patients a rash develops 3-5 days after the onset of symptoms and begins on the extremities and spreads centripetally. It may be maculopapular or petechial and classically involves the palms and soles. Focal neurological signs, seizure, and meningismus may be seen in more severe cases.

Ehrlichial infection has a similar but generally less severe presentation and can be asymptomatic. Children present with fever, headache, myalgia, nausea, or rarely neurologic symptoms such as altered mental status and meningismus. Despite being known as "spotless RMSF," ehrlichiosis in children may present with a maculopapular or petechial rash in 50% of patients.

Laboratory Tests/Radiographs

Although RMSF and erhlichiosis are clinical diagnoses, classic laboratory abnormalities may be seen with both diseases. RMSF has been associated with thrombocytopenia, mild hyponatremia, and mild transaminitis. In severe cases, prolonged coagulation studies, hypoalbuminemia, and azotemia may be seen. CSF studies in RMSF typically demonstrate mildly elevated WBC (< 100 WBCs/μL) with a slight lymphocytic or polymorphonuclear predominance, mildly elevated protein, and normal glucose. Diagnosis of RMSF is best accomplished through the use of serologic testing, with antibodies appearing 1 week after initial infection. Skin biopsy with direct immunofluorescence is highly specific but is not sensitive enough to be used routinely.

Leukopenia, thrombocytopenia, and a mild transaminitis are frequently seen with ehrlichial infection. CSF studies may be normal or show a mildly elevated WBC count with a lymphocytic predominance, normal glucose, and slightly elevated protein. PCR for ehrlichia has become the preferred mode of diagnosis and blood or CSF samples may be used. The peripheral blood smear may be examined for the presence of intracytoplasmic bacterial inclusions known as morulae, but this method is highly insensitive. Serodiagnosis is also possible but is complicated by the high rate of previous infection in the general population.

Treatment

Prompt diagnosis and management of RMSF is critical as delays in treatment are associated with seizures, coma, disseminated intravascular coagulation, and death. Patients who are moderately or severely ill with suspected RMSF should be monitored closely and admitted to an ICU. Mildly ill children with suspected RMSF should be admitted until clinical improvement is documented; however, outpatient therapy with close follow-up is possible in select cases. Fever and headache should prompt an evaluation for meningitis, and empiric antibiotics to cover for bacterial meningitis should be started until CSF studies are available. Doxycycline, 2 mg/kg/dose every 12 hours, should be started as empiric treatment of RMSF in children, and the risk of dental staining is remote if a short course of therapy is used.

Though generally less severe than RMSF, ehrlichoisis in children must be treated promptly to prevent complications. Doxycycline is the drug of choice and is dosed at 2 mg/kg/dose every 12 hours. Mildly ill children may be managed as outpatients provided close follow-up is arranged. Moderately or severely ill children should be monitored in the ICU if necessary; admission is required until clinical improvement on doxycycline is documented.

Buckingham SC, Marshall GS, Schutze GE, et al: Clinical and laboratory features, hospital course, and outcome of Rocky Mountain Spotted Fever in children. *J Pediatr.* 2007;150:180 [PMID: 17236897].

Dumler JS, Madigan JE, Pusterla N, et al: Ehrlichioses in humans: Epidemiology, clinical presentation, diagnosis, and treatment. *Clin Infect Dis.* 2007;45:S45 [PMID: 17582569].

Graham J, Stockley K, Goldman RD: Tick-borne illnesses: a CME update. *Pediatr Emerg Care.* 2011;27(2):141 [PMID: 21293226].

Schutze GE, Buckingham SC, Marshall GS, et al: Human monocytic ehrlichiosis in children. *Pediatr Infect Dis J.* 2007;26(6):475 [PMID: 17529862].

LYME DISEASE

 ESSENTIALS OF DIAGNOSIS

▶ Erythema migrans.

▶ Fever.

▶ Malaise.

▶ Tick exposure.

Treat with amoxicillin 14-21 days.

General Considerations

Lyme disease is a common tick-borne illness caused by a spirochete, *Borrelia burgdorferi*. It is transmitted by the *Ixodes scapularis* tick and is most common in the northeastern and upper midwestern regions of the United States. The majority of cases occur in the summer months, and symptoms typically develop within 2-3 weeks of a tick bite. After inoculation into a human host the bacteria proliferates rapidly and spreads hematogenously throughout the body. Most symptoms of infection result from the immune response to the bacteria rather than specific bacterial toxins. The disease has a bimodal age distribution, with the most infections occurring in children aged 5-14 years and in adults aged 40-60 years. Lyme disease is capable of causing late findings if it is not treated effectively, but the existence of chronic-treated Lyme disease has never been proven and remains a controversial entity in adults and children.

Clinical Findings

Early finding of Lyme disease is characteristic skin rash erythema migrans, an erythematous annular macule which may exhibit central clearing. The lesion is generally flat, without scale, and is not painful. The rash represents bacterial invasion of the skin and spreads rapidly if not treated. Children most commonly exhibit the rash on the head, neck, extremities, back. Associated systemic symptoms include fever, headache, malaise, and arthralgias. Left untreated, children may develop disseminated disease manifested by multiple areas of erythema migrans, carditis, facial nerve palsy, meningitis. Rarely, children develop monoarticular arthritis of the large joints, most commonly the knee, up to 2 years after initial infection.

Laboratory Tests/Radiographs

Routine laboratory tests are not indicated for diagnosis of Lyme disease. Serologic testing is not recommended for early-stage disease manifested by erythema migrans because antibodies are not apparent early in the disease course. Evidence of disseminated disease should prompt an evaluation of IgG and IgM antibodies against *B. burgdorferi*, but the results must be interpreted with caution because IgG and IgM antibodies have been shown to persist for years following initial infection. CSF analysis in children with suspected Lyme meningitis may reveal a modestly elevated WBC count with a lymphocytic or monocytic predominance, elevated protein, and normal glucose. Synovial fluid in Lyme arthritis is characterized by a WBC of 20-40,000 cells/mm³ with a neutrophilic predominance and with mildly elevated serum inflammatory markers.

Treatment

Children with Lyme disease may be managed as outpatients, with admission and IV antibiotics reserved for children with severe disseminated disease, heart block, or arthritis. Lumbar puncture is recommended for children with facial palsy or nuchal rigidity. Children older than 8 years may be treated with doxycycline (4 mg/kg/d in 2 divided doses) and those younger than 8 years may be given amoxicillin (50 mg/kg/d in 3 divided doses) or a second-generation cephalosporin such as cefuroxime (30 mg/kg/d in 2 divided doses). Treatment duration is 10-21 days, with 28 days recommended for treatment of arthritis.

Feder HM: Lyme disease in children. *Infect Dis Clin North Am.* 2008;22(2):315 [PMID: 18452804].

O'Connell S: Lyme borreliosis: Current issues in diagnosis and management. *Curr Opin Infect Dis.* 2010;23(3):231 [PMID: 20407371].

Puius YA, Kalish RA: Lyme arthritis: Pathogenesis, clinical presentation, and management. *Infect Dis Clin North Am.* 2008;22(2):289 [PMID: 18452802].

Endocrine & Metabolic Emergencies

Matthew N. Graber, MD, PhD, FAAEM

Ruqayya Gill, MBS, DO

DIABETES MELLITUS

General Considerations

Diabetes mellitus (DM) is one of the most common chronic diseases of the pediatric population accounting for more than 150,000 current US cases. Traditionally, DM in the pediatric patient is generally thought to be diabetes mellitus type 1 (DM1), previously referred to as juvenile onset DM. However, diabetes mellitus type 2 (DM2) is increasingly common among children and adolescents. Previously referred to as adult-onset DM, the disease is becoming increasingly common among children due to dietary and obesity issues.

DM1 accounts for approximately two of every three childhood cases of DM. The presentation of DM1 varies greatly among patients but often falls into two distinct groups: (1) approximately 20–40% of new-onset DM1 present with diabetic ketoacidosis (DKA) and, (2) most of the remainder present with classic signs and symptoms of new-onset DM (Table 42–1). The difference between the two groups is that those presenting with DKA have often progressed to complete or near complete β-cell dysfunction. A third less common group includes children diagnosed early due to historical information such as relatives with DM or via an incidental finding as other concerns are evaluated.

HYPERGLYCEMIA

Clinical Presentation

Children with hyperglycemia often present with a recent history of polyuria and polydipsia and with clinical dehydration. In younger children, the history may be difficult to elicit but suspicion should be raised by an increasing numbers of wet diapers, especially in the dehydrated child and in child with unexplained weight loss.

Laboratory evaluation may include studies to evaluate for DKA (Table 42–2) and glycated hemoglobin A_{1c} (HbA_{1c}). The test may not be helpful in the emergency department; however, it is an integral part of the hyperglycemia workup and may hasten the patient's long-term treatment plan.

It is difficult to make a diagnosis of hyperglycemia in children younger than 6 years; therefore, a child presenting with a classic finding (see Table 42–1) or yeast infection in children should have a glucose level obtained.

Treatment

Pediatric patients determined to be hyperglycemic will present in a range of dehydrated states that require intravenous (IV) fluids. In the patient with significant dehydration, resuscitation should begin with repeated 10-20 mL/kg boluses of normal saline (NS) until normal perfusion is attained. Fluid is continued with ½ NS to allow for rehydration and maintenance to replace total fluid deficit over 24 hours. An easy way to calculate fluid deficit as follows:

$$\text{Fluid deficit}_{mL} = \text{weight}_{kg} \times \% \text{ deficit} \times 10$$

so that total fluids to be administered = maintenance fluids + deficit correction.

After resuscitation, the patient's glucose is likely to have decreased but may still be elevated. If the patient is on an acceptable home insulin regimen, it may be instituted at this time. Patients with DM2 on oral medications may be restarted on their usual medications. The clinical scenario may require that subcutaneous (SQ) insulin be instituted for the first time; a number of regimens are available to start the process but the goal is to avoid DKA and metabolic decomposition rather than tight glucose control. There is no role for IV insulin in most hyperglycemic pediatric patients not in DKA and no role for IV bolus insulin for hyperglycemic complications.

Table 42–1. Classic diabetes mellitus presentation.

Lethargy/fatigue
Polydipsia
Polyuria[a]
Polyphagia
Weight loss
Candidiasis

[a]History may be unclear, but concerns such as recurrent bed wetting and increased number of wet diapers.

Disposition

Pediatric patients with new-onset DM presenting with hyperglycemia are generally admitted. It is difficult if not impossible to confirm diagnosis of DM1 or DM2 in a new pediatric patient in the emergency department. All DM1 will require insulin therapy and associated patient and family education prior to discharge. The patient receiving insulin for the first time may be admitted for these reasons. However, the patient with DM who presents with hyperglycemia but not DKA may be discharged if rehydrated, hyperglycemia is correcting with SQ insulin, able to take oral fluids, has access to medications and acceptable family and social support, and if there is an inciting cause to the hyperglycemia (infection) that may be addressed as outpatient.

DIABETIC KETOACIDOSIS

Clinical Presentation

Children in DKA usually present with lethargy, dehydration, tachypnea, and a recent history similar to that for hyperglycemia. The fruity smell of acetone may be on their breath. It is more difficult to make the diagnosis in infants and younger children who may be misdiagnosed as having a common airway infection such as bronchiolitis due to their tachypnea, viral upper airway infection, or pneumonia; therefore, the diagnosis is often made later and in a sicker child. DKA may be exacerbated by the treatment with steroids or β-agonists for asthma or bronchiolitis.

Risk factors for patients with known DM presenting to the emergency department in recurrent DKA include noncompliance with insulin regimen (most common in adolescents), decreased access to health care, lower family socioeconomic status and lower parental education levels, unstable family dynamics, and complications with insulin pump therapy (as pumps use short-acting insulins, dysfunction quickly leads to insulinopenia and symptoms).

Diagnosis of DKA is based on findings commonly, but not always found during the laboratory workup (see Table 42–2). Patients may present with laboratory abnormalities that are not classic but still in DKA. A common diagnostic strategy includes diagnosis from an elevated β-hydroxybutyrate plus abnormalities in two of the following three areas: serum bicarbonate, anion gap, and venous pH.

Hyponatremia often reported by the laboratory for patients in DKA is usually an artifact due to hyperglycemia (and occasionally hypertriglyceridemia) and sodium level needs to be corrected before any attempt to supplement:

$$Na_{corrected} = [measured\ Na] + (measured\ Glu - 100) \times 1.6/100)$$

Potassium homeostasis is an important consideration in evaluation of the pediatric DKA patient. Although patients will often present with hyperkalemia, DKAs associated acidosis and hyperosmolality causes a shift of potassium from the intracellular to the extracellular space allowing for the continued osmotic diuresis of DKA to deplete potassium stores. An ECG may be helpful to assess the clinical level of hypokalemia. Phosphate and magnesium levels may also be low.

Cerebral edema complicating DKA is generally an unpredictable phenomenon that occurs in children who seem to be metabolically returning to normal, generally 3-12 hours after the initiation of therapy. Less than 1% of children with DKA will experience catastrophic cerebral edema, however, subclinical cerebral edema has been described as common during treatment of DKA children. Signs and symptoms include headache, vomiting, abrupt changes to respiration, and any sign of increased intracranial pressure. Risk factors have included elevated blood urea nitrogen (BUN), low pCO_2, treatment with bicarbonate, failure of serum sodium concentration to rise with correction, young age (usually < 3 yr). Although commonly believed, there does not appear to be any causative association between the rate of fluid administration or glucose decrease and the occurrence of symptomatic cerebral edema. Instead, cerebral edema may be associated with degree of presenting dehydration and acidosis; that is, cerebral edema appears to be associated with

Table 42–2. Common laboratory findings used to make the diagnosis of diabetic ketoacidosis.

[a]Elevated serum β-hydroxybutyrate: > 2.0 mmol/L
Hyperglycemia (glucose > 250 mg/dL)
Elevated anion gap > 16
Venous pH: < 7.30
Serum HCO$_3$: < 15 mEq/L

[a]Many laboratories assay for serum acetoacetate and most urine studies also assay for acetoacetate. Acetoacetate is not sensitive or specific enough for DKA to use diagnostically.

the degree of DKA present in the patient. The treatment for symptomatic cerebral edema is mannitol at 0.25-1 g/kg as an IV bolus. Reports of treatment with 3% hypertonic NS have also been used for management of cerebral edema. Hyperventilation to decrease pCO_2 should be avoided as it likely worsens outcomes. If intubated, the patient should be hyperventilated to the pCO_2 at which they presented on arrival prior to intubation. This is performed to prevent subsequent increase in cerebral blood flow and ultimate further increase in intracranial pressure. Consultation with the pediatric intensivist is recommended.

Treatment

Pediatric patients in DKA are typically about 10% dehydrated although the length of time in DKA and degree of disease may increase the level. Fluid resuscitation should commence with judicious administration of 10-20 ml/kg boluses of NS until normal perfusion is attained. Normally only 1-2 fluids boluses are required. Fluid is continued with at least ½ NS to NS to allow for rehydration and maintenance to replace the total fluid deficit over 24-48 hours.

Insulin is commonly used to treat hyperkalemia and therefore is no surprise that in the pediatric DKA patient with a significant total body potassium deficit, its administration can lead to a dangerous drop in potassium levels. Therefore, hypokalemia must be addressed prior to initiation of insulin therapy. Potassium is replaced IV starting at 40 mEq/L as a combination of potassium acetate and potassium phosphate. Magnesium and phosphate may also be supplemented. There are many institutional "DKA protocols" which may vary in their treatment management of DKA. Consult with a pediatric endocrinologist if needed.

Insulin therapy is an important component of the treatment plan but must be used with adverse effects of hypokalemia and hypoglycemia in mind. There is no indication for IV bolus insulin in the treatment of hyperglycemia or DKA. After the patient is resuscitated and hypokalemia addressed, insulin infusion may be started at 0.1 units regular insulin/kg/hour IV. During this therapy, hourly glucose levels and every other hour chemistries for potassium levels are required. If the patient's glucose level falls below 300 mg/dL, IV fluids should be changed to D5½ NS with electrolytes to maintain acceptable glucose levels. Occasionally, D10 or D12.5% is required to maintain acceptable glucose levels during insulin therapy. Insulin infusion should not be discontinued if hypoglycemia develops as long as the patient remains acidotic. As stated, the glucose concentration in the IV fluids should be increased.

Once the anion gap has normalized (≤ 16) the patient may be transitioned to SQ insulin. If the patient has an appropriate home insulin regimen, it may be reinstituted at this time. If the patient has not been on insulin, a number of regimens may be considered. Consultation with an endocrinologist is recommended. Note that IV insulin infusion should overlap SQ insulin by 1 hour for rapid-acting SQ insulins and by 2 hours for longer-acting insulins.

Pediatric DKA patients who can tolerate it may be allowed oral fluids and food if they are clinically well and desire them. This intake may partially guard against the adverse treatment effects of hypoglycemia and hypokalemia. Caution should be used in a patient who may require later intubation or is at risk for aspiration.

There is no role for bicarbonate therapy in the treatment of pediatric DKA, although some have suggested that significant cardiac dysrhythmias due to severe acidosis may be an indication. Bicarbonate leads to a paradoxical cerebral acidosis. It has been postulated that the combination of worsening cerebral acidosis and hyperosmolarity of bicarbonate may increase the risk for cerebral edema.

Disposition

Pediatric patient in DKA should be admitted to a closely monitored unit where regular glucose levels and serum chemistries can be drawn and the patient can be watched closely for clinical signs of hypoglycemia, hypokalemia, and cerebral edema. Additionally, the patient and family members may benefit from this time for additional education about DM and how to guard against future DKA episodes.

Bangstad HJ, Danne T, Deeb L, et al: ISPAD Clinical Practice Consensus Guidelines 2009 Compendium: Insulin treatment in children and adults with diabetes. *Ped Diabetes.* 2009;10:8 [PMID: 19754612].

Centers for Disease Control. Children and diabetes. Bethesda, MD; 2012. Also available at http://www.cdc.gov/diabetes/projects/cda2.htm. Accessed August 30, 2012.

Clark L, Preissig C, Rigby M, et al: Endocrine issues in the pediatric intensive care unit. *Pediatr Clin North Am.* 2008;55:805 [PMID: 18501767].

Orlowski JP, Cramer CL, Fiallos MR: Diabetic ketoacidosis in the pediatric ICU. *Pediatr Clin North Am.* 2008;55:577 [PMID: 18501755].

HYPOGLYCEMIA

Clinical Presentation

Hypoglycemia is a common pediatric concern (Table 42–3), especially in the first 30 days of life. The definition of hypoglycemia in the pediatric patient is poorly delineated. A glucose greater than 40 mg/dL in neonates older than 2 days and glucose greater than 30 mg/dL in premature neonates in the first day of life is often considered normal. Therefore, the glucose level should be interpreted in light of the patient's clinical picture. Glucose levels less than 60 mg/dL in the child with signs or symptoms of hypoglycemia warrant evaluation and treatment. Glucose level may increase to 70 mg/dL in adolescents and those approaching adulthood (see Chapter 17).

Table 42–3. Common causes of hypoglycemia.

- Increased Insulin
  - Islet cell adenoma or hyperplasia
  - Infant of diabetic mother
  - Exposure to oral hypoglycemic medication or exogenous insulin
- Infection
- Hypothermia
- Asphyxia
- Inborn errors of metabolism
- Decreased glucose availability
  - Malnutrition
  - Malabsorption
  - Low glycogen stores (prematurity and congenital liver disease)
- Poisoning
  - Salicylates
  - Alcohols
  - Trimethoprim/sulfamethoxazole
  - β-blockers

Responses to hypoglycemia are divided into two categories: autonomic response symptoms are due to the surge of counter-regulatory hormones such as epinephrine and neuroglycopenic symptoms are due to decreased glucose uptake by the brain (Table 42–4).

With gradual hypoglycemia autonomic responses may be blunted, whereas during an acute hypoglycemic episode (such as due to an insulin reaction) responses usually dominate. Autonomic symptoms may be decreased or absent in patients with advanced neuropathy, in those with the syndrome of hypoglycemic unawareness (blunting of the autonomic response to hypoglycemia attributable to the brain and specifically the paraventricular nucleus of the hypothalamus), and those experiencing frequent hypoglycemia. Patients with uncontrolled DM and therefore chronic hyperglycemia may experience neuroglycopenic symptoms at higher glucose levels than others and even at "normal glucose levels."

A search for the cause of hypoglycemia is essential. Although a common cause is the administration of insulin or oral hypoglycemic without proper calorie intake, diagnosis should be made only after other, more concerning etiologies, are excluded. History and physical examination should evaluate for an infection that might increase glucose metabolism. Urinalysis negative for ketones in the face of documented hypoglycemia may provide clue to diagnosis of inborn errors of metabolism or hyperinsulinemia. Urine testing for drug ingestions and organic acids should be considered. Therefore, in infants, testing is often expanded. If appropriate, before glucose is administered, hold blood testing for the following: glucose, comprehensive metabolic panel, lactate, insulin, cortisol, growth hormone, pyruvate, β-hydroxybutyrate, and acetoacetate. Because insulin is metabolized by both kidneys and liver, it is appropriate to evaluate for decreased function of these organs with chemistry (creatinine) and liver functions testing (prothrombin time [PT]).

Treatment

The first action upon determination of hypoglycemia is the administration of IV glucose for any patient with altered mental status. If the patient is able, IV administration of glucose should be followed by oral complex carbohydrates. The concentration and amount of glucose solution given is based upon the patient's age (Table 42–5). A second glucose bolus may be necessary in some patients. An infusion of glucose-containing fluids should be continued after the bolus. Glucose levels should be checked frequently while on the infusion.

Neonates have a decreased ability to store glycogen and produce glucose via gluconeogenesis and therefore continued infusion of a glucose-containing solution following the bolus

Table 42–4. Signs and symptoms of hypoglycemia.

Autonomic Response	Neuroglycopenia
Sweating	Dizziness
Tremor	Headache
Tachycardia	Visual changes
Anxiety	Confusion/altered mental status
Hunger	Loss of fine motor skills
	Abnormal behavior
	Seizures
	Loss of consciousness

Responses to hypoglycemia may be divided into two categories: Autonomic response symptoms due to the surge of counter-regulatory hormones such as epinephrine. Neuroglycopenic symptoms due to decreased glucose uptake by the brain.

Table 42–5. Zimmerman rule of 50 (glucose administration for hypoglycemia).*

Age	Glucose Concentration	Amount
Neonates	D10	5 cc/kg
Infants < 2 y	D25	2 cc/kg
Children/adolescents	D50	1 cc/kg

*Zimmerman rule of 50: Glucose concentration x cc/kg always equals 50.

is important in this age group. The usual glucose requirement in the neonate is approximately 8-10 mg/kg/min.

Adjunct treatments include the following:

Glucagon (0.1-0.2 mg/kg up to 1 mg IV or IM) may be given for persistent hypoglycemia or when an IV cannot be obtained. Glucagon is not helpful in those without glycogen stores (glycogen storage diseases, significant malnutrition, neonates).

Octreotide is used as an antidote for sulfonylurea overdose. It is a somatostatin analogue that directly inhibits the secretion of insulin from pancreatic β-cells (see Chapter 46). Dose is 4-5 mcg/kg/day SQ divided every 6 hours (max 50 mcg every 6 hr).

Unless the patient has a known preexisting diagnosis of an endocrine disorder, such as congential adrenal hyperplasia, steroids should not be used. Steroids provide minimal initial resolution of hypoglycemia and may delay the diagnosis.

Disposition

Patients with the following conditions require admission:

- Recurrent or refractory hypoglycemia.
- Infection that is the likely cause of hypoglycemia.
- Renal or liver dysfunction to the extent that it may be the cause of hypoglycemia.
- Taking long-acting insulin (glargine) or long-acting oral hypoglycemic medications.
- Hypoglycemia due to an unknown cause (presenting in infancy).

Patients who are well-appearing, have had one episode of hypoglycemia due to a readily reversible cause (such as not eating after taking insulin), and have appropriate social and family support may be discharged home.

It is appropriate to admit a patient who may be at risk for recurrent hypoglycemia because of the following: patient's or family's lack of understanding of medication and required calorie needs, information cannot be given confidently and in an expedited manner, and patient does not have appropriate supervision or support.

DIABETES INSIPIDUS

General Considerations

Vasopressin (antidiuretic hormone [ADH], arginine vasopressin) is a hormone that acts to increase water permeability in the renal collecting system therefore increasing water reabsorption. It is produced by the hypothalamus and released from the pituitary gland. A lack of vasopressin effect may be due to central diabetes insipidus (DI) caused by either improper hormone formation or release, or be due to nephrogenic DI caused by a hormone-receptor issue in the kidney. Either mechanism can cause reduced water reabsorption in the renal collecting system and therefore increased diuresis and dehydration.

Clinical Presentation

Patients usually present with clinical dehydration and polyuria. Patients who have a functional thirst mechanism and are able to drink water will also have polydipsia. However, infants and those without the ability to drink water often present with profound dehydration. Historical clues to diagnosis include polydipsia, polyuria, and overwhelming thirst in individuals who can express it. Physical examination may suggest a range of dehydration states. When the exam reveals abnormal visual fields, pituitary tumor is a possibility. Severe dehydration due to DI may lead to lethargy, seizures, and death.

There are a number of causes of DI and most require extensive workup outside the emergency department to determine the cause. However, a few possible causes should be considered in the emergency department (Table 42–6). Laboratory findings include: hypernatremia (Na+ greater than 145 mmol/L), serum hyperosmolality (greater than 300 mOsm/L), low urine osmolarity (less than 600 mOsm/L).

Treatment

Patients in whom the diagnosis of DI is suspected most likely will require hydration. IV NS should be given in 20 cc/kg bolus until patient resuscitated and then admitted for further testing. Replace free water deficit over 48 hours to avoid complications such as development of cerebral edema (see Chapter 17).

Patients with a known diagnosis of central DI should be treated currently with DDAVP (available intranasally, orally, or via SQ or IV injection). Those with known nephrogenic DI are usually treated with diuretics and a salt-restricted diet.

Table 42–6. Important emergency department causes of diabetes insipidus.

Central Diabetes Insipidus	Nephrogenic Diabetes Insipidus
Head trauma	Urinary tract obstruction/renal disease
Suprasellar brain tumors	
Hypoxic brain injury	Significant disturbance in K+ or Ca2+
Encephalitis/Meningitis	Multiple drug ingestions
Wolfram syndrome	Sex-linked recessive
	Sickle cell disease
	Idiopathic

Disposition

Patients in whom diagnosis is suspected require admission for a water deprivation test. Additional tests include a morning urinary osmolality compared to the morning serum sodium and osmolality, and MRI to search for tumors or pituitary abnormalities.

HYPONATREMIA

Clinical Presentation

Hyponatremia, serum sodium less than 135 mEq/L, is due to various causes (Table 42–7). Symptoms usually do not appear until sodium levels fall below 120 mEq/L. This can result from excess free water intake or the inability of the kidneys to excrete free water. Etiologies include GI losses due to vomiting and diarrhea and renal losses due to diuretics and renal tubular acidosis. Other causes are CHF, nephrotic syndrome, cirrhosis, SIADH, and adrenal insufficiency. Pseudohyponatremia is due to hyperglycemia, hyperlipidemia, or hyperproteinemia (see Chapter 17).

Treatment

It is important to determine the etiology of the hyponatremia and begin aggressive treatment. In the acute setting of seizures or coma, 3% hypertonic NS should be initiated. A dose of 5 mL/kg over 10-20 minutes should raise sodium level by approximately 5 mEq/L; additional lesser doses of 2-3 mL/kg can be considered if there is no clinical improvement.

Sodium deficit can be calculated as follows:

$$mEq\ Na\ needed = 0.6 \times weight\ (kg)$$
$$\times (Na\ desired - Na\ measured)$$

When sodium level is 125 mEq/L, symptoms should improve. The goal is to raise the sodium level slowly at a rate of 0.5 mEq/L/hr (maximum 12 mEq/L/day) by using 0.9% NS infusion. If SIADH or other causes are suspected, treatment includes fluid restriction and administration of furosemide 1-2 mg/kg. If chronic hyponatremia is corrected rapidly, the patient can develop central pontine myelinolysis, a potentially devastating outcome. Therefore, unless the acuteness of hyponatremia is ascertained, assume a chronic condition and correct slowly.

Disposition

Admission should be considered for children with symptomatic hyponatremia, sodium level below 126 mEq/L with comorbid conditions, and a patient with a sodium level less than 120 mEq/L. Any child with hyponatremia should be considered for observation or admission.

SIADH

Syndrome of inappropriate secretion of antidiuretic hormone (SIADH) is the inability to excrete free water caused by excessive secretion of ADH with normal or low plasma osmolarity, or an inappropriate sodium concentration. Causes of SIADH are summarized in Table 42–8.

Classic diagnostic criteria are:

- Evolemic hyponatremia and low plasma osmolality.
- Failure of kidney to dilute urine in the presence of reduced serum osmolality (urine concentration >100 mOsmol/kg).
- Continued urinary sodium excretion (> 20 mEq/L) despite hyponatremia.
- Absence of conditions such as hypothyroidism, adrenal insufficiency, renal disease, congestive heart failure.

Treatment

Therapy for SIADH includes treatment of the underlying disorder (or discontinuation of an offending drug) and fluid restriction. Replacement of sodium loss may also be necessary, but can usually be achieved by means of normal dietary salt intake. Severe hyponatremia (serum sodium < 120 mEq/L) may be associated with central nervous system (CNS) abnormalities, including seizures, and may require treatment with hypertonic (3%) IV sodium chloride solution. Fosphenytoin has been advocated for use in SIADH as it inhibits ADH release and may be helpful in seizures secondary to SIADH. Additional treatment regimen include loop diuretics and vasopressin-2 receptor antagonists. If SIADH and hyponatremia are chronic (> 48 hr), overzealous treatment can result in CNS damage, including central pontine myelinolysis.

Table 42–7. Common causes of hyponatremia.

Abnormal sodium/free water intake (incorrect formula water to powder ratio)
Hyperglycemia
Mannitol, glycerol therapy
Congestive heart failure
Acute renal failure
Nephrosis
Gastrointestinal losses (diarrhea, emesis)
Renal losses (diuretic, renal tubular acidosis, renal interstitial disease)
Adrenal causes
Third spacing
SIADH
Water intoxication
Pseudohyponatremia

Chung CH, Zimmerman D: Hypernatremia and hyponatremia: Current understanding and management. *Clin Pediatr Emerg Med.* 2009;10:4.

Table 42–8. Causes of SIADH.

Tumors
Hodgkin disease
Neuroblastoma
Thymoma
Pancreatic carcinoma
Small cell lung carcinoma
CNS disorders
Stroke
Hemorrhage
Infection
Trauma
Drugs
Antidepressants
Antipsychotics
Anticonvulsants
Sulfonylureas
ACE inhibitors
Narcotics
MDMA (Ectasy)
Antineoplastic agents
Pulmonary disorders
Tuberculosis
Pneumonia
Abscess
Bronchiectasis
Mechanical ventilation

Reproduced, with permission, from Stone CK, Humphries RL: Current Diagnosis & Treatment Emergency Medicine, 7th ed. New York: McGraw-Hill, 2011. Copyright © McGraw-Hill Education LLC.

Ghirardello S: The diagnosis of children with central diabetes insipidus. *J Ped Endrocinol Metab.* 2007;20:359 [PMID: 17451074].

Ranadive S, Rosenthal S: Pediatric disorders or water balance. *Pediatr Clin North Am.* 2011;58(5):1271 [PMID: 21981960].

Patra S, Nadri G, Chowdhary H, et al: Idiopathic Fanconi's syndrome with nephrogenic diabetes insipidus in a child who presented as vitamin D resistant rickets: A case report and review of literature. *J Pediatr Endocrinol Metab.* 2011;24:755 [PMID: 22145469].

HYPOPARATHYROIDISM PRESENTING AS HYPOCALCEMIA

Clinical Presentation

Hypocalcemia is defined by a total serum Ca^{2+} less than 7 mg/dL or an ionized Ca^{2+} less than 1.1 mmol/L. This usually occurs in premature and low-birth-weight infants and in neonates born to mothers who have diabetes. Calcium levels decline when the infant no longer receives the maternal supply through the placenta. Parathyroid hormone (PTH) secretion is then stimulated, however the gland responds slowly and calcium concentrations fall more quickly during the first 2 days of life. Because of this, decreased PTH concentrations are common in early hypocalcemia (see Chapter 17).

Infants can also develop hypocalcemia after 3 days of life. Causes can include excessive intake of phosphate in the diet, chronic renal insufficiency, low magnesium levels, and vitamin D deficiency associated with maternal vitamin D insufficiency. The parathyroid gland in the infant can take longer to mature or have dysembryogenesis. Classic DiGeorge syndrome infants have the triad of hypocalcemia caused by parathyroid gland hypoplasia, defective T-lymphocyte function, and impaired cell-mediated immunity caused by impaired thymic differentiation. Autoimmune states, as Addison disease and lymphocytic thyroiditis are associated with hypoparathyroidism.

Infants present clinically with clonic seizures, jerking, and tetany. Additional signs and symptoms include laryngospasm, stridor, a weak cry, and prolonged QT interval on ECG.

The following laboratory tests need to be drawn in the emergency department: serum total and ionized calcium, magnesium, phosphorous, creatinine, and PTH. Magnesium is required for PTH release. To rule out DiGeorge syndrome obtain a CBC, a T (CD4)-lymphocyte count, and a chest x-ray. Since the thymus is hypoplastic or absent in DrGeorge syndrome, a chest x-ray with a normal neonatal thymic shadow would not be consistent with the diagnosis.

Treatment

Treatment of infants who have acute or symptomatic hypocalcemia, as with prolonged QT or calcium level less than 7 mg/dL, should receive an IV bolus of 100-200 mg/kg of 10% calcium gluconate followed by repeat boluses every 6 hours and/or a continuous calcium infusion if needed. If a neonate is asymptomatic, no treatment is necessary unless the total serum calcium concentration is less than 6 mg/dL in the preterm infant and less than 7 mg/dL in the term infant. Calcium supplementation is important after the acute episode, addition of calcium to a low-phosphorous diet. Neonates may also need vitamin D supplementation and magnesium to correct hypocalcemia.

CONGENITAL ADRENAL HYPERPLASIA

Clinical Presentation

Congenital adrenal hyperplasia (CAH) is an autosomal recessive disorder. CAH is caused in 95% of cases by 21-hydroxylase enzyme deficiency. This results in a glucocorticoid deficiency, low measured cortisol levels, and excess ACTH secretion. This results in adrenal hyperplasia and increased production of androgens. In the neonate, CAH is a major cause of primary adrenal insufficiency.

Classically, female infants present to the emergency department with ambiguous genitalia, clitoral enlargement or fusion of the labial folds. Male genitalia may look normal at birth with a hyperpigmented scrotum as the only sign. Typically, male neonates present to the emergency department within the first 2 weeks of life. Infants may feed poorly, have vomiting, and signs of dehydration. They may deteriorate rapidly, developing altered mental status and hypotension.

Chemistries, specifically blood glucose, sodium, and potassium, assist in the diagnosis of CAH. Classically, hyponatremia, hypoglycemia, and hyperkalemia are seen on laboratory results. Salt wasting can be seen early with elevated potassium. Hypotensive patients unresponsive to IV fluid boluses may be steroid deficient. Up to 75% of affected neonates have the classic salt-losing virilizing variant, associated with aldosterone deficiency and androgen overproduction (17-hydroxyprogesterone).

If a child with CAH presents to the emergency department, treatment must be initiated immediately. Parents and the older child are likely to be familiar with the disease and the steroid treatment or regimen. If the child is able to tolerate oral fluids, it is recommended that the steroid dosing be doubled or tripled. With additional history of vomiting, the child should be given hydrocortisone intramuscularly or intravenously; (25 mg for < 1 yr, 50 mg for 1-5 yr, 100 mg for > 5 yr). The ill child or those who do not have a normalization of vital signs and chemistries in the emergency department posttreatment should be admitted.

In severe cases, such as loss of consciousness, severe dehydration, or circulatory collapse, the stress IV dose of hydrocortisone is 25-50 mg/m^2 (~ 2-3 mg/kg), followed by 100 mg/m^2/day in divided doses. Hydrocortisone is the steroid of choice because it has equal glucocorticoid and mineralocorticoid effects. Patients should also be given aggressive fluid resuscitation with a 20-mL/kg 0.9% sodium chloride bolus. Electrolytes including urea and glucose should be monitored closely and aggressive hydration continued until patient blood pressure stabilizes. Hypoglycemia should be treated with administration of 0.25 g/kg of dextrose IV.

Dehydration should be corrected and input and output monitored. Sodium should be corrected to 120-125 mmol/L at a rate of 0.5 mmol/L/h, thereafter correction to normal values should take place over several days. Dexamethasone does not interfere with ACTH stimulation testing; however, it has no mineralocorticoid effect. Fludrocortisone, an oral mineralocorticoid, can be started after initial stabilization with IVF and glucocorticoids. Hyperkalemia should correct with fluids and steroid therapy. Calcium gluconate should be used for arrhythmias associated with hyperkalemia. Avoid therapy with glucose and insulin as hypoglycemia may result.

In the neonate, serum should be drawn for adrenal etiology, to include cortisol, 17-hydroxyprogesterone, dehydroepiandrosterone, androstenedione and testosterone. It is best to draw these before administration of hydrocortisone if possible.

A pediatric endocrinologist should be consulted early in these crises. Parent and patient education about CAH is paramount and the child's wearing of a medical alert bracelet should be strongly encouraged. It is imperative that parents know how to give hydrocortisone and recognize when to bring child to the emergency department. The glucocorticoid, hydrocortisone, is vital in blocking secretion of corticotropin-releasing hormone (CRH) and ACTH and decreasing the release of androgens. CAH is a chronic disease and patients will require lifelong monitoring.

Hindmarsh PC: Management of the child with congenital adrenal hyperplasia. *Best Pract Res Clin Endocrinol Metab.* 2009;23:2 [PMID: 19500763].

CUSHING SYNDROME

General Considerations

Cushing syndrome results when the body is exposed to excessive levels of cortisol.

There are several etiologies for Cushing syndrome in children. In children younger than 4 years, ACTH-independent adrenocortical tumors are the most common. In children older than 4 years, Cushing disease is the most common endogenous cause of hypercortisolism, and 75-80% is caused by an ACTH-secreting pituitary adenoma. Male predominance is more common in young or prepubertal children, whereas female predominance is more common in the postpubertal period.

Clinical Presentation

Classic presentation is of patients with a cushingoid appearance. The young child can present with weight gain, poor growth, or short stature. Symptoms such as hypertension, hirsutism, striae, and muscular weakness are subtle, and the disease can go unrecognized. This disease can chronically expose patients to glucocorticoids, which results in hypertension.

Treatment

Anti glucocorticoid drugs and antihypertensive agents should be used to treat blood pressure and the associated increased cardiovascular risk and mortality. Consultation with a endocrinologist is recommended. Surgical excision is ultimately the treatment; postsurgery, patients will need long-term steroids and regular visits with endocrinologist. Transsphenoidal pituitary surgery, which selectively removes the adenoma, is first-line therapy for pediatric Cushing disease. Children and adolescents show complete resolution of hypertension within 1 year after surgical treatment.

Table 42–9. Diagnostic characteristic of selected inborn errors of metabolism.

Laboratory Findings	Disorder	Treatment
Respiratory alkalosis	Urea cycle defects	Hyperammonia
Hyperammonemia	Urea cycle defects Organic Acidemias	Hyperammonia Hypoglycemia Acidosis
Lactic acidosis	• Mitochondrial disorders • Glycogen storage disease • Organic acidemias • Fatty acid oxidation disorders • Aminoaciduria • Disorders of glyconeogenesis/or pyruvate metabolism	Hypoglycemia Acidosis
Hypoglycemia	Glycogen storage	Hypoglycemia Acidosis
Hypoglycemia + ketosis	Organic acidemias	Hypoglycemia Acidosis
Hypoglycemia w/o ketosis	Maple syrup urine disease Fatty acid oxidation disoders Disorders of ketogenesis	Hypoglycemia Acidosis

Goncalves da Silva RM, Pinto E, Goldman SM, et al: Children with Cushing's syndrome: Primary pigmented nodular adrenocortical disease should always be suspected. *Pituitary.* 2011;14:61 [PMID: 20924687].

Sharma ST, Nieman LK: Cushing's syndrome: All variants, detection, and treatment. *Endocrinol Metab Clin.* 2011;40:2 [PMID: 21565673].

Savage MO, Chan LF, Grossman AB, et al: Work-up and management of paediatric Cushing's syndrome. *Curr Opin Endocrinol Diabetes Obes.* 2008;15:346 [PMID: 18594275].

INBORN ERRORS OF METABOLISM

Inborn errors of metabolism are usually caused by single gene defect resulting in abnormalities in protein, carbohydrate, fat, or complex molecule metabolism. Most have a defect or deficiency in an enzyme, enzyme cofactor, transport protein which leads to a block in their metabolic pathway leading to toxic metabolites (Figure 42-1).

HYPERAMMONEMIA

Clinical Presentation

Conditions that lead to hyperammonemia in the infant or child are a group of disorders that prevent the conversion of ammonia to urea. Prematurity and perinatal hypoxia may lead to temporary liver dysfunction and hyperammonemia. Neonatal illnesses such as sepsis may also lead to the condition. Congenital causes include deficiencies in the enzymes argininosuccinic acid synthetase, ornithine transcarbamylase, and arginase, urea cycle defects, as well as in the mechanisms of fatty acid oxidation. Infants may present with poor feeding, vomiting, altered activity levels (from disinterest in feeding, to abnormal tone, to coma), unwillingness to intake orally, and bulging fontanelles due to increased intracranial pressure. These undiagnosed inborn errors are often life-threatening when presenting in the neonatal period. Symptoms often develop after the initiation of feeds containing protein or carbohydrates, which they are unable to breakdown and lead to toxic metabolites. Older children may present with significant vomiting, developmental delay, tachypnea, and occasionally ataxia.

Laboratory findings are consistent with hyperammonemia; however, the exact level is a poor predictor of clinical illness (usually not diagnosed unless ammonia > 100 μmol/L). Patients classically present with a low BUN and a normal pH; however, findings of a normal BUN and acidosis do not rule this process out. Other abnormalities may include: hypoglycemia, elevated lactate, increased anion gap, and elevated transaminases.

Treatment

Initial management of the hyperammonemic patient includes assessment of airway and breathing as elevated levels of ammonia directly affect the central respiratory function, IV boluses of NS to correct dehydration and/or shock, and dextrose containing fluids (10% dextrose in ½ NS at 1.5 times maintenance). Glucose should be administered to provide 8-10 mg/kg/min to prevent catabolism. Patients should be kept nothing by mouth (NPO) to prevent worsening of the condition by consumption of protein that may act as ammonia precursors. Hemodialysis should be strongly considered in a neonate with an ammonia level greater than 120 μmol/L. For urea cycle defects, consider administration of sodium phenylacetate, sodium benzoate, and arginine. Cofactors which may be administered include pyridoxine, folinic acid, biotin, and carnitine. Additional treatments in consultation with pediatric metabolism specialists may include amino acid supplements and special diet. Children often present to the emergency department with personalized protocol in hand provided by the caretaker.

- ABC—as usual, Airway, Breathing, Circulation
- Stops feeds
- Isotonic fluid boluses to correct dehydration (do not use Lactated Ringers though)
- No hypotonic fluid load-risk of cerebral edema ($\uparrow NH_4$)
- Consult a Pediatric Genetics or Metabolic specialist urgently
- Consider sepsis, obtain appropriate cultures and administer IV antibiotics if sepsis remains in the differential diagnosis
- Provide enough glucose to prevent catabolism
  - Glucose for hypoglycemia
  - D_{10}-D_{15} + lytes at 1.5 times maintenance
  - If needed, treat hyperglycemia with insulin
- Lab studies to consider in patients with IEM
- Blood: CBC, CMP, lactate, ammonia (arterial or venous without a tournequet used and put on ice), Uric acid, blood gas
- Urine: UA, pH, color, specific gravity, ketones, reducing substances
- Correct metabolic acidosis (pH < 7.0 slowly and cautiously)
  - 1-2 mEq/kg/hour $NaHCO_3$
  - If intractable, consider hemodialysis
- Eliminate toxic metabolites
  - Hyperammonia therapy
    - NH4 > 100 micromol/mL
      - Consider Sodium phenylacetate, sodium phenylbutarate as Ammonul
      - Arginine hydrochoride 210 mg/kg in D_{10} over 90 minutes, then 210 mg/kg/d as a continuous infusion
      - Consider Sodium phenylacetate/benzonate 250 mg/kg IV
      - If no IV, may give both in $D_{10}W$ via NG
    - NH4 > 300 micromol/mL
      - Consider hemodialysis
- Administer cofactors if indicated
  - Pyridoxine (B_6): 100 mg IV (pyridoxine deficiency seizures)
  - Folinic acid (Leucovorin): 2.5 mg IV
  - Biotin: 10 mg IV, po or NG tube (organic acidopathy)
  - L-Carnitine: 400 mg IV for presumed carnitine deficiency if life-threatening manifestations of organic acidopathies (fatty acid oxidation defect)

▲ **Figure 42–1.** Management of unknown or suspected IEM.

Dispostion

Hyperammonemic patients presenting to the emergency department are almost universally admitted for further care, often to the intensive care unit. The rare discharge should be considered only in consultation with the pediatric metabolism specialist and with the patient's primary care physician.

METABOLIC ACIDEMIAS

Clinical Presentation & Treatment

Organic acidemias and acidurias are disorders of amino acid metabolism in which high levels of nonamino organic acids accumulate in serum and urine resulting in metabolic acidemia. Hypoglycemia, elevated transaminases, elevated lactate, and ketonuria are common.

Maple syrup urine disease is named because of its sweet sugar odor. The CNS is affected with signs of lethargy, failure to thrive, and poor feeding. Worsening of symptoms include ketoacidosis and coma. If not treated with branch chain amino acid restriction and thiamine, neonates will develop mental retardation.

Propionic and methylmalonic acidemia present with a fruity odor, similar to DKA. Methylmalonic acidemia is a disorder of amino acid metabolism, involving a defect in the conversion of methylmalonyl-coenzyme A (CoA) to succinyl-CoA. Episodes occur with increased protein intake or increased protein catabolism. Both disorders affect the CNS and present with severe acidosis and hyperammonemia. Acidosis often requires administration of sodium bicarbonate. If not treated, developmental delay and mental retardation will ensue. Methylmalonic acidemia patients can have movement disorders, whereas propionic acidemia patients can have speech defects.

Patients need to be treated with a vitamin cofactor, such as biotin and vitamin B_{12}. Consultation with a metabolic specialist is imperative.

- Remember that many inborn errors of metabolism become symptomatic in association with an acute infection—evaluate appropriately.
- Consider antibiotics for a serious bacterial infection.

CONGENITAL HYPOTHYROIDISM

Clinical Presentation

Congenital hypothyroidism can be prevented and treated before children develop mental retardation. This is the most common congenital endocrine disorder and early neonate screening of hormone levels will identify neonates with this disorder. This condition results from mutations of genes involved in the many steps of thyroid hormone synthesis, storage, secretion, delivery, or utilization.

Infants present clinically with lethargy, hypotonia, poor feeding, and constipation. On physical examination, they may have a large tongue, hoarse cry, mottled dry skin and hair, and an umbilical hernia. Children will show failure to thrive, respond slowly, and have delayed development as later signs.

Treatment

Treatment should be started within the first 2 weeks of life. An initial dosage of 10-15 mcg/kg/day levothyroxine (T4) per os is recommended. T4 and TSH should be normalized in 2-4 weeks of T4 therapy, respectively. Serum total T4 or free T4 should be maintained in the upper half of the reference range (130-204 nmol/L or 18-30 pmol/L) during the first 3 years of life, with a low normal serum TSH concentration.

Neonatal screening is crucial in preventing developmental delay, and must be treated immediately when detected in children. The pediatrician plays a central role in providing care and life long disease management in a child with congenital hypothyroidism.

Kambj M: Clinical approach to the diagnoses of inborn errors of metabolism. *Pediatr Clin North Am.* 2008;55(5):1113 [PMID: 18929055].

Kwon KT, Tsai VW: Metabolic Emergencies. *Emerg Med Clin North Am.* 2007;25:1041-1060 [PMID: 17950135].

Waisbren SE: Expanded newborn screening: Information and resources for the family physician. *Am Fam Physician.* 2008;77:7 [PMID: 18441864].

GRAVES' DISEASE

Clinical Presentation

Graves' disease, a diffuse autoimmune thyroid hyperplasia, develops as T lymphocytes become sensitized and stimulate B lymphocytes to produce antibodies to the TSH receptor. This is the most common cause of hyperthyroidism in children, and female adolescents are affected significantly more often than male adolescents.

Clinically, patients present with palpitations, insomnia, weight loss, and heat intolerance. On physical examination, patients are tachycardic, have a widened pulse pressure, hypertension, overactive precordium, tremor, and brisk deep tendon reflexes. They may have exophthalmos or pretibial myxedema. A goiter is present in nearly 100% of patients.

If a child presents with these signs and symptoms, the following laboratory tests should be ordered: TSH, free T_4, T_3, thyroid antibodies, complete blood count, and complete metabolic panel including liver function tests. TSH will be suppressed and T_3 will be elevated; free T_4 may be increased or normal.

Treatment

The initial treatment for Graves' disease is antithyroid medication. Methimazole and propylthiouracil (PTU) inhibit thyroid hormone biosynthesis. PTU has the added benefit of inhibiting the extrathyroidal conversion of T_4 to T_3. However, PTU is contraindicated for pediatric use stemming from reports of liver failure in children. Methimazole can be given once daily, in a dose of 0.4–0.6 mg/kg/day. Maximum effect of the medications is seen after 4-6 weeks of treatment. However, this medication can have significant adverse effects, including rash and agranulocytosis. Agranulocytosis under these conditions commonly presents with fever and sore throat. At this time medication should be held, broad spectrum antibiotics started, and patient placed in isolation. Methimazole can cause cholestatic jaundice. Patients on methimazole are given strict instructions to report to the emergency department in case they develop a fever.

Propranolol is typically used in children who develop tachycardia or hypertension due to Graves' disease. In patients with asthma, atenolol can be substituted because it is a cardioselective β-blocker.

Antithyroid medication treatment requires 2-5 years of therapy, with close medical follow-up. Remission is achieved in 30-70% of patients. Definitive therapy includes thyroidectomy in adults or radioactive iodine treatment (RAI), however, it is controversial in children due to the high-dose radiation and its adverse effects. Education and discussions with a pediatric endocrinologist should follow any emergency stabilization.

THYROTOXICOSIS (THYROID STORM)

Clinical Presentation

Thyrotoxicosis is a severe and life-threatening form of hyperthyroidism. Thyroid storm is typically found in a patient with underlying thyrotoxicosis in whom a crisis is precipitated by severe illness, injury, or surgery. Other causes include abrupt discontinuation of antithyroid medications and patients receiving iodine-containing materials such as radiocontrast dye or amiodarone.

Thyroid storm must be diagnosed clinically without waiting for laboratory results. Moderate presentations typically include fever, tachycardia out of proportion to the fever, vomiting, diarrhea, and lethargy. Severe presentations include seizures, altered mental status, pulmonary edema, and vascular compromise.

Laboratory findings will have elevated total and free serum T_4 and T_3. The following may also be elevated: calcium, glucose, white cell count, lactate dehydrogenase, liver function studies, and bilirubin. The cortisol level may also be elevated as patients may have developed a relative adrenal insufficiency. Also obtain T3 resin uptake and TSH to make the diagnosis.

Treatment & Disposition

Patients must be admitted to the intensive care unit and the emergency department physician should initially focus on resuscitation and aggressive medical management. Mortality rates for hospitalized patients with thyroid storm are estimated from 10 to 75%. Patients should receive IV fluids, glucose, and oxygen. ECG monitoring for arrhythmias and heart rate is recommended. Treatment is similar to other hyperthyroid disease including the need for antithyroid medications. A β-adrenergic antagonist, propranolol, or esmolol infusion helps resolve the tachycardia and hypertension. Methimazole or PTU inhibits thyroid hormone synthesis. As previously stated, PTU is contraindicated for pediatric use. Potassium iodide, Lugol solution, iopanoic acid, sodium ipodate, or lithium carbonate if iodine is contraindicated, can be used to decrease thyroid hormone secretion. Note that iodine-containing solutions should not be given until at least 1 hour after medications to prevent the synthesis of thyroid hormones are administered; otherwise the iodide may add fuel to the fire. Inhibition of the peripheral conversion of T_4 to T_3 can be achieved with PTU, glucocorticoids (hydrocortisone or dexamethasone) and β-antagonists. T_4 and T_3 can also be removed from the body through plasmapheresis, cholestyramine treatment, hemodialysis, or hemoperfusion. Patients may need a thyroidectomy, but this is considered when patients are hemodynamically stable.

NEONATAL GRAVES' DISEASE

Clinical Presentation

Autoimmune or transient neonatal hyperthyroidism (neonatal Graves' disease) occurs in 1-5% of the offspring of mothers with active or inactive Graves' disease. Maternal thyroid receptor stimulating antibodies (TRSAb) pass through the placenta, and elevated levels can cause hyperthyroidism in the neonate. During pregnancy, mothers with Graves' disease should be treated to prevent this disease.

Neonates present with cardiac abnormalities including tachycardia (heart rate > 160/min), arrhythmias, cardiac failure, and hyperthermia. Infants can be hyperactive, irritable, diaphoretic, and have poor weight gain. On physical examination, patients have hyperreflexia, goiter, exophthalmos, narrow sutures, craniosynostosis, advanced bone age, vomiting/diarrhea, icterus, and hepatosplenomegaly. Laboratory tests will show the following: Serum T_3, free T_3, free triiodothyronine, and triiodothyronine are higher, and serum thyrotropin level is lower than the normal range of the same gestational age, and thrombocytopenia. This disease can be life-threatening, with a reported mortality rate of up to 20%, usually from heart failure.

Treatment

Treatment of the mother with antithyroid medications can prevent neonatal hyperthyroidism. Treatment is the same in neonates as it is in children and adolescents. Antithyroid medications are used, methimazole 0.5-1.0 mg/kg/day or propylthiouracil 5-10 mg/kg/day in divided doses, but this is effective only after 1-2 weeks. The recovery occurs after 2-5 months of antithyroid drug treatment. Again, caution should be used with PTU as it has been associated with pediatric liver failure. Note that a maternal overdose of antithyroid medications may lead to an iatrogenic fetal hypothyroidism and goiter. Extended use of maternal β-blockers may cause fetal growth retardation, postnatal bradycardia, of hypoglycemia of the neonate. Neonatal Graves' disease resolves when maternal TRSAb in the neonate is degraded, which usually occurs at 3-12 weeks.

NEONATAL THYROTOXICOSIS

Clinical Presentation

Neonatal thyrotoxicosis is rare affecting children from birth to 6 weeks of age. Maternal Graves' disease is the most common cause, which results in transplacental passage of thyroid-stimulating hormone receptor antibodies, which leads to an increase in thyroid hormone secretion.

Diagnosis is made by measuring neonatal levels of serum-free thyroxine (T4) and TSH shortly after birth. Clinically, neonates will present with irritability, tachycardia, tremors, sweating, and excessive appetite but failure to thrive. Complications include arrhythmias, heart failure, goiter, exophthalmos, thrombocytopenia, and advanced skeletal maturation.

Treatment

If a neonate presents with hyperthyroidism or thyrotoxicosis, early consultation with a pediatric endocrinologist is recommended. Propylthiouracil has been administered orally at a dose of 5-10 mg/kg/day divided into three doses. PTU not only blocks thyroid hormone synthesis, but also decreases the conversion of T4 to T3, which methimazole does not. Caution should be used with PTU as it has been associated with pediatric liver failure. A saturated solution of potassium iodide ([SSKI], 48-mg iodine per drop) 1 drop/day or Lugol solution (8-mg iodine per drop) 1-3 drops/day may be added in severe cases to decrease thyroglobulin proteolysis and thyroid hormone secretion. Propranolol (1-2 mg/kg/day in 2-4 divided doses) helps resolve the tachycardia. Glucocorticoids (prednisone 2 mg/kg/day) have been used to decrease thyroid hormone release and to inhibit T4 to T3 conversion, in severe cases. Iodine should be started at least 1 hour after administering an antithyroid medication to avoid increasing thyroid gland stores before the antithyroid effect occurs.

Furthermore, the treatment of hyperthyroidism in the neonate may include sedatives (midazolam as a single dose, 50-100 mcg/kg, or by continuous infusion at a rate of 0.4-0.6 mcg/kg/min; phenobarbital 5-10 mg/kg/day in 2 divided doses) and digoxin if cardiac failure is present. The neonate should also receive a high fluid and caloric intake.

Neonatal thyrotoxicosis is transient, but patients should still be treated aggressively to avoid short- and long-term complications. Breast-feeding can transfer TRSAb from mother to infant through milk, resulting in transient infant hyperthyroidism.

Finlayson C, Zimmerman D: Hyperthyroidism in the emergency department. *Clin Pediatr Emerg Med.* 2009;10:4.

Kratzsch J, Pulzer F: Thyroid gland development and defects. *Best Pract Res Clin Endocrinol Metab.* 2008;22:1 [PMID: 18279780].

Peter F, Muzsnai A: Congenital disorders of the thyroid: Hypo/hyper. *Endocrinol Metab Clin.* 2009;38:3 [PMID: 19717001].

Glaser NS, Ghetti S, Casper TC, et al: Pediatric diabetic ketoacidosis, fluid therapy, and cerebral injury: The design of a factorial randomized controlled trial. *Pediatri Diabetes.* 2013;14:435-46 [PMID: 23490311].

Hyman SJ, Novoa Y, Holzman I: Perinatal endocrinology: Common endocrine disorders in the sick and premature newborn. *Endocrinol Metab Clin.* 2009;38:3 [PMID: 19717002].

Kim UO, Brousseau DC, Konduri GG: Evaluation and management of the critically ill neonate in the emergency department. *Clin Pediatr Emerg Med.* 2008;9:3.

Orthopaedics: Non-Traumatic Disorders

Alicia Shirakbari, MD

Michael Feldmeier, MD

INTRODUCTION

Pediatric orthopedics is a unique area of pediatric emergency medicine as children are not "little adults." The growth process of infants, children, and adolescents differentiates them from adults. Whether treating congenital, developmental, or injury-related problems in children, the constant change in structure and size of the skeletal system determines the plan of treatment. It is important to become familiar with the different appearance of growth plates, ossification centers, and appearance of bones at the various stages of development. This chapter focuses on non-traumatic orthopedic disorders encountered in the emergency department.

DISORDER OF THE NECK

ACQUIRED MUSCULAR TORTICOLLIS

Torticollis, or wryneck, is stiff neck associated with muscle spasm in previously normal children. There are congenital causes but discussion will focus on acquired muscular torticollis, which is often seen in the emergency department. Most common symptoms are neck muscle pain, and inability to turn the head, holding the head in an awkward position with a slight chin tilt. The sternocleidomastoid and trapezius muscles are usually involved. Sleeping on the side, drafts (sleeping under a fan), and colds are commonly described historical factors but often there are no specific causes. The neck is usually "stiff" and pain is elicited with movement of the head. Patient will have complaint of pain with turning the head toward the side of the spasm. There is limited published data on the best treatment in the pediatric population; however, there are options. Muscle relaxers are often used in adults, but in children diazepam is a good medication choice because dose can be weight based. Nonsteroidal anti-inflammatory agents (NSAIDs) or narcotic pain medications may also be of benefit to alleviate discomfort. Physical therapists

may advise heat or ultrasound (US) therapy. Patients and parents can be reassured that torticollis is usually a self-limiting process that will resolve in 1-4 weeks.

The immediate or life-threatening associated conditions could be atlantoaxial rotary subluxation, which is secondary to trauma. Posterior fossa tumors can cause torticollis and further investigation may be necessary if this is suspected. Infections in the posterior pharynx such as retropharyngeal abscess may also present with torticollis. A reported history of fever, sore throat, or difficulty swallowing may be an indication of a more serious etiology. Grisel syndrome, subluxation of the upper cervical joints can be a major cause. In neonates, a tightening and shortening of one sternomastoid muscle results in torticollis. Usually at 3 weeks of age, a visible palpable swelling develops, known as sternomastoid tumor. Treatment with physical therapy is often initiated.

Diagnostic testing such as cervical spine radiographs may need to be obtained to rule out bony abnormalities. Magnetic resonance imaging (MRI) should be considered if there is concern for structural problems or an infectious soft tissue process.

COMMON DISORDERS OF THE UPPER EXTREMITIES

There are a number of open growth plates in the shoulders and elbows of children and adolescents. Growth plates are the weak link in the joints during sporting activities, in contrast to ligaments in adults. This makes the growth plates susceptible to injury. Excessive and repetitive stress during certain activities can cause these injuries.

PROXIMAL HUMERAL EPIPHYSEOLYSIS (LITTLE LEAGUER SHOULDER)

Proximal humeral epiphyseolysis (Little leaguer shoulder) is an overuse injury. Young athletes who are involved in sports associated with repetitive throwing. Baseball pitchers may present with pain to the lateral shoulder of the dominant or throwing arm. Patients will have complaint of increasing pain over time as well as decreased velocity or control of their pitches. There may be a recent history of increased frequency of pitches or a change from their normal regimen such as throwing a different type of pitch.

Diagnostic workup should include bilateral shoulder imaging. The nondominant shoulder should appear normal in comparison to epiphyseal widening of the injured shoulder. Repeated throwing and stress to the immature growth plate can lead to epiphyseal widening, an indication of the diagnosis.

Treatment is rest from all stressful activities to the shoulder, especially throwing or pitching for 3 months. After a restful period, the patient can gradually return to pitching as long as he or she is absent from pain or any or any other symptoms. The appearance of the growth plate on imaging should not influence the decision of a patient's return to pitching as the abnormal widening of the growth plate may take several months to resolve. The decision to return to competitive play should be based clinically.

Brennan B, Kelly M. Little Leaguer's shoulder: *Clin Pediatr.* 2011;50(5):462-463 [PMID: 20837624].

ELBOW

Annular Ligament Displacement

Annular ligament displacement (radial head subluxation, nursemaid elbow) is the most common elbow injury in young children (1-4 years). It occurs when the annular ligament becomes displaced into the radial-humeral joint. History is important in establishing the diagnosis. A young child may incur injury from someone pulling on the extended arm which pulls the radius through the annular ligament. It is most often an accidental occurrence. The child will hold the arm closely by the side with slight elbow flexion and pronation. The child often quietly refuses to use the arm. However, if there is an attempt to bend or straighten the elbow, the child will often cry out in pain. Tenderness may be present with palpation over the joint but there is no swelling, redness, or ecchymosis. Diagnosis is by history and examination. Radiographs are not necessary and often, the movements of the arm by the radiology technician to get the radiographs will inadvertently reduce the subluxation. Manual reduction is performed by the physician's pronating the arm (hyperpronation reduction technique) (see Chapter 29). This technique is reportedly less painful and more successful than a previous maneuver of supporting the radial head followed by supination and flexion (flexion/supination technique). Once the reduction is performed, the child will often use the arm shortly thereafter. There is no indication for immobilization. Parents should be informed there is a high incidence of recurrence and be shown the mechanism of

injury (usually traction on the forearm with on an extended elbow) as well as the simple reduction method to correct this injury should their child experience a reoccurrence of radial head subluxation.

Crowther M: Elbow pain in pediatrics: *Curr Rev Musculoskelet Med.* 2009;2(2):83-87 [PMID: 19468873].

Krul M, van der Wouden JC, van Suijlekom-Smit LWA, Koes BW: Manipulative interventions for reducing pulled elbow in young children. *Cochrane Database Syst Rev.* 2009;7:(4):CD007759, and 2012;18:1:CD007759 [PMID: 22258973] [PMID: 19821438].

Rudloe TF, Schutzman S, Lee LK, et al: No longer a nursemaid's elbow: Mechanisms, caregivers, and prevention. *Pediatr Emerg Care.* 2012;28(8):771-774 [PMID: 22858743].

Tendinitis

Tendinitis occurs as a result of injury, overuse, or aging as the tendon loses elasticity. An action that places prolonged repetitive strain on the forearm muscles can cause tendinitis of the elbow. Two common causes of tendinitis in the elbow are lateral epicondylitis and medial epicondylitis.

Lateral Epicondylitis (Tennis Elbow)

This is one of the most common conditions affecting the elbow of athletic children and adolescents. Although it frequently occurs in tennis players who use a single-handed backhand or have poor technique, it can also occur from repetitive use of the wrist and forearm muscles such as using a hammer or painting. Patients often present with inability to fully extend the elbow secondary to pain, tightness of the muscles in the forearm, and decreased grip strength. There is tenderness over the lateral epicondyle on examination. The medial epicondyle should also be examined for injury. Treatment is rest for 4-6 weeks and slow reintroduction through physical therapy after the recovery period. A brace may be used to relieve symptoms during continued activities.

Medial Epicondylitis (Golfer Elbow, Little Leaguer Elbow)

Medial epicondylitis is an overuse syndrome frequently caused by playing golf, throwing a baseball, or from a tennis forehand injury. It may be the result of repetitive use of the wrist and forearm muscles, even nonsporting injuries. Medial epicondylitis is a chronic inflammation of the growth plate. It can occur in up to 40% of pitchers or baseball throwers secondary to throwing too many pitches in a game and pitching on too many days in a short period of time. The cumulative number of throws is more stress than the medial elbow can tolerate. On physical examination, there is tenderness over the medial epicondyle but the patient will still have full range of motion (ROM). The lateral side of the elbow should also be palpated for possible injury or pain with palpation as concurrent injuries are common. Plain radiographs should be obtained to exclude a stress fracture; however, they will be normal in 85% of patients. If an abnormality is present, there will be an irregularity of the growth plate of the medial epicondyle. Treatment is complete rest from the inciting activity for 4-6 weeks. A slow reintroduction can occur under the direction of a physical therapist. The total recovery time is approximately 12 weeks.

CHART—USA Baseball Medical & Safety Advisory Committee: *Youth baseball pitching injuries.* Nov 2008. Also available at USA Baseball.com. http://mlb.mlb.com/usa_baseball/article.jsp?story=medsafety11. Accessed July 12, 2012.

COMMON DISORDERS OF THE LOWER EXTREMITIES

GAIT EVALUATION

Development of gait is a complicated process of physical development and external learning. Familiarity with the normal motor milestones in a child is essential when performing a pediatric physical examination.

Delay in motor milestones does not always indicate pathology as a large range of normal variation can be present. A motor milestone history is essential when evaluating a child with possible neurological or musculoskeletal disorders. A developmental delay can be suggestive of neurologic or musculoskeletal disorders (Table 43–1).

NORMAL GAIT

Normal gait requires an intact neuromusculoskeletal system to develop properly. In order to recognize abnormalities in gait, one must be familiar with normal gait patterns and normal variations of gait in comparison to abnormal gait patterns.

The toddler has a broad-base gait which appears to be flat-footed and high-stepping with arms out for balance. Heel striking gait develops approximately 15-18 months of age with reciprocal arm swinging.

The school-aged child will demonstrate an increase in step length and a decrease in step frequency. There is a significant variation in normal gait patterns and ages at which they occur but most children achieve an adult pattern by 8 years of age and some as early as 3 years. Family history influences normal gait patterns.

NORMAL VARIATIONS OF GAIT

Flatfoot (pes planus) is usually a normal variant of gait. Baby fat and looser ligaments can give this appearance until 3-5 years of age when baby fat disappears and ligaments tighten.

Table 43–1. Normal motor milestones.

Sit without support	6-8 mo
Creep on hands and knees	9-11 mo
Cruise or bottom shuffle	11-12 mo
Walk independently	12-14 mo
Climb up stairs on hands and knees	15 mo
Run stiffly	16 mo
Walk down steps (nonreciprocal)	20-24 mo
Walk up steps, alternate feet	3 yr
Hop on one foot, broad jump	4 yr
Skipping	5 yr
Balance on one foot, 20 sec	6-7 yr

(Reproduced, with permission, from Foster H, Drummond P, Jandial S. Assessment of gait disorders in children. BMJ Best Practice. March 2013. http://bestpractice.bmj.com/best-practice/monograph/709.html Last accessed 30 July 2014.)

Toe walking is a habitual condition more common in boys than in girls. There is often a family history of toe walking, and it tends to be a learned behavior more than an indication of abnormality. Idiopathic toe walking usually resolves spontaneously during childhood.

Intoeing is characterized by the child walking with the patella and feet pointing inward and is common between 3 and 8 years of age. It is due to persistent femoral anteversion.

Internal tibial torsion is similar to intoeing but the patella is facing forward while the toes are pointing inward. This commonly resolves by 3 years of age.

Metatarsus adductus is characterized by a flexible "C-shaped" lateral border of the foot. This usually resolves by 6 years of age.

Bowlegs (genu varus) are common from birth and often resolve by 18 months of age.

Knock knees (genu valgus) most often resolve by 7 years of age.

Concern is raised when normal variations persist beyond the expected age range, if there is pain or functional limitation, or there are other indications of neurologic diseases.

ABNORMAL GAIT PATTERNS

Antalgic gait (limp) is gait in which there is a predominance of weight-bearing on the normal leg in order to minimize or avoid pain in the affected leg.

Circumduction is gait in which the knee stays extended and stiff, foot is rotated outward and moves in a semicircle pattern. This is referred to as a hemiplegic or hemiparetic gait (unilateral spastic gait). It is seen in children with upper motor neuron lesions.

Spastic gait of both legs (paraparetic) is gait in which both legs are stiff and the patient appears to be wading in waist-deep water as the arms move much more than the legs.

Ataxic gait is a wide-based gait with truncal instability and often, incoordination of upper extremities. Steps taken are irregular which result in veering laterally and if severe, patients can fall. This is associated with cerebellar disease or in the case of sensory ataxia, due to a loss of proprioception.

Toe-walking gait (equinus) with absent heel contact is a common abnormality in children with cerebral palsy, and is discriminated from habitual toe walking often seen in toddlers.

Evaluation of Patient With a Limp

Limp is defined as any asymmetric deviation from a normal gait pattern. Appropriate assessment requires an understanding of the normal and abnormal gait patterns as findings may be subtle early in a disease process. Causes can vary from benign to potentially life threatening; therefore, a thorough history and examination should be obtained. Evaluation can be challenging as the history is often unclear and vague. The differential diagnosis is age-specific and includes congenital, developmental, trauma, infectious, inflammatory, and neoplastic diseases.

A head-to-toe evaluation is essential to avoid missing any possible etiology. It is important to get the child to walk or attempt to walk in order to observe the abnormality. Encouraging a young child to walk from the examiner to the parent can provide this opportunity. Observing a child run may also demonstrate a gait abnormality not otherwise seen with walking alone. The examination should include observing the child walking on the toes, heels, and hopping on one foot. The neurological examination includes testing for deep tendon reflexes and clonus.

The child should also bend forward to identify asymmetry of the spine with flexion. Pain with spinal flexion or palpable tenderness along the spine may suggest diskitis. The child should also extend the back by leaning backward. Spondylolysis or spondylolisthesis will cause lumbosacral pain with this maneuver.

The Galeazzi test is performed to test for developmental dysplasia or leg-length discrepancy. The test is performed by having the child lay supine, placing the feet adjacent to the buttocks with maximum flexion at the knees and hips. The test is abnormal if there is a difference in the height of one knee in comparison with the other (Figure 43–1).

Evaluation of the Hip

Examination of the hip is the most important part of the physical examination of a child with a limp. Hip pain is often

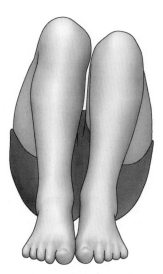

▲ **Figure 43–1.** The Galeazzi test demonstrates a difference in knee height and leg length.

difficult to illicit, and patients have complaint of referred pain to the thigh or knee. A refusal to ambulate is common in toddlers. Hip abduction can be observed by having the child lay supine (face up) with hips flexed and extended. Any asymmetry in hip abduction may be an indication of inflammatory pathology or developmental dysplasia of the hip. Another examination technique is to have the child lay prone (face down) on the stretcher, flex the knees up toward the back, and then allow the ankles to fall away from the body to each side. Asymmetry of internal rotation can be an indication of an inflammatory condition in the hip (Figure 43–2).

Hip flexion, abduction, and external rotation (FABER) test causes pain in the sacroiliac joint (SIJ). The test is performed by having the patient lie supine with the ipsilateral ankle on the contralateral knee. The examiner exerts a small amount of downward pressure on the knee. The test is positive when there is pain at the SIJ (Figure 43–3).

Joints should be evaluated for a loss of ROM, both actively and passively. Full ROM should include abduction, adduction, flexion and extension is possible. All joints should be palpated for tenderness and warmth.

Laboratory Studies

If infectious etiology is considered, a CBC with differential, blood culture, erythrocyte sedimentation rate (ESR), and C-reactive protein (CRP) should be obtained. The CRP is more sensitive and will rise earlier in an acute infection than an ESR but will decrease more rapidly than the ESR. Orthopedic specialists use the ESR and CRP as markers for clinical response to treatment and baseline values are of importance.

If an infectious process is being considered, joint aspiration of synovial fluid should be performed. Gram stain,

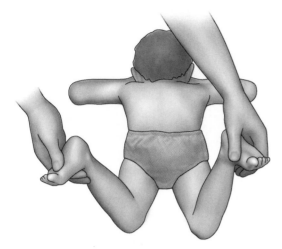

▲ **Figure 43–2.** Have a child lay in the position shown. Asymmetry of internal rotation can be an indication of an inflammatory condition in the hip.

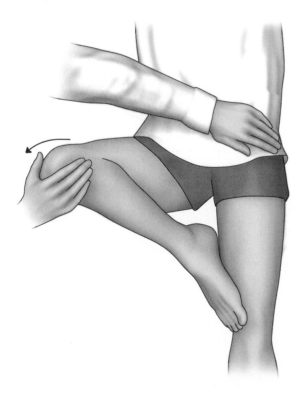

▲ **Figure 43–3.** Faber test is performed by having the patient lie supine with the ipsilateral ankle on the contralateral knee. The examiner places a small amount of downward pressure on the knee. A positive test causes pain at the SIJ when test is performed.

anaerobic and aerobic cultures, protein, and glucose should be ordered. A white blood cell count (WBC) greater than 50,000 per mm³ indicates infection. Negative cultures do not exclude an infected joint as up to one-third of patients will not have organism growth in cultures. If the patient is sexually active, the fluid should be sent for gonorrhea culture.

Serum rheumatoid factor, antinuclear antibody, and HLA typing should not be part of the emergency workup.

Imaging

Plain radiographs of the areas of concern should be ordered before any other films. At least two views (anteroposterior [AP] and lateral) should be performed as a single view is inadequate. If hip films are ordered, AP and frog-leg lateral views are necessary. If the child is nonverbal, then screening radiographs from the hips to feet should be performed.

If a septic hip is being considered, US is a noninvasive test that can easily be performed to identify an effusion. US can also be extended to looking for soft tissue infections such as abscess (see Chapter 2).

Bone scans are infrequently ordered in an emergency setting but should be considered if easily obtained. CT scans are best for identifying bony lesions, whereas MRI is best for soft tissue abnormalities and inflammatory conditions.

DISORDERS OF THE HIP

Developmental Dysplasia of the Hip

Developmental dysplasia of the hip (DDH) is often seen in infants younger than 2 months. Congenital hip dislocations are commonly seen in firstborn females. The Ortolani maneuver tests for this abnormality. It is performed by having the infant in a supine position. The physician flexes the hips and knees to 90 degrees while applying anterior pressure on the greater trochanters and gently abducting the legs. This motion results in an upward to outward rotation of the hip and tests for posterior dislocation of the hip. The presence of a "click" (feeling the dislocation) is a positive test. The Ortolani maneuver will frequently be negative in an infant older than 2 months. The Barlow maneuver is another test of DDH and is performed by adducting the hip while applying pressure posteriorly on the knees and listening or feeling for the click. All cases of DDH should prompt consultation with an orthopedist (Figure 43–4).

Storer SK, Skaggs DL: Developmental dysplasia of the hip. *Am Fam Physician.* 2006;74 (8):1310-1316 [PMID: 17087424].

Legg-Calvé-Perthes Disease

Legg-Calvé-Perthes disease (LCPD) is an idiopathic osteonecrosis of the capital femoral epiphysis. It commonly occurs in children aged 3-12 years; however, it occurs often in

Barlow test

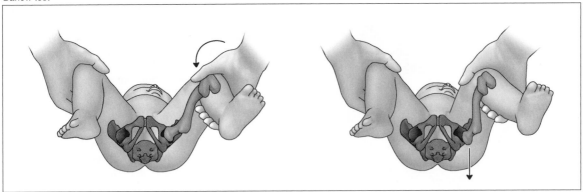

Ortolani test

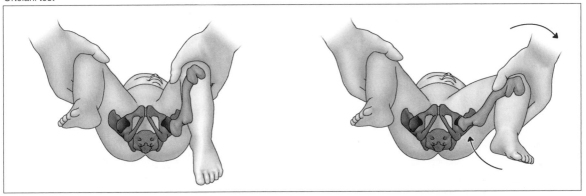

▲ **Figure 43–4.** Comparison of Barlow with the Ortolani test.

4- to 8-year-old boys with delayed skeletal maturity. Males are more often affected than females. LCPD is bilateral in 10-20% of patients. The patient may have complaint of hip or groin pain but often reports knee pain that is insidious and may be ongoing for weeks or months. Patient will be afebrile and nontoxic in appearance. Physical examination may show atrophy of the thigh muscles and an antalgic gait secondary to pain with limited ROM. X-ray findings are dependent on the duration of the disease process. There may be flattening of the femoral head giving the appearance of a small femoral epiphysis, slight widening of the hip joint, and later in the disease, collapse and even fragmentation. A CT scan may be useful when radiographs are inconclusive or normal, especially early in the disease. MRI and bone scan are more useful for staging of the disease and can be done as outpatient. Referral to an orthopedist is necessary when LCPD is diagnosed or suspected. The age of the child at time of diagnosis is a prognostic indicator as younger children have more favorable long-term outcome (Figure 43–5).

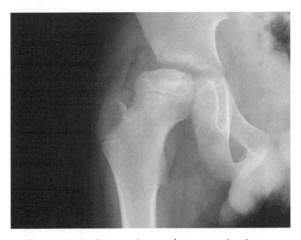

▲ **Figure 43–5.** An x-ray image demonstrating Legg-Calvé-Perthes disease; note the small and irregularly shaped femoral head.

Kim HK: Legg-Calvé-Perthes disease. *J Am Acad Orthop Surg.* 2010;18(11):676-686 [PMID: 21041802].

Slipped Capital Femoral Epiphysis

Slipped capital femoral epiphysis (SCFE) is a common disorder in adolescents. The femoral neck moves in relation to the femoral epiphysis due to a weakness in the physis (growth plate). The epiphysis, thus, stays in the acetabulum. It commonly occurs in boys aged 14-16 years, and in girls aged 11-13 years. Obesity is a risk factor due to mechanical forces, but there is also relation to the rapid growth spurt in adolescents. Additionally, endocrinopathies, such as hypothyroidism, hypogonadal conditions, and growth hormone deficiency are reported in patients with SCFE. The disorder occurs more often in males than in females and involves the left hip more commonly than the right. Bilateral hip involvement occurs in 25% of patients. Patient will have complaint of hip pain or referred pain to the knee. The patient may demonstrate an antalgic gait. Radiographs in AP and "frog leg" views demonstrate displacement of the femoral head in a posterior and inferior direction relative to the femoral neck. It is described as the appearance of "ice cream slipping off the cone." On an AP x-ray, use of Klein line, a line drawn along the lateral aspect of the femoral neck which should intersect a portion of the femoral epiphysis in a normal hip but not in SCFE, is valuable. Suspected cases should be non–weight-bearing until evaluation by an orthopedist can be performed. Definitive treatment is operative internal fixation. Chronic complications can develop from severe misplacement and result in avascular necrosis, leg length discrepancy, and chondrolysis (Figure 43–6).

Peck D: Slipped capital femoral epiphysis: Diagnosis and management. *Am Fam Physician.* 2010;82(3):258 [PMID: 20672790].

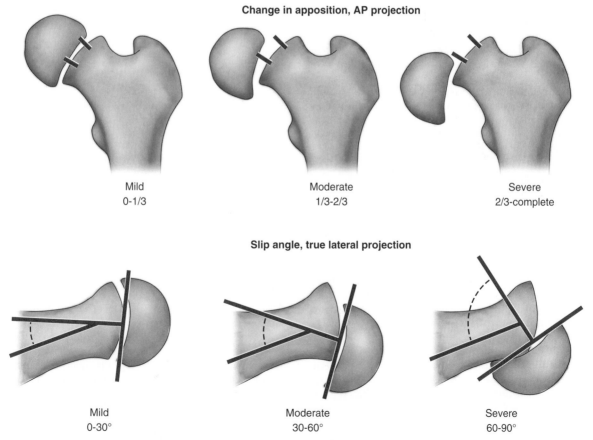

Change in apposition, AP projection

| Mild | Moderate | Severe |
| 0-1/3 | 1/3-2/3 | 2/3-complete |

Slip angle, true lateral projection

| Mild | Moderate | Severe |
| 0-30° | 30-60° | 60-90° |

▲ **Figure 43–6.** The figure demonstrates the degrees of severity of SCFE.

Transient Synovitis

Transient synovitis (toxic synovitis) is the most common cause of unilateral hip pain in children and often affects children 3-10 years of age. Transient synovitis is a result of inflammation of the synovium of the hip joint and as the name implies, is present only for a short period of time. The child will have pain in the hip and often presents to the emergency department with a limp. The cause is often unknown and may be related to a recent minor trauma or viral infection. Up to 50% of children may have a history of a recent upper respiratory infection or otitis media. The child is generally nontoxic in appearance with no history of fever. It is important to distinguish this clinical entity from a septic arthritis. The modified log roll test can help discriminate transient synovitis from a septic hip. The patient lays supine with legs outstretched. The physician hold onto the big toe and rolls the leg from medial to laterally which is in effect, rotating the hip. If an arc of 30 degrees or greater of hip rotation is able to be performed without pain, diagnosis of transient synovitis is more likely than septic hip joint. If further evaluation is necessary, radiographs, CBC, ESR, and CRP should be performed as transient synovitis is a diagnosis of exclusion. Values are generally normal or slightly elevated. If septic arthritis still suspected, MRI or needle aspiration with US guidance should be performed. CT scans are not beneficial in this setting and should not be ordered. Treatment is with NSAIDs (ibuprofen) or acetaminophen and parents instructed to limit weight-bearing of the child. Recheck within 24 hours is suggested although this is a self-limiting illness that resolves in 7-10 days. Discharge instructions should include immediate return to emergency department for an increase of pain or development of fever.

Kocher MS, Mandiga R, Zurakowski D, et al: Validation of a clinical prediction rule for the differentiation between septic arthritis and transient synovitis of the hip in children. *J Bone Joint Surg Am.* 2004;86:1629-1635 [PMID: 15292409].

Septic Arthritis of the Hip

Septic arthritis of the hip is often diagnosed in children younger than 4 years. The child has complaint of pain in the groin area which gradually increases in severity. He or she is generally toxic in appearance with fever and irritability. The child often demonstrates a limp on the affected side. When the child is supine, the hip will often be flexed, abducted, and externally rotated. Palpate the SIJ for local tenderness. X-rays may show the presence of an effusion and joint space widening when compared to the contralateral hip. US may detect an effusion or a distended capsule (positive when the capsule is distended 2 mm more than the contralateral side) (see Chapter 2). MRI will demonstrate the effusion and increased joint inflammation.

The Kocher criteria can help establish the likelihood of a diagnosis. The original four criteria included non-weight bearing on the affected side, ESR greater than 40 mm/hr, fever, and WBC greater than 12,000 mm^3. CRP greater than 20 mg/L has been added to this list of predictors. Most recent reports suggest that the likelihood of a child having septic arthritis is 2% with no positive criteria, 5% with 1 positive criteria, 11% with 2 positive criteria, 22% with 3 positive criteria, 40% with 4 positive criteria, and 60% with all 5 criteria positive. WBC is often obtained but is not reliable to exclude septic arthritis. A CRP less than 1 has been shown to have a negative predictive value of 87% in a study by Levine. The ESR and CRP are not only useful for making the diagnosis, but also for following response to treatment. A blood culture must be obtained to aid in identifying an organism and existence of bacteremia. The Gram stain and culture of the synovial fluid are the ultimate diagnostic tests. Emergent drainage in the operating room by an orthopedist is the definitive treatment.

Pathogens vary by age and immunization status. Pathogens in the neonate include *Staphylococcus aureus,* Group B *Streptococcus,* and gram-negative bacilli. Pathogens in children aged 6-24 months include *Haemophilus influenzae, Streptococcus,* and *S. aureus.* Pathogens in children older than 2 years include *S. aureus, Streptococcus,* and gram-negative bacilli. Choice of antibiotic should be based on the likely pathogen (see Chapter 41).

McKenzie M, Carlson B, Carlson WO: Evaluating hip pain in children. *S D Med.* 2012;65(8):303 [PMID: 22924207].

Levine MJ, et al: Assessment of the test characteristics of C-reactive protein for septic arthritis in children. *J Pediatrc Orthop.* 2003;23:373 [PMID: 12724603].

Sultan J, Hughes PJ. Septic arthritis or transient synovitis of the hip in children. *J Bone and Joint Surg.* 2010;92(9):1289-1293 [PMID: 20798450].

DISORDERS OF THE KNEE

When children or adolescents present with knee pain, it is commonly caused by one of the following disorders.

Tibial Apophysitis

Tibial apophysitis (Osgood-Schlatter disease [OSD]) is a common condition seen in adolescent boys who have recently undergone a growth spurt. Pain is to the anterior knee and localized to the area where the patellar tendon inserts into the anterior tibia. It occurs after repetitive injury to the tibial tuberosity and commonly seen in young athletes. Patients have complaint of pain with running, jumping, and climbing stairs. On examination, patient will have pain with extension against resistance. There may be a palpable mass or lump to the anterior tibial apophysis. The area may have some mild erythema. Effusions of the knee are absent. Up to 25%

of patients will have bilateral lesions. Diagnosis is clinical; however, radiographs may be beneficial in excluding other causes of pain. The condition is self-limited and resolves in a few months, or up to a few years. NSAIDs and rest from an aggravating activity or sport can improve the condition.

Gholve PA, Scher DM, Khakharia S, et al: Osgood-Schlatter syndrome. *Curr Opin Pediatr.* 2007;19(1):44-50 [PMID: 17224661].

Patellofemoral Dysfunction

There are a number of causes of patellofemoral dysfunction but this section will focus on the most frequent problems seen in the emergency department.

Pain in the patellofemoral joint secondary to dysfunction is one of the most common knee disorders. It is a prevalent problem in athletes but the type and duration of sporting activities are contributing factors. Patients have complaint of anterior knee pain. Pain exacerbated by activity is typical of chondral pathology. If the patella is tracking improperly along the patellofemoral groove (trochlea), the chondral surface of the patella can become inflamed and begin to degenerate. When the condition progresses with premature erosion of the cartilage, it is known as chondromalacia patellae. Knee pain that improves during physical activity but returns at rest suggests tendonitis. Osgood-Schlatter disease should be considered in a child with patellofemoral pain.

Patellar Subluxation

Patellar subluxation is a condition that commonly affects adolescents and occasionally, younger children. The patella normally slides up and down, centrally in a groove (trochlea). In some individuals, the patella does not slide centrally because it is pulled to the side with flexion of the knee. There are variations of severity but improper tracking along the trochlea may lead to pain or even dislocation. The apprehension test is performed to test for subluxation. The knee is placed at 30 degrees of flexion. The examiner places lateral pressure to the patella. Medial instability results in apprehension by the patient as this causes pain, and the patient will often grab the examiner's hands to stop the maneuver, hence the name, apprehension. Diagnostic imaging is not always necessary but CT scanning is more sensitive than radiography if indicated. Acute management initially should be conservative: protecting the affected knee, rest, ice, and elevation (PRICE). Patients may return to physical activities and sports when there is resolution of pain and return of ROM of the knee joint. Patients with continued pain and problems should be referred to an orthopedist for further evaluation.

Patellar Tendonitis (Jumper Knee)

Patellar tendonitis is an overuse syndrome and results from repetitive microtrauma, most often, sporting activities. It commonly occurs in athletes involved in jumping sports such as basketball or volleyball, but also occurs in soccer players or long-distance novice runners. Pain is usually directly to the patellar tendon, and tenderness can be produced with palpation. Many athletes resume activities before healing has occurred, which can cause chronic patellar tendonitis. Treatment is conservative with PRICE therapy. Use of patellar bands has not proven beneficial in the literature, although a number of therapists advise the use and many athletes report pain relief from its use.

Osteochondritis Dissecans

Osteochondritis dissecans (OCD) is a disorder most commonly seen in adolescents. A focal area of subchondral bone becomes necrotic and the overlying cartilage loses its supporting structure and subsequently displaces into the joint space; 20-30% of cases are bilateral. The knee is involved in about 75% of patients; however, OCD can occur in the elbow. The etiology is unclear but repetitive and compressive forces play a significant role. Repetitive microtrauma in the athlete is believed to be a contributing factor in addition to increased susceptibility of adolescents during growth spurts. Patients have complaints of subtle and vague knee discomfort with sensations of "catching" and "giving way." Pain increases with weight-bearing and patients have periods of stiffness after rest. Patients are often unable to fully extend at the knee, and this restriction of motion is an important clinical finding. Physical examination may demonstrate effusion, crepitus, and tenderness along the joint line.

OCD is a radiologic diagnosis and if suspected, tunnel view (knee in flexion) with AP and lateral views are ordered. If a lesion is found, the contralateral knee should also be examined and radiographed as OCD often is bilateral. If the diagnosis is made in the emergency department, the patient should be referred to an orthopedist for further evaluation including MRI for stability, staging, and possible surgical intervention.

DISORDERS OF THE LOWER LEG

Medial Tibial Stress Syndrome

Medial tibial stress syndrome (MTTS) is a painful condition, commonly known as shin splints. It is a cumulative stress disorder common in runners or in sporting activities played on hard surfaces (tennis). Patients have complaint of pain along the side of the tibia, palpable tenderness, and possible swelling. Pain usually resolves after activity, but pain may become constant. Treatment involves

PRICE therapy. NSAIDs or acetaminophen may alleviate pain. Proper shoes for the sporting activity are essential in prevention and treatment. Arch supports may be helpful and can be custom made or bought over-the-counter. Encourage cross-training with less impact sports during recovery periods.

Differential diagnosis should include stress fractures, chronic exertional compartment syndrome, nerve entrapment, and popliteal artery entrapment syndrome. These syndromes can have symptoms similar to MTTS, so confirmation of diagnosis is essential.

Radiographs may be indicated to exclude stress fractures. Bone scans, MRI, MRA, compartmental pressures, and arteriograms may be indicated to evaluate for more serious aforementioned conditions.

Carr K, Seveton E: Clinical Inquiries: How can you help athletes prevent and treat shin splints? *J Fam Pract.* 2008;57(6),406-408 [PMID: 18544325].

Edwards PH Jr., Wright ML, Hartman JF: A practical approach for the differential diagnosis of chronic leg pain in the athlete. *Am J Sports Med.* 2005;33(8),1241-1249 [PMID: 16061959].

Galbraith M, Lavallee M: Medial tibial stress syndrome: Conservative treatment options. *Curr Rev Musculoskelet Med.* 2009;2(3):127-133 [PMID: 19809896].

Tibia Vara (Blount Disease)

Tibia vara (Blount disease) is a growth abnormality of the tibia in which the tibia turns inward, giving the child or adolescent the appearance of bow legs. The cause is unknown but believed to be related to excessive weight on the growth plate. It is associated with obesity, short stature, and early walking. Tibia vara seen at birth tends to improve with age, whereas Blount disease gradually worsens as a child gets older, which may result in permanent disability if the disease is allowed to progress. Children and adolescents with Blount disease should be referred to an orthopedist as bracing is indicated in children younger than 3 years and surgery may be indicated in older children.

SPINAL PATHOLOGY

SCOLIOSIS

Lateral curvature of the spine of 10 degrees or greater in the coronal plane defines scoliosis. The deformity may be secondary to another pathologic process, such as neuromuscular disease or a connective tissue disorder. It may also be congenital. When no predisposing factor is identified, idiopathic scoliosis may be diagnosed. Although idiopathic scoliosis may occur at any time from birth, most cases appear during adolescence. Though not a frequent cause of emergency department visits, scoliosis can result in significant morbidity if ignored.

Patients with adolescent idiopathic scoliosis are often asymptomatic at diagnosis, although they may present when asymmetry is noticed by themselves or their parents in shoulders, ribs, or gait. Although musculoskeletal back pain is more common in individuals with scoliosis than in the general population, back pain is an uncommon way for the patient to present. More likely, physical examination by physician will detect signs of scoliosis and prompt further investigation. If concern about scoliosis in an emergency department patient, referral to the primary care physician for more detailed evaluation is appropriate.

Standing plain radiographs of the spine remain the gold standard for diagnosis and evaluation of scoliosis. The goal of the physician is to assess severity of disease and risk of progression of the curvature. In short, the more severe the curve and the more skeletally immature the patient, the greater the risk of curve progression. Most patients with adolescent idiopathic scoliosis will require no treatment and suffer no significant morbidity. In patients where curvature becomes severe, there is risk of chronic pain, functional limitations, and restrictive lung disease. Treatment options include observation, bracing, and surgical correction. Decisions on which plan is best are best left to the patient, the parents, and the primary care physician in consultation with an orthopedic surgeon when necessary. Treatment plans are individualized based on the psychological implications of bracing and surgery and the data available on the efficacy of bracing techniques.

Dolan LA, Weinstein SL: Surgical rates after observation and bracing for adolescent idiopathic scoliosis: An evidence-based review. *Spine (Phila, Pa 1976).* 2007;32:S91 [PMID: 17728687].

Kim HJ, Green DW: Adolescent back pain. *Curr Opin Pediatr.* 2008;20:37 [PMID: 18197037].

Malfair D, Flemming AK, Dvorak MF, et al: Radiographic evaluation of scoliosis: Review. *AJR Am J Roentgenol.* 2010;194:S8 [PMID: 20173177].

KYPHOSIS (SCHEUERMANN KYPHOSIS)

Scheuermann kyphosis is defined radiographically as anterior wedging of three or more adjacent vertebrae by 5 degrees or greater on lateral radiographs of the spine. It most frequently becomes evident near the onset of puberty. Patients may present due to the deformity produced; however, in the emergency department it is more likely patients will present with pain. The pain is often aching in nature and insidious at onset, with exacerbation by activity and relief with rest. Very rarely, the kyphosis can cause a compressive myelopathy. The exact etiology of Scheuermann kyphosis is not clear, but genetic factors have been implicated as well as a role for repetitive trauma.

Plain radiographs are needed for the diagnosis of Scheuermann kyphosis, and can generally be deferred to the primary care physician. Treatment is conservative in the majority of cases and consists of strengthening and stretching exercises. Bracing and surgery are reserved for more severe deformity or debilitation. Patients are at risk for chronic back pain in adulthood, but the pain is generally not severe and the prognosis is good for these patients.

Lowe TG, Line BG: Evidence based medicine: Analysis of Scheuermann kyphosis. *Spine (Phila Pa 1976)*. 2007;32:S115 [PMID: 17728677].

SPONDYLOLISTHESIS

Spondylolysis describes a defect in the vertebral pars interarticularis, often acquired from repetitive trauma conveyed during flexion and extension of the lumbar spine. When the defect is bilateral, the vertebral body may slip anteriorly, termed spondylolisthesis. Most cases occur during adolescence, and athletes engaged in sports such as football, dance, weightlifting, and gymnastics are at highest risk. The patient will usually present with subacute or acute low back pain, and the pain is often exacerbated by hyperextension of the lumbar spine. True weakness or radicular pain is rare.

In the emergency department, plain radiographs with oblique views of the lumbar spine should be sufficient for initial evaluation. The oblique view will show the posterior elements overlapping the vertebral body to form a "Scotty

dog" outline on the radiograph. For patients with spondylolysis, the radiograph may demonstrate a pars defect in the lamina corresponding to a "broken neck" on the Scott dog figure (Figure 43-7). Spondylolisthesis can also be graded based on the severity of slippage. In very early disease without complete development of the pars defect, the plain films may be negative. If suspicion remains high, the patient can follow up with their primary care physician for further diagnostic imaging, usually MRI. Once diagnosed, treatment is generally conservative with activity restriction, targeted exercises, and sometimes bracing. Surgery is generally reserved for high-grade spondylolisthesis or refractory pain.

Leone A, Cianfoni A, Cerase A, et al: Lumbar spondylolysis: A review. *Skeletal Radiol.* 2011;40:683 [PMID: 20440613].

ANKYLOSING SPONDYLITIS

Ankylosing spondylitis is a chronic inflammatory disease with involvement of the sacroiliac and axial skeletal joints. Although classically diagnosed in young adults, ankylosing spondylitis can occur in children, typically during adolescence. Presentation differs from that seen in adult-onset disease. Juvenile-onset ankylosing spondylitis generally lacks the spine symptoms seen in adults. Instead, patients first develop a polyarthritis of the extremities. It may be years before the sacroiliitis

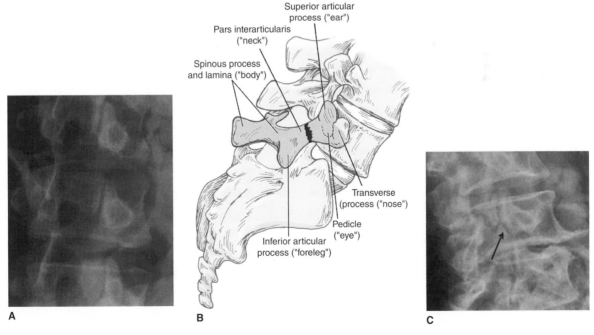

Superior articular process ("ear")
Pars interarticularis ("neck")
Spinous process and lamina ("body")
Transverse (process ("nose")
Pedicle ("eye")
Inferior articular process ("foreleg")

A   B   C

▲ **Figure 43–7.** The Scotty dog appearance of the posterior elements on the oblique view of the lumbar spine. A. Normal oblique radiograph. B. Schematic. C. Spondylolysis on radiograph (arrow). (Reproduced, with permission, from Simon RR, Sherman SC. *Emergency Orthopedics*, 6th ed. New York: McGraw-Hill, 2011. Copyright © McGraw-Hill Education LLC.)

required for diagnosis of adult-onset disease becomes radiographically apparent. Multisystem involvement may occur as with other inflammatory spondyloarthopathies. Inflammatory bowel disease and uveitis are relatively common, although cardiac manifestations such as aortic insufficiency are rare.

Treatment involves symptom control with NSAIDs, physical therapy, and judicious use of corticosteroids. Care of the patient in the emergency department with exacerbations of juvenile-onset ankylosing spondylitis should be closely coordinated with the child's pediatric rheumatologist. If a new diagnosis of ankylosing spondylitis or other spondyloarthropathy is suspected, consultation with a pediatric rheumatologist is important to establish a close follow-up as extensive serologic and genetic testing will likely be required.

DISCITIS

Inflammation of the intervertebral disc (discitis) is usually self-limited. It occurs in children approximately 3-5 years of age. Presenting symptoms can be vague and gradual in onset, making accurate diagnosis difficult. Children may present with refusal to walk, limp, back pain, irritability, low-grade fevers, and vomiting. Symptoms have usually been present for approximately 3 weeks at time of diagnosis. Physical examination may reveal tenderness with percussion over the spine, refusal to flex the spine, and hip stiffness. Neurologic findings are rare but include decreased reflexes and muscle weakness. Laboratory evaluation should include complete blood count (CBC), CRP, ESR, and blood cultures. The ESR is usually elevated, but WBC is generally normal, and blood cultures are rarely positive. Plain radiographs show narrowing at the disc space after 2-3 weeks of disease. MRI with contrast is the study of choice to diagnose and identify the extent of discitis.

Once diagnosed, treatment is initiated with intravenous (IV) antibiotics [ceftazidine (50 mg/kg q8h), ceftriaxone (50 mg/kg 12h), vancomycin (10 mg/kg q6h)], including a third-generation cephalosporin and an antistaphylococcal agent. Bacterial isolates are uncommly recovered but when cultures are positive, the most common bacteria isolated are *S. aureus* and *Kingella kingae*. Once clinical improvement occurs, IV antibiotics may be transitioned to oral agents. Pain control is an essential aspect of care, and bed rest with limitation of movement may be helpful. Some advocate for spinal immobilization with casting. Serious complications are rare, but can include vertebral osteomyelitis and spinal epidural abscess. Anterior fusion of the vertebral bodies above and below the involved disc is not uncommon, but is generally asymptomatic.

Garron E, Viehweger E, Launay F, et al: Nontuberculous spondylodiscitis in children. *J Pediatr Orthop.* 2002;22:321 [PMID: 11961447].

Kayser R, Mahlfeld K, Greulich M, et al: Spondylodiscitis in childhood: Results of a long-term study. *Spine (Phila Pa 1976).* 2005;30:318 [PMID: 15682013].

Nussinovitch M, Sokolover N, Volovitz B, et al: Neurologic abnormalities in children presenting with diskitis. *Arch Pediatr Adolesc Med.* 2002;156:1052 [PMID: 12361454].

SPINAL EPIDURAL ABSCESS

Spinal epidural abscess is a true emergency that requires prompt identification and treatment to prevent serious morbidity and mortality. Because of its rarity and vague presentation, diagnosis of spinal epidural abscess is often delayed. In adults, it has been proposed that inflammatory markers be used in combination with risk factor assessment as a screening tool for spinal epidural abscess in the emergency department. Adults with spinal epidural abscess often display a minimum of one risk factor such as medical comorbidities, recent spinal instrumentation, trauma, or intravenous drug abuse; however, in children, no predisposing factors are likely to be found. Classic triad of fever, back pain, and neurologic deficit is uncommon as well. Symptoms may progress in a stepwise fashion, from aching back pain to neuropathic-type pain, followed by weakness and sensory changes until finally paralysis develops.

Initial laboratory studies should include CBC, ESR, CRP, and blood cultures. Although a leukocytosis with elevated inflammatory markers may raise suspicion for spinal epidural abscess, they cannot be relied upon solely. WBC is insensitive, and inflammatory markers are not specific. MRI is the imaging modality of choice and should be obtained as quickly as possible. When spinal epidural abscess is most likely diagnosis, antibiotic treatment should begin without delay. Broad-spectrum coverage is generally advocated with care to cover for MRSA (Vancomycin 10 mg/kg q6h). Once radiographic confirmation of abscess is obtained, immediate consultation with a spinal surgeon for definitive drainage is necessary.

Darouiche R: Spinal epidural abscess. *N Engl J Med.* 2006;55:2012 [PMID: 17093252].

Davis DP, Wold RM, Patel RJ, et al: The clinical presentation and impact of diagnostic delays on emergency department patients with spinal epidural abscess. *J Emerg Med.* 2004;26:285 [PMID: 15028325].

OTHER ORTHOPAEDIC DISORDERS PRESENTING IN EMERGENCY DEPARTMENT

PSOAS ABSCESS

A psoas (iliopsoas) abscess is a collection of purulence in the iliopsoas muscle compartment. The incidence is rare but there is increased frequency of diagnosis with use of computed tomography (CT) or MRI. Primary psoas abscess tends to occur in children and adolescents. Signs and symptoms include back, hip or flank pain, fever, inguinal mass, and limp. Children may present with abdominal pain or genitourinary complaints. The "psoas sign," pain with extension of the hip, may be present.

Primary causes of psoas abscess include idiopathic, hematogenous seeding from an occult cutaneous source, and suppurative lymphadenitis. Secondary causes less likely in children include Crohn disease, ruptured appendicitis, periappendicular abscess, pyelonephritis, renal tuberculosis, tuberculous spondylitis, and complication of spinal surgery. Tuberculous etiologies of psoas abscess occur most often in developing countries.

Microbiology of the abscess will vary with geography and pathogenesis of the infection. Primary psoas abscess is most often caused by infection with a single organism. The most common bacterial pathogen is *S. aureus*, including MRSA.

Laboratory studies should include a CBC, ESR, CRP, and blood cultures. An elevated aspartate aminotransferase has also been described.

CT is the diagnostic study of choice as it is accurate, rapid, and noninvasive. MRI is acceptable alternative for diagnosis. Plain radiographs and US are not reliable in this setting.

Management of psoas abscess includes surgical drainage and antibiotic therapy. Empiric antibiotic therapy should include coverage for MRSA (Vancomycin 10 mg/kg q6h).

Complications and serious sequelae can include septic shock, DVT secondary to extrinsic compression of the iliac vein, hydronephrosis due to ureteric compression, and bowel ileus.

Atkinson C, Morris SK, Ng V, et al: A child with fever, hip pain and limp. *Can Med Assoc J.* 2006;174(7):924 [PMID: 16567754].

Mallick IH, Thoufeeq MH, Rajendran TP: Iliopsoas abscess. *Postgrad Med J.* 2004;80(946):459-462 [PMID: 15299155].

Navarro López V, Ramos JM, Meseguer V, et al: Microbiology and outcome of iliopsoas abscess in 124 patients. *Medicine (Baltimore).* 2009;88:120 [PMID: 19282703].

GROWING PAINS

Growing pains are a benign and self-limited process of unknown etiology. Despite the name, growing pains do not occur during the time of most rapid growth, they do not affect the growth of children who have them, and do not occur at specific sites of growth. Many clinicians hold that growing pains do not exist, rather pain is caused by overuse during the day. Growing pains, most common 2-12 years, are described as aching or throbbing sensation in the front of the thighs or the posterior calves. Pain is intermittent and may last for months or years. It generally resolves without intervention. Three criteria must be met for the diagnosis: (1) bilateral leg pain; (2) pain occurs only at night and; (3) patient has no pain, limp, or symptoms

during the day. The diagnosis of growing pains is unlikely if there are other symptoms such as fever, weight loss, pain to a specific joint, increasing pain over time, limping, decreased ROM to joints, the presence of tenderness, redness, swelling, or warmth to a specific area.

Evans A: Growing pains: Contemporary knowledge and recommended practice. *J Foot Ankle Res.* 2004;1:4 [PMID: 18822152].

OSTEOGENESIS IMPERFECTA

Children may present to the emergency department with unexplained fractures. Health care workers, social workers, and law enforcement officials often suspect child abuse. Undiagnosed osteogenesis imperfecta (OI) should be considered in such children but not at the expense of the safety of a child.

OI is genetic abnormality that may be inherited or the result of a spontaneous mutation, which causes a structural or quantitative defect in type I collagen. Clinical features of OI vary between types, within types, and within the same family. Fractures may occur during ordinary activities such as changing diapers or when infant tries to crawl or pull up to stand. There may be no obvious abnormality other than crying or refusing to bear weight on a limb. All types of fractures may occur, including rib fractures and spiral fractures, even with no history of trauma. The child may bruise easily. X-rays may reveal old fractures that were undetected or fractures in various stages of healing. The OI child may not have blue sclera, bone deformities, or brittle teeth. Children with mild or moderate OI may have normal-appearing bones on x-rays. Diagnosis of OI is made by clinical presentation. Prenatal US may show bony abnormalities. Laboratory confirmation is made by collagen and genetic testing. Laboratory tests are not required for emergency department evaluation.

It is important to obtain a family history in suspected cases. Ask if parents, siblings, or extended family members have a history of multiple fractures, hearing loss, spinal curvature, or brittle teeth. Severity of OI can vary, even within the same family.

It has been estimated that 7% of children who have signs suggestive of child abuse have an underlying medical condition that explain the injuries. In addition to OI, disorders with fragile bones and bruising include Ehlers-Danlos syndrome, glutaric acidemia type 1, hypophosphatasia, disorders of vitamin D metabolism, disorders of copper metabolism, and premature birth.

BENIGN TUMORS

Various soft tissue and bony tumors may be found when evaluating the pediatric patient in the emergency department. Although the tumors often cause symptoms such as local pain or swelling, it is likely that the lesion is found incidentally on physical examination or radiographs. By recognizing common benign tumors, the emergency physician can provide appropriate referrals to follow the lesion and avoid expensive workups that increase cost and anxiety.

Lipomas

Lipomas are the most common benign soft tissue tumors. They are comprised of mature adipose tissue. Most are located superficially in subcutaneous tissues of the neck, back, upper arms, and abdomen. Asymptomatic, lipomas may cause local tenderness or neuropathic type pain. They are often brought to the attention of the physician in connection with cosmetic issues or concerns about cancer. Lipomas are generally palpable, soft, and mobile. Although diagnosis is clinical, imaging may be useful to discriminate lipomas from other soft tissue masses. Larger lipomas will appear radiolucent on plain radiographs. Bedside US will reveal an elliptical mass that is hyperechoic compared to the adjacent muscle. No emergent treatment is necessary, and patients can be referred to a surgeon for resection of the mass if desired.

Wu J, Hochman M: Soft-tissue tumors and tumorlike lesions: A systematic imaging approach. *Radiology.* 2009;253:297 [PMID: 19864525].

Ossifying Fibroma

Ossifying fibroma is a fibro-osseous lesion found in children younger than 10 years. It affects the tibia in 90% of patients. Although not painful, it carries the risk of pathologic fracture. Plain radiographs will show an elliptical, lytic bubble-like lesion with anterolateral bowing. Patients should be referred to a pediatric orthopedist. They are generally followed with serial radiographs until skeletal maturity, at which time excision and bone graft may be performed for symptomatic lesions or deformity.

Nonossifying Fibroma

Nonossifying fibromas are the most common benign bone lesions in children. An area of bone that would normally have ossified is replaced by fibrous tissue. Most common locations are the tibia and femur, often near a growth plate. Diagnosis is usually incidental when radiograph of the extremity is ordered for another reason. Nonossifying fibromas appear as elongated, sclerosing lesions with scalloping of adjacent cortex. If large enough, the integrity of the bone is compromised and pathologic fracture may result; however, this is rare. In general, no further evaluation or follow-up is required.

Osteochondroma

Osteochondromas are cartilage-producing tumors that present most often during the second decade of life. The area of cartilaginous growth expands during childhood and ossifies

as the child reaches skeletal maturity. The most common location of lesions is the distal femur. The bony spur produced by the osteochondroma is often palpable, and patients may present with an asymptomatic mass. Pain at the site is a common presenting symptom, and lesions may be found incidentally on radiographs taken for another reason. Plain radiographs show a metaphyseal bony spur that is usually directed away from the joint. Small and asymptomatic osteochondromas can be followed by the primary care physician, while large or bothersome lesions should be referred to an orthopedist. Surgery is indicated for osteochondromas when they produce complications such as pain, decreased ROM, deformity. If diagnosed in childhood, the lesion should be followed into adulthood due to the rare chance of malignant transformation to chondrosarcoma.

Levine SM, Lambiase RE Petchprapa CN: Cortical lesions of the tibia: Characteristic appearances at conventional radiography. *RadioGraphics.* 2003;23:157-177 [PMID: 12533651].

Wright JG, Yandow S, Donaldson S, et al: A randomized clinical trial comparing intralesional bone marrow and steroid injections for simple bone cysts. *J Bone Joint Surg Am.* 2008;90:722 [PMID: 18381307].

Bone Cysts

Unicameral bone cysts, simple bone cysts, are common lesions that usually present in the late childhood to early adolescent years. The most frequent sites are the proximal humerus and femur. Patients may present because of localized pain, limp, or pathologic fracture. Unicameral bone cysts are seen on plain radiographs as a sharply defined cystic structure within metaphysis of bone; there is generally very little surrounding sclerosis. No further diagnostic workup is warranted, and the cyst may be followed on an outpatient basis. Most cysts will spontaneously resolve, although sometimes corticosteroid injections are used to hasten resolution. Curettage and grafting are used for large lesions that threaten the integrity of the bone.

Aneurysmal bone cysts are vascular lesions that occur mainly in adolescents. Frequent sites include the spine, femur, and tibia. They can present with localized pain and swelling or pathologic fracture. Spinal lesions may cause neurologic symptoms such as radiculopathy. Plain radiographs reveal sharply circumscribed lytic lesions with aneurysmal dilation of the bone. Although benign, aneurysmal bone cysts are locally aggressive and destructive lesions. Treatment is with curettage and grafting, although recurrence rates can be as high as 50%.

Novais EN, Rose PS, Yaszemski MJ, et al: Aneurysmal bone cyst of the cervical spine in children. *J Bone Joint Surg Am.* 2011;93:1534 [PMID: 22204009].

MALIGNANT TUMORS

Primary malignant tumors of the bone are a rare cause of visits to the emergency department. It is important to recognize the constellation of signs and symptoms indicating presence of such a tumor so that diagnosis is not delayed. Ewing sarcoma, osteosarcoma, and rhabdomyosarcoma are the most common pediatric bony malignancies.

Ewing Sarcoma

The Ewing sarcoma family of tumors can have a wide variance in location, but most commonly presents in the pelvis or femur with pain as the primary symptom. Pain is usually intermittent and often worse at night. The history of minor trauma preceding the onset of symptoms is not unusual and can lead to a misdiagnosis of musculoskeletal injury rather than neoplasm. Systemic symptoms of fever and weight loss are present in a small number of patients, so their absence is not helpful in lowering clinical suspicion. Most common examination findings are localized tenderness to palpation and a soft tissue mass; therefore, this combination should prompt radiographic evaluation.

Plain radiographs are the mainstay of initial diagnosis for Ewing sarcoma. Classic findings include a poorly marginated, destructive bony lesion. Displacement of the bony cortex by tumor produces the phenomenon of Codman triangle. Unfortunately, it is not uncommon for initial films to be misinterpreted as normal and thus delay diagnosis. Once a tentative diagnosis is made based on plain radiographs, more exhaustive radiographic evaluation is required; however, not as part of emergency department workup.

Patients with established diagnoses of Ewing sarcoma may present to the emergency department with complaints related to the disease. Chemotherapy is a routine treatment since metastatic disease is common, with associated complications. Patients have the risk of pathologic fractures, so there should be a low threshold to order radiographs in the setting of increased pain, especially at the sites of known lesions. Close communication with the patient's oncologist is helpful in providing good emergency department care.

Osteosarcoma

Osteosarcoma is a rare childhood tumor with peak incidence in the second decade of life. It is the most common primary bone malignancy in children. The most frequent site is the distal femur, followed by the proximal tibia and proximal humerus. Symptoms at presentation are similar to Ewing sarcoma, with localized pain often associated with a soft tissue mass. Systemic symptoms are often absent. Time from onset of symptoms to diagnosis may be prolonged by delayed presentation as well as initial misdiagnosis.

In the emergency department, plain radiographs are the initial imaging modality of choice to evaluate localized bony tenderness. Osteosarcomas can display both lytic and sclerotic areas, with a soft tissue mass often described as a sunburst pattern caused by its radial pattern of ossification. Codman triangle may be formed in a manner similar to that in Ewing sarcoma. Suspected diagnosis on plain films should prompt immediate consultation with a pediatric oncologist. Treatment involves both surgical and chemotherapeutic approaches, as metastatic disease is common, though often subclinical.

Mirabello L, Troisi RJ, Savage SA: Osteosarcoma incidence and survival rates from 1973 to 2004: Data from the Surveillance, Epidemiology, and End Results Program. *Cancer.* 2009;115:1531 [PMID: 19197972].

Rhabdomyosarcoma

Rhabdomyosarcoma is the most common soft tissue sarcoma in children. Common sites include head and neck, genitourinary tract, and extremities. Presenting symptoms vary by tumor location. Head and neck tumors produce clinical pictures including proptosis, ophthalmoplegia, nasal obstruction, or aural obstruction. Genitourinary tumors result in hematuria, urinary obstruction, scrotal swelling, and vaginal discharge. Primary tumor in the extremities usually presents as localized, painful swelling.

Rhabdomyosarcoma in the head and neck or genitourinary tract is most often found in children younger than 6 years; tumor of the extremities is most prevalent in adolescents. It is the most common soft tissue sarcoma of adolescents and young adults. Evaluation in the emergency department when rhabdomyosarcoma is suspected should include plain films of the affected extremity as well as CBC and basic chemistries. Serum calcium should be measured as there is a risk of hypercalcemia in those with bony metastasis. Metastatic disease is found in approximately 20% of cases at time of initial staging and carries a poor prognosis. Treatment for rhabdomyosarcoma involves a combined approach with local resection, chemotherapy, and radiation.

Ilaslan H, Schils J, Nageotte W, Lietman SA, Sundaram M: Clinical presentation and imaging of bone and soft-tissue sarcomas. *Cleve Clin J Med.* 2010;77(suppl 1):S2 [PMID: 20179183].

Thermal Injury & Smoke Inhalation

Margaret Strecker-McGraw, MD, FACEP

Khylie McGee, MD

Ian Taylor McGraw, MS, MS1

GENERAL CONSIDERATIONS

Burn injury results from exposure to heat, chemical, or electricity. The extent of the injury is dependent upon temperature and duration of exposure, as well as the vascular supply and the thickness of the injured skin. At the center of the exposure there is an irreversible tissue necrosis. Surrounding the area of central necrosis is a zone of ischemia in which there is a reduction in dermal microcirculation. This ischemic zone may progress to full necrosis unless the ischemia is reversed. At the periphery of the burn is a third zone of hyperemia characterized by a reversible increase in blood flow.

In the United States in 2012, there were approximately 450,000 emergency department/urgent care/outpatient visits resulting in 40,000 acute hospitalizations for burn injuries. There were 2,550 deaths from residential fires and an additional 550 deaths from other sources including motor vehicle crashes, aircraft crashes, and contact with electricity, chemicals or hot liquids. The World Health Organization (WHO) states a high percentage of patients admitted to burn units worldwide are children younger than 12 years. Fortunately, most burns are superficial and involve less than 5% of total body surface area (TBSA).

Superficial burns in children result most from scalding with hot liquids. Deeper burns are usually secondary to direct contact with flame, hot objects, chemicals, and electricity. Smoke inhalation is seen in 18% of reported injuries and has a significant impact on mortality and length of hospital stay.

American Burn Association: Burn incidence and treatment in the United States: 2012 Fact Sheet. Chicago, IL, 2012. Also available at http://www.ameriburn.org/resources_factsheet.php. Accessed August 15, 2013.

American Burn Association: Facts about injuries: Burns. Chicago, IL, 2012. Also available at http://ameriburn.org/WHO-ISBIBurn Factsheet.pdf. Accessed August 15, 2013.

BURN CLASSIFICATION

Burns are classified by depth and surface area of skin involved:

- **First-degree burns** involve the epidermal layer only. This results in pain and erythema but the burn usually heals in a few days without scarring.

- **Second-degree burns** involve the epidermis and part of the underlying dermis. They are further classified based on the depth of injury:

  - **Superficial partial-thickness burns** are characterized by erythema, blister formation, and weeping. They are painful but generally heal in 1-2 weeks with minimal to no scarring.

  - **Deep partial-thickness burns** involve the reticular and the papillary layers of the dermis and the burn does not blanch with pressure. A nonelastic red or white layer on top of the burn characterizes these burns. They require up to 3-4 weeks to heal and will often have significant scarring.

- **Third-degree (full-thickness) burns** are characterized by an injury with a thick white, brown, or tan overlying layer with a leathery texture. They are insensate and do not blanch. The surrounding area may have painful, deep partial-thickness burn. These burns require excision and skin grafting.

- **Fourth-degree burns** are characterized by involvement of all layers of the skin and involve structures below the skin, such as tendons, bone, ligaments, and muscles. These burns are insensate.

Depth of the burn may be underestimated in the first 24 hours and may reveal itself to be deeper than originally estimated as time progresses. The TBSA of the burn is also used for classification. The "rule of nines" can be used to gain a rough estimate of the TBSA but there is high interrater

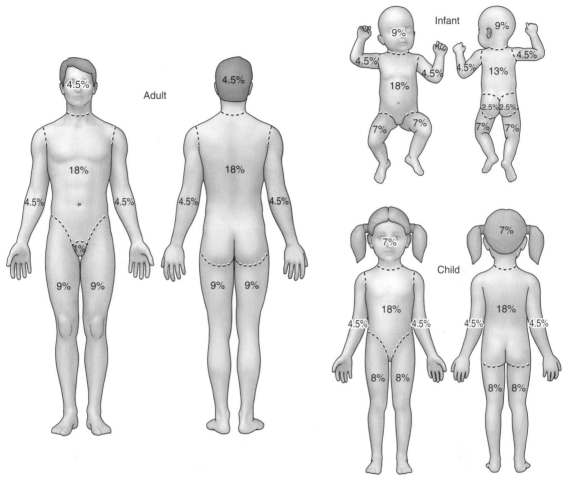

▲ **Figure 44–1.** Classic rule of nines chart to estimate percentage of total body surface area burned (TBSA%).

variability and frequent overestimation using this method (Figure 44–1). In addition, the rule must be modified in children and infants because of the disproportionate size of the head compared to the head of adults. A more accurate calculation of burn injury size can be obtained by using a standardized burn chart such as the Lund-Browder chart (Figure 44–2).

BURN RESUSCITATION

INITIAL EVALUATION

Prehospital Care

Prehospital physicians should minimize delay of patient transportation to an appropriate emergency care facility or burn center. Immediate cooling of the burn wound with cool running water for 20 minutes improves outcomes and reduces the extent of the injury, but must be kept within the context of minimizing patient transport times, and may not be appropriate for prehospital care. Cooling of the wound with cool running water may be efficacious up to 3 hours after injury. Optimal temperature for cool running water is 12-18°C (53.6-64.4°F) and should not contain ice or be less than 8°C (46.4°F), as these have been shown to further necrosis and tissue injury. Submersion of burn wounds in standing water increases the risk of infection and is not recommended.

The pediatric patient should be provided basic life support care. Emergency medical services (EMS) personnel should administer supplemental oxygen, unless the burn injury is isolated, minimal, and does not involve an inhalation injury or upper airway component. Clothing and accessories should be removed to minimize ongoing injury, unless they are adherent to the patient's skin.

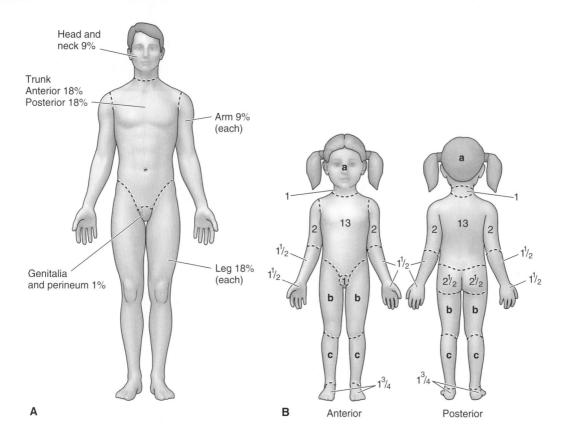

Relative percentage of body surface area (% BSA) affected by growth

Body Part	Age				
	0 yr	1 yr	5 yr	10 yr	15 yr
a = $\frac{1}{2}$ of head	$9\frac{1}{2}$	$8\frac{1}{2}$	$6\frac{1}{2}$	$5\frac{1}{2}$	$4\frac{1}{2}$
b = $\frac{1}{2}$ of 1 thigh	$2\frac{3}{4}$	$3\frac{1}{4}$	4	$4\frac{1}{4}$	$4\frac{1}{2}$
c = $\frac{1}{2}$ of 1 lower leg	$2\frac{1}{2}$	$2\frac{1}{2}$	$2\frac{3}{4}$	3	$3\frac{1}{4}$

▲ **Figure 44–2.** Lund-Browder chart. Relative percentages of areas affected by growth

EMS personnel should be advised to begin intravenous (IV) fluid resuscitation if transport time is expected to exceed 1 hour, or if the burn injury is ≥ 25% of TBSA.

Pediatric patients are particularly susceptible to hypothermia and precautions to prevent hypothermia should be provided, including covering of the patient with a clean sheet or blanket.

Emergency Department

Pediatric patients may have difficulty expressing themselves making initial assessment difficult. Burned patients should be treated as any other traumatic injury, recognizing the possibility of additional or occult traumatic injury.

Approximately 10% of patients with burn injuries present with concomitant trauma. Because of the variety of mechanisms associated with burn injuries, a thorough examination is necessary. Airway, breathing, and circulation (ABC) should be evaluated as well as cervical spine stabilization during the initial assessment.

▶ Airway Management

Airway management is critical due to a smaller cross-sectional diameter of the pediatric airway, which may be effected by postburn injury edema. The emergency physician should evaluate for signs of inhalation injury, which include facial burns, stridor, dysphonia, dysphagia, tachypnea, history of burn injury in an enclosed space, unconsciousness, carbonaceous sputum, drooling, and singed facial hair. If inhalation injury is suspected or confirmed, intubation should be performed immediately before airway edema can progress to full obstruction. Cervical spine precautions should be followed.

Breathing

Burn patients are subjected to a multifactorial physiological insult. Inhalation injury, inhaled toxins from burning substances, and thermal burns to the chest wall and abdomen have potential to result in inadequate ventilation and perfusion. Pediatric patients who have sustained burn injuries involving the chest wall or abdomen, especially circumferential burns, may require escharotomy to relieve the restrictive nature of their dysfunction. Pulse oximetry and capnography should be utilized to determine the effectiveness of the patient's ventilation and perfusion.

Circulation

Unstable or dysfunctional circulation in a pediatric patient should prompt a thorough evaluation to rule out other injuries that result in hemodynamic instability. Communication with EMS personnel may help determine the mechanism of injury and the possibility of additional injuries. Tachycardia, hypotension, or weak distal pulses in a patient presenting acutely with a burn injury may be signs of circulatory compromise for reasons not related to the burn. Patients who sustain burn injuries and do not immediately seek emergency care may have circulatory dysfunction directly related to burn injuries and the ensuing distributive and hypovolemic shock.

EMERGENCY DEPARTMENT MANAGEMENT

After the rapid initial assessment of the patient, a thorough physical examination should be performed to determine the extent of injuries. Accurate measurement of the patient's weight and determination of the TBSA burn are required for the initial estimation for fluid resuscitation. Second- and third-degree burns only are factored into the TBSA calculation. Pediatric patients have disproportionately larger heads and smaller proximal lower extremities, so the use of a modified Lund-Browder chart is recommended. Pediatric patients 5 years of age or younger are more at risk for deeper burns than older children because of thinner skin layers.

Intravenous Access

IV access is essential for pediatric patients with major burns. IV access should be obtained with use of large-bore IV catheters, preferably at a site away from the burn injury. If obtaining IV access away from the burn injury is not possible, central venous catheters may be placed in pediatric burn patients, or through the burn injury itself. High-fluid resuscitation volumes may require two sites of IV access with large-bore IV catheters.

Additional Considerations

Circumferential burns have a high likelihood of causing compartment syndrome in pediatric burn patients. Compartment syndrome in extremities results in inadequate perfusion, leading to more serious complications. Burn patients who have a TBSA ≥ 30% have a high likelihood of developing ileus and increased intra-abdominal pressures that may progress to abdominal compartment syndrome, with a mortality of 100% if untreated. These considerations warrant insertion of nasogastric tube for stomach decompression, reducing the risk of abdominal aspiration and compartment syndrome. Insertion of a Foley catheter is also useful to decompress the bladder by further reducing intra-abdominal pressures and is required to monitor the effectiveness of fluid resuscitation via urine output.

Children who have sustained full-thickness burns or worse should receive tetanus immunization if their last booster was greater than 5 years. If they have not yet received a complete tetanus immunization, tetanus immune globulin should be administered.

Pediatric patients should be checked regularly for hypoglycemia, and appropriate action taken. Strict glycemic control appears to improve outcomes for pediatric burn patients.

Diagnostic Studies

Pediatric patients who have sustained major thermal burns should have thorough diagnostic studies performed to anticipate problems as well as the extent of injury. Mechanism and severity of injury, as well as possible or confirmed inhalation injury indicate the need for various studies. Obtain a complete blood count, metabolic panel with renal function, lactate, type and Rh, carboxyhemoglobin, urinalysis, and two-view chest radiograph. Renal function is particularly useful in anticipation of major fluid shifts secondary to metabolic changes. Urinalysis is important as glycosuria may falsely give the impression of adequate perfusion by causing an osmotic diuresis. Additional laboratory studies and trauma body imaging should be obtained as dictated by history and physical examination.

Fluid Resuscitation

Apart from maintaining the patient's airway, fluid resuscitation is the most important therapeutic intervention for the severely burned patient. Organs are not properly perfused without proper fluid resuscitation, and end-organ failure may develop rapidly. Injured tissue in the "zone of ischemia or stasis" progresses to an ischemic state, resulting in further tissue damage and death. Aggressive fluid resuscitation helps to support tissue perfusion and mitigates microvascular damage following thermal burn injuries.

Fluid resuscitation is required for patients with burns of TBSA $\geq$ 10%. Consensus is lacking on when IV fluid resuscitation is necessary. A recent survey of burn care providers showed a clear majority (81.8%) believe that a TBSA less than 15% could receive oral fluid resuscitation. The American Burn Association (ABA) recommends that patients with burns greater than 10% of TBSA should be referred to a specialized burn treatment center. Burn care specialists may have recommendations and preferences for fluid resuscitation, and this should be discussed during the consultation or prior to transfer.

Burn resuscitation formulas are an approximation of fluid requirements for supportive care in the postburn injury period. Children younger than 5 years have insufficient hepatic glycogen reserves, requiring maintenance fluid in the form of dextrose 5% in water (D_5W) in addition to the primary fluid resuscitation. The most common estimation formulas are the Parkland burn formula and the Galveston Shriners Hospital formula, which estimate fluid requirements in the form of Ringers Lactate (RL) otherwise specified.

- Parkland burn formula (adapted for pediatric use): 4 mL/kg per % TBSA Ringers Lactate solution with additional D_5W for maintenance of blood glucose.
- Galveston Shriners Hospital formula: 5000 mL/m^2 per % burned BSA plus 2000 mL/m^2 total BSA (BSA is the body surface area in square meters).

These fluid estimations represent a generalized estimate of fluid needed for a 24-hour period. One-half of the fluid in the estimations is given over the first 8-hour period, and the remaining one-half is administered over the following 16 hours. Each burned child is unique, and fluid resuscitation therapy must be monitored diligently and adjusted for the individual patient. Failure to do so may result in underresuscitation or overresuscitation. Specific mechanisms of injury, especially inhalation injuries, may increase the fluid requirements dramatically.

Overresuscitation is as dangerous to the patient as underresuscitation. Severe thermal burns result in fluid shifts that cause generalized edema, which can cause vascular insult to extremities and body compartments in the form of compartment syndrome. Overresuscitation of the patient further adds to compartment pressures. Each patient should be carefully observed for signs of developing complications.

Monitoring

Evaluating the efficacy of fluid resuscitation is achieved by monitoring of the patient. One of the most common endpoints to monitoring burn patients is urine output measured through a Foley catheter. For pediatric burn patients weighing less than 30 kg, urine output should be maintained at 1-2 mL/kg per hour, and for those weighing $\geq$ 30 kg, urine output should be maintained at 0.5-1 mL/kg per hour.

Trend monitoring of vital signs is equally important in determining adequacy of resuscitation.

Pain Control

Burn injuries are exquisitely painful and adequate control of pain and anxiety is a fundamental part of burn care. Children typically receive opiate pain medications for pain, and fentanyl may be a good choice for hemodynamically unstable patients. Consider intranasal fentanyl as a useful adjunct until IV access is obtained. Anxiety may be alleviated with use of a benzodiazepine. Children receiving narcotic analgesics or benzodiazepines should be placed on end-tidal carbon dioxide (CO_2) monitoring if they are not intubated.

CRITERIA FOR REFERRAL TO A BURN CENTER

Criteria according to the American College of Surgeons (ACS) and American Burn Association (ABA):

1. Greater than 10% TBSA partial-thickness burns.
2. Burns that involve the face, genitalia, perineum, hands, feet, major joints.
3. Third-degree burns in any age group.
4. Electrical burns including lightning injury.
5. Chemical burns.
6. Inhalation injury.
7. Burn injuries in patient with preexisting medical conditions that could complicate management, prolong recovery, or affect mortality.
8. Patient with burns and concomitant trauma such as fractures in which burn injury poses the greatest risk of morbidity or mortality. In such patients, trauma poses the greater immediate risk; the patient may be stabilized in a trauma center before being transferred to a burn unit. Physician judgment will be necessary in such situations and should be in concert with the regional medical central plan and triage protocols.
9. Burned children in hospitals without qualified personnel or equipment for the care of children.
10. Burn injury in patients who will require special social, emotional, or rehabilitative interventions.

If the patient is being transferred to dedicated burn center, wounds should be covered with dry sterile dressings without application of topical agents.

OUTPATIENT CARE OF BURNS

GENERAL CONSIDERATIONS

More than 95% of burns can be successfully managed in the outpatient setting. Referral to a burn center does not necessarily mean admission to the burn center. Close monitoring and follow-up are important aspects of outpatient management because of the dynamic and fragile progression of burn injuries.

Outpatient management of burns predicates careful selection of children capable of taking fluids by mouth, a family or support system that can follow instructions, the capability to manage dressing changes at home, the ability to obtain early and frequent follow-up visits, as well as clearly defined instructions to return if any problems are encountered. Adequate control of pain and anxiety in the child during dressing changes is also necessary. Judicious use of narcotics will help the patient tolerate the wound debridement. Child with a burn greater than 10% TBSA should not be discharged home from the emergency department. Outpatient management should not be undertaken in a child who may have airway compromise, risk of aspiration, or other injuries requiring inpatient management.

DEBRIDEMENT

Most authors agree that small blisters (< 6 mm) with clear fluid underneath can be left intact, although controversy exists. Larger blisters and dead tissue should be debrided using sterile water rather than providing iodine or chlorhexidine that may delay wound healing. Scrubbing and sharp dissection with scissors may be necessary to remove debris that is adherent to the underlying tissue. Pain control and/or sedation will be necessary for the young patient to tolerate debridement.

TOPICAL AGENTS

Topical burn care involves multiple pharmacological options. Fortunately, most superficial burns heal well under any agent or membrane if wounds are kept clean and desiccation is avoided.

Silver Sulfadiazine

Silver sulfadiazine is a common topical wound treatment that both prevents desiccation due to a viscous carrier and has broad-spectrum bactericidal activity. It is also painless upon application. Some authors question whether silver sulfadiazine hinders healing, but most burn centers continue to use this formulation.

Other Ointments

Bacitracin and triple antibiotic ointment are clear ointments that are used on superficial wounds on the face and hands without the worry of silver staining (argyria) and are readily available. Burns around the eye can be treated with topical ophthalmic antibiotic ointments. Significant ear burns should be treated with mafenide acetate as it is the only topical that has significant penetration into a relatively avascular area.

Wound Membranes

Wound membranes such as Biobrane (Dow Hickham, Sugar Land Texas) or a silver-impregnated membrane such as Acticoat (Smith & Nephew, UK) provide a physiologic covering of the wound until natural healing takes place. These membranes have revolutionized burn wound care by covering the wound, diminishing pain, and protecting from mechanical trauma and bacterial contamination.

LONG-TERM MANAGEMENT

Close follow-up for outpatient burns is advisable. The absence of complete healing in 7-10 days suggests the burn is deep or infected and warrants prompt referral to a burn specialist.

American Burn Association/American College of Surgeons: Guidelines for the operation of burn centers. *J Burn Care Res.* 2007;28(1):134-141 [PMID: 17211214].

Balogh ZJ, Butcher NE: Compartment syndromes from head to toe. *Crit Care Med.* 2010;38:S445-S451 [PMID: 20724877].

Ejike JC, Mathur M: Abdominal decompression in children. *Crit Care Res Pract.* 2012:180797 [PMID: 22482041].

Gauglitz GG, Herndon DN, Jeschke MG: Emergency treatment of severely burned pediatric patients: Current therapeutic strategies. *Pediatric Health.* 2008;2(6):761-775.

Greenhalgh DG: Burn resuscitation: The results of the ISBI/ABA survey. *Burns.* 2010;36(2):176-182 [PMID: 20018451].

Kasten KR, Makley AT, Kagan RJ: Update on the critical care management of severe burns. *J Intensive Care Med.* 2011;26(4): 223-236 [PMID: 21764766].

Kim LK, Martin HC, Holland AJ: Medical management of paediatric burn injuries: Best practice. *J Paediatr Child Health.* 2012;48(4):290-295 [PMID: 21679339].

Latenser BA: Critical care of the burn patient: The first 48 hours. *Crit Care Med.* 2009;37(10):2819-2826 [PMID: 19707133].

Lloyd EC, Rodgers BC, Michener M, et al: Outpatient burns: Prevention and care. *Am Fam Physician.* 2012;85(1):25-32 [PMID: 22230304].

Medscape: Burn resuscitation and early management. New York, NY, 2012. Also available at http://emedicine.medscape.com/article/1277360-overview. Accessed August 15, 2013.

O'Brien SP, Billmire DA: Prevention and management of outpatient pediatric burns. *J Craniofac Surg.* 2008;19(4):1034-1039 [PMID: 18650728].

Orgill DP, Piccolo N: Escharotomy and decompressive therapies in burns. *J Burn Care Res.* 2009;30(5):759-768 [PMID: 19692906].

Peddy SB, Rigby MR, Shaffner DH: Acute cyanide poisoning. *Pediatr Crit Care Med.* 2006;7(1):79-83 [PMID: 16395080].

Sargent RL: Management of blisters in partial thickness burns: An integrative research review. *J Burn Care Res.* 2006;27(1):66-81 [PMID: 16555539].

Sheridan RL, Weber JM: Mechanical and infectious complications of central venous cannulation in children: Lessons learned from a 10-year experience placing more than 1000 catheters. *J Burn Care Res.* 2006;27(5):713-718 [PMID: 16998405].

Singer AJ, Brebbia J, Soroff HH: Management of local burn wounds in the ED. *Am J Emerg Med.* 2007;25(6):666-671 [PMID: 17606093].

SMOKE INHALATION INJURY

Smoke inhalation injury is a significant cause of increased morbidity and mortality in burn victims. It can be associated with concomitant thermal or chemical burns, or may be an isolated injury. Smoke inhalation injury is grouped into three types of damage: thermal injury, localized chemical injury, and systemic chemical poisoning.

THERMAL INJURY

Mechanism

Thermal injury occurs when superheated air, smoke, or flames are inhaled into the respiratory tract. The upper respiratory tract is very efficient at heat exchange and therefore injury below the larynx is uncommon in most patients. The caveat is when a patient has potentially inhaled steam or another superheated liquid gas formulation, in which case direct thermal injury may occur below the carina. Once the heat contacts the mucosal surface or lung tissue, it causes damage by increased blood flow secondary to increased microvasculature permeability, increased bronchial blood flow, and decreased hypoxic pulmonary vasoconstriction. There can also be direct destruction of the mucosal surface, inactivation of surfactant, and activation of neutrophils. The insults can lead to significant edema within the tissues.

Clinical Findings

Initial physical examination findings of thermal inhalation injury include burns to the face and neck, soot in the mouth, carbonaceous sputum, singed nostrils, stridor, rhonchi, and dysphonia. A high level of suspicion based on the history is important as thermal injury to the upper airway may not yet be evident due to delayed tissue swelling. Significant injury will cause progression of swelling, ultimately resulting in macroglossia, macrouvula, heat-induced epiglottitis, and croup. If severe, burn-induced edema can cause acute or subacute airway obstruction. In addition, airway obstruction may be aggravated by edema-induced laryngospasm and bronchospasm.

CHEMICAL INJURY

Mechanism

Smoke is a dynamic combination of carbonaceous material laced with toxic compounds created by the combustion of the contents of a fire. Localized chemical injury occurs primarily in the lower airways and lung parenchyma. Common causes of chemical lung injury in children are related to the toxins within flammable building materials and household contents such as wood, cotton, polyvinyl chloride (PVC), and polyurethane. The burning of PVC alone produces more than 50 potentially hazardous compounds including hydrochloric acid, phosgene, and chlorine.

Hydrochloric acid causes denaturation of proteins and cell death within the airways. It may also cause tearing or irritation of the eyes, mucosal inflammation, and dyspnea.

Acrolein is a toxic compound frequently encountered in inhalation injury. It is a product of the combustion of wood, papers, and cotton. Like hydrochloric acid, acrolein causes protein denaturation that can result in ocular-related complaints at low concentrations. At higher concentrations or with prolonged exposure, it can result in death secondary to significant pulmonary edema and hypoxia.

Other compounds most commonly cause damage via activation of inflammatory mediators that cause bronchoconstriction, bronchospasm, pulmonary edema, and cast formation. Many irritants inactivate surfactant directly upon contact, further contributing to ventilation-perfusion mismatch.

Clinical Findings

A thorough history may raise suspicion of chemical inhalation injury despite minimal or absent signs of disease initially in emergency department. Clinical course is progressive and symptoms are often delayed.

Water-soluble irritants are readily absorbed into the lung parenchyma and may result in dyspnea, wheezes, rhonchi, and rales. However, findings are often absent in the presence of lung damage. Lipid-soluble compounds may take many hours to absorb and symptoms may be delayed up to 48 hours. The current gold standard for diagnosis of chemical inhalation injury is fiberoptic bronchoscopy for direct visualization of the airways, but its use is limited to the upper airways. Bronchoscopy is readily used at burn centers but is not available in all emergency departments, making the diagnosis of chemical inhalation injury difficult.

Computed tomography of the chest can be obtained quickly in most emergency departments and may show ground glass opacities and consolidation to adjacent large airways. Chest x-ray is often normal in the emergency department but should be obtained as a baseline.

SYSTEMIC CHEMICAL POISONING

Systemic chemical poisoning is caused by inhalation of carbon monoxide and cyanide. These toxic compounds represent important causes of morbidity and mortality associated with pediatric inhalation injury. They should be suspected in children with inhalation injury or burns by a substantial mechanism.

Mechanism

▶ **Carbon Monoxide**

Carbon monoxide is an invisible, odorless gas and one of the leading causes of immediate mortality associated with fires. Carbon monoxide is produced by incomplete combustion of materials when matter is burned. After inhalation, it binds to all compounds that contain heme. Carbon monoxide affinity for hemoglobin is greater than 200 times that of oxygen, resulting in production of carboxyhemoglobin. Formation of carboxyhemoglobin shifts the oxygen dissociation curve to the left, resulting in more tightly bound oxygen and exponentially decreasing oxygen delivery to tissues. It also binds to myoglobin, reducing oxygen delivery to skeletal muscle and cardiac muscle, which may result in rhabdomyolysis and cardiac dysfunction. Finally, carbon monoxide also causes hypoxia by binding to cytochrome oxidase and decreasing aerobic respiration at the cellular level.

► Cyanide

Hydrogen cyanide is a poisonous compound formed when heat from a fire is exposed to nitrogen-containing polymers, such as the glue that holds together laminate. Once inhaled, hydrogen cyanide binds with high affinity to mitochondrial cytochrome oxidase. This association causes immediate arrest of oxidative phosphorylation resulting in conversion of aerobic metabolism to anaerobic metabolism. With impairment of cellular respiration, hypoxia ensues, resulting in lactic acidosis that can progress to cardiovascular and neurologic dysfunction.

Clinical Findings

► Carbon Monoxide

Serum carboxyhemoglobin level should be measured in a child potentially exposed to carbon monoxide. Normal carboxyhemoglobin level is 1-3% but may be slightly elevated in children who are regularly exposed to tobacco smoke. A carboxyhemoglobin level greater than 15% directly correlates with severity of symptoms. Minor toxicity often presents as light-headedness, headache, nausea, and vomiting. More than 50% of symptoms progress to neurologic dysfunction, including confusion, ataxia, seizure, coma, and death.

Infants are particularly difficult to diagnose, as they may only be irritable and mildly lethargic until more grave signs appear. The classic cherry red pigmentation of the skin is present in less than 40% of patients with carbon monoxide poisoning and should not be used as a single indicator. Most pulse oximeters and equipment used to measure arterial and venous blood gases cannot discriminate oxyhemoglobin from carboxyhemoglobin, and are inaccurate to assess hypoxemia. To obtain accurate tissue oxygenation, the carboxyhemoglobin must be subtracted from the total oxygenation saturation.

Inhalation of 100% oxygen reduces the half-life of carboxyhemoglobin from 4-5 hours to approximately 1 hour. It is important to remember this as many patients are transported by EMS to the emergency department and have been breathing 100% oxygen prior to arrival. The interval of prehospital treatment may lead to inaccuracy in the initial carboxyhemoglobin level and should be considered on a case-by-case basis.

► Cyanide

Similar to carbon monoxide, cyanide poisoning should be suspected in a child who had a potential exposure. Unfortunately, symptoms are often vague and no specific test is readily available in the emergency department to confirm the diagnosis of cyanide toxicity. Patients may show signs and symptoms including headache, confusion, dyspnea, seizures, pulmonary edema, coma, and death. Lactic acidosis not resolved after supplemental oxygen and high venous oxygen saturations may aid in the diagnosis, but both may also occur in many other burn-related pathologies.

Treatment

► Airway Management

Suspicion of significant smoke inhalation injury warrants endotracheal intubation. This includes children with facial or neck burns, carbonaceous sputum, stridor, dyspnea, abnormal lung examination, or significant surface burns. A secure, definitive airway is critical in children with suspected inhalation injury. Compared with adults, airway resistance is more notably increased with relatively less edema due to the smaller diameter of the airway. Even in children with patent airways and moderate injury, endotracheal intubation should be considered. Progressive edema in the subacute phase can lead to difficult intubations and the need for possible surgical airway management.

Succinylcholine is a safe paralytic to use for rapid sequence intubation within 24 hours of initial injury without concern for hyperkalemia. It should not be utilized after 24 hours. The use of cuffed endotracheal tubes is now recommended, a change from prior recommendations. This is a result of an attempt to decrease the number of uncuffed endotracheal tubes that need to be exchanged for cuffed tubes in order to adequately ventilate children. There is significant risk of distortion of the airway associated with exchanging the tube after edema is present. There are documented cases of cardiac arrest in uncomplicated tube exchange lasting less than 30 seconds, secondary to the patient's critically ill status and fragile cardiopulmonary balance.

► Additional Management

Once a definitive airway has been secured or deemed unnecessary, high-flow oxygen should be initiated. Arterial blood gas evaluation and carboxyhemoglobin levels should be obtained. Venous blood gas and lactate levels may also be helpful. Patients with thermal or localized chemical inhalation injury should receive inhaled bronchodilators such as albuterol. An aggressive pulmonary toilet should also be instituted. In the emergency department, suction secretions aggressively, and avoid oversedation to allow for coughing. These measures will be continued and augmented by chest physiotherapy and bronchoscopy once in the intensive care unit.

Carbon Monoxide–Specific Therapy

Elevated carboxyhemoglobin levels or suspected carbon monoxide poisoning should be treated with high-flow 100% oxygen by an appropriate route. Oxygen alone reduces the half-life of carboxyhemoglobin to less than one-third of the corresponding half-life while breathing room air as noted previously.

Hyperbaric oxygen therapy further reduces the half-life and may be considered as a treatment if readily available or possible with transport. It should be considered in patients who are hemodynamically stable with ongoing neurologic dysfunction or unresolved metabolic acidosis. Benefit from hyperbaric treatment for carbon monoxide poisoning is not completely clear, and the decision to institute this therapy should be made on a case-by-case basis. Take into account the small amount of space within the chamber for medical equipment and stability of the patient.

Cyanide–Specific Therapy

Cyanide toxicity has been treated in the past with many different compounds, most notably sodium thiosulfate and hydroxycobalamin. Sodium thiosulfate is no longer routinely recommended in children secondary to the production of the byproduct methemoglobin. Children are especially susceptible to methemoglobinemia due to lower levels of methemoglobin reductase and the ease at which fetal hemoglobin converts to methemoglobin. Hydroxycobalamin combines with cyanide to form the nontoxic compound cyanocobalamin and is treatment of choice in children with suspected cyanide poisoning. Prophylactic treatment of cyanide toxicity is not recommended and hydroxycobalamin should be administered in suspected poisoning only.

Disposition

Children with suspected inhalation injury should be observed in the hospital for at least 24 hours to monitor for delayed onset of signs and symptoms. Patients who are intubated or for whom there is concern for likely intubation should be monitored in an intensive care unit. Patients with carboxyhemoglobin level of 20% or higher should be admitted for observation.

Duke J, Wood F, Semmens J, et al: A study of burn hospitalizations for children younger than 5 years of age: 1983-2008. *Pediatrics.* 2011;127(4):e971-e977 [PMID: 21382945].

Fidkowski CW, Fuzaylov G, Sheridan RL, et al: Inhalation burn injury in children. *Paediatr Anaesth.* 2009;19:147-154 [PMID: 19143954].

Hall AH, Dart R, Bogdan G: Sodium thiosulfate of hydroxycobalamin for the empiric treatment of cyanide poisoning? *Ann Emerg Med.* 2007;49(6):806-813 [PMID: 17098327].

Mlcak RP, Suman OE, Herndon DN: Respiratory management of inhalation injury. *Burns.* 2007;33(1):2-13 [PMID: 17223484].

Toon MH, Maybauer MO, Greenwood JE, et al: Management of acute smoke inhalation injury. *Crit Care Resusc.* 2010;12(1): 53-61 [PMID: 20196715].

CHEMICAL BURNS

General Considerations

Caustic ingestion is the most frequent mechanism for chemical burns in children, compared with occupational exposures in adults. Children younger than 6 years often go through a physical exploratory phase that includes touching and sometimes tasting items within their reach. Many household items are toxic when they contact skin or mucosa. A number of substances have been implicated in pediatric chemical burns, and generally fall into two types: acids and alkalis. Factors that contribute to the mortality and morbidity associated with such ingestions include pH and preparation of the chemical, tissue contact time, and exposed location (especially if location impairs irrigation).

Burns caused by acidic substances cause coagulative necrosis, limiting the depth of the burn. Commonly ingested household acids include toilet bowl cleaners, battery acids, and drain cleaners. In contrast, alkali burns produce liquefactive necrosis that leads to a deeper burn and increased mortality and morbidity. Alkaline substances also induce thrombosis in surrounding vasculature, which causes additional tissue ischemia. Common household alkalis are drain cleaner, lye-containing soaps, and oven cleaners. Each type of chemical burns can cause gastrointestinal injury including perforation and esophageal and pyloric strictures.

Clinical Findings

Children presenting to the emergency department following chemical ingestion or skin exposure can have a wide range of presentations, from asymptomatic to sepsis secondary to a perforated viscus. Studies have attempted to define signs and symptoms that put a patient at increased risk for significant gastrointestinal injury after ingestion, but no clear guidelines exist. History and physical examination should be directed to complaints of nausea, vomiting, dysphagia, difficulty handling secretions, stridor, visible mucosal injury or ulcerations, and abdominal pain. Absence of visible injury in the oropharynx does not exclude possible esophageal or gastrointestinal pathology. Substantial ingestions can lead to disseminated intravascular coagulation, acute renal failure, and acute liver failure.

Treatment

The mainstay of treatment for a cutaneous chemical-related burn is irrigation with large amounts of water. Ingested caustic agents require a more complicated treatment plan. Irrigating the esophagus and stomach with large quantities can lead to emesis of the offending toxic substance, which should be avoided to limit reexposure of the esophageal and oral tissues. A considerable amount of liquid within the stomach also obstructs the view of gastric mucosa during endoscopy, which is currently the gold standard for diagnosis of esophageal and gastric damage.

Antiemetics should be used to prevent or limit emesis. Poison Control should be contacted (in the United States, call (800) 222-1222) for more information about specific chemical exposures and to report the ingestion to the national databank. The airway should be assessed upon initial examination and secured if necessary.

▶ Disposition

A child presenting with what appears to be a surgical abdomen secondary to perforated esophagus or viscus warrants emergent evaluation by a surgeon. Endoscopy may be needed to determine extent of injury. Significant symptoms or worsening clinical condition indicates the need for further emergency department observation or admission.

ELECTRICAL BURNS

See Chapter 45.

CONTACT BURNS

Contact burns are the second most common cause of pediatric burns that present to emergency departments nationwide. Contact burns occur when skin touches a hot surface, including irons, ovens, stovetops, curling irons, motorcycle exhaust pipes, and related heat sources. An additional mechanism for contact burns is prolonged exposure to an object with a lesser temperature, such as a heating pad.

▶ Clinical Findings

Contact burns occur predominately on the upper extremities secondary to the mechanism of injury. Burns are usually limited to a small percent of body surface area but can extend quite deep. As with all pediatric injuries, close examination for patterns should be conducted to help rule out non-accidental trauma as a cause (see Chapter 5).

▶ Treatment

Treatment of contact burns varies upon the degree of dermal involvement and correlates with the treatment regiments for pediatric thermal burns. Local wound care and analgesia are the primary emergent treatments. Most contact burns are accidental in nature. Caregiver and patient education should also be provided in an effort to prevent future contact burns.

▶ Disposition

Minor contact burns can be managed similarly to thermal burns with local wound care, oral analgesia, and outpatient follow-up. More extensive contact burns should be managed as major thermal burns with admission and possible transfer to a burn center.

SUNBURNS

Sunburns are caused by an inflammatory response within the skin in reaction to ultraviolet (UV) ray exposure. They are more prominent in fair-skinned individuals but can occur with any skin type. Sunburns are usually limited to first-degree and minor second-degree burns but can be more extensive with prolonged exposure to UV rays and underlying predisposition. Tanning beds are now a significant cause of sunburn and have been implicated in the sunburns of even young children but are more common in adolescents.

▶ Clinical Findings

Sunburns are very common and easy to recognize clinically by a basic history and physical examination. Skin inflammation peaks in approximately 12-24 hours and declines in clinical significance thereafter. Sunburns are staged with the same criteria as all other thermal burns based on physical examination findings.

▶ Treatment

The primary treatment for most sunburns is supportive care with analgesia by oral nonsteroidal agents. Although uncommon, more serious sunburns may be treated like thermal burns with fluid resuscitation and parenteral analgesia. Patient and caregiver education should be provided while in the emergency department as an endeavor to prevent future sunburns and the long-term sequelae of skin cancers.

▶ Disposition

Most patients with sunburns evaluated and treated within the emergency department can be discharged home to follow-up with their primary care physician as needed. More extensive burns and requiring fluid resuscitation or parenteral analgesia should be admitted for additional observation and treatment.

Faurschou A, Wulf HC: Topical corticosteroids in the treatment of acute sunburn. *Arch Dermatol.* 2008;144(5):620-624 [PMID: 18490588].

Salzman M, O'Malley RN: Updates on the evaluation and management of caustic exposures. *Emerg Med Clin North Am.* 2007;25(2):459-476 [PMID: 17482028].

Smollin CG: Toxicology: Pearls and pitfalls in the use of antidotes. *Emerg Med Clin North Am.* 2010;28(1):149-161 [PMID: 19945604].

Toon MH, Maybauer DM, Arceneaux LL, et al: Children with burn injuries: Assessment of trauma, neglect, violence and abuse. *J Inj Violence Res.* 2011;3(2):98-110 [PMID: 21498973].

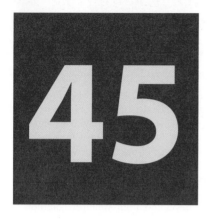

Environmental Emergencies

Dorian Drigalla, MD, FACEP

Tyler McSpadden, MD

HEAT EXPOSURE EMERGENCIES

GENERAL CONSIDERATIONS

Heat-related illnesses occur when the body's ability to dissipate heat is overcome by endogenous and/or environmental heat burdens. As the core body temperature (CBT) rises, a continuum of disease occurs from mild cutaneous findings to coma and death. Mild heat disorders such as heat edema and heat cramps are sequelae of the body's compensatory mechanisms to dissipate heat. Treatment principles are aimed primarily at supportive care for mild disease, and cooling plus hydration for more serious hyperthermic injuries. Children are at no increased risk due to anatomic or physiologic reasons compared with adults. However, infants and very young children can be at greater risk of heat-related illness in settings of abandonment, neglect, and inability to rehydrate.

The body uses four mechanisms to dissipate heat: radiation, conduction, convection, and evaporation. The body attempts to thermoregulate by two physiologic methods. Shunting of blood from core to dilated peripheral vessels allows conduction and convection, if ambient temperature and air movement allow for a heat gradient. Sweating allows for skin surface evaporation and is effective up to a relative humidity of about 75%. Very high temperatures, prolonged exposures, and high relative humidity can overwhelm the body's heat dissipation efforts and lead to heat-related illness.

HEAT RASH (MILIARIA RUBRA)

Clinical Findings

Heat rash occurs when sweat saturates the skin, mixes with sebum and dead skin cells, and clogs the sweat ducts. It is characterized by a papulovesicular rash, which may be pruritic or mildly painful. Small pustules or vesicles may appear as the obstructed ducts continue to produce sweat, infiltrating the dermis and epidermis. Outbreaks usually occur in clothed areas where clothing traps the sweat against the skin, preventing sweat from evaporation or run off.

Treatment

Keeping the area cool and dry should provide resolution within a week. Lotions such as calamine and topical corticosteroids may provide symptomatic relief if the rash is uncomfortable. Rarely, staphylococcal or streptococcal superinfection may result from the vesicular rash. Secondary infections should be treated with appropriate topical or oral antibiotics.

Disposition

In the absence of severe cellulitis or rapidly spreading infection, patients with heat rash may be discharged home. Precautions should be given to parents regarding signs of spreading infection.

HEAT EDEMA

Clinical Findings

Heat edema is more typical in older persons but can occur in children. It is a benign bilateral swelling of the (typically lower) extremities due to peripheral vasodilation. It is seen almost exclusively in nonacclimatized individuals during the first few days of exposure to very hot conditions. The interstitial fluid will usually resolve spontaneously as acclimatization occurs.

Treatment

Compressive stockings and elevation of the extremities should hasten resolution. Do not administer diuretics as they are not needed and could lead to volume depletion and more serious heat injury in an already susceptible patient.

Disposition

Patients can be discharged home with precautions and appropriate follow-up.

HEAT SYNCOPE

Clinical Findings

Heat syncope is a possible deleterious effect of peripheral vasodilation and venous pooling. Seen most commonly in children who are playing sports or exercising, then cease activity temporarily, perhaps to sit down, allowing blood to pool in the extremities. Upon standing or resumption of activity, syncope results from transient cerebral hypoperfusion.

Treatment

Symptoms should resolve quickly once the patient is in the supine position with legs elevated to increase venous return. Emergency department evaluation should aim at ruling out potential causes of syncope in the child's age group, especially if the circumstances surrounding the event are unclear. Hypovolemia and orthostasis are the most likely etiologies. Orthostatic vital signs should be measured and oral or intravenous (IV) hydration should occur until the patient is no longer orthostatic. Consider an electrocardiogram (ECG).

Disposition

Discharge home is appropriate when the patient is tolerating fluids by mouth, no further symptoms have occurred, vital signs have normalized, and additional serious etiologies have been excluded.

HEAT CRAMPS

Clinical Findings

Heat exposure with excessive sweating, usually in the setting of physical activity, may lead to painful spasm/contracture of muscles. Water and sodium depletion from sweating coupled with inadequate rehydration during activity is the usually setting. The large muscle groups of the lower extremities (calves, quadriceps) are most commonly involved followed by the arms and abdominal muscles.

Treatment

Symptoms typically respond well to passive stretching of the affected muscles and oral rehydration with an electrolyte solution. In cases of refractory or persistently recurrent cramps, IV hydration with a 20 mL/kg bolus of normal saline (NS) is indicated and often rapidly curative.

Disposition

Patients with heat cramps can typically be discharged home with precautions and further hydration instructions. If symptoms persist in the emergency department, consider laboratory evaluation and the possibility of other underlying etiologies (rhabdomyolysis).

HEAT EXHAUSTION

General Considerations

More serious illnesses occur with the rise of CBT and failure of the body's own thermoregulation. Intrinsic heat and environmental exposure to heat can play a role in worsening a clinical picture. Hyponatremia may result from excessive dehydration, and may persist or worsen when oral rehydration is accomplished with water rather than electrolyte solutions. Hyponatremia and dehydration are the precipitating causes of the symptoms of heat exhaustion. Without recognition or adequate treatment, heat exhaustion easily and rapidly progresses to heat stroke.

Clinical Findings

Heat exhaustion may present as malaise, fatigue, dizziness, cramps, nausea, vomiting, weakness, and/or syncope in the setting of heat exposure. Patients will likely have profuse sweating with cold and clammy skin. Keys to diagnosis are normal mental status and a CBT less than 40°C (104°F) with a known exposure to a hot environment. Children can progress rapidly to heat stroke, therefore close observation and frequent reassessment of CBT and mental status are crucial.

Treatment

The patient with normal neurologic status and CBT between 37-40°C (98.6-104°F) may need supportive treatment only. Move the patient to a cool environment and provide oral or IV hydration allowing the CBT to normalize and reverse symptoms. Laboratory evaluation is indicated to assess for electrolyte disturbance, especially hyponatremia. If the patient exhibits a decline in cognition or other evidence of central nervous system (CNS) disturbance, initiate treatment for heat stroke immediately while evaluating for other potential causes.

Disposition

Children with heat exhaustion should be hospitalized to observe for normalization of symptoms and clinical findings.

HEAT STROKE

With prolonged elevation of the CBT above 41-42°C (104-106°F), direct cellular injury begins to occur. Proteins are denatured and precipitate causing cell lysis and accumulation of toxins. Cytokines are produced that initiate inflammatory cascades. Vascular endothelium is damaged causing impaired circulation and possibly disseminated intravascular coagulation. Ensuing ischemia and inflammation may lead to multisystem organ failure. Without prompt treatment, death or permanent disability is possible.

Clinical Findings

Heat stroke may present with signs or symptoms of heat exhaustion coupled with neurologic dysfunction and a CBT greater than 40°C (104°F). Keep in mind that some cooling may have occurred during transportation and the temperature may be less than 40°C at the time of presentation. Patients with heat stroke due to high environmental heat exposure may exhibit warm, dry skin, whereas those with exertional heat stroke may still be sweaty. Although the appearance of the skin and absence of sweat (anhidrosis) are conventionally part of the diagnosis of heat stroke, they have no bearing on management. Neurologic symptoms may be subtle such as sluggishness or confusion, but in children tend to be more profound such as delirium, hallucination, seizure, or coma. If the time of exposure is very long or there is a delay in seeking care, the patient may exhibit signs of organ failure at initial presentation. A classic scenario is an infant or toddler locked in a hot car for a long period of time, presenting in extremis. Without a clear history, heat stroke may easily be confused with sepsis, toxic ingestion, or status epilepticus.

Treatment

Upon arrival and identification of possible heat injury, move the patient into a cool environment. Assess airway, breathing, and circulation (ABC) and control the airway if necessary. If the patient is seizing, use benzodiazepines to control seizure activity. Assess CBT by performing a rectal temperature immediately. Begin external cooling immediately. Blood should be drawn for laboratory evaluation but not at the expense of delaying cooling. If possible, ice-water immersion provides the most efficient cooling and should be the first choice for rapid reduction of CBT. Ice-water immersion may not be feasible due to mechanical ventilation or other constraints related to the patient or facility. Dousing with water and fanning the patient combined with ice pack application to the groin, neck, and axilla is an alternative method until more advanced cooling means can be used. Peritoneal lavage with cold, potassium-free dialysate solution, and continuous bladder irrigation with refrigerated saline may aid cooling efforts. Frequently reassess the rectal temperature and continue cooling measures until a CBT less than 39°C is reached, ideally in the first 30-60 minutes. Once cooling strategies are initiated, evaluation for evidence of end-organ failure should occur. Obtain an arterial blood gas (ABG) or venous

blood gas (VBG) to determine acid-base status, especially if the child exhibits respiratory distress. Blood glucose should be checked to assess for hypoglycemia. CBC, complete metabolic profile (CMP), prothrombin time (PT), international normalized ratio (INR), creatine kinase (CK), and urinalysis will be useful to evaluate for DIC, liver injury, electrolyte derangement, rhabdomyolysis, and renal failure. In the setting of respiratory distress, a chest radiograph should be ordered to evaluate for pulmonary edema. Persistent neurologic symptoms or apparent increased intracranial pressure (ICP) despite cooling efforts warrant a heat CT. In the setting of an arrhythmia, delay electrical cardioversion until the CBT is less than 39°C (102°F).

The remainder of management is targeted at supportive care and addressing organ injury or failure that has occurred. IV fluid therapy will not only be beneficial in the treatment of rhabdomyolysis, hypovolemia, and renal failure but will also contribute to cooling. Benzodiazepines can be beneficial by reducing the shivering that may accompany cooling strategies and slow the cooling process.

Disposition

Any child presenting with heat stroke should be admitted to pediatric intensive care unit (PICU) or a similar level of care following cooling and resuscitation. Delayed manifestation of organ failure is possible and close observation is paramount due to the high potential for morbidity and mortality.

Adams T, Stacey E, Stacey S, et al: Exertional heat stroke. *Br J Hosp Med.* 2012;73(2):72-78 [PMID: 22504748].

Bouchama A, Dehbi M, Chaves-Carballo E: Cooling and hemodynamic management in heatstroke: Practical recommendations. *Crit Care.* 2007;11:R54 [PMID: 17498312].

Howe AS, Boden BP: Heat-related illness in athletes. *Am J Sports Med.* 2007;35(8):1384-1395 [PMID: 17609528].

McDermott BP, Casa DJ, Ganio MS, et al: Acute whole-body cooling for exercise-induced hyperthermia: A systematic review. *J Athl Train.* 2009;44:84 [PMID: 19180223].

Rowland T: Thermoregulation during exercise in the heat in children: Old concepts revisited. *J Appl Physiol.* 2008;105(2):718-724 [PMID: 18079269].

COLD EXPOSURE EMERGENCIES

CHILBLAINS (PERNIO)

Clinical Findings

Chilblains (pernio or perniosis) is an inflammatory skin condition thought to be caused by an abnormal vascular response to cold exposure. Chilblains are characterized by erythematous to violaceous painful lesions noted most commonly on the distal extremities, ears and nose in the setting of repeated cold exposure. Patients may experience a prodrome of tingling or itching in the affected area shortly after cold exposure followed 12-24 hours later by painful lesions which typically resolve spontaneously after 1-3 weeks. Although rare, in some patients these lesions can progress to bullae or ulcerations and chronic reexposure can lead to fibrosis or scarring of the affected area.

Treatment

Treatment is supportive and aimed primarily at prevention. Affected areas should be wrapped in warm dry material with care taken to avoid mechanical trauma. Counsel the patient and parents about avoiding cold exposure and using extra garments for protection as a prevention strategy. Some success has been reported using nifedipine in acute treatment and prophylaxis of chilblains. Additionally, topical and oral corticosteroids may provide symptomatic relief.

Disposition

Because chilblains is a clinical diagnosis of exclusion and there is a reported association with rheumatologic disease, referral from the emergency department to the child's pediatrician or a rheumatologist for further workup should be considered.

Prakash S, Weisman MH: Idiopathic chilblains. *Am J Med.* 2009; 122(12):1152-1155 [PMID: 19958897].

Vano-Galvan S, Martorell A: Chilblains. *CMAJ.* 2012;184(1):67 [PMID: 22025653].

FROSTBITE

Frostbite is caused by exposure of tissue to freezing temperature resulting in the formation of ice crystals within the intracellular and extracellular spaces. Vasoconstriction, endothelial damage, and cell lysis lead to a prothrombotic state resulting in capillary occlusion. Ischemia is the major factor in permanent tissue loss due to frostbite. In the pediatric patient, an immobilizing injury, inadequate clothing,

and prolonged exposure to a cold environment are major contributing factors. Initial cold sensation progresses to painful or numb areas of skin blanching, and ends with firm, insensate tissue and white or waxy skin.

Clinical Findings

In initial assessment of frostbite, the two most important variables are the time from injury and clinical appearance of the tissue. Because many frostbite injuries occur on recreational trips (hiking, climbing) and medical attention is distant, it is important to establish the chronicity of injury because timing will affect treatment strategies. Frostbite injuries are classified based on four clinical features: depth of tissue freezing, color of tissue, blistering/necrosis, and tissue edema (Table 45–1). The full extent of the injury and clear demarcation may not be apparent for days after the insult.

Treatment

Treatment of frostbite has four primary goals:

- Treatment of life-threatening comorbid conditions.
- Rewarming.
- Prevention of infection and further injury.
- Restoration of blood flow to ischemic areas.

Traumatic immobilizing injury is a common underlying cause of pediatric frostbite and should be suspected. Systemic hypothermia should also be suspected and treatment prioritized before focusing on localized injury.

Once life-threatening conditions are addressed, begin rewarming the affected areas by immersion in a whirlpool bath or other water source containing chlorhexidine or another antiseptic agent at 40-41°C (104-106°F) for 30 minutes or until all tissues are warm, red, and pliable. A commercial foot spa may be an acceptable alternative to whirlpool, although warm water will likely need to be added periodically because these devices do not operate at

Table 45–1. Classification of frostbite.

Class	Depth of Skin Freezing	Color of Tissue	Blistering/Necrosis	Tissue Edema
1	Partial thickness	Erythematous/hyperemic	None	Little or none
2	Full thickness	Erythematous	Clear, fluid-filled bullae	Moderate
3	Full thickness *and* subcutaneous involvement	Blue or black	Hemorrhagic blisters; small areas of necrosis possible	Significant
4	Full thickness, *and* subcutaneous tissue, muscle, tendon, and bone involvement	Initial: mottled or red Later: black, mummified	Extensive necrosis	Little or none

the recommended 40°C. Rewarming should be performed 30 minutes twice daily until there is evidence of tissue healing or clear demarcation of necrosis. Prehospital rewarming should not be initiated if there is a possibility of refreezing as freeze-thaw-freeze injuries are more damaging than single freeze events. Do not massage the affected area as this will cause further tissue damage.

Necrotic tissue is a potential nidus for infection. A patient with evidence of nonviable tissue should be treated with broad-spectrum antibiotics and a tetanus vaccine. Early surgical debridement of necrotic-appearing tissue is not recommended because of the time interval for clear demarcation to occur. Clear, nontense blisters may be left alone but some sources recommend sterile aspiration of tense or hemorrhagic bullae due to increased risk of infection. Affected areas should be kept warm and dry with loose protective bandaging to prevent further damage to this friable tissue. In the case of lower extremity frostbite, the patient should be kept non–weight-bearing. Treatment with ibuprofen may limit prostaglandin production in inflamed tissue and may prove beneficial.

There is evidence to support the use of intra-arterial tissue plasminogen activator (tPA) for patients presenting within 24 hours of injury and with evidence of severe frostbite in which tissue loss is expected. Although there has been no pediatric study to date, there is no contraindication for use of this strategy in children who otherwise have no contraindication to thrombolysis. A leading cause of frostbite in the pediatric population is immobilizing trauma and therefore a high percentage of children will have contraindication to tPA. If the patient presents within 24 hours of injury and has evidence of Class 3-4 frostbite, consider ordering magnetic resonance angiography (MRA) or computed tomography angiography (CTA) of the affected limb(s) to assess for intra-arterial thrombosis. If an area of occlusion is identified, consider consultation with an interventional radiologist for intra-arterial tPA administration. In one small study, the incidence of digital amputation following frostbite was reduced from 41% without tPA administration to 10% with thrombolysis. Reperfusion will likely cause increased edema to the area and may result in compartment syndrome.

Disposition

Patients with nonextensive Class 1 frostbite may be discharged home after rewarming with outpatient follow-up. Children with Class 2 or above injury or extensive Class 1 frostbite involving two or more extremities or a large surface area should be admitted for further observation. As mentioned, distinguishing among classifications and demarcating frostbite can be very difficult and sometimes take many days. If significant tissue destruction occurs, rhabdomyolysis, secondary infection, or sepsis may complicate the course.

Pain control is important both in the acute phase and in the long term and will likely be better facilitated as an inpatient.

Bruen KJ, Ballard JR, Morris SE, et al: Reduction of the incidence of amputation in frostbite injury with thrombolytic therapy. *Arch Surg.* 2007;142:546-551 [PMID: 17576891].

Hallam MJ, Cubison T, Dheansa B: Managing frostbite. *BMJ.* 2010;341:c5864 [PMID: 21097571].

Imray C, Grieve A, Dhilon S: Cold damage to the extremities: Frostbite and non-freezing cold injuries. *Postgrad Med J.* 2009;85:481-488 [PMID: 19734516].

HYPOTHERMIA

General Considerations

Accidental hypothermia is an unintended decrease in CBT less than 35°C (95°F). Hypothermia results from exposure to a low enough temperature for a sufficient amount of time to overwhelm the body's ability to compensate. Hypothermia is classified as: mild 32-35°C (90-95°F), moderate 28-32°C (82-90°F), and severe less than 28°C (82°F). Although there are predicted clinical features within each temperature range, the disease process represents a continuum from mild compensatory symptoms (shivering) to fatal disturbances in physiology (asystole, ventricular fibrillation.) Treatment principles for hypothermia are guided by the degree of hypothermia and clinical features of the patient. Treatment consists primarily of rewarming, fluid resuscitation, and cardiopulmonary resuscitation.

Key physiologic differences in children make them more susceptible to hypothermia. Infants do not have the ability to shiver. Younger children have limited glycogen stores to increase metabolism. Also, children have a higher ratio of body surface area to mass leading to increased heat loss to the environment. Hypovolemia, blood sludging due to cold, bradycardia, and decreased cardiac contractility contribute to decreased cardiac output and circulatory collapse.

Clinical Findings

Mild hypothermia: 32-35°C (90-95°F). This stage is characterized by the body's attempt to generate and preserve heat. Peripheral vasoconstriction causes cyanosis of the hands, lips, and feet, as well as pallor and prolonged capillary refill time. If older than 1 year, the child will likely be shivering and skin will exhibit piloerection. Mental status should be intact.

Moderate hypothermia: 28-32°C (82-90°F). In this stage the body's compensatory mechanisms are overwhelmed and physiologic disturbance ensues. Shivering stops and mental status begins to be depressed. Children may initially appear agitated and clumsy giving way to somnolence and confusion. Respiratory rate and heart rate may fluctuate before slowing. Fatal arrhythmias are possible.

Severe hypothermia < 28°C (82°F): Below 28°C, enzymatic disturbance gives rise to severe manifestations of hypothermia. The child may appear stuporous or comatose. In extreme cases the pupils may be fixed and signs of life absent. Muscle filament dysfunction may cause rigidity even though the tissue is well above freezing temperature. Respiration may be severely depressed or absent and arrhythmias are likely.

Treatment

▶ Prehospital Care

Avoid rough handling of the patient and maintain the patient in a horizontal position, in consideration of the potentially unstable myocardium that may be easily irritated into a fatal arrhythmia. Wet clothing should be removed, and the patient wrapped in blankets or warm dry clothes during transport. Further attempts at rewarming should be delayed until the child is brought to the emergency department. This is to avoid core temperature after drop that can result from mobilization of cold, acidotic blood from the extremities to the central circulation.

▶ Initial Evaluation

Assess the ABC. Some variances to the normal treatment of primary survey abnormalities exist and are discussed below. Traumatic immobilizing injury is a leading cause of hypothermia in children, and a careful secondary survey should be undertaken, especially if the child is altered or unable to provide a clear history. Remove remaining wet clothing, and wrap the patient in warm dry blankets. Core temperature should be measured with a low reading thermometer. Rectal temperature readings are the most widely used but rectal temperature may lag behind core temperature, especially stool is present in the rectal vault. Esophageal probes carry the risk of myocardial agitation during placement and may be falsely elevated by warm air in the trachea. Central venous probes may be affected by the administration of warm fluids. Bladder probes via a temperature-sensing Foley are accurate and will be adversely affected only if patient is receiving warm peritoneal lavage.

Laboratory and imaging studies are indicated but should not delay rewarming. Electrolytes, blood count, glucose, lipase, and coagulation studies are of particular interest in management. ECG analysis may reveal J point elevation (see Figure 45–1), slowed conduction with prolonged intervals, or a variety of arrhythmias. Imaging should include chest x-ray to assess for aspiration or pulmonary edema, especially if the patient has respiratory symptoms. Additional imaging may be indicated in the setting of trauma but should not interfere with rewarming efforts.

▶ Management

Rewarming is guided by the degree of hypothermia, cardiopulmonary status of the patient, and availability of each

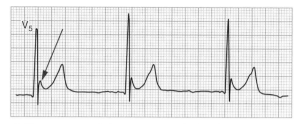

▲ **Figure 45–1.** Osborn wave (marked with an arrow), noted immediately after the QRS complex, in hypothermia.

modality. Extensive supportive care may be necessary during rewarming and is discussed below. Rapid institution of rewarming is the most crucial element of treatment, and other measures may not be effective until core temperature begins to rise.

▶ Rewarming Modalities

- Passive rewarming. Remove wet clothing, dry the patient, and insulate with warm blankets. This allows for the body to warm itself while preventing further heat loss.

- Forced air rewarmers. Available in most institutions as they are used frequently in the operating room setting. They are efficacious but can cause peripheral vasodilation and shunting of cold, acidotic blood to the central circulation causing core temperature afterdrop.

- Heat lamps or radiant heat devices. Adjunct to other therapies, also keep the treatment area warm.

- Heating pads/packs. Apply to the chest or abdomen. Frequent reassessment of the underlying skin is necessary as these may produce burns to underperfused skin.

- Warm, humidified oxygen via non-rebreather. Safe and acceptable for most patients as an adjunct, prevents further heat loss via respiration.

- Warmed IV fluid. Indicated for most hypothermic children. Special delivery systems are required for the delivery of warm IV fluid (normal IV tubing and equipment will result in cooling of the fluid prior to infusion and may worsen the situation).

- Warm saline lavage. Very effective at raising the CBT. Without the capability to heat large quantities of saline quickly, heated tap water may be substituted. Fluid warmed to 40-44°C (104-111°F) may be utilized by

  - Bladder irrigation: Insert a three-way Foley catheter and provide continuous bladder irrigation with warmed fluid.

  - Gastric lavage: Easily applied through a nasogastric or orogastric tube, may increase aspiration risk and is best used in the intubated patient.

- Peritoneal lavage: A large-caliber catheter may be easily inserted to peritoneal space and warm saline or potassium-free dialysate solution periodically infused and withdrawn. This carries the potential for internal organ damage via traumatic insertion or thermal injury and should be used with caution.

- Pleural lavage: The most effective warmed-fluid method. This involves placement of one or more chest tubes through which warm saline is infused and drained. A number of strategies exist for accomplishing pleural lavage, none of which has proven clinically superior. The simplest method involves placing one large gauge left-sided chest tube, inserting 500-mL warm saline, clamping the tube for 2-3 minutes, and then allowing the fluid drain out. This can also be performed with bilateral chest tubes and alternating the side of infusion with each application. Alternatively, place two chest tubes on the same side, one anterior and one posterior which allow for almost continuous infusion of warm fluid. Theoretically, the heart will be warmed more efficiently by left-sided pleural lavage; however, there is possible increased risk of inducing cardiac arrhythmia by irritating the left ventricle during tube placement. No evidence exists to recommend one method over the other.

- Extracorporeal warming: In extreme cases and when available, extracorporeal warming may be necessary. Cardiac bypass and extracorporeal membrane oxygenation (ECMO) are the most effective means of raising CBT and also provide circulatory support and oxygenation. The primary contraindication to using these modalities is trauma due to risk of bleeding with heparin but this may be avoided by using nonheparinized bypass circuits when available.

▶ Hypothermia

Mild hypothermia: Children with mild hypothermia may respond well to passive rewarming alone. It is important to continually monitor the CBT to assess for effectiveness of treatment and to assure that no afterdrop occurs. Forced-air rewarmers and warm, humidified oxygen are also appropriate for both comfort and to speed rewarming.

Moderate hypothermia: In this temperature range (28-32°C), serious pathology is a possibility and close extended monitoring is necessary. If respiratory status is intact, warm humidified oxygen should be applied and warm saline infusion begun. A warm fluid bolus of 20 mL/kg should precede other measures due to the potential for rewarming shock when peripheral vasodilation occurs. The combination of warm IV fluids and a forced air rewarmer may be sufficient to treat children in this stage of hypothermia, however cardiopulmonary involvement is possible and more invasive

measures may be required. Regardless of temperature, circulatory collapse should be treated as severe hypothermia.

Severe hypothermia: Treatment for severe hypothermia depends largely on circulatory status. In many cases, pulse and respiration may be very slow and difficult to detect. If the child has no detectable pulse, extracorporeal warming is indicated and should be instituted if available. If unavailable or in the setting of significant delay, pleural lavage in combination with warm fluid boluses and other warming modalities should be started immediately. Advanced life-support measures including CPR should be initiated. There are two key advanced life-support modifications for the hypothermic child. First, the hypothermic myocardium is unlikely to respond to defibrillation. If a shockable rhythm is present (ventricular fibrillation or pulseless ventricular tachycardia), attempt defibrillation but note that repeated shocks will be unlikely to succeed until rewarming occurs. Second, the cold liver does not metabolize medications as rapidly so consider increasing the spacing of doses. Continue chest compressions until return of spontaneous circulation or the availability of cardiac bypass. If the child has or regains a pulse, pleural lavage, warm saline fluid resuscitation, and other warming methods should be instituted without delay. Bradyarrhythmias are common in hypothermia but are well tolerated due to the cerebral protective effects of the cold. Refrain from cardiac pacing or chest compressions in the presence of a pulse.

Intensive supportive care will likely be required. Respiratory support may be necessary and intubation should be accomplished in the gentlest manner possible to avoid irritating the myocardium. Venous access is crucial and two large-bore IVs are a minimum. Consider placing a femoral line early as vasoconstriction may make peripheral lines difficult to obtain. Internal jugular and subclavian lines should be avoided to prevent inducing arrhythmia.

Hypoglycemia is common in hypothermia and should be treated with 0.5-g/kg dextrose. Comorbid traumatic injury or underlying medical conditions should be evaluated and treated appropriately.

Hypothermia can have a profound protective affect on the body, particularly the brain. A number of cases report complete neurologic recovery in hypothermic patients following prolonged cardiac arrest. For this reason, resuscitative measures should not be withdrawn until a patient has reached a CBT of 35°C and is still refractory to advanced life-support measures.

Disposition

After assessment for underlying conditions or injury that may have led to hypothermia, children with mild hypothermia may be safely discharged home if they have achieved normothermia and baseline mental status. Children with moderate or severe hypothermia should be admitted for extended monitoring and continued therapy. Pulmonary edema, coagulopathy, and renal failure are possible following rewarming. Severe cases and patients with significantly invasive treatment strategies should be cared for in an intensive care setting.

Avellanas ML, Ricart A, Botella J, et al: Management of severe accidental hypothermia. *Med Intensiva.* 2012;36:200-212 [PMID: 22325642].

Brown DJ, Brugger H, Boyd J, et al: Accidental hypothermia. *N Engl J Med.* 2012;367(20):1930-1938 [PMID: 23150960].

Gordon L, Peek GJ, Ellerton JA: Extracorporeal life support is recommended for severe accidental hypothermia. *BMJ.* 2010;341:c7411 [PMID: 21193508].

Hughes A, Riou P, Day P: Full neurological recovery from profound (18.0 degrees C) acute accidental hypothermia: Successful resuscitation using active invasive rewarming techniques. *Emerg Med J.* 2007;24(7):511-512 [PMID: 17582054].

Kjaergaard B, Bach P: Warming of patients with accidental hypothermia using warm water pleural lavage. *Resuscitation.* 2006;68(2):203-207 [PMID: 16378671].

Waibel BH, Durham CA, Newell MA, et al: Impact of hypothermia in the rural, pediatric trauma patient. *Pediatr Crit Care Med.* 2010;11(2):199-204 [PMID: 19794329].

HIGH-ALTITUDE ILLNESS

General Considerations

High-altitude illness is a collective term for the systemic, cerebral, and pulmonary pathologies that occur following ascent to high altitude. Most manifestations of high-altitude illness may be prevented by gradual ascent with adequate time for acclimatization. There are three types of high-altitude illness: acute mountain sickness (AMS), high-altitude cerebral edema (HACE), and high-altitude pulmonary edema (HAPE). The conditions result from the hypoxic stress of high-altitude and are characterized by excessive extravascular fluid accumulation. Cerebral and pulmonary manifestations of high-altitude illness may be fatal if untreated, but all types respond to descent from altitude and oxygen therapy. Children with a high-altitude illness should halt ascending and descent from altitude should be considered.

Prevention

Although not studied in children, some authors recommend prophylactic medications to prevent or lessen disease. Acetazolamide is used as prophylaxis for AMS and HACE in the absence of sulfa allergy. It speeds acclimatization by enhancing renal excretion of bicarbonate to combat respiratory alkalosis. It can be given in a pediatric dose of 2.5 mg/kg twice daily up to 125 mg per dose beginning the day before ascent and again the next 2 days or until maximum altitude is reached. Dexamethasone is useful for treatment of moderate to severe AMS or HACE and is dosed at 0.15 mg/kg

every 6 hours. It does not aid in acclimatization and should be reserved for symptomatic patients. Nifedipine is used for HAPE prevention and may be given to children in a dose of 0.5 mg/kg up to 20 mg every 8 hours beginning the day prior to ascent and continuing for 3-5 days at maximum altitude. Nifedipine is not universally recommended in children, and further studies regarding its use in altitude illness are warranted.

It is impossible to predict if otherwise healthy children will suffer from high-altitude illness, but some underlying factors may predispose them. Rapid ascent to high-altitude is a common historical finding. History of high-altitude illness at a similar altitude would likely warrant prophylaxis. Recent or current upper respiratory infection, pneumonia, or other infection are independent risk factors for HAPE. Children with congenital cardiac defects or Down syndrome are at higher risk for HAI. Chronic medical conditions such as sickle cell anemia, cystic fibrosis, and obstructive sleep apnea may be relative contraindications to high-altitude travel when slow, gradual ascent is not possible.

ACUTE MOUNTAIN SICKNESS

Clinical Findings

Acute mountain sickness (AMS) is the most common form of high-altitude illness and is thought to be on a continuum of disease with HACE. In children with AMS, headache will likely be the first symptom combined with nausea, vomiting, or anorexia, light-headedness, weakness, and fatigue. Time to onset can vary widely from 1-2 hours to 3-4 days. In younger children and infants, AMS may be more difficult to recognize, presenting only as fussiness, poor appetite, vomiting, or decreased sleep. Emergency department physicians should have a low threshold for suspecting AMS in younger children because it may be easily mistaken for travel-associated behavioral changes and if unrecognized may progress to potentially fatal HAPE or HACE.

Treatment

Mild cases of AMS may be treated with cessation of ascent, rest, supplemental oxygen, and symptomatic therapy such as NSAIDs for headache and antiemetics for nausea. Symptoms should resolve as acclimatization occurs. In patients with worsening symptoms, decreased mental status, or suspicion of developing HACE or HAPE, rapid descent to a level at or below 1500 m (4000 ft) or at least down 1000 m (3281 ft) from the current altitude is indicated. If descent is not possible or will be delayed, administration of supplemental oxygen via facemask or CPAP, or use of a portable hyperbaric chamber (Gamow bag) will serve as temporizing measures.

Pharmacologic treatment with acetazolamide may improve symptoms but is better for prophylaxis. Dexamethasone 0.15 mg/kg may be given every 6 hours and is more reliable in more significant cases. Emergency department evaluation of children recently ascended to high altitude should include a chest x-ray in the setting of pulmonary signs or symptoms.

Disposition

Cessation of ascent to higher altitude may allow for acclimatization. Parents should be advised to limit exertional activity and avoid airline flights early in recovery. If the patient is being treated at an emergency department or other site at high altitude, and in the setting of persistent clinical findings, descent is the key to management and disposition. Once symptoms resolve and the patient is not taking dexamethasone, continued ascent is acceptable. Prophylaxis with acetazolamide is recommended.

HIGH-ALTITUDE PULMONARY EDEMA

Clinical Findings

High-altitude pulmonary edema (HAPE) is the altitude illness with highest mortality and is noncardiogenic in nature. In older children, HAPE presents as persistent cough, shortness of breath with minimal exertion that may not respond to rest, and occasionally, frothy pink or rusty sputum. In younger children and infants, signs may not be readily apparent and they may exhibit only fussiness, pallor, lethargy, or progressive respiratory distress. Time to onset following ascent varies widely and may be insidious or sudden. Florid pulmonary edema and respiratory collapse may ensue if HAPE goes unrecognized.

A chest radiograph may demonstrate patchy infiltrates, dilated pulmonary arteries, and normal cardiac size. More generalized pulmonary edema will be noted in severe cases. An echocardiogram is indicated when HAPE is unclear, in the presence of a heart murmur without known history, or when underlying cardiac abnormalities are thought to be contributing to illness.

Treatment

Suspicion of developing HAPE in the appropriate historical setting is important. Early respiratory support with supplemental oxygen is warranted and should continue after descent. CPAP may be useful to further improve symptoms. Intubation may be necessary for respiratory support in severe cases. When descent is delayed or impossible, a Gamow bag acts as a temporizing measure. Nifedipine may be considered in significant cases.

Disposition

Descent to lower altitude and hospitalization is indicated in patients with HAPE.

HIGH-ALTITUDE CEREBRAL EDEMA

Clinical Findings

High altitude cerebral edema (HACE) can present similarly to AMS, with worsening or additional symptoms. Neurologic symptoms discriminate HACE from AMS, and may occur in the setting or absence of HAPE. Patients will exhibit truncal ataxia, confusion, or other neurologic disturbance. Ataxia is often an early finding and should be considered serious. Cranial nerve palsies and papilledema indicate increased cranial pressure, and potential impending cerebral herniation. Retinal hemorrhages may be seen. A comatose patient with recent history of rapid altitude ascent should be considered to have HACE until proven otherwise.

Treatment

In the presence of altitude exposure and altered mental status or other neurologic findings, a head CT in the emergency department is warranted. Consider conditions such as dehydration, hypoglycemia, and hyponatremia. MRI will allow for detailed evaluation of structural insult and increased ICP. Cranial nerve abnormalities likely signify herniation and indicate the need for urgent decompression. Descent should occur when possible, or a portable hyperbaric chamber considered. Supplemental oxygen and dexamethasone should be provided until asymptomatic.

Disposition

Patients with HACE should be admitted for monitoring and continued therapy. When no clinic or hospital is available: stop ascent, descend when possible, and utilize a portable hyperbaric chamber if available. If significant neurologic abnormalities are present, or radiographic evidence of impending brainstem herniation is apparent, neurosurgical consultation should be obtained. Patients with severe symptoms at the time of presentation likely warrant admission regardless of resolution. ICU level monitoring may be necessary for persistent severe symptoms, especially in the setting of ongoing altered mental status.

Imray C, Wright A, Subudhi A, et al: Acute mountain sickness: Pathophysiology, prevention, and treatment. *Prog Cardiovasc Dis.* 2010;52(6):467-484 [PMID: 20417340].

Luks LM, McIntosh SE, Grissom CK, et al: Wilderness Medical Society consensus guidelines for the prevention and treatment of acute altitude illness. *Wilderness Environ Med.* 2010;21(2)146-155 [PMID: 20591379].

Ritchie ND, Baggott AV, Andrew Todd WT: Acetazolamide for the prevention of acute mountain sickness: A systematic review and meta-analysis. *J Travel Med.* 2012;19(5):298-307 [PMID: 22943270].

Stream JO, Grissom CK: Update on high-altitude pulmonary edema: Pathogenesis, prevention, and treatment. *Wilderness Environ Med.* 2008;19(4):293-303 [PMID: 19099331].

VENOMOUS ANIMAL INJURIES

Children are naturally curious about animals and new things in nature. Envenomations, bites, and stings are common in the pediatric population and require awareness by the emergency physician of standard treatments and antivenins, to appropriately treat this group of patients. Common envenomations and treatments are discussed below.

SNAKEBITES

General Considerations

Snakes worldwide vary greatly among species, including the presence or lack of venom and the resultant toxicity. In rural areas and underdeveloped nations, snakebite prevalence is higher, as is morbidity and mortality. Travelers and individuals regularly exposed to undeveloped wilderness should wear protective clothing including long pants and sleeves, and boots when possible, particularly if vegetation is dense or visibility is low. Modern medical knowledge has afforded specific treatment indications and options dependent on the type of snake reported. Snakebites in the United States have notably lower rates of fatality, thought to be due to less lethal venom in native snakes. Nonindigenous species are sometimes involved, often as pets, which may or not be legal to own. When possible, identification of the snake will guide the emergency physician in therapeutic options.

Two main families of venomous snakes are native to the United States. The family *Viperidae* includes three snakes of the subfamily *Crotalinae* (pit vipers): the copperhead, the water moccasin (or cottonmouth), and the rattlesnake. The family *Elapidae* includes only the coral snake in the United States, although the Texas species *Micrurus tener* has been shown to differ from the eastern coral snake, *Micrurus fulvius.*

Clinical Findings

Snakebites most frequently occur on the extremities. The exposed leg is a target to the snake at ground level, and the upper extremity is often bitten as a result of attempting to touch or handle the snake. Instant localized pain and bleeding at the puncture sites are likely. Edema, tenderness, discoloration, and spread of swelling up the extremity tend to follow when significant envenomation has occurred. Systemic symptoms may also result, including nausea and vomiting, headache, and malaise.

▶ *Elapidae*

In general, these snakes are known for severe venom effects from many species in Africa and Asia. Their venom is known primarily as neurotoxic, and effects may be delayed several hours. Paralysis of muscle groups, especially those involving respiratory function, the face, and neck may pose significant airway and respiratory concerns. Severe tissue injury including bullous lesions and sloughing of necrotic skin may occur. Hematologic and muscle effects may also be seen, including rhabdomyolysis.

▶ *Crotalinae* (pit vipers)

Envenomation may range from mild extremity involvement to adjoining truncal involvement. Children can experience whole-body effects. Bruising and blistering may occur in the first several hours. Hemodynamic instability may occur, as may hemorrhage to include bleeding from the gastrointestinal tract, lungs, mouth, nose, and skin. Thrombocytopenia, hemolysis, coagulopathy, and severe cardiopulmonary compromise have been described.

Treatment

Previously described first-aid measures such as tourniquet application, local incisions, cryotherapy, electric shock, and suctioning have been discouraged. Transport the patient to the nearest hospital with the bitten extremity immobilized with a traditional splint. Many authors also advocate the pressure-immobilization (constriction band) method in conjunction with splinting in the setting of severe envenomation and presence of systemic symptoms. Studies have reported compressions of 20-55 mm Hg in using such bands, and these should be left intact until hospital arrival. Outlining apparent swelling or discoloration and denoting the time are helpful for assessment of progression.

In the emergency department, initial assessment should begin with airway and cardiopulmonary function. Resuscitation with vasopressors, IV fluids, and possibly blood products may be indicated. Document progression of swelling and ecchymosis, including further outlining and timing. Compartment syndrome is infrequent, but the emergency physician should be aware of this possibility and consult the appropriate surgeon as indicated. A general, trauma, orthopedic, or plastic surgeon may be required depending on the location of the compartment syndrome. Laboratory evaluation includes a complete blood count, coagulation profile, electrolytes, type and screen or crossmatch, and serum chemistry.

Antivenin is the mainstay of treatment for venomous snakebite. When indicated, CroFab (crotalidae polyvalent immune Fab) is current standard therapy in the United States and has been demonstrated to be safe for use in children. Particular attention to dosing and reconstituting instructions is required. CroFab was initially approved for the treatment of rattlesnake bites and has also been shown to be effective and appropriate for copperhead bites.

An initial, slow IV trial should precede full treatment, as allergic reactions have been reported. Manufacturer-specific guidelines for therapy should be followed based on the patient's level of symptoms; dosing is adjusted for severity of envenomation rather than weight based. Volume overload is a potential concern for the child less than 10 kg or with other comorbid conditions limiting fluid intake. The usual dose of CroFab is diluted in 250 mL of NS. Continued administration is indicated until symptom progression is controlled. Maintenance dosing may be indicated according to included instructions.

Other antivenins are potentially available in geographic regions where specific species are prevalent. Eastern coral snake antivenin exists and is used to treat coral snakebites in adults when indicated. The Texas variety of coral snake has shown least toxicity in most patients, requiring antivenin less frequently. Limited data is available regarding the use of this treatment in children; risks and benefits of antivenin should be weighed against severity of presentation.

Indications for antivenin

- Hemorrhage/coagulopathy
- Hemolysis
- Shock/hypotension
- Neurotoxicity
- Rhabdomyolysis
- Rapid swelling
- Severe tissue damage including blistering and bruising

Additional appropriate wound care and tetanus immunization should be provided when indicated.

Dispostion

Patients receiving antivenin should be admitted to the hospital for hemodynamic monitoring and observation of the injury. Most institutions utilize the intensive care unit (ICU) for these admissions. Potential rebound effects of the venom or reaction to antivenin may occur, and serial examinations and laboratory evaluations are warranted. The asymptomatic patient with a normal laboratory evaluation and no worsening symptoms may be discharged home after a period of observation of 6-8 hours.

Goto CS, Feng S: Crotalidae polyvalent immune Fab for the treatment of pediatric crotaline envenomation. *Pediatr Emerg Care.* 2009;25:273-279 [PMID: 19369845].

Morgan DL, Borys DJ, Stanford R, et al: Texas coral snake (Micrurus tener) bites. *South Med J.* 2007;100:152-156 [PMID: 17330685].

Warrell DA: Venomous bites, stings, and poisoning. *Infect Clin Dis North Am.* 2012;26:207-223 [PMID: 22632635].

MARINE ENVENOMATIONS

STINGRAYS

General Considerations

Worldwide distribution of marine life varies with vast numbers of species. Toxic effects can be seen by physical exposure or consumption of certain marine animals. Stingray exposure occurs approximately 1500-2000 times per year in the United States, although specific pediatric numbers are not known. Stingrays have venom-containing glands along their barbed elongated tails. Venom is complex and includes peptides, histamine, and enzymes. Most exposures occur to the distal lower extremity of people walking in shallow waters along beaches or reefs. Sliding feet along the sand and protective footwear is recommended to minimize risk of exposure.

Clinical Findings

Stingray envenomation results in sudden spreading heat and pain that ascends the affected limb. Stingray spines may cause a single puncture wound, or depending on the size and if the patient falls, a laceration or penetrating injury may be present. Dependent on the timing of presentation, apparent infection from *Vibrio* species or other bacteria may be present. Systemic effects including gastrointestinal upset, hemodynamic instability, and neurologic findings may occur.

Treatment

Irrigate the wound extensively. Hot water immersion of the affected limb is recommended. Any remaining stinger spine or barb should be removed. A radiograph to evaluate for retained foreign body, as well as local anesthesia of the wound may help the physician assure appropriate exploration of the wound. Antibiotic therapy should be instituted for suspected bacterial infections and should be appropriate coverage for marine species. Large wounds should be closed loosely or packed open. Hemodynamic instability should be managed with appropriate advance life-support measures, including epinephrine or atropine when indicated.

Disposition

A stingray envenomation with systemic effects or significant wound should be observed for at least 4-6 hours. Hemodynamically stable patients may be discharged home. Prompt outpatient follow-up for wound care and reassessment is necessary.

JELLYFISH

General Considerations

Jellyfish envenomations occur frequently along beaches and in shallow waters. Species vary by geographic location and include box jellyfish, Irukandji jellyfish, and Portuguese man-of-war. The US Atlantic coast is a known exposure region for *Chrysaora* species. Local skin inflammation is most common, but several significant systemic effects may occur. Wet suits and protective clothing may prevent stings from the capsulated cysts (nematocysts) along the jellyfish tentacles.

Clinical Findings

Jellyfish envenomation usually results in immediate significant pain, and skin wheals frequently appear. More severe syndromes are described based on jellyfish type.

▶ Box Jellyfish

Chironex fleckeri is the Australian region species noted for causing fatalities, especially in children. The jellyfish may cause respiratory distress and cough, nausea, vomiting, sweating, myalgias, and cardiopulmonary arrest. Mental status changes may occur and proceed to coma. Significant banded erythema occurs along the skin and may progress to necrotic or vesicular eruptions.

▶ Irukandji Jellyfish

Severe muscle and joint pain, hypertension, shaking chills and piloerection occur, typically delayed to approximately 30 minutes after exposure. Pulmonary edema and cardiac dysfunction are known later complications.

▶ Portuguese Man-of-War

Skin welts often resemble a string-of-beads. Severe systemic effects may occur as described above. Intravascular hemolysis, kidney injury, and vascular spasm may also occur.

Treatment

▶ Box Jellyfish

Manage all severe presentations with appropriate basic and advanced life-support measures. Commercial vinegar of 3-10% acetic acid will inactivate the nematocysts. Antivenom is available and is indicated in severe envenomations; however, availability may be limited and its effectiveness is unclear. IV analgesics will likely be needed. Hot water treatment will relieve the pain.

▶ Irukandji Jellyfish

Vinegar or acetic acid should be used as above. A razor can be used to shave off tentacles still attached to the skin. IV analgesia and blood pressure control, as well as monitoring for worsening systemic effects are needed. Heart failure and respiratory compromise may occur gradually and should be considered.

▶ Portuguese Man-of-War

Hot water treatment is indicated, but vinegar is not effective. Further pain control will likely be required.

▶ *Chrysaora* Species

Baking soda and water mixed 1:1 results in a wet paste and is useful in relieving the sting of these species noted along the eastern US coast.

Disposition

Patients with ongoing severe systemic effects after envenomation should be admitted for further evaluation and management of progressive symptoms. Severe exposures should be otherwise observed in the emergency department for 6-8 hours, or admitted for further monitoring based on the potential delayed progression of symptoms. Smaller children should be considered at higher risk for progressive worsening.

ARTHROPOD ENVENOMATIONS

General Considerations

Hymenoptera species include many varieties of bees, wasps, hornets, yellow jackets, and ants. Anaphylactic reactions are potential with a single sting from any of these insects. African killer bees have been noted in the United States for roughly two decades and are the most common source of multiple stings. The collective venoms include amines, phospholipases, hyaluronidase, and neurotoxins. Allergic reactions and direct effects of the venoms are possible. Systemic allergic reactions are relatively rare, but may occur in up to 4% in the United States. Desensitization with purified venoms is an option for the patient with known allergy.

Clinical Findings

Localized reaction forming a painful, pruritic wheal or pustule is common. Urticaria and other allergic symptoms may occur, or progress to anaphylaxis. Children with prior sting exposure resulting in urticaria have a 10% likelihood of significant reaction. Patients with prior anaphylaxis have a 50-60% likelihood of reaction with the subsequent sting.

Anaphylaxis is a rapidly progressing state that includes flushing, dizziness, wheezing, oral and facial angioedema, gastrointestinal upset, and hypotension. Hemolysis, renal failure, disseminated intravascular coagulopathy, and rhabdomyolysis are possible.

Treatment

Removal of the stinger or barb is recommended, as continued envenomation is possible with bee stings. Yellow jackets and hornets can sting more than once. Cold packs and oral analgesia, as well as diphenhydramine are sufficient for confined local reactions. Significant local reactions may require steroids and histamine (H_1) blockers. Systemic anaphylaxis should be treated with intramuscular epinephrine 0.01 mg/kg of 0.1% (1:1000 solution). Bronchodilators, pressors, and intubation may be required. Additional management will be guided by the results of other systemic effects.

Disposition

Isolated local reactions can be discharged home. For children with more significant reactions and all cases of anaphylaxis, 24-hour admission and monitoring should occur. A patient size-appropriate emergency epinephrine auto injector should be prescribed and anaphylaxis precautions given.

SCORPION ENVENOMATION

General Considerations

Most scorpion stings result in localized reactions that are extremely painful. *Centruroides exilicauda*, a North American species, common to Arizona, New Mexico, and Texas is known for neurotoxicity that may cause significant symptoms. Severity of symptoms varies among species worldwide.

Clinical Findings

An initially painful sting is followed by rapid progression of systemic symptoms. Initial cholinergic symptoms include vomiting, sweating, abdominal pain, and piloerection. Later adrenergic symptoms may lead to cardiopulmonary disturbances including hypertension, shock, arrhythmias, and pulmonary edema. Neurotoxic effects are often seen in children with *C. exilicauda* envenomation and include fasciculations, spasticity, and rapid eye movements. Respiratory distress may occur.

Treatment

Local anesthetics and systemic pain control are recommended. Cold packs may improve localized pain reaction. Children with severe reactions should be managed according to symptoms. Medical therapy for hypertension, shock, and progressive or persisting symptoms is warranted.

Disposition

Most children will do well without significant intervention. Patients requiring vasoactive medications or ongoing neurologic monitoring should be managed in the ICU.

BLACK WIDOW SPIDER BITES

Clinical Findings

The black widow spider, *Latrodectus mactans*, is known for its neurotoxic venom and characteristic appearance. The dangerous female is shiny black with a ventral red hourglass pattern and occasionally dorsal red dots. The male is typically gray or brown and not dangerous. The bite is typically painful but localized. Sweating and piloerection at the site is characteristic of this bite, and systemic symptoms follow. Lymphadenopathy, spreading extremity pain, diffuse sweating, hypertension, irritability, priapism, and muscle spasms may occur. Rigidity of the masseters may progress to trismus, and rigidity in the abdominal musculature can mimic a surgical or "acute" abdomen. Infants are at greatest risk of mortality.

Treatment

Narcotic analgesics are recommended. Immobilization is thought to be helpful, and antivenom is available for seriously affected patients, especially infants. Allergic reaction has been frequently reported with antivenom and should be used with caution.

Disposition

Children bitten by a black widow spider should be observed for progressive symptoms at least 12 hours. Most recommendations indicate admission for children with a confirmed or suspected bite and any progressive symptoms.

BROWN RECLUSE SPIDER BITES

Clinical Findings

The brown recluse spider, *Loxosceles reclusa*, has a brown body with a darker violin-shaped marking on its dorsal side. It is known for its spingomyelinase D–containing venom. The venom is cytotoxic and known to cause necrotic lesions. The bite is usually painless but eventual burning pain ensues. The classic lesion is described as a target or red, white, and blue lesion: erythema forms, surrounded by a halo of vasoconstriction. Cyanotic appearing tissue may surround the red and white areas. A necrotic blackened eschar follows this initial reaction over the following few days and may leave a significant ulcerated area. Approximately 10% of patients develop systemic symptoms including fever, rash, headache, intravascular hemolysis, and kidney injury. Smaller-sized children are at higher risk for severe symptoms.

Treatment

Minor wounds can be managed expectantly with local wound care and appropriate tetanus prophylaxis. More severe or progressive lesions may require surgical follow-up. Delayed surgical debridement is preferred over immediate surgical exploration, given the progressive worsening of most wounds.

Disposition

Most bites can be managed outpatient with appropriate follow-up and precautions. Systemic toxicity and severe wounds are indications for admission for further management.

Forrester JA, Holstege CP, Forrester JD: Fatalities from venomous and nonvenomous animals in the United States (1999-2007). *Wilderness Environ Med.* 2012;23:146-152 [PMID: 22656661].
Warrell DA: Venomous bites, stings, and poisoning. *Infect Clin Dis North Am.* 2012;26:207-223 [PMID: 22632635].

ELECTRICAL ENERGY EMERGENCIES

ELECTRICAL INJURIES

General Considerations

Electrical injury (electrical shock or burn) ranges from minor to devastating dependent upon a number of factors. Thermal injury or burn size is often misleading and may underestimate possible deeper tissue damage of shock. The term electrocution refers to execution or death by electricity, and is not clinically appropriate for most pediatric patients presenting with an electrical shock injury. Severity of injury will vary by voltage, current type, exposure time, and resistance. Most pediatric electrical injuries result from household exposures to AC (alternating current) at 120 volts. Some higher consuming appliances require 240 volts but are not as frequently associated. Approximately, 60-70% are associated with electrical cords, and 10-15% with residential electrical outlets. High-voltage injuries (> 1000 volts) are rare. Exposure duration correlates directly with increasing temperature and electrical arc formation. AC exposures may be very brief, physically "throwing" a victim from the source, or initiate tetanic contraction causing prolonged contact. The skin is relatively protective against current passage with its higher resistance, compared to nervous, vascular, and muscle tissues. Moisture and open wounds are factors that lower resistance. Deeper tissues such as tendon and bone tend to have the highest resistance and gain the highest amount of heat during exposures, whereas skin resistance is surpassed. In addition to internal body tissue exposure and potential injury, thermal burns may result from clothing or material ignited by the electrical source.

Clinical Findings

A detailed history combined with protocol-driven advanced life support should guide the emergency physician's initial evaluation. Brief or prolonged loss of consciousness may indicate a history of more severe exposure. Apparent injuries should be surveyed, and clinical estimation of potential deep tissue injuries should occur. Consideration must be made for traumatic injuries such as dislocations, compression fractures, and head injuries from being thrown and from tetanic contraction. Central nervous system effects may occur acutely or delayed. Arrhythmias may occur and include ventricular fibrillation, atrial fibrillation, sinus tachycardia or bradycardia, QT-prolongation, heart block of varying degree, nonspecific ST-segment abnormalities, and asystole. Overall physical effects are related to the site of exposure and the often unclear path through the body from which the current is passed. Perioral burns after mouth-to-electrical-cord exposure are relatively unique to pediatric patients. Oral commissure contracture, hypertrophic scarring, or delayed labial artery bleeding (at 10-14 days) may be significant complications of this type of burn.

Treatment

The initial treatment of electrical injury should begin with evaluation for potential or ongoing life threats. In the field, the rescuer should ensure personal protection via clothing or gear and remove the patient from the electrical source. Disconnect the power source or move the patient to a safe location. ABC should be assessed and treated accordingly. Visible surface burns should be treated in the usual manner (see Chapter 44), as well as suspected for deep tissue injury. Extent of injury may not be realized for several days. Assess renal function and evaluate for rhabdomyolysis. In burns and rhabdomyolysis, adequate fluid resuscitation should be initiated. Any complaint of pain may indicate internal organ or musculoskeletal injury, and should prompt further laboratory or radiographic evaluation.

In the setting of high-voltage exposure, an ECG should be obtained on all patients, and should be considered in certain low-voltage household electrical exposures. A recent evidence-based review recommends no ECG or inpatient monitoring for otherwise healthy, asymptomatic children exposed to household current (without water involvement). Documented cardiac arrest or ventricular arrhythmia in the field after household exposure are exceptions and should be monitored. The review indicated that pediatric patients with a normal initial ECG do not demonstrate delayed arrhythmias. Those with nonfatal ECG abnormalities or abnormal rhythms return to normal spontaneously over 24 hours. Typical medical management is appropriate for significant ECG abnormalities. Some authors recommend ongoing telemetry monitoring for the patient with cardiac arrest, an ECG abnormality or documented dysrhythmia (in the emergency department or in the field), or loss of consciousness. Cardiac injury may result in as myocardial contusion. Cardiac biomarkers such as CK-MB and troponin are of uncertain value in assessing such injury. Permanent damage to conduction pathways, myocardium, and coronary arteries has been described.

Serial examinations of the electrical-injured extremity are indicated to assess for signs of deep tissue injury and compartment syndrome. Neurologic and vascular status should be documented as well as tissue appearance. Absence of pulse is usually the last clinical indication to appear in compartment syndrome. Prompt consultation with a surgeon should be considered if developing compartment syndrome is suspected.

Oral burns should prompt telephone consultation with a plastic or oral surgeon. Dependent on the extent of apparent burn and injury, a personal evaluation in the emergency department or hospital may be warranted.

Disposition

Historically, all patients with electrical injury were admitted for monitoring for at least 24 hours. Studies of adult patients began to question the need for this practice in low-voltage exposures, and more recent reviews have documented evidence pertinent to children. Children with history of low-voltage (most household) exposures can be discharged home safely from the emergency department if no indication for telemetry monitoring is present. Disposition of a patient exposed to high voltage is frequently institution specific and unclear; some facilities admit all high-voltage exposure patients, whereas other facilities admit only those with injuries requiring ongoing in hospital management or cardiac monitoring.

Superficial burns should be dressed appropriately (typically with mafenide acetate and/or silver sulfadiazine) and be followed as an outpatient in 48-72 hours for wound reassessment and possible debridement. Physical and occupational therapy will likely be utilized as outpatient. Patients with significant burns may require admission or transfer to a burn center. Parents should be cautioned about the potential for severe bleeding if a labial artery injury is suspected from oral burns (often delayed to 10-14 days after initial injury), and referral to an oral surgeon provided. If no other indication for admission is present, follow-up with the appropriate surgeon should be arranged as part of the discharge plan. Patients with traumatic injuries resulting from electrical exposure should be admitted or discharged as appropriate.

Arnoldo BD, Purdue GF: The diagnosis and management of electrical injuries. *Hand Clin.* 2009;25:469-479 [PMID: 19801121].
Chen EH, Sareen A: Do children require ECG evaluation and inpatient telemetry after household electrical exposures? *Ann Emerg Med.* 2007;49:64-67 [PMID: 17141143].
Toon MH, Maybauer DM, Arceneaux LL, et al: Children with burn injuries-assessment of trauma, neglect, violence, and abuse. *J Inj Violence Res.* 2011;3:98-110 [PMID: 21498973].

CONDUCTED ELECTRICAL WEAPON INJURIES

General Considerations

Law enforcement personnel utilize conducted electrical weapons (frequently TASER branded models) to deal with dangerous or uncooperative individuals, including minors in some jurisdictions. Standard devices are shaped like a gun, and fire two barbs attached by wires to contact the subject. Others are designed as direct-contact devices. The device is further designed to emit electrical pulses upon deployment, stunning the suspect when an electric circuit is completed. Electrical exposure is considered mild and brief in comparison to household and electric currents. Most episodes involving children described include adolescents older than 12 years.

Clinical Findings

Minor injuries are typically reported; most common are puncture wounds resulting from the barbs when contact is made. Abrasions, superficial laceration, and trauma related to falls comprise most recorded injuries. Limited research exists on this topic pertinent to children, but available data suggests that ECG and cardiac rhythm abnormalities are rare. The patient may have complaint of palpitations, lightheadedness, or chest pain if prolonged electrical stimulus is used. Because of the potential for transthoracic current to affect the cardiac rhythm, all related complaints should be considered legitimate.

Treatment

Given limited study of these devices in children, general recommendations include treating wounds as in normal practice, and removal of electrical barbs similar to fishhooks. The symptomatic patient should receive symptom-driven treatment and assessment, including a screening ECG or telemetry monitoring if indicated.

Disposition

Available data suggests most patients will have limited, self-resolving symptoms after exposure. Asymptomatic patients can be discharged with standard emergency department precautions.

Gardeer AR, Hauda WE, Bozeman WP, et al: Conducted electrical weapon (TASER) use against minors: A shocking analysis. *Pediatr Emerg Care.* 2012;28:873-877 [PMID: 22929134].

LIGHTNING INJURIES

General Considerations

Lightning injuries occur approximately 400 times per year in the United States; approximately 10% are fatal. Most deaths occur in young adults. Summer months, afternoon time, and southern US locations predominate in most cases.

Injury is classified as one of four types:

1. Direct strike injury is rare and results when a person is stricken without interruption by an object or source.

2. Contact injury results when lightning strikes an object in direct contact with the person.

3. Side splash injury results from the tremendous amount of current jumping from a stricken object to the person.

4. Ground current injury results when lightning first strikes the ground, then travels via ground to the person.

Lightning injury prevention measures include seeking the largest possible indoor shelter available away from doors or windows, and avoid being near high-elevation points or towers. Insulation from the ground with a nonconductive object, standing with feet together to minimize ground contact points, and sitting with feet elevated from the ground are also recommended.

Clinical Findings

▶ Cardiopulmonary

Sudden cardiac and respiratory arrest are the mechanisms of fatal lightning injury. Asystole is thought to be the most common rhythm, although ventricular fibrillation has been described. A return of rhythm, usually bradycardia, usually occurs before respiratory function. Unlike the victims of other mass casualty situations, the apparent deceased at the scene of a lightning strike may have significant chance of recovery if advanced life-support protocols are performed and respiratory function is supported as soon as feasible. Other dysrhythmias in the nonarrested patient may be present, or may present in delayed fashion up to 72 hours.

▶ Burns

Lightning burns may occur as a result of "flashover" of the skin, rather than penetrating the skin as in other electrical burns. Linear burns along lines of sweat are partial thickness in nature. Punctate burns are thought to be evidence of lightning current exiting the body from deeper tissues. Skin burns resultant from heated objects or melted/ignited clothing may also result and require burn care. Lichtenberg

figures are pathognomonic for lighting injury, thought to result from electron showers. A feather-like pattern appears on the skin and is not a burn, resolving in 24 hours.

▶ Neurologic

Altered mental status, headache, loss of consciousness, seizure, and paresthesias may occur. Symptoms are often temporary, but may last for prolonged periods. Keraunoparalysis is typically a temporary paralysis after lightning injury, affecting the lower extremities more frequently than the upper. Symptoms of compartment syndrome may seem apparent, due to loss of pulse and autonomic overstimulation. Spinal injury and cardiac arrest may also be apparent; spinal precautions and checking a central pulse before CPR are indicated. The paralytic effects may last several hours. CNS injury from the massive nature of the strike may result and may be permanent, including hypoxic injuries and intracranial bleeding. Delayed neurologic findings have been described.

▶ Musculoskeletal

Traumatic injury, and those associated with electrical injuries described above are possible. A thorough evaluation for fractures, compartment syndrome, truncal injury, and rhabdomyolysis is warranted.

▶ Facial

Optic nerve and lens are vulnerable to lightning injury, and cataract formation is a frequent ophthalmic complication. "Blown" or dilated pupils may be transient and should not be considered an initial indicator of devastating neurologic injury. Tympanic membrane rupture is considered a high-incidence injury (~ 60%). Deafness, partial hearing loss, and other ear injuries are also noted.

Treatment

At the scene, "reverse field triage" is recommended. Patients in cardiac arrest have a higher survival after lightning injury compared with the general category of cardiac arrest. These patients should be treated before the more stable, responsive patients. Ventilatory support should begin rapidly for any patient who is pulseless and advanced life-support measures initiated.

ECG and echocardiogram are recommended for all victims of direct lightning strike and for those patients presenting with chest pain, loss of consciousness, focal neurologic findings, or apparent major trauma. If either is abnormal, or if direct lighting strike is reported, further telemetry monitoring in the emergency department should ensue. Cardiac markers are considered to be of limited value and are likely to be abnormal.

Detailed evaluation should include search for traumatic injury, assessment for deep tissue injury or burn, and detailed neurologic examination. Radiographic evaluation for underlying injury is appropriate. Routine trauma and burn care should proceed in parallel with other considerations. Consultation with an ophthalmologist, otolaryngologist, neurologist, or other specialist may be indicated dependent on presenting findings.

Disposition

Many authors recommend admitting all victims of lightning strike for cardiac and neurologic monitoring. Direct strike victims, as well as those with an abnormal ECG or echocardiogram should be admitted for further monitoring for at least 24 hours.

Davis C, Engeln A, Johnson E, et al: Wilderness Medical Society practice guidelines for the prevention and treatment of lightning injuries. *Wilderness Environ Med.* 2012;23:260-269 [PMID: 22854068].

Toxic Ingestions & Exposures

Sing-Yi Feng, MD
Collin S. Goto, MD

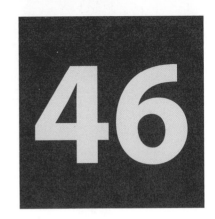

GENERAL MANAGEMENT OF THE INTOXICATED PATIENT

POISON CONTROL CENTERS

Poison control centers were developed to provide immediate advice from trained specialists in poison information to aid in the management of poisonings. In the United States, 1(800) 222-1222 is the nationwide toll-free number to a regional poison center. A clinical toxicologist is available to provide expert consultation.

PRINCIPLES OF MANAGEMENT OF THE POISONED PATIENT

PATIENT EVALUATION

History

Obtaining an accurate history is of critical importance.

▶ Nature of the Toxin(s)

Obtain the trade, brand, generic, or chemical name(s). It is important to be precise because products with similar names may have different compositions. Concentrations or amounts of various constituents from the label are useful. Unknown tablets and capsules can frequently be identified from the imprint code on the item along with the color and shape.

▶ Magnitude of Exposure

Estimate the volume of liquid or number of tablets or capsules ingested. In cases of intentional ingestion, the history can be inaccurate, frequently underestimating the amount and the nature of what has been consumed. When the exact amount ingested is not known, it is prudent to manage the patient according to the worst-case scenario.

▶ Time of Exposure

Signs and symptoms of toxicity usually occur within a few hours of ingestion for most overdoses. However, some poisons demonstrate delayed onset of toxicity. Examples of delayed toxicity include acetaminophen, methanol, ethylene glycol, and modified-release pharmaceuticals.

▶ Progression of Symptoms

The severity and progression of toxicity are determinants of the need for therapy.

▶ Other Medical Conditions (both acute and chronic)

Preexisting medical conditions may increase susceptibility to a specific toxin. Unwanted pregnancy may precipitate an attempted suicide. In addition, the effect of the toxin on the fetus should be considered.

TOXIDROMES

Toxidromes are toxic syndromes (characteristic signs and symptoms caused by a particular toxin) and may facilitate diagnosis when the toxin is unknown. They are also useful for anticipating signs and symptoms that are likely to occur when the toxin is known. Table 46–1 describes commonly encountered toxidromes.

Toxidromes have several limitations. Many poisonings will not present with a recognizable syndrome. Toxidromes may be confounded when multiple drugs with competing pharmacological effects are involved or when the patient has comorbidities that alter the predicted effects of a toxin.

Table 46–1. Common toxic syndromes.

Syndrome	Signs and Symptoms	Sources
Anticholinergic	**Anticholinergic mnemonic:** Mad as a hatter (delirium, hallucinations), Hot as a hare (hyperthermia), Dry as a bone (dry mouth and skin), Blind as a bat (mydriasis), Red as a beet (flushed skin), Also tachycardia, ileus, urinary retention.	Belladonna alkaloids (such as atropine, scopolamine, hyoscyamine, and others found in certain plants and medicinals), antihistamines, tricyclic antidepressants, antiparkinson agents, antipsychotic agents.
Cholinergic (muscarinic and nicotinic)	**Muscarinic mnemonic: DUMBELLS** D: Diarrhea, Diaphoresis U: Urination M: Miosis B: Bronchorrhea, Bronchospasm, Bradycardia E: Emesis L: Lacrimation L: Lethargy S: Salivation **Nicotinic mnemonic: Days of the week** Sunday: Somnolence Monday: Mydriasis Tuesday: Tachycardia Wednesday: Weakness Thursday: Hypertension Friday: Fasciculations Saturday: Seizures	Organophosphates and carbamate insecticides, nerve agents, nicotine
Extrapyramidal	**Acute dystonia:** Involuntary muscle contraction, oculogyric crisis, facial grimacing, torticollis, dysphonia **Akathisia:** Restlessness **Neuroleptic malignant syndrome (NMS):** Altered mental status, hyperthermia, autonomic instability, motor abnormalities including lead pipe rigidity **Parkinsonism:** Rigidity, bradykinesia, mask-like facies, resting tremor **Tardive dyskinesia:** Orobuccolingual masticatory movements, chorea, tics	Antipsychotic agents (the extrapyramidal syndromes occur more commonly with the typical antipsychotics compared to the newer atypical antipsychotics)
Serotonin syndrome	Altered mental status, hyperthermia, autonomic instability, motor abnormalities including tremor, myoclonus, hyperreflexia, and rigidity	Serotonergic agents: Serotonin precursors or agonists Serotonin release enhancers Serotonin reuptake inhibitors Serotonin breakdown inhibitors
Opioid/sympatholytic	Decreased mental status, respiratory depression, miosis, hypotension, bradycardia, hypothermia	Opioids: Clonidine and other imidazolines, methyldopa, guanabenz, guanfacine
Sympathomimetic	Agitation, hyperthermia, tachycardia, hypertension, mydriasis, diaphoresis, increased bowel sounds	Cocaine, amphetamines, other stimulants

LABORATORY EVALUATION

Toxicology Screens

Toxicology screens should be ordered only when the results will alter patient management. The laboratory turnaround time may be longer than the critical intervention period for a poisoning. The history, physical examination, and common laboratory tests will usually narrow the differential diagnosis to allow adequate patient management. The most common toxicology screens are the drugs of abuse screen (urine) and the comprehensive drug screen (blood or urine). The results must be interpreted in the clinical context of the patient because the qualitative presence of a drug does not confirm that it is contributing to the symptoms. In addition, false-positive and false-negative results may occur.

The urine drugs of abuse screen has a rapid turnaround time and may help support the clinical diagnosis. It is a limited immunoassay that only detects a panel of several common drugs of abuse. Synthetic designer drugs, however, are usually not detected. Comprehensive blood and urine toxicology screens have a longer turnaround time and are not helpful with the initial management of the patient. In severe cases with an unclear diagnosis, they may assist in the management of the patient after hospital admission. These screens typically utilize gas chromatography and mass photospectrometry techniques to detect a large but selected group of common drugs.

Toxicity Calculations

▶ The Anion Gap

The anion gap is the difference between measured serum cations and anions and represents unmeasured anions.

$$\text{Anion gap} = [Na] - ([Cl] + [HCO_3])$$

The normal range is 8-12 mEq/L. The mnemonic LA MUD PIES is used to remember the toxins or diseases associated with a metabolic acidosis with an elevated anion gap include:

<u>L</u>actic acidosis, <u>A</u>lcoholic ketoacidosis, <u>M</u>ethanol and <u>M</u>etformin, <u>U</u>remia, and <u>D</u>iabetic ketoacidosis. In addition, <u>P</u>araldehyde and <u>P</u>henformin can also cause an elevated anion gap, along with <u>I</u>ron, <u>I</u>buprofen, <u>I</u>soniazid (when seizures have occurred), certain <u>I</u>nborn errors of metabolism. <u>E</u>thylene glycol, <u>S</u>alicylates, and <u>S</u>tarvation ketosis. Many toxins or conditions that interfere with normal oxygen transport or utilization will produce lactic acidosis, including carbon monoxide, cyanide, methemoglobinemia, hypoxemia, prolonged seizures, sepsis, shock, and many other illnesses.

▶ The Osmol Gap

The osmol gap is the difference between the measured serum osmolality and the calculated serum osmolarity. A sample of the patient's blood is sent to the laboratory to determine the measured serum osmolality, sodium, glucose, and BUN.

$$\text{Osmol gap} = \text{Osm (measured)} - \text{Osm (calculated)}$$
$$\text{Osm (calculated)} = 2[Na] + [\underline{glucose}]/18 + [\underline{BUN}]/2.8$$

The normal gap is less than 10 mOsm.

Substances that produce an increased osmol gap include alcohols (such as methanol, ethanol, and isopropyl alcohol), glycols (such as ethylene glycol), and ketones (such as acetone).

Gelbakhiani G, Ebralidze K, Zedania Z, Tugushi M: Osmolar gap in the clinical practice and the way of decrease the quantative data of osmolar gap by using fundamentally new method measuring of osmolality. *Georgian Med News.* 2009;(169):48-51 [PMID: 19430044].

RADIOLOGY

Abdominal radiographs aid in the visualization of certain substances such as bezoars, radio-opaque medications, metals, and drug-filled packets. Radio-opaque medications include chloral hydrate, iron-containing preparations, calcium carbonate, iodinated compounds, acetazolamide, busulfan, and potassium preparations. Antihistamines, phenothiazines, and tricyclic antidepressants have varying radiopacity. Serial abdominal radiographs are useful to assess gastrointestinal (GI) decontamination in such patients.

DECONTAMINATION

GI Decontamination

GI decontamination techniques such as gastric lavage, activated charcoal, cathartics or whole-bowel irrigation are not routinely recommended for each patient who presents to the hospital with an overdose. These techniques are reserved for selected patients such as those with a recent life-threatening ingestion, especially if no antidote or effective treatment is available. The decision to perform GI decontamination must be individualized, and may be discussed with the regional poison control center.

Activated charcoal is an effective adsorbent for many drugs and chemicals. Activated charcoal does not bind metals, low-molecular-weight alcohols, mineral acids, alkalis, cyanide, boric acid, most organic solvents, hydrocarbons, and certain insecticides.

Activated charcoal may be considered if a patient has ingested a potentially toxic amount of a poison (which is known to be adsorbed to charcoal) up to 1 or 2 hours previously.

The dose for activated charcoal is 10-30 g in small children and 50-100 g in older children and adults (~1-2 g/kg), administered orally or via nasogastric tube. Activated charcoal should not be administered to a patient with altered mental status and an unprotected airway. The repeated use of cathartics (most commonly sorbitol) with activated charcoal is not recommended.

Whole-bowel irrigation is the enteral administration of polyethylene glycol electrolyte (PEG) solution to irrigate the intestinal contents, including any unabsorbed toxins. The rate of administration via nasogastric tube is 25-40 mL/kg/hr in children up to 2 L/hr in adolescents and adults. The endpoint is a clear rectal effluent, which may take 6-10 hours. Indications include overdose of sustained-release products and substances not adsorbed by activated charcoal such as iron and lithium. Contraindications include unprotected airway or presence of GI disease or ileus.

Skin Decontamination

Dermal exposure may result in absorption of the toxin as well as dermal injury. Removal of contaminated clothing decreases exposure by up to 80%. Personnel who decontaminate and treat the patient should wear appropriate protective apparel, including gloves. Affected skin should be cleansed with copious amounts of water or mild soap and water. Avoid using abrasives because they may increase dermal absorption. Other solvents such as petroleum jelly, alcohol, and PEG may be used to remove specific substances not readily removed by water.

Ocular Decontamination

Most chemicals are irritating to the eye. However, caustic agents such as acids and alkalis may result in devastating eye injuries. Ocular decontamination should be started immediately after exposure. Initial decontamination involves flooding the eye with copious quantities of water. Contact lenses should be removed. Immediate medical attention is required for caustic exposures.

In the emergency department, further ocular irrigation is indicated until the pH of the tears in the palpebral sulcus returns to the neutral range as measured by litmus paper.

Respiratory Decontamination

Acute inhalation exposures may result in airway irritation, bronchospasm, pulmonary injury, asphyxia, or systemic toxicity. Victims should be moved to fresh air and oxygen provided. First responders must take precautions to avoid inhalational exposure.

Benson BE, Hoppu K, Troutman WG, et al: Position paper update: Gastric lavage for gastrointestinal decontamination. *Clin Toxicol (Phila)*. 2013;51:140-146 [PMID: 23418938].

Hojer J, Troutman WG, Hoppu K, et al: Position paper update: Ipecac syrup for gastrointestinal decontamination. *Clin Toxicol (Phila)*. 2013;51:134-139 [PMID: 23406298].

ENHANCED ELIMINATION

Enhanced elimination procedures increase the excretion rate of toxins from the systemic circulation. Interventions include multiple-dose activated charcoal, urinary alkalization, and hemodialysis.

Multiple-Dose Activated Charcoal

Multiple-dose activated charcoal (MDAC) is a technique which enables both decontamination and enhanced elimination by (1) disrupting enterohepatic recirculation of the toxin; (2) utilizing the intestinal mucosa as a dialysis membrane (gut dialysis) by drawing the toxin from the bloodstream into the intestinal lumen; and (3) binding a toxin present in the intestinal lumen. It may enhance the elimination of phenobarbital, salicylate, quinidine, theophylline, carbamazepine, dapsone or any other drug that undergoes enterohepatic recirculation. The dose of activated charcoal without cathartic is 0.5-1 g/kg by mouth or via nasogastric or orogastric tube every 4 hours. Contraindications include ileus, persistent vomiting, altered mental status with an unprotected airway, and GI disease. Complications include aspiration, bezoars, and intestinal obstruction.

Urinary Alkalinization

Urinary alkalinization enhances renal elimination of drugs that are weak acids. Ionized drug is trapped in the renal tubule and eliminated in the urine. Salicylate poisoning is the most common indication and the intravenous (IV) administration of sodium bicarbonate for urinary alkalinization is discussed with salicylate poisoning.

Hemodialysis

Hemodialysis is used to correct fluid, electrolyte, and acid-base imbalances, and to increase the elimination of specific toxins from the blood. It is effective for toxins with small volumes of distribution (< 1 L/kg), low molecular weight, and low protein binding. Additional indications include a blood level of the toxin associated with severe toxicity or death, impairment of the natural mechanism of elimination, deteriorating clinical condition despite maximal supportive care, and toxins with severe delayed effects.

ANTIDOTES

An antidote prevents or reverses the effects of poisoning. Antidotes can decrease toxicity by altering absorption, distribution, metabolism, or elimination, competing with the toxin for receptor sites or altering the physiologic effect of the toxin. Antidotes are only available for a limited number of toxins and do not replace supportive care and good clinical judgment. The risks and benefits of an antidote must be carefully considered prior to administration. Table 46–2 outlines the indications and dosing of selected antidotes.

DISPOSITION

Asymptomatic patients are observed long enough to determine whether toxic effects will occur, based on the known onset of action of the agent involved. If symptoms develop, the patient is admitted to the hospital for further management. A patient with severe toxicity will require admission to an intensive care unit. A longer observation period is required for toxins with delayed onset of action, agents that are converted into toxic metabolites, and drugs with delayed distribution.

Table 46–2. Selected antidotes with pediatric dose.

Antidote	Indication	Pediatric Dose
N-acetylcysteine	Acetaminophen	IV: 150 mg/kg over 1 hr, 50 mg/kg over 4 hr, 100 mg/kg over 16 hr Oral: 140 mg/kg followed by 70 mg/kg every 4 hr for 17 doses
Atropine	Cholinesterase inhibitors	50 µg/kg IV (minimum dose 0.1 mg) doubled every 3-5 min until bronchorrhea resolves
L-carnitine	Valproic acid–induced hyperammonemia or transaminitis	100 mg/kg (max 6g) IV over 30 min followed 15 mg/kg IV every 4 hr
Crotaline Fab antivenom	Crotaline snakebite	Symptom control dose: 4-6 vials IV Maintenance: 2 vials every 3 hr × 3 doses
Deferoxamine	Iron	5 mg/kg/h and titrate up to 15 mg/kg/h. Maximum daily dose 6 g/d
Digoxin-specific antibody fragments (Fab)	Digoxin	Empiric dosing: Acute poisoning: 10 vials IV Chronic poisoning: 1-2 vials IV and repeat as needed
Dimercaprol (BAL)	Lead encephalopathy	75 mg/m^2 IM every 4 hr. Contraindicated in peanut allergy
Edetate calcium disodium (CaNa$_2$EDTA)	Lead encephalopathy	1500 mg/m^2/d (max 3 g/d) IV continuously
Ethanol	Ethylene glycol/methanol	800 mg/kg IV loading dose, followed by 100-150 mg/kg/hr infusion. Dilute pharmaceutical grade ethanol (96%) to 10% solution with D5W
Fomepizole	Ethylene glycol/methanol	15 mg/kg IV over 30 min, next 4 doses at 10 mg/kg every 12 hr, additional doses at 15 mg/kg every 12 hr. Administer every 4 hr while patient is on dialysis
Glucagon	β-Blocker/calcium channel blocker	50 µg/kg IV over 1-2 min
Hydroxycobalamin	Cyanide	70 mg/kg up to 5 g. Repeat second dose as needed
Hyperinsulinemic euglycemic (HIE) therapy	Calcium channel or β-blockers	1 U/kg IV bolus regular human insulin and follow with 0.5 U/kg/hr, and titrate to adequate blood pressure. Monitor blood glucose every 30 min until stable, then check every hour. Maintain blood glucose at 100-200 mg/dL. May need to bolus with 25% dextrose followed by continuous dextrose infusion to maintain adequate blood sugar
Lipid 20%	Cardiac arrest from lipophilic drugs (calcium channel blockers, local anesthetics)	1.5 mL/kg over 1 min followed with IV infusion 0.25 mL/kg/min. Repeat bolus every 3-5 min up to total dose of 3 mL/kg until circulation is restored. If BP decreases, increase rate to 0.5 mL/kg/min. Max total dose 8 mL/kg
Methylene blue	Methemoglobinemia	1-2 mg/kg IV over 5 min. May repeat × 1
Naloxone	Opioids	0.4-2 mg IV, repeat at 2-3 min intervals until desired response is achieved. Synthetic opioids may requires higher doses. If 10 mg produces no response, other etiologies need to be considered
Nitrites and sodium thiosulfate (cyanide antidote kit)	Cyanide	Sodium nitrite: 6-8 mL/m^2 (max 300 mg) IV over 2-5 min Sodium thiosulfate: 7 g/m^2 (max 12.5 g) IV over 10-30 min
Octreotide	Sulfonylurea-induced hypoglycemia	1.25 µg/kg (max 50 µg) SQ or IV every 6 hr
Physostigmine	Anticholinergic syndrome	20 µg/kg IV (max 0.5 mg). Repeat as needed
Pralidoxime (2-PAM)	Cholinesterase inhibitors	20-50 mg/kg (max 1-2 g) infused over 30-60 min and then 10-20 mg/kg/hr (max 500 mg/h)
Pyridoxine	Isoniazid	1 g for each g of isoniazid ingested up to 70 mg/kg (max 5g) IV infusion at 0.5 g/h until seizure desists
Succimer	Lead, mercury	350 mg/m^2 orally every 8 hr for 5 d followed by every 12 hr for 14 d

All poisonings in children require social evaluation to determine home safety and provide poison prevention education. Patients may have been intentionally poisoned as a form of physical abuse or sexual exploitation. An intentional overdose warrants psychiatric evaluation to evaluate suicidal intent. Patients with chemical dependency should be referred to an appropriate treatment program.

PHARMACEUTICAL AGENTS

ACETAMINOPHEN

Mechanism of Toxicity

Acetaminophen undergoes hepatic metabolism to a highly reactive metabolite via the cytochrome P450 system. The toxic metabolite is normally inactivated by hepatic glutathione. After a large overdose, hepatic glutathione stores are overwhelmed, resulting in hepatocellular necrosis.

Clinical Presentation

A single acute ingestion of greater than 150-200 mg/kg in children or 7.5 g total in adults is potentially hepatotoxic. Patients who have taken supratherapeutic doses of acetaminophen over the course of consecutive days should also be evaluated for hepatotoxicity. Table 46–3 delineates the stages of acetaminophen toxicity.

Diagnostic Evaluation

A plasma acetaminophen concentration should be obtained no sooner than 4 hours following the acute ingestion. Plot the acetaminophen concentration on the Rumack Matthew nomogram (Figure 46–1) to estimate potential for hepatotoxicity.

Evaluate for liver injury with serum AST and ALT. If significant injury has occurred, other indicators of liver function should be checked such as PT/INR, bilirubin, and ammonia.

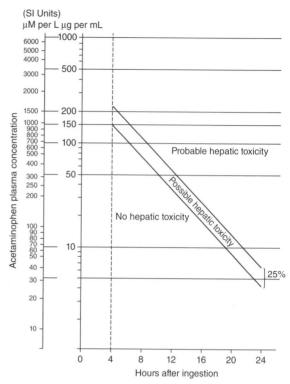

▲ Figure 46–1. Treatment protocol for acetaminophen. (Adapted from Rumack BH, Peterson RC, Koch GG, Amara IA. Acetaminophen overdose: 662 cases with evaluation of oral acetylcysteine treatment. *Arch Intern Med.* 1981;141:382 [PMID: 7469629]. Copyright © 1981 American Medical Association. All rights reserved.)

Treatment

N-acetylcysteine (NAC) is the antidote for acetaminophen toxicity and works by replenishing glutathione stores as well as being a potent free radical scavenger. It is most efficacious if given within 8 hours of an acute ingestion. NAC should be administered if the plasma acetaminophen concentration is in the toxic range (see Table 46–2 for dosing).

Emmett M: Acetaminophen toxicity and 5-oxoproline (pyroglutamic acid): A tale of two cycles, one an ATP-depleting futile cycle and the other a useful cycle. *Clin J Am Soc Nephrol.* 2014; 9:191-200 [PMID: 242335282].

Green JL, Heard KJ, Reynolds KM, Albert D: Oral and intravenous acetylcysteine for treatment of acetaminophen toxicity: A systematic review and meta-analysis. *West J Emerg Med.* 2013;14:218-226 [PMID: 23687539].

Kanji HD, Mithani S, Boucher P, Dias VC, Yarema MC: Coma, metabolic acidosis, and methemoglobinemia in a patient with acetaminophen toxicity. *J Popul Ther Clin Pharmacol.* 2013;20:e207-211 [PMID: 24077426].

Table 46–3. Stages of acetaminophen toxicity.

Stage	Time of Onset (post-ingestion)	Signs and Symptoms
1	0-24 hr	Epigastric pain, nausea, vomiting, diaphoresis, malaise.
2	24-36 hr	Hepatotoxicity, RUQ abdominal tenderness.
3	72-96 hr	Maximal hepatotoxicity, encephalopathy, cerebral edema, coagulopathy, renal insufficiency, and fatal hepatic failure.
4	3-5 d	Hepatic recovery.

ANTICONVULSANTS

CARBAMAZEPINE

Mechanism of Toxicity

Carbamazepine is structurally related to the tricyclic antidepressants, resulting in similar inhibitory effects on sodium channels and cholinergic neurotransmission. However, most of carbamazepine's toxicity is related to its central nervous system (CNS) depressant and anticholinergic activity.

Clinical Presentation

Following acute ingestion, carbamazepine results in anticholinergic effects, CNS depression, and cardiovascular (CV) toxicity. Cerebellar signs, unusual posturing, increased seizures, ataxia, coma, and respiratory depression may occur. CV toxicity includes widening of the QRS complex, cardiac dysrhythmias, atrioventricular (A-V) block, and hypotension. Hyponatremia can result from carbamazepine's antidiuretic hormone-like effect.

Diagnostic Evaluation

Carbamazepine serum levels are widely available. Normal therapeutic serum concentration is 4-12 mg/L. In general, mild toxicity is observed with serum concentrations in excess of 12 mg/L. Levels greater than 25 mg/L are associated with more severe toxicity.

Treatment

The need for intensive monitoring and supportive care should be anticipated following substantial ingestions. Seizures are treated with benzodiazepines. Fluids and inotropes are indicated for hypotension. Significant QRS widening greater than 120 milliseconds may respond to IV sodium bicarbonate. Consider multidose charcoal administration to counteract potential enterohepatic circulation in patients with severe carbamazepine toxicity.

PHENOBARBITAL

Mechanism of Toxicity

Phenobarbital increases the inhibitory action of gamma-aminobutyric acid (GABA), resulting in CNS depression. Large overdoses can result in direct myocardial depression.

Clinical Presentation

Initial signs and symptoms include CNS depression with decreased coordination, speech, and cognition. In severe overdose, coma, respiratory failure and CV collapse can occur. Deep tendon and brain stem reflexes are depressed, and the patient may be bradycardic and hypothermic.

Diagnostic Evaluation

Most hospital laboratories quantitate serum phenobarbital concentrations rapidly. Toxicity is typically manifested at phenobarbital levels above 30 mg/L. Deep coma usually occurs with levels greater than 60 mg/L.

Treatment

Respiratory depression often requires endotracheal intubation and mechanical ventilation in patients with severe phenobarbital overdose. Hypotension usually responds initially to intravascular volume expansion and inotropes. Hemodialysis may be considered for life-threatening toxicity that does not respond to supportive care. Consider multidose charcoal administration to counteract potential enterohepatic circulation in patients with severe phenobarbital toxicity.

PHENYTOIN

Mechanism of Toxicity

Phenytoin inhibits voltage-dependent sodium channels. Phenytoin is also categorized as a class Ib antidysrhythmic but cardiotoxicity from oral overdose is not reported. The IV formulation of phenytoin contains propylene glycol as a diluent that may cause myocardial depression and cardiac arrest when infused rapidly. IV phenytoin also causes tissue necrosis when subcutaneously infiltrated. IV fosphenytoin is a water-soluble prodrug, which does not contain propylene glycol and does not cause cardiac toxicity with rapid IV administration or local tissue necrosis with infiltration.

Clinical Presentation

Phenytoin does not produce the dose-related respiratory and central CNS depression seen with other anticonvulsant drugs. Most phenytoin toxicity results from accumulation of the drug due to inappropriate dosing or drug-drug interactions. Serum phenytoin levels greater than 15 mg/L are associated with nystagmus. Concentrations greater than 30 mg/L are associated with ataxia and poor coordination. Lethargy, slurred speech, and pyramidal and extrapyramidal symptoms are seen at concentrations greater than 50 mg/L.

Diagnostic Evaluation

Serum concentrations of phenytoin are readily available in most laboratories and should be obtained in all cases of phenytoin overdose. Toxic levels (> 20 mg/L) should be monitored until trending downward.

Treatment

Treatment of phenytoin toxicity is mainly supportive. Fortunately, mortalities are rare.

Gupta V, Yadav TP, Yadav A: Phenytoin toxicity presenting as acute meningo-encephalitis in children. *Neurol India.* 2011;59:66-67 [PMID: 21339662].

VALPROIC ACID

Mechanism of Toxicity

Valproic acid (VPA) is a broad-spectrum anticonvulsant with three primary mechanisms: (1) inhibition of the voltage-dependent sodium channel; (2) inhibition of voltage activated calcium channels; (3) prevention of the breakdown of GABA.

The metabolism of VPA consists of glucuronidation, which accounts for 80% of its metabolism, mitochondrial β-oxidation (14%), and cytosolic β-oxidation (6%). β-Oxidation depletes both carnitine and acetyl CoA stores. Depletion of carnitine stops β-oxidation leading to hepatic steatosis. Depletion of acetyl CoA leads to impaired ureogenesis and hyperammonemia.

Valproate-induced hyperammonemic encephalopathy is thought to be due to elevated ammonia concentrations from elevated concentrations of neurotoxic VPA metabolites.

Clinical Presentation

Common effects associated with VPA toxicity include sedation, ataxia, nausea, and tremors. Metabolic complications include hypernatremia, hypocalcemia, elevated anion gap metabolic acidosis, and hyperammonemia. Bone marrow suppression can be seen 3-5 days after a massive acute overdose but is usually self-limited. Complications such as pancreatitis, hepatotoxicity, and renal insufficiency are rare in acute overdoses of VPA but can be associated with chronic VPA therapy. Valproate-induced hyperammonemic encephalopathy presents with altered mental status, increased seizure frequency, and coma.

Diagnostic Evaluation

Serum VPA levels are widely available. Therapeutic VPA levels are defined as 50-100 mg/L. Serum VPA concentrations in excess of 150 mg/L are considered to be toxic. Serum VPA levels should be repeated every 4-6 hours until a downward trend is documented. Electrolytes, blood gas, liver function tests, complete blood count (CBC), serum ammonia, and lactate levels should be monitored in patients with VPA overdoses who exhibit neurologic impairment.

Treatment

In addition to supportive care, L-carnitine should be given to patients with elevated serum ammonia or hepatotoxicity. L-carnitine can be administered as IV (see Table 46–2 for dosing). Hemodialysis is recommended for patients with severe VPA toxicity to remove metabolites and ammonia and to correct life-threatening metabolic disturbances.

Chateauvieux S, Morceau F, Dicato M, Diederich M: Molecular and therapeutic potential and toxicity of valproic acid. *J Biomed Biotechnol.* 2010;2010:ID number 479364 [PMID: 20798865].

Lheureux PE, Hantson P: Carnitine in the treatment of valproic acid-induced toxicity. *Clin Toxicol (Phila).* 2009;47:101-111 [PMID: 19280426].

ANTIPSYCHOTICS

Mechanism of Toxicity

Toxicity of the antipsychotics results from inhibition of dopaminergic, muscarinic, and α receptors as well as myocardial sodium and potassium channels. Predominant effects vary among agents.

Clinical Presentation

Extrapyramidal syndromes include acute dystonic reactions, akathisia, akinesia, neuroleptic malignant syndrome, and tardive dyskinesia. Dystonic reactions have been seen at therapeutic doses, although overdoses produce dystonia more often. Extrapyramidal toxicity is much less common with the newer atypical antipsychotic agents.

Acute overdose often results in sedation, tachycardia, and other anticholinergic effects, and may progress to coma, seizures, and respiratory depression. Hypotension is attributable to peripheral α-adrenergic blockade. Inhibition of myocardial sodium channels leads to widening of the QRS interval, ventricular tachycardia, and CV collapse. Inhibition of myocardial potassium channels leads to prolongation of the QT interval and polymorphic ventricular tachycardia (torsade de pointes).

Diagnostic Evaluation

Quantitative serum levels are not of value and are not recommended.

Treatment

Dystonic reactions respond to anticholinergics such as diphenhydramine. Akathisia (restlessness) is treated with benzodiazepines and anticholinergics. Neuroleptic malignant syndrome is a life-threatening condition characterized by altered mental status, rigidity, tremor, hyperthermia, and autonomic instability. It must be treated aggressively with cooling, sedation with benzodiazepines, dantrolene, and bromocriptine. The dose for dantrolene is 1 mg/kg IV up to 2.5 mg/kg. This may be repeated as needed every 5-10 minutes to a cumulative dose of 10 mg/kg. The pediatric dose for bromocriptine is not well defined. In adults, give 2.5-10 mg orally or by gastric tube 3-4 times daily. Tardive dyskinesia is a delayed-onset movement disorder with long-term antipsychotic therapy that is treated with anticholinergics and cessation of the offending agent. Hypotension is treated with IV fluids and inotropic/vasoactive agents. Sodium channel toxicity is treated with IV sodium bicarbonate. Torsade de pointes is treated with IV magnesium sulfate or overdrive pacing.

Aggarwal S, Burnett P: Tardive dyskinesia with atypical antipsychotics in youth. *Australas Psychiatry*. 2013:21:507-508 [PMID: 24085720].

β-BLOCKERS

Mechanism of Toxicity

These drugs block β-adrenergic receptors with varying degrees of β-receptor selectivity. β-Receptor selectivity is often lost after overdose. In addition, several β-blockers have additional toxicities. For example, propranolol has sodium channel blocking effects and is lipid soluble, resulting in CNS penetration, with coma and seizures.

Clinical Presentation

Bradycardia and hypotension are common and may lead to shock. Bronchospasm may occur in patients with asthma. Other effects include CNS depression, seizures respiratory depression, hypoglycemia, and hyperkalemia.

Diagnostic Evaluation

Quantitative serum levels are not rapidly available and are of no clinical value.

Treatment

Bradycardia and hypotension may respond to standard supportive measures such as IV fluid boluses, atropine, and catecholamine infusions. However, significant β-blocker overdoses should be treated with the specific antidote, glucagon. Refer to Table 46–2 for dosing. Hemodialysis is helpful to enhance elimination only of acebutolol, atenolol, nadalol, and sotalol.

CALCIUM CHANNEL BLOCKERS

Mechanism of Toxicity

Calcium channel blockers inhibit the influx of calcium through calcium channels in the heart and vascular smooth muscle, resulting in systemic and coronary vasodilation, impaired cardiac conduction, slowed velocity of cardiac electric impulses, and depression of myocardial contractility. The selectivity of specific agents for cardiac versus vascular smooth muscle calcium channels may be lost with large overdoses.

Clinical Presentation

Calcium channel blocker overdose causes hypotension and bradycardia, which may be severe, resulting in intractable shock, A-V dissociation, sinus arrest, and asystole. CNS depression occurs from poor cerebral perfusion. Hyperglycemia results from inhibition of calcium-dependent insulin release from the pancreas.

Diagnostic Evaluation

Specific plasma concentrations are not rapidly available.

Treatment

Patients with severe calcium channel blocker overdose may not respond to standard supportive measures, including IV fluids, atropine, cardiac pacing, catecholamine infusions, calcium or phosphodiesterase inhibitors such as milrinone. Glucagon is a specific antidote for β-blocker overdose and is usually of little benefit for calcium channel blockade.

Hyperinsulinemic euglycemia (administration of high-dose insulin simultaneously with sufficient dextrose to maintain normal serum glucose) is recommended to improve cardiac contractility in severe calcium channel blocker overdose (see Table 46–2 for dosing). In addition, there is mounting evidence for the use of IV lipid emulsion (see Table 46–2 for dosing). Extraordinary measures such as intra-aortic balloon pump, cardiopulmonary bypass, and extracorporeal membrane oxygenation (ECMO) have been reported to be successful in case reports. For patients with severe calcium channel blocker toxicity, high-dose insulin, lipid emulsion therapy, or ECMO should be considered early before intractable shock and multi-organ failure have occurred.

Arroyo AM, Kao LW: Calcium channel blocker toxicity. *Pediatr Emerg Care*. 2009;25:532-538 [PMID: 19687715].

CLONIDINE

Mechanism of Toxicity

Clonidine is an α_2-adrenergic receptor agonist that inhibits central sympathetic outflow, resulting in bradycardia, hypotension, sedation, and respiratory depression.

Clinical Presentation

Symptoms typically appear within 30-60 minutes after ingestion. CNS signs of toxicity are most common with miosis, lethargy, coma, which may be accompanied by respiratory depression. This clinical presentation mimics opioid overdoses. CV signs include bradycardia and hypotension.

Diagnostic Evaluation

Serum measurements of these agents are not clinically useful.

Treatment

There is no specific antidote and treatment is primarily supportive.

Naloxone has been recommended due to the similarities of clonidine and opioid overdose and theoretical interactions of clonidine with opioid receptors. However, results are inconsistent. Patients with significant respiratory depression require endotracheal intubation. Symptomatic bradycardia may be treated with atropine, while hypotension is treated with IV fluids and pressors. Activated charcoal and whole-bowel irrigation are recommended for the patient who has ingested a clonidine patch once airway protection has been assured.

Farooqi M, Seifert S, Kunkel S, Johnson M, Benson B: Toxicity from a clonidine suspension. *J Med Toxicol.* 2009;5:130-133 [PMID: 19655285].

CYCLIC ANTIDEPRESSANTS

Mechanism of Toxicity

Tricyclic antidepressant (TCA) toxicity is manifested by anticholinergic effects, sodium channel blockade, α receptor blockade, and inhibition of catecholamine reuptake.

Clinical Presentation

Early signs and symptoms include drowsiness, dry mucous membranes, mydriasis, hyperreflexia, and tachycardia rapidly progressing to coma, seizures, wide-QRS complex dysrhythmias, and CV collapse.

Diagnostic Evaluation

An electrocardiogram (ECG) revealing a widened QRS complex together with a consistent history and clinical presentation may establish the diagnosis of TCA toxicity. Some urine drug screens detect TCAs. Serum levels are not helpful in treatment of acute ingestion.

Treatment

Hypotension is treated with IV fluids and catecholamine infusions. Patients with QRS widening greater than 120 milliseconds, cardiac dysrhythmias, and hypotension benefit from treatment with IV sodium bicarbonate, which reduces toxicity by alkalinizing the serum and provision of a sodium

load to overcome the sodium channel blockade. Seizures are treated with benzodiazepines. Patients with severe TCA toxicity require endotracheal intubation to protect the airway. Extraordinary measures such as ECMO may be considered in extreme cases. IV lipid emulsion therapy has also been effective in limited case reports.

Gheshlaghi F, et al: Evaluation of serum sodium changes in tricyclic antidepressants toxicity and its correlation with electrocardiography, serum pH, and toxicity severity. *Adv Biomed Res.* 2012;1:68 [PMID: 23326798].

Suksaranjit P, Ratanapo S, Srivali N, et al: Electrocardiographic changes in tricyclic antidepressant toxicity. *Am J Emerg Med.* 2013;31:751-752 [PMID: 23399330].

DIGOXIN & CARDIAC GLYCOSIDES

Mechanism of Toxicity

Cardiac glycosides inhibit the Na^+/K^+ ATPase pump. This mechanism is used to treat congestive heart failure because it increases the intracellular calcium in myocardial cells, resulting in improved contractility. During repolarization, the Na^+/K^+ ATPase pump restores the resting membrane potential by pumping potassium ions into the myocardial cell in exchange for sodium ions out of the cell. When this pump is inhibited by cardiac glycosides, the result is an increase in intracellular sodium and an increase in extracellular potassium. The increased intracellular sodium inhibits efflux of calcium through the Na^+/Ca^{2+} antiporter at the cell membrane. With digoxin poisoning, excessive increases in intracellular calcium cause disturbances of membrane potential, resulting in ectopy and tachydysrhythmias. In addition, digoxin enhances vagal tone, decreasing the rate of depolarization and conduction through the sinoatrial (SA) and A-V nodes.

Clinical Presentation

The clinical presentation of acute digoxin poisoning includes cardiac and noncardiac features. The noncardiac effects include GI manifestations such as nausea, vomiting, and diarrhea; neurologic manifestations such as confusion, headaches, weakness, and seizures; and visual manifestations such as blurred vision, scotoma, and xanthopsia (predominance of yellow vision).

The cardiac effects of digoxin poisoning are the primary concern, but life-threatening cardiac symptoms may be delayed up to 18 hours due to a prolonged distribution phase to the intracellular compartment. Early ECG changes include prolonged PR interval, shortened QT interval, depressed ST segment, and flattened or inverted T waves. Bradycardia and varying degrees of AV block may occur. This is often followed by increased myocardial automaticity and excitability, resulting in atrial, junctional, and ventricular ectopy and tachydysrhythmias. Death occurs due to intractable dysrhythmias, hypotension, and ventricular fibrillation.

Diagnostic Evaluation

Measurement of serum digoxin concentration is an important aspect of diagnosis and management. However, the digoxin level must be interpreted carefully. Digoxin demonstrates a biphasic distribution pattern following acute overdose. Serum levels will initially be elevated without clinical toxicity because distribution into the tissues occurs over many hours. Serum digoxin concentrations then decline as the drug is distributed into the tissues and eliminated by the kidneys, and it is during this phase that toxicity may begin. With chronic digoxin poisoning, the serum digoxin concentration is reflective of steady-state concentration and therefore a better predictor of toxicity. Although the therapeutic range for serum digoxin is usually 0.5-2 ng/mL, up to 10% of patients in this range may demonstrate toxicity. Most patients with toxicity have serum concentrations greater than 2 ng/mL for digoxin when measured at least 6 hours after the last dose. When interpreting the significance of these levels, it is also important to take into consideration the overall status of the patient in addition to the serum concentration. Healthy children tolerate much higher levels than adults and patients with underlying cardiac disease. Most laboratories measure total digoxin concentration. Following administration of digoxin-specific Fab, total serum digoxin levels increase dramatically because digoxin is pulled from the tissue compartment into the intravascular space, where it is bound by the Fab fragments and inactivated. Therefore, continued measurement of total serum digoxin concentration is not helpful following administration of digoxin-specific Fab.

In addition to the serum digoxin concentration, it is important to frequently assess the serum chemistries, especially potassium, calcium, magnesium, and creatinine. Hyperkalemia is an expected consequence and a marker of acute digoxin toxicity due to inhibition of the Na^+/K^+ ATPase pump. In this setting a serum potassium concentration greater than 5.5 mEq/L is predictive of severe cardiotoxicity. In contrast, hypokalemia may be present with chronic digoxin poisoning due to long-term potassium loss, especially in patients who are also on diuretic therapy. Hypokalemia also worsens digoxin toxicity. Continuous monitoring of the ECG is necessary to detect conduction abnormalities, ectopy, and dysrhythmias.

Treatment

Management of potassium, magnesium, and calcium homeostasis is of critical importance. Hyperkalemia is a consequence of digoxin poisoning and may be treated with sodium bicarbonate or glucose and insulin to shift potassium into the cells. Administration of calcium is contraindicated because digoxin has already caused an excessive influx of calcium into myocardial cells. Administration of additional calcium increases the incidence of dysrhythmias. Although digoxin initially causes an elevated extracellular potassium concentration, increased renal elimination leads to depleted total body stores. Serum potassium concentrations often fall precipitously following digoxin-specific Fab and must be checked frequently.

Hypokalemia is especially dangerous in digoxin poisoning because it exacerbates cardiotoxicity. Patients with chronic digoxin toxicity are often hypokalemic due to concomitant treatment with diuretics. Significant hypokalemia should be corrected cautiously, especially in the patient with renal insufficiency.

Magnesium plays an important role in digoxin toxicity because it is a cofactor for the Na^+/K^+ ATPase pump. Hypomagnesemia potentiates digoxin-induced cardiotoxicity and inhibits correction of hypokalemia. Patients who are on chronic digoxin therapy may be hypomagnesemic due to concurrent diuretic use. Intracellular magnesium depletion may be present despite a normal serum magnesium concentration. Magnesium replacement is indicated for patients with digoxin-related cardiotoxicity, hypokalemia, and documented hypomagnesemia. Caution is again advised in the patient with renal insufficiency.

The treatment of choice for serious digoxin (or other cardioactive steroid) poisoning is IV administration of digoxin-specific Fab antibody fragments. Indications include life-threatening dysrhythmia, conduction delay, hyperkalemia (> 5 mEq/L), cardiogenic shock, or cardiac arrest due to digoxin overdose. Other indications are based on a high likelihood of progression to life-threatening digoxin toxicity, serum digoxin level equal to or greater than 15 ng/mL at any time or equal to or greater than 10 ng/mL 6 hours after ingestion, or progressive signs and symptoms of digoxin poisoning.

Formulas are available to calculate the dose of digoxin-specific Fab based on the serum digoxin concentration or the known amount of digoxin that was ingested. However, the history of the amount ingested is notoriously inaccurate, and after an acute exposure, the serum digoxin concentration does not reflect steady-state distribution. It is more practical to administer an empiric dose of 10-20 vials of digoxin-specific Fab for acute overdose, repeating as needed to reverse life-threatening toxicity. A lower dose is recommended for chronic digoxin poisoning to neutralize a fraction of the digoxin while maintaining therapeutic benefits in the patient with underlying cardiac disease. Empiric dosing of digoxin-specific Fab for chronic poisoning is 1-2 vials for children and 3-6 vials for adults, titrated to clinical effect. Adverse effects are rare and include hypersensitivity reactions, hypokalemia, and worsening of preexisting congestive heart failure.

Ip D, Syed H, Cohen M: Digoxin specific antibody fragments (Digibind) in digoxin toxicity. *BMJ.* 2009;339:b2884 [PMID: 19729422].

Levine M, Nikkanen H, Pallin DJ: The effects of intravenous calcium in patients with digoxin toxicity. *J Emerg Med.* 2011;40: 41-46 [PMID: 19201134].

IRON

Mechanism of Toxicity

The toxicity of iron poisoning is multifactorial, resulting from direct corrosive effects of iron salts in the GI tract and widespread cellular toxicity after systemic absorption. Excess iron (exceeding the iron-binding capacity) is widely distributed throughout the vasculature and deposited in all major organs, where cellular toxicity ensues. Iron participates in redox reactions that generate free radicals, resulting in oxidative damage to cell membranes and cellular necrosis. Injury to the vasculature results in vasodilation and increased vascular permeability and fluid loss, with subsequent hypotension and metabolic acidosis. Fatty degeneration and necrosis are seen in hepatocytes, renal tubules, and myocardial cells. Mitochondrial oxidative phosphorylation is disrupted, resulting in decreased cellular energy production and increased metabolic acidosis.

Clinical Presentation

Acute iron poisoning characteristically follows a biphasic course. GI toxicity occurs first, followed by systemic toxicity. Vomiting usually occurs within 30 minutes to 1 hour after ingestion. Vomitus may be bloody and may continue for several hours. Enteric-coated tablets may pass into the small intestine without causing gastric symptoms. Abdominal pain, tarry stools or bloody diarrhea, lethargy, and, in severe cases, acidosis and shock may occur within the first 6-12 hours. The child may appear to improve clinically as the GI symptoms subside, and then develop profound CV collapse hours later. This phase of systemic toxicity may include hypovolemia, vasodilation, decreased cardiac contractility, metabolic acidosis, renal failure, coma, seizures, coagulopathy, hepatic failure, acute respiratory distress syndrome, and death. Patients who survive severe iron poisoning with GI corrosive injury may develop the delayed complication of gastric outlet obstruction and intestinal scarring several weeks later.

In contrast to patients with severe poisoning, those who manifest no GI symptoms within 6 hours of iron salt ingestion have not been exposed to a significant amount of elemental iron and will uniformly do well. Patients with mild to moderate iron toxicity will manifest GI distress and mild acidosis, but will not progress to severe systemic toxicity and shock.

Diagnostic Evaluation

The serum iron concentration should be obtained within 4-6 hours of ingestion. Peak serum iron concentrations less than 300 mg/dL are usually nontoxic, whereas levels of 300-500 μg/dL often result in mild to moderate toxicity. Peak serum iron concentrations greater than 500 μg/dL are associated with severe toxicity, and those greater than 1000 μg/dL may be lethal. Other helpful laboratory studies include a CBC, blood gas analysis, electrolytes, glucose, BUN, creatinine, liver function tests, ammonia, lactate, and coagulation studies to evaluate for anemia, metabolic acidosis, hypoglycemia, liver failure, renal insufficiency, and coagulopathy. Abdominal radiographs may identify iron tablets, concretions, or free air in the abdomen.

Treatment

Deferoxamine is a specific chelating agent for iron. Deferoxamine binds ferric iron with high affinity, forming ferrioxamine, which is eliminated by the kidneys. The classic *vin rosé* coloration of the urine does not always occur even in the presence of significant iron toxicity. Indications for deferoxamine after iron overdose include patients with serum iron levels equal to or greater than 500 μg/dL, with or without symptoms, and patients with significant symptoms of hypotension and metabolic acidosis regardless of the serum iron level (see Table 46–2 for dosing of deferoxamine). Therapy should be discontinued when systemic toxicity resolves and serum iron levels return to normal. Rapid infusion of deferoxamine may result in hypotension, and prolonged deferoxamine therapy has been associated with ARDS and *Yersinia enterocolitica* sepsis. Rapid boluses of deferoxamine should be avoided, and deferoxamine therapy should be discontinued after 24 hours in all but the most severe cases.

Valentine K, Mastropietro C, Sarnaik AP: Infantile iron poisoning: challenges in diagnosis and management. *Pediatr Crit Care Med.* 2009;10:e31-33 [PMID: 19433938].

ISONIAZID

Mechanism of Toxicity

Isoniazid (INH) and its metabolites deplete CNS pyridoxine (vitamin B_6) and inhibit the formation of pyridoxal 5-phosphate (the active form of vitamin B_6). Pyridoxal 5-phosphate is a necessary cofactor for the enzyme glutamic acid decarboxylase, which converts glutamate to the inhibitory neurotransmitter GABA. A decrease in GABA results in seizures. Isoniazid also inhibits the conversion of lactate to pyruvate, resulting in lactic acidosis.

Clinical Presentation

Typical clinical picture consists of coma, seizures, and metabolic acidosis. Initial clinical signs include vomiting, blurred vision, ataxia, and decreased mental status.

Diagnostic Evaluation

Isoniazid is not detected in routine drug screens, and serum levels are generally not available. Blood gas analysis may demonstrate severe anion gap metabolic acidosis after only one or two seizures.

Treatment

Pyridoxine hydrochloride given IV is the specific antidote for INH-induced seizures. Pyridoxine should be administered until the seizures are well controlled (see Table 46–2 for pyridoxine dosing). Benzodiazepines alone may not terminate seizures because they require the presence of GABA. Metabolic acidosis is treated with sodium bicarbonate, while ensuring adequate ventilation.

Gokhale YA, Vaidya MS, Mehta AD, Rathod NN: Isoniazid toxicity presenting as status epilepticus and severe metabolic acidosis. *J Assoc Physicians India.* 2009;57:70-71 [PMID: 19753763].

LITHIUM

Mechanism of Toxicity

The exact mechanism of action of lithium is not well understood although several complex theoretical mechanisms have been postulated.

Clinical Presentation

Lithium toxicity can be categorized as acute, chronic, and acute-on-chronic.

▶ Acute Toxicity

Acute ingestions of lithium produce GI irritation, nausea, vomiting, and diarrhea. Dehydration and hyponatremia decrease renal elimination of lithium. Neurologic manifestations are delayed due to the slow redistribution of lithium into the CNS. Elevated lithium levels are associated with T-wave flattening or inversion, prolonged QT intervals, sinoatrial dysfunction, and bradycardia.

▶ Chronic Toxicity

Lithium has a very narrow therapeutic range. Serum concentrations of 0.6-1.2 mmol/L are therapeutic and higher levels can result in chronic toxicity with neurologic symptoms such as ataxia, choreoathetoid movements, clonus,

dysarthria, fasciculations, hyperreflexia, nystagmus, tremors, rigidity, agitation, confusion, coma, and seizures. Chronic lithium therapy is associated with the development of nephrogenic diabetes insipidus and chronic tubulointerstitial nephropathy, and is also associated with thyroid and parathyroid gland dysfunction.

▶ Acute-on-Chronic Toxicity

Patients on maintenance lithium therapy who acutely overdose will manifest signs and symptoms of acute and chronic toxicity.

Diagnostic Evaluation

A serum lithium concentration should be obtained immediately and repeated serially, especially in situations of extended release preparations. Blood samples must be placed in lithium-free tubes to avoid a false-positive result. Other laboratory evaluation includes serum electrolytes, BUN, creatinine, and a CBC. An ECG should also be obtained for QT prolongation and dysrhythmias.

Treatment

Emphasis is placed on optimizing intravascular volume status, sodium homeostasis, and evaluation of renal function. Renal lithium elimination is impaired by hypovolemia, hyponatremia, and renal insufficiency. Patients are treated with normal saline boluses to restore the normal volume followed by normal saline at 1.5-2 times maintenance. Care is taken to avoid fluid overload, resulting in congestive heart failure and pulmonary edema. Hemodialysis or continuous venovenous hemofiltration (CVVH) are recommended for patients with severe neurologic signs and symptoms, patients with renal failure exhibiting signs and symptoms of lithium toxicity, and patients with lithium toxicity who can not tolerate sodium repletion, such as those with congestive heart failure.

Whole-bowel irrigation is recommended in the elimination of extended-release preparations of lithium. Activated charcoal does not bind lithium.

Dennison U, Clarkson M, O'Mullane J, Cassidy EM: The incidence and clinical correlates of lithium toxicity: A retrospective review. *Ir J Med Sci.* 2011;180:661-665 [PMID: 21516355].
McKnight RF, Adida M, Budge K, Stockton S, Goodwin GM, Geddes JR: Lithium toxicity profile: A systematic review and meta-analysis. *Lancet.* 2012;379:721-728 [PMID: 22265699].
Wells JE, Cross NB, Richardson AK: Toxicity profile of lithium. *Lancet.* 2012;379 (9834):2338 [PMID: 22726509].

LOCAL ANESTHETICS

Mechanism of Toxicity

Local anesthetics inhibit sodium channels in peripheral nerves. CV and CNS toxicity occurs with overdose.

Methemoglobinemia has been associated with certain local anesthetics, including lidocaine, tetracaine, and prilocaine. These local anesthetics are metabolized to oxidizing agents resulting in methemoglobinemia.

Clinical Presentation

An awake but toxic patient will have complaints of auditory and visual disturbances, circumoral numbness, confusion, disorientation, lethargy, and light-headedness.

As the serum concentration increases, shivering, tremors, and seizures will develop. At higher levels, respiratory and cardiac arrest can occur.

The mechanism of CV toxicity is usually caused by sodium channel blockade. Shock and CV collapse are related to dysrhythmias, poor inotropy and decreased vascular tone. CV toxicity usually occurs at higher serum concentrations than CNS symptoms.

Refer to the section on methemoglobinemia for diagnosis and treatment of that particular toxicity.

Diagnostic Evaluation

An ECG should be obtained as soon as local anesthetic systemic toxicity is suspected to evaluate for cardiac dysrhythmias. Serum assays of local anesthetic concentrations are not available rapidly to aid in clinical management. A methemoglobin level should be obtained in patients with suspected methemoglobinemia.

Treatment

At the first sign of toxicity, administration of local anesthetic should be stopped immediately. Airway compromise and seizure should be treated quickly because the hypoxia and acidosis worsens the CNS and CV toxicity. IV benzodiazepines are used to treat seizure activity. Standard advanced cardiac life support protocols are used to treat CV toxicity. There is strong evidence for the use of IV fat emulsions (IFE) for the treatment of local anesthetic toxicity. This therapy should be started immediately for life-threatening local anesthetic toxicity (see Table 46–2 for dosing). The main mechanism is thought to be trapping the drug in an intravascular lipid "sink," removing it from the sodium channels.

Dix SK, Rosner GF, Nayar M, et al. Intractable cardiac arrest due to lidocaine toxicity successfully resuscitated with lipid emulsion. *Crit Care Med.* 2011;39:872-4 [PMID: 21263316].

OPIOIDS

Mechanism of Toxicity

Opioids bind to specific receptors in the CNS producing desired effects such as analgesia or euphoria. Excessive doses result in coma, respiratory depression, and hemodynamic compromise.

Clinical Presentation

The classic toxidrome consists of miosis, coma, and respiratory depression. Bradycardia, hypotension, hypothermia, and noncardiogenic pulmonary edema also occur.

Specific opioids can have unique toxic effects. For example, meperidine, pentazocine, and propoxyphene may not present with miosis. Seizures are associated with meperidine, propoxyphene, and tramadol. Rapid IV infusion of fentanyl causes chest wall rigidity and inability to ventilate. Propoxyphene has sodium channel antagonism resulting in wide-complex dysrhythmias. Methadone increases the QT interval and risk for torsade de pointes.

Diagnostic Evaluation

In most cases, the diagnosis is made clinically in patients presenting with the opioid toxidrome and a positive response to naloxone. Although many opioids are detected on the urine drugs of abuse screen, certain drugs such as synthetic opioids are not detected. A positive urine drug screen only implies recent use and may not be completely relied upon to explain the patient's presentation.

Treatment

Patients with respiratory depression will often require support with bag-valve-mask ventilation until naloxone can be administered. Naloxone is an opioid antagonist that reverses the CNS and respiratory depression associated with opioid intoxication (see Table 46–2 for naloxone dosing). Larger than usual naloxone doses may be required to reverse the effects of synthetic opioids. Smaller doses are usually effective at reversing the effects of heroin, and are often titrated until only the respiratory depression is reversed, avoiding the full awakening of the patient and precipitation of withdrawal symptoms. Regardless of the availability of naloxone, certain patients with opioid toxicity will require endotracheal intubation such as those with pulmonary edema, aspiration, hemodynamic instability, seizures, and ingestion of multiple drugs, trauma, or other comorbidities.

Bektas F, Eken C, Sayrac V: Opioid toxicity as a result of oral/transmucosal administration of transdermal fentanyl patch. *Eur J Emerg Med.* 2009;16:344-345 [PMID: 19904081].

Madadi P, Ross CJ, Hayden MR, et al: Pharmacogenetics of neonatal opioid toxicity following maternal use of codeine during breastfeeding: A case-control study. *Clin Pharmacol Ther.* 2009;85:31-35 [PMID: 18719619].

SALICYLATES

Mechanism of Toxicity

Salicylates inhibit cyclooxygenase (COX), resulting in analgesic, anti-inflammatory, and antipyretic effects. Salicylates directly stimulate the respiratory center in the brain causing hyperventilation and respiratory alkalosis. They also inhibit Krebs cycle enzymes, which decreases the production of ATP. Salicylates uncouple oxidative phosphorylation resulting in hyperthermia and lactic acidosis. Last but not least, salicylates increase fatty acid metabolism, which contributes to the anion gap metabolic acidosis.

In addition, aspirin is a gastric irritant, decreases platelet adhesiveness, and inhibits the synthesis of clotting factor VII, increasing the risk of bleeding.

Ingestion of oil of wintergreen is especially dangerous for toddlers. One milliliter of oil of wintergreen (99% methylsalicylate) contains the equivalent quantity of salicylate as 1.4 g of aspirin.

Clinical Presentation

Nausea, vomiting, and abdominal pain occur soon after ingestion. Tinnitus is an early symptom of rising serum salicylate concentration. Respiratory alkalosis results from respiratory stimulation and hyperventilation, while metabolic acidosis occurs due to the accumulation of lactic acid and other organic acids. Combined respiratory and metabolic acidosis indicates severe salicylate poisoning and is usually a preterminal finding. Dehydration and electrolyte disturbances are common. Fever and sweating contribute to dehydration. CNS symptoms include headache, irritability, delirium, convulsions, coma.

Transient hyperglycemia and glycosuria are common; small children may develop hypoglycemia. Other complications include hemorrhagic diathesis from inhibition of prothrombin synthesis or platelet dysfunction, and pulmonary, or cerebral edema. Death results from respiratory failure, CV collapse, and cerebral edema.

Diagnostic Evaluation

Determine serum salicylate concentration initially and serially every 4 hours until a downward trend to nontoxic levels has been recorded. Salicylate absorption from the GI tract is notoriously delayed and erratic. Patients with salicylate toxicity should also have serum electrolytes, glucose, BUN, creatinine, and blood gas analysis checked every 4 to 6 hours as well as urine pH to monitor adequate urine alkalinization.

Treatment

Fluids, electrolytes, and dextrose are administered as required to correct dehydration, acidosis, hypoglycemia, and electrolyte imbalance. A good urine flow should be established. Alkalinization of the urine increases the clearance of salicylates. Start with an initial dose of 1-2 mEq/kg of sodium bicarbonate IV followed by a continuous infusion of 150 mEq sodium bicarbonate in 1 L D5W at twice maintenance rate. Urine pH should be maintained at 7.5 to 8. Hypokalemia must be corrected because hypokalemia inhibits urinary alkalinization. When urine output is adequate, potassium chloride should be added to the IV fluids at a concentration of 30 to 40 mEq/L. Administration of sodium bicarbonate also corrects metabolic acidosis favoring movement of salicylate from the tissues to the serum compartment. Care should be taken to avoid excess alkalinization (serum pH > 7.55).

Multiple-dose activated charcoal (MDAC) is recommended to decrease GI absorption of salicylate especially if a pharmacobezoar or extended release preparation is suspected.

Hemodialysis is effective in removing salicylate as well as correcting fluid, acid-base, and electrolyte disturbances. Hemodialysis should be considered early in patients with severe toxicity, extremely high or progressively increasing serum salicylate concentration, renal failure, inadequate clinical improvement with supportive care and administration of sodium bicarbonate.

Endotracheal intubation of the patient with severe salicylate poisoning must be undertaken with extreme caution. These patients have severe metabolic acidosis and any increase in pCO$_2$ during or after intubation worsens acidosis, often resulting in CV collapse. If at all possible, fluid and electrolyte derangements should be corrected prior to intubation. Preoxygenation and meticulous preparation to ensure first-pass success is critical and the most experienced person available should attempt intubation to avoid prolonged apnea time. Immediately following intubation, attention must be given to hyperventilation to decrease pCO$_2$. Subsequent adjustment of ventilation can be guided by serial blood gas analysis, patient condition and response to therapy.

Bora K, Aaron C: Pitfalls in salicylate toxicity. *Am J Emerg Med.* 2010;28(3):383-384 [PMID: 20223401].

O'Malley P: Sports cream and arthritic rubs: The hidden dangers of unrecognized salicylate toxicity. *Clin Nurse Spec.* 2008;22:6-8 [PMID: 20223401].

SULFONYLUREAS

Mechanism of Toxicity

The sulfonylureas bind to receptors on pancreatic β cells, resulting in insulin release with resultant hypoglycemia. A single tablet of sulfonylurea has the potential to produce hypoglycemia in a toddler.

Clinical Presentation

Early manifestations of hypoglycemia result from increased catecholamine release, including anxiety, diaphoresis, tachycardia, tremor, and vomiting. Progressive neuroglycopenia may result in focal neurologic deficits, confusion, lethargy, coma, seizures, permanent neurologic injury, and death. Hypoglycemia usually begins within 4 hours and peaks within 12 hours after ingestion. However, rare cases of delayed onset of hypoglycemia are reported. Large ingestions result in severe and prolonged hypoglycemia. Sulfonylurea overdose should be suspected in patients presenting with altered mental status and unexplained hypoglycemia that is resistant to treatment.

Diagnostic Evaluation

It is essential to check the serum glucose concentration serially to detect hypoglycemia. Evaluation of serum concentration of sulfonylureas is not immediately available and does not assist in acute management. However, blood may be sent to a reference laboratory for qualitative or quantitative detection of sulfonylureas in unusual cases of hypoglycemia in which malicious or surreptitious administration is suspected.

Treatment

IV access is needed so the patient will not require multiple needle punctures for serial blood testing, and to provide a route for administration of dextrose and other treatments. Rapid serum glucose determination at the bedside with glucose reagent strips provides immediate confirmation of hypoglycemia so that treatment can be initiated without delay.

Asymptomatic patients should be observed with serial serum glucose determinations, and normal access to food and liquids. Prophylactic administration of dextrose is not recommended for asymptomatic patients with normal blood sugar, because it masks the onset of hypoglycemia, and prolongs the observation period. Excessive dextrose will stimulate the release of insulin. Most authorities recommend 24-hour hospitalization for all patients due to the possibility of delayed onset hypoglycemia.

Patients who become hypoglycemic require IV dextrose and hospital admission. Children with hypoglycemia should receive 2-4 mL/kg of 25% dextrose IV, repeated as needed to normalize serum glucose. This should be followed by a continuous IV infusion of 5% or 10% dextrose in ½ normal saline with 20 mEq/L of potassium chloride per liter at one times maintenance rate, titrated to maintain normal serum glucose. Patients with severe hypoglycemia may require central venous access for infusion of dextrose at concentrations of 25% or greater to maintain euglycemia.

Patients with large dextrose requirements should also be treated with octreotide, a semisynthetic long-acting somatostatin analog. Octreotide binds to a distinct receptor on pancreatic β cells that inhibits insulin release. Refer to Table 46-2 for dosing. Most significant sulfonylurea poisonings will require 24 hours of octreotide therapy and another 24 hours of observation after therapy is discontinued to monitor for recurrent hypoglycemia.

Rowden AK, Fasano CJ: Emergency management of oral hypoglycemic drug toxicity. *Emerg Med Clin North Am.* May 2007;25:347-356 [PMID: 17482024].

WARFARIN-BASED ANTICOAGULANTS

Mechanism of Toxicity

The emergence of warfarin-resistant strains of rats has led to the development of "superwarfarins," or long-acting warfarin-based rat poisons. These derivatives include brodifacoum and related second-generation 4-hydroxycoumarins which block the synthesis of vitamin K–dependent clotting factors (II, VII, IX, and X). Peak effects are not seen for 2-3 days due to long half-lives of factors IV and X. Superwarfarins may result in coagulopathy for weeks to months after large or repeated ingestions.

Clinical Presentation

A single small unintentional ingestion of superwarfarin is unlikely to cause prolongation of the international normalization ratio (INR). It is even less likely to cause clinically significant anticoagulation. Most children with unintentional superwarfarin ingestions are asymptomatic with a normal coagulation profile. However, clinically significant coagulopathy can result especially with repeated, intentional or surreptitious ingestion. Intracranial bleeding, GI hemorrhage, retroperitoneal bleeding, hemorrhagic shock, hemarthroses, and epistaxis have all been reported.

Diagnostic Evaluation

Routine measurement of the PT or INR is unnecessary for most children with a single small unintentional ingestion of superwarfarin rodenticide. If coagulation tests are recommended, the optimal time is 2-3 days after a single exposure.

If bleeding is present or a large or repeated exposure to rodenticide has occurred, determine the PT/INR and hemoglobin/hematocrit at presentation, 24 hours, and 48 hours after ingestion. Partial thromboplastin time (PTT) is generally not prolonged except in severe poisonings.

Treatment

Patients presenting with active blood loss and hemodynamic instability will require packed red cell blood (PRBC) transfusion. Although PRBC transfusion helps to replace blood loss, it does not correct the coagulopathy. Fresh frozen plasma (FFP) and other factor concentrates are also necessary.

Vitamin K is indicated for patients who present with significant coagulopathy. Hematology consultation is recommended to optimize treatment of coagulopathic patients. The long-acting superwarfarins may result in prolonged coagulopathy requiring weeks to months of close monitoring and treatment.

Altay S, Cakmak HA, Boz GC, Koca S, Velibey Y: Prolonged coagulopathy related to coumarin rodenticide in a young patient: Superwarfarin poisoning. *Cardiovasc J Afr.* 2012;23:e9-e11 [PMID: 23108575].

Fang Y, Ye D, Tu C, et al: Superwarfarin rodent poisons and hemorrhagic disease. *Epidemiology.* 2012;23:932-934 [PMID: 23038123].

Watson KS, Mills GM, Burton GV: Superwarfarin intoxication: Two case reports and review of pathophysiology and patient management. *J La State Med Soc.* 2012;164:70-72 [PMID: 22685854].

DRUGS OF ABUSE

AMPHETAMINES

Mechanism of Toxicity

Amphetamines are sympathetic nervous system stimulants. They increase the release of catecholamines and serotonin, the relative activity of which depends on the specific compound and dose; for example, methylenedioxymethamphetamine (Ecstasy) has more serotoninergic properties. A large number of amphetamine-like compounds have been synthesized, such as the street drugs known as "bath salts" (cathinones).

Clinical Presentation

Initial CNS effects of euphoria and stimulation may progress to severe agitation, combativeness, seizures, and coma. Tachycardia, hypertension, tremor, and diaphoresis are common. More severe toxicity includes hyperthermia, acute myocardial ischemia and infarction, dysrhythmias, intracranial hemorrhage, rhabdomyolysis, multi-organ failure, CV collapse, and death.

Diagnostic Evaluation

Diagnosis and management of stimulant toxicity is based on the identification of the sympathomimetic toxidrome. Serum electrolytes should be checked especially in seizing patients. "Ecstasy" can cause syndrome of inappropriate secretion of antidiuretic hormone (SIADH) and hyponatremia. Urine drugs of abuse testing can confirm recent amphetamine exposure. However, certain compounds are not detected by the routine urine drug screen. For example, confirmation of "bath salts" (cathinones) exposure may require sending blood or urine samples to a reference laboratory therefore results will not be immediately available for clinical management of the patient. False-positive results on the urine drugs of abuse screen may also be caused by pharmaceuticals that have an amphetamine-like structure.

Treatment

Treatment of severe amphetamine toxicity requires aggressive supportive care with emphasis on control of agitation, hyperthermia, and hypertension. Initial physical restraint followed by large doses of benzodiazepines may be required. Patients who are extremely hyperthermic, combative, or hemodynamically unstable may require immediate rapid sequence intubation and continued neuromuscular paralysis. Severe hypertension is usually improved by such measures but occasionally a short-acting vasodilator such as nitroprusside or nitroglycerine is indicated. β-Blockers are discouraged because unopposed α-adrenergic stimulation may worsen hypertension. External cooling and intravascular volume resuscitation are important aspects of management.

Spiller HA, Hays HL, Aleguas A: Overdose of drugs for attention-deficit hyperactivity disorder: Clinical presentation, mechanisms of toxicity, and management. *CNS Drugs.* 2013;27:531-543 [PMID: 23757186].

CANNABINOIDS

Mechanism of Toxicity

Marijuana contains delta-9-tetrahydrocannabinol (THC) and other homologues that bind to specific cannabinoid receptors in the brain and other parts of the body. Action at these receptors can result in stimulation, sedation, and hallucinations. Synthetic cannabinoids with street names such as "spice" and "K9" have similar actions although they appear to produce more stimulation and CV toxicity.

Clinical Presentation

Smoking or ingesting marijuana usually produces a state of euphoria and relaxation, compromising the ability to perform complex psychological and motor tasks such as driving. High doses may cause paranoid behavior or psychosis with hallucinations and bizarre behavior. Coma may occur following large ingestions in small children.

Tachycardia and postural hypotension may occur. Chest pain and myocardial infarction have been reported in young healthy patients who have used synthetic cannabinoids.

Diagnostic Evaluation

Diagnosis of cannabinoid intoxication is based on history of use and the presence of signs and symptoms such as altered mental status, conjunctival injection, and tachycardia.

THC is detected in most routine urine drugs of abuse screens. Positive urine screens only reflect prior usage and they do not correlate with clinical effects. THC may be detected up to several days following the smoking of a single marijuana cigarette and up to 4 weeks after the last exposure in chronic users. Synthetic cannabinoids are not detected on urine drugs of abuse screens. Blood or urine samples can be sent to reference laboratories for detection of certain synthetic cannabinoids. However, results are not immediately available to aid in management of the patient.

Treatment

Treatment is limited to supportive care.

Lewis TF, Mobley AK: Substance abuse and dependency risk: The role of peer perceptions, marijuana involvement, and attitudes toward substance use among college students. *J Drug Educ.* 2010;40:299-314 [PMID: 21313988].

Stanger C, Budney AJ, Kamon JL, Thostensen J: A randomized trial of contingency management for adolescent marijuana abuse and dependence. *Drug Alcohol Depend.* 2009;105:240-247 [PMID: 19717250].

Thoma RJ, Monnig MA, Lysne PA, et al: Adolescent substance abuse: The effects of alcohol and marijuana on neuropsychological performance. *Alcohol Clin Exp Res.* 2011;35:39-46 [PMID: 20958330].

Wu LT, Pan JJ, Blazer DG, et al: An item response theory modeling of alcohol and marijuana dependences: A National Drug Abuse Treatment Clinical Trials Network study. *J Stud Alcohol Drugs.* 2009;70:414-425 [PMID: 19371493].

COCAINE

Mechanism of Toxicity

Cocaine causes sympathetic stimulation by increasing neuronal release of catecholamines and inhibiting their reuptake. Cocaine inhibits sodium channels, resulting in local anesthesia, but large doses inhibit myocardial sodium channels and lead to QRS prolongation and impaired contractility.

Clinical Presentation

CNS effects include initial euphoria followed by agitation, delirium, coma, and seizures. Severe psychomotor agitation leads to hyperthermia, rhabdomyolysis, metabolic acidosis, and multi-organ failure. CV effects include hypertension, tachycardia, and vasoconstriction. Large doses of cocaine inhibit myocardial sodium channels resulting in QRS prolongation, ventricular dysrhythmias, and CV collapse. Severe hypertension in cocaine patients can lead to hemorrhagic stroke or aortic dissection. Chest pain and myocardial infarction result from coronary artery spasm and thrombosis. Similarly, infarction of the brain, kidney, or intestine can

occur. Snorting or smoking cocaine can result in pneumomediastinum, pneumothorax, pulmonary edema, and alveolar hemorrhage. Pulmonary infiltrates ("crack lung") are reported in patients who smoke crack.

Diagnostic Evaluation

Diagnosis is usually made clinically based on patient history and the typical symptoms of cocaine intoxication. Urine drugs of abuse screens detect benzoylecgonine. Cocaine undergoes rapid metabolism and hydrolysis, but its metabolite benzoylecgonine may be detected 2-3 days after exposure.

Treatment

Treatment of severe cocaine toxicity requires aggressive supportive care with emphasis on control of agitation, hyperthermia, and hypertension. Initial physical restraint followed by large doses of benzodiazepines may be required. Patients who are extremely hyperthermic, combative, or hemodynamically unstable may require immediate rapid sequence intubation and continued neuromuscular paralysis. Severe hypertension usually improves with such measures but occasionally short-acting vasodilators such as nitroprusside or nitroglycerine are indicated. β-Blockers are discouraged because unopposed α-adrenergic stimulation may worsen hypertension. External cooling and intravascular volume resuscitation are important aspects of management.

Supraventricular dysrhythmias typically improve with cooling, fluids, and benzodiazepines. Rapid atrial fibrillation and narrow complex reentry tachycardias may require diltiazem. Evaluation for myocardial ischemia or infarction is routine.

Toxicity secondary to cardiac sodium channel blockade, such as QRS prolongation, decreased inotropy, and ventricular tachycardia, usually responds to IV sodium bicarbonate. Refractory ventricular dysrhythmias may respond to lidocaine or electrical cardioversion.

Goldstein RA, DesLauriers C, Burda A, Johnson-Arbor K: Cocaine: history, social implications, and toxicity: A review. *Semin Diagn Pathol.* 2009;26:10-17 [PMID: 19292024].

Heard K, Palmer R, Zahniser NR: Mechanisms of acute cocaine toxicity. *Open Pharmacol J.* 2008;2:70-78 [PMID: 19568322].

INHALANTS

Mechanism of Toxicity

Most inhalants are lipophilic hydrocarbons, which permit their rapid diffusion into the CNS, resulting in altered states of consciousness.

Clinical Presentation

Inhalants produce initial euphoria followed by CNS depression. Hydrocarbons sensitize the myocardium to endogenous catecholamines, leading to spontaneous ventricular tachydysrhythmias and fibrillation ("sudden sniffing death"). There are unique effects associated with particular inhalants: methemoglobinemia (nitrites), peripheral neuropathy (chronic *n*-hexane abuse), and carbon monoxide (methylene chloride). Toluene abuse can result in renal tubular acidosis, hypokalemia, and severe muscle weakness. Products such as carburetor cleaners contain methanol, resulting in metabolic acidosis and blindness when inhaled. Chronic abuse of inhalants can result in debilitating leukoencephalopathy.

Diagnostic Evaluation

Diagnosis of inhalant abuse may be difficult, unless clinical clues are present, such as solvent odor, paint stains, or dermatitis around the mouth and hands. Urine drugs of abuse screens do not detect inhalants.

Treatment

Treatment is supportive. Specific toxicities such as hypokalemia, methemoglobinemia, and carbon monoxide poisoning should be sought and treated in the appropriate clinical setting. Patients with cardiac dysrhythmias secondary to myocardial sensitization to catecholamines may benefit from treatment with β-blockers.

Gupta SK, Bali S, Jiloha RC: Inhalant abuse: An overlooked problem. *Indian J Psychiatry.* 2009;51:160-161 [PMID: 19823642].

Kerridge BT, Saha TD, Smith S, et al: Dimensionality of hallucinogen and inhalant/solvent abuse and dependence criteria: Implications for the diagnostic and statistical manual of mental disorders, 5th ed. *Addict Behav.* 2011; 36(9):912-916 [PMID: 21621334].

Konghom S, Verachai V, Srisurapanont M, et al: Treatment for inhalant dependence and abuse. *Cochrane Database Syst Rev.* 2010(12):CD007537 [PMID: 21154379].

Marsolek MR, White NC, Litovitz TL: Inhalant abuse: monitoring trends by using poison control data, 1993-2008. *Pediatrics.* 2010;125:906-913 [PMID: 20403928].

Perron BE, Howard MO: Adolescent inhalant use, abuse and dependence. *Addiction.* 2009;104:1185-1192 [PMID: 19426292].

LYSERGIC ACID DIETHYLAMIDE (LSD) & OTHER HALLUCINOGENS

Mechanism of Toxicity

LSD and other hallucinogens alter the activity of serotonin and dopamine in the CNS and increase sympathetic stimulation.

Clinical Presentation

Patients often appear anxious and fearful and may exhibit bizarre behavior. They may be combative or self-destructive. Mydriasis, tachycardia, and diaphoresis are common. Severe intoxication results in hyperthermia, hyperreflexia, muscle rigidity, seizures, cardiac dysrhythmias, hypertension or hypotension, and rhabdomyolysis.

Diagnostic Evaluation

Diagnosis is usually based on history and presenting symptoms. Routine urine drugs of abuse screens do not detect LSD and other hallucinogens.

Treatment

Anxiety and agitation are best treated with sensory isolation and reassurance. If a pharmacologic agent is needed, benzodiazepines are the agents of choice. Treatment of more severe toxicity is supportive with control of agitation and correction of hyperthermia, dehydration, electrolyte disturbances, and CV instability.

Iaria G, Fox CJ, Scheel M, et al: A case of persistent visual hallucinations of faces following LSD abuse: A functional magnetic resonance imaging study. *Neurocase.* 2010;16:106-118 [PMID: 19927262].

ENVIRONMENTAL & HOUSEHOLD TOXINS

CARBON MONOXIDE

Mechanism of Toxicity

Carbon monoxide (CO) toxicity results from several mechanisms: (1) CO binds to hemoglobin with an affinity 250 times greater than that of oxygen, decreasing oxygen-carrying capacity, (2) CO shifts the oxyhemoglobin dissociation cure to the left, decreasing oxygen release to the tissues, (3) CO binds to cytochrome oxidase, adversely affecting the ability of tissues to utilize oxygen.

Clinical Presentation

The signs and symptoms of CO poisoning relative to carboxyhemoglobin (CoHb) levels are listed in Table 46-4. Signs and symptoms do not always correlate with measured CoHb levels, reflecting the multiple mechanisms of CO poisoning. Furthermore, once an individual is removed from exposure, CoHb levels in blood diminish rapidly and may not reflect insults to high-demand tissues of the CV and CNS.

Table 46–4. Carboxyhemoglobin blood concentration and clinical presentation.

CoHb Level (%)	Clinical Presentation
0-10	Most persons are asymptomatic. Mild headache, decreased exercise tolerance. May impair driving skills.
10-20	Headache, fatigue, nausea.
20-30	Severe headache, syncope, dizziness, visual changes, weakness, nausea, vomiting.
30-40	Headache, syncope, confusion, loss of consciousness, tachycardia, nausea, vomiting.
40-50	Coma, convulsions, tachycardia, tachypnea.
50-60	Coma, convulsions, cardiorespiratory collapse.
> 60	Death.

Diagnostic Evaluation

An arterial or venous CoHb level should be obtained via co-oximetry. A low level does not rule out poisoning if the measurement is obtained several hours after the exposure. Oxygen saturation will be low if it is directly measured. Many blood gas analyzers calculate the oxygen saturation rather than directly measuring the saturation. Blood gas analysis will demonstrate metabolic acidosis if significant impairment of oxygen delivery and utilization has occurred.

Treatment

Administer 100% oxygen via a non-rebreathing mask or endotracheal tube. The half-life of CO is approximately 4-6 hours in room air but is shortened to 1-2 hours in 100% oxygen and 20-30 minutes in 3 atmospheres of hyperbaric oxygen (HBO). Potential indications for HBO treatment are a CoHb concentration of greater than 25% (lower if the patient is pregnant); major symptoms, including loss of consciousness, seizures, or cardiac dysrhythmias; or symptoms unresponsive to 100% oxygen therapy.

Kealey GP: Carbon monoxide toxicity. *J Burn Care Res.* 2009;30: 146-147 [PMID: 19060737].

Laing C: Acute carbon monoxide toxicity: The hidden illness you may miss. *Nursing.* 2010;40:38-43 [PMID: 20890232].

Prockop LD: Carbon monoxide brain toxicity: Clinical, magnetic resonance imaging, magnetic resonance spectroscopy, and neuropsychological effects in 9 people. *J Neuroimaging.* 2005;15(2):144-149 [PMID: 15746226].

Suner S, Partridge R, Sucov A, et al: Non-invasive pulse CO-oximetry screening in the emergency department identifies occult carbon monoxide toxicity. *J Emerg Med.* 2008;34: 441-450 [PMID: 18226877].

CAUSTIC OR CORROSIVES

Mechanism of Toxicity

Alkalis produce liquefactive necrosis with deeper tissue injury and risk of perforation. Acids produce coagulation necrosis with a lower perforation risk. Additional corrosive agents cause injury by alkylating, denaturing, oxidizing or reducing cellular proteins, and defatting surface tissues. Metal salts from leakage of ingested button batteries and possibly from discharge of the electrical current may also result in corrosive injuries.

Clinical Presentation

Oral burns may manifest as whitish lesions with associated burning pain. Retrosternal pain, salivation, dysphagia, and vomitus containing mucous and blood suggest esophageal injury. Gastric or intestinal injury presents with abdominal pain and hematemesis.

Hypotension may develop due to GI hemorrhage. Perforation of the alimentary tract can result in mediastinitis or peritonitis with resultant septic shock. Long-term sequelae include esophageal strictures or gastric outlet obstruction. Dermal and ocular burns may also occur.

Diagnostic Evaluation

Diagnosis of caustic burns is usually made clinically. X-rays of the chest and abdomen may reveal the button battery.

Treatment

After ingestion, do not induce vomiting or perform gastric lavage. The patient's mouth should be rinsed thoroughly and clear liquids swallowed as tolerated to dilute the caustic agent. Activated charcoal does not bind caustic agents and obscures the view of the endoscopist.

If a significant ingestion is suspected, admit the patient and consult a gastroenterologist for endoscopy. Surgical consultation should be obtained for all patients with suspected perforation.

Antibiotic therapy is not indicated unless there is perforation or evidence of infection.

Ocular and dermal decontamination should be performed rapidly to decrease the length of contact time with the offending agent. Remove contaminated clothing and irrigate the skin with tepid water for 15 minutes. Do not attempt to neutralize the alkali or acid. Ocular exposures to caustic agents especially alkalis may result in severe eye injuries and blindness. The eyes should be irrigated immediately with water or saline for at least 15 minutes. The pH of the tears in the conjunctival sac should then be measured using litmus paper. Further irritation is indicated until the pH returns to the neutral range of 7.4. Topical ophthalmic anesthetic drops prior to irrigation facilitate patient comfort and compliance. Fluorescein dye with Wood lamp and slit lamp examination are indicated to evaluate eye injuries. Consultation with an ophthalmologist is advised.

Button batteries located in the esophagus must be removed. Once the battery has passed into the stomach, spontaneous passage is expected and removal is not needed unless complications of obstruction or perforation are present.

Bicakci U, Tander B, Deveci G, Rizalar R, Ariturk E, Bernay F: Minimally invasive management of children with caustic ingestion: Less pain for patients. *Pediatr Surg Int.* 2010;26:251-255 [PMID: 19936762].

Chang JM, Liu NJ, Pai BC, et al: The role of age in predicting the outcome of caustic ingestion in adults: A retrospective analysis. *BMC Gastroenterol.* 2011;11:72 [PMID: 21672200].

Karagiozoglou-Lampoudi T, Agakidis CH, Chryssostomidou S, Arvanitidis K, Tsepis K: Conservative management of caustic substance ingestion in a pediatric department setting, short-term and long-term outcome. *Dis Esophagus.* 2011;24:86-91 [PMID: 20659141].

Kumaraaguru N, Haddad M: Multiple button battery ingestion. *Arch Dis Child.* 2010;95:213 [PMID: 20308338].

Rafeey M, Shoaran M: Clinical characteristics and complications in oral caustic ingestion in children. *Pak J Biol Sci.* 2008;11:2351-55 [PMID: 19137870].

CYANIDE

Mechanism of Toxicity

Cyanide (CN) inhibits cellular respiration by interfering with oxygen use in the electron transport chain, specifically inhibiting cytochrome oxidase.

Clinical Presentation

CN gas inhalation can be fatal within minutes with the appearance of anxiety, headache, hypertension, and hyperpnea, followed rapidly by confusion, coma, profound metabolic acidosis, seizures, and finally, respiratory and CV arrest. Venous blood may appear bright red in color, and retinal veins and arteries may appear similarly red. Cardiac monitoring may show evidence of myocardial ischemia.

Lethal ingestions of CN salts produce a similar but less rapid progression of symptoms. Nausea, vomiting, and hemorrhagic gastritis are followed by progressive symptoms of systemic toxicity as described previously.

Diagnostic Evaluation

Routine drug screen does not detect CN. A whole blood or plasma CN determination can be diagnostic but is not rapidly available, and therefore is not clinically helpful. Also, CN levels may not be accurate because CN is an intracellular toxin. Laboratory evaluation demonstrates severe anion gap metabolic acidosis, increased lactate, elevated venous oxygen saturation and a narrow arterial-venous oxygen difference because the tissues are unable to utilize oxygen.

Treatment

Administer 100% oxygen and institute life support measures. Treatment of choice is hydroxocobalamin, which binds CN to form cyanocobalamin (vitamin B_{12}), which is then eliminated by the kidneys (see Table 46-2 for dosing of hydroxocobalamin and the older cyanide kit). If hydroxocobalamin is not available, the older cyanide kit may be used.

The cyanide antidote kit contains three agents administered in the following order:

1. An amyl nitrite ampule (crushed and inhaled for 30 seconds while the other agents are being prepared)
2. Sodium nitrite for IV use
3. Sodium thiosulfate for IV use

The nitrites produce methemoglobin which binds CN, thus freeing tissue cytochrome oxidase to resume cellular respiration. Nitrite-induced methemoglobinemia can be dangerous and nitrites should not be given if the symptoms are mild or diagnosis is uncertain. Nitrites are vasodilators and therefore should not be given to hypotensive patients. Methemoglobin levels should not exceed 30% (70% is fatal). Thiosulfate acts as a sulfhydryl donor to increase the activity of rhodanese, the rate limiting enzyme in CN detoxification. This enzyme converts CN to thiocyanate, which is then excreted in urine.

Because methemoglobin does not transport oxygen, therapy with nitrites may be omitted in patients likely to already have high methemoglobin levels or in patients with mixed CN and CO exposure (such as in a fire in a closed space), cyanotic patients, or those with severe CV disease who may not tolerate hypotension. Sodium thiosulfate alone, without prior nitrite administration, may be an effective antidote.

Barillo DJ: Diagnosis and treatment of cyanide toxicity. *J Burn Care Res.* 2009;30:148-152 [PMID: 19060738].

Thomas C, Svehla L, Moffett BS: Sodium-nitroprusside-induced cyanide toxicity in pediatric patients. *Expert Opin Drug Saf.* 2009;8:599-602 [PMID: 19645589].

HYDROCARBONS

Mechanism of Toxicity

Most deaths following ingestion of hydrocarbons result from pulmonary aspiration. Products with low viscosity, high volatility, and low surface tension pose a high aspiration hazard. Chemical pneumonitis results direct tissue injury, inflammation, and disruption of surfactant, resulting in decreased gas exchange and pulmonary compliance. Most common hydrocarbons are poorly absorbed from the GI tract and do not result in systemic toxicity. However, certain compounds such as aromatic or halogenated hydrocarbons may result in systemic toxicity including CNS depression, seizures, or cardiac dysrhythmias.

Clinical Presentation

Ingestion of hydrocarbons can lead to immediate coughing or choking with pulmonary aspiration. Ingestion produces significant gastric irritation with the risk of vomiting and further aspiration. Significant aspiration may lead to the rapid development of severe chemical pneumonitis with coughing, grunting, nasal flaring, tachypnea, retractions, rales, hypoxemia, cyanosis, and decreased mental status, rapidly progressing to respiratory failure.

Diagnostic Evaluation

Routine toxicology screening does not identify these agents. Pulse oximetry, blood gas analysis, and chest radiography are important studies in patients with pulmonary aspiration.

Treatment

Administer 100% oxygen and institute life support measures. Patients with severe chemical pneumonitis will require endotracheal intubation and mechanical ventilation. However, high positive end-expiratory pressure (PEEP) requirements increase the risk of barotrauma. In such patients, high-frequency jet ventilation and ECMO may be required. If cardiac dysrhythmias develop, a short-acting β-blocker may be effective. If vasopressors are indicated, a pure α-agonist such as norepinephrine is less dysrhythmogenic than other catecholamines.

Solvents on the skin should be removed with large volumes of soap and water. Eyes should be copiously rinsed with water for at least 10-15 minutes.

LEAD

Mechanism of Toxicity

Lead causes multisystem toxicity by disrupting numerous cellular functions. Mechanisms include binding sulfhydryl groups and other ligands on receptors, enzymes, and structural proteins as well as interacting with calcium and other cations to disrupt enzymes, secondary messenger systems, membrane function, energy production, neurotransmitter release, and many other biological processes.

Clinical Presentation

Children with lead exposure may be asymptomatic or demonstrate a spectrum of toxicity that generally correlates with increasing blood lead concentration (Table 46–5). The most

Table 46–5. Childhood lead poisoning.

Severity	BLL (μg/dL)*	Chelation
Severe (Encephalopathy) Pallor, vomiting, ataxia, lethargy, coma, seizure, cranial nerve palsies, cerebral edema, increased intracranial pressure, death.	> 70	Intensive care unit. Parenteral BAL and CaNa₂EDTA.
Mild to Moderate Loss of developmental milestones, apathy, irritability, anorexia, colicky abdominal pain, vomiting, constipation, anemia. May be asymptomatic.	45-70	Hospital admission for significant symptoms. Parenteral BAL and CaNa₂EDTA. Outpatient management if asymptomatic. Oral succimer.
Asymptomatic Subtle neurocognitive impairment.	< 45	Outpatient management. Chelation usually not required.

*BLL (Blood lead level or concentration) does not correlate exactly with severity. Expert toxicology consultation is advised.

severe consequence is acute lead encephalopathy, resulting in coma, cerebral edema, increased intracranial pressure, and death.

Consultation with toxicologist is advised.

Diagnostic Evaluation

A venous blood lead level or concentration (BLL) should be obtained, although results may not be immediately available. Capillary blood lead levels may be falsely elevated and must be confirmed with a venous sample. Supportive laboratory data include an elevated erythrocyte protoporphyrin concentration and a CBC demonstrating anemia due to inhibition of heme synthesis. Basophilic stippling of erythrocytes may be seen on the blood smear due to clumping of damaged RNA. Urinalysis and serum chemistries are helpful to evaluate for renal injury. Lead is radiopaque and may be detected on an abdominal radiograph. Radiographs of long bones of growing children may demonstrate metaphyseal densities of "lead lines." Head CT is indicated for patients with encephalopathy and suspected cerebral edema.

Treatment

All patients should be removed from the source of lead exposure. Whole-bowel irrigation may be used to decontaminate the GI tract when lead is seen on abdominal radiographs.

The cornerstone of treatment is chelation therapy with agents that bind lead in the vascular compartment, with subsequent elimination in the urine (see Table 46–2 for dosing). Patients with significant symptoms or BLL greater than 70 µg/dL should be hospitalized. Asymptomatic patients with very high BLL should be considered for hospital admission if parental compliance, a lead-free environment, or close outpatient monitoring and follow-up cannot be ensured. Asymptomatic patients with BLL less than 45 µg/dL usually do not require chelation. Outpatient management guidelines for lead screening and follow-up are available from the American Academy of Pediatrics (AAP) and the Centers for Disease Control and Prevention (CDC).

Flora G, Gupta D, Tiwari A: Toxicity of lead: A review with recent updates. *Interdisc Toxicol.* 2012;5:47–58 [PMID: 23118587].

MERCURY

Mechanism of Toxicity

Mercury distributes throughout the body resulting in multiorgan toxicity. Interaction with ligands such as sulfhydryl, phosphoryl, and other functional groups leads to disruption of membrane function, structural proteins, transport systems, enzymes, and additional biological processes. The toxicity of mercury is determined by whether it is elemental (metallic), an inorganic salt, or organic mercury. Route of absorption, dose, chronicity of exposure, and other factors also determine toxicity.

Clinical Presentation

▶ Elemental Mercury

Metallic mercury is poorly absorbed from the GI tract. The main risk of elemental mercury is inhalation because it is a volatile liquid at room temperature. Acute inhalation of elemental mercury causes chemical pneumonitis with cough and fever, which may be followed by GI distress, neurological symptoms, and kidney dysfunction. Chronic exposure to elemental or inorganic mercury can result in neurasthenia, characterized by fatigue, weakness, depression, and headaches. Patients may demonstrate erethism with frequent blushing and redness of the skin, extreme shyness, anxiety, irritability, and insomnia. Gingivostomatitis, hypertension, tachycardia, and tremor may also be present.

▶ Inorganic Mercury

Acute ingestion of mercuric salts (mercury chloride) is caustic to the GI tract, which leads rapidly to hemorrhagic gastroenteritis with oral burns, abdominal pain, vomiting, GI bleeding, intestinal perforation, CV collapse, acute tubular necrosis, and renal failure.

Chronic exposure to inorganic mercury can result in neurasthenia and erethism as discussed previously. In addition, an idiosyncratic syndrome called acrodynia (pink disease) has been described as an erythematous acral rash, irritability, tremors, weakness, diaphoresis, tachycardia, and hypertension. Renal dysfunction, including nephritic syndrome, may also occur.

▶ Organic Mercury

Ingestion of organic mercury compounds (methylmercury) typically results in profound neurotoxicity, which is apparent a few weeks after exposure. Symptoms include paresthesias, tremor, ataxia, weakness, hyperreflexia, blindness, and dementia. Children born to mothers who were exposed to methylmercury in Minamata, Japan had severe spastic quadriparesis, developmental delay, deafness, blindness, and seizures.

Diagnostic Evaluation

Laboratory evaluation for mercury poisoning must be interpreted within the clinical context, including patient symptoms, form of mercury, and chronicity of exposure. A 24-hour urine collection for heavy metals is sometimes used as a screening test for mercury, arsenic, and lead. When mercury specifically is suspected, whole blood and urine mercury concentrations should be obtained. The urine collection may be over 24 hours or a spot collection corrected for creatinine excretion. Other helpful studies include serum chemistries and urinalysis to evaluate renal function.

Treatment

Management consists of supportive care and chelation therapy. Patients with elemental or inorganic mercury poisoning are treated with parenteral dimercaprol (British anti-lewisite [BAL]) when toxicity is severe, or succimer (2,3-dimercaptosuccinic acid, DMSA) when the patient is stable enough to tolerate oral therapy (see Table 46–2 for dosing). Patients with organic mercury poisoning usually have irreversible neurologic damage and do not benefit from chelation therapy. Succimer may be considered, but BAL is contraindicated due to redistribution of mercury to the brain.

Tezer H, Kaya A, Kalkan G, et al: Mercury poisoning: A diagnostic challenge. *Pediatr Emerg Care.* 2012;28:1236-1237 [PMID: 23128656].

METHANOL & ETHYLENE GLYCOL

Mechanism of Toxicity

Methanol and ethylene glycol are rapidly absorbed from the GI tract and very small quantities can result in toxicity. The parent compounds cause inebriation similar to other alcohols but are converted to more toxic metabolites.

Methanol is metabolized by alcohol dehydrogenase to formaldehyde, which is then converted to formic acid by aldehyde dehydrogenase, resulting in an increased anion gap metabolic acidosis. Formate inhibits oxidative phosphorylation, particularly affecting the optic nerve and certain areas of the CNS, such as the basal ganglia.

Ethylene glycol is metabolized by alcohol dehydrogenase to glycoaldehyde, and then via aldehyde dehydrogenase and other enzymes to glycolic acid, glyoxal, glyoxylic acid, and oxalic acid. The metabolites cause an increased anion gap metabolic acidosis. Oxalic acid complexes with calcium to form calcium oxalate, which then precipitates in the kidneys and other organs. This results in renal failure and cerebral edema. Resultant hypocalcemia may cause cardiac dysrhythmias.

Clinical Presentation

Methanol and ethylene glycol poisoning are characterized by initial inebriation and gastritis, followed by a delay until more severe toxicity occurs as the parent alcohol is slowly converted to more toxic metabolites. Severe anion gap acidosis is the hallmark of methanol and ethylene glycol poisoning.

Methanol poisoning presents after a delay as long as 24-30 hours with progressive metabolic acidosis, Kussmaul respirations, visual disturbances, blindness, coma, and seizures. Fundoscopic examination may demonstrate venous engorgement and optic disc hyperemia or edema.

Ethylene glycol poisoning can present after a latent period of 4-12 hours. Symptoms include increasing metabolic acidosis, Kussmaul respirations, renal failure, coma, seizures, and hypocalcemia with tetany or cardiac dysrhythmias.

Diagnostic Evaluation

Serum concentrations of methanol and ethylene glycol should be obtained, but treatment decisions are usually made before results are available due to delayed laboratory turnaround time. Furthermore, if the patient is presenting late in the poisoning, the serum concentration of methanol or ethylene glycol may be low due to metabolism of the parent compound. Supporting laboratory data include an early osmol gap caused by the alcohol, followed by an increased anion gap metabolic acidosis caused by the toxic metabolites (Figure 46–2).

See toxic calculations section for calculation of osmol gap and anion gap. Useful laboratory evaluation includes serum electrolytes, serum osmolality, hepatic transaminases, ethanol level, and blood gas analysis. Hypocalcemia, renal failure and calcium oxalate crystals in the urine suggest ethylene glycol poisoning. In addition, if ethylene glycol toxicity is the result of ingestion of fluorescein-containing antifreeze, the urine may fluoresce under a Wood lamp.

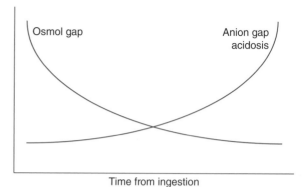

▲ **Figure 46–2.** Reciprocal relationship of acidosis and osmol gap over time.

Treatment

Cornerstones of treatment are supportive care; blockade of the alcohol dehydrogenase enzyme to prevent formation of toxic metabolites; and hemodialysis to remove methanol, ethylene glycol, and their metabolites; as well as correcting acid-base, electrolyte, and fluid abnormalities.

Fomepizole (4-methlpyrazole 4-MP) is the drug of choice to block alcohol dehydrogenase (see Table 46–2 for dosing). Initiation of fomepizole early in the poisoning before toxic metabolites have formed may obviate the need for dialysis. Conversely, fomepizole is not beneficial late in the poisoning after all of the parent alcohol has been metabolized. If fomepizole is not available, ethanol may be used to block alcohol dehydrogenase, but this therapy is less reliable and more cumbersome (see Table 46–2 for dosing.

Indications for fomepizole or ethanol include serum methanol or ethylene glycol concentrations greater than 20 mg/dL, or suspected ingestion with unexplained osmol gap greater than 10 mOsm/L, and metabolic acidosis with serum bicarbonate less than 20 mEq/L or arterial pH less than 7.3. Calcium oxalate crystals in the urine also suggest ethylene glycol poisoning and the need for therapy in this setting.

Indications for hemodialysis include renal failure, severe metabolic acidosis, serum methanol or ethylene glycol level greater than 50 mg/dL (unless the patient is asymptomatic and receiving fomepizole), and visual disturbances in the setting of methanol overdose.

Administration of pyridoxine, folate, and thiamine may favor conversion to less toxic metabolites.

Brent J: Fomepizole for the treatment of pediatric ethylene and diethylene glycol, butoxyethanol, and methanol poisonings. *Clin Toxicol (Phila).* 2010;48:401-406 [PMID: 20586570].

METHEMOGLOBINEMIA

Mechanism of Toxicity

Methemoglobin is the oxidized form of hemoglobin, which is incapable of carrying oxygen. Methemoglobinemia is usually caused by an inducer, which oxidizes ferrous (Fe^{2+}) hemoglobin into ferric (Fe^{3+}) hemoglobin. In addition, the oxygen-hemoglobin dissociation curve is shifted to the left, inhibiting release of oxygen to the tissues.

Clinical Presentation

Symptoms of methemoglobinemia are due to cellular hypoxia and include headache, dizziness, and nausea. Mild methemoglobinemia is well tolerated, but concentrations greater than 20% will result in cyanosis. The skin discoloration can be significant at lower methemoglobin levels and is described as "chocolate cyanosis." Patients with mild to moderate methemoglobinemia appear profoundly cyanotic but may be relatively asymptomatic. As methemoglobin levels increase, symptoms become more severe with dyspnea, confusion, seizures, and coma. Methemoglobin levels greater than 70% are usually lethal.

Diagnostic Evaluation

Methemoglobin is suspected if the patient's blood is "chocolate brown." The discoloration is observable when methemoglobin levels are greater than 15%. Diagnosis is confirmed with an arterial blood gas via co-oximeter analyzer. A co-oximeter analyzer directly measures oxygen saturation and methemoglobin percentages. Methylene blue, the antidote for methemoglobinemia, can cause falsely elevated levels of methemoglobin on the co-oximeter. A routine blood gas analyzer should not be used to direct clinical care in methemoglobinemia because it will calculate a falsely normal oxygen concentration. Pulse oximetry is also not reliable because it does not accurately reflect the degree of hypoxemia in a methemoglobinemia patient. Pulse oximetry will be falsely abnormal in patients who have been given methylene blue.

Treatment

The antidote, methylene blue, is indicated for symptomatic patients (see Table 46–2 for dosing). Methylene blue can worsen methemoglobinemia if given in excessive amounts. Since methylene blue is a dye, it will interfere with pulse oximetry. In patients with G6PD deficiency, methylene blue can aggravate methemoglobinemia and cause hemolysis. Ascorbic acid, which can reverse methemoglinemia via an alternate metabolic pathway, has been used in patients unable to tolerate methylene blue. However, its slow onset of action precludes its use acutely. If methylene blue is contraindicated or is ineffective, exchange transfusion or hyperbaric oxygen therapy may be considered.

Lehr J, Masters A, Pollack B: Benzocaine-induced methemoglobinemia in the pediatric population. *J Pediatr Nurs.* 2012;27: 583-588 [PMID: 22819745].

MUSHROOMS

Mechanism of Toxicity

Poisonous mushrooms are categorized according to the toxins they contain and the toxic syndromes they produce. Mechanism of toxicity depends on the toxins involved, as outlined in Table 46–6.

Clinical Presentation

Gastroenteritis may be the only complaint of an otherwise benign ingestion, or may be a sign of many other syndromes. If gastroenteritis occurs, identification of the mushroom should be pursued. Other syndromes of poisoning include potentially lethal hepatotoxicity, (cyclopeptides; monomethylhydrazine), a disulfiram reaction (coprine), cholinergic crisis (muscarine), delirium or hallucinations (muscimol, ibotenic acid, psilocybin), anticholinergic syndrome (ibotenic acid, muscimol), and renal failure (orelline) (see Table 46–6 for categories of mushroom poisoning).

Diagnostic Evaluation

Mushroom identification should be attempted in all symptomatic cases. Specimens should be kept in a paper bag in the refrigerator. Gastric contents and stools that are saved and refrigerated may be useful for spore identification. Definitive identification of the mushroom should be made in consultation with a mycologist and the regional poison control center. Often, no specimen is available and a presumptive diagnosis is based on the geographic location, history, and clinical presentation. Laboratory evaluation, such as liver function or renal function tests, also depends on the clinical presentation.

Treatment

In addition to supportive care, specific treatments and antidotes as listed in Table 46–6. Treatment with activated charcoal may prevent further absorption of the toxin if used early. However, most patients present late after onset of symptoms. Furthermore, the presence of vomiting and diarrhea often precludes the administration of charcoal.

Eren SH, Demirel Y, Ugurlu S, Korkmaz I, Aktas C, Guven FM: Mushroom poisoning: Retrospective analysis of 294 cases. *Clinics (Sao Paulo).* 2010;65:491 [PMID: 20535367].

Trabulus S, Altiparmak MR: Clinical features and outcome of patients with amatoxin-containing mushroom poisoning. *Clin Toxicol (Phila).* 2011;49:303 [PMID: 21563906].

Table 46–6. Mushroom poisoning syndromes.

Toxin/Mechanism	Representative Species	Onset	Clinical Presentation	Treatment
Amatoxins (amanitine)/ interferes with RNA polymerase II–mediated transcription	Amanita phalloides Galerina autumnalis	6-24 hr 36-48 hr	Abdominal pain, vomiting, diarrhea Hepatitis	IV fluids electrolyte replacement, penicillin G 300,000-1,000,000 U/kg/d Silibinin (investigational) N-acetylcysteine, Liver transplantation
Orelline, cortinarin A and B/tubulo-interstitial nephritis due to alkaline phosphatase inhibition	Cortinarius orellanus	36 hr-20 d	Nausea, vomiting, and progressive renal failure	Supportive care Hemodialysis
Muscimol, ibotenic acid, muscazone/ mimics GABA at receptor site, peripheral anticholinergic activity	Amanita muscaria Amanita pantherina	30-90 min	Decreased mental status, delirium, hallucinations, ataxia	Supportive care, symptomatic treatment
Monomethyl hydrazine/ inhibits pyridoxine-dependent step in GABA synthesis	Gyromitra esculenta	5-10 hr	Seizures, nausea, vomiting, hepatorenal failure	Pyridoxine 25 mg/kg for neurological symptoms, benzodiazepines
Muscarine, histamine/ attaches strongly to acetylcholine receptor site causing prolonged stimulation	Inocybe geophylla Omphalotus olearius	30-120 min	Muscarinic effects: Diarrhea Urination, Miosis, Bronchorrhea Bronchospasm, Emesis Lacrimation, Salivation	Atropine
Coprine/inhibits aldehyde dehydrogenase	Coprinus atramentarius	20 min-2 hr	Disulfuram-like if alcohol ingested before or within 72 hr mushroom ingestion	Supportive care, symptomatic treatment
Psilocybin, psilocin/stimulates autonomic nervous system and serotonin receptors	Psilocybe caerulipes Psilocybe cubensis Gymnopilus spectabilis	30-60 min	Ataxia, nausea, vomiting, hallucinations	Supportive care

ORGANOPHOSPHATE & CARBAMATE INSECTICIDES

Mechanism of Toxicity

These compounds interfere with enzymes that break down acetylcholine, thus allowing continued transmission of impulses in muscarinic and nicotinic nerve fibers. Affected enzymes include acetylcholinesterase (principally found in red blood cells and neurons), pseudocholinesterase (present in serum, hepatocytes, and other organs), and neurotoxic esterase in the CNS.

Organophosphate compounds interfere noncompetitively with the degradation of acetylcholine. Initially their activity is reversible. For many of the organophosphates, "aging" of the bond between the organophosphate and the active site of the enzyme occurs, rendering the bond permanent and the blockade of enzyme activity irreversible. Aging can occur from a few minutes to greater than 48 hours following exposure. The specific chemical compound and the host determine the duration of time to permanent inhibition. Once aging has occurred, enzyme activity is permanently abolished and it can be restored only upon synthesis of new enzyme, a process typically requiring weeks to months. Although carbamates also bind to cholinesterase, this bond is reversible over a period of hours and aging does not occur.

Clinical Presentation

Characteristic signs and symptoms of cholinergic excess are summarized in the muscarinic and nicotinic toxidromes (see Table 46–1). Exocrine gland hypersecretion usually results in increased salivation and diaphoresis. Vomiting and diarrhea are common. Excess cholinergic stimulation of the neuromuscular junction results in muscle fasciculations and weakness. CNS effects include agitation, coma, and seizures. Respiratory failure is the usual cause of death due to the combination of bronchorrhea, bronchospasm, weakness of the muscles of respiration, CNS depression, and seizures.

Diagnostic Evaluation

Rapid metabolism makes detection of organophosphates and carbamates in the blood difficult. Detection of metabolites in the urine may be possible up to 48 hours after exposure, depending on individual kinetics and the extent of exposure.

Cholinesterase activity may be measured in serum or red blood cells. Serum cholinesterase (pseudocholinesterase) measurements generally reflect recent exposure over the past several days to weeks. Red blood cell cholinesterase (RBC acetylcholinesterase) activity, on the other hand, may continue to fall for several days after a single acute exposure, and remain depressed for 1-3 months. Factors that may depress enzyme activity include malnutrition, liver dysfunction, pregnancy, oral contraceptives, and hemolytic anemias.

Treatment

Cornerstones of management include decontamination, supportive care, atropine, and pralidoxime (2-PAM). Immediate decontamination of the patient is essential to preventing further absorption of toxin and protecting those caring for the patient. Emergency personnel should wear protective gear while decontaminating patients because these agents are dermally absorbed. Patients should be decontaminated prior to entering the treatment facility. Remove contaminated clothes and place in sealed plastic bags away from patients care areas. Wash exposed skin with soap and water. If a recent ingestion has occurred, gastric lavage and activated charcoal may be considered if the airway is adequately protected. Good air circulation must be ensured and personnel should avoid inhalation of vapors. Symptomatic personnel should be replaced and decontamination safety procedures reconsidered.

Atropine is the first antidote to consider for organophosphate or carbamate poisoning. It is readily available in the resuscitation cart and emergency practitioners are familiar with its use. The most important indication for atropine is respiratory distress and the alleviation of bronchorrhea and bronchospasm. Extremely large doses may be required to overcome the cholinergic excess (see Table 46–2 for dosing). The endpoint of treatment is reversal of respiratory distress. Atropine reverses the muscarinic excess but has no effect on the nicotinic effects of muscle fasciculations and weakness.

The second antidote to consider for organophosphate poisoning is pralidoxime (2-PAM), which regenerates the anticholinesterase enzyme activity, and therefore has an atropine-sparing effect (see Table 46–2 for dosing). Restoration of the enzyme function improves both muscarinic and nicotinic effects, including muscle weakness. However, pralidoxime must be given early before the aging process renders the enzyme inhibition irreversible. Pralidoxime is not usually indicated for carbamate poisoning because the cholinesterase inhibition is reversible and self-limited, and patients can be managed with supportive care and atropine.

Jokanovic M: Medical treatment of acute poisoning with organophosphorus and carbamate pesticides. *Toxicol Lett.* 2009;190:107-115 [PMID: 19651196].

PLANTS

Mechanism of Toxicity

Mechanism of toxicity depends on the specific plant involved and the toxin it contains. Many plant exposures result in no symptoms or cause only mild local irritation, gastroenteritis, or dermatitis. However, certain plants contain potent systemic toxins that cause severe or life-threatening poisoning.

Clinical Presentation

Most pediatric plant exposures are unintentional and do not result in serious poisoning because the plant is nontoxic or only a small quantity was ingested. Severe toxicity is usually the result of misuse, intentional abuse, or suicide attempts. Toxicity of selected common or dangerous plants is summarized in Table 46–7.

Diagnostic Evaluation

Most plant constituents cannot be measured in body fluids. Diagnostic evaluation is guided by the specific plant involved and the symptoms present. Plant identification can be aided by contacting the regional poison center or botanical expert.

Treatment

Patients with exposure to plants causing systemic toxicity require supportive care and specific treatments as outlined in Table 46–7. Consultation with the regional poison center is recommended. Activated charcoal may be considered for recent ingestions if the airway is protected.

Glatstein MM, Alabdulrazzaq F, Garcia-Bournissen F, Scolnik D: Use of physostigmine for hallucinogenic plant poisoning in a teenager: Case report and review of the literature. *Am J Ther.* 2010;19:384-388 [PMID: 20861718].

Schep LJ, Slaughter RJ, Beasley DM: Nicotinic plant poisoning. *Clin Toxicol (Phila).* 2009;47:771-781 [PMID: 19778187].

NATURAL TOXINS & ENVENOMATIONS

SNAKEBITES

Mechanism of Toxicity

Approximately 20 species of venomous snakes are indigenous in the United States. These include crotalines, such as rattlesnakes, cottonmouths (water moccasins), and copperheads and Elapidae (coral snakes).

Table 46–7. Selected poisonous plants.

Toxin	Symptoms and Special Treatment	Plants	Scientific Name
Abrin	Burning sensation of the mouth and throat, delayed gastroenteritis, depression of vasomotor center, vascular collapse	Precatory bean (rosary pea)	*Abrus precatorius*
Aconitine	Restlessness, salivation, cardiac dysrhythmias	Monkshood Larkspur	*Aconitum* sp *Delphinium* sp
Aglycone	Irritation to mucous membranes, gastroenteritis	Anemone	*Anemone* sp
Anticholinergic alkaloids: Atropine, solanine, and related glycoalkaloids	Dry mouth; mydriasis and loss of accommodation; hot, flushed skin; hyperthermia; convulsions. Treatment: physostigmine for severe anticholinergic symptoms (seizures, hallucinations, hypertension, dysrhythmias) (see Table 46-2 for dosing)	Black nightshade Climbing nightshade (also called woody or deadly) Deadly nightshade Henbane Horse nettle Jimson weed Jerusalem cherry	*Solanum nigrum* *Solanum dulcamara* *Atropa belladonna* *Hyoscyamus niger* *Solanum carolinense* *Datura* sp *Solanum pseudocapsicum*
Capsicum	Strong irritant; stinging and burning of mucous membranes	Christmas pepper	*Capsicum annum*
Cardiac glycosides	CV toxicity. Treatment: measure serum potassium level and treat if high digoxin-specific Fab fragments [Digibind]	Lily-of-the-valley Foxglove Oleander	*Convallaria majalis* *Digitalis purpurea* *Nerium oleander*
Cicutoxin	Seizures. Treatment: benzodiazepines, salivation, vomiting, and diarrhea	Water hemlock	*Cicuta maculata*
Colchicine	GI, respiratory, renal, and CNS toxicity	Autumn crocus Glory lily	*Colchicum autumnal* *Gloriosa* sp
Coniine	Nicotinic excess: Salivation, nausea, vomiting, diarrhea, sensory disturbances, seizures, coma; death may occur from respiratory paralysis	Poison hemlock	*Conium maculatum*
Cyanogenic glycosides (in fruit pits)	Dyspnea, paralysis, convulsions, coma, and death	Cherry trees Apple trees Peach trees Apricot trees Choke cherry trees	*Prunus* sp *Malus sylvestris* *Prunus persica* *Prunus armeniaca* *Prunus virginiana*
Dihydrocoumarin	Burning and irritation GI tract, bloody diarrhea, stupor, weakness, and convulsions	Daphne	*Daphne* sp
Grayanotoxin	Local and GI irritation, respiratory and CV depression	Mountain Laurel Rhododendrons	*Kalmia latifolia* *Rhododendron* sp
Ilexanthin and ilex acid	Vomiting and diarrhea	English holly	*Ilex aquifolium*
Lysergic acid	CNS and psychic stimulation, hallucinations	Morning glory	*Ipomoea leptophylla*
Lycorine	Vomiting and diarrhea	Narcissus Amaryllis Daffodil	*Amaryllidaceae* sp
Nicotine	Nicotinic toxidrome (see Table 46-1)	Tobacco	*Nicotiana* sp

(Continued)

Table 46–7. Selected poisonous plants. (*Continued*)

Toxin	Symptoms and Special Treatment	Plants	Scientific Name
Oxalates	Irritation of the buccal mucosa, edema of the pharynx, gastroenteritis; large ingestions may result in hypocalcemia. Treatment: rinse the mouth with milk; use calcium salts for systemic hypocalcemia	Philodendron Caladium Dumb cane Elephant ear Peace lily Pothos Jack-in-the-pulpit Wild calla Skunk cabbage	*Philodendron* sp *Caladium* sp *Dieffenbachia* sp *Colocasia* sp *Spathiphyllum* sp *Epipremnum aureum* *Arisaerna triphyllum* *Calla palustris* *Symplocarpus foetidus*
Phoratoxin	Gastroenteritis and CV collapse	Mistletoe	*Phoradendron flavescens*
Pohophyllotoxin-like resins	Vomiting, sweating, colic, diarrhea, CNS depression	Pokeweed	*Phytolacca* sp
Podophyllotoxin	May produce peripheral neuropathy, vomiting, colic, diarrhea, drowsiness, impaired vision	May apple	*Podophyllum* sp
Protoanemonin	GI irritation	Buttercup	*Ranunculus* sp
Pyrethrins	Skin reactions	Chrysanthemum	*Chrysanthemum* sp
Pyrrolizodine alkaloids	Weakness, debilitation, vomiting, and tremors. Also can present with liver failure. Treatment; *N*-acetylcysteine	Snakeroot	*Ageratina altissima*
Ricin	Burning sensation of the mouth and throat, delayed gastroenteritis depression of vasomotor center, hepatic injury, hemolysis, convulsions and death	Castor bean	*Ricinus* sp
Taxine	AV block, hypotension, wide QRS	Yew	*Taxus* sp
Urushiol	Dermatitis manistested by red, itchy and clear blisters that exude serum, if ingested causes severe mucosal irritation	Poison ivy Poison oak Poison sumac	*Toxicodendron* sp
Veratrum alkaloids	GI irritation, respiratory and cardiac depression	Green hellebore False hellebore Death camus	*Veratrum viride* *Veratrum californicum* *Zygadonus venerious*

Crotaline venoms are complex mixtures of proteins with enzymatic activity. These enzymes are capable of causing injury to most organ systems. Elapidae venom is primarily a neurotoxin, affecting both the central and peripheral nervous systems.

Clinical Presentation

Crotaline envenomations usually produce local pain, ecchymosis, necrosis, and ascending swelling. In addition, fasciculations and paresthesias may be noted. Systemic signs include coagulopathy, thrombocytopenia, hypotension, respiratory paralysis, pulmonary edema, and renal dysfunction. Elapidae envenomation produces light-headedness, weakness, tremors, nausea, vomiting, and cranial nerve dysfunction with respiratory insufficiency.

Diagnostic Evaluation

No laboratory test is readily available to confirm a suspected snakebite. Diagnosis is based on history and clinical presentation of the patient. Useful laboratory tests for patients with crotaline envenomation include CBC, PT/INR, and fibrinogen.

Treatment

Patients with crotaline bites should be monitored for development of symptoms for at least 6-8 hours. If patients are asymptomatic following the observation period, they can be safely discharged home. If symptoms develop during the observation, then antivenom treatment should be considered, along with poison center consultation.

An ovine Fab fragment antivenom is available in the United States for the treatment of crotaline envenomation (see Table 46–2 for dosing). The antivenom is safe and highly efficacious for the treatment of local and systemic effects in children. Patients receiving antivenom should be monitored closely for allergic reactions and treated appropriately. True muscle compartment syndrome is unusual and the need for fasciotomy is rare. Aggressive antivenom therapy often obviates the need for fasciotomy, but if compartment swelling and pressures continue to increase despite medical management, surgical consultation should be obtained expeditiously.

There is no FDA-approved antivenom available currently in the United States for treatment of coral snake envenomation. However, there is an equine-based Fab2 antivenom produced in Mexico for *Micrurus nigrocinctus* that has shown cross reactivity with North American *Micrurus* species. The regional poison center should be contacted in the case of coral snake envenomation to aid in obtaining the antivenom if needed. If antivenom is unavailable, patients with progressive muscle weakness may require endotracheal intubation and mechanical ventilation.

Prior to the use of an antivenom, notify your regional poison center for consultation with the toxicologist.

Ashton J, Baker SN, Weant KA: When snakes bite: The management of North American Crotalinae snake envenomation. *Adv Emerg Nurs J.* 2011;33:15-22 [PMID: 21317694].

Norris RL, Pfalzgraf RR, Laing G: Death following coral snake bite in the United States—first documented case (with ELISA confirmation of envenomation) in over 40 years. *Toxicon.* 2009;53:693-697 [PMID: 19673084].

HYMENOPTERA ENVENOMATION

Mechanism of Toxicity

Hymenoptera is a group of arthropods including bees, wasps, and ants. Hymenoptera stings are associated with two mechanisms of toxicity: envenomation and hypersensitivity reactions. Hymenoptera venom contains a number of peptides that cause histamine release, muscle necrosis, and intravascular hemolysis.

Clinical Presentation

Acute hypersensitivity reactions include typical signs of angioedema, upper airway obstruction, hypotension, respiratory failure, hives, flushing, and pruritus. Delayed serum sickness reactions also occur. Envenomations involving large, multiple doses of venom exhibit edema, respiratory

failure, hypotension, and renal failure. Widespread damage to muscle can occur, causing rhabdomyolysis and renal failure. Intravascular hemolysis has also been reported.

Diagnostic Evaluation

No specific diagnostic test is available for the effects of venom.

Treatment

Stingers that are retained in the skin should be scraped off rather than removed with forceps or by other methods. Scraping the stinger avoids compression of the venom sack, and prevents further venom exposure. Wash the affected area with soap and an antiseptic.

Treatment for multiple stings is largely supportive, because there is no antivenom available. Because of the possibility of non–IgE-mediated histamine release complicating the acute massive exposure to venom, antihistamine therapy should be considered in the absence of other manifestations of a hypersensitivity reaction.

Hypersensitivity reactions can be treated with epinephrine. β_2-Agonist aerosols may be useful for the management of acute bronchospasm. Antihistamines and corticosteroids should be administered for any systemic manifestations. Referral to an allergy-immunology specialist is appropriate. Patients should be sent home with an epinephrine autoinjector.

Broides A, Maimon MS, Landau D, Press J, Lifshitz M: Multiple hymenoptera stings in children: Clinical and laboratory manifestations. *Eur J Pediatr.* 2010;169:1227-1231 [PMID: 20461529].

Friedman LS, Modi P, Liang S, Hryhorczuk D: Analysis of hymenoptera stings reported to the Illinois Poison Center. *J Med Entomol.* 2010;47:907-912 [PMID: 20939389].

Golden DB, Kelly D, Hamilton RG, Craig TJ: Venom immunotherapy reduces large local reactions to insect stings. *J Allergy Clin Immunol.* 2009;123:1371-1375 [PMID: 19443022].

Jennings A, Duggan E, Perry IJ, Hourihane JO: Epidemiology of allergic reactions to hymenoptera stings in Irish school children. *Pediatr Allergy Immunol.* 2010;21:1166-1170 [PMID: 20408970].

MARINE ENVENOMATIONS

Mechanism of Toxicity

Many marine species are capable of envenomation, particularly in the Indo-Pacific waters. Physicians in North America are more likely to encounter envenomations from species living in marine aquariums or in shallow waters near the East and West coasts, including lionfish, stingray, jellyfish, and sea urchins. Toxic effects of marine envenomations are due to complex mechanisms that vary depending on the species.

Table 46–8. Selected marine envenomation.

Species	Examples	Toxicity	Signs and Symptoms	Treatment
Invertebrates				
Cnidaria	*Chironex fleckeri* (Box jellyfish) *Physalia utriculus* (Portuguese man-of-war)	Nematocysts releasing venom. Venom depends on species	Severe pain, linear rash, nausea, vomiting, muscle spasms, headache, fever, chills	Nematocyst removal, antivenom if needed Immerse wound in vinegar or hot water
Mollusca	Cephalopoda: *Hapalochlaena maculosa* (Blue ringed octopus)	Tetrodotoxin: blocks sodium conductance in neurons	Paresthesias, muscle paralysis, respiratory failure	Supportive care
	Gastropoda: *Conus* sp (cone snail)	Nematocysts inject conotoxin: antagonizes voltage and ligand-gated ion channels	Severe pain, tissue ischemia, numbness	Nematocyst removal Pain control Hot water immersion
Vertebrates				
Scorpaenidae	*Pterois volitans* (lionfish) *Scorpaena guttata* (stonefish)	Venomous spines. Venom depends on species	Severe pain headache, vomiting, abdominal pain, delirium	Remove retained spines Antivenom if needed Pain control
Chondrichthyes	*Dasytidae* sp (stingrays)	Venomous spines. Venom depends on species	Severe pain	Remove retained spines Hot water immersion Pain control
Reptilia (sea snakes)	*Enhydrina schistose* (Beaked sea snake)	Venomous fangs. Venom depends on species	Painful muscular rigidity, myoglobinuria ascending flaccid paralysis, dysphagia, trismus	Antivenom, if available

Clinical Presentation

Signs and symptoms of envenomation depend on the type of animal. Table 46–8 describes clinical presentation and treatment of selected marine envenomation.

Diagnostic Evaluation

Marine animal venom cannot be measured in body fluids. Diagnostic evaluation is dependent on the specific animal involved and the symptoms present.

Treatment

Wounds should be thoroughly cleansed, with careful attention to removing residual spines. Systemic symptoms are treated with supportive care.

Antivenom treatment is only available for sea snakes, box jellyfish, and stonefish. These species are generally found in the Indo-Pacific region and are unlikely to be found in the United States. Contact the regional poison center or aquarium for consultation regarding marine envenomations.

SPIDER BITES

Mechanism of Toxicity

Two species in particular are capable of significant toxicity: *Latrodectus* species (black widow spider) and *Loxosceles* species (brown recluse spiders). The α-latrotoxin of black widow spiders is a neurotoxin that causes the rapid release of several endogenous neurotransmitters from presynaptic nerve membranes. The venom from the brown recluse spider contains several tissue-destructive enzymes capable of producing local injury and allowing the spread of venom. The tissue necrosis that develops is the result of liposomes released by polymorphonuclear cells attracted to the area of the bite. Venom components also cause lysis of red blood cells.

Clinical Presentation

Bites from widow spiders cause pain and muscle spasms. The bite may not be immediately painful, and local inflammatory symptoms are mild or absent. Pain starts as muscle cramping which progresses to chest pain, or abdominal cramping that is easily confused with acute appendicitis.

Pain can be severe and associated with hypertension and tachycardia. Symptoms usually peak within a few hours of the envenomation and subside over a period of hours to days. Death is rare.

Bites from brown recluse spiders are usually painless until local symptoms develop. Typical lesions develop within a few hours with a central bleb surrounded by concentric rings of pale ischemic tissue and erythema. The bleb can enlarge slowly and turn purple to black over a few days. Breakdown of the bleb may lead to a central ulcer that heals slowly over weeks. Necrotic areas may become large and sometimes require skin grafting. A systemic reaction (loxoscelism) occurs in a small number of patients characterized by fever, hypotension, chills, nausea, myalgia, renal failure, seizures, hemolysis, and occasionally disseminated intravascular coagulation (DIC). Systemic symptoms may progress over a period of several days after envenomation.

Diagnostic Evaluation

Diagnosis is based on the clinical presentation and evidence of envenomation. No specific diagnostic test is available.

Treatment

Pain control with opioids is the preferred treatment for *Lactrodectus* (black widow spider) bites. An equine antivenom is commercially available. The dose is one to two vials given over 1 hour. It is associated with the risk of serum sickness and anaphylaxis, and should be reserved for severe cases only.

There is no available antivenom for brown recluse spider bites in the United States. Treatment is wound care, opioids for pain control, and antipruritic agents. Excision of the bite early does not improve outcome and steroids are also of no proven value. Limited data in humans have suggested the use of dapsone, an agent that inhibits leukocyte migration. The dose is 0.5 mg/kg/d for 2 days, increasing to 1 mg/kg/d if tolerated. Side effects from dapsone include methemoglobinemia and hemolytic anemia (particularly in patients with G6PD deficiency) and it should be considered for severe cases only.

Gaisford K, Kautz DD: Black widow spider bite: A case study. *Dimens Crit Care Nurs.* 2011;30:79-86 [PMID: 21307681].

Dermatologic Emergencies

Craig T. Carter, DO
Timothy R. Howes, MD
Evan Moore, MD

▼ INTRODUCTION & GENERAL CONSIDERATIONS

Although the title of this chapter is Dermatologic Emergencies, patients with rashes who make their way to the emergency department although certainly dermatologic, almost never present as emergencies. Few rashes are emergent; however, emergency physicians will never be without a steady stream of rashes in their examination rooms and should have a working knowledge of the most common rashes. It is important to identify if the rash is emergent, indicative of an emergent process, or requiring specific treatment.

INITIAL EVALUATION

As with any complaint that presents to the emergency department, it is important to first assess the patient's airway, breathing, and circulation (ABC). After initial assessment, a full history and physical will provide the most useful information to make a diagnosis.

HISTORY

A thorough history should be performed including exposure to foods, chemicals, animals, plants, medications, insects, immunizations, toxins, and sick contacts. Attention should be paid to medications, allergies, past medical history (especially history of the same or similar rash in the past), social history, and sexual history. Associated symptoms should be elicited and are necessary in most rashes to make a clinical diagnosis.

EXAMINATION

Patient should be gowned and examined in a room with adequate lighting. Care should be taken to thoroughly expose all pertinent areas of skin including the scalp, nails, and mucous membranes. Take note of the distribution, pattern, arrangement, morphology, extent, and evolutionary changes of the lesions. For an accurate diagnosis, be careful to discriminate

primary lesion from secondary lesions. Finally, document your findings using descriptive terminology. Tables 47–1 and 47–2 list descriptors and morphology of lesions.

Humphries RL, Stone C.: Dermatologic emergencies. In: Humphries RL, Stone C, eds. *Current Diagnosis & Treatment Emergency Medicine*. 7th ed. New York: McGraw-Hill; 2011.

Thomas JJ, Perron AD, Brady WJ: Approach to skin disorders in the emergency department. In: Tintinalli JE, Kelen GD, Stapczynski JS, eds. *Tintinalli's Emergency Medicine: A Comprehensive Study Guide*. 7th ed. New York: McGraw-Hill; 2011.

COMMON FUNGAL RASHES

 ESSENTIALS OF DIAGNOSIS

► Superficial fungal infections.

► Flat, scaly patches.

► Erythematous, pruritic lesions.

General Considerations

Dermatophytes include a group of fungi that infect the nonviable keratinized cutaneous structures such as the stratum corneum, nails, and hair. The infections are generally superficial in immunocompetent hosts.

Clinical Findings

▶ Tinea Capitis

Tinea capitis is a common scalp lesion caused by various dermatophytes. Tinea capitis commonly affects children aged

Table 47–1. Lesion configuration descriptors.

Descriptor	Configuration
Annular	Ring-like or pertaining to the outer edge
Arcuate	Curved or pertaining to the curve
Circinate	Circular
Confluent	Blending together
Dermatomal	Belt-like or limited to one side of the body in anatomic dermatome
Discoid	Solid, round, slightly raised, or pertaining to a disk
Discrete	Separate or individual
Grouped	Clustered
Guttate	Scattered
Gyrate	Coiled or winding
Herpetiform	Creeping
Iris	Concentric circles
Linear	In a line
Polycyclic	Overlapping circles or borders of irregular curves
Retiform	Net-like
Serpiginous	Snake-like

(Reproduced, with permission, from Tintinalli JE, Stapczynski JS, Ma OJ, Cline DM, Cydulka RK, Meckler GD: *Tintinalli's Emergency Medicine: A Comprehensive Study Guide*, 7th ed. New York, McGraw-Hill, 2011. Copyright © McGraw-Hill Education LLC.)

6-10 years; however, individuals of any age can be affected. Lesions generally present with dry scaly patches which may resemble seborrheic or atopic dermatitis. Findings may include alopecia with broken off hairs with the appearance of "black dots." Lesions may progress to folliculitis or a severe painful inflammatory mass known as a kerion (Figure 47–1).

Treatment

Topical treatment is ineffective for tinea capitis and systemic treatment with griseofulvin (children over 12 months of age, 10-20 mg/kg/day divided bid to qid; consider checking baseline CBC and CMP prior to initiating the drug) for 6-8 weeks is first-line therapy. Second-line treatments include terbinafine, itraconazole, and fluconazole. Selenium sulfide 2.5% shampoo may be used as an adjunct to systemic treatment. The kerion will resolve with conservative oral antifungal medication. No incision or drainage is necessary for the treatment of a kerion.

▶ Tinea Corporis

Tinea corporis is a dermatophyte infection which involves the body, excluding the feet, hands, and groin. Tinea corporis is most commonly caused by *Trichophyton rubrum*. Ringworm, or *T circinatum*, is the most common form of tinea corporis that usually begins as a flat scaly patch with a raised, palpable border. Ringworm gradually advances its border outward leaving an area of central clearing. Tinea corporis may present as well-demarcated, erythematous, pruritic scaly patches (Figure 47–2).

Treatment

Mild cases of tinea corporis can usually be treated with over-the-counter topical preparations, such as miconazole nitrate or clotrimazole. Prescription agents include ketoconazole 2% cream or econazole nitrate. Topical remedies should be continued for 1-2 weeks after resolution of symptoms. Extensive disease or difficult cases may require oral therapy. Oral therapies include griseofulvin, itraconazole, terbinafine, and fluconazole.

▶ Tinea Cruris

Tinea cruris, or "jock itch," affects the groin area, sparing the genitalia. Men are affected more commonly than women, and the condition is more common in the summer months (Figure 47–3).

Treatment

Tinea cruris can often be treated with topical antifungal therapies used for 2-3 weeks (see Treatment under Tinea Corporis). The area should be kept dry, because moisture and maceration are typical. Antifungal powders and loose-fitting clothing are often useful adjuncts. A mild topical corticosteroid (1% hydrocortisone cream) may be used cautiously for a short time to help relieve the pruritus, which is often severe. Corticosteroids may be used only for 48-72 hours; longer use is contraindicated. As with tinea corporis, resistant disease may require oral therapy.

▶ Tinea Pedis

Tinea pedis is a dermatophytic infection of the feet, commonly known as athlete's foot. It causes erythema, scaling, maceration and sometimes, bulla formation. In most cases it is caused by *T. rubrum*. It is divided into three subtypes. The most prevalent type is interdigital, a chronic condition that occurs with fissuring and maceration between the toes. The second type, moccasin tinea pedis, has a plantar distribution in which the plantar surface is tender and erythematous. Tinea pedis infections are usually covered with a silvery scale. The third type is the wet, vesicular type. Occasionally the lesions of tinea pedis can become secondarily infected (Figure 47–4).

Table 47–2. Lesion morphology.

Descriptor	Morphology	Lesion Nature	Height Relative to Adjacent Skin	Image
Excoriation	Linear marks from scratching	Secondary	Flat	
Erosion	Ruptured vesicle or bulla with denuded epidermis	Secondary	Depressed	
Fissure	Linear cracks on skin surface	Secondary	Flat	
Ulcer	Epidermal or dermal tissue loss	Secondary	Depressed	

(Continued)

Table 47–2. Lesion morphology. (*Continued*)

Descriptor	Morphology	Lesion Nature	Height Relative to Adjacent Skin	Image
Macule	Flat, circumscribed discoloration ≤ 1 cm in diameter; color varies	Primary	Flat	
Petechiae	Nonblanching purple spots < 2 mm in diameter	Primary	Flat	
Sclerosis	Firm, indurated skin	Secondary	Flat or elevated	
Telangiectasia	Small, blanchable superficial capillaries	Primary	Flat	
Purpura	Nonblanching purple discoloration of the skin	Primary	Flat	

(*Continued*)

Table 47–2. Lesion morphology. (*Continued*)

Descriptor	Morphology	Lesion Nature	Height Relative to Adjacent Skin	Image
Abscess	Tender, erythematous, fluctuant nodule	Primary	Elevated	
Cyst	Sack containing liquid or semisolid material	Primary	Elevated	
Nodule	Palpable solid lesion < 1 cm in diameter	Primary	Elevated	
Tumor	Palpable solid lesion > 1 cm in diameter	Primary	Elevated	

(Continued)

Table 47–2. Lesion morphology. (*Continued*)

Descriptor	Morphology	Lesion Nature	Height Relative to Adjacent Skin	Image
Scar	Sclerotic area of skin	Secondary	Flat or elevated	
Wheal	Transient, edematous papule or plaque with peripheral erythema	Primary	Flat or elevated	
Vesicle	Circumscribed, thin-walled, elevated blister < 5 mm in diameter	Primary	Elevated	
Bulla	Circumscribed, thin-walled, elevated blister > 5 mm in diameter	Primary	Elevated	

(*Continued*)

Table 47–2. Lesion morphology. (*Continued*)

Descriptor	Morphology	Lesion Nature	Height Relative to Adjacent Skin	Image
Pustule	Vesicle containing purulent fluid	Primary	Elevated	
Papule	Elevated, solid, palpable lesion < 1 cm in diameter; color varies	Primary	Elevated	
Plaque	Flat-topped elevation formed by confluence of papules > 0.5 cm in diameter	Primary	Elevated	
Comedo	Papule with an impacted pilosebaceous unit	Primary	Elevated	

Reproduced, with permission, from Tintinalli JE, Stapczynski JS, Ma OJ, Cline DM, Cydulka RK, Meckler GD: *Tintinalli's Emergency Medicine: A Comprehensive Study Guide,* 7th ed. New York: McGraw-Hill, 2011. Copyright © McGraw-Hill Education LLC.

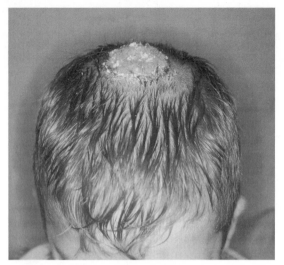

▲ **Figure 47–1.** Tinea capitis with kerion. (Source: Centers for Disease Control and Prevention.)

Treatment

Mild cases of tinea pedis can be treated successfully with 1-4 weeks of therapy with an over-the-counter preparation, in conjunction with the use of drying powders (tolnaftate or butenafine spray, cream or powder). Severe cases may require oral therapy. Drugs such as griseofulvin, fluconazole, and itraconazole are effective. Cases are often recurrent if concomitant nail disease is present.

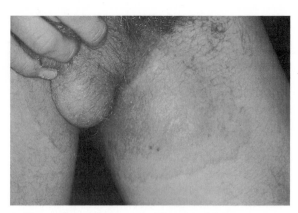

▲ **Figure 47–3.** Tinea cruris. (Photo contributor: James J. Nordlund, MD. Reproduced, with permission, from Knoop KJ, Stack LB, Storrow AB, Thurman R: *The Atlas of Emergency Medicine,* 3rd ed. New York: McGraw-Hill, 2010. Copyright © McGraw-Hill Education LLC.)

▶ Tinea Versicolor

Tinea versicolor affects a deeper layer of the skin than the previously described infections. It is caused by the yeast *Malassezia furfur* and is often associated with multiple hypopigmented macular lesions distributed over the trunk and extremities. Most common colors are brown (hyperpigmented) and whitish-tan (hypopigmented). Exposure to sunlight accentuates the lesions, which do not tan normally like the surrounding skin. A fine scale is often present (Figure 47–5).

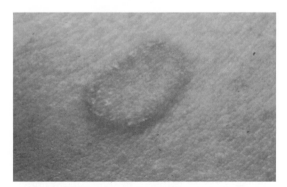

▲ **Figure 47–2.** Tinea corporis (ringworm). (Photo contributor: the Department of Dermatology, Wilford Hall USAF Medical Center and Brooke Army Medical Center, San Antonio, TX. Reproduced, with permission, from Knoop KJ, Stack LB, Storrow AB, Thurman R: *The Atlas of Emergency Medicine*, 3rd ed. New York: McGraw-Hill, 2010. Copyright © McGraw-Hill Education LLC.)

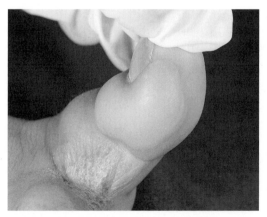

▲ **Figure 47–4.** Tinea pedis with secondary bullous impetigo. (Photo contributor: Binita R. Shah, MD. Reproduced, with permission, from Shah BR, Lucchesi M, eds: *Atlas of Pediatric Emergency Medicine*, 2nd ed. New York: McGraw-Hill, 2013. Copyright © McGraw-Hill Education LLC.)

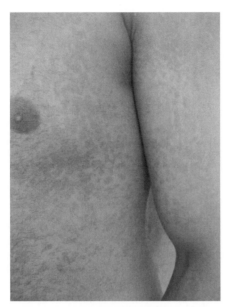

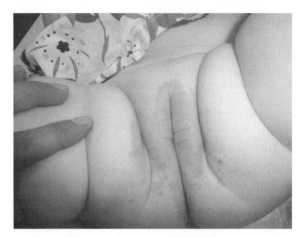

▲ **Figure 47–6.** Candidal diaper dermatitis. Involvement of perianal and inguinal creases with classic satellite papules. (Photo contributor: Julie Cantatore, MD. Reproduced with permission from Shah BR and Lucchesi M (Eds). *Atlas of Pediatric Emergency Medicine*, 2ed. McGraw-Hill, Inc., 2013. Fig 7-116. Copyright © McGraw-Hill Education LLC.)

▲ **Figure 47–5.** Tinea versicolor. (Photo contributor: Sharon A. Glick, MD. Reproduced, with permission, from Shah BR, Lucchesi M, eds: *Atlas of Pediatric Emergency Medicine*, 2nd ed. New York: McGraw-Hill, 2013. Copyright © McGraw-Hill Education LLC.)

Treatment

Limited tinea versicolor can be treated with topical selenium sulfide 2.5%. Multiple regimens have been advocated for use of selenium sulfide 2.5% shampoo. One method is to apply topically and leave on 15 minutes before rinsing, 3-4 times a week until resolved. Daily application of ketoconazole to the affected areas for 3 days is an alternative regimen. Recurrence of the disease may be prevented with the use of a once-monthly bedtime application of selenium sulfide 2.5%.

▶ *Candida* Perineal Dermatitis

Candida perineal dermatitis generally presents as a secondary infection to diaper dermatitis. Diaper dermatitis usually is caused by irritation but spares the skin folds. *Candida* overgrowth resulting in *Candida* perineal dermatitis can be differentiated from irritant diaper dermatitis by involvement of the skin folds as well as satellite lesions which extend beyond the area of erythema. *Candida* dermatitis is a common side effect of antibiotic use. Typical presentation includes diffuse erythema in the perianal area with scaling and satellite lesions (Figure 47–6).

Treatment

Treatment for *Candida* perianal dermatitis is topical nystatin, ketoconazole, or clotrimazole.

Bonfante G, Rosenau AM. Chapter 134. Rashes in infants and children. In: Tintinalli JE, Kelen GD, Stapczynski JS, eds. *Tintinalli's Emergency Medicine: A Comprehensive Study Guide*. 7th ed. New York: McGraw-Hill; 2011.

Hardin J: Cutaneous conditions. In: Knoop KJ, Stack LB, Storrow AB, Thurman RJ, eds. *The Atlas of Emergency Medicine*. 3rd ed. New York: McGraw-Hill; 2010.

Mendez-Tovar LJ: Pathogenesis of dermatophytosis and tinea versicolor. *Clin Dermatol*. 2010;28:185 [PMID: 20347661].

Shah BR: Dermatology. In: Shah BR, Lucchesi M, eds. *Atlas of Pediatric Emergency Medicine*. New York: McGraw-Hill; 2006.

Wolff K, Johnson RA, Suurmond D: Fungal infections of the skin and hair. In: Wolff K, Johnson RA, Suurmond D, eds. *Fitzpatrick's Color Atlas and Synopsis of Clinical Dermatology*. 6th ed. New York: McGraw-Hill; 2009.

COMMON BACTERIAL RASHES

SCARLET FEVER

 ESSENTIALS OF DIAGNOSIS

- ▶ Acute febrile illness.
- ▶ Sore throat.
- ▶ Group A or group C *Streptococcus* species.
- ▶ Red sandpaper rash.
- ▶ Strawberry tongue.

General Considerations

Scarlet fever is an acute febrile illness, caused by erythrogenic toxin (ET). Group A *Streptococcus* is the most commonly associated species to produce ET; however, other strains of bacteria such as group C *Streptococcus* and *Staphylococcus aureus* are capable of producing ET. Scarlet fever is most common in children.

Clinical Findings

Scarlet fever begins as an acute febrile illness with symptoms of fever, sore throat, headache, flushing, tachycardia, and cervical lymphadenopathy. An exanthem of rough, "sandpaper," finely punctate erythematous rash appears first on the upper trunk 1-2 days after onset of fever and can spread to the abdomen and extremities, usually sparing the palms and soles. The rash can sometimes be accentuated in skin folds such as the axilla or groin forming Pastia lines. Rash lasts 4-5 days, followed by desquamation of skin including the palms and soles. Patients may have a mild or subclinical pharyngitis and rash and present due to desquamation. Scarlet fever is also generally associated with an enanthem of a beefy red pharynx, small red macules on the hard and soft palates called Forchheimer spots, and a white strawberry tongue which becomes a red strawberry tongue after the fourth to fifth day (Figure 47–7).

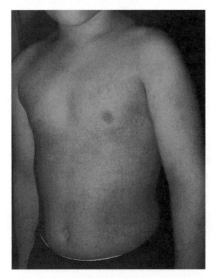

▲ **Figure 47–7. Scarlet fever.** (Photo contributor: Lawrence B. Stack, MD. Reproduced, with permission, from Knoop KJ, Stack LB, Storrow AB, Thurman R: *The Atlas of Emergency Medicine*, 3rd ed. New York: McGraw-Hill, 2010. Copyright © McGraw-Hill Education LLC.)

Diagnosis

Scarlet fever is a clinical diagnosis; however, antistreptolysin O (ASO) antibodies will generally be elevated. Culture of the pharynx may be performed although rapid point-of-care screen tests have sensitivity reported to be between 85-90% and even higher specificity. The Centor criteria of (1) history of fever, (2) tender anterior cervical lymphadenopathy, (3) lack of cough and (4) tonsillar exudates may also be helpful in determining a patient's pretest probability of *Streptococcus* and informing the physician's decision to screen/culture or treat a patient for *Streptococcus* pharyngitis.

Treatment

Penicillin VK (15-17 mg/kg/dose q8h) or amoxicillin (45 mg/kg/dose q12 h) for a 10-day course. Benzathine penicillin G IM (25,000-50,000 units/kg, max 1.2 million units) once. Clindamycin (10 mg/kg q8h) or azithromycin (12 mg/kg/dose q24h for 5 days) are choices for penicillin-allergic patients. Acetaminophen or ibuprofen for symptomatic treatment of fever. Emollients and anti histamines are recommended for the rash. Antibiotic treatment for 24 hours is recommended before return to school. Follow-up is recommended to ensure resolution of symptoms.

Bonfante G, Rosenau AM: Rashes in infants and children. In: Tintinalli JE, Kelen GD, Stapczynski JS, eds. *Tintinalli's Emergency Medicine: A Comprehensive Study Guide.* 7th ed. New York: McGraw-Hill; 2011.

Wiebe RA, Shah MV: Exanthems. In: Wiebe RA, Ahrens WR, Strange GR, Schafermeyer RW, eds. *Pediatric Emergency Medicine.* 3rd ed. New York: McGraw-Hill; 2009.

Wolff K, Johnson RA, Suurmond D: Bacterial infections involving the skin. In: Wolff K, Johnson RA, Suurmond D, eds. *Fitzpatrick's Color Atlas and Synopsis of Clinical Dermatology.* 6th ed. New York: McGraw-Hill; 2009.

CELLULITIS & ERYSIPELAS

 ESSENTIALS OF DIAGNOSIS

▶ **Cellulitis**

▶ Deeper infection involving skin and deep subcutaneous tissues.

▶ **Erysipelas**

▶ Well-demarcated, elevated, palpable, superficial, erythematous infection.

▶ Often affects face and lower extremities.

General Considerations

Cellulitis and erysipelas are infections involving subcutaneous tissues with breaks in the skin barrier. Erysipelas is a more superficial infection of the upper dermis and lymphatics (Figure 47–8), whereas cellulitis is associated with deeper structures including subcutaneous tissue and fat. About 80% of cellulitis is caused by gram-positive bacteria (β-hemolytic streptococci, S. aureus). Erysipelas is commonly caused by group A β-hemolytic streptococci, but may also be caused by non-A *Streptococcus* strains.

If left untreated, cellulitis and erysipelas may cause septicemia. Other complications include abscesses, gangrene with cellulitis, and cavernous sinus thrombosis.

Clinical Findings

Erysipelas and cellulitis present as areas of swollen skin that contain erythema, edema, and warmth. Erysipelas involves superficial layers of the skin and as a result the borders are more clearly demarcated with indurated plaques and occasionally palpable borders. In contrast, cellulitis involves the dermal layer of the skin as well as the deeper layers of tissue such as the subcutaneous fat. Facial erysipelas may result in a "butterfly" appearance. A distinguishing feature of erysipelas includes involvement of the ear (Milian ear sign) as the ear

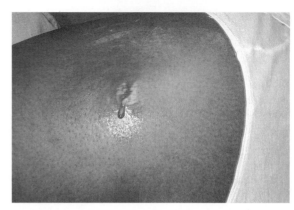

▲ **Figure 47–9.** Cutaneous abscess caused by MRSA. [Public Health Image Library (PHIL). Department of Health and Human Services. Centers for Disease Control and Prevention.]

does not contain deeper dermal tissue. Fever and chills are more commonly associated with erysipelas. Cellulitis has a more indolent course taking a few days to produce symptoms. Characteristics found in both include vesicles, bullae, ecchymosis, and orange peel texture ("peau d'orange") around hair follicles due to dimpling of the skin from edema. Cellulitis borders are not usually well defined or palpable. Areas of infection are warm with painful swelling.

Diagnosis

The diagnosis is made clinically for both. Occasionally cellulitis is accompanied by fluid collections indicative of abscess (Figure 47–9). Ultrasound is used more commonly in the emergency department to identify this clinical situation and direct appropriate therapy.

Treatment

General treatment involves rest, elevation of affected area, antibacterial soaks, and target specific antibiotics. Treat dry skin with topical agents such as moisturizers containing emollients. Cellulitis presenting with purulent drainage is often associated with methicillin-resistant *Staphylococcus aureus* (MRSA) and may be treated with oral clindamycin (10 mg/kg/dose q8h), trimethoprin-sulfamethoxazole (3-5 mg/kg trimethoprin q12h) or linezolid (10 mg/kg/dose q8h) for 7-10 days. IV antibiotics are indicated for patients with high fever, rapidly spreading cellulitis, immunocompromised state or inability to take oral antibiotics, IV antibiotics with clindamycin (15-25 mg/kg/day divided q6 or q8h)

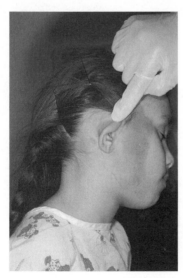

▲ **Figure 47–8.** Erysipelas. (Photo contributor: Binita R. Shah, MD. Reproduced, with permission, from Shah BR, Lucchesi M, eds: *Atlas of Pediatric Emergency Medicine*, 2nd ed. New York: McGraw-Hill, 2013. Copyright © McGraw-Hill Education LLC.)

or vancomycin (10-15 mg/kg/dose q6-8h with max dose 1 gram/dose) are reasonable choices. Cellulitis in neonates is treated with IV vancomycin with either cefotaxime or gentamicin. Antibiotic dosing in neonates is determined by age in days and weight. Erysipelas can be treated with oral antibiotics (penicillin, amoxicillin, erythromycin) or IV antibiotics [ceftriaxone (50 mg/kg/dose q12h) or cefazolin (30 mg/kg/dose q8h)].

Baddour LM: Cellulitis and erysipelas. In: Rose B, ed. *UpToDate*. 2012. Available at http://www.uptodateonline.com.

Kelly EW, Magilner D: Soft tissue infections. In: Tintinalli JE, Kelen GD, Stapczynski JS, eds. *Tintinalli's Emergency Medicine: A Comprehensive Study Guide*. 7th ed. New York: McGraw-Hill; 2011.

Shah BR: Infectious diseases. In: Shah BR, Lucchesi M, eds. *Atlas of Pediatric Emergency Medicine*. New York: McGraw-Hill; 2006.

Wolff K, Johnson RA, Suurmond D: Bacterial infections involving the skin. In: Wolff K, Johnson RA, Suurmond D, eds. *Fitzpatrick's Color Atlas and Synopsis of Clinical Dermatology*. 6th ed. New York: McGraw-Hill; 2009.

STAPHYLOCOCCAL SCALDED SKIN SYNDROME & BULLOUS IMPETIGO

 ESSENTIALS OF DIAGNOSIS

▶ The skin is scalded, bright red, with a blistering appearance.

▶ Rough sandpaper feel.

▶ Acute pain with pressure to the skin.

General Considerations

Staphylococcal scalded skin syndrome (SSSS) (Figure 47–10) and bullous impetigo (Figure 47–11) represent a spectrum of the same disease process. Lesions in bullous impetigo are localized to the site of infection and those in SSSS are distant and more widespread (*F*. staphylococcal SSSS) commonly affecting children younger than 5 years. Both result from an exfoliative exotoxin produced by certain strains of *S. aureus*. Strains producing exfoliative exotoxin are found primarily in the nasopharynx, but can also be found in abscesses and the sinuses. The toxin (exfoliatin) circulates in the blood binding to desmoglein-1 in the granular layers of the skin leading to separation of cells. Mucous membranes are spared in SSSS discriminating it from Stevens-Johnson syndrome (SJS) and toxic epidermal necrolysis (TEN).

Mortality rates in children are (11%) with severe skin involvement. Exfoliation of the skin can cover a large surface

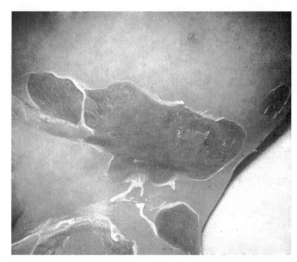

▲ **Figure 47–10.** Staphylococcus scalded skin syndrome. (Reproduced, with permission, from Shah BR and Laude TL: *Atlas of Pediatric Clinical Diagnosis*. Philadelphia: WB Saunders, 2000. Copyright Elsevier.)

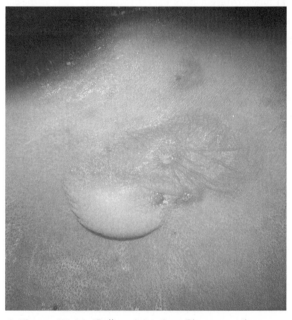

▲ **Figure 47–11.** Bullous impetigo. (Photo contributor: Binita R. Shah, MD. Reproduced, with permission, from Shah BR, Lucchesi M, eds: *Atlas of Pediatric Emergency Medicine*, 2nd ed. New York: McGraw-Hill, 2013. Copyright © McGraw-Hill Education LLC.)

area leading to significant fluid loss and electrolyte imbalance. Infants with large surface area coverage can be susceptible to hypothermia. Loss of the skin barrier can lead to secondary infections.

Clinical Findings

Initial presentation is with fever, malaise, irritability, and poor feeding. Bullous impetigo may not have systemic symptoms. Patient may present following an upper respiratory infection including rhinorrhea, conjunctivitis, or pharyngitis. The skin will develop an erythematous rash with possible crusting near the eyes, mouth, and neck similar to a sunburn appearance usually starting on the face, neck, axillae, and groin. The rash will become tender to palpation and in 2-3 days skin will start to fall off; pressure on the bullae will cause extension bullous lesions (Nikolsky sign). As SSSS progresses flaccid bullae appear.

Diagnosis

For the diagnosis of SSSS, cultures are taken from blood and all orifices. Biopsies of the skin may be taken at the border of blisters as well as normal skin, if required. Bullous impetigo requires no cultures; it is a clinical diagnosis.

Treatment

Direct therapy to treat *S. aureus* and eliminate toxin production. Nafcillin (25 mg/kg/dose q6h) is the IV drug of choice. Other antibiotics include IV clindamycin, first-generation cephalosporins, or semisynthetic penicillinase-resistant penicillins (dicloxacillin). Electrolytes should be closely monitored. Treat pain with narcotics if needed. Corticosteroids are contraindicated. Patients with extensive involvement of lesions should be cared for in a burn unit. Bullous impetigo is treated with oral antibiotics, such as cephalexin (25-50 mg/kg/day divided twice a day), dicloxacillin (12.5 mg/kg/day divided 4 × d), amoxicillin-clavulanate (40 mg/kg/day), or clindamycin (10-25 mg/kg/day divided every 6-8 hours) for penicillin-allergic children.

Brown L: Rashes in infants and children. In: Cline DM, Ma OJ, Cydulka RK, Meckler GD, Handel DA, Thomas SH, eds. *Tintinalli's Emergency Medicine Manual.* 7th ed. New York: McGraw-Hill; 2012.

Mittiga MR, Gonzalez del Rey JA, Ruddy RM: Pediatric conditions. In: Knoop KJ, Stack LB, Storrow AB, Thurman RJ, eds. *The Atlas of Emergency Medicine.* 3rd ed. New York: McGraw-Hill; 2010. Available at http://www.accessemergencymedicine.com/content.aspx?aID=6004422. Accessed October 12, 2012.

Morelli JG: Skin. In: Hay WW, Levin MJ, Sondheimer JM, Deterding RR, eds. *Current Diagnosis & Treatment: Pediatrics.* 20th ed. New York: McGraw-Hill; 2011. Available at http://www.accessmedicine.com/content.aspx?aID=6580202. Accessed October 12, 2012.

Shah BR: Infectious diseases. In: Shah BR, Lucchesi M, eds. *Atlas of Pediatric Emergency Medicine.* New York: McGraw-Hill; 2006.

Welsch MJ, Laumann AE: Dermatologic conditions. In: Hall JB, Schmidt GA, Wood LD, eds: *Principles of Critical Care.* 3rd ed. New York: McGraw-Hill; 2005. Available at http://www.accessmedicine.com/content.aspx?aID=2281907. Accessed October 12, 2012.

Wiebe RA, Shah MV: Superficial skin infections. In: Wiebe RA, Ahrens WR, Strange GR, Schafermeyer RW, eds. *Pediatric Emergency Medicine.* 3rd ed. New York: McGraw-Hill; 2009. Available at http://www.accessemergencymedicine.com/content.aspx?aID=5344406. Accessed October 12, 2012.

TOXIC SHOCK SYNDROME

ESSENTIALS OF DIAGNOSIS

▶ Fever.

▶ Desquamative rash on the palms and soles.

▶ Hypotension.

▶ Multisystem organ involvement of three or more systems.

General Considerations

Toxic shock syndrome (TSS) is caused by exotoxins (A, B, C) that act as a superantigen causing massive T-cell activation with a mortality rate of 10-15%. Originally TSS was associated with tampon use but can be caused by many other types of packing including wound, nasal, and abscess packing.

Clinical Findings

TSS is described as hypotension, headache, confusion, nausea, vomiting, watery diarrhea, high fever, a desquamative rash on the palms and soles (Figure 47–12), with multiorgan involvement in three or more organ systems. There are multiple definitions but one includes the isolation of group A streptococci or *S. aureus* with hypotension plus at least two of the signs listed: diarrhea, vomiting, renal impairment, elevated liver enzymes, respiratory distress syndrome, disseminated intravascular coagulation, cutaneous erythema, soft tissue inflammation, or necrosis. Blood cultures are negative in 85% of patients.

Differential Diagnosis

Symptoms of TSS may overlap those of acute pyelonephritis, septic shock, pelvic inflammatory disease, hemolytic uremic syndrome, Reye syndrome, TEN, scarlet fever, scalded skin

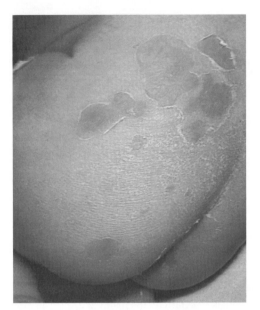

▲ **Figure 47–12.** Staphylococcus toxic shock syndrome. (Reproduced, with permission, from Tintinalli JE, Stapczynski JS, Ma OJ, Cline DM, Cydulka RK, Meckler GD: *Tintinalli's Emergency Medicine: A Comprehensive Study Guide*, 7th ed. New York: McGraw-Hill, 2011. Copyright © McGraw-Hill Education LLC.)

syndrome, erythema multiforme, viral exanthema, rickettsial disease, Kawasaki syndrome, and leptospirosis.

Diagnosis

General laboratory tests to order are blood and urine cultures, blood gas, CBC, electrolytes with magnesium, calcium, coagulation studies, urinalysis, chest x-ray and ECG. TSS may produce lymphocytopenia, leukocytosis, thrombocytopenia, azotemia, myoglobinuria, anemia, elevated liver enzymes, metabolic acidosis, hypocalcemia, hypophosphatemia, hyponatremia, and hypokalemia.

Treatment

Treatment involves emergent removal of the source of infection followed by supportive care, fluids, vasopressors, and IV antibiotics. Typical antibiotic treatment includes IV clindamycin and vancomycin.

Cunningham FG, Leveno KJ, Bloom SL, Hauth JC, Rouse DJ, Spong CY: Puerperal infection. In: Cunningham FG, Leveno KJ, Bloom SL, Hauth JC, Rouse DJ, Spong CY, eds. *Williams Obstetrics*. 23rd ed. New York: McGraw-Hill; 2010.

Hoffman BL, Schorge JO, Schaffer JI, Halvorson LM, Bradshaw KD, Cunningham FG, Calver LE: Gynecologic infection. In: Hoffman BL, Schorge JO, Schaffer JI, Halvorson LM, Bradshaw KD, Cunningham FG, Calver LE, eds. *Williams Gynecology*. 2nd ed. New York: McGraw-Hill; 2012.

Laumann AE: Dermatologic conditions. In: Hall JB, Schmidt GA, Wood LD, eds. *Principles of Critical Care*. 3rd ed. New York: McGraw-Hill; 2005.

Mackay G: Sexually transmitted diseases & pelvic infections. In: DeCherney AH, Nathan L, Laufer N, Roman AS, eds. *Current Diagnosis & Treatment: Obstetrics & Gynecology*. 11th ed. New York: McGraw-Hill; 2013.

Perry SJ, Reid RD: Toxic shock syndrome and streptococcal toxic shock syndrome. In: Tintinalli JE, Stapczynski JS, Cline DM, Ma OJ, Cydulka RK, Meckler GD, eds. *Tintinalli's Emergency Medicine: A Comprehensive Study Guide*. 7th ed. New York: McGraw-Hill; 2011.

Schwartz BS: (2013). Chapter 33. Bacterial & chlamydial infections. In Papadakis MA, McPhee SJ, Rabow MW, eds. *Current Medical Diagnosis & Treatment*; 2013.

MRSA CELLULITIS & RELATED SKIN INFECTIONS

MRSA

 ESSENTIALS OF DIAGNOSIS

▶ Cause of cellulitis, furuncles, carbuncles, abscesses, and other infections.

▶ Community-acquired MRSA (CA-MRSA) is more aggressive than health associated, hospital-acquired MRSA (HA-MRSA).

▶ Warm, erythematous, painful lesions.

▶ Clinical diagnosis.

General Considerations

CA-MRSA is prevalent in all age groups and causes most skin abscesses in children. CA-MRSA contains a virulence factor which makes it more aggressive than HA-MRSA.

CA-MRSA and HA-MRSA may each cause severe and invasive infections. CA-MRSA is more aggressive with more frequent serious complications including sepsis, osteomyelitis, joint infections, and death. Most infections caused by CA-MRSA are skin and soft tissue infections including cellulitis, abscesses (see Figure 47–9), furuncles, and carbuncles.

Diagnosis

CA-MRSA must be identified early for proper treatment and for this reason it is a clinical diagnosis. Infections in which *S. aureus* or *Streptococcus* species could be the responsible bacteria should be treated as MRSA due to the high prevalence of MRSA in the community.

Treatment

Antibiotic choice for treatment of MRSA is difficult because of the resistance of MRSA to cephalexin, dicloxacillin and increasing resistance to clindamycin. MRSA abscesses can be treated with incision and drainage (I&D) alone. Treatment with antibiotics is optional. Antibiotics are advised for the treatment of immunocompromised patients and those with surrounding cellulitis after I&D. Mild cellulitis may be treated with clindamycin or trimethoprim-sulfamethoxazole (TMP-SMX). Moderate cellulitis should be treated with IV vancomycin or linezolid. Severe infections or cellulitis should be treated with vancomycin in addition to meropenem or piperacillin-tazobactam.

Of note, cellulitis may also be caused by *Streptococcus pyogenes* (group A strep), and for this reason, if TMP-SMX is prescribed, addition of cephalexin or amoxicillin will be required in children.

FOLLICULITIS, FURUNCLE, & CARBUNCLE

ESSENTIALS OF DIAGNOSIS

▶ Folliculitis is inflammation of hair follicles related to infection, chemical irritation or physical injury.

▶ Folliculitis is a superficial bacterial infection.

▶ A furuncle can result from more extensive infection of hair follicles.

▶ A carbuncle is a collection of furuncles.

FOLLICULITIS

General Considerations

Folliculitis is most commonly caused by *S. aureus* but can also have a fungal, viral, candidal, or pseudomonal cause. "Hot tub folliculitis" is attributed to pseudomonas and occurs with pools or hot tubs that have not been adequately treated with chlorine. *Candida* folliculitis is more common in patients receiving broad-spectrum antibiotics, glucocorticoids, or who are immunocompromised.

Clinical Findings

Folliculitis most commonly involves the upper back, chest, buttocks, hips, and axilla but can develop anywhere where hair follicles exist. Folliculitis presents as a cluster of erythematous and pruritic lesions which occasionally have central pustules (Figure 47–13). "Hot tub folliculitis" or

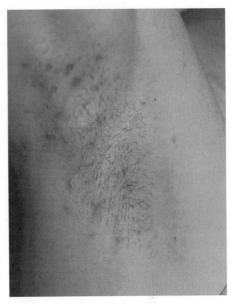

▲ **Figure 47–13. Folliculitis.** (Reproduced, with permission, from Wolff K, Johnson RA, Suurmond D. In: Wolff K, Johnson RA, Suurmond D, eds: *Fitzpatrick's Color Atlas and Synopsis of Clinical Dermatology*, 6th ed. New York: McGraw-Hill, 2009. Copyright © McGraw-Hill Education LLC.)

pseudomonal folliculitis develops in areas which are exposed to contaminated water.

Diagnosis

Folliculitis is a clinical diagnosis.

Treatment

Simple cases of folliculitis are treated by removing the offending or predisposing agent and twice daily cleansing with mild soap. Warm compresses may be applied for symptomatic treatment, and topical antibiotic ointment can be used. Oral antibiotics with coverage of *Streptococcus* and *Staphylococcus*, such as cephalexin, dicloxacillin, or azithromycin, should be used for more extensive or painful folliculitis.

FURUNCLE & CARBUNCLE

General Considerations

Furuncles and carbuncles are infections involving the epidermis which delineates them from abscesses which involved deeper soft tissue. Furuncles or carbuncles can occur in patients with no risk factors.

Clinical Findings

Furuncles or carbuncles are caused by a number of organisms including methicillin-sensitive *Staphylococcus aureus*

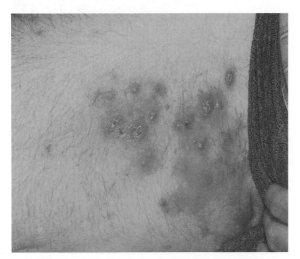

▲ **Figure 47–14. Furuncle.** (Reproduced, with permission, from Wolff K, Johnson RA, Suurmond D. In: Wolff K, Johnson RA, Suurmond D, eds: *Fitzpatrick's Color Atlas and Synopsis of Clinical Dermatology*, 6th ed. New York: McGraw-Hill, 2009. Copyright © McGraw-Hill Education LLC.)

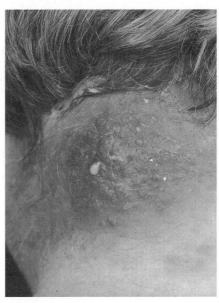

▲ **Figure 47–15. Carbuncle.** (Reproduced, with permission, from Wolff K, Johnson RA, Suurmond D. In: Wolff K, Johnson RA, Suurmond D, eds: *Fitzpatrick's Color Atlas and Synopsis of Clinical Dermatology*, 6th ed. New York: McGraw-Hill, 2009. Copyright © McGraw-Hill Education LLC.)

(MSSA), MRSA, *Pseudomonas*, *Candida*, and other pathogens. Furuncles rarely present with systemic symptoms. Carbuncles may be associated with fevers and malaise.

Diagnosis

Diagnosis of furuncles (Figure 47–14) and carbuncles (Figure 47–15) is clinical and can be discriminated from abscess with ultrasound or needle aspiration.

Treatment

Small furuncles can be treated with a warm compress or hot water soak. While uncommon, large furuncles and carbuncles behave more like abscesses and require I&D for resolution. Antibiotics are unnecessary after I&D but are indicated in extensive cellulitis or systemic symptoms. IV or oral antibiotics should be used with coverage of MRSA.

Disposition

Most patients with furuncles or carbuncles can be managed as outpatients with clear instructions to practice frequent hand washing and good hygiene. Patients with systemic symptoms or extensive cellulitis should be hospitalized for IV antibiotics.

Bonfante G, Rosenau AM: Rashes in infants and children. In: Tintinalli JE, Kelen GD, Stapczynski JS, eds. *Tintinalli's Emergency Medicine: A Comprehensive Study Guide*, 7th ed. New York: McGraw-Hill; 2011.

Kelly EW, Magilner D: Soft tissue infections. In: Tintinalli JE, Kelen GD, Stapczynski JS, eds. *Tintinalli's Emergency Medicine: A Comprehensive Study Guide*, 7th ed. New York: McGraw-Hill; 2011.

Tubbs RJ, Savitt DL, Suner S: Extremity conditions. In: Knoop KJ, Stack LB, Storrow AB, Thurman RJ, eds. *The Atlas of Emergency Medicine*, 3rd ed. New York: McGraw-Hill; 2010.

Wolff K, Johnson RA, Suurmond D: Bacterial infections involving the skin. In: Wolff K, Johnson RA, Suurmond D, eds. *Fitzpatrick's Color Atlas and Synopsis of Clinical Dermatology*, 6th ed. New York: McGraw-Hill; 2009.

Wolff K, Johnson RA, Suurmond D: Disorders of hair follicles and related disorders. In: Wolff K, Johnson RA, Suurmond D, eds. *Fitzpatrick's Color Atlas and Synopsis of Clinical Dermatology*, 6th ed. New York: McGraw-Hill; 2009.

IMPETIGO

 ESSENTIALS OF DIAGNOSIS

▶ Superficial erythematous lesion with crusted vesicles.

▶ Honey-colored yellow crust.

▶ *S. aureus* or *S. pyogenes*.

▶ Large flaccid bullae in bullous impetigo.

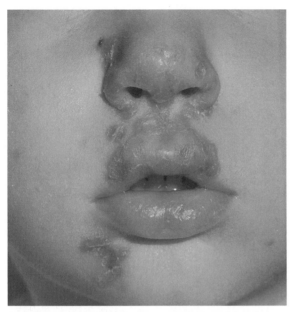

▲ **Figure 47–16.** Impetigo. (Reproduced, with permission, from Wolff K, Johnson RA, Suurmond D. In: Wolff K, Johnson RA, Suurmond D, eds: *Fitzpatrick's Color Atlas and Synopsis of Clinical Dermatology*, 6th ed. New York: McGraw-Hill, 2009. Copyright © McGraw-Hill Education LLC.)

Clinical Findings

Impetigo is a superficial bacterial skin infection which is caused by S. aureus or S. pyogenes. In some geographic regions, MRSA is the cause of most impetigo infections. Impetigo can be bullous or nonbullous (Figure 47–16) with bullous impetigo always caused by S. aureus, phage II type 71 which targets desmoglein 1 in the granular layer. Diagnosis is clinical. Bullous impetigo commonly has systemic symptoms; however, nonbullous impetigo does not.

Treatment

Topical mupirocin is an effective treatment for most impetigo infections. Mupirocin ointment should be applied 2-3 times per day until lesions resolve. Infections that involve a larger area may be treated with oral antibiotics. For systemic treatment, local resistance patterns should be followed; however, a 10-day course of cephalexin is generally sufficient. Clindamycin may be used in areas with high rates of MRSA. Patients should be encouraged to use good hand hygiene to limit its spread.

Bonfante G, Rosenau AM: Rashes in infants and children. In: Tintinalli JE, Kelen GD, Stapczynski JS, eds. *Tintinalli's Emergency Medicine: A Comprehensive Study Guide*, 7th ed. New York: McGraw-Hill; 2011.

Mittiga MR, Gonzalez del Rey JA, Ruddy RM: Pediatric conditions. In: Knoop KJ, Stack LB, Storrow AB, Thurman RJ, eds. *The Atlas of Emergency Medicine*, 3rd ed. New York: McGraw-Hill; 2010.

Shah BR: Infectious diseases. In: Shah BR, Lucchesi M, eds. *Atlas of Pediatric Emergency Medicine*. New York: McGraw-Hill; 2006.

Wiebe RA, Shah MV: Superficial skin infections. In: Wiebe RA, Ahrens WR, Strange GR, Schafermeyer RW, eds. *Pediatric Emergency Medicine*, 3rd ed. New York: McGraw-Hill; 2009.

MENINGOCOCCEMIA

See Chapter 41.

 ESSENTIALS OF DIAGNOSIS

▶ Fever and petechial rash in 70% of patients presenting with meningococcemia.

▶ Acute febrile illness with rapid onset and marketed toxicity.

▶ Rapid progression to hypotension, DIC, and multisystem organ failure.

General Considerations

Meningococcemia is a rapidly progressing systemic bacterial illness which is caused by the gram-negative diplococcus *Neisseria meningitidis*. Acute meningococcemia can present as pharyngitis, bacteremia, or meningitis. Meningococcemia is most common in patients younger than 20 years with most patients presenting younger than 5 years. *N. meningitidis* is transmitted by aerosolized droplets. A low white blood cell count less than 10,000 cells/mm³ or coagulopathy may indicate a poor prognosis.

Clinical Findings

Clinical infection develops 3-4 days after exposure with rapid onset to severe illness. Initial presenting symptoms are headache, fever, nausea, vomiting, myalgias, altered mental status, joint pain, stiff neck, or a rash. The rash in meningococcemia classically includes petechiae (Figure 47–17), urticaria, or palpable purpura. Purpura may rapidly progress and develop gray necrotic centers which is a pathognomonic finding for a meningococcal infection. The rash is present in 70% of patients.

Management

Meningococcal disease may rapidly progress to purpura fulminans (Figure 47-18) so once the diagnosis is suspected,

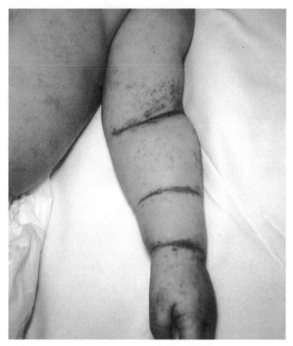

▲ Figure 47–17. An infant presenting with petechiae, septic shock and DIC with meningococcemia. (Photo contributor: Binita R. Shah, MD. Reproduced, with permission, from Shah BR, Lucchesi M, eds: *Atlas of Pediatric Emergency Medicine*, 2nd ed. New York: McGraw-Hill, 2013. Copyright © McGraw-Hill Education LLC.)

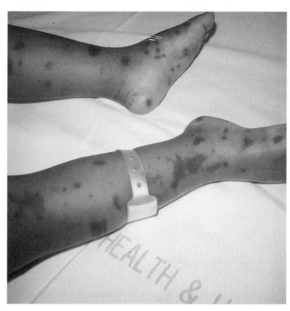

▲ Figure 47–18. Meningococcemia. (Photo contributor: Binita R. Shah, MD. Reproduced, with permission, from Shah BR, Lucchesi M, eds: *Atlas of Pediatric Emergency Medicine*, 2nd ed. New York: McGraw-Hill, 2013. Copyright © McGraw-Hill Education LLC.)

emergent interventions should proceed rapidly. ABC of resuscitation should be performed with IV fluid resuscitation for signs of shock. Parenteral antibiotics should be administered as soon as there is suspicion for meningococcemia. Cultures from blood, skin lesions (if indicated), and CSF should be obtained in patients with suspected meningococcemia. The treatment of choice includes cefotaxime (200 mg/kg/day) or ceftriaxone (100 mg/kg/day). Penicillin G (300,000 units/kg/day) is a drug of choice after susceptibility testing has been performed.

Mittiga MR, Gonzalez del Rey JA, Ruddy RM: Pediatric conditions. In: Knoop KJ, Stack LB, Storrow AB, Thurman RJ, eds. *The Atlas of Emergency Medicine.* 3rd ed. New York: McGraw-Hill; 2010.

Shah BR: Infectious diseases. In: Shah BR, Lucchesi M, eds. *Atlas of Pediatric Emergency Medicine.* New York: McGraw-Hill; 2006.

Thomas JJ, Perron AD, Brady WJ: Serious generalized skin disorders. In: Tintinalli JE, Kelen GD, Stapczynski JS, eds. *Tintinalli's Emergency Medicine: A Comprehensive Study Guide,* 7th ed. New York: McGraw-Hill; 2011.

SYPHILIS

ESSENTIALS OF DIAGNOSIS

▶ Spirochete infection (*Treponema pallidum*).

▶ Painless ulcers (chancre).

▶ Episodes of active disease with intermittent episodes of latency.

General Considerations

Increased incidence of syphilis has been noted among the adolescent population. Syphilis has an incubation period of 2-6 weeks prior to the appearance of the first primary lesions. A latency period (time may vary) occurs followed by a second stage of infection. One-third of untreated patients in second stage may progress to a tertiary stage. There are high rates of infection among men who have sex with men with other risk factors including substance abuse and decreased condom use. Transmission occurs in 30-50% of unprotected sex with an infected person.

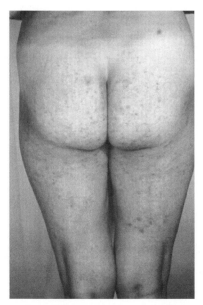

▲ **Figure 47–19. Syphilis.** (From the CDC, Public Health Image Library.)

Clinical Findings

Syphilis is divided into three stages: primary, secondary, and tertiary. The primary stage is characterized by nontender lymphadenopathy and painless ulcers located on the genitalia, tongue, lip, pharynx, and rectum. The second stage can present with fever, lymphadenopathy, a generalized rash (Figure 47–19) including the palms and soles, condyloma lata, and lesions involving mucous membranes. Less common signs during the second stage are meningitis, arthritis, hepatitis, and iritis. Tertiary stage may present with a number of signs but gumma formation is the most characteristic of this stage. This stage also involves cardiovascular and CNS changes. Vascular signs include aortitis, aneurysms, and aortic regurgitation. CNS findings include dementia, psychosis, paresthesias, shooting pains, and abnormal reflexes.

Differential Diagnosis

Chancroid, genital herpes, cancer, lymphogranuloma venereum, trauma, Reiter syndrome, erythema multiforme, and pityriasis rosea.

Diagnosis

Diagnosis can be performed with laboratory evaluations including VDRL, RPR, Treponemal antibody test, and dark-field microscopy.

Treatment

Primary, secondary, and tertiary treated with benzathine penicillin G 2.4 million units IM. An inflammatory response, resembling bacterial sepsis, known as the Jarisch-Herxheimer reaction is a common side effect of treatment and can be treated with antipyretics.

Katz KA: Syphilis. In: Goldsmith LA, Katz SI, Gilchrest BA, Paller AS, Leffell DJ, Dallas GJ, eds, *Fitzpatrick's Dermatology in General Medicine*. 8th ed. New York: McGraw-Hill; 2012. Available at http://www.accessmedicine.com/content.aspx?aID=56090705. Accessed April 2, 2013.

Lukehart SA: Syphilis. In: Longo DL, Fauci AS, Kasper DL, Hauser SL, Jameson JL, Loscalzo J, eds. *Harrison's Principles of Internal Medicine*. 18th ed. New York: McGraw-Hill; 2012. Available at http://www.accessmedicine.com/content.aspx?aID=9102029. Accessed April 2, 2013.

Nobay F, Promes SB: Sexually transmitted diseases. In: Tintinalli JE, Kelen GD, Stapczynski JS, eds. *Tintinalli's Emergency Medicine Manual*. 7th ed. New York: McGraw-Hill; 2011. Available at http://www.accessemergencymedicine.com/content.aspx?aID=6364645. Accessed April 2, 2013.

Papadakis MA, McPhee SJ: Syphilis. *Quick Medical Diagnosis & Treatment*. Available at http://www.accessmedicine.com/quickam.aspx.

Shah BR, Rawstron S, Suss A: Sexual abuse, gynecology, and sexually transmitted diseases. In: Shah BR, Lucchesi M, eds. *Atlas of Pediatric Emergency Medicine*. New York: McGraw-Hill; 2006. Available at http://www.accessemergencymedicine.com/content.aspx?aID=78599. Accessed April 2, 2013.

COMMON VIRAL RASHES

ENTEROVIRUSES: COXSACKIE VIRUS INFECTIONS

Coxsackie viruses are a large subgroup of enteroviruses divided into groups A and B with more than 50 serotypes. They cause a variety of clinical syndromes occurring most during the summer and transmitted primarily by fecal-oral route as well as respiratory aerosols.

Clinical Findings

Syndromes associated with Coxsackie virus infections are nonspecific febrile illness, herpangina, epidemic pleurodynia, aseptic meningitis, acute nonspecific pericarditis, myocarditis, hand, foot, and mouth disease, and epidemic conjunctivitis.

▶ Herpangina (A2-6, 10:B3)

Herpangina presents with sudden onset of a high fever (40.6°C) with a sore throat, headache, and malaise. Oral vesicles will then form on the soft palate, uvula, and tonsillar pillars which will rupture to form shallow painful ulcers. Buccal mucosas, tongue, gingiva, and usually the lips are

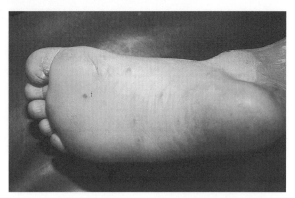

▲ Figure 47–20. Coxsackie: Hand-foot-and-mouth disease. (Photo contributed by Raymond C. Baker, MD. Reproduced, with permission, from Knoop K, Stack L, Storrow A, Thurmond RJ: *Atlas of Emergency Medicine*, 3rd ed. New York: McGraw-Hill, 2010. Copyright © McGraw-Hill Education LLC.)

spared separating it from herpes infection. The viral infection is self-limited and treatment is symptomatic.

▶ Hand-Foot-and-Mouth Disease (A5, 10, 16)

Hand-foot-and-mouth disease is a viral infection with oral and pharyngeal ulcerations presenting with a vesicular rash on the palms and soles that spread to surrounding limbs (Figure 47–20). The vesicles of the rash heal without crusting which discriminates it from herpesviruses and poxviruses. Hand-foot-and-mouth disease commonly affects toddlers and school-aged children. Infected children should remain home until lesions are gone. Supportive therapy is suggested. Complications include myocarditis, pneumonia, and meningoencephalitis. Several serotpyes present with lesions on the buttocks in addition to palms, soles, and mouth.

Laboratory Findings

None, as this is a clinical diagnosis.

Treatment & Prognosis

Treatment is mainly symptomatic. Children often present with poor feeding or signs of dehydration which may require IV fluids.

Brooks GF, Carroll KC, Butel JS, Morse SA, Mietzneron TA: Picornaviruses (enterovirus & rhinovirus groups). In: Brooks GF, Carroll KC, Butel JS, Morse SA, Mietzneron TA, eds. *Jawetz, Melnick, & Adelberg's Medical Microbiology*. 25th ed. New York: McGraw-Hill; 2010. Available at http://www.accessmedicine.com/content.aspx?aID=6431439. Accessed February 18, 2013.

Go S: Oral and dental emergencies. In: Cline DM, Ma, OJ, Cydulka RK, Meckler GD, Handel DA, Thomas SH, eds. *Tintinalli's Emergency Medicine Manual*. 7th ed. New York: McGraw-Hill; 2011. Available at http://www.accessemergencymedicine.com/content.aspx?aID=56279753. Accessed February 18, 2013.

Levinson W: RNA Nonenveloped viruses. In: Levinson W, ed. *Review of Medical Microbiology & Immunology*. 12th ed. New York: McGraw-Hill; 2010. Available at http://www.accessmedicine.com/content.aspx?aID=56759812. Accessed February 18, 2013.

Mittiga MR, Gonzalez del Rey JA, Ruddy RM: Pediatric conditions. In: Knoop KJ, Stack LB, Storrow AB, Thurman RJ, eds. *The Atlas of Emergency Medicine*. 3rd ed. York: McGraw-Hill; 2010. Available at http://www.accessemergencymedicine.com/content.aspx?aID=6004422. Accessed February 18, 2013.

HERPES SIMPLEX

 ESSENTIALS OF DIAGNOSIS

▶ Erythematous base with vesicles.

▶ HSV-1, mostly oral cavity; HSV-2, usually genital.

▶ Contagious with spread through direct contact.

General Considerations

Herpes simplex virus (HSV) is a double-stranded DNA virus which is spread by direct contact and is a major cause of recurrent oral, facial, and genital lesions. HSV may also cause keratitis and encephalitis. The primary infection is usually the worst infection in terms of symptoms. After a primary infection, the virus may permanently remain in sensory neurons where it can be reactivated. HSV is associated with two types: HSV-1 and HSV-2. HSV-1 occurs commonly with more oral lesions and spreads through contact with saliva. HSV-2 commonly causes genital lesions and spreads through sexual contact; however, HSV-1 and HSV-2 can cause either oral or genital infections.

Herpes in neonates occurs in 1:3,000-1:20,000 births. Congenital HSV infections are rare and usually present result in premature birth with microcephaly, vesicular rash, and retinitis. Herpetic whitlow is also commonly seen in children and is caused by a secondary infection from mouth to fingers (children who suck their fingers or thumbs).

Clinical Findings

▶ Primary Herpes Simplex Infection

A primary infection with HSV is more severe and usually lasts 2-3 weeks with some lasting as long as 6 weeks. A child typically presents with irritability, arthralgias, malaise, fever, loss of appetite, and lymphadenopathy. The lesions present as

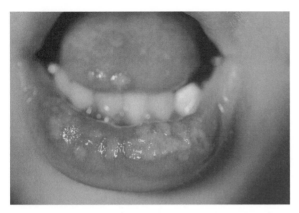

▲ **Figure 47–21.** Herpes simplex virus. (Photo contributor: Lawrence B. Stack, MD. Reproduced, with permission, from Knoop KJ, Stack LB, Storrow AB, Thurman R: *The Atlas of Emergency Medicine*, 3rd ed. New York: McGraw-Hill, 2010. Copyright © McGraw-Hill Education LLC.)

a group of vesicles which will erode, punctate, or denudate on to a swollen tender erythematous base. Vesicles will rupture to form ulcers, and pain with adenopathy is usually common. HSV-1 manifests most often as gingivostomatitis (Figure 47–21), whereas HSV-2 manifests as genital lesions (on the penis, vulva, vagina, anus, and perineum). Evaluation for abuse must be undertaken in a child who presents with vesicular lesions in the genital area.

▶ Recurrent HSV Infection

Infections that lay dormant may reactivate by triggers. Studies have suggested fever, stress, fatigue, trauma from sexual intercourse, menstruation, and ultraviolet (UV) light are potential causes for reactivation. Patients may present with focal pain, itching, and aching which will occur before the appearance of vesicles. Vesicles will rupture and heal within a week. Patients should avoid skin-to-skin contact while lesions are moist or until the lesions have been completely dried and healed. The incidence of reactivation decreases with age.

Diagnosis

Diagnosis can be made clinically, but a more definitive diagnosis can be made for both primary and recurrent herpes infections by culture or antigen detection. In cases of herpes encephalitis, HSV PCR or viral culture of cerebrospinal fluid will determine the diagnosis. HSV can be discriminated from Coxsackie virus enanthems by the presence of intense gingivitis or location. Herpetic stomatitis typically presents on the anterior lips in contrast to herpangina which often is seen in the posterior pharynx and tonsillar pillars.

Table 47–3. Primary HSV Infection treatment for adolescents 13 years and older.

Antiviral	Dose	Amount	How long
Acyclovir	400 mg PO	3 × daily	10 d
Famiciclovir	250 mg	3 × daily	7-10 d
Valacyclovir	1 g	2 × daily	7-10 d

Treatment

▶ Primary Infection

Symptomatic relief is obtained by antipyretics or analgesics. Acyclovir, valacyclovir, and famciclovir may be given for 7-10 days. Severely ill patients with HSV encephalitis or neonatal disease should be given IV acyclovir 10 mg/kg every 8 hours. Outpatient treatment for primary and recurrent infections for adolescents are outlined in Tables 47-3 and 47-4. For children one to twelve years old with severe symptoms able to be treated as outpatients use acyclovir 40-80 mg/kg/day po in 3 divided doses (max dose 1 g) for 5-10 days, or valacyclovir 20 mg/kg/dose po 3 times a day for 5-10 days.

Antibiotics are not necessary unless bacterial infection is suspected. Adolescent females with primary genital herpes may also have *Candida* vaginitis.

Acyclovir, valacyclovir, and famciclovir will reduce healing time and duration of the virus shedding when given at the onset of the lesion. Patients should avoid skin-to-skin contact with active lesions.

Disposition

In severely ill patients, hospitalizations can occur mostly with primary genital herpes that have systemic symptoms or other complications (aseptic meningitis, neuropathic bladder). Pregnant patients with newly diagnosed genital herpes should consult an obstetrician.

Complications

Dehydration is the most common complication seen in children with herpetic stomatitis. Patients, especially women

Table 47–4. Recurrent HSV Infection treatment for adolescents 13 years and older.

Antiviral	Dose	Amount	How long
Acyclovir	400 mg PO	3 × daily	5 d
Famiciclovir	125 mg	2 × daily	5 d
Valacyclovir	500 mg	2 × daily	3 d

with genital herpes, may develop aseptic meningitis. Most severe complications of HSV occur in immunocompromised patients and neonates.

Beaudreau RW: Oral and dental emergencies. In: Tintinalli JE, Kelen GD, Stapczynski JS, eds, *Tintinalli's Emergency Medicine: A Comprehensive Study Guide.* 7th ed. New York: McGraw-Hill; 2011. Available at http://www.accessemergencymedicine.com/content.aspx?aID=6388278. Accessed December 2, 2012.

Drugge JM, Allen PJ. A nurse practitioner's guide to the management of herpes simplex virus-1 in children. *Pediatr Nurs.* 2008;34:310-18 [PMID: 18814565].

Ray CG, Ryan KJ: Herpesviruses. In: Ray CG, Ryan KJ, eds. *Sherris Medical Microbiology.* 5th ed. New York: McGraw-Hill; 2010. Available at http://www.accessmedicine.com/content.aspx?aID=6939841. Accessed December 2, 2012.

Rothman RE, Marco CA, Yang S: Human immunodeficiency virus infection and acquired immunodeficiency syndrome. In: Cline DM, Ma, OJ, Cydulka RK, Meckler GD, Handel DA, Thomas SH, eds. *Tintinalli's Emergency Medicine Manual.* 7th ed. New York: McGraw-Hill; 2011. Available at http://www.accessemergencymedicine.com/content.aspx?aID=6365597. Accessed December 2, 2012.

Wiebe RA, Shah MV: Exanthems. In: Wiebe RA, Ahrens WR, Strange GR, Schafermeyer RW, eds. *Pediatric Emergency Medicine.* 3rd ed. New York: McGraw-Hill; 2009. Available at http://www.accessemergencymedicine.com/content.aspx?aID=5344456. Accessed December 2, 2012.

PRIMARY VARICELLA INFECTION (CHICKENPOX)

 ESSENTIALS OF DIAGNOSIS

▶ Most patients are children younger than 10 years.

▶ Much less common now that varicella vaccination is common.

▶ Rash appears as pruritic "teardrop" vesicles on a red base that spread completely over body; described as "dewdrop on a rose petal."

▶ Extremely contagious with airborne and contact spread days prior to developing rash.

General Considerations

Varicella zoster virus (VZV) is highly contagious double-stranded DNA virus. The initial transmission of the VZV occurs through airborne and personal contact with respiratory secretions and occasionally fluid from the vesicles of herpes zoster patients.

Clinical Findings

Patients usually have a constellation of non-specific symptoms including fever, malaise, cough, coryza and sore throat

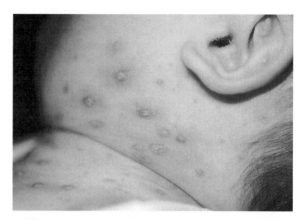

▲ **Figure 47–22. Varicella.** (Photo contributor: Lawrence B. Stack, MD. Reproduced, with permission, from Knoop KJ, Stack LB, Storrow AB, Thurman R: *The Atlas of Emergency Medicine,* 3rd ed. New York: McGraw-Hill, 2010. Copyright © McGraw-Hill Education LLC.)

which typically precede the development of the characteristic rash by 1-2 days.

Diagnosis

Diagnosis is generally clinical. The pruritic rash is vesicular on an erythematous base and usually begins on the trunk, face, and scalp before spreading; however, the distal extremities are rarely involved (Figure 47–22). Mucous membranes are often involved. The vesicles break easily and scab over. Three stages of lesions, erythematous macule, macule with central vesicle, and scabbed lesion, are often seen at the same time as the rash develops. A Tzanck smear can be performed looking for multinucleated giant cells but is not usually necessary. PCR or viral culture can be done for a definite diagnosis. Patients can also develop varicella after immunization but this is not common and the rash is generally mild with much fewer lesions than would be expected after a primary infection with varicella (Figure 47–23). Herpes zoster is the latent reactivation of the varicella virus which lay dormant in the cutaneous nerves. The vesicular rash is painful and localized to a specific dermatome (Figure 47–24).

Treatment

Treatment is generally symptomatic with antihistamines for itching not relieved by oatmeal baths and antipyretics (nonaspirin) for control of fever. For immunocompromised patients, acyclovir (<12 years: 20 mg/kg/dose IV q8h for 7 days; >12 years: 10 mg/kg/dose IV q8h for 7 days) is indicated. Parents should be instructed to keep infectious children (those still developing new lesions) away from immunocompromised patients or pregnant mothers without primary immunity to varicella.

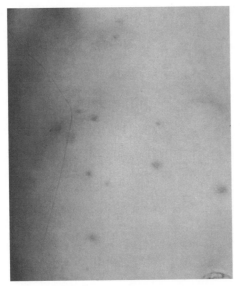

▲ **Figure 47–23.** Varicella immunization 10 days prior in a 1-year-old boy. (Reproduced, with permission, from Wolff KL, Johnson R, Suurmond R: *Fitzpatrick's Color Atlas & Synopsis of Clinical Dermatology*, 6th ed. New York: McGraw-Hill, Inc., 2009. Copyright © McGraw-Hill Education LLC.)

Cline DM: Occupational exposures, infection control, and standard precautions. In: Tintinalli JE, Kelen GD, Stapczynski JS, eds. *Tintinalli's Emergency Medicine: A Comprehensive Study Guide.* 7th ed. New York: McGraw-Hill; 2011. Available at http://www.accessemergencymedicine.com/content.aspx?aID=6375423. Accessed December 2, 2012.

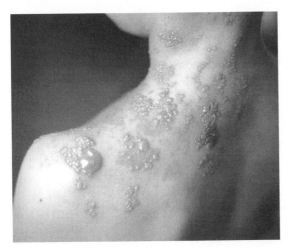

▲ **Figure 47–24.** Herpes zoster. (Reproduced, with permission, from Weinberg S, Prose NS, Kristal L, eds: *Color Atlas of Pediatric Dermatology*, 4th ed. New York: McGraw-Hill, 2008. Copyright © McGraw-Hill Education LLC.)

Hardin J. Cutaneous conditions. In: Knoop KJ, Stack LB, Storrow AB, Thurman RJ, eds. *The Atlas of Emergency Medicine.* 3rd ed. New York: McGraw-Hill; 2010. Available at http://www.accessemergencymedicine.com/content.aspx?aID=6003676. Accessed December 2, 2012.

Hess MR, Hess SP: Skin disorders common on the trunk. In: Tintinalli JE, Kelen GD, Stapczynski JS, eds. *Tintinalli's Emergency Medicine: A Comprehensive Study Guide.* 7th ed. New York: McGraw-Hill; 2011. Available at http://www.accessemergencymedicine.com/content.aspx?aID=6367974. Accessed December 2, 2012

Humphries RL, Stone C: Dermatologic emergencies. In: Humphries RL, Stone C, eds. *Current Diagnosis & Treatment Emergency Medicine.* 7th ed. New York: McGraw-Hill; 2011. Available at http://www.accessemergencymedicine.com/content.aspx?aID=55759117. Accessed December 2, 2012.

Varicella vaccine information sheet. Available at www.cdc.gov/vaccines/pubs/vis/downloads/vis-varicella.pdf. Accessed March 13, 2008.

Wiebe RA, Shah MV: Exanthems. In: Wiebe RA, Ahrens WR, Strange GR, Schafermeyer RW, eds. *Pediatric Emergency Medicine.* 3rd ed. New York: McGraw-Hill; 2009. Available at http://www.accessemergencymedicine.com/content.aspx?aID=5344456. Accessed December 2, 2012.

ERYTHEMA INFECTIOSUM (FIFTH DISEASE)

 ESSENTIALS OF DIAGNOSIS

▶ Prodrome with mild upper respiratory symptoms.

▶ Rash begins as erythema of cheeks, macular first, then reticular.

▶ Rash lasts 1-3 weeks.

General Considerations

Erythema infectiosum, fifth disease, is a common acute childhood infection that rarely causes significant disease.

Pathogenesis

Fifth disease is caused by a single-stranded DNA virus, parvovirus B19, transmitted mainly by respiratory secretion contact. The virus can target red cell precursors causing a decrease in red blood cell formation. Fifth disease occurs sporadically primarily in the spring and is seen most often in children aged 5-15 years. Children are infectious during the prodromal stage. The rash is not infectious and is an immune-mediated phenomenon that occurs after the infection.

Clinical Findings

Fifth disease starts with a prodromal stage with upper respiratory infection symptoms, headache, and low-grade fever. The rash begins with facial flushing (slapped cheek) leading

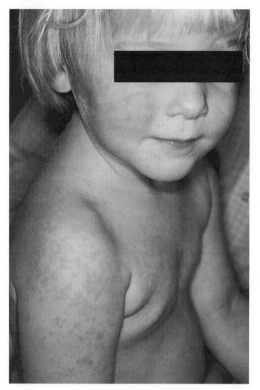

▲ **Figure 47–25.** Erythema infectiosum (5th disease, parvovirus B19). (Photo contributed by Anne W. Lucky, MD. Reproduced, with permission, from Knoop K, Stack L, Storrow A, Thurman RJ: *Atlas of Emergency Medicine*, 3rd ed. New York: McGraw-Hill, 2010. Copyright © McGraw-Hill Education LLC.)

to a macular rash (Figure 47–25), followed by a lacy reticular rash on the extremities and trunk. The rash will resolve in a few days but can reappear especially with after sun exposure or a warm bath.

Differential Diagnosis

Rubella, enteroviral infections, scarlet fever, measles, roseola infantum, collagen vascular diseases (SLE, JRA), and drug eruptions.

▶ Complications

Pregnant women are at risk of fetal hydrops fetalis especially in the first trimester. Patients with chronic hemolytic anemias (such as sickle cell disease) may have rapid cell turnover which can cause severe anemia. Other complications are rare and include arthritis, arthralgias, thrombocytopenic purpura, and aseptic meningitis.

Treatment & Prognosis

Care is supportive in immunocompetent patients. Patients with hemolytic anemia may need blood transfusions.

Bonfante G, Rosenau AM: Rashes in infants and children. In: Tintinalli JE, Kelen GD, Stapczynski JS, eds. *Tintinalli's Emergency Medicine: A Comprehensive Study Guide.* 7th ed. New York: McGraw-Hill; 2011. Available at http://www.accessemergencymedicine.com/content.aspx?aID=6383200. Accessed February 18, 2013.

Place R, Lagoc AM, Mayer TA, Lawlor CJ: Oncology and hematology emergencies in children. In: Tintinalli JE, Kelen GD, Stapczynski JS, eds. *Tintinalli's Emergency Medicine: A Comprehensive Study Guide.* 7th ed. New York: McGraw-Hill; 2011. Available at http://www.accessemergencymedicine.com/content.aspx?aID=6383506. Accessed February 18, 2013.

Shah BR: Infectious diseases. In: Shah BR, M. Lucchesi M, eds. *Atlas of Pediatric Emergency Medicine.* New York: McGraw-Hill; 2006. Available at http://www.accessemergencymedicine.com/content.aspx?aID=77310. Accessed February 18, 2013.

Wiebe RA, Shah MV: Exanthems. In: Wiebe RA, Ahrens WR, Strange GR, Schafermeyer RW, eds. *Pediatric Emergency Medicine.* 3rd ed. New York: McGraw-Hill; 2009. Available at http://www.accessemergencymedicine.com/content.aspx?aID=5344456. Accessed February 18, 2013.

ROSEOLA (EXANTHEM SUBITUM, (SIXTH DISEASE)

 ESSENTIALS OF DIAGNOSIS

▶ High fever with sudden onset.

▶ Children 6-36 months of age.

▶ Exanthem develops 3-4 days after fever breaks.

Pathogenesis

Roseola, sixth disease, is in the human herpes virus (HHV) family with most cases caused by HHV-6A, HHV-6B, and HHV7. Infection is rarely seen in infants younger than 3 months due to passive immunity from antibodies, or in children older than 4 years. Most patients present 6-12 months of age; roseola occurs year round. Primary infection comes from oropharyngeal secretions.

Clinical Findings

Roseola classically presents with abrupt onset of fever between 38.9 and 41.1°C that remains high until about the fourth day when the temperature drops and a rash appears. Additional symptoms are usually absent. The rash will be blanchable, pink macules and papules with distribution along the trunk which spreads to arms, neck, face, and legs.

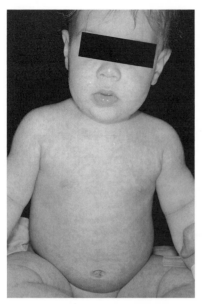

▲ **Figure 47–26.** Roseola (6th disease). (Photo contributor: Binita R. Shah, MD. Reproduced, with permission, from Shah BR, Lucchesi M, eds: *Atlas of Pediatric Emergency Medicine*, 2nd ed. New York: McGraw-Hill, 2013. Copyright © McGraw-Hill Education LLC.)

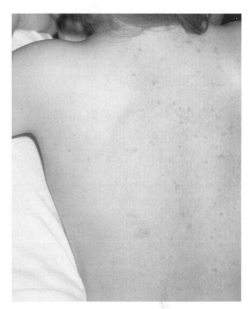

▲ **Figure 47–27.** Roseola (6th disease). (Reproduced, with permission, from Karen Wiss, MD.)

self-limited infection. Often, previous investigation for the fever source had been performed.

The rash will usually disappear in 3 days (Figures 47–26 and 47–27). Children presenting with fever will appear well with possible mild signs of an upper respiratory infection, abdominal discomfort, and anorexia.

Laboratory Findings

No laboratory investigation is needed. It is a clinical examination.

Differential Diagnosis

Morbilliform exanthem, measles, rubella, parvovirus B19, infectious mononucleosis, papular urticarial, and scarlet fever.

Complications

There are rare cases of encephalitis or fulminant hepatitis, but the most common complication is febrile seizures which can occur in up to one-third of patients.

Treatment & Prognosis

Symptomatic treatment is suggested. Unless the patient develops a rare complication, the disease is a benign,

Bonfante G, Rosenau AM: Rashes in infants and children. In: Tintinalli JE, Kelen GD, Stapczynski JS, eds. *Tintinalli's Emergency Medicine: A Comprehensive Study Guide*. 7th ed. New York: McGraw-Hill; 2011. Available at http://www.accessemergencymedicine.com/content.aspx?aID=6383200. Accessed February 18, 2013.

Levin MJ, Weinberg A: Infections: viral & rickettsial. In: Hay Jr WW, Levin MJ, Deterding, RR, Ross JJ, Sondheimer JM, eds. *Current Diagnosis & Treatment: Pediatrics*. 21st ed. New York: McGraw-Hill; 2012. Available at http://www.accessmedicine.com/content.aspx?aID=56833136. Accessed February 18, 2013.

Mittiga MR, Gonzalez del Rey JA, Ruddy RM: Pediatric conditions. In: Knoop KJ, Stack LB, Storrow AB, Thurman RJ, eds. *The Atlas of Emergency Medicine*. 3rd ed. New York: McGraw-Hill; 2010. Available at http://www.accessemergencymedicine.com/content.aspx?aID=6004422. Accessed February 18, 2013.

Suurmond D: Viral infections of skin and mucosa. In: Suurmond D, ed. *Fitzpatrick's Color Atlas & Synopsis of Clinical Dermatology*. 6th ed. New York: McGraw-Hill; 2009. Available at http://www.accessmedicine.com/content.aspx?aID=5195325. Accessed February 13, 2013.

Wiebe RA, Shah MV: Exanthems. In: Wiebe RA, Ahrens WR, Strange GR, Schafermeyer RW, eds. *Pediatric Emergency Medicine*. 3rd ed. New York: McGraw-Hill; 2011. Available at http://www.accessemergencymedicine.com/content.aspx?aID=5344456. Accessed February 18, 2013.

INFECTIOUS MONONUCLEOSIS/ EPSTEIN-BARR VIRUS

ESSENTIALS OF DIAGNOSIS

▶ Classically presents with fever, exudative pharyngitis, and cervical adenopathy.

▶ Lymphadenopathy, splenomegaly.

▶ Positive monospot test (heterophile agglutination test).

▶ Blood smear with atypical large lymphocytes.

General Considerations

Infectious mononucleosis is a primary infection of Epstein-Barr virus (EBV) that is characterized by fever, exudative pharyngitis, and adenopathy. Children with EBV may have no symptoms or a minor febrile illness. Older children and adolescents are more likely to present with symptoms. EBV is commonly transmitted through oral secretion.

Clinical Findings

EBV has an incubation period of 30-50 days with symptoms of fatigue, malaise, sore throat, tonsillar enlargement, and low-grade fever. Pharyngitis may be present as exudative or nonexudative. Bilateral posterior cervical lymphadenopathy is a characteristic sign. Further findings can include splenic tenderness in early stages to splenomegaly in later stages. Other reported signs include maculopapular rash (Figure 47–28) or bilateral periorbital edema.

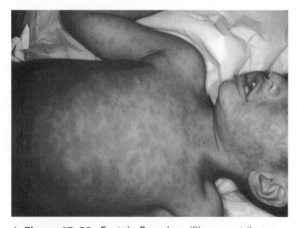

▲ **Figure 47–28.** Epstein-Barr virus. (Photo contributor: Binita R. Shah, MD. Reproduced, with permission, from Shah BR, Lucchesi M, eds: *Atlas of Pediatric Emergency Medicine*, 2nd ed. New York: McGraw-Hill, 2013. Copyright © McGraw-Hill Education LLC.)

Laboratory Findings

Peripheral blood smear may show atypical enlarged lymphocytes in more than 10% of patients. The monospot antibody test detects IgM antibody to viral capsid antigen. The monospot test in ideal conditions is 85% sensitive and almost 100% specific. Early stages of the disease lower the sensitivity, and children younger than 2 years will have a negative monospot test. A significant positive titer suggests EBV but does not prove the infection. False positive may be present in patients with CMV, rubella, SLE, RA, HIV, and herpes simplex. PCR for EBV DNA is the method of choice for CNS and ocular infections. It may be necessary to measure specific antibody titers and/or EBV PCR when the monospot antibody fails to appear as in young children.

Differential Diagnosis

Cytomegalovirus, acute HIV infection, mycoplasma infection, peritonsillar abscess, influenza, chronic fatigue syndrome, viral hepatitis, toxoplasmosis, rubella, and pertussis.

Complications

Reported complications include, splenic rupture (0.5-1%), hepatitis, fulminant hepatitis, acalculous cholecystitis, uvular edema, Bell palsy, optic neuritis, encephalitis, Guillain-Barré syndrome, transverse myelitis, and aseptic meningitis. Epstein-Barr virus infections are linked to B-cell lymphoma, Hodgkin disease, Burkitt lymphoma, and nasopharyngeal carcinoma.

Treatment

The infection is self-limited and treatment is primarily symptomatic for uncomplicated cases. Acetaminophen may be used to treat fever and throat discomfort. Cautioned use of acetaminophen when EBV hepatitis is present. Steroid treatment is controversial with insufficient evidence to support its use. Patients should eliminate strenuous physical activity including sports for 3 weeks. Patients infected with EBV treated with amoxicillin or ampicillin mistaken for streptococcal pharyngitis may form a morbilliform rash.

Belazarian LT, Lorenzo ME, Pearson AL, Sweeney SM, Wiss K: Exanthematous viral diseases. In: Goldsmith LA, Katz SI, Gilchrest BA, Paller AS, Leffell DJ, Dallas NA, eds. *Fitzpatrick's Dermatology in General Medicine*. 8th ed. New York: McGraw-Hill; 2012. Available at http://www.accessmedicine.com/content.aspx?aID=56087223. Accessed February 18, 2013.

Levin MJ, Weinberg A. Infections: viral & rickettsial. In: Hay Jr WW, Levin MJ, Deterding RR, Ross JJ, Sondheimer JM, eds. *Current Diagnosis & Treatment: Pediatrics*. 21st ed. New York: McGraw-Hill; 2012. Available at http://www.accessmedicine.com/content.aspx?aID=56833136. Accessed February 18, 2013.

Shah BR: Infectious diseases. In: Shah BR, Lucchesi M, eds. *Atlas of Pediatric Emergency Medicine.* New York: McGraw-Hill; 2006. Available at http://www.accessemergencymedicine.com/content.aspx?aID=77310. Accessed February 18, 2013.

Shandera WX, Roig IL: Viral & rickettsial infections. In: Papadakis MA, McPhee SJ, Rabow MW, eds. *Current Medical Diagnosis & Treatment 2013.* New York: McGraw-Hill; 2013. Available at http://www.accessmedicine.com/content.aspx?aID=17051. Accessed February 19, 2013.

Takhar SS, Moran GJ: Disseminated viral infections. In: Tintinalli JE, Kelen GD, Stapczynski JS, eds. *Tintinalli's Emergency Medicine: A Comprehensive Study Guide.* 7th ed. New York: McGraw-Hill; 2011. Available at http://www.accessemergency-medicine.com/content.aspx?aID=6365448. Accessed February 18, 2013.

ZeigerRoni F: McGraw-Hill's Diagnosaurus 2.0. Available at http://www.accessmedicine.com/diag.aspx.

RUBEOLA (MEASLES)

ESSENTIALS OF DIAGNOSIS

▶ Three Cs: Cough, coryza, conjunctivitis.

▶ Fever, malaise, Koplik spots, photophobia.

▶ Rash appears 3-4 days after onset.

▶ Red irregular maculopapular rash that spreads from face to the extremities.

Pathogenesis

Measles is an acute infection caused by a single-stranded RNA paramyxovirus transmitted primarily from person to person by respiratory droplets. The virus is highly contagious and peaks in the winter to spring. It enters the respiratory tract and incubates for 10 days with the prodromal phase lasting 3 days, followed by a rash. Patients are contagious for the first 5 days of symptoms. Incidence is low in the United States due to vaccinations but is rising due to a large number of unvaccinated children. Measles infections have significant morbidity and mortality among pediatric patients.

Clinical Findings

Measles presents classically with the three Cs of cough, coryza, and conjunctivitis along with fever. Three days after the onset of symptoms a maculopapular erythematous rash appears that starts on the face (Figure 47–29) and spreads to the trunk and extremities. Characteristic Koplik spots (small irregular whitish dots with a red base on the buccal mucosa near Stensen duct) appear at early stages of the infection. Fever will end 3 days from the onset of the rash and most symptoms resolve in 7-8 days.

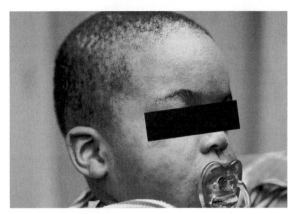

▲ **Figure 47–29.** Measles. (Photo contributor: Javier A. Gonzalez del Rey, MD. Reproduced, with permission, from Knoop KJ, Stack LB, Storrow AB, Thurman R: *The Atlas of Emergency Medicine,* 3rd ed. New York: McGraw-Hill, 2010. Copyright © McGraw-Hill Education LLC.)

Laboratory Findings

Leukopenia is commonly present. Other laboratory values include thrombocytopenia and proteinuria. Detection of IgM antibodies using ELISA can support diagnosis. If rubeola is clinically suspected, confirmatory test should be done by contacting public health officials.

Differential Diagnosis

Scarlet fever, rubella, erythema infectiosum, exanthema subitum, and infectious mononucleosis.

Complications

Otitis media is the most common complication occurring in 25% of children. Other complications include pneumonia and diarrhea. Serious complications include encephalitis, blindness, and subacute sclerosing panencephalitis (SSPE). SSPE is a late CNS degenerative disease occurring 5-15 years later.

Treatment & Prognosis

Supportive care is suggested for uncomplicated cases. Vitamin A has been used to help prevent corneal ulcerations and blindness in nutrition poor children. Exposed children susceptible to measles should get IVIG 0.25 mL/kg within 6 days of exposure. The suggested dose for exposed immunodeficient children is 0.5 mL/kg.

Bonfante G, Rosenau AM: Rashes in infants and children. In: Tintinalli JE, Kelen, GD Stapczynski JS, eds. *Tintinalli's Emergency Medicine: A Comprehensive Study Guide.* 7th ed. New York: McGraw-Hill; 2011. Available at http://www.accessemergencymedicine.com/content.aspx?aID=6383200. Accessed February 19, 2013.

Cline DM: Occupational exposures, infection control, and standard precautions. In: Tintinalli JE, Kelen GD, Stapczynski JS, eds. *Tintinalli's Emergency Medicine: A Comprehensive Study Guide.* 7th ed. New York: McGraw-Hill; 2011. Available at http://www.accessemergencymedicine.com/content.aspx?aID=6375423. Accessed February 19, 2013.

Galbraith JC, Verity R, Tyrrell LD: Encephalomyelitis. In: Hall JB, Schmid GA, Wood LD, eds. *Principles of Critical Care.* 3rd ed. New York: McGraw-Hill; 2005. Available at http://www.accessmedicine.com/content.aspx?aID=2291508. Accessed February 19, 2013.

Mittiga MR, Gonzalez del Rey JA, Ruddy RM: Pediatric conditions. In: Knoop KJ, Stack LB, Storrow AB, Thurman RJ, eds. *The Atlas of Emergency Medicine.* 3rd ed. New York: McGraw-Hill; 2010. Available at http://www.accessmedicine.com/content.aspx?aID=6004422. Accessed February 19, 2013

MMR vaccine information sheet. Available at www.cdc.gov/vaccines/pubs/vis/downloads/vis-mmr.pdf. Accessed April 20, 2012.

Shandera WX, Roig IL (2013). Chapter 32. Viral & rickettsial infections. In Papadakis MA, McPhee SJ, Rabow MW, eds. *Current Medical Diagnosis & Treatment 2013.* New York: McGraw-Hill; 2013. Available at http://www.accessmedicine.com/content.aspx?aID=17051. Accessed February 19, 2013.

RUBELLA (GERMAN MEASLES)

 ESSENTIALS OF DIAGNOSIS

▶ No prodrome in children.

▶ Lymphadenopathy in posterior cervical and posterior auricular lymph nodes.

▶ Maculopapular rash, spreading from face to extremities.

Pathogenesis

Rubella virus is a single-stranded RNA virus which is part of the Togaviridae family of viruses which spreads by respiratory droplets. Primary infection begins in the nasopharynx and spreads to local lymph nodes. Generally the infection is mild and self-limited. Patients are contagious 1 week before and usually only 5-7 days after the onset of the rash, however, infants with congenital rubella syndrome may shed the virus for up to a year. Rubella is dangerous to pregnant woman especially in the first 20 weeks in which it can cause great morbidity and mortality to the fetus. According to the CDC, Rubella was last reported in 2004 but outbreaks still occur in developing countries and physicians still need to be aware of the disease.

Clinical Findings

A rubella infection is often mild and asymptomatic. It presents with cough, coryza, conjunctivitis, low-grade fever,

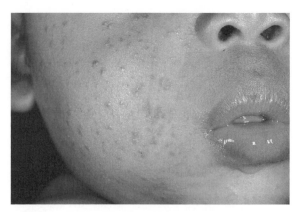

▲ **Figure 47–30.** Rubella. (Photo contributor: Binita R. Shah, MD. Reproduced, with permission, from Shah BR, Lucchesi M, eds: *Atlas of Pediatric Emergency Medicine*, 2nd ed. New York: McGraw-Hill, 2013. Copyright © McGraw-Hill Education LLC.)

and rash. The erythematous irregular pink maculopapular rash begins on the face (Figure 47–30) and spreads to the extremities. Rubella differs from rubeola on the start of the rash: Rubella rash appears at or near the onset of symptoms. Symptoms will clear in 3-4 days. Additional clinical findings include posterior auricular lymphadenopathy, polyarthralgias, and polyarthritis.

Infants who acquire the infection through the mother can get congenital rubella syndrome which is recognized by hepatosplenomegaly, "blueberry muffin rash," microcephaly, and low birth weight. Congenital abnormalities include patent ductus arteriosus, cataracts, glaucoma, and hearing loss.

Laboratory Findings

Detection of rubella is done by specific IgM antibody titers. Congential rubella is detected by the measurement of specific IgG antibodies. In most patients it is diagnosed as another viral exanthema. No laboratory investigation is needed unless diagnosis is required in certain cases, as in immunosuppressed children.

Differential Diagnosis

Measles, erythema infectiosum, exanthema subitum, infectious mononucleosis, enteroviral infection, adenovirus infection, and Rocky Mountain spotted fever.

Complications

Most common complications that occur are thrombocytopenia and encephalitis. In pregnant women, acquired infection can lead to fetal death and congenital rubella syndrome.

Treatment & Prognosis

For most patients, no specific therapy is used and symptomatic treatment is used in this self-limited infection. Rubella is highly contagious and patients should remain out of contact for 7 days after rash onset. IVIG (0.55 mL/kg) has been used to reduce viral load and to treat exposed pregnant women.

Bonfante G, Rosenau AM: Rashes in infants and children. In: Tintinalli JE, Kelen GD, Stapczynski JS, eds. *Tintinalli's Emergency Medicine: A Comprehensive Study Guide*. 7th ed. New York: McGraw-Hill; 2011. Available at http://www.accessemergencymedicine.com/content.aspx?aID=6383200. Accessed February 20, 2013.

Brown L: Rashes in infants and children. In: Cline DM, Ma OJ, Cydulka RK, Meckler GD, Handel DA, Thomas SH, eds. *Tintinalli's Emergency Medicine Manual*. 7th ed. New York: McGraw-Hill; 2012. Available at http://www.accessemergencymedicine.com/content.aspx?aID=56274747. Accessed February 20, 2013.

Shah BR: Infectious diseases. In: Shah BR, Lucchesi M, eds. *Atlas of Pediatric Emergency Medicine*. New York: McGraw-Hill; 2006. Available at http://www.accessemergencymedicine.com/content.aspx?aID=77310. Accessed February 20, 2013.

Shandera WX, Roig IL: Viral & rickettsial infections. In: Papadakis MA, McPhee SJ, Rabow MW, eds. *Current Medical Diagnosis & Treatment 2013*. New York: McGraw-Hill; 2013. Available at http://www.accessmedicine.com/content.aspx?aID=17051. Accessed February 19, 2013

Zimmerman LA, Reef SE: Rubella (German measles). In: Longo DL, Fauci AS, Kasper DL, Hauser SL, Jameson JL, Loscalzo J, eds. *Harrison's Principles of Internal Medicine*. 18th ed. New York: McGraw-Hill; 2012. Available at http://www.accessmedicine.com/content.aspx?aID=9124501. Accessed February 20, 2013

MOLLUSCUM CONTAGIOSUM

ESSENTIALS OF DIAGNOSIS

▶ Viral infection.

▶ Small, well-circumscribed, domed pearly pink papules with a central depression.

General Considerations

Molluscum contagiosum is common viral infection of the skin caused by the poxvirus typically through direct skin contact. It is commonly seen in children aged 3-16 years. The virus can cause multiple lesions on the skin distributed throughout the body. In most cases, it is self-limited and will resolve in approximately 8 weeks. Patients who are immunocompromised (HIV) can present with large widespread lesions for a longer duration. It is generally spread by direct skin contact which includes sexual contact; however, fomites can also transmit the disease.

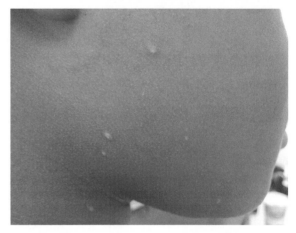

▲ **Figure 47–31.** Molluscum contagiosum. (Photo contributor: Sharon A. Glick, MD. Reproduced, with permission, from Shah BR, Lucchesi M, eds: *Atlas of Pediatric Emergency Medicine*, 2nd ed. New York: McGraw-Hill, 2013. Copyright © McGraw-Hill Education LLC.)

Clinical Findings

Molluscum contagiosum typically presents as rounded domed flesh-colored papules with a central umbilication, and can also appear as pearly pink (Figure 47–31). The papules are generally 1-5 mm in diameter but can be larger in immunocompromised patients. Lesions can be found anywhere on the skin but rarely on the palms or the soles. The papules tend to be in groups with fewer than 20 present.

Diagnosis

Diagnosis can be made clinically by the identification of lesions.

Treatment

In most patients lesions will resolve in time without treatment. Children are typically observed but can be treated with imiquimod cream 5%, cantharidin, freezing, or curettage. Lesions located in the perineum and genitalia are typically treated to avoid spread by sexual contact. Treatment for lesions is either cryosurgery or curettage. Topical therapies have limited effect (lactic acid, podophyllin, cantharidin, silver nitrate). Patients should be educated to avoid swimming pools and activities involving multiple contacts until the lesions have healed.

Morrell DS, Nelson K: Disorders of the groin and skinfolds. In: Tintinalli JE, Kelen GD, Stapczynski JS, eds. *Tintinalli's Emergency Medicine: A Comprehensive Study Guide*. 7th ed. New York: McGraw-Hill; 2011.

Shah BR: Dermatology. In: Shah BR, Lucchesi M, eds. *Atlas of Pediatric Emergency Medicine.* New York: McGraw-Hill; 2006.

Wolff K, Johnson RA, Suurmond D: Disorders of the genitalia, perineum, and anus. In: Wolff K, Johnson RA, Suurmond D, eds. *Fitzpatrick's Color Atlas and Synopsis of Clinical Dermatology.* 6th ed. New York: McGraw-Hill; 2009.

COMMON BENIGN INFANT RASHES

MILIA

Milia are tiny white epidermal cysts filled with keritinous material limited to the face and scalp (Figure 47–32). The cysts come from sebaceous glands at the base of hair follicles. The rash is self-limited and no treatment is necessary. Lesions resolve in weeks to months.

MILIARIA

Miliaria, heat rash, is an obstruction of eccrine sweat glands which leads to lesions on the skin. Miliaria is comprised of several groups including miliaria crystallina, miliaria rubra, miliaria pustulosa, and miliaria profunda. Miliaria rubra are erythematous papules and macules found on the head and upper trunk of febrile overheated infants (heat rash). Miliaria pustulosa (Figure 47–33) is a progression from M. rubra (Figure 47–34) as a result of longer duration of sweat duct occlusion. Miliaria crystallina (Figure 47–35) is a superficial sweat gland obstruction causing tiny clear vesicles on the skin. Miliaria profunda is a less frequent obstruction of the sweat glands deeper in the skin that leaves papules. In

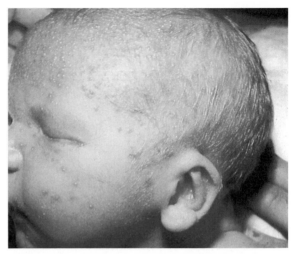

▲ **Figure 47–33.** Miliaria pustulosa. (Reproduced, with permission, from Weinberg S, Prose NS, Kristal L, eds: *Color Atlas of Pediatric Dermatology*, 4th ed. New York: McGraw-Hill, 2008. Copyright © McGraw-Hill Education LLC.)

general, parental reassurance is the most important part of treatment because miliaria crystallina and miliaria rubra are benign conditions. Management and prevention are accomplished by the following recommendations: 1) avoidance of overheating, 2) removal of excess clothing, and 3) cooling baths, and air conditioning.

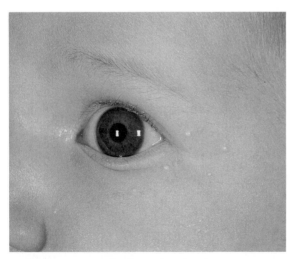

▲ **Figure 47–32.** Milia. (Reproduced, with permission, from Weinberg S, Prose NS, Kristal L, eds: *Color Atlas of Pediatric Dermatology*, 4th ed. New York: McGraw-Hill, 2008. Copyright © McGraw-Hill Education LLC.)

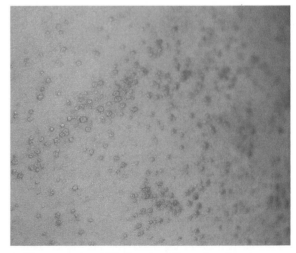

▲ **Figure 47–34.** Miliaria rubra. (Reproduced, with permission, from Weinberg S, Prose NS, Kristal L, eds: *Color Atlas of Pediatric Dermatology*, 4th ed. New York: McGraw-Hill, 2008. Copyright © McGraw-Hill Education LLC.)

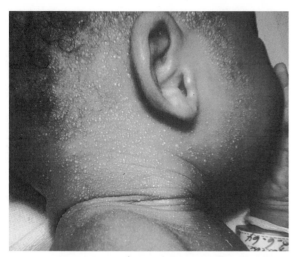

▲ **Figure 47–35.** Miliaria crystallina. (Reproduced, with permission, from Weinberg S, Prose NS, Kristal L, eds: *Color Atlas of Pediatric Dermatology*, 4th ed. New York: McGraw-Hill, 2008. Copyright © McGraw-Hill Education LLC.)

ERYTHEMA TOXICUM

Erythema toxicum occurs in 50% of neonates occurring 24-48 hours after discharge and lasts 1 week. The rash is described as pinpoint papulopustular lesions on a red base that appear on the face, trunk, and extremities (Figure 47–36). Using a Wright stain on scrapings of the rash will reveal eosinophils characteristic of the rash. In general,

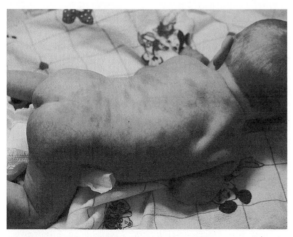

▲ **Figure 47–36.** Erythema toxicum. (Photo contributed by Kevin J. Knoop, MD. Reproduced, with permission, from Knoop K, Stack L, Storrow A, Thurman RJ: *Atlas of Emergency Medicine*, 3rd ed. New York: McGraw-Hill, Inc., 2010. Copyright © McGraw-Hill Education LLC.)

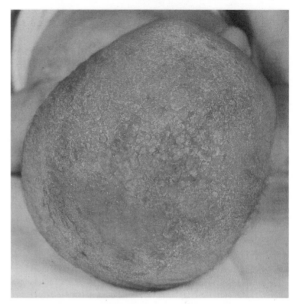

▲ **Figure 47–37.** Seborrheic dermatitis. (Reproduced, with permission, from Fleischer AB Jr, Feldman SR, McConnell CF et al: *Emergency Dermatology: A Rapid Treatment Guide.* New York: McGraw-Hill, 2002. Copyright © McGraw-Hill Education LLC.)

parental reassurance of the benign and transient nature of the rash is all that is needed.

Seborrheic Dermatitis

Seborrheic dermatitis exists in infants and adults. In infants the rash usually appears during the first 4 weeks of life (Figure 47–37). Rash appears as sharply demarcated greasy yellow, red, and brown patches or plaques. Cause is unclear, but the overproduction of sebum leaves the greasy scales. Low potency corticosteroids, such as 1% hydrocortisone cream, are used to treat inflammation. Additional treatment includes oatmeal baths. Ketoconazole shampoo (over-the-counter shampoo) appears to be a safe and efficacious treatment for infants with cradle cap. Some have recommended massaging mineral oil to the scalp and a soft brush to loosen the scale prior to shampoo.

Diaper Dermatitis

Diaper dermatitis is an irritant dermatitis in the diaper area. The dermatitis originates from prolonged skin exposure to urine, feces, soaps, and chemicals in the diaper. The rash appears as macular or papular scaling erythema of the skin excluding skin folds (Figure 47–38). *Candida* can be a source of secondary infection involving skin

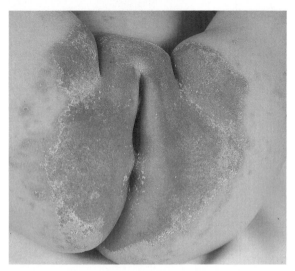

▲ **Figure 47–38.** Diaper dermatitis. (Reproduced, with permission, from Wolff KL, Johnson R, Suurmond R: *Fitzpatrick's Color Atlas & Synopsis of Clinical Dermatology*, 6th ed. New York: McGraw-Hill, Inc., 2009. Copyright © McGraw-Hill Education LLC.)

folds. Superinfection in the perineal and perianal areas is commonly caused by *S. aureus* or group A *Streptococcus* (Figure 47–39) and requires oral antibiotics. Perianal *Streptococcus*, another complication of diaper dermatitis, presents with erythema around the anus and is treated with oral antibiotics. Topical antifungals such as nystatin, ketoconazole, or clotrimazole are used to treat the secondary infection with *Candida*. Thorough drying of the skin before diapering is a good preventive measure because it is the excess moisture, either from urine and feces, or from

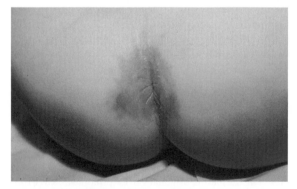

▲ **Figure 47–39.** Perianal strep. (Photo contributor: Raymond C. Baker, MD. Reproduced, with permission, from Knoop K, Stack L, Storrow A, Thurman RJ: *Atlas of Emergency Medicine*, 3rd ed. New York: McGraw-Hill, 2010. Copyright © McGraw-Hill Education LLC.)

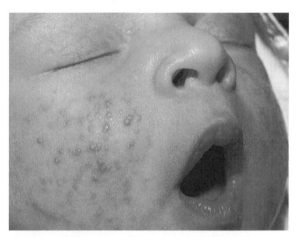

▲ **Figure 47–40.** Neonatal acne. (Reproduced, with permission, from Wolff K, Goldsmith LA, Katz SL, et al: *Fitzpatrick's Dermatology in General Medicine*, 7th ed. New York: McGraw-Hill, Inc., 2008. Copyright © McGraw-Hill Education LLC.)

sweating, that sets the conditions for a diaper rash to occur. Blocking moisture from reaching the skin through the use of barrier creams available over-the-counter (zinc oxide creams, petroleum jelly, is a useful method to reduce skin susceptibility to Candida infection).

Neonatal Acne

Neonatal acne occurs in up to 20% of infants usually during the third week of life due to maternal hormones stimulating sebaceous glands. Acne presents as erythematous papules and pustules mostly around the face and sometimes the trunk (Figure 47–40). Diagnosis is clinical and treatment is not necessary because lesions will resolve usually during the third month of life.

Bonfante G, Rosenau AM: Rashes in infants and children. In: Tintinalli JE, Stapczynski JS, Cline DM, Ma OJ, R.K. Cydulka RK, Meckler GD, eds. *Tintinalli's Emergency Medicine: A Comprehensive Study Guide*. 7th ed. New York: McGraw-Hill; 2011. Available at http://www.accessmedicine.com/content.aspx?aID=6383200. Accessed February 20, 2013.

Collins CD, Hivnor C: Seborrheic dermatitis. In: Goldsmith LA, Katz SI, Gilchrest BA, Paller AS, Leffell DJ, Dallas NA, eds. *Fitzpatrick's Dermatology in General Medicine*. 8th ed. New York: McGraw-Hill; 2012. Available at http://www.accessmedicine.com/content.aspx?aID=56027072. Accessed February 20, 2013.

Laumann AE: Dermatologic conditions. In: Hall JB, Schmidt GA, Wood LD, eds. *Principles of Critical Care*. 3rd ed. New York: McGraw-Hill; 2005. Available at http://www.accessmedicine.com/content.aspx?aID=2281907. Accessed February 20, 2013.

Morelli JG, Prok LD: Skin. In: Hay Jr WW, Levin MJ, Deterding RR, Ross JJ, Sondheimer JM, eds. *Current Diagnosis & Treatment: Pediatrics.* 21st ed. New York: McGraw-Hill; 2006. Available at http://www.accessmedicine.com/content.aspx?aID=56816195. Accessed February 20, 2013.

OConner NR, McLaughlin MR, Ham P. Newborn Skin: Part I. Common Rashes. 2008;77:47-52 [PMID:18236822].

Tintinalli JE, Kelen GD, Stapczynski JS. Neonatal emergencies and common neonatal problems. In: Tintinalli JE, Kelen GD, Stapczynski JS, eds. *Tintinalli's Emergency Medicine: A Comprehensive Study Guide.* 7th ed. New York: McGraw-Hill; 2011.

HYPERSENSITIVITY REACTIONS

URTICARIA

ESSENTIALS OF DIAGNOSIS

▶ Urticaria, often called hives, are raised; red/pink, pruritic wheals often associated with an allergic trigger.

▶ Confirm that the patient does not exhibit systemic symptoms from the allergic trigger that requires early and aggressive intervention.

Urticaria, often called hives, are comprised of erythematous pale red/pink-colored raised patches in the skin known as wheals, which are pruritic in nature, and often a sign of an allergic reaction (Figure 47–41). Urticaria affects up to 20% of the population and can be confused with eczema, contact dermatitis, insect bites/stings, and erythema multiforme. Because urticaria is often triggered by an allergic exposure,

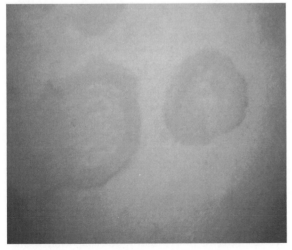

▲ **Figure 47–41.** Urticaria. (Reproduced, with permission, from Weinberg S, Prose NS, Kristal L, eds: *Color Atlas of Pediatric Dermatology,* 4th ed. New York: McGraw-Hill, 2008. Copyright © McGraw-Hill Education LLC.)

evaluate immediately for systemic symptoms such as shortness of breath, airway compromise, angioedema, vomiting, and cardiovascular compromise. Upon confirmation that the urticarial is cutaneous and not systemic, perform a thorough history to identify previous episodes, treatments, and outcomes, and attempt to identify the offending allergen. Common triggers include medications, specific foods (nuts, eggs, shellfish), and any known new exposures (cleaning detergents/soaps, pets, chemicals). If systemic symptoms are present, intramuscular (IM) epinephrine 0.01 mg/kg 1:1000 up to a dose of 0.3 mg may be required emergently. Moderate to severe urticaria treatment includes H_1 blocker therapy such as diphenhydramine (1.25 mg/kg po/IV/IM) or hydroxyzine (0.5 mg/kg po or IM), and H_2 blocker therapy such as ranitidine (1 mg/kg IV) or famotidine (0.5 mg/kg IV). Glucocorticoids are used for moderate to severe cases such as prednisone (1-2 mg/kg) for older children, and prednisolone (1-2 mg/kg) for younger children. Ingested allergens can cause a prolonged effect; therefore, continued medications dosing after the initial treatment may be warranted. Depending on the severity of the allergic reaction, prescription of an Epi-Pen may be warranted, as well as a referral to an allergist.

Frigas E, Park MA: Acute urticaria and angioedema: Diagnostic and treatment considerations. *Am J Clin Dermatol.* 2009;10(4):239 [PMID: 19489657].

Poonawalla T, Kelly B: Urticaria: A review. *Am J Clin Dermatol.* 2009;10(1):9 [PMID: 19170406].

Simons FE: Anaphylaxis. *J Allergy Clin Immunol.* 2010;125 (2 suppl 2):S161 [PMID: 20176258].

ANGIOEDEMA

ESSENTIALS OF DIAGNOSIS

▶ Acute edema of deep dermis, often involving face, mouth, and intraoral structures.

▶ Angioedema can be a life-threatening emergency due to airway obstruction. Aggressive, early definitive management may be required.

Angioedema is an acute reaction involving swelling of the deep dermal layers of the skin, but often involving the face, lips, intraoral structures, or deep airway. Other names include Quincke edema and angioneurotic edema. Allergic angioedema, an IgE and histamine-related reaction, usually occurs with an acute allergen exposure and is associated with urticaria. There are two types of nonallergic angioedema: hereditary and acquired. They involve diminished function of C1-inhibition either by hereditary basis or immune complex autoantibody production. The primary cause of nonallergic angioedema is ACE inhibitor medication.

Treatment, regardless of etiology, is aggressive airway management and maintenance of breathing and circulation. Severe angioedema can result in rapid airway obstruction that may require patient intubation or performance of an emergent surgical airway. If etiology of angioedema can be identified, the varied treatment options can be modified. Allergic angioedema is treated similar to urticaria with intravenous antihistamine, H_2 blockers, and steroids and often IM epinephrine. With nonallergic angioedema, the above treatments have been shown to have limited improvement in symptoms. Fresh frozen plasma (FFP) has shown benefit in some patients. Ecallantide (Kalbitor), Icatibant (Firazyr), and C1-INH infusion (Berinert) are approved for the treatment of hereditary angioedema.

Craig T, Aygören-Pürsün E , Bork K, et al: WAO guideline for the management of hereditary angioedema. *World Allergy Organ J.* 2012;5(12):182 [PMID: 23282420].

Kumar SA, Martin BL: Urticaria and angioedema: Diagnostic and treatment considerations. *J Am Osteopath Assoc.* 1999;99 (suppl 3):S1 [PMID: 10217914].

Marx J, Hockberger R, Walls R: Urticaria and angioedema. *Rosen's Emergency Medicine.* 7th ed. Mosby; 2009.

Contact Dermatitis

Contact dermatitis is defined by hives, a characteristic localized, raised, pruritic skin erythema, and is triggered by a dermal irritant. Contact dermatitis can present as papules, macules, vesicles, or a plaque. The reaction to the dermis is an inflammatory response with direct damage to the skin. This differs from allergic contact dermatitis (ACD) which is a dermal reaction due to a patient's sensitivity to a particular allergen.

PLANTS: POISON IVY, OAK, SUMAC

ESSENTIALS OF DIAGNOSIS

► Poison ivy, oak, and sumac cause severe contact dermatitis via oil resin (urushiol).

► Can be spread from direct plant contact, inhalation, ingestions, or by contact with pets, tools, and clothing that had been exposed.

► Classic linear vesicles are a hallmark sign.

► Treatment is symptomatic and systemic steroids for severe cases.

The most common cause of contact dermatitis in the summer months is urushiol, an oil-based resin, from plants from the Toxicodendron class including poison ivy, oak, and sumac. Poison ivy is a three-leafed plant that grows throughout the United States and Southern Canada, except the West coast of the United States. However, the West coast has poison oak. The urushiol oil that comes from contact with the plant directly, or by indirect contact with the oil found on shoes, gloves, clothing, tools, pets will cause an extremely pruritic rash that can last 1-3 weeks. Initially, the rash presents with linear or singular papules that evolve into vesicles. Smoke from plants that are burned can be inhaled and be a significant lung irritant and if accidentally ingested, can cause the same reaction to the mucosal lining of the gastrointestinal tract. If exposure occurs, rinse the area with warm water immediately, as well as all clothing and anything that may have been exposed. The rash can present over a variable duration, which can be indicative of how much urushiol was exposed to the skin, or that the patient continues to spread the oil from a source, such as oil on the shoes that have not been cleaned. The rash itself, and vesicular fluid that follows, is not infective after the initially skin cleaning. Treatment includes symptomatic relief with antihistamines, topical steroid cream, oatmeal baths, calamine lotion, and cool compresses. Oral steroids (prednisone 0.5-1 mg/kg/day for 7-10 days followed by a taper of 7-10 days) are indicated with facial, genitalia, or diffuse involvement of the skin. On occasion, the patient may have a diffuse dermal allergic reaction to this chemical contact dermatitis. Over-the-counter preparations such as Ivy Block can be applied similar to sunscreen to prevent skin absorption of the urushiol oil if exposed, and Zanfel may be of benefit to relieve symptomatic pruritus and bind the urushiol in the dermis after exposure.

American Academy of Dermatology, 2013. Available at http://www.aad.org/skin-conditions/dermatology-a-to-z/poison-ivy#.UVEUEY6EPGs.

DRUG HYPERSENSITIVITY/DRUG ERUPTIONS

ESSENTIALS OF DIAGNOSIS

► Medication or drug-induced hypersensitivity is commonly a type 4 reaction.

► A morbilliform rash is the most commonly found skin lesion.

► Drugs most often involved are antimicrobials, anticonvulsants, and NSAIDs.

A number of medications have been identified that cause a drug hypersensitivity reaction that results in a rash. Surprisingly, the majority of these reactions to medications are type 4 delayed type cell-mediated hypersensitivity reactions. Only a small number are the classic IgE-mediated reactions that cause urticaria and anaphylaxis. Most type 4 reactions occur 7-15 days after medication is started and present with a classic morbilliform type rash (Figure 47–42) that spares the palms

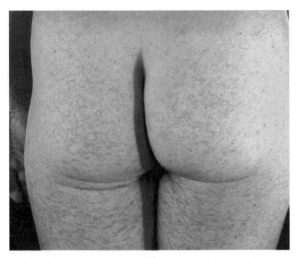

▲ **Figure 47–42.** Drug eruption. (Reproduced, with permission, from Weinberg S, Prose NS, Kristal L, eds: *Color Atlas of Pediatric Dermatology*, 4th ed. New York: McGraw-Hill, 2008. Copyright © McGraw-Hill Education LLC.)

of the hands and soles of the feet; however, the rash can have varying presentations. Most offending agents fall into a few drug categories: antimicrobial with penicillin and sulfa-based antibiotics are most prevalent, NSAIDs, anticonvulsants such as phenytoin and valproic acid, and antihypertensives such as ACE inhibitors or diuretics. Treatment may include some symptomatic relief with antipruritic therapy and steroids. However, because most reactions are type 4 hypersensitivity reactions, the actual treatment is removal of the offending agent with resolution of the rash in 2-3 days. Because severity of the rash falls under a spectrum, mucosal body areas and dermal areas consistent with desquamation must be evaluated for progression into SJS and TEN.

Gendernalik SB, Galeckas KJ: Fixed drug eruptions: A case report and review of the literature. *Cutis.* 2009;84(4):215 [PMID: 19911677].

Greenberger PA: Drug allergy. *J Allergy Clin Immunol.* 2006;117 (2 Suppl Mini-Primer):S464 [PMID: 16455348].

ATOPIC/ECZEMATOUS DERMATITIS

 ESSENTIAL OF DIAGNOSIS

▶ Dry, scaly patches usually located over flexor surfaces of joints or face.

▶ Unknown etiology but triggers include hereditary, dry skin, allergen induced, and cold climate.

Atopic dermatitis presents with scaly erythematous raised patches that can evolve into chronic thickening of the dermis or lichenification. It is often found on the face and flexor surfaces of the joints such as the antecubital fossa. It is often associated with a positive family history, known allergen sensitivities and asthma. Onset in children is usually 2-12 months of age and most resolve by adulthood. Although etiology of atopic dermatitis is unknown, factors known to exacerbate symptoms include stress, dry cool climates, and allergen exposures. The goal for treatment is skin management to avoid the acute flares of atopic dermatitis. Keys to treatment include skin-moisturizing products (Cetaphil, Aveeno, Aquaphor, petroleum-based products) and avoidance of soaps that cause drying of the skin. Topical steroids can be utilized in varying potency depending on severity of atopic dermatitis. Avoidance of topical steroids to the face and periorbital region is recommended to prevent thinning of skin. Secondary superficial skin infections can be common with atopic dermatitis; close evaluation of the dermis to identify inflammatory versus infectious ideology is recommended with the use of oral antibiotics in the event of secondary cellulitis. Additional treatments include coal tar preparations, topical NSAIDs, and topical calcineurin inhibitors such as pimecrolimus and tacrolimus.

Boguniewicz M: Topical treatment of atopic dermatitis. *Immunol Allergy Clin North Am.* 2004;24:631-644 [PMID: 15474863].

Kvenshagen B, Jacobsen M, Halvorsen R: Atopic dermatitis in premature and term children. *Arch Dis Child.* 2009;94:202-205 [PMID: 18829619].

Ong PY, Boguniewicz M: Atopic dermatitis. *Prim Care.* 2008;35: 105-117 [PMID: 18206720].

ERYTHEMA MULTIFORM/STEVENS-JOHNSON SYNDROME/TOXIC EPIDERMAL NECROLYSIS

 ESSENTIALS OF DIAGNOSIS

▶ Type 4 hypersensitivity reaction that results in a "bulls eye" lesion.

▶ EM is mild form, with severity of symptoms progressing to SJS, then TEN based on mucosal involvement and BSA desquamation.

Erythema multiforme (EM) is an acute type 4 hypersensitivity reaction with known triggers that include infectious ideology and certain medications. Skin lesions appear initially as small papules located on the extremities and quickly evolve into the classic target-appearing lesions with concentric rings of erythema (Figure 47–43) within the first 72 hours. Medication triggers include barbiturates, penicillins, phenytoin, and sulfamides. Infectious sources include HSV, mycoplasma,

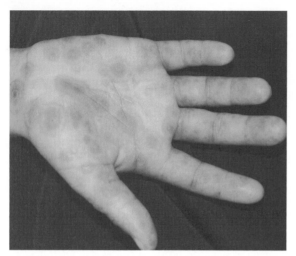

▲ **Figure 47–43.** Erythema multiforme. (Reproduced, with permission, from Weinberg S, Prose NS, Kristal L, eds: *Color Atlas of Pediatric Dermatology*, 4th ed. New York: McGraw-Hill, 2008. Copyright © McGraw-Hill Education LLC.)

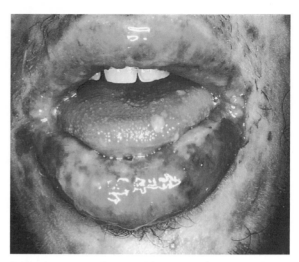

▲ **Figure 47–44.** Stevens-Johnson syndrome. (Reproduced, with permission, from Weinberg S, Prose NS, Kristal L, eds: *Color Atlas of Pediatric Dermatology*, 4th ed. New York: McGraw-Hill, 2008. Copyright © McGraw-Hill Education LLC.)

and EBV and other viruses. If only target lesions are present, the rash is considered EM minor. EM minor converts to EM major when one or more mucous membranes that encompass less than 10% of total body surface area (TBSA) are present with typical target lesions. The progression from EM major to SJS consists of inclusion of widespread blistering in the trunk face to greater than 10% TBSA involvement with associated dermal desquamation (Figures 47–44 and 47–45). Mucous membranes are affected in more than 90% of patients, usually involving two or more sites (ocular, oral, genital). TEN is now considered a more severe version of SJS. TEN is diagnosed when the desquamation encompasses greater than 30% body surface area. Most cases of EM minor are self-limiting with lesions resolving within 2-3 weeks. Treatment for EM minor is symptomatic and includes analgesics, skin care for mild desquamation, and mouthwashes to help with intraoral pain. Evaluation for the underlying cause of the EM is key and involves elimination of the offending medication or treatment of the underlying infectious trigger. EM major and TEN require inpatient care and management with IV fluid for rehydration, pain management, and wound care for the mucosal and dermal desquamation. Severe TEN may require admission to a burn unit for definitive management and care.

Hazin R, Ibrahimi OA, Hazin MI, Kimyai-Asadi A. Stevens-Johnson syndrome: Pathogenesis, diagnosis, and management. *Ann Med.* 2008;40(2):129-38. PMID: 18293143

Sokumbi O, Wetter DA. Clinical features, diagnosis, and treatment of erythema multiforme: A review for the practicing dermatologist. *Int J Dermatol.* 2012;51(8):889 [PMID: 22788803].

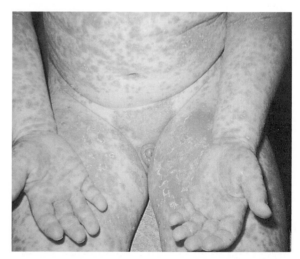

▲ **Figure 47–45.** Stevens-Johnson syndrome. (Reproduced, with permission, from Weinberg S, Prose NS, Kristal L, eds: *Color Atlas of Pediatric Dermatology*, 4th ed. New York: McGraw-Hill, 2008. Copyright © McGraw-Hill Education LLC.)

PHOTOSENSITIVITY

ESSENTIALS OF DIAGNOSIS

▶ UV light causing direct injury to dermis can result in superficial burn.

▶ Pain, warmth, and blistering can occur based on severity, often resolving into superficial desquamation.

▶ Drug-induced photosensitivity results in a superficial burn with appearance of contact dermatitis in exposed skin areas. Specific medications lower the dermis threshold to have a reaction.

▶ Acute Sun Damage

UV light from the sun can cause direct injury to the dermis leading to a superficial burn, known as first-degree burn. Common in younger children with fair or sensitive skin, the superficial layers of the dermis become erythematous, warm to touch, within 3-4 hours of exposure, and peak about 24 hours. Risk factors include certain medications, living in higher altitude, alcohol, and male gender. The skin usually heals within 4-7 days, often followed by desquamation of the superficial dermis. In severe cases, it can cause superficial partial-thickness burns which present with vesicles or blisters. Treatment is cool water soaks and NSAIDs. Dehyration, if present, may need to be addressed in severe cases. Topical emollients such as aloe vera can provide symptomatic relief. Topical steroids have not shown benefit in improvement or shortening the course of the burn symptoms.

Brown TT, Quain RD, Troxel AB, Gelfand J: The epidemiology of sunburn in the US population in 2003. *J Am Acad Dermatol.* 2006;55(4):577 [PMID: 17010735].

Cokkinides V, Weinstock M, Glanz K, Albano J, Ward E, Thun M: Trends in sunburns, sun protection practices, and attitudes toward sun exposure protection and tanning among US adolescents, 1998-2004. *Pediatrics.* 2006;118(3):853 [PMID: 16950974].

▶ Drug-Induced Photosensitivity

A number of medications can cause acute photosensitivity when combined with sun (UV) exposure. Medications specific and common to the pediatric population include antibiotics (sulfonamides, tetracyclines, fluoroquinolones), NSAIDs (ibuprofen), and antifungals (griseofulvin). Classes of drugs less commonly utilized in pediatrics are oral hypoglycemics, diuretics, and neuroleptics. Classically, drug-induced hypersensitivity will have characteristics similar to combining a first-degree sunburn with a contact dermatitis, and be present on sun-exposed surfaces only. Treatment includes discontinuation of the medication, avoidance of sun exposure, and liberal use of sunscreen to avoid UV light exposure. Of note, on occasion, the sunscreen can be the offending or exacerbating agent.

Onoue S, Seto Y, Gandy G, Yamada S: Drug-induced phototoxicity; an early in vitro identification of phototoxic potential of new drug entities in drug discovery and development. *Curr Drug Saf.* 2009;4(2):123-36. [PMID: 19442106].

VASCULTIS & AUTOIMMUNE RASHES

ERYTHEMA NODUSUM

ESSENTIALS OF DIAGNOSIS

▶ Tender 2-3 cm nodules located anterior to lower extremities.

▶ Etiology includes streptococcal and mycoplasma bacteria, sulfa-based drugs, and enteropathic diseases: Crohn disease, ulcerative colitis, and Hodgkin lymphoma.

Erythema nodosum (EN) is a hypersensitivity reaction from disease or drug-induced etiology that results in tender, nodular eruptions, usually located on the anterior tibial regions of the lower extremities. It is more prevalent in females and in adolescents and young adults. Onset of the tender, erythematous, or ecchymotic-appearing 2-3 cm nodules (Figure 47–46)

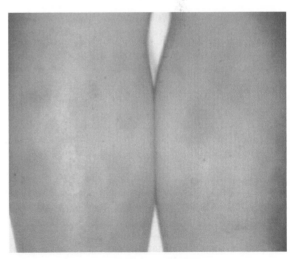

▲ **Figure 47–46.** Erythema nodosum. (Reproduced, with permission, from Weinberg S, Prose NS, Kristal L, eds: *Color Atlas of Pediatric Dermatology*, 4th ed. New York: McGraw-Hill, 2008. Copyright © McGraw-Hill Education LLC.)

is usually preceded by a flu-like illness. The lesions can last up to 2 weeks and are commonly seen with myalgias and arthralgias. Specific pediatric causes include bacterial etiologies, often streptococcal and mycoplasma pneumonia, fungal infections, commonly coccidiomycosis, drug-induced reaction from sulfonamides, and enteropathic diseases such as Crohn disease and ulcerative colitis, tuberculosis, sarcoidosis, and Hodgkin disease. Patients suspected with EN should have blood cultures performed, ESR, CBC with differential, *Streptococcus* screen or culture, and, if warranted, stool studies. Treatment of the underlying disease trigger is all that is required with symptomatic relief from NSAIDs, elevation, and rest needed for the nodules.

Mert A, Ozaras R, Tabak F, Pekmezci S, Demirkesen C, Ozturk R: Erythema nodosum: An experience of 10 years. *Scand J Infect Dis.* 2004;36(6-7):424-7 [PMID: 15307561].

ERYTHEMA CHRONICUM MIGRANS

See Parasitic/Vector Rashes.

HENOCH-SCHÖNLEIN PURPURA

 ESSENTIALS OF DIAGNOSIS

▶ Acute vasculitis with fever, purpura of lower extremities, abdominal pain, and gastrointestinal bleeding.

▶ 50% of patients can have renal involvement.

▶ Intussusception can be associated with syndrome.

Henoch-Schönlein purpura (HSP) is an acute immunoglobulin A (IgA)-mediated vasculitis that presents with a constellation of symptoms in children aged 2-11 years. It is often associated with arthralgia, fever, cutaneous purpura usually located on the lower extremities (Figure 47–47), abdominal pain and cramping, gastrointestinal (GI) bleeding, and acute nephritis. Scrotal pain and swelling can be found in affected males. The purpuric rash can begin as a macular rash that evolves into a 0.5- to 2-cm purpuric lesion that can coalesce into areas that appear ecchymotic. As the vasculitis progresses, up to 50% of patients can have renal involvement. Another serious complication can be intussusception in up to 3% of patients. Because abdominal pain is a common finding, discriminating simple abdominal pain from intussusception can be difficult. No laboratory test is diagnostic. Evaluation includes a CBC that can show a leukocytosis and thrombocytosis, a guaiac test for fecal occult blood, a urinalysis to evaluate for blood and protein, and a metabolic profile to evaluate renal function. Consider coagulation profile is the rash is petechial. Treatment is supportive. Many children will need hospital admission to

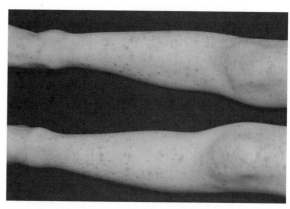

▲ **Figure 47–47.** Henoch-Schönlein purpura. (Reproduced, with permission, from Kane KS, Lio PA, Stratigos AJ, Johnson RA, eds: *Color Atlas & Synopsis of Pediatric Dermatology,* 4th ed. McGraw-Hill, Inc., 2009. Copyright © McGraw-Hill Education LLC.)

monitor GI bleeding, abdominal pain, and renal function. Patients with mild HSP and no systemic symptom involvement can be dispositioned home with close follow-up. NSAIDs are recommended for pain with arthralgias.

Ebert EC: Gastrointestinal manifestations of Henoch-Schönlein Purpura. *Dig Dis Sci.* 2008;8:2011 [PMID: 18351468].
Nong BR, Huang YF, Chuang CM, Liu CC, Hsieh KS: Fifteen-year experience of children with Henoch-Schönlein purpura in southern Taiwan, 1991-2005. *J Microbiol Immunol Infect.* 2007;40(4):371 [PMID: 17712473].

PITYRIASIS ROSEA

 ESSENTIALS OF DIAGNOSIS

▶ A 2- to 10-cm red, round/oval lesion (Herald patch).

▶ Herald patch is followed by outbreak of multiple 1- to 2-cm lesions in groups on trunk, back, and abdomen that can appear in a "Christmas tree" pattern.

▶ Symptomatic treatment for pruritus, can utilize UV light to speed resolution.

Pityriasis rosea (PR) has a hallmark exanthem, herald patch, which is round or oval from 2-10 cm in size with an erythematous center and raised scaly borders (Figure 47–48). Herald patch is often confused with eczema or tinea corpora (Figure 47–49). Days to weeks after the initial solitary lesion presentation, the patient will break out in 1- to 2-cm salmon-colored patches in groups on the trunk, abdomen, and extremities. This secondary outbreak is known as a "Christmas tree" appearance because of the alignment of the

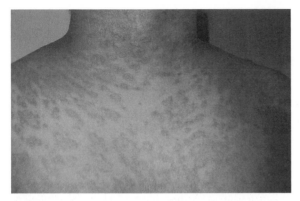

▲ **Figure 47–48.** Pityriasis rosea. (Reproduced, with permission, from Kane KS, Lio PA, Stratigos AJ, Johnson RA, eds: *Color Atlas & Synopsis of Pediatric Dermatology*, 4th ed. McGraw-Hill, Inc., 2009. Copyright © McGraw-Hill Education LLC.)

lesions on the back. Pruritus occurs in up to 75% of patients. The rash can last up to 8 weeks, then spontaneously resolve. The cause of PR is unknown but felt to be an immune response to a viral trigger. Treatment includes symptomatic relief with diphenhydramine and topical application of hydrocortisone and moisturizing creams. UV light treatment can aid in resolution of the rash. PR is more common in the spring and winter months and occurs more often in adolescents. PR has been shown to cause skin hypopigmentation at the sites of the lesions and has been associated with an increased risk in miscarriage if symptoms occur in the first 15 weeks of pregnancy.

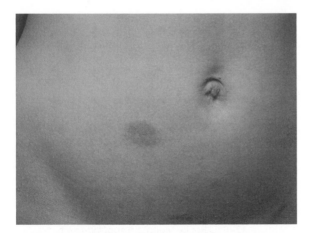

▲ **Figure 47–49.** Pityriasis rosea, herald patch. (Reproduced, with permission, from Kane KS, Lio PA, Stratigos AJ, Johnson RA, eds: *Color Atlas & Synopsis of Pediatric Dermatology*, 4th ed. McGraw-Hill, Inc., 2009. Copyright © McGraw-Hill Education LLC.)

Browning JC: An update on pityriasis rosea and other similar childhood exanthems. *Curr Opin Pediatr.* 2009;21(4):481 [PMID: 19502983].

Drago F, Broccolo F, Zaccaria E, et al: Pregnancy outcome in patients with pityriasis rosea. *J Am Acad Dermatol.* 2008;58 (5 suppl 1):S78 [PMID: 18489054].

Lim SH, Kim SM, Oh BH, et al: Low-dose ultraviolet A1 phototherapy for treating pityriasis rosea. *Ann Dermatol.* 2009;21(3):230 [PMID: 20523795].

KAWASAKI DISEASE

 ESSENTIALS OF DIAGNOSIS

▶ Onset with fever greater than 5 days.

▶ Including fever, 4 of 5 criteria: cervical lymphadenopathy, bilateral conjunctivitis, hand and feet edema, erythema and desquamation, oral mucosal dry cracked lips with strawberry-appearing tongue, body red rash usual of groin and lower extremities.

▶ High risk of coronary artery vasculitis including aneurysms and thrombosis if untreated.

Kawasaki disease (mucocutaneous lymph node syndrome, infantile polyarthritis) is an acute pediatric illness that causes an inflammatory vasculitis. It occurs almost exclusively (90-95%) in children younger than 10 years, with most children younger than 5 years. Considere to be immune-mediated, it begins with a high, persistent fever for at least 5 days that is difficult to control with normal antipyretic therapy. In addition to fever for 5 days, criteria required for a Kawasaki diagnosis per the American Heart Association (AHA) include four of the following five symptoms: acute painless bilateral conjunctivitis; oral mucosal involvement with dry, cracked lips and strawberry tongue; erythematous and edematous hands and feet often with skin desquamation (Figure 47–50); swollen cervical lymphadenopathy usually unilateral and greater than 1.5 cm; and a nonvesicular generalized rash usually located in the groin and lower extremities. Additional findings include joint pain and effusions, irritability, vomiting and diarrhea, and cough with nasal congestion, myocarditis, and pericarditis. Laboratory evaluations can show elevated levels of ESR, CRP, and α_1-antitripsyn, as well as thrombocytosis, and sterile pyuria on urinalysis evaluation. Diagnosis and early treatment are essential as 20-25% of untreated patients will develop cardiovascular complications ranging from coronary artery aneurysms, coronary artery thrombosis, acute myocardial infarctions, and death; therefore, an ECG should be obtained at presentation. Serial evaluation with echocardiography for the above complications is recommended. Inpatient treatment, which entails intravenous gamma globulin and aspirin therapy, should begin within

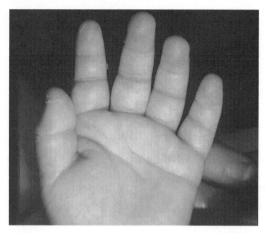

▲ **Figure 47–50.** Kawasaki disease, hand edema with desquamation. (Reproduced, with permission, from Weinberg S, Prose NS, Kristal L, eds: *Color Atlas of Pediatric Dermatology*, 4th ed. New York: McGraw-Hill, 2008. Copyright © McGraw-Hill Education LLC.)

10 days of onset of fever. Kawasaki disease is now the leading cause of acquired heart disease in the United States in children younger than 5 years.

Baker AL, Lu M, Minich LL, et al: Associated symptoms in the ten days before diagnosis of Kawasaki disease. *J Pediatr.* 2009;154(4):592. e2 [PMID: 19038400].

Heuclin T, Dubos F, Hue V, et al: Increased detection rate of Kawasaki disease using new diagnostic algorithm, including early use of echocardiography. *J Pediatr.* 2009;155(5):695. e1 [PMID: 19595368].

Rowley AH, Shulman ST: Pathogenesis and management of Kawasaki disease. *Expert Rev Anti Infect Ther.* 2010;8(2):197 [PMID: 20109049].

Satou GM, Giamelli J, Gewitz MH: Kawasaki disease: Diagnosis, management, and long-term implications. *Cardiol Rev.* 2007;15(4):163 [PMID: 17575479].

PARASITIC/VECTOR RASHES

ROCKY MOUNTAIN SPOTTED FEVER

 ESSENTIALS OF DIAGNOSIS

▶ Tick-borne illness from the parasite Rickettsia rickettsii.

▶ Infection causes an acute systemic vasculitis that often presents with a petechial rash; most infected patients present with fever and headache.

▶ Hallmark finding of RMSF is progression of rash to petechia on the palms of the hands and soles of the feet.

Rocky Mountain spotted fever (RMSF) is a tick-borne illness caused by the parasite *Rickettsia rickettsii*. The vector is primarily the dog tick, *Dermacentor variabilis*, found primarily in the Eastern United States, and *Dermacentor andersoni*, found in the Rocky Mountain region. This gram-negative coccobacilli is transmitted via tick bite which needs a minimum of 6 hours of attachment to the host before the rickettsiae is transferred. Incubation period can vary from 3-12 days. Most infected patients present with fever and headache with less than 25% presenting with neurological deficits. This parasitic infection causes an acute systemic vasculitis that often presents with a petechial rash anywhere from days 2-8 post-tick bite. A maculopapular rash begins on the wrists and ankles and can be blanching initially. Hallmark finding of RMSF is progression of the rash to petechia on the palms of the hands and soles of the feet, which can be present in 30-80% of patients (Figure 47–51). The face is usually spared. Interestingly, up to 15% of patients may not have this classic rash distribution during their illness. Additional findings include conjunctivitis with periorbital edema, chest pain with myocarditis which can lead to congestive heart failure, and bradycardia, pneumonitis, abdominal pain with hepatosplenomegaly and jaundice, severe myalgias, altered mental status with meningoencephalitis, and sepsis. Laboratory findings often include leukocytosis and thrombocytopenia, anemia, hyponatremia, elevated bilirubin and aminotransferase (AST), and a pleocytosis of cerebral spinal fluid with increase of monocytes. Treatment consists of early antibiotic therapy which has shown to decrease the mortality rate from

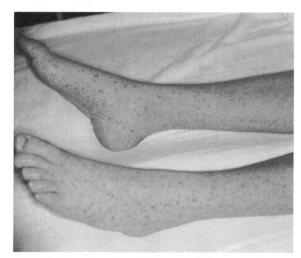

▲ **Figure 47–51.** Rocky Mountain spotted fever. (Reproduced, with permission, from Weinberg S, Prose NS, Kristal L, eds: *Color Atlas of Pediatric Dermatology*, 4th ed. New York: McGraw-Hill, 2008. Copyright © McGraw-Hill Education LLC.)

20 to 5%. Antibiotic drug of choice includes doxycycline followed by chloramphenicol. Short courses of doxycycline do not cause teeth staining and are now the recommended first-line therapy by the AAP. Aggressive supportive treatment in the setting of sepsis is a necessity.

Buckingham SC, Marshall GS, Schutze GE, et al: Clinical and laboratory features, hospital course, and outcome of Rocky Mountain spotted fever in children. *J Pediatr.* 2007;150(2):180,184.e1 [PMID: 17236897].

Chapman AS, Bakken JS, Folk SM, et al: Diagnosis and management of tickborne rickettsial diseases: Rocky Mountain spotted fever, ehrlichioses, and anaplasmosis—United States: A practical guide for physicians and other health-care and public health professionals. *MMWR Recomm Rep.* 2006;55:1 [PMID: 16572105].

LYME DISEASE

ESSENTIALS OF DIAGNOSIS

▶ Deer tick-borne infection from the spirochete *Borrrelia burgdorferi.*

▶ Classic "bulls-eye" or "target" looking rash named erythema chronicum migrans (ECM).

▶ Systemic symptoms include fatigue, myalgias, flu-like symptoms, headache, and fever.

Lyme disease is an infection from the spirochete *Borrrelia burgdorferi* transmitted from the bite of a deer tick, specifically of the *Ixodes* species. The likelihood of infection is clearly correlated to the duration of tick attachment to the host, and although the host is unlikely to contract the infection if the tick is attached less than 24 hours, it is possible. Twenty five percent of patients are children with the same percentage of patients infected that do not recall a tick bite. Early localized infection occurs commonly at the site of the tick bite from days 7 to 10, with a classic "bulls-eye" or "target" appearance, erythema chronicum migrans (ECM) (Figure 47–52) in 90% of infected patients. Most lesions are flat, erythematous macules with central clearing from 2- to 15- cm or larger; 40% of patients will develop secondary ECM lesions. Additional systemic symptoms include fatigue, myalgias, flu-like symptoms, headache, and fever. Treatment for early disease, with absent neurologic or cardiac findings, is doxycycline, amoxicillin, or cefuroxime for 14 days. If arthritic symptoms are present, the duration of therapy is increased to 30 days. If neurologic symptoms are present, or the patient is younger than 8 years, 14 days of parenteral antibiotics are recommended.

Centers for Disease Control and Prevention, Division of Vectorborne Infectious Diseases. *Lyme disease statistics*: 2009. Available at http://www.cdc.gov/ncidod/dvbid/lyme/ld_statistics.htm.

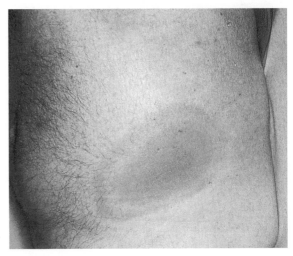

▲ **Figure 47–52.** Erythema chronicum migrans (Lyme disease). (Reproduced, with permission, from Weinberg S, Prose NS, Kristal L, eds: *Color Atlas of Pediatric Dermatology*, 4th ed. New York: McGraw-Hill, 2008. Copyright © McGraw-Hill Education LLC.)

Dandache P, Nadelman RB: Erythema migrans. *Infect Dis Clin North Am.* 2008;22(2):235, vi [PMID: 18452799].

Halperin JJ, Shapiro ED, Logigian E, et al: Practice parameter: Treatment of nervous system Lyme disease (an evidence-based review): Report of the Quality Standards Subcommittee of the American Academy of Neurology. *Neurology.* 2007;69(1):91 [PMID: 17522387].

ARTHROPODS

SCABIES

ESSENTIALS OF DIAGNOSIS

▶ Arthropod *Sarcoptes scabiei var hominis* is an extremely common parasitic infection that causes highly pruritic skin eruptions.

▶ Transmission of the small mite is through direct skin-to- skin contact.

▶ Scabies presents with lesions consisting of burrows, which are tortuous, elevated, pink tracts 2-3 mm in length, along the superficial epiderm, with a small vesicle at the end.

The arthropod *Sarcoptes scabiei* var *hominis* is an extremely common parasitic infestation that causes highly pruritic skin eruptions and affects over 300 million individuals worldwide each year. Transmission of the small mite is through direct skin-to-skin contact with humans being the only host who can provide an environment to foster the living cycle for this parasite. Scabies can survive only 72 hours away from a human host. In classic scabies infestations, the host can be asymptomatic for up to 4 weeks and carry anywhere from 5 to 50 mites. Norwegian scabies, a much more severe form of infestation, primarily affects immunocompromised, elderly, and developmentally disabled persons. The mites are smaller in size and can number from the thousands to the millions on the host. This also makes the host more contagious to others. Classic scabies presents with highly pruritic skin lesions consisting of burrows, which are tortious elevated pink tracts 2-3 mm in length, along the superficial epidermis with a small vesicle at the end (Figure 47–53). They can appear with pustules, papules, nodules, and even plaques, often located in skin folds such as the digital web spaces, or flexor surfaces of the wrist, arms, legs, and groin. Lesions can be present on the abdomen and genital areas. In children younger than 2 years, lesions typically occur on the head, neck, palms, soles, and axilla. The burrow can also present as secondary cellulitis or have the appearance of impetigo due to the child's severe scratching of the infected area. Norwegian scabies, due to the high number of mites, presents with crusting, scabbing, and plaques over the flexor joint surfaces. Diagnosis can be made from skin scraping of burrows, followed by microscopic evaluation for the mite, ova, and feces. However, lack of microscopic findings does not rule out the diagnosis; therefore, a simple good clinical history and physical examination are required to make the diagnosis. Treatment consists of topical lindane or permethrin, as well as symptomatic relief of the pruritus with oral antihistamines or a short course or steroid therapy. Lindane is not recommended in young children secondary to concerns of neurotoxicity. Permethrin is the topical treatment of choice for children and infants older than 2 months. In severe cases or Norwegian scabies, ivermectin, although not FDA approved for scabies treatment, is often utilized successfully in children greater than 15 kg.

Currie BJ, McCarthy JS: Permethrin and ivermectin for scabies. *N Engl J Med.* 2010;362(8):717 [PMID: 20181973].

Gunning K, Pippitt K, Kiraly B, Sayler M: Pediculosis and scabies: Treatment update. *Am Fam Physician.* 2012;86(6):535-541 [PMID: 23062045].

Hicks MI, Elston DM: Scabies. *Dermatol Ther.* 2009;22(4):279 [PMID: 19580575].

Scheinfeld N: Controlling scabies in institutional settings: A review of medications, treatment models, and implementation. *Am J Clin Dermatol.* 2004;5(1):31 [PMID: 14979741].

SPIDER BITE

ESSENTIALS OF DIAGNOSIS

▶ Most spider bites present as a simple focal, single papule, erythematous and pruritic.

▶ The female Black Widow is shiny black and has a red hourglass on the underside of the abdomen and produces a neurotoxin.

▶ The black widow's alpha-latrotoxin affects the patient within 1 hour after the bite and causes severe abdominal muscle spasms, muscle cramps or spasms, nausea, vomiting, headache, and anxiety.

▶ The Brown Recluse is a 1-3 cm long, brown-toned spider with a characteristic "fiddle" shape on its back.

▶ The Brown Recluse bite is initially painless, but the venom has cytotoxic and hemolytic properties and causes tissue ischemia. Initially, it is a small vesicle that evolves into a darkening eschar over 2-3 days.

▶ The hobo spider found in the Pacific Northwest is brown with yellow markings on its abdomen, and the bite causes tissue necrosis secondary to ischemia and hemolysis.

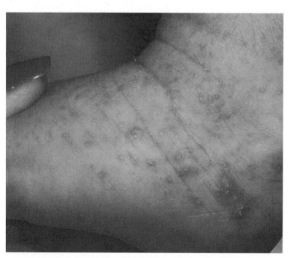

▲ **Figure 47–53.** Scabies. (Reproduced, with permission, from Weinberg S, Prose NS, Kristal L, eds: *Color Atlas of Pediatric Dermatology*, 4th ed. New York: McGraw-Hill, 2008. Copyright © McGraw-Hill Education LLC.)

Patients often present with primary complaint of spider bite as the etiology of their rash. Most "spider bites" are actually MRSA abscesses, and the patient's perception of the rash should not cloud the physician's judgment. There are hallmark differences that can identify the two distinct lesions. If the patient visually sees the spider on their skin in the location of the rash of lesion or if patient brings in a specimen of the arthropod for evaluation, then highly suspect a spider bite as the source. Most spider bites present as a simple focal, single papule, erythematous and pruritic. They can have an allergic urticarial wheel as a finding as well. However, there are three poisonous spiders in the United States one must consider if a spider bite is likely and specific symptoms are present.

Black Widow Spider

The Black Widow is endemic to the United States but is more prevalent in the Southern and Western regions of the country. It is 1-2 cm in length, and only the female, which is shiny black and has a red hourglass on the underside of the abdomen and produces a neurotoxin, is problematic. The bite site will be erythematous and swollen with possibly a halo or target appearance and pain to the local region. The alpha-latrotoxin begins to affect the patient within 1 hour after the bite and causes symptoms of muscle cramps or spasms, nausea, vomiting, headache, and anxiety. Severe abdominal muscle spasms can present similar to an acute abdomen. Treatment includes benzodiazepine and antihistamines. Antivenom is a choice for a patient with severe symptoms if it is available. Calcium gluconate is no longer recommended for treatment.

CDC: www.cdc.gov/niosh/topics/spiders/

The Brown Recluse

The Brown Recluse is a 1-3 cm long, brown-toned spider with a characteristic "fiddle" shape on its back. It is endemic to the entire United States but is more prevalent in the midwestern and southern regions. The bite is initially painless, but due to venom which has cytotoxic and hemolytic properties, pain at the site begins a few hours after the bite due to tissue ischemia. Initially, one can have a small vesicle that evolves into a darkening eschar over 2-3 days (Figure 47–54). As the tissue becomes necrotic, the ulcer can begin to form. Systemic response to the venom can include nausea, vomiting, chills, fever, hemolysis, seizures, and renal failure. Wound treatment includes minimal wound debridement and basic wound care. There are no studies to support a specific line of therapy, but dapsone and steroids have been utilized as well as hyperbaric oxygen for wound treatment.

Hobo Spider

The Hobo spider is a large spider found in the Pacific Northwest, with its body measuring 1-1.5 cm in addition to long thin protruding legs. It has brown with yellow markings on its abdomen and builds a funnel web to catch its prey. The bite has nearly the same effect as the Brown Recluse

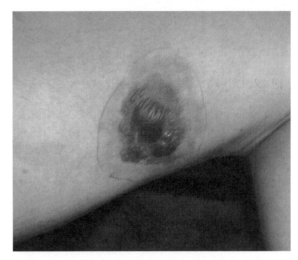

▲ **Figure 47–54.** Brown recluse bite. (Reproduced, with permission, from Weinberg S, Prose NS, Kristal L, eds: *Color Atlas of Pediatric Dermatology*, 4th ed. New York: McGraw-Hill, 2008. Copyright © McGraw-Hill Education LLC.)

bite as it causes tissue necrosis secondary to ischemia and hemolysis. Local and systemic symptoms are similar as is the treatment listed above.

PETECHIAL RASHES

THROMBOCYTOPENIA

 ESSENTIALS OF DIAGNOSIS

▶ Thrombocytopenia occurs when platelet production is decreased, or there is an increased breakdown of circulating platelets, or an increased breakdown or sequestration of platelets by the spleen or liver.

▶ Defined as a platelet count of less than 50,000/μL.

▶ Low platelets can result in a petechial rash that appears as small nonraised, dark purple/red scattered dots on the skin.

Platelets in the blood assist with coagulation to create hemostasis. Normal blood serum contains 150,000-450,000 platelets/μL of blood. Thrombocytopenia occurs when not enough platelets are being made by the bone marrow, or there is an increased breakdown of circulating platelets in the vascular system, or an increased breakdown or sequestration of platelets by the spleen or liver. It is often defined as a platelet count less than 50,000/μL. Regardless of the etiology, low platelets can result in a petechial rash that appears as small nonraised, dark purple/red scattered dots on the skin. Petechiae, aside from indicating a low platelet count, can be indicative of many diseases or pathophysiology problems in a pediatric patient. If petechiae coalesce and enlarge under the dermis, the large spot or patch is called purpura.

IDIOPATHIC THROMBOCYTOPENIA PURPURA

ESSENTIALS OF DIAGNOSIS

▶ ITP is an autoimmune response creating a bleeding disorder via antibody mediated platelet destruction.

▶ Found primarily in children aged 2-4 years.

Idiopathic thrombocytopenia purpura (ITP) is an autoimmune response that creates a bleeding disorder via antibody-mediated platelet destruction. It is often found primarily in children aged 2-4 years, with approximately 50 patients per 1,000,000 per year, following an acute viral illness. It can also be associated with medications that can induce thrombocytopenia. Common presenting symptoms include petechiae (Figure 47–55), purpura (Figures 47–56 and 47–57), oral bleeding, GI bleeding, or more severe findings like intracranial bleeding and retinal hemorrhages. Coagulation studies are usually normal with isolated thrombocytopenia on a complete blood count (CBC). Treatment includes hemostasis, platelet transfusion if life-threatening

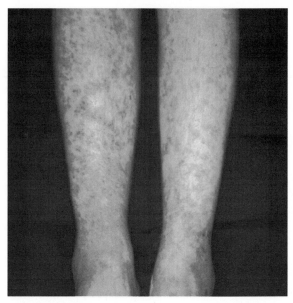

▲ **Figure 47–56.** Purpura. (Reproduced, with permission, from Weinberg S, Prose NS, Kristal L, eds: *Color Atlas of Pediatric Dermatology*, 4th ed. New York: McGraw-Hill, 2008. Copyright © McGraw-Hill Education LLC.)

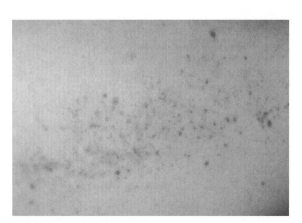

▲ **Figure 47–55.** Idiopathic thrombocytopenic purpura. (Reproduced, with permission, from Kane KS, Lio PA, Stratigos AJ, Johnson RA, eds: *Color Atlas & Synopsis of Pediatric Dermatology*, 4th ed. McGraw-Hill, Inc., 2009. Copyright © McGraw-Hill Education LLC.)

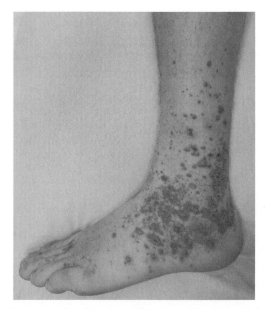

▲ **Figure 47–57.** Purpura with surrounding petechial. (Source: James Heilman, MD/CC-BY-SA-3.0. http://upload. wikimedia.org/wikipedia/commons/5/5e/Vasculitis.JPG.)

hemorrhage is present, parenteral IV immunoglobin (IVIg), steroid therapy, anti-Rho(D) immune globulin, and pediatric hematology consultation and admission. Approximately 90% of children will recover with about a 2% mortality rate.

Arnold DM, Kelton JG. Current options for the treatment of idiopathic thrombocytopenic purpura. *Semin Hematol.* Oct 2007; 44(4 Suppl 5):S12-S23. [PMID: 18096468].

THOMBOTIC THROMBOCYTOPENIC PURPURA/HEMOLYTIC UREMIC SYNDROME

ESSENTIALS OF DIAGNOSIS

▶ TTP entails the clotting of small blood vessels that lead to thrombocytopenia.

▶ It results in purpura, altered mental status and seizures, renal involvement, fever, and a hemolytic anemia.

▶ Childhood variant (hemolytic uremic syndrome [HUS]) has more renal disease involvement.

▶ HUS is associated with an infectious colitis trigger from pathogens *E. coli* O157:H7 and *Shigella*.

▶ A peripheral blood smear will show schistocytosis.

Thrombotic thrombocytopenic purpura (TTP) occurs much less commonly than ITP, and differs in its etiology, which entails the clotting of small blood vessels that lead to TTP. It results in purpura on the skin, neurologic sequela, such as altered mental status and seizures, renal involvement, fever, and a hemolytic anemia. Although TTP primarily occurs in adults, and has a predominance of neurological involvement, the childhood variant of TTP is known as hemolytic uremic syndrome (HUS) and has more renal disease involvement. HUS is often associated with an infectious colitis trigger from pathogens *Escherichia coli* O157:H7 and *Shigella*. When evaluating, the CBC may show an elevated WBC, but a low hemoglobin and platelet count. A peripheral blood smear will show schistocytosis. Renal involvement is confirmed with an elevated BUN and creatinine. Lactate dehydrogenase (LDH) is also often elevated in HUS. Treatment options overlap for TTP and HUS, but plasma exchange with FFP is utilized more frequently in TTP, whereas renal dialysis is often the chosen treatment for HUS.

Bouw MC, Dors N, van Ommen H, Ramakers-van Woerden NL: Thrombotic thrombocytopenic purpura in childhood. *Pediatr Blood Cancer.* 2009;53(4):537 [PMID: 19544391].
Marn Pernat A, Buturovic-Ponikvar J, Kovac J, et al: Membrane plasma exchange for the treatment of thrombotic thrombocytopenic purpura. *Ther Apher Dial.* 2009;13(4):318 [PMID: 19695067].

CHILDHOOD CANCER/LEUKEMIA/BONE MARROW SUPPRESSION

ESSENTIALS OF DIAGNOSIS

▶ Leukemia accounts for 25% of the overall total pediatric cancers.

▶ Acute lymphoblastic leukemia (ALL) accounts for 80% of leukemia cases.

▶ New-onset leukemia will often have significant lymphocytic leukocytosis and severe anemia, thrombocytopenia, and neutropenia.

Childhood cancer is seen in about 16 children and adolescents per 100,000 with leukemia accounting for 25% of the total, closely followed by tumors of the CNS, neuroblastoma, non-Hodgkin lymphoma, Wilms tumor, and Hodgkin lymphoma. Acute lymphoblastic leukemia (ALL) accounts for 80% of leukemia cases primarily in children younger than 5 years. Patient presenting with new-onset leukemia will often have significant lymphocytic leukocytosis and severe anemia, thrombocytopenia, and neutropenia. As the bone marrow becomes infiltrated with lymphocytes, the precursors to forming red blood cells and platelets are rendered incapacitated. With this severe thrombocytopenia, the presenting pediatric complaint with leukemia can be petechiae, easy bruising, fatigue due to anemia, fever, or even spontaneous bleeding. Chemotherapy is the primary treatment, which can lead to bone marrow suppression, resulting in pancytopenia, which in turn can lead to petechiae, purpura, and spontaneous bleeding.

US Cancer Statistics Working Group. United States Cancer Statistics: 1999–2005 Incidence and Mortality Web-based Report. Atlanta (GA): Department of Health and Human Services, Centers for Disease Control and Prevention, and National Cancer Institute; 2009 National Cancer Institute, 2008. Available at www.cancer.gov/cancertopics/factsheet/Sites-Types/childhood.

PHYSIOLOGIC/TRAUMATIC PETECHIA

ESSENTIALS OF DIAGNOSIS

▶ Children can present with periorbital petechia and palatal petechia from conditions such as vomiting, straining, breath-holding spells, and coughing.

▶ Children who have been abused from a choking mechanism around the neck will also have neck abrasions from direct trauma and petechia above the area being compressed.

Petechia can also be found in patients with normal platelet counts for a variety of reasons. Children can present with periorbital petechia and palatal petechia from symptoms such as vomiting, straining, breath-holding spells, and coughing. Any of these can lead to an unintentional Valsalva effect that increases intrathoracic pressure, which in turn leads to microvascular pressure increases that cause rupture of capillary beds resulting in a petechia. Children who have been abused from a choking mechanism around the neck will also have neck abrasions from direct trauma and petechia above the area being compressed. Trauma, including falls, direct blows, twisting injuries, and compression injuries, can result in petechia. Petechia can also be found in the sclera in any of the above scenarios from Valsalva effect or trauma.

PETECHIA ASSOCIATED WITH INFECTIOUS ETIOLOGY

ESSENTIALS OF DIAGNOSIS

▶ Group A streptococcal pharyngeal infections can cause petechial rash located along the posterior soft palate arches.

▶ Petechiae of the extremities/hands/feet are a common finding with infective endocarditis.

▶ Streptococcal Pharyngitis

Acute pharyngitis secondary to group A streptococcal infections (*S. pyogenes*) can cause fever, tender anterior cervical lymphadenopathy, posterior pharyngeal exudate, and petechia located along the posterior soft palate arches (Figure 47–58). Primary treatment for group A *Streptococcus* is penicillin.

▶ Infective Endocarditis

Infective endocarditis can be seen in the pediatric population, especially in rheumatic heart disease, congenital heart disease, patent ductus arteriosus, ventricular-septal defects, and mitral valve prolapse. IV drug use in adolescents can lead to infective endocarditis. Causative organisms include *Streptococcus viridans* and *bovis*, enterococci, and *Staphylococcus* species. Petechia of the extremities is a common finding with initial infective endocarditis, along with splinter hemorrhages of the nail beds which appear as dark red subungual linear lesions. Heart murmurs, septic emboli which lead to neurologic changes and pulmonary abscess, pallor, pericardial rub, chest pain, fever, and arrhythmias are also found in infective endocarditis. Cardiac echogram

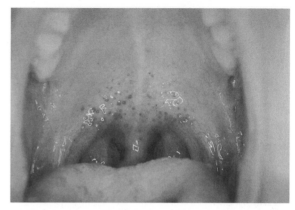

▲ **Figure 47–58.** Palatal petechial from streptococcal pharyngitis. (Source: Heinz Eichenwald, MD, CDC Public Health Image Library.)

will identify vegetation of cardiac valves or lesions, as well as serial blood cultures to identify the causative organism. Treatment with oxygen and management of possible congestive heart failure and renal failure may be required in the acute phase of treatment. Long-term IV antibiotics are required and cardiac surgical intervention may be needed for valve destruction by the bacterial organism.

Murdoch DR, Corey GR, Hoen B, et al: Clinical presentation, etiology, and outcome of infective endocarditis in the 21st century: The International Collaboration on Endocarditis-Prospective Cohort Study. *Arch Intern Med.* 2009;169(5):463 [PMID: 19273776].

DISSEMINATED INTRAVASCULAR COAGULOPATHY/PURPURA FULMINANS

ESSENTIALS OF DIAGNOSIS

▶ DIC is the activation of blood coagulation resulting in microvascular thrombi.

▶ Consumption of platelets with depletion of coagulation factors leads to petechia which can form on any part of the skin.

▶ Purpura fulminans can be seen with cutaneous hemorrhage and tissue necrosis.

Disseminated intravascular coagulopathy (DIC) is the activation of blood coagulation resulting in microvascular thrombi in multiple organs, resulting in a depletion of

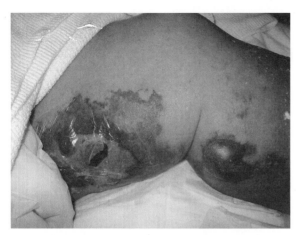

▲ **Figure 47–59.** Disseminated intravascular coagulation, purpura fulminans. (Reproduced, with permission, from Kane KS, Lio PA, Stratigos AJ, Johnson RA, eds: *Color Atlas & Synopsis of Pediatric Dermatology*, 4th ed. McGraw-Hill, Inc., 2009. Copyright © McGraw-Hill Education LLC.)

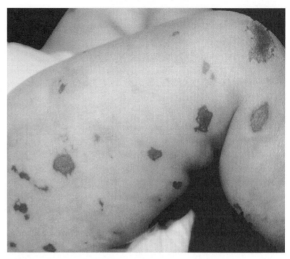

▲ **Figure 47–60.** Meningococcemia. (Reproduced, with permission, from Kane KS, Lio PA, Stratigos AJ, Johnson RA, eds: *Color Atlas & Synopsis of Pediatric Dermatology,* 4th ed. McGraw-Hill, Inc., 2009. Copyright © McGraw-Hill Education LLC.)

coagulation factors and platelets which can cause severe intractable bleeding. Causes include sepsis, trauma, malignancy, transfusion reactions, hepatic failure, and obstetric complications. With the consumption of platelets coupled and the depletion of coagulation factors, petechia can form on any area of the skin. As DIC progresses from sepsis, purpura fulminans can be seen with cutaneous hemorrhage and tissue necrosis (Figure 47–59). It can also occur from protein C or S deficiency. Treatment entails correction of the coagulopathy, performing hemostasis if needed, correction of hypervolemia and aggressive treatment of the underlying etiology of the DIC.

MENINGOCOCCEMIA

See section above on meningoccemia.

 ESSENTIALS OF DIAGNOSIS

▶ *Neisseria meningitidis*, a gram-negative diplococcus, is the bacterial organism that causes meningococcemia.

▶ As meningococcemia can present with a classic petechial rash, it can quickly evolve into purpura.

▶ Rapid treatment includes parenteral antibiotics with third-generation cephalosporin, management of shock with IV fluid replacement, and hypotensive management with inotropic pressors.

N. meningitidis, a gram-negative diplococcus, is the bacterial organism that causes meningococcemia. It presents initially with classic viral symptoms such as fever, vomiting, headache, myalgias and abdominal pain, but quickly progresses to bacteremia and/or meningitis. As meningococcemia rapidly progresses, it can lead to hypotension, shock, a classic petechial rash that, in a matter of hours, can evolve into purpura (Figure 47–60), followed by meningitis, DIC, and death if not aggressively treated. With mortality up to 10%, rapid treatment includes parenteral antibiotics with third-generation cephalosporin, management of shock with IV fluid replacement, and possible hypotensive management with inotropic pressors such as norepinephrine, dobutamine, or dopamine. Community isolation and treatment to persons exposed to *N. meningitidis* should be performed within 24 hours

Kaplan SL, Schutze GE, Leake JA, et al: Multicenter surveillance of invasive meningococcal infections in children. *Pediatrics.* 2006;118(4):e979 [PMID: 17015517].

Pollard AJ, Nadel S, Ninis N, Faust SN, Levin M: Emergency management of meningococcal disease: Eight years on. *Arch Dis Child.* 2007;92(4):283 [PMID: 17376933].

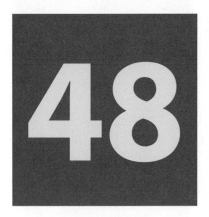

Psychiatric Emergencies

Brian Wagers, MD
Selena Hariharan, MD, MHSA

INTRODUCTION & DEMOGRAPHICS OF PEDIATRIC MENTAL ILLNESS

Children present in increasing numbers to the emergency department with psychiatric-related complaints. An estimated 21% of children aged 9-17 years have an identifiable mental health disorder. There are several drivers behind the increase in psychiatric cases presenting to the emergency department, including increased demand for pediatric psychiatric services unable to be met in the outpatient arena, decreased comfort by primary care physicians with psychiatric conditions, decreased practitioners of child and adolescent psychiatry, and various cultural phenomena. The increase in children presenting with psychiatric disorders is also leading to an increase in children admitted for mental health reasons.

Many children who present to the emergency department live in environments with risk factors for poor mental health. These include poverty, single parenthood, witnessed domestic abuse, parental mental illness, and substance abuse in the home. As primary care physicians are increasingly less comfortable with psychiatric complaints and the pool of child/adolescent psychiatrists has not been able to match demand, the emergency department is increasingly viewed as the patient's access point to the mental health system.

Because emergency department physicians are thrust into the role of evaluating children with psychiatric needs, it is imperative that they have the proper knowledge to screen children appropriately for organic causes of their symptoms and identify psychiatric illness when it presents. Indications that an organic disorder may be causing a patient's symptoms include a relatively new onset of symptoms, substance use/abuse, and abnormal vital signs or physical examination findings.

A key aspect of the history and physical examination of the pediatric psychiatric patient is the mental status examination (Table 48–1).

After determining the mental status of the patient, it is imperative to have a systematic approach to obtain a psychiatric history of present illness. Special care must be taken to inquire about events leading up to the situation for which the child is presenting, school performance, family status, stressors, relationships, and previous psychiatric diagnoses and care. A family history of mental illness is also important. The physician should screen each child for the presence of suicidal or homicidal ideation, and this can be accomplished using any of several rapid screens (Tables 48–2 and 48–3).

Initial workup of the child presenting with a psychiatric complaint includes a toxicology screen and, in females, a urine pregnancy screen, although procurement of either of these studies should not delay the patient's evaluation and treatment in the emergency department as there is little the emergency department physician will do with these results. In addition, if obtaining these tests will agitate the patient, they should be deferred. The results of these tests do provide valuable information for the physicians who will undertake long-term care of the child. Additional imaging or testing should be done based on concerning historical or physical examination findings. In pediatrics, there is no standard laboratory panel to evaluate for organic causes of symptoms, although some have suggested that in the truly undifferentiated patient, helpful adjuncts may include a complete blood count, glucose, renal panel, alcohol level, thyroid studies, electrocardiogram, intracranial imaging, or lumbar puncture. This information is drawn from adult literature, and no true standard for a medical screening laboratory evaluation exists in pediatrics.

Children and adolescents who present to the emergency department for psychiatric complaints rarely require restraint, but in the case of violent or agitated patients, restraints may be necessary. In a recent evaluation, 1 in 15 children with psychiatric illness required restraint in the emergency department. The emergency department physician should be comfortable with both physical and

Table 48–1. Essential elements of the mental status examination.

Element	Description
Orientation	Determine level of consciousness and orientation in all spheres: person, place, time, and situation
Appearance	Assess physical size, personal hygiene, clothing, neatness, grooming, posture, and gait
Memory	Evaluate both short- and long-term memory
Cognition	Assess gross level of intelligence, fund of knowledge, and ability to think or reason according to age
Behavior	Observe activity to determine age appropriateness for goal directedness and speed. Assess degree of distraction and ability to manage anger
Relating ability	Assess the ability to relate to the examiner based on eye contact, spontaneous conversation, trust, and desire to seek approval
Speech	Evaluate speech for spontaneity, coherence, articulation, content (vocabulary), and the quality of the thought process
Affect	Determine overall state of affect and observe for fluctuations
Thoughts	Determine content and process, looking for predominant themes as well as hallucinations, delusions, grandiosity, ideas of reference, and past or present suicidal or homicidal tendencies
Insight and judgment	Evaluate degree of understanding of the current problem and the ability of the child to think before acting
Strengths	Determine areas of interest, competence, and motivation as a prelude for developing positive interventions
Synthesis	Integrate the above information to form a comprehensive description of the child

Reproduced, with permission, from Baren, JM, Mace SE, Hendry PL, et al: Children's mental health emergencies—part 2: Emergency department evaluation and treatment of children with mental health disorders. *Pediatr Emerg Care.* 2008;24:485 [PMID: 18633314].

chemical restraints; however, the physician should always attempt to de-escalate the situation prior to using restraints. This can include a show of force with security personnel, isolation of the patient from acute stressors (often caretakers), dimming the lights, reducing external stimuli, and speaking to the patient in a continuous, soft manner. If de-escalation fails and the physician must employ restraints in the care of an agitated or violent patient, it is imperative that adequate documentation accompany this decision and

Table 48–2. Suicidal behavior in children younger than 12: A diagnostic challenge for emergency department personnel.

Assessment for risk of suicide

1. Do you ever think about hurting yourself?
2. Do you ever feel sad enough to want to go away and not come back?
3. Do you want to hurt/kill yourself now?
4. Have you ever hurt yourself/attempted suicide in the past?
5. Do you want to die?
6. Do you think you would die by doing *X*?
7. Has anyone you know ever killed themselves?
8. Have you been under stress lately?
9. Will you be safe?
10. In the past week, have you thought about hurting yourself?
11. Previous emergency department visits for unexplained accidents
12. Substance abuse
13. Cognitive ability of child
14. Family circumstances

Data from Tishler CL, Reiss NS, Rhodes AR: Suicidal behavior in children younger than twelve: A diagnostic challenge for emergency department personnel. *Acad Emerg Med.* 2007;14:813 [PMID: 17726127].

encompass the reasoning behind restraints, the mechanisms employed, regular reassessment of the need for as well as patient safety during restraint use, and personnel who used the restraints. It is recommended that trained security staff employ physical restraints and assist nurses in delivering chemical restraints. A minimum of 5:1 ratio of personnel to patient should be used to facilitate safe restraint of each limb and head during the application process (physical or chemical restraint). Table 48–4 provides detail regarding the use of restraints.

Table 48–3. Assessment of psychiatric patients' risk of violence toward others.

Assessment for risk of harm to others

1. Is there a past history of violence?
2. Assess the patient's perception of his/her situation—does he/she feel helpless or distressed?
3. Is there a loss of reality like feeling controlled by an outside force or paranoia?
4. Is the patient also suicidal?
5. Is there drug/alcohol abuse?
6. What is the patient's outpatient situation like?
7. Make sure you warn anyone against whom the patient makes a credible threat.

Data from Theinhaus OJ, Piasecki M. Assessment of psychiatric patients' risk of violence toward others. *Psychiatr Serv.* 1998;49:1129 [PMID: 9735952].

Table 48–4. Use of physical or mechanical restraints.

(A) Indications for the Use of Seclusion and Restraint
- When the patient is a danger to harm himself/herself or others (to prevent dangerous behavior)
- To prevent serious disruption of the treatment program including significant property damage
- When less restrictive measures have failed or are impractical

(B) Seclusion/Restraint Practices that are Contraindicated and/or Dangerous
- Use as punishment
- Use for convenience
- Use by untrained personnel
- Use when prohibited by state guidelines/law
- Use that results in medical compromise of the patient
- Physical or mechanical restraints that cause airway obstruction (eg, choke holds)*
- Covering the patient's face with a towel, bag or other object*
- "Prone wrap-up" (immobilizing a patient in a face-down position)*
- "Hobble position" (arms and legs restrained behind the patient)*
- Avoid restraints in unstable patients who need close monitoring
- Avoid positions that cause alteration of respiratory mechanics and airway obstruction
- Avoid prone restraints
- Avoid airway obstruction—do not bury patient's face/neck into pillow, mattress, etc.
- Do not restrict the patient's lungs by excessive pressure on the back

(C) Appropriate Methods of Physical or Mechanical Restraints
- Use professional non-threatening attitude (the show of force alone by enough trained calm personnel may cause the violent person to decompress)
- Have enough personnel ("restraint team") (≥5 people needed to restrain a violent individual)
- If a female patient is to be restrained, have at least 1 female on restraint team
- Have a restraint team leader and a restraint protocol
- The restraint team leader (often the physician) explains calmly in an organized way why the restraints are needed and what will be occurring (eg, psychiatric evaluation, medical examination), and instructs the patient to cooperate
- Never negotiate with the patient
- Each team member restrains 1 extremity by controlling the major joint (eg, knee or elbow) while the team leader controls the head
- Apply restraints securely to each extremity and tie restraints to the stretcher's solid frame not to the side rails
- Two mattresses can be used to immobilize (by "sandwiching") a violent patient
- Allow the patient's head to rotate freely
- Elevate head of bed, if possible, to decrease risk of aspiration
- Remember cocaine or stimulant intoxicated patients who are restrained are at an increased risk for adverse outcomes
- Document specific reasons (actual violent behavior, threats, etc., such as threatened nurse he would hit her, tried to hit physician) rather than general indication ("was violent")
- Have a colleague also document the need for restraints (≥2 health care personnel should document the need)

*May cause increased risk of positional asphyxia/respiratory compromise as well as other complications of physical restraints such as rhabdomyolysis.
Reproduced, with permission, from Baren, JM, Mace SE, Hendry PL, et al: Children's mental health emergencies—part 2: Emergency department evaluation and treatment of children with mental health disorders. *Pediatr Emerg Care*. 2008;24:485 [PMID: 18633314].

Physical and chemical restraints have important side effects that must be considered. In physical restraint, one must consider rhabdomyolysis, skin necrosis, asphyxia, and neurovascular impediment in the restrained limb(s). In chemical restraints the side effects are those effects known to be associated with the chosen agent, although one must consider interactions between drugs the patient was taking and the agent chosen as chemical restraint. Table 48–5 lists drugs commonly used as chemical restraints. The type of restraint used is at the discretion of the physician, but commonly, physical restraints are used first followed by chemical restraints, unless the patient's behavior precludes the safe placement of physical restraints.

In most instances, children and adolescents presenting to the pediatric emergency department for psychiatric complaints are dispositioned with the assent of both the caregivers and the patient. Occasionally, it is necessary to employ a medical hold on a patient to ensure treatment and safety of the patient or the safety of individuals known to the patient. Laws regarding the circumstances and requirements for placing children in an involuntary psychiatric admission or "hold" vary from state to state, and the physician should consult his or her state's revised code for specific requirements for locale of practice. This information is readily available to physicians at the point of care through internet portals, social services at the institution in which they practice, or local law enforcement offices.

Table 48–5. Medications commonly used for chemical restraint.

Drug	Usual Indication	Contraindication	Route of Administration	Dose for Agitation (maximum)	Complications	Notes
Ziprasidone	Bipolar disorder Tics Autism Pervasive developmental disorder-Not otherwise specified (PDD-NOS)	Allergy Prolonged QT History of arrhythmia Drugs that may interact	PO IM	5-11 yr: 10 mg ≥ 12 yr: 10-20 mg Adult max: 40 mg/d	Prolonged QTc Neuroleptic malignant syndrome Extrapyramidal symptoms Hyperglycemia Allergic reaction	FDA advised may be effective for children 10-17 yr but did not conclude it was safe
Haloperidol	Agitation Tourette disorder Psychosis	Allergy Narrow angle glaucoma Bone marrow suppression CNS depression Coma Severe liver or cardiac disease Parkinsonism	PO IM	3-12 yr: 0.01-0.03 mg/kg/d 6-12 yr: Can use IM 1-3 mg/dose Adult usual max: 30 mg/d	Prolonged QTc Extrapyramidal symptoms Bone marrow suppression Allergic reaction	
Midazolam	Sedation Anxiolysis Seizures	Allergy Narrow angle glaucoma	PO IM IV Intranasal Rectal	IM/IV: 0.1 mg/kg PO/PR: 0.25-0.5 mg/kg Intranasal: 0.2-0.3 mg/kg IM/IV max 10mg PO max 20 mg	Respiratory depression/arrest Allergic reaction	Flumazenil as reversal agent
Lorazepam	Sedation Anxiolysis Seizures	Allergy CNS depression Narrow angle glaucoma Pain Hypotension	PO IM IV	PO/IM/IV: 0.05-0.1 mg/kg Single dose max: 4 mg Total max: 8 mg	Respiratory depression/arrest Allergic reaction	SLOW IV push Flumazenil as reversal agent

Data from Lexi-Comp Online, Pediatric & Neonatal Lexi-Drugs Online, Hudson, Ohio: Lexi-Comp, Inc. 2012;7.

American Academy of Pediatrics, Committee on Pediatric Emergency Medicine; American College of Emergency Physicians and Pediatric Emergency Medicine Committee. Pediatric mental health emergencies in the emergency medical services system. *Pediatrics.* 2006;118:1764-1767 [PMID: 17015573].

Baren JM, Mace SE, Hendry PL, et al: Children's mental health emergencies—part 1: Challenges in care: definition of the problem, barriers to care, screening, advocacy, and resources. *Pediatr Emerg Care.* 2008;24:399-408 [PMID: 18562887].

Baren JM, Mace SE, Hendry PL, et al: Children's mental health emergencies—part 2: Emergency department evaluation and treatment of children with mental health disorders. *Pediatr Emerg Care.* 2008;24:485-498 [PMID: 18633314].

Dorfman DH, Mehta SD: Restraint use for psychiatric patients in the pediatric emergency department. *Pediatr Emerg Care.* 2006;22:7 [PMID: 16418605].

Grupp-Phelan J, Mahajan P, Foltin GL: Referral and resource use patterns for psychiatric-related visits to pediatric emergency departments. *Pediatr Emerg Care.* 2009;25:217 [PMID: 19382317].

Lexi-Comp Online: Pediatric & Neonatal Lexi-Drugs Online, Hudson, Ohio: Lexi-Comp, Inc. Accessed July 7, 2012.

DEPRESSION

Background

Depression in children is very common and can lead to significant reductions in functioning for the individual and the family. As with most psychiatric disorders, there is a wide range in the severity of symptoms that a child may manifest, but depression can be observed even in young children. There are equal rates of depression in males and females prior to puberty; but after puberty, there is a 2:1 ratio of female to male. Several conditions are commonly found to be comorbid with depression, including attention deficit hyperactivity disorder (ADHD), substance use, oppositional

Table 48–6. Commonly used psychiatric medications in pediatrics.

Drug Class	Drug Name	Common Uses in Children/Adolescents	Potential Risks	Notes
Selective serotonin reuptake inhibitor (SSRI)	Fluoxetine	Depression Obsessive compulsive disorder Elective mutism	Abnormal bleeding Weight loss Vomiting Mydriasis (increased risk of acute narrow angle glaucoma) Decreased growth SSRI syndrome	May worsen depression/suicidal ideation Other SSRI not FDA approved in children
Selective serotonin reuptake inhibitor	Sertraline	Depression Obsessive compulsive disorder	Abnormal bleeding Weight loss Vomiting Decreased growth SSRI syndrome	May worsen depression/suicidal ideation
Selective serotonin reuptake inhibitor	Escitalopram	Depression	Abnormal bleeding Vomiting (especially in younger children) Mental and motor impairment SSRI syndrome	May worsen depression/suicidal ideation
Tricyclic antidepressants	Amitriptyline	Depression Pain Migraine prophylaxis	Anticholinergic effects Sedation Cardiac conduction problems	Increase suicidal thinking
Atypical antipsychotics	Olanzapine	Bipolar disorder (acute mania or mixed episodes) Schizophrenia Anorexia nervosa Tourette syndrome Tic disorder	Neuroleptic malignant syndrome Extrapyramidal reactions Hyperglycemia Blood dyscrasias Sedation	May worsen depression/suicidal ideation
Atypical antipsychotics	Aripiprazole	Bipolar disorder (acute mania or mixed episodes) Schizophrenia Autism Tourette syndrome Tic disorder	Neuroleptic malignant syndrome Extrapyramidal reactions Hyperglycemia Blood dyscrasias Sedation	May worsen depression/suicidal ideation Not FDA approved for treatment of pediatric depression
Atypical antipsychotics	Quetiapine	Bipolar disorder (mania) Autism (off-label use) Schizophrenia	Neuroleptic malignant syndrome Extrapyramidal reactions Hyperglycemia Cardiac arrhythmias Anticholinergic effects Blood dyscrasias	May worsen depression/suicidal ideation
Atypical antipsychotics	Risperidone	Autism Bipolar disorder Schizophrenia Tourette syndrome	Neuroleptic malignant syndrome Extrapyramidal reactions Hyperglycemia Blood dyscrasias	
Atypical antipsychotics	Ziprasidone	Bipolar I disorder Tourette syndrome Tic disorder Autism PDD-NOS irritability Acute agitation	Prolonged QTc Neuroleptic malignant syndrome Extrapyramidal reactions Hyperglycemia Blood dyscrasias	See section on chemical restraints

(Continued)

Table 48–6. Commonly used psychiatric medications in pediatrics. (*Continued*)

Drug Class	Drug Name	Common Uses in Children/Adolescents	Potential Risks	Notes
Dopamine reuptake inhibitor	Bupropion	Depression ADHD	Seizures CNS stimulation Anorexia	May increase depression and suicidal thinking Not FDA approved for use in children.
Serotonin/norepinephrine reuptake inhibitor	Venlafaxine	ADHD Autism Depression	Seizures Mydriasis Anxiety Nervousness Insomnia Mania Anorexia Growth problems Bleeding problems	May increase depression and suicidal thinking Not FDA approved Based on single, small studies *Not Recommended*
Antianxiety agent	Buspirone	Anxiety	CNS effects (low risk)	Limited information Do *not* use with MAO inhibitors
Benzodiazepines	Diazepam	Anxiety Seizures Sedation	Respiratory depression Hypotension Sedation Paradoxical reactions	Flumazenil is a reversal agent
Stimulant	Dextroamphetamine/amphetamine	ADHD Narcolepsy	Cardiac complications Hypertension Growth problems Psychosis Mania Drug abuse Tics	Recent studies have not shown association with cardiac complications
Stimulant	Methylphenidate hydrochloride	ADHD	Cardiac complications Hypertension Growth problems Psychosis Mania Drug abuse	Recent studies have not shown association with cardiac complications
Selective norepinephrine reuptake inhibitor	Atomoxetine	ADHD	Mania (if bipolar) Cardiac complications Psychosis Hypertension Urinary retention Raynaud	Increased risk of suicidal thinking Recent studies have not shown association with cardiac complications
α_2-adrenergic agent	Guanfacine	ADHD Hypertension	Bradycardia Hypotension Syncope Rash	Causal relationship to rash unknown but discontinue drug
α-adrenergic agonist	Clonidine	Neonatal abstinence syndrome Hypertension ADHD Neuropathic pain Tic disorder Tourette syndrome	Cardiac complications Rebound sympathetic over activity Hypotension Bradycardia Sedation	

Data from Lexi-Comp Online, Pediatric & Neonatal Lexi-Drugs Online, Hudson, Ohio: Lexi-Comp, Inc.; 2012;7.

defiant disorder (ODD), or conduct disorder (CD). One should also seek out self-inflicted injuries in a patient who presents with a complaint of depression.

Clinical Findings

Symptoms of major depressive disorder in children include depressed or irritable mood, anhedonia, weight loss or failure to make expected weight gains, sleep disturbances, observable psychomotor agitation or retardation, fatigue, diminished ability to concentrate or focus, and recurrent thoughts of death. Some children even develop psychotic features, such as delusions or hallucinations or symptoms of anxiety including social withdrawal. Prevalence estimates have ranged from up to 2% of prepubertal children to 3-8% of adolescents experiencing depression's constellation of symptoms. Another review placed the prevalence rates of depression at 0.9% in preschool-aged children, 2.5% in school-aged children, and 4.7-6.1% in adolescents. It is important to search for stressors in the child's life as the presence of a significant stressor as well as the duration of the symptoms will determine the depressive disorder diagnosis that is assigned to the patient. The physician must inquire about suicidal and homicidal ideation and plan in any patient who presents with symptoms of depression.

Differential Diagnosis

As with many psychiatric disorders, the differential diagnosis of depression includes both psychiatric and nonpsychiatric disorders. Posttraumatic stress disorder (PTSD), bipolar disorder, adjustment disorder, anxiety disorder, substance use, psychosis, endocrinopathies (diabetes, thyroid disorders, parathyroid disorders), drug intoxication or withdrawal, hepatic abnormalities, and electrolyte abnormalities must be considered when faced with a patient presenting with symptoms of depression.

Treatment

Once the determination has been made that the patient is suffering from depression, one must decide on treatment. Ideally, the treatment is completed under the auspices of a trained child/adolescent psychiatrist, but given the shortage of these specialists, much of the treatment burden falls on the primary care physician. Currently, selective serotonin reuptake inhibitors (SSRIs) and cognitive behavioral therapy (CBT) are the primary modalities of treatment (see Table 48-6). There is a black box warning on several SSRIs indicating an increase in suicidal ideation and suicide attempts after starting treatment, but no increased risk of completed suicide. Cognitive behavioral therapy (CBT) is the second arm in what should be a two-pronged treatment regimen for depressive disorders. A large study of adolescents demonstrated that a combination of SSRIs (fluoxetine) and CBT was the most efficacious treatment regimen, followed by fluoxetine alone. CBT alone was the least efficacious of the treatments.

Disposition

The disposition of depressed children depends on the risk for their committing self-harm. If it is deemed that they are not at high risk for self-harm, meaning they contract for safety, have no history of self-injurious behavior, and have not taken a drug overdose, they can then be discharged home after consultation with a psychiatrist. It is important to realize that no evidence demonstrates the efficacy of a contract for safety, and this should only be used as part of a total risk assessment of the child's intent/ability to attempt and complete suicide. If a child makes a suicide attempt with little hope of rescue and does not inform anyone that he or she made an attempt, one must assign higher risk than the patient who threatens suicide after an argument with a parent but does not have means or a plan by which to carry this out. The pediatric emergency department physician must arrange follow-up for patients so that they can receive the treatment they require. If a child does not meet the criteria for a safe discharge, then he or she must be admitted to either a psychiatric facility or a medical bed pending psychiatric service availability.

Baren JM, Mace SE, Hendry PL, et al: Children's mental health emergencies—part 2: Emergency department evaluation and treatment of children with mental health disorders. *Pediatr Emerg Care*. 2008;24:485-498 [PMID: 18633314].

Nischal A, Tripathi A, Nischal A, et al: Suicide and antidepressants: What current evidence indicates. *Mens Sana Monogr*. 2012;10:33-44 [PMID: 22654381].

Prager LM: Depression and suicide in children and adolescents. *Pediatr Rev*. 2009;30:199-205 [PMID: 1948742].

BIPOLAR DISORDER

Background

Bipolar disorders are increasingly thought to be a real phenomenon in children, although this was in debate as recently as 5-10 years ago. Two-thirds of adults with bipolar disorder report that the onset of their illness began in childhood and approximately 16% of children who present with psychiatric complaints to tertiary hospitals demonstrate evidence of mania. In recent surveys of adults with bipolar disorders, 10-20% of respondents indicate the symptoms of their bipolar disorder began prior to 10 years of age. In recent studies, approximately 1.8% of children demonstrate findings consistent with a bipolar spectrum disorder. Pediatric bipolar disorder is well documented in families and as such a large genetic component is thought to play a role, although the specific gene(s) responsible have not been elucidated. A family member with the disease is the most significant risk factor for a child to develop pediatric bipolar disorder.

Clinical Findings

Bipolar disorder in children is diagnosed using the same criteria as that in adults. Essentially, a person needs to have one episode of mania to qualify for a diagnosis of bipolar disorder, but this must be a part of new symptoms that persist for at least 2 weeks. The symptoms that adolescents most commonly manifest during times of mania include distractibility, speech that is both pressured and grandiose, decreased desire and need for sleep, and increased energy. Children and adolescents demonstrate the presence of both manic and depressed symptoms simultaneously more often than do adults. Children with bipolar disorder spend longer periods of time in manic and/or depressive periods compared with adults. In order to have the diagnosis definitively made, one symptom during the 2-week period must include depressed mood.

Pediatric bipolar disorder is often comorbid with other psychiatric conditions and treatment for these conditions must be offered. Particularly, ADHD and ODD are often found in children with bipolar disorder. In a recent study, 62% of children with bipolar disorder demonstrated symptoms of ADHD and 53% demonstrated symptoms of ODD. The presence of ADHD or ODD significantly complicates the treatment of bipolar disorder in that the drugs used to treat ADHD or ODD can precipitate mania, and these children often manifest the mania as psychosis concomitant with depression. The severity of the presentation in these children often necessitates that the child be hospitalized for intensive treatment and further evaluation. Children with ADHD or anxiety disorders and bipolar disorder demonstrate reduced efficacy of mood stabilizers.

Recent estimates state that approximately 28-36% of children with bipolar disorder have medical comorbidities. Hypertension, diabetes mellitus, and obesity are the most common; however, epilepsy, migraine headaches, and asthma occur in higher rates in children with bipolar disorder than occur in children with other psychiatric disorders. A discussion of pediatric bipolar disorder would not be complete without drawing attention to the increased risk of suicide attempt and completion in children with this disorder. Approximately 75% of children with bipolar disorder endorse suicidality and between 20 and 50% will attempt suicide. Children with bipolar disorder are at approximately double the risk of suicide attempt as those children with major depressive disorder and have a much higher risk of suicide than healthy children. Importantly, pediatric bipolar disorder leads to increased numbers of suicide attempts, more lethal attempts, and a younger age at first attempt of suicide versus nonaffected children.

Differential Diagnosis

Differential diagnosis of bipolar disorder includes many of the commonly comorbid conditions one may find in a patient with bipolar disorder. These conditions include ADHD, anxiety disorder, substance intoxication or withdrawal, major depressive disorder, ODD, and obsessive compulsive disorder (OCD). Organic disorders such as endocrinopathies, metabolic derangements, infectious causes, and delirium must also be considered. In children, irritability can be a diagnostic symptom for bipolar disorder, and the subjective nature of this symptom can lead to a very broad differential diagnosis when considering potential causes of irritability in children.

Treatment

Treatment of bipolar disorder is primarily focused on treating acute mania and not depressive manifestations of the disease. Pharmacologic treatment is the first-line therapy for pediatric bipolar disorder. Studies have demonstrated that newer antipsychotic drugs, such as olanzapine, aripiprazole, quetiapine, risperidone, and ziprasidone have greater efficacy than older mood stabilizers such as lithium or divalproate (see Table 48-6). This treatment effect is not seen in adults and seems to be unique to children. Side effects, particularly sedation and weight gain, seem more prevalent in children compared with adults treated with newer antipsychotics; children, however, demonstrate less akathisia than adults treated with similar drugs. Acute stabilization of the individual is paramount, with benzodiazepines or antipsychotics such as ziprasidone commonly used drugs for this purpose in the emergency department setting. Because of the complex nature of pediatric bipolar disorder, long-term pharmacologic treatment is best left to a primary care physician or pediatric therapist, especially if comorbid condition such as ADHD or ODD exists. Psychotherapeutic modalities are best as an adjunct to pharmacologic treatment. Psychotherapeutic strategies focus on medication adherence and incorporating the family structure into support for the child in addition to reinforcement of stress reduction and coping mechanisms.

Disposition

Disposition of children with an acute manifestation of bipolar disorder usually includes admission as they carry significant risk to themselves and others. Admission can be either to a psychiatric service or to a medical service and consultation with a psychiatrist.

Goldstein BI: Recent progress in understanding pediatric bipolar disorder. *Arch Pediatr Adolesc Med.* 2012;166:362-371 [PMID: 22213607].

Nanagas MT: Bipolar disorders. *Pediatr Rev.* 201;32:502-503 [PMID: 22045900].

ANXIETY DISORDERS

Background

Anxiety disorders are widespread in the general population and may underlie or be comorbid conditions for many children that present to the emergency department. The lifetime prevalence of anxiety disorders is estimated to be 29% and responsible for approximately 42.3-46.6 billion dollars of health care costs annually. The average age of onset for children with anxiety disorders is 11 years. Children who suffer from anxiety disorders often display social problems and school failure. They also have an increased risk of adult psychiatric problems. These children are often treated by primary care physicians, but frequently present to the emergency department for evaluation and treatment, especially if they have never been formally diagnosed. In fact, these children often present to the pediatric emergency department a number of times for various somatic complaints, and only after the pattern is discerned and no organic reasons are found on workup can the physician posit a diagnosis of an anxiety disorder. The most common somatic complaints children present with include chest pain, fatigue, headache, insomnia, abdominal pain, nausea, and vomiting. The more nonspecific the symptomatology a child manifests, the more likely that anxiety is playing a part in the presentation.

Clinical Findings

There are several types of anxiety disorders, including generalized anxiety disorder (GAD), social anxiety disorder (SAD), PTSD, panic disorder, OCD, and separation anxiety disorder. GAD manifests as a fear of harm to the child's self or family and is all encompassing in the child's world. If untreated, GAD can progress to agoraphobia. SAD is the typical "shy" child, but the pathology of the disorder is that it affects the child's ability to function. A child who has SAD may refuse to go to school or play with other children. PTSD is unique among the anxiety disorders in that it requires an inciting event and differs from acute stress disorder in its longevity (> 1 month). These children manifest a heightened sense of arousal, re-experience the event repeatedly, and avoid situations that remind them of the traumatizing event to such a degree that normal functioning is impaired. There is physiologic evidence that children with higher sympathetic activity immediately following a traumatic event are at increased risk for PTSD. In OCD, children form an obsession that then becomes associated with a compulsion

that requires specific rituals to reduce the anxiety surrounding the obsession. Ultimately, these rituals and compulsions interfere with normal child functioning. SAD is very common in younger children who are often described as clingy, but eventually the disorder interferes with normal development because they are fearful to explore and experience new things.

Diagnosis of an anxiety disorder is usually fairly apparent after taking a detailed history. The prime obstacle to obtaining a proper history is the fast-paced environment of the emergency department! Various questionnaires exist to help the physician determine whether an anxiety disorder is at the heart of what is ailing the patient. These scales focus on questions of physical symptoms, harm avoidance, social anxiety, and separation anxiety. The physician must also seek out a family history of similar disorders or other psychiatric problems and look for potential triggers, especially in the case of PTSD.

Many psychiatric disorders can be comorbid with anxiety disorders, including ADHD, ODD, Tourette syndrome, substance abuse, eating disorders, and autism spectrum disorders.

Differential Diagnosis

As with most psychiatric disorders, the differential diagnosis for anxiety disorders includes many medical conditions. The physician must determine that thyroid and parathyroid function is normal. A careful history of medications taken must be elicited to ensure that a medication side effect is not responsible for the symptoms observed. Sleep disorders, seizure disorders, substance abuse, other endocrine disorders, and cardiac problems must be considered and ruled out by history, physical examination, and limited testing.

Treatment

Cognitive behavioral therapy (CBT) is the first-line, non-pharmacologic treatment with the primary goal of changing the thought patterns of the child. The treatment often attempts to desensitize the child to fear-inducing situations through visualization and actual exposure once coping mechanisms are mastered. Randomized controlled trials demonstrate the sustained benefit of CBT in treating anxiety disorders.

In the emergency department, the physician often must provide children with therapy to help them acutely calm themselves, and benzodiazepines are effective short-term pharmacologic medications for these conditions. These medications do nothing for the long-term treatment of the child, but do allow safe evaluation of the child who is undergoing an acute crisis. After management, the first-line pharmacologic therapy is an SSRI, although SSRI use for treatment of anxiety is not FDA approved. The use of

SSRI carries FDA approval for use in obsessive compulsive disorder only. One must instruct the family and patient to be vigilant about signs of suicidality and react promptly if any is suspected as these drugs can cause an increase in suicidal thoughts, especially if depression is a comorbid condition in the patient. Selective norepinephrine reuptake inhibitors (SNRIs), such as venlafaxine, have also treated anxiety disorders successfully, but they are not as efficacious as SSRIs and carry similar warnings of increased suicidality (see Table 48-6). Tricyclic antidepressants are a less expensive option, but carry a lethal risk in overdose and also have significant side effects of sedation and other anticholinergic effects. Several drugs have demonstrated success in anxiety disorders, including buspirone, bupropion, gabapentin, D-cycloserine, and propranolol, but drugs often are not approved for use in children. In fact, D-cycloserine is efficacious only as an adjunct to other psychopharmacologic treatments.

Disposition

Disposition of most children with anxiety disorders will be home with outpatient follow-up, unless they manifest symptoms that concern the physician for their personal or others' safety. All patients discharged home from the emergency department should have a follow-up plan in place so that formal psychiatric treatment may begin. A crisis plan should also be discussed with the patient and family, should the safety of the individual come into question. As with all psychiatric patients, a discussion of firearms in the home or other easily accessible and lethal means should be carried out with the family to improve the environment into which the patient is being discharged.

DeVane CL, Chiao E, Franklin M, Kruep EJ: Anxiety disorders in the 21st century: Status, challenges, opportunities, and comorbidity with depression. *Am J Manag Care.* 2005;11:S344-S353 [PMID: 16236016].

Herrick SE, Purcell R, Garner B, Parslow R: Combined pharmacotherapy and psychological therapies for post traumatic stress disorder (PTSD). *Cochrane Database Syst Rev.* 2010;7:CD007316 [PMID: 20614457].

Kirsch V, Wilhelm FH, Goldbeck L: Psychophysiological characteristics of PTSD in children and adolescents: A review of the literature. *J Trauma Stress.* 2011;24:307 [PMID: 21438015].

Kodish I, Rockhill C, Varley C: Pharmacotherapy for anxiety disorders in children and adolescents. *Dialogues Clin Neurosci.* 2011;13:439-452 [PMID: 22275849].

Ramsawh HJ, Chavira DA, Stein MB: The burden of anxiety disorders in pediatric medical settings: Prevalence, phenomenology, and a research agenda. *Arch Pediatr and Adolesc Med.* 2010;164:965-972 [PMID: 20921356].

Seligman LD, Ollendick TH: Cognitive-behavioral therapy for anxiety disorders in youth. *Child Adolesc Psychiatr Clin N Am.* 2011;20:217 [PMID: 21440852].

PSYCHOSIS

Background

Pediatric psychosis is a relatively rare phenomenon and affects more males than females. Most pediatric patients who have psychosis will have their first psychotic break in late adolescence, often between 16 and 30 years of age. Many subtle elements are present in the history of children affected by psychosis, including mild delay in achieving developmental milestones, diminished educational achievement, decreased social competence, and decreased cognitive function. A major risk factor for the development of psychosis is a first-degree relative with psychotic symptoms. Psychosis often goes undiagnosed for some time with most children having subtle symptoms for at least 5 years prior to their first psychotic break and with frank psychotic symptoms for approximately 1 year prior. It is important to screen all children with symptoms of psychosis for suicidality, as they are at increased risk for suicide attempt and completion.

Differential Diagnosis

Differential diagnosis is a broad term for pediatric psychosis and many conditions must be considered. Neurodegenerative disorders like Huntington disease and multiple sclerosis, infectious causes like HIV and syphilis, delirium of unknown etiology, nutrient deficiencies like B_{12} or folate deficiencies, inheritable disorders such as Wilson disease, primary and metastatic tumors, endocrinopathies such as diabetes mellitus and thyroid/parathyroid disorders, vasculitides, rheumatologic diseases like lupus, neurologic conditions including migraines, and other developmental and psychiatric conditions must be considered when presented with a pediatric psychosis patient.

Clinical Findings

Symptoms of psychosis are similar to those seen in pediatric schizophrenia and include positive symptoms (hallucinations, delusions, and thought disorders) and negative symptoms (anhedonia, flat affect). As in adults, the negative symptoms are more difficult to treat compared with the positive symptoms. In pediatric psychosis, auditory hallucinations are the most common symptom and often command the child to perform tasks or think in a certain manner. In the early stages, the symptoms are often viewed as behavioral problems, but then progress to frank psychosis.

Treatment

Treatment of pediatric psychosis carries a high risk of failure with one study demonstrating recurrence of symptoms in 80% of patients who stopped taking their medication. Studies demonstrate that approximately 10-20% of first psychotic episodes are refractory to treatment. As children have more relapses of symptoms, the prognosis for successful treatment decreases. Medication compliance is limited by the side effects of the drugs used to treat pediatric psychosis and is bolstered by maintaining a therapeutic alliance with the patient and family, although this is difficult to forge in a crisis period. Several studies have demonstrated successful initiation of treatment during a "prodromal" phase of the illness, in which the patient begins to feel positive or negative symptoms and immediately begins treatment. This strategy reduces the consequences of side effects because the patient is not on the medications continuously; however, the strategy requires intensive monitoring by the caregivers and a patient with excellent self-awareness, both of which can be difficult to achieve with psychosis patients. The mainstays of treatment are atypical antipsychotics such as olanzapine, quetiapine, risperidone, and aripiprazole (see Table 48-6). These drugs have fewer side effects than older generation antipsychotics such as haloperidol and chlorpromazine. One benefit of the atypical antipsychotics is that they treat the negative symptoms more effectively than older generation antipsychotics. One negative of the atypicals is that they are associated with significant weight gain which can exacerbate or even cause metabolic syndrome. It is important to tell the family that medications will not take effect right away; rather, they require a titration period of approximately 1-2 weeks with dosing adjustments made every 1-2 weeks until the desired effect is achieved. The older antipsychotics (haloperidol, chlorpromazine, droperidol) have a number of side effects, including extrapyramidal symptoms, tardive dyskinesia, gynecomastia, galactorrhea, cardiac conduction changes, and a risk of neuroleptic malignant syndrome.

Disposition

The necessity for titration of medications is important for the emergency physician to be aware of so that proper discharge instructions and counseling can take place, although, in practice, the emergency physician will not likely prescribe these medications and most children with psychotic symptoms will be admitted to the hospital for stabilization and treatment.

Berger G, Fraser R, Carbone S, McGorry P: Emerging psychosis in young people–Part 1. Key issues for detection and assessment. *Aust Fam Physician.* 2006;35:315-321 [PMID: 16680211].

Berger G, Fraser R, Carbone S, McGorry P: Emerging psychosis in young people–Part 2. Key issues for acute management. *Aust Fam Physician.* 2006;35:323-327 [PMID:16680212].

Berger G, Fraser R, Carbone S, McGorry P: Emerging psychosis in young people–Part 3. Key issues for prolonged recovery. *Aust Fam Physician.* 2006;35:329-333 [PMID: 16680213].

Messias E, Chen C: Epidemiology of schizophrenia: Review of findings and myths. *Psychiatr Clin North Am.* 2007;30(3): 323-338 [PMID: 17720026].

Robinson DG, Woerner MG, Delman HM, Kane JM: Pharmacological treatments for first-episode schizophrenia. *Schizophr Bull.* 2005;31:705-722 [PMID: 16006592].

Young CM, Findling RL: Pharmacologic treatment of adolescent and child schizophrenia. *Expert Rev Neurother.* 2004;4:53-60 [PMID: 15853615].

SCHIZOPHRENIA

Background

Schizophrenia is a disorder of cognition that affects the social ability of an individual. It is relatively rare prior to puberty, but is documented in children as young as 5 years of age. Most cases in children present after the age of 13 years and incidence increases with age. Approximately 10-20% of children diagnosed with schizophrenia have intelligence quotients at or near 2 standard deviations below the mean intelligence level.

Clinical Findings

Schizophrenia in children is diagnosed using the same criteria as in adults. Diagnostic criteria include two of the following symptoms for a significant part of at least 1 month: delusions, hallucinations, disorganized speech patterns, catatonic or disorganized behavior, and negative symptoms of flat affect, decreased thoughts or speech. The diagnosis of schizophrenia can also be made if the patient experiences only one of the following: bizarre delusions, auditory hallucinations that are a running commentary on behavior or thought, or two or more voices that converse with one another.

Most children who have schizophrenia are male and have significant comorbid medical or psychiatric conditions. Childhood-onset schizophrenia carries a poor prognosis as the younger the child at diagnosis, the more severe the presentation.

Differential Diagnosis

A number of disorders can be comorbid with or present similarly to schizophrenia. Psychiatric disorders such as bipolar disorder and PTSD must be considered and ruled out prior to the diagnosis of schizophrenia. Organic disorders that can cause schizophrenia-like symptoms include epilepsy, brain malignancies, traumatic brain injury, Huntington disease, Wilson disease, lysosomal storage disorders, substance use and abuse (both prescribed and recreational), heavy-metal intoxication, withdrawal from substances, encephalitis, and HIV. Focused history, physical examination, and testing can reduce the myriad of possibilities for schizophrenic-like symptoms in the emergency department. A urine toxicology screen and appropriate imaging or other studies indicated by the history and/or physical are appropriate. The urine toxicology screen is especially appropriate in that approximately 50% of individuals with schizophrenia have a history of alcohol or drug use.

Treatment

Treatment of schizophrenia is primarily by psychopharmacology with psychotherapy as an adjunct. Atypical antipsychotics are the medications of choice in children (see Table 48-6). As with most psychiatric disorders, treatment of schizophrenia should ideally be undertaken by a trained child and adolescent psychiatrist as there are significant side effects associated with atypical antipsychotics and treatment must be followed long term as medication changes are the norm. Most common side effects include extrapyramidal effects, weight gain, and development of metabolic syndrome.

Disposition

The disposition of most schizophrenic patients in the pediatric emergency department, particularly in times of active symptoms will be admission to the hospital, either to a psychiatric service or to a medical service, pending transfer to a psychiatric facility capable of inpatient treatment. In rare circumstances the schizophrenic patient can be discharged home, but this should be done only after the child has been evaluated by psychiatric providers and they agree on the appropriateness of discharge for the patient.

Messias E, Chen C: Epidemiology of schizophrenia: Review of findings and myths. Psychiatr *Clin North Am.* 2007;30(3): 323-338 [PMID: 17720026].

Robinson DG, Woerner MG, Delman HM, Kane JM: Pharmacological treatments for first-episode schizophrenia. *Schizophr Bull.* 2005;31(3):705-722 [PMID: 16006592].

Young CM, Findling RL: Pharmacologic treatment of adolescent and child schizophrenia. *Expert Rev Neurother.* 2004;4(1):53-60 [PMID: 15853615].

AGGRESSIVE BEHAVIOR (OPPOSITIONAL DEFIANT DISORDER, CONDUCT DISORDER)

Background

Recent estimates suggest the prevalence of aggressive behavior is between 3 and 7% of the pediatric population. The diagnostic criteria are included in successive revisions of the Diagnostic and Statistical Manual (DSM) of the American Psychiatric Association. The DSM IV-TR defines ODD as a disorder in a child who, younger than 8 years, demonstrates, "negativistic, defiant, disobedient, and hostile behaviors toward authority figures." The prevalence of ODD in general pediatric samples ranges from 2 to 15%, but 28 to 65% in samples of children with known psychiatric disorders. ODD

demonstrates a higher prevalence in males relative to females in childhood, but this difference disappears during adolescence. ODD is a significant risk factor for the development of comorbid conditions such as mood disorders and more severe behavioral disorders such as antisocial personality disorder and CD. In a recent study investigating ODD, 92.4% of the participants met criteria for another psychiatric disorder (mood 45.8%, anxiety 62.3%, impulse-control 68.2%, and substance use 47.2%). Not all children and adolescents diagnosed with ODD will progress to CD.

Low socioeconomic status, rigid parental discipline, and poor parental supervision are associated with both ODD and CD. Maltreatment of the child, particularly younger than 2 years, demonstrates a correlation with later aggressive behavior, as does intimate partner violence witnessed by the child. In patients with ODD or CD, the physician must consider substance use as a possible cause for the behavior, as well as evaluate for other psychiatric disorders that may be comorbid or the root cause for the aggressive behavior.

Clinical Findings

Aggressive behavior is best thought of as a spectrum that ranges from normal developmental stage to pathologic, such as ODD and CD. If the behavior in question lasts for a short time only, it can be considered as part of the child's normal development, whereas prolonged demonstration of symptoms indicates the likelihood of an underlying aggression disorder. On the mild side, temper tantrums, sibling rivalry, and striking or biting of other children can be normal developmental behaviors, whereas theft, vandalism, property destruction, and continued, willful opposition to authority figures can present familial and societal problems for the individual who manifests these behaviors. Most acts of aggression can place stress on the family, but children with mild symptoms rarely present to the pediatric emergency department for evaluation. The emergency department physician is much more likely to encounter a child with severe symptoms.

The DSM IV-TR defines CD as "[a] repetitive and persistent pattern of behavior in which the basic rights of others or major age appropriate societal norms or rules are violated." In children, the definitive behaviors fall into four general categories: aggression toward people/animals; deceit and theft; disregard for societal norms; and disregard for other's property. Diagnostic criteria differ for children younger and for those older than 10 years. A child younger than 10 years must demonstrate longstanding behaviors (> 6 months) of one of the categories described above. A child older than 10 years must demonstrate long-standing behavior of at least three of the four categories. Prevalence estimates vary widely (0.8-16%) for CD with 2-4% in school-aged children as the most commonly quoted rates. There are persistent gender differences in CD, with males approximately twice as likely as females to display symptoms. CD is linked with later development of antisocial personality disorder and does not exhibit the predilection for other comorbid psychiatric conditions that ODD demonstrates.

Differential Diagnosis

The differential diagnosis of aggressive behavior includes a number of psychiatric illnesses such as depression, bipolar disorder, anxiety disorder, substance use, adjustment disorder, and PTSD. Nonpsychiatric illnesses are included in the differential diagnosis. Endocrine abnormalities such as thyroid/parathyroid disorders and pheochromocytomas, delirium, seizure disorders, Wilson disease, pervasive developmental disorders, cognitive impairment, traumatic brain injury, and metabolic disorders must be considered as possible etiologies for aggressive behavior in children.

Treatment

Mainstays of treatment for both ODD and CD are cognitive behavioral therapy, specifically focused on problem-solving skills, and parent management training. A combination of these two modalities has shown increased efficacy compared with either modality alone. Only after these modalities have been fully explored with the patient should pharmacotherapy be considered. In order to treat ODD or CD effectively with medication, the physician must evaluate for underlying comorbid conditions that can exacerbate aggressive tendencies. It is important to note that pharmacologic treatment should be viewed as an adjunct to therapy and not as a comprehensive solution in itself. Pharmacotherapy should focus on comorbid conditions to minimize the exacerbating effects of aggression from organic or psychiatric conditions, thus allowing cognitive behavioral therapy to focus on the ODD and CD. From this perspective, it is recommended that standard therapies be employed for psychiatric conditions (SSRIs for depression, medication for ADHD, or atypical antipsychotics for aggression).

Disposition

Disposition of these children is dependent on the severity of their aggressive behavior and their antinormative behavior. Children will often present to the pediatric emergency department in police custody and should be discharged to proper authorities after medical screening has occurred. Ultimately, many children will be admitted to the hospital for further psychiatric treatment and evaluation.

American Psychiatric Association: *Diagnostic and Statistical Manual of Mental Disorders*, 4th ed. Text-Revision (DSM IV-TR). Washington, DC: American Psychiatric Association. 83, 1994.

Loeber R, Burke J, and Pardini DA: Perspectives on oppositional defiant disorder, conduct disorder and psychopathic features. *J Child Psychol Psychiatry.* 2009;50:133-142 [PMID: 19220596].

Nock MK, Kazdin AE, and Hiripi E, et al: Lifetime prevalence, correlates, and persistence of oppositional defiant disorder: Results from the National Comorbidity Survey Replication. *J Child Psychol Psychiatry.* 2007;48:703-713 [PMID: 17593151].

Sanders LM, Schaechter J: Conduct disorder. *Pediatr Rev.* 2007;28:433-434 [PMID: 17974708].

Turgay A: Psychopharmacological treatment of oppositional defiant disorder. *CNS Drugs.* 2009;23:1-17 [PMID: 19062772].

Zahrt DM, Melzer-Lange MD: Aggressive behavior in children and adolescents. *Pediatr Rev.* 2011;32:325-332 [PMID: 21807873].

ATTENTION DEFICIT HYPERACTIVITY DISORDER

Background

Attention deficit hyperactivity disorder (ADHD) is a disorder of children defined by inappropriate levels of hyperactivity, inattentive behavior, and impulsivity. Prevalence of ADHD in school-aged children is estimated at 5-8%, with a 2.5:1 male to female predominance. No predilection for ADHD has been determined based on social or demographic information such as ethnicity, race, or socioeconomic status; however, biologic factors such as prematurity and conditions that lead to a low birth weight, as well as environmental factors such as toxin exposure (lead, cigarette smoke, ethanol) can increase a child's risk of manifesting symptoms consistent with ADHD.

Clinical Findings

Clinical findings of ADHD are divided into three categories: those considered to be impulsive, those that demonstrate inattentiveness, and those that indicate hyperactivity. The definition of ADHD has changed throughout the years as the mental health community's views on the disease have evolved. The most recent iteration of the diagnostic criteria in the DSM IV-TR is "a persistent pattern of inattention and/or hyperactivity-impulsivity that is more frequent and severe than is typically observed in individuals of comparable levels of development." There are three types of ADHD: predominately hyperactive, predominantly inattentive, and combined type. In order for a child to be diagnosed with either the hyperactive or the inattentive type, they must meet six of nine of the diagnostic criteria delineated in the DSM IV-TR; to be diagnosed with the combined type, they must demonstrate six of nine symptoms from the hyperactive and the inattentive categories.

Although children with ADHD will present to the emergency department (however, they are more likely to have significant physical injuries), the disorder is best diagnosed and monitored in the setting of a patient–primary care physician relationship as longitudinal observation of the patient and medication effects are warranted. Because vulnerable populations may not have primary care physician, the pediatric emergency physician must recognize the symptoms of such a common disorder and be able to make referrals as necessary for proper management and care. In the emergency department one must attempt to elucidate findings that may suggest a disorder with more potential for immediate harm (psychosis, trauma/abuse, depression, bipolar disorder) and should features of more worrisome diagnoses be present, treat the child accordingly.

Differential Diagnosis

As discussed above, a number of mental health disorders in children can manifest with symptoms similar to ADHD. ODD, CD, PTSD, schizophrenia/psychosis, mood disorders (depression and bipolar disorders), pervasive developmental disorders, adjustment disorders due to stressors, learning disabilities, anxiety disorders, and intellectual deficiencies may have symptoms that closely resemble features of ADHD. One must also consider other disorders such epilepsy, sleep disorders, unreasonable parental/school expectations, and, in older children, drug use/abuse. In up to two-thirds of children with ADHD, one can expect to find a comorbid condition, making it essential to elicit any suggestive symptoms of a comorbidity to allow effective treatment of the patient.

Treatment

ADHD should be thought of as a chronic medical condition that will require long-term treatment. Many children will continue to have symptoms as adults, necessitating indefinite treatment. The mainstay of ADHD treatment is with medication. Medication alone is more effective in the treatment of ADHD than therapy or a combination of medication and therapy (unless a comorbid psychiatric condition is present, in which case a combination of medication and therapy is the more efficacious regimen). There are two types of medications prescribed for ADHD: stimulant and nonstimulant. Stimulant medications are considered the first-line treatment for ADHD. More than 150 studies have demonstrated the benefit of stimulant medications.

There are two main agents for treatment of ADHD: methylphenidate and amphetamine derivatives. If methyphenidate is not effective, the patient may be changed to a trial of an amphetamine medication. In the emergency department setting, one should be aware that stimulant drugs can have significant effects on appetite for children and as such should be considered as a potential cause for children who present with acute weight loss. This side effect should be discussed with caregivers prior to initiating treatment with stimulant drugs and weight should be followed

closely to ensure adequate growth. Sleep disturbances can also occur with stimulants and can be ameliorated by using the shortest-acting preparation that demonstrates efficacy. More worrisome side effects of mania or hallucinations occur rarely, but stimulants must be considered as a potential cause of symptoms in a child treated with stimulants for ADHD. All children should have a thorough history and physical examination for cardiac risk factors prior to beginning stimulant drugs and should have blood pressure screened regularly to monitor for significant elevations. If significant hypertension occurs, an underlying medical problem should be suspected.

Nonstimulant drugs should be considered as second-line therapy and only three are currently approved for treatment of ADHD: atomoxetine, guanfacine, and clonidine (see Table 48-6). Atomoxetine has a longer half-life than stimulants and can take up to 6 weeks to demonstrate effect. There is a black box warning on atomoxetine secondary to a potential increase in suicidality. Other side effects of atomoxetine include gastrointestinal (GI) upset and somnolence. Guanfacine can cause low blood pressure, headache, and somnolence. Clonidine can cause side effects similar to guanfacine except that it can also cause insomnia. Although a full discussion of side effects of various drugs is beyond the scope of this chapter, these are the main symptoms that patients have complaint about when presenting to the emergency department.

Nonmedical interventions are important in the school setting. Children with ADHD qualify for individualized learning plans to accommodate the various symptoms a child might manifest as part of the disorder. Children and adolescents with ADHD are likely to have academic underachievement or failure, making it imperative to intervene in a timely fashion to allow the child to reach full potential. Impulsive and hyperactive behavior can place significant stress on the family; successful treatment can greatly improve family dynamics. In later years, self-medication for feelings of restlessness can cause harm and further impair functioning of the individual. Appropriately treated individuals demonstrate lower risks of substance abuse than do nontreated peers.

Disposition

Children who present to the pediatric emergency department with symptoms of ADHD usually are safe to discharge home, unless comorbid psychiatric or medical conditions do not allow this to be accomplished in a safe manner. Appropriate referral to a psychiatrist should be initiated.

American Academy of Pediatrics Subcommittee on Attention-Deficit/Hyperactivity Disorder Committee on Quality Improvement. Clinical Practice Guideline: Treatment of the school-aged child with attention deficit/hyperactivity disorder. *Pediatrics.* 2001;108:1033-1044 [PMID: 11581465].

American Psychiatric Association: *Diagnostic and Statistical Manual of Mental Disorders*, 4th ed. Text-Revision (DSM IV-TR). Washington DC: American Psychiatric Association. 83, 1994.

Perrin JM, Friedman RA, Knilans TK; Black Box Working Group, Section on Cardiology and Cardiac Surgery: Cardiovascular monitoring and stimulant drugs for attention-deficit/hyperactivity disorder. *Pediatrics.* 2008;122:451-453 [PMID: 18676566].

Polanczyk G, Jensen P: Epidemiologic considerations in attention deficit hyperactivity disorder: A review and update. *Child Adolesc Psychiatr Clin N Am.* 2008;17:245-260 [PMID: 18295145].

Stein MT, Perrin JM: Diagnosis and treatment of ADHD in school-age children in primary care settings: A synopsis of the AAP practice guidelines. *Pediatr Rev.* 2003;24:92-98 [PMID: 12612186].

Wilms Floet AM, Schneider C, Grossman L: Attention deficit/hyperactivity disorder. *Pediatr Rev.* 2010;31:56-69 [PMID: 20124275].

Special Needs & High-Tech Children

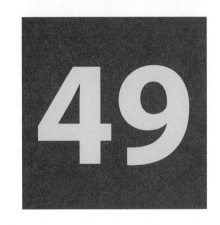

Julie Phillips, MD
Cristina M. Estrada, MD

Recent medical advances have led to longer survival of chronically ill children, often referred to as the "high-tech" child. As a result, emergency departments are seeing these medically-fragile patients more frequently. Patients with a cerebrospinal fluid (CSF) shunt, a tracheostomy tube, the need for chronic oxygen therapy, invasive or noninvasive ventilatory support, chronic dialysis, a gastrostomy tube (GT), or an indwelling central venous catheter (CVC), among others, are defined as technology dependent. Review of available previous medical records and contacting the medical home or primary care physician early in the patient's course can provide information that may help guide the decision-making process.

CEREBROSPINAL FLUID SHUNTS

GENERAL CONSIDERATIONS

Cerebrospinal fluid (CSF) is made and absorbed by the body at a constant rate. Mainly made at the choroid plexus, it flows from the lateral ventricles into the third and fourth ventricles where it passes to the subarachnoid space. It is reabsorbed through one-way valve into the venous system. When excess fluid is present either from overproduction, blockage of circulation, or diminished absorption, hydrocephalus occurs. These patients become symptomatic when this increase in CSF increases intracranial pressure (ICP). The most common neurosurgical procedure in children is the placement of a CSF shunt. The role of a CSF shunt is to divert CSF from the brain to another portion of the body. The proximal portion of the catheter may be in the cerebral ventricle, an intracranial cyst, or the lumbar subarachnoid space. Most commonly the CSF is shunted into the peritoneal cavity via a ventriculoperitoneal (VP) shunt. Occasionally the distal end drains into the vascular system via a ventriculoatrial (VA) shunt. Most CSF shunts are made of three components: proximal shunt tubing, a reservoir system, and distal shunt tubing.

SHUNT OBSTRUCTION

Clinical Findings

Obstruction of the catheter lumen or disconnection of the component parts of a CSF shunt leads to malfunction. Shunt obstructions are most common within 6 months of shunt placement. Headache, visual disturbances, vomiting, and lethargy are the most common signs and symptoms of a mechanical shunt obstruction. In infants who have an open fontanel, there may be an increase in head circumference or a bulging fontanel. Parents may report that the child is "not acting right" or is less active than usual. Seizures may be seen in those patients with predisposing brain lesions; however, they are uncommonly the sole manifestation of a CSF shunt malfunction.

On physical examination, signs of shunt malfunction include papilledema, an enlarging head, bulging fontanel, and engorged head veins. Abnormalities on neurologic examination include increased deep tendon reflexes, increased lower extremity tone, and a positive Babinski sign. Cranial nerve palsies of either the sixth cranial nerve leading to lateral gaze deviation or the fourth cranial nerve leading to limitation of upward gaze, also known as "sunsetting" gaze.

As obstruction continues, the patient's ICP continues to rise. Cushing triad of hypertension, bradycardia, and an abnormal respiratory pattern may develop.

Treatment

When a CSF shunt malfunction is suspected, a noncontrasted CT of the head is needed for evaluation of ventricle size for comparison with previous scans if possible. Many pediatric centers have instituted the use of a rapid sequence brain magnetic resonance imaging (MRI) for evaluation of shunted hydrocephalus. It avoids the deleterious effects of radiation while allowing adequate evaluation of the ventricles. This method has been used successfully in infants and young children without the use of sedation. Some programmable VP shunts may be affected by MRI so clinicians should be aware of this possibility and consult a neurosurgeon if there are any questions. A shunt series, which includes plain radiographs of the skull, chest, and abdomen, can assess the integrity of the shunt components and ensure there are no kinks, breaks, or discontinuities in the tubing. A shunt aspiration may be performed to assess for infection, as well as to evaluate ICP. It should also be performed if the patient is in extremis, deteriorating neurologically, or has signs of herniation on the computed tomography (CT) scan.

It is recommended that a neurosurgeon be consulted and given the first option to perform the procedure (Figure 49–1). The neurosurgeon may have already manipulated the hardware multiple times and will ultimately be responsible for any shunt revisions and follow-up. A lumbar puncture should never be performed in lieu of tapping the shunt. Obstruction of the shunt system can result in obstructive hydrocephalus. Lumbar puncture in a patient with obstructive hydrocephalus can cause a significant pressure differential and precipitate brain herniation.

Plain radiographs may be helpful if the reservoir is difficult to identify upon palpation. To prepare the patient, surrounding hair should be shaved or trimmed. The scalp is cleaned first with alcohol and then with three applications of povidone-iodine solution. The skin should be given time to dry between each application. A 23- or 25-gauge needle is inserted obliquely into the shunt reservoir. The butterfly tubing should be held vertically perpendicular to the floor. Measuring the height in centimeters of the CSF within the tubing represents the patient's ICP. A pressure of greater than 20 cm is consistent with a distal shunt malfunction. A proximal shunt malfunction is suspected when there is slow

or absent flow from the proximal reservoir. However, slit ventricles can also lead to slow flow. Although aspirating a shunt can alleviate the symptoms of increased ICP, it is advised to remove only enough CSF to decrease ICP to 20 cm. A larger volume of CSF removal can lead to disruption of subdural vessels related to abrupt fluid shifts. Medical management of increased ICP is a temporizing treatment until operative repair can be performed. Interventions include acetazolamide 30-80 mg/kg/day in nonemergency situations. In those patients with unstable vital signs and signs of increased ICP, 3% normal saline (NS) 3-5 mL/kg or mannitol 0.25-2 g/kg can be given intravenously (IV). Hyperventilation in an intubated patient can be used. The target PCO_2 is 30-35 mm Hg. If there are signs of hypovolemia, consider a bolus of 20 mL/kg of NS.

If immediate surgical repair is not available and the patient is unresponsive to medical management, consider burr hole puncture. This is a high-risk procedure that should be performed only if a patient has life-threatening symptoms of a proximal shunt malfunction. Palpation of the posterior aspect of the skull can identify the position of the burr hole that was created during placement of the shunt. After cleansing the scalp with povidone-iodine, insert a 3½-in spinal needle perpendicular to the skull. The needle should be advanced through the burr hole to a maximum depth of 5 cm. Removing the stylet from the needle allows fluid to drain spontaneously. Continue to drain CSF until the flow slows down. This procedure will tear the proximal shunt catheter. Therefore, it is used as a temporizing measure until operative treatment can be performed.

Disposition

Definitive management of CSF shunt obstruction is operative revision. Patients should be transferred to a facility with a neurosurgeon.

SHUNT INFECTIONS

Clinical Findings

CSF shunt infections are most often seen in the perioperative period. Most are seen within 2 months of placement. The highest incidence of shunt infection is seen in children younger than 4 years. Infections within the first few weeks of shunt placement are commonly caused by *Staphylococcus* species and other gram-positive organisms. After the shunt is in place for 6 months, gram-negative organisms are more commonly seen.

Classic meningeal signs are often not seen because the shunt prevents communication between the infected ventricle and the meninges. Shunt infection may present without symptoms. Signs and symptoms of shunt infection include fever, a change in sensorium, irritability, vomiting, or abdominal pain. However, as infection progresses, a shunt

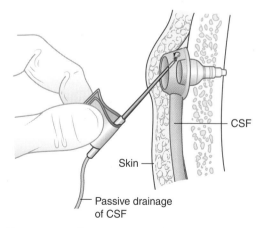

▲ **Figure 49–1.** Shunt aspiration. (Reproduced, with permission, from Reichman EF, Simon RR: *Emergency Medicine Procedures.* New York: McGraw-Hill, 2004. © McGraw-Hill LLC.)

obstruction or malfunction may occur, leading to a patient with clinical signs of increased ICP.

Skin and soft tissue infections overlying the hardware can also develop. Without prompt treatment, these may be treated before the shunt becomes infected. Signs of a wound infection include erythema, tenderness, or swelling overlying any portion of the shunt reservoir or tubing. A linear, erythematous tract along the skin paralleling the shunt tubing from head to chest is highly suspicious for a CSF shunt infection. Furthermore, any breakdown of the skin exposing the internal hardware of a shunt is considered a shunt infection.

A primary peritoneal infection or the passage of infected CSF through the shunt can lead to distal shunt infection. Pseudocysts, which are infected, loculated cysts, may develop around the terminal portion of the catheter. These patients will exhibit signs of peritonitis which includes fever, abdominal pain, and anorexia. In distal shunt infections, CSF obtained from the reservoir may not show signs of infection.

Shunt infections in the setting of a VA shunt can lead to bacteremia when infected CSF is shunted to the bloodstream, endocarditis, and septic emboli.

Treatment

Diagnosis of CSF shunt infections requires direct aspiration of CSF. A CSF shunt aspiration should be performed as described in the previous section. If there is evidence of overlying skin infection, this should be avoided to prevent introduction of bacteria into the shunt system. When possible, this procedure should be performed by a neurosurgeon. Sampled fluid should be sent for culture, Gram stain, cell count with differential, and glucose and protein concentrations. Cell count abnormalities may be subtle because infections of CSF shunts often result in less inflammation than bacterial meningitis. Patients without infection can have up to 500 white blood cell count (WBC) per mm³. The CSF WBC differential may be helpful in making the diagnosis. Patients with greater than 10% neutrophils are likely to have a shunt infection.

In patients who present with abdominal pain, with or without fever, consider abdominal radiographs and ultrasound to evaluate for a pseudocyst.

Medical therapy alone typically has low success rates for the treatment of shunt infections. Broad-spectrum antibiotics should be selected while awaiting results of the CSF Gram stain and culture. Vancomycin and a third-generation cephalosporin (cefotaxime/ceftriaxone) provide coverage for coagulase negative staphylococci and endogenous gram-negative flora.

Disposition

The ultimate management of a CSF shunt infection is operative. Neurosurgery should be consulted for removal of infected hardware, placement of a temporary external drain, and parenteral antibiotics. Once the CSF is sterile, a new CSF shunt can be placed.

OVERDRAINAGE

Clinical Findings

Overdrainage of CSF can result in low ICP. This most commonly occurs in infants younger than 6 months in whom the shunt was placed. Infants with overdrainage may present with a sunken fontanel, microcephaly, or overriding parietal bones. Intermittent complaints of headaches, nausea, vomiting, and lethargy may be seen in older children. CSF drainage is improved by being in an upright position. Therefore, the symptoms of intracranial hypotension may be worse when the patient is in the standing position or after being awake for several hours. Lying for several hours slows drainage and may relieve symptoms.

Treatment

A noncontrasted CT or MRI scan is typically obtained. Small ventricles are often seen. Only a small number of patients will have slit ventricle syndrome in which the proximal catheter port is blocked by a collapsed ventricle. This blocks further drainage of CSF. Oral analgesics and placing the patient in a supine position can treat mild cases of overdrainage. Recurrent episodes of slit ventricle syndrome can be corrected surgically. Options for management include upgrading the resistance of the drainage valve or inserting an antisiphon device, which are performed at the discretion of a neurosurgeon.

Disposition

If pain, discomfort and nausea can be controlled, the patient can be discharged with outpatient neurosurgical follow-up. Operative management of overdrainage is performed electively.

Horton C, Byrd L, Lucht L, et al: Emergency care of children with high-technology neurological disorders. *Clin Pediatr Emerg Med.* 2012;13(2):114-124.

Wait S, Lingo R, Boop F, Einhaus S: Eight-second MRI scan for evaluation of shunted hydrocephalus. *Child Nerv Syst.* 2012;28:1237-1241.

TRACHEOSTOMY TUBES

GENERAL CONSIDERATIONS

A diverse number of diseases result in chronic respiratory insufficiency (CRI) that requires a tracheostomy and mechanical ventilation. Frequently inadequate airway protection, such as frequent aspiration events, absent gag reflex, or poor oromotor control, is the primary indication for tracheostomy in pediatric patients. Children with airway obstruction, as the result of anatomical abnormality, subglottic stenosis, or tumor, chronic lung disease, central hypoventilation, neuromuscular disease, or a combination of these may also be managed with a tracheostomy tube. Most tracheostomy tubes are made of polyvinylchloride or silicone which conforms to the shape of the trachea without collapsing. There are many types of tracheostomy tubes, and it is important to know which are available to the physician, as well as how to convert from one brand to another (Table 49–1). Each tube is variable in terms of the inner diameter, outer diameter, and length. The inner diameter of the tube is typically standardized and imprinted on the flange of the tube regardless of the manufacturer. However, most often external diameter and length of tube are more variable.

The tube also may be cuffed or uncuffed. Cuffs create a seal around the trachea, which limits air leak in patients with mechanical ventilation and reduces aspiration. Cuffs also stabilize the tracheostomy tube within the airway. If a cuffed tracheostomy tube is to be manipulated, the cuff should be deflated. Some tracheostomy tubes have dual cannula. The advantage of a dual cannula is the inner cannula can be removed for cleaning, while the outer cannula maintains the airway. However, the inner cannula has a smaller internal diameter, making it susceptible to obstruction. In this type of tracheostomy tube, only the proximal portion of the inner cannula can be connected to a manual resuscitation bag. Therefore it must be in place prior to attempt at bag-mask ventilation. For vocalization in a patient with a tracheostomy, air must move upward through the vocal cords. Fenestration of some tracheostomy tubes allows exhaled air to enter into the larynx to facilitate speech. The end of the tracheostomy tube can be attached to a swivel. The role of a swivel is to allow a child to move without placing traction on the tracheostomy tube if attached to a ventilator. In normal respiration, the nose is responsible for warming and humidifying air. Since tracheostomy tubes bypass the nose, a humidification system is added. A heat-moisture exchanger that traps the patient's exhaled moisture and heat for inhalation with the next breath may be added to the end of a tracheostomy tube. It is important if the patient is going to have prolonged bag-valve ventilation performed to have the heat-moisture exchanger in place to prevent drying of the mucosa.

TRACHEOSTOMY OBSTRUCTION/ DECANNULATION

Clinical Findings

Decannulation or obstruction of the tracheostomy tube is the most life-threatening emergency in a patient with an artificial airway. Pediatric patients are particularly at risk

Table 49–1. Tracheostomy tube conversion.

Bivona			
Size	Internal Diameter	External Diameter	Length mm
2.5 Neo	2.5	4.0	30
3.0 Neo	3.0	4.7	32
3.5 Neo	3.5	5.3	34
4.0 Neo	4.0	6.0	36
2.5 Ped	2.5	3.0	38
3.0 Ped	3.0	4.7	39
3.5 Ped	3.5	5.3	40
4.0 Ped	4.0	6.0	41
4.5 Ped	4.5	6.7	42
5.0 Ped	5.0	7.3	44
5.5 Ped	5.5	8.0	46
Shiley			
Size	Internal Diameter	External Diameter	Length mm
3.0 Neo	3.0	4.5	30
3.5 Neo	3.5	5.2	32
4.0 Neo	4.0	5.9	34
4.5 Neo	4.5	6.5	36
3.0 Ped	3.0	4.5	39
3.5 Ped	3.5	5.2	40
4.0 Ped	4.0	5.9	41
4.5 Ped	4.5	6.5	42
5.0 Ped	5.0	7.1	44
5.5 Ped	5.5	7.7	46
Jackson			
Size	Internal Diameter	External Diameter	Length mm
00	2.4	4.5	33
0	2.8	5.0	36/38
1	3.0	5.5	40/44
2	3.4	6.0	44/51
3	4.3	7.0	48/58
4	5.3	8.0	52/62
5	6.2	9.0	56/6.8

for obstruction or decannulation because of the size of their tracheostomy tubes. The length of the tracheostomy tube in an infant may be as short as 3-4 cm. The overall risk for obstruction of a tracheostomy tube in the pediatric patient is greater than in adults. The internal diameter of the tracheostomy tube, as well as the patient's trachea is smaller than an adult. Additionally, younger children have weaker and less effective cough, making clearance of an obstructed tube more difficult. The patient may present with signs of respiratory distress. Accessory muscle use, nasal flaring, tachypnea, and cyanosis are all possible. If there has been a prolonged period of respiratory distress, the patient may tire, and therefore present obtunded or lethargic.

Evaluate the position of the tracheostomy tube. The tube should be fully inserted to the level of the hub and secured in place with tracheal ties. Although the tube may be in the stoma, it may not terminate in the trachea. If a tracheostomy tube exchange was attempted prior to presentation, a false tract into the soft tissues of the neck may have been created. The neck should be palpated. Crepitus in the neck can indicate the presence of subcutaneous air introduced from a dislodged tracheostomy tube. Auscultation should evaluate for symmetric air entry.

Treatment

When a patient with a tracheostomy tube presents in respiratory distress, the patient should be immediately placed on high-flow humidified oxygen. The tracheostomy tube should be suctioned. This procedure will serve two functions: it can clear airway secretions, as well as assess patency of the tube. Caregivers can often provide information about the usual size of suction catheter utilized and the depth it should be passed. If caregivers are not present, select a suction catheter that is less than one-half the internal diameter of the tracheostomy tube. The suction catheter should be inserted to the end of the tracheostomy tube. Insertion beyond the tracheostomy tube can result in mucosal damage or trigger vagal stimulation. Suction should be applied as the catheter is withdrawn in a rotating motion.

If the patient is ventilator dependent, he or she should be taken off of the ventilator and a self-inflating bag-valve should be used. If there is continued respiratory distress, attach a self-inflating bag to the tracheostomy tube. Giving several positive pressure breaths can dislodge a mucus plug. If there is significant resistance felt with ventilated breaths, additional breaths should not be delivered. This finding is concerning for a tube that has become dislodged. The tracheostomy tube should be replaced in this case. Additionally, if suctioning a tracheostomy does not relieve an obstruction, the tracheostomy tube should be changed. In the case of a recent tracheostomy (< 7 days from tube insertion), the new tracheostomy tube should be the same size or smaller than the original. Fresh tracheostomies are more likely to

create a false tract with replacement than those with mature tracts. If cuffed, the replacement tracheostomy tube should be assessed prior to placement. The stylet should be inserted into the tracheostomy tube. Two individuals should perform this procedure. The first person should deflate the cuff, if present, on the old tracheostomy tube. The hub should be grasped on both sides, and the tube should be removed in a smooth motion. The second person is prepared with the new tube. The tip of the new tube should be lubricated with a sterile, water-soluble lubricant. It should be held in the same manner and inserted with gentle pressure in the posterior and inferior direction. Introduce the tube to the level of the hub and secure with tracheostomy ties. If the appropriate size tracheostomy tube is not available, an endotracheal tube that is one-half size smaller than the tracheostomy tube should be placed. If there is significant resistance to the placement of either the tracheostomy or endotracheal tube, do not force the tube forward, as this can create a false tract, which leads to subcutaneous emphysema and can cause additional airway compromise. In these patients, attempt bag-mask ventilation with a self-inflating bag. Additionally, a suction catheter can be used as a guidewire for the tracheostomy tube. Feed a large suction catheter through the tracheostomy tube. Insert the catheter into the stoma and guide the tracheostomy tube into place. If unable to ventilate the patient, oral intubation should be attempted. All providers should wear a facial shield and eye protection as this can force secretions out of the open stoma.

If the patient also has a GT in place, it should be vented. This allows for decompression of the abdomen which may have been contributing to the patient's increased work of breathing.

Disposition

Patients with increased respiratory support or an increased oxygen requirement need admission to the hospital. In the case of dislodgement within 7 days of placement, the service responsible for tube placement should be contacted. All patients with "fresh" tracheostomies should be observed in either the emergency department or hospital after successful recannulation. An otolaryngologist should be contacted for any difficulty in tracheostomy issues.

TRACHEOSTOMY INFECTION

Clinical Findings

Infections associated with tracheostomy tubes include localized peristomal cellulitis, tracheitis, and pneumonia. Tracheostomy tubes, ventilator tubing, and humidifier circuits often become colonized with bacteria. Organisms that commonly colonize tracheostomy tubes include gram-positive cocci, gram-negative bacilli, and anaerobes. Mucosal injuries related to airway cannulation allow these same organisms to lead to infection.

The risk of peristomal cellulitis is in patients with poor hygiene or inadequate padding surrounding the tracheostomy tube. The tracheostomy site should be evaluated for signs of infection. Erythema alone is typically the result of irritation. Evaluate the area beneath the tracheostomy ties for signs of inflammation. If there is associated warmth, tenderness, fever, or purulent drainage, this should be considered peristomal cellulitis. The presence of erythematous changes and satellite lesions is concerning for a fungal infection.

It is difficult to distinguish between tracheal colonization and tracheal infection (tracheitis). Patients often present with changes in the quality, volume, or color of their tracheal secretions. Additionally, caregivers may report the need for changes in the amount of oxygen supplied or in the mechanical ventilator settings. If patients are hypercarbic or hypoxemic, they may present with somnolence or be combative. The diagnosis should be considered when the patient presents with signs of respiratory distress or systemic illness including assessment of oxygenation by pulse oximetry is important.

Treatment

If the patient is not on humidified oxygen, it should be applied. Humidified oxygen reduces the risk of occluding the tube by keeping mucus thin and preventing secretions from drying. Tracheal secretions should be suctioned to clear the airway. Secretions can be sent for Gram stain, culture, and rapid viral detection assay. Predominance of one organism on Gram stain and leukocytosis are suggestive of bacterial tracheitis. If available, review the results of previous tracheal aspirates for culture results and sensitivities. A chest x-ray (CXR) should be obtained. The presence of a new infiltrate is suggestive of bacterial pneumonia.

In patients with irritated skin around the stoma, increasing the frequency of tracheostomy care at home may be effective. The area should be cleaned regularly with a dilute hydrogen peroxide solution. If erythema is present beneath tracheal ties, additional padding should be placed and effort should be made to keep the tracheal ties dry. The presence of fungal infection should be treated with topical antifungals. Mild cases of peristomal cellulitis can be treated with oral antibiotics. Oral antibiotics, such as sulfamethoxazole/trimethoprim or clindamycin, should be used. In children, trimethoprim/sulfamethoxazole (TMP-SMX) dosing is 8 mg/kg of the trimethoprim component/day orally divided twice daily. Clindamycin dosing is 8-16 mg/kg/day orally divided every 6-8 hours.

Disposition

Well-appearing patients with adequate follow-up can be treated as an outpatient. If there is an increased oxygen requirement or there is increased ventilator support, the patient should be hospitalized. IV antibiotics, chosen based on previous culture data and local susceptibility, and aggressive pulmonary toilet should be started.

TRACHEOSTOMY BLEEDING

Clinical Findings

Although not a common complication, a tracheostomy tube may cause bleeding. The timing of a bleed compared to tracheostomy placement can indicate the source. Within 6 weeks of placement, a tracheal-innominate artery fistula must be ruled out. Although formation of a fistula is rare, it is associated with high mortality. One-half of patients will have a small sentinel bleed prior to catastrophic hemorrhage. Sentinel bleeding may present as hemoptysis, bleeding from the stoma, or the presence of blood in tracheal secretions. Patients presenting with bleeds more than 6 weeks from initial tracheostomy placement are more likely to have tracheobronchitis, granulation tissue, or friable mucosa. Granulation tissue develops as a result of chronic inflammation. When air is not adequately humidified, the mucosa becomes dry and friable. Irritation from the tube can lead to bleeding, especially at the stoma, level of the cuff, and adjacent to the tip. Additionally, suctioning with elevated pressures (> 150 mm Hg) and frequent suctioning can lead to bleeding.

Treatment

Increased humidification of the inspired air is usually effective in management of small volume tracheal bleeding. Suctioning should be minimized in small volume bleeds to reduce irritation, and the suction pressure should be maintained between 100 and 150 mm Hg. The persistence of small volume bleeding is often the result of granuloma. Direct visualization by an otolaryngologist can identify and treat granulomas. Small volume bleeds within 6 weeks of tracheostomy should be evaluated by an otolaryngologist as this may represent sentinel bleed.

Large volume tracheostomy bleeding is a surgical emergency. Prior to airway manipulation or bronchoscopy, obtain IV access and begin volume replacement. A type and screen should be obtained and blood products should be available. The tracheostomy tube should be left in place to ensure a definitive airway is present. Perform frequent suctioning of the tube to clear blood and reduce the risk of aspiration. If the site of bleeding is identified, direct pressure can be applied. Hyperinflation of the cuff of the tracheostomy tube may tamponade the bleeding vessel. Consultation with an otolaryngologist should be obtained early so that the bleeding vessel can be identified and ligated.

Disposition

Small bleeds can be managed as an outpatient with referral to an otolaryngolist for evaluation of the presence of granulomas. Large volume bleeds need emergent surgical intervention.

Bassham BS, Kane I, MacKeil-White K, et al: Difficult airways, difficult physiology and difficult technology: Respiratory treatment of the special needs child. *Clin Pediatr Emerg Med.* 2012;13(2):81-90.

Bradley PJ: Bleeding around a tracheostomy wound: What to consider and what to do? *J Laryngol Otol.* 2009;123(9):952-956 [PMID: 19374781].

Engels PT, Bagshaw SM, et al: Tracheostomy: From insertion to decannulation. *Can J Surg.* 2009;52(5):427-433 [PMID: 19865580].

Graf J, Stein F: Tracheitis in pediatric patients. *Semin Pediatr Infect Dis.* 2006;17(1):11-13 [PMID: 16522500].

Graf J, Montagnino B, et al: Pediatric tracheostomies: A recent experience for one academic center. *Pediatr Crit Care Med.* 2008;9(1):96-100 [PMID: 18477921].

Joseph R: Tracheostomy in infants: Parent education for home care. *Neonatal Netw.* 2011;30(4):231-242 [PMID: 20636760].

Mitchell R, Hussey H, et al: Clinical consensus statement: Tracheostomy care. *Otolaryngol Head Neck Surg.* 2013;148(1):6-20 [PMID: 22990518].

Peterson-Carmichael S, Cheifetz I: The chronically critically ill patient: Pediatric considerations. *Respir Care.* 2012;57(6):993-1003 [PMID: 22663972].

INDWELLING CENTRAL VENOUS CATHETER (CVC)

GENERAL CONSIDERATIONS

CVCs are placed in patients who need semipermanent vascular access. Indications for placement include chemotherapy, renal replacement therapy, total parenteral nutrition (TPN), poor peripheral access, or prolonged antibiotic therapy. The types of CVCs include tunneled and nontunnelled, single- or multilumen, and peripherally inserted central catheter (PICC). The goal of CVC placement is placement of the tip in the largest vein possible. Ideally, the tip should lie within the superior vena cava or inferior vena cava, but outside the pericardial sac. Nontunneled catheters are typically 12-15 cm in length. They are typically inserted into the subclavian, internal jugular, or femoral vein. This type of catheter is suited for short-term access, such as for IV antibiotic administration. PICCs are up to 40 cm in length. They are inserted into the cephalic, brachial, or basilica vein with the tip lying in the superior vena cava. In tunneled catheters, a large-bore catheter is tunneled several centimeters under the skin and terminates in a central vein. It is anchored in the skin by a Dacron cuff, which stimulates fibrosis in the surrounding tissues and prevents migration of bacteria into the vessel. Tunneling a catheter decreases the risk of infection because the entry into the skin is several centimeters from the venous entry site. A female Luer lock tip is located at the proximal end of the CVC.

An additional type of CVC is the totally implantable venous access device which is entirely under the skin. The proximal end of the catheter is attached to a subcutaneous, silicone reservoir chamber which is anchored to the muscle wall with sutures. A noncoring needle (Huber needle) is used to puncture the reservoir.

CATHETER OCCLUSION

Clinical Findings

The catheter may become partially or totally occluded making it difficult to flush and infuse the line or draw blood. This is most commonly the result of thrombus formation. The clot may be the result of fibrin deposition within the CVC, surrounding the tip, or as a sheath outside the catheter. Additional causes for occlusion include kinking of the catheter, the tip abutting the vessel wall or valve, and crystallization of medication, like diazepam or phenytoin, within the tubing. TPN may occlude a catheter with waxy precipitates or particulate precipitates of calcium and phosphorus due to their poor solubility. Silicone catheters are at risk for obstruction, as lipid emulsions are more likely to adhere to the catheter wall.

Treatment

The catheter should be closely inspected to determine if a mechanical obstruction is suspected. Possible obstructions include kinking of the tubing, a suture that is too tight, a malpositioned Huber needle, or a clamp that is inadvertently closed. A dye study may be used to evaluate for an internal kink in the catheter. In the case of mechanical obstruction from the tip abutting the vessel wall or valve or internal kink, surgery should be consulted for possible catheter exchange. After evaluation for mechanical obstruction, nonthrombotic internal occlusions like precipitates must be considered. These are mainly secondary to precipitations of medications or parenteral nutrition constituents. The appropriate treatment depends on the properties of the suspected offending agent. Drugs with a low pH are at risk of precipitation in a basic solution. Some institutions suggest infusion of hydrochloric acid (0.1 mol/L). However, several facilities have banned this practice because of concerns about damage to the integrity of the catheter. It is important to review your institutional policy regarding the volume and duration of infusion. Conversely, drugs with a high pH may be cleared with use of sodium bicarbonate (1.0 mol/L) or sodium hydroxide (0.1 mol/L). Again, refer to your institutional policy regarding administration. Treatment of occlusion from a thrombotic etiology is with the use of tissue plasminogen activator (tPA). This catalyzes the conversion of clot-bound plasminogen to plasmin, which then activates the fibrinolysis cascade. There are a number of tPA products available for this use with varying dosing and administration guidelines. Again, refer to your institutional policy regarding drug choice and administration.

Phlebotomy can be facilitated by increasing the venous pressure gradient along the catheter. Techniques for increasing the pressure gradient include having the patient cough or perform Valsalva maneuvers, placing the patient in reverse Trendelenburg position, or holding his or her arms above the head. If these fail, the catheter should be gently irrigated with 3 mL of NS. This may dislodge the clot, which should then be aspirated into the syringe. Avoid pushing the clot into the venous system by flushing 2-3 mL of fluid into and out of the catheter. Too much force can dislodge the clot into the blood stream or rupture the catheter.

Disposition

Once patency of the catheter lumen is restored, the patient can be discharged home. If patency cannot be restored and the patient requires venous access, consider placement of a peripheral IV and admission for further interventions on a nonemergent basis.

CATHETER BREAKAGE

Clinical Findings

Patients with a broken catheter typically present with leakage of fluid or blood from the externalized portion of the catheter. For indwelling catheters, leakage leads to the accumulation of fluid or blood in the subcutaneous tissues. These patients present with swelling over the catheter port. Breakage most often occurs during routine care, although trauma during playtime can also lead to a damaged catheter.

Treatment

Clamp the externalized catheter immediately proximal to the break. Clean the area with a povidone-iodine solution and cover with a sterile dressing until repair. If the externalized catheter is too short to clamp, apply direct pressure over the site of venous entry. To establish the site of venous entry, palpate along the catheter from the exit site until it can no longer be felt and apply pressure at that site.

Each catheter size has an available repair kit, which contains a new external catheter segment with a hollow male connection, a syringe, needle, and glue. Using sterile technique, slice the proximal end of the catheter and glue into place within the male connector of the new segment. Ideally, the catheter should be repaired by a person familiar with the procedure.

In patients with implantable catheters, a CXR should be obtained to evaluate for the broken segment. Surgical management is necessary for repair.

Disposition

Once the catheter is repaired, it should be evaluated for patency by drawing blood and flushing the system. If the catheter is functional, the patient can be discharged from the emergency department. An indwelling catheter needs surgical repair.

CATHETER DISPLACEMENT & MIGRATION

Clinical Findings

The venous portion of the catheter can be dislodged from the vessel, often as the result of inadvertent tugging on the externalized catheter. The greatest risk for dislodgement occurs within a few weeks of placement before fibrosis occurs around the catheter cuff. Implanted catheters can dislodge at both ends. However, it takes a large amount of tension to create enough force to dislodge the distal tip from the vein. When the distal tip migrates, it often is located in the surrounding soft tissue. However, the catheter tip may be in the arterial systems, mediastinum, pleura, or pericardium. When the tip displaces through the wall of the vein, bleeding into the soft tissue is usually minimal. This is because the low-pressure venous system is tamponaded by the surrounding structures. However, if the tip has entered another low-pressure body cavity, massive bleeding can occur. A tip displaced into the pleural can result in massive hemothorax or pleural effusion. Catheters migrating through the right side of the SVC, the azygous, hemiazygos, or internal thoracic vein can access the pleural space. A CVC that erodes through the right atrium or distal portion of the superior vena cava can lead to cardiac tamponade, either from bleeding or infusion. Erosion of a CVC through the femoral vein can access the peritoneal space. Complications include migration of the catheter tip, cardiac arrhythmias, pneumothoraces, and superior vena cava syndrome.

Treatment

In externalized CVCs, the presence of the cuff outside the surface of the skin is concerning for a dislodged catheter. For an implanted catheter, difficulty obtaining free flowing blood when drawing back is concerning for a dislodged catheter. The catheter should not be used until its location has been confirmed. Clamp the catheter and secure it close to the skin. A chest x-ray can be used to visualize the location of the catheter tip. If there is doubt about the position of the CVC, a small amount of water-soluble contract can be injected under fluoroscopy to identify the position of the tip.

After thoracic trauma, dislodgement of the implantable catheter should be suspected if the device is not functioning. A collection of blood or fluid leads to a bulge or painful swelling overlying the reservoir. Surgical management is required for repair. It is generally safest to leave the CVC in place while awaiting surgical management, as it may traverse a great vessel.

When the CVC is displaced into another low-pressure system, such as the pleural space, peritoneal space, or pericardial sac, the catheter should be left in position. This helps to plug the hole into these spaces. Additional venous access should be obtained for volume resuscitation. Infusion into the pericardium can lead to cardiac tamponade. If tamponade is confirmed, leave the CVC in place and attempt to aspirate fluid through it. If this is unsuccessful, a pericardiocentesis should be performed. Emergent consultation with a surgeon or interventional radiology is needed.

Disposition

A dislodged catheter requires immediate surgical or interventional consultation with a radiologist.

CENTRAL LINE INFECTION

Clinical Findings

Catheter colonization, catheter-related bloodstream infections, and exit site infections are the most common types of CVC infection. Colonization usually results from contamination of the hub or the migration of bacteria along the interface between the skin and the catheter. Long-standing catheters increase the risk for both bacteremia and fungemia. There is higher risk for catheter infection in an externalized CVC than an indwelling catheter. Femoral CVCs become infected more often than subclavian and internal jugular CVCs. In early infection, localized changes may be the only signs. Symptoms of an exit site infection include pain, swelling, induration, and erythema present within 2 cm of site where the catheter exits the skin. If there is concern for infection at a catheter site, the entire dressing needs to be removed so that the exit site and catheter tract may be examined. Bacteremia can occur without signs of skin infection. Fever is more likely when there is bacteremia or sepsis. Chills, hypotension, and delayed capillary refill may be seen in a patient with bacteremia or sepsis.

Treatment

Most common pathogens in these infections are gram-positive organisms, especially methicillin-resistant *Staphylococcus aureus* (MRSA) and *Enterococcus*. Fungal, gram-negative, and polymicrobial organisms are more commonly seen in immunocompromised patients. Patients receiving TPN are at increased risk for gram-negative infections.

Exit site infections often appear similar to cellulitis. If there is purulent drainage at the catheter site, it should also be cultured and sent for Gram stain. When there are signs of sepsis, the catheter should be removed, and the tip of the catheter sent for culture. If an additional CVC is needed, it should be placed at a distal site. Oral antibiotics, such as TMP-SMX or clindamycin, should be used. In children, TMP-SMX dosing is 8 mg/kg of the trimethoprim component/day orally divided twice daily. Clindamycin dosing is 8-16 mg/kg/day orally divided every 6-8 hours. In well-appearing patients, it is difficult to determine if a positive culture represents catheter colonization or true catheter-related bloodstream infection. Therefore, a blood culture from the catheter and culture from a peripheral site should be obtained. One to 2 mL of blood should be drawn for each culture. In a catheter with multiple ports, the distal port should be used to obtain the culture. Fungal cultures should be obtained in immunocompromised patients with a history of invasive fungal disease. Ideally, cultures should be obtained prior to the initiation of antibiotics. A CBC with differential can be useful, but normal results can be seen in invasive bacterial infection. In patients who are ill-appearing, consider additional testing such as coagulation studies.

While in the emergency department, the initial treatment is IV antibiotics, as well as supportive measures. Broad-spectrum antibiotics should be started (Table 49–2). Although oxacillin and gentamicin are often first-line choices, some institutions use vancomycin and gentamicin based on local resistance patterns. Ill-appearing neutropenic patients should have coverage for *Pseudomonas* with ceftazidime or cefepime. Patients on broad-spectrum antibiotics and or TPN, with solid organ or stem cell transplant, or hematologic malignancy are at greater risk for *Candida* infection.

Short-term CVC, such as a PICC line, should be removed in the case of a bloodstream infection. Long-term CVC or port may be retained as long as the patient remains stable. The catheter may be changed over a wire if there is no sign of associated exit tunnel infection or sepsis. In the setting of sepsis, the catheter should be removed and replaced at a different site. If the catheter is removed, the tip should be cultured. If a venous access port is removed, the subcutaneous reservoir should be sent for culture. A positive culture from the reservoir is more sensitive than a culture from the tip. Additional indications for catheter removal include infection of the subcutaneous tunnel, persistent infection, critical illness, endocarditis, and thrombophlebitis.

TABLE 49–2. Antibiotic dosing for central line infections.

Antibiotic	Dosing and Frequency	Maximum Dosing
Oxacillin	150-200 mg/kg/d IV divided Q6-8 hr	2 g per dose
Gentamicin	2.5 mg/kg IV Q8 hr	
Vancomycin	10 mg/kg IV Q6 hr	2 g per day
Ceftazidime	30-50 mg/kg IV Q8 hr	6 g per day
Cefepime	50 mg/kg IV Q8 hr	2 g per dose

Disposition

Patients with presumed CVC infections require admission to the hospital for further antibiotic therapy. Patients with signs of sepsis may need admission into the pediatric intensive care unit for close monitoring.

Baskin JL, Pui CH, Reiss U, et al: Management of occlusion and thrombosis associated with long-term indwelling central venous catheters. *Lancet.* 2009;374(9684):159-169 [PMID: 19595359].

Chopra V, Anand S, Krein SL, et al: Bloodstream Iinfection, venous thrombosis, and peripherally inserted central catheters: Reappraising the evidence. *Am J Med.* 2012;125(8):733-741 [PMID: 22840660].

Gibson F, Bodenham A: Misplaced central venous catheters: Applied anatomy and practice management. *Br J Anaesth.* 2013;110(3):333-346 [PMID: 23384735].

Meek ME: Diagnosis and treatment of central venous access-associated infections. *Tech Vasc Interv Radiol.* 2011;14(4):212-216 [PMID: 22099013].

Ogston-Tuck S: Intravenous therapy: Guidance on devices, management and care. *Brit J Community Nurs.* 12012;7(10)474-483.

Weber DJ, Rutala WA: Central line-associated bloodstream infections: Prevention and management. *Infect Dis Clin North Am.* 2011;25(1):77-1102 [PMID: 21315995].

Zaghal A, Khalife M, Mukherji D, et al: Update on totally implantable venous access devices. *Surg Oncol.* 2012;21(3):207-215 [PMID: 22425356].

GASTROSTOMY TUBE

GENERAL CONSIDERATIONS

Gastrostomy tubes (GT) are placed in a surgically or endoscopically created stoma into the stomach, typically for the delivery of nutrition or medications. Indications for placement of a GT include neurologic impairment, severe gastroesophageal reflux, chronic malabsorptive syndromes, esophageal atresia, esophageal burns, and significant craniofacial malformations. Jejunostomy tubes (J-tube) are placed into a surgically created stoma that brings the jejunum to the skin surface to allow for postpyloric feedings. Indications for J-tube placement include delayed gastric emptying, recurrent aspiration pneumonia, and severe gastroesophageal reflux. A gastrojejunostomy tube (GJ-tube) is used when there is a need for postpyloric feeding as well as the delivery of medications to the stomach. There are a variety of enteric tubes with different lengths, number of ports, types of catheter tips, and number of lumens. Most GTs are low profile gastrostomy tubes (Mic-Key, Bard) which are skin-level tubes with either a balloon or mushroom tip. The tube was introduced for the pediatric patient and known as a "button," and is now also used in the adult patient. The advantage of this tube is there is less chance of it being pulled out, and is easier to conceal under clothing. The tube is usually placed once the stoma tract has matured, replacing the original GT.

DISLODGED ENTERIC TUBE

Clinical Findings

Accidental removal of an enteric tube is the most common complication, especially in young children and in combative or confused patients. Enteric tubes can become dislodged when tension is applied to the external tubing, the balloon ruptures, or there is occult deflation of the balloon. It is important to assess the stoma site. In most patients there will be no stomal injuries. There may be active bleeding at the site secondary to trauma.

Treatment

The goal of management of a displaced enteric tube is to maintain the stomal tract without inflicting additional trauma. It is important to know the time of initial placement of the enteric tube. GTs with mature tracts can be replaced at the bedside. The replacement GT should be matched in size and length to properly fit in the stomal tract. If the tube size is unknown or an appropriate size tube is not available, a Foley catheter can be placed to maintain the stoma tract. Prior to insertion of the new GT, the balloon should be tested. It should then be deflated. Surgical lubrication may be applied to the GT. Gentle but consistent downward pressure should be applied to the GT as it is slid into the stomal tract. Avoid using excessive force in replacement of a GT as it may lead to a false tract into the peritoneal cavity. The balloon should be inflated with the package recommended amount of NS to anchor the GT in place. The tract can close quickly. The longer the tract has been without a GT present, the more likely it is that the appropriate size GT may not pass. Therefore, a replacement tube or Foley catheter one or two sizes smaller than the original should be inserted. If there is resistance, abort the attempt for passage of Foley catheter and use a smaller size. Serial dilation with sequentially larger Foley catheters can restore the stoma to the appropriate size and allow the proper GT to be placed. Once the GT is in place, attempt to aspirate stomach contents. If this is successful, flush the tube. If there is difficulty in either flushing or drawing from the GT or concern that it is not appropriately positioned, fluoroscopy after instilling water-soluble dye can confirm the placement of the tip. Of note, the Bard type low-profile GT will require an obturator for placement and thus use caution to avoid perforation. Surgeons or gastroenterologists may aid in the replacement of this type of GT.

A GT that was initially placed less than 4 weeks prior to presentation is treated different from one in a patient with a mature stoma tract. The GT should not be blindly replaced at the bedside. In this time period the tract has not matured, allowing the abdominal wall and gastric wall to separate.

Blind placement may result with the tip in the peritoneal cavity. Temporary placement of a smaller Foley catheter into the stoma may prevent the separation of the stomach and the anterior abdominal wall. A gastroenterologist or surgeon should be consulted for definitive management.

If a J-tube or GJ-tube is displaced, it needs to be replaced by the subspecialist who placed it. While awaiting subspecialist intervention, a GT of the same size can be inserted in the stoma to maintain the tract. Interventional radiologists use fluoroscopy to replace a J-tube inserted via the GT. Surgically placed J-tubes need a surgeon for replacement.

Disposition

If there is concern about the positioning of a GT after replacement, a water-soluble contrast should be injected through the GT for radiographic confirmation. This should be performed prior to the initiation of feeding. If the GT is in the proper position, the patient can be discharged from the emergency department.

CLOGGED ENTERIC TUBE

Clinical Findings

Clogging of an enteric tube from medications or formula is one of the most common types of enteric tube dysfunction. It can also be caused by twisting or kinking of the tube. Caregivers will report an inability to flush the patient's enteric tube.

Treatment

If formula clogs the tube, aspiration and gentle flushing should first be attempted. Warm water is the best irrigant for a clogged enteric tube. Flushing of the tube with a 60 mL syringe is recommended. Extension tubing should be removed if possible before flushing. Avoid placing a stylet into the tubing to dislodge the clot. This can perforate the tubing beneath the skin. Specially designed declogging brushes can be used if these techniques fail. If the tube remains clogged, remove the old GT and replace with a new one. If the gastrostomy was placed within the previous month or if there is a J-tube component, a gastroenterologist or surgeon should be consulted prior to removal.

Disposition

When flow through the enteric device is restored, the patient can be discharged from the emergency department.

ENTERIC TUBE LEAKAGE

Clinical Findings

Enteric tube leaks can arise from the peristomal area or from the lumen of the tube. If the stoma becomes too wide, fluid contained in the stomach is able to leak around the tube. Peristomal leakage typically occurs within the first few days after tube placement. Patients with poor wound healing, such as those who are malnourished or on corticosteroids, are at higher risk for leakage. Leakage may also be seen in patients where the external bolster is secured too tightly, leading to diminished blood flow to this area, skin breakdown, and ultimately peristomal leakage. Additionally, a balloon that is underinflated can also lead to leakage around the tube. Leakage from the lumen of the tube can indicate that the valve is no longer patent.

Peristomal skin should be cleaned and dried prior to assessment. Irritant dermatitis may be present if there is chronic leakage of fluid. The stoma may have small vesicular lesions with surrounding erythema.

Treatment

Skin breakdown can be addressed with the addition of powdered absorbing agents or zinc oxide paste. Loosening of the external bolster can allow for improved blood flow, which promotes wound healing. Placing a larger sized GT in the tract is not helpful, as it will further distend the tract, which does not promote healing.

Patients with mature tracts (GT placed > 4 weeks ago) may benefit from removal of the GT temporarily (24-48 hours). Place a Foley catheter at least two sizes smaller than the GT into the stoma. This allows the stomal tract to close slightly. Another approach is to remove the GT entirely for several hours. Take caution though, stomal tracts close at different rates, and some may close within 24 hours. After allowing the tract to contract, a GT the same size as the previous tube can be inserted. Remember that GJ-tubes or J-tubes should not be removed at the bedside, as these require subspecialists for replacement. Leakage from these types of tubes can be managed on an outpatient basis by the service responsible for the enteric tube.

Disposition

If there are no signs of associated stomal infection, most GT leaks can be treated on an outpatient basis. However, if there is concern that the stoma has been disrupted, consultation with a surgeon should be obtained.

GASTRIC ULCERATION

Clinical Findings

If tip of the GT is too long, it can scratch the gastric mucosa on the opposite side. Continued irritation of the mucosa can lead to the formation of a gastric ulcer. Some GTs are anchored with an internal and external bolster. When excessive tension between the two is exerted, there can be erosion into the mucosa. Also, when the balloon is overinflated, it can lead to friction that irritates the mucosa. Balloon over-dilation may result from infusion of medications or flushes into the wrong GT port.

Patients with gastric ulceration present with complaints of abdominal pain, irritability, hematemesis, hematochezia, or coffee-ground drainage from the GT.

Treatment

If there is concern for gastric ulceration, a saline lavage should be performed. If the fluid is nonbloody, consider starting the patient on medication to reduce additional damage. H_2-blockers, sucralfate, or antacids should be considered. Acid reduction should be continued for 4-6 weeks. Because most gastric ulcers in this population are related to the GT, it should be changed and the balloon should be inflated as instructed in the packet. If the GT is anchored with bolsters, they should be secured so that gentle traction on the GT creates 0.5-1 cm of space beneath the other bolster.

Disposition

With no signs of active bleeding, patients with gastric ulceration should be scheduled for an upper endoscopy on an outpatient basis.

STOMAL CELLULITIS

Clinical Findings

Irritation, often caused by chronic or intermittent exposure to drainage, surrounding the stoma can lead to cellulitis. Infection typically begins as erythematous changes, warmth, or tenderness surrounding the GT. As the infection progresses, the patient may exhibit systemic signs such as fever. Manipulation of the tube can cause pain as it moves along irritated skin; parents may report the patient with difficulty tolerating feeds. Localized infection may lead to peristomal abscess formation. When an abscess is present, an area of fluctuance is often present. Cellulitis can also be caused by fungal infection. In this case, fiery red plaques can be seen surrounding the stoma.

Treatment

Cellulitis should be treated with systemic antibiotics. Most often these infections are caused by gram-positive organisms, including *Staphylococcus* and *Streptococcus*. Therefore, a 5- to 7-day course of first-generation cephalosporins or fluoroquinolones are often adequate. However, if there is evidence of abscess, an incision and drainage should be performed prior to administration of antibiotics. When there is concern for fungal infection, the area should be kept dry when possible. Topical clotrimazole or nystatin ointments are effective in most patients. If there is concern for MRSA, treat appropriately.

Disposition

Most GT infections can be treated as outpatient with oral antibiotics or topical antifungals as the case indicates. However, if the patient has signs of systemic illness, consider admission for IV antibiotics.

GASTRIC OUTLET OBSTRUCTION

Clinical Findings

Migration of the internal bolster into the pylorus or small bowel can lead to gastric outlet obstruction. The small internal diameter of the intestine places the pediatric population at greater risk for this. Often the external is too loose, allowing distal migration of the tube. Signs of obstruction include cramping abdominal pain, and intermittent emesis. The internal bolster position should be documented with a radiograph.

Treatment

Obstruction is typically relieved at the bedside. Tension on the tube is used to move the internal bolster back toward the gastric mucosa. The external bolster should be secured in a position that anchors the tube in the appropriate position.

Disposition

When the tube is repositioned and confirmed to be in the proper position (either through aspiration of gastric contents or administration of radio-opaque contrast followed by a radiograph), the tube should be used. If there is no recurrence of emesis or abdominal pain, the patient can be discharged and GT use can resume.

Bogie AL, Guthrie C: High-technology gastroenterology disorders in children. *Clin Pediatr Emer Med*. 2012;13(2):106-111.

Covarrubias DA, O'Connor OJ, McDermott S, et al: Radiologic percutaneous gastrostomy: Review of potential complications and approach to managing the unexpected outcome. *AJR Am J Roentgenol*. 2013;200(4):921-931 [PMID: 23521471].

Stayner JL, Bhatnagar A, McGinn AN, et al: Feeding tube placement: Errors and complications. *Nutr Clin Pract*. 2012;27(6):738-748 [PMID: 23064019].

COLOSTOMY & ILEOSTOMY

GENERAL CONSIDERATIONS

In a colostomy, a portion of the colon is brought to the level of the skin and an outflow tract is created. The patient continues to have semiformed stools as the colon continues to absorb water and store fecal material. The ileum is brought to the skin in an ileostomy. The patient will have frequent, loose stools since large bowel function is missing. There are multiple indications for the creation of a colostomy or ileostomy. Congenital gastrointestinal lesions that may lead to gastrointestinal diversions include Hirschsprung disease or an imperforate anus. Patients with inflammatory bowel disease, necrotizing enterocolitis, or traumatic injuries to the bowel may also have a colostomy or ileostomy. The location of disease and the predicted duration of need of conduit influence the surgical method used. An ostomy pouch is typically placed over the stoma to collect the effluent.

STOMAL STENOSIS

Clinical Findings

Patients may present with reduced or absent stool output, diarrhea, or cramping abdominal pain. Severe stenosis can lead to a bowel obstruction. A careful digital examination of the stoma should be performed for assessment of the degree of stenosis. However, in patients where the stoma is too small for digital examination, a catheter should be passed. When there is concern for a bowel obstruction, abdominal x-rays should be performed.

Treatment

If there is concern for bowel obstruction, prompt consultation with a surgeon is needed.

Disposition

Stomal stenosis needs operative revision. A surgeon should be consulted for management.

STOMAL PROLAPSE

Clinical Findings

Increase in the size of the stoma after it matures leads to stomal prolapse. Most stomal prolapses are not an emergency. Emergent complications of prolapse include incarcerated bowel. In this case, the prolapse may be painful with decreased output. Dusky discoloration of the prolapsed stoma indicates that there is ischemia or strangulation, and immediate surgical management is necessary. Skin excoriation and bleeding can also occur.

Treatment

In order to reduce a stomal prolapse, it should be grasped with both hands. Gentle pressure should be applied with the thumbs to reduce the prolapsed area back into the stoma. This may need to be done a number of times while awaiting definitive surgical treatment. When the prolapsed stoma is difficult to reduce, osmotic therapy can be attempted. Granulated sugar is applied to the prolapsed stoma and left in place for 30 minutes. Osmotic shifts of fluid can reduce the edematous changes allowing manual reduction. If there

are signs of ischemia, consultation with a surgeon should be obtained.

Disposition

In patients with no signs of incarceration, and manual reduction is successful, the patient can be discharged. When incarceration is present, urgent consultation with a surgeon and management is necessary.

PERISTOMAL CONTACT DERMATITIS

Clinical Findings

Frequent, watery stools are produced by patients with ileostomies. Irritation occurs when the alkaline effluent and proteolytic enzymes come in contact with the skin. When the ostomy is retracted, the risk of irritation increases. Obese patients are at increased risk for skin irritation when the ostomy is positioned along an abdominal crease. An ileostomy pouch that is not emptied frequently allows the effluent to pool, irritating the skin further.

Contact dermatitis leads to erythema surrounding the ostomy, often in the outline of the ostomy pouch. Irritated skin increases the risk for fungal infection. The erythema will have associated satellite lesions in this case.

Treatment

Peristomal fungal infections respond well to topical antifungal agents. Because of the associated dermatitis, a sealant should be applied over the antifungal. Sufficient time for drying should be allowed before the pouch is reapplied. If the erythema matches the outline of the ostomy devices, there is concern for allergic reaction. Topical steroids can be applied to reduce inflammation and protect the skin from further irritation.

Disposition

Contact dermatitis, allergic dermatitis, and fungal dermatitis all respond well to topical treatments in the outpatient setting.

Brandt AR, Schouten O: Sugar to reduce a prolapsed ileostomy. *N Engl J Med.* 2011;364:1855 [PMID: 21561351].
Martin ST, Vogel JD: Intestinal stomas: Indications, management, and complications. *Adv Surg.* 2012;46:19-49 [PMID: 22873030].
Shabbir J, Britton DC: Stoma complications: A literature overview. *Colorectal Dis.* 2010;12(10):958-964 [PMID: 19604288].

URINARY DIVERSIONS

A number of types of urinary diversion are employed. The most common long-term diversions include ureterostomies (dilated ureter brought to the level of the skin), vesicostomies (bladder opens to the skin), pyelostomies (dilated renal pelvis brought to the level of the skin), and ileal conduits (ureters are attached to a short segment of externalized ileum). In addition, temporary conduits, including percutaneous drainage catheters are employed, which are outside the scope of this chapter. Imperforate anus, cloacal extrophy, bladder extrophy, posterior urethral valves, and neurogenic bladder either from myelomeningocele or the result of traumatic injury are all indications for the creation of genitourinary diversion. Many of these diversions are low enough on the abdomen that the effluent can be collected in a diaper.

BLADDER PROLAPSE

Clinical Findings

Posterior aspect of the bladder can prolapse through the stoma. This presents as a red mass. The longer it is externalized, the greater the risk of vascular compromise resulting in purple discoloration.

Treatment

Apply pressure to the bladder with an index finger and gently push the bladder into the stoma. Many children with bladder extrophy develop latex allergies; therefore, this procedure should be performed with nonlatex gloves. The procedure may be easier if the patient receives sedatives. Those prolapses that cannot be manually reduced need emergent surgical revision.

Disposition

Patients with successfully reduced prolapses may be discharged home. Prolapses that cannot be manually reduced need emergent surgical revision.

STOMAL STENOSIS

Clinical Findings

Patients may report unwanted voiding or symptoms of urinary tract infections. The storage pressure continues to rise as the bladder fails to empty which can lead to increased chance of bacteria seeding the upper urinary tract. Patients may report that the stoma appears smaller. If a patient with a vesicostomy has stomal stenosis, the bladder may be palpable. The stoma may also appear pinpoint in size.

Treatment

A small urinary catheter should be placed into the bladder to decompress it. Typically a 6F or 8F catheter can be used. If this is unsuccessful and the patient has an intact urethra, bladder catheterization via the urethra should be attempted. If catheterization is successful, it should be left in place while awaiting surgical revision. Stomal contamination leads many vesicostomies to be colonized with bacteria. Because of the association with urinary tract infection, a sample of urine should be obtained for urinalysis and culture if there is a fever or other systemic signs. If no source for the fever is found, antibiotic treatment should be started.

Disposition

Stomal stenosis needs operative revision. Consultation with a urologist is needed for management.

Floyd S, Gray M: Managing the cutaneous vesicostomy. *J Wound Ostomy Continence Nurs.* 2009;36(1):94-99 [PMID: 19155829].

INTRATHECAL PUMPS (Baclofen Pump)

Implantable pump devices, specifically intrathecal baclofen pumps, have become a therapeutic option in children for the treatment of spasticity, athetosis, and dystonia, associated with cerebral palsy; spinal cord injuries; and anoxic brain injuries.

Although the delivery of baclofen via an implantable pump device offers significant benefits, and improves the quality of life, serious complications can occur (Table 49–3). These complications are associated with an increased risk of morbidity and mortality. If the continuous infusion of baclofen via intrathecal pump requires interruption,

Table 49–3. Complications of intrathecal baclofen infusion.

Hypotension
Bradycardia
Apnea
Oversedation
Respiratory depression
Pump pocket effusions
Mechanical failure
Catheter extrusion
Catheter dislodgement
Local infection
Meningitis
Cerebrospinal fluid fistula formation

Reproduced, with permission, from Tintinalli JE, Stapczynski JS, Ma OJ, Cline DM, Cydulka RK, Meckler GD: *Tintinalli's Emergency Medicine: A Comprehensive Study Guide,* 7th ed. New York: McGraw-Hill, 2011. © McGraw-Hill LLC.

baclofen, withdrawal symptoms can occur. These include hypertonicity and spasms that may lead to rhabdomyolysis. Oral baclofen, dantrolene, and oral or parenteral benzodiazepines may be used to alleviate the symptoms.

Most common clinical presentations in patients with superficial infections are local inflammation, purulence, erythema, and tenderness. Patients with fevers, altered mental status, lethargy, and severe pain or erythema, should be evaluated for sepsis and meningitis. Organisms identified include methicillin-sensitive *Staphylococcus aureus* (MSSA) and MRSA, *Enterococcus fecalis*, and *Corynebacterium* species. A neuorologist should be consulted on all issues regarding baclofen pumps.

Dickey M, Rice M, Kinnett D, et al: Infectious complications of intrathecal baclofen pump devices in a pediatric population. *Pediatr Infect Dis J*. 2013;32(7):715-722 [PMID: 23429557].

VAGAL NERVE STIMULATOR

Vagal nerve stimulation (VNS) has been in use for the treatment of refractory epilepsy in pediatric patients since the 1990s. The spectrum of seizure type that has been treated by VNS includes both partial and rapidly generalizing seizures and epilepsy syndromes such as Lennox-Gastaut syndrome. Stimulation of the vagus nerve is provided by a device that consists of a pulse generator and a set of wire leads that terminate around the vagus nerve by means of a wire coil. The stimulator and battery pack are placed in a subcutaneous pocket, usually in the infraclavicular fossa.

Common adverse effects are intermittent voice alteration during stimulation. This has been described as a hoarseness or vibration of the voice. Other, less common adverse effects that have been described by patients are pharyngeal paresthesias, coughing, increased drooling, sensation of shortness of breath, headache, nausea, and skin breakdown over the device and infections. More significant adverse events include lead fracture and device malfunction. Although pocket infections of the VNS device are uncommon, they can cause considerable morbidity. Infections superficial to the device may be treated successfully with antibiotics alone. However, deep pocket infections are uncommon, and occur in approximately 3-8% of devices placed. Organisms responsible include MSSA and MRSA. Management of VNS-related pocket infections, as with other device-associated infections, may require the removal of device in addition to treatment with IV antibiotics requiring hospital admission. Neurologic consultation is recommended on all issues concerning the VNS.

Patel N, Edwards M: Vagal nerve stimulator pocket infections. *Pediatr Infect Dis J*. 2004;23(7):681-683 [PMID: 15247613].
Sunny O, Chandrasekaran K: Vagal nerve stimulator: Evolving trends. *J Nat Sci Biol Med*. 2013;4(1):8-13 [PMID: 23633829].

Index

Page references followed by *f* indicate figures; page references followed by *t* indicate tables.

O

obstipation, 152
obstruction
   airway, 126–127, 127f, 133–135
   of CSF shunt, 458, 725–726, 726f
   gastric outlet, 736
   GI, 158–162, 164
   of tracheostomy tube, 728–729
obstructive shock, 115
obturator sign, 153, 416
occlusion, of catheter, 731–732
OCD. *See* osteochondritis desiccans
octreotide, 197, 580, 635t, 646
Ocuflox. *See* ofloxacin
ocular decontamination, 634
ocular ultrasound, 24–25, 24f, 25f
ODD. *See* oppositional defiant disorder
odontogenic infections, 393
odontoid fracture, 277–278, 278f
ofloxacin (Ocuflox), 375t, 510t, 510t–511t
OI. *See* osteogenesis imperfecta
ointments
   eye applications, 374, 376
   wound care with, 354–355
olanzapine, 714t, 717, 720
oliguria, 467–469, 468t
OM. *See* otitis media
omeprazole, 161
oncologic emergencies
   fever and neutropenia, 533–534, 533f, 534t
   hematologic malignancies, 530, 530t, 531f
   hypercalcemia, 532
   hyperleukocytosis, 531
   lymphoma, 530, 531f
   solid tumors, 530–531
   superior vena cava syndrome/ superior mediastinal syndrome, 532
   tumor lysis syndrome, 532
ondansetron, 163
OPA. *See* oropharyngeal airway
open fractures, 225–226, 225f, 286–287
open injuries, hand, 334–336
open pneumothorax, 217, 243
ophthalmic medications, 374, 375t
Ophthetic Alcaine. *See* proparacaine
opiates/opioids
   for burn patients, 608–609

for chest trauma patients, 242, 245, 249
for gastrointestinal emergencies, 417
for head trauma patients, 223
for migraines, 208
for PSA, 56–58, 56t
for SCD pain, 524t
toxic ingestion/exposure of, 197, 632t, 635t, 644
oppositional defiant disorder (ODD), 721–722
oral contraceptive pills, 499
oral emergencies
   epiglottitis, 134, 388–390, 390f, 392t, 549
   immediate management of, 378–379
   infection, 380–383
   obstruction, 378–379
   odontogenic infections, 393
   peritonsillar abscesses, 387–388, 387f, 392t, 541–542
   postoperative complications, 390–391
   retropharyngeal abscesses, 134, 388, 389f, 392t, 541–542
   sore throat, 391, 392t
oral rehydration therapy
   for diarrhea, 165, 168–169
   for gastroenteritis, 419, 558–559
   for heat exposure emergencies, 615
   technique of, 177
   for vomiting, 162–163
oral wounds, 356–357
orbital cellulitis, 365–366, 548–549, 548t
orbital fractures, 238
orbital hemorrhage, 373
orbital trauma, 372
orchitis, 427t, 470–471, 471t
organic mercury, 653
organophosphate poisoning, 656–657
orogastric tube, 220
oropharyngeal airway (OPA), 85, 101, 102f, 215
orthopedic disorders
   benign tumors, 601–602
   growing pains, 601
   of lower extremities, 591–598, 591t, 592f, 593f, 594f, 595f
   malignant tumors, 603
   of neck, 589
   osteogenesis imperfecta, 601

psoas abscess, 600–601
   of spine, 598–600, 599f
   of upper extremities, 589–591
orthopedic injuries. *See* extremity trauma
orthostatic hypotension, 188
OSD. *See* Osgood-Schlatter disease
oseltamivir, 401
Osgood-Schlatter disease (OSD), 313, 596–597
osmol gap, 633
osmotic agents
   for coma, 192, 196
   for headache, 210
   for increased ICP, 218
ossifying fibroma, 602
osteochondritis desiccans (OCD), 597
osteochondroma, 602
osteogenesis imperfecta (OI), 601
osteomyelitis, 560–561
osteosarcoma, 603
otitis externa, 380–381
otitis media (OM), 170, 381–382, 545, 546t
otorhinolaryngology emergency procedures
   EAC foreign body removal, 46–47
   epistaxis management, 48–49
   nasal foreign body removal, 47–48
Ottawa Ankle Rules, 318
ovarian cyst, 505
ovarian torsion, 151t, 157, 436, 502
overdrainage, of CSF shunts, 727
oxacillin, 561, 562, 733, 733t
oxcarbazepine, 453t–455t
oxygen administration
   for asthma, 128–129
   for carbon monoxide exposure, 650
   for cardiac arrest, 85, 87
   for cardiac emergencies, 406–407
   for chest trauma patients, 243, 245
   for compromised airway, 101–103
   for cyanosis, 124
   for endotracheal intubation, 106, 215
   for GI emergencies, 413
   for headache, 209
   for high altitude illness, 621–622
   of hypothermia patients, 619–620
   for respiratory distress, 126, 128–135
   for shock, 116, 117f